Calculations for determining the amount of local anesthetic and/or vasoconstrictor in dental cartridges

Typical local anesthetic concentrations

Strength		mg/ml Equivalent
0.5%	=	5 mg/ml
1.5%	=	15 mg/ml
2.0%	=	20 mg/ml
3.0%	=	30 mg/ml
4.0%	=	40 mg/ml

Typical vasoconstrictor concentrations

Strength		mg/ml (or µg/ml) Equivalent
1:20,000	=	0.05 mg/ml (50 µg/ml)
1:50,000	=	0.02 mg/ml (20 µg/ml)
1:100,000	=	0.01 mg/ml (10 µg/ml)
1:200,000	=	0.005 mg/ml (5 µg/ml)

General calculation guidelines:

1) Convert % solution to mg/ml (or µg/ml) as shown above.
2) Multiply mg/ml (or µg/ml) × cartridge volume × number of cartridges = quantity of drug. *Note:* Cartridge volumes may vary between products.

Example: Two cartridges of a 2% lidocaine HCl and 1:100,000 epinephrine HCl solution were administered. The cartridge volume was 1.8 ml for each. What quantity of each drug was given?

Answer:
for lidocaine HCl: 20 mg/ml × 1.8 ml × 2 cartridges = 72 mg
for epinephrine HCl: 0.01 mg/ml × 1.8 ml × 2 cartridges = 0.036 mg or 10 µg/ml × 1.8 ml × 2 cartridges = 36 µg

Mosby's
Dental
Drug
Reference

Mosby's **Dental Drug Reference**

Sixth Edition

Tommy W. Gage, RPh, DDS, PhD

Director of Curriculum, Academic Services
Professor, Department of Oral and Maxillofacial
Surgery and Pharmacology
Baylor College of Dentistry
The Texas A&M University System Health Science Center
Dallas, Texas

Frieda Atherton Pickett, RDH, MS

Formerly, Associate Professor
Caruth School of Dental Hygiene
Baylor College of Dentistry
The Texas A&M University System Health Science Center
Dallas, Texas
Adjunct Associate Professor
Department of Dental Hygiene
East Tennessee State University
Johnson City, Tennessee

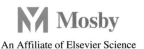

An Affiliate of Elsevier Science

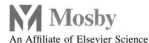
Mosby
An Affiliate of Elsevier Science

11830 Westline Industrial Drive
St. Louis, Missouri 63146

DENTAL DRUG REFERENCE   ISBN 0-323-02477-7
Copyright © 2003 by Mosby, Inc.

A NOTE TO THE READER

The authors and publisher have made every attempt to check dosages and
dental content for accuracy. Because the science of pharmacology is
continually advancing, our knowledge base continues to expand. Therefore we recommend that the reader always check product information for
changes in dosage or administration before administering any medication.
This is particularly important with new or rarely used drugs.

THE PUBLISHER

SIXTH EDITION
Previous editions copyrighted 1994, 1996, 1997, 1999, 2001

Publishing Director: Linda Duncan
Senior Acquisitions Editor: Penny Rudolph
Developmental Editor: Kimberly Alvis
Project Manager: Linda McKinley
Production Editor: Jim Rygelski
Designer: Julia Dummitt

Printed in the United States of America

03   04   05   06   07   /   9   8   7   6   5   4   3   2   1

Editorial Review Board

Authors' Comments

Our goal of creating a quick and concise drug reference resource remains steadfast. We are excited to present this sixth edition, trusting it will serve you even better than previous editions. We have added two new appendixes to this edition. One contains a listing of drugs and related cytochrome P450 (CYP450) enzymes and the other, which we hope you will like, features sample prescriptions. Your acceptance of this drug information resource has been extremely gratifying and supports our vision of the need for such a volume. Because the book is revised every two years, new drug information is posted as periodic updates on Mosby's web site at http://www. mosby.com/dental. You are encouraged to access this web site for updated drug information and for information about new drugs approved after the publication date for this volume.

We are excited to include a CD-ROM with the sixth edition. The CD features over 100 patient education sheets that you can customize to include your practice information before you give them to patients. These sheets will provide your patients with invaluable drug information, and all are available in both English and Spanish.

Another feature of the CD-ROM is the inclusion of 30 oral pathologic conditions that may result from drugs patients are taking. These conditions, shown in full color, are representative of those the dentist or members of the dental team may see in patients. Each condition is cross-referenced to the page in this book where the drug is discussed.

The pharmacologic and therapeutic index has been maintained in the front section of this volume. This index has been well accepted in assisting both users and patients, and especially students, in the identification of drugs by class or therapeutic usefulness.

In addition to updating each monograph, additional herbal and nonherbal remedies were added. We are continually working to keep the book as small as possible for convenience in handling, but the number of new drugs and drug products approved for marketing each year presents a considerable challenge. Our focus is on the most frequently prescribed medications, dental specialty products, and new products. Because of these reasons, not every drug that is available in the market place is listed. However, it does include the majority of new drugs marketed through December 2001.

This book is only as good as it is able to assist the practitioner to quickly locate drug facts. The authors are hopeful this edition will be equally acceptable and useful. Your comments for improvements are solicited.

Preface

Mosby's Dental Drug Reference is designed to be used chairside in the dental office and by the student or resident as a quick, concise drug reference resource. Its purpose is to assist in the rapid identification of drugs patients may be taking as they present for dental care. The easy-to-use design provides rapid access to essential drug information to facilitate completion of the medical history review and patient evaluation.

This book is not intended to be a comprehensive drug compendium or to make specific recommendations about selecting and prescribing dental drugs. It contains concise and easy-to-read "micro" drug monographs with basic information about each drug.

Selected herbal and nonherbal remedies have been placed in a separate appendix to aid the dental practitioner in identifying dental implications of these products. Drugs are presented alphabetically by generic name in a succinctly ordered and standardized format with pertinent drug information for the dentist, dental hygienist, dental assistant, or student. A user-friendly cross index is the key to using the book for both brand and generic name identification. A second index, based on a therapeutic and pharmacologic classification, also can be used to quickly locate drug monographs. In addition, this index will aid in identifying drugs when the patient cannot recall the name or spelling of a drug being taken. This index also groups drugs by classes or use so the reader can easily identify other drugs within a given class or application. Information is provided on more than 1600 drug products, including the most recently approved drugs and new drug products through 2001.

A feature new to the sixth edition is an appendix with sample prescriptions. These samples are suitable to use as a guide in writing prescriptions.

A special feature of this book is an emphasis on drug interactions of dental interest and the highlighting of oral side effects. The dental considerations section includes information that will be useful in developing patient management strategies. Useful fact tables with information about dose calculations are located on the front inside covers and in the appendix. This volume also contains the 1997 AHA drug and dose recommendations for antibiotic prophylaxis for patients at risk for bacterial endocarditis and the 1997 ADA advisory statement for those patients with prosthetic joints. We have also revised the tables listing drugs that can alter salivary flow and affect taste.

Each drug monograph is designed to include the following information:

GENERIC NAME of the drug

PRONUNCIATION of the generic name

COMMON BRAND NAMES for the generic drug as sold in the United States and Canada (drugs available in Canada only are designated by a maple leaf)

DRUG CLASS to facilitate drug identification

CONTROLLED SUBSTANCES schedule as appropriate for the United States and Canada

ACTION, with a brief description of the mechanism of action of the drug

USES or indications for the drug, including those approved by the FDA (unapproved uses are identified as appropriate for selected drugs)

DOSES AND ROUTES OF ADMINISTRATION to assist the dental professional in assessing the dose in relationship to the seriousness of the patient's disease and predicting potential side effects and drug interactions

SIDE EFFECTS/ADVERSE REACTIONS are grouped according to body systems; common side effects listed in italics, and life-threatening reactions listed in boldface type; information regarding oral manifestations of side effects highlighted separately

CONTRAINDICATIONS are identified for instances in which the medication should absolutely not be given or when risk benefit criteria must be established

PRECAUTIONS to be considered when prescribing and using the drug and identification of pregnancy categories

PHARMACOKINETICS, with brief descriptions for each drug

DRUG INTERACTIONS OF CONCERN TO DENTISTRY listed for the purpose of determining whether a given interaction is beneficial or harmful. This section is organized so that the response is given followed by a colon. This is followed by the drug(s) interacting with the monograph drug. For example, increased hypoglycemia: aspirin. When the monograph drug alters the effects of another drug the interaction is stated as the effect "with" or "of" another drug. For example, increased nausea with codeine, hydrocodone. Another example is: increased blood levels of carbamazepine. Few drug interactions are absolute; therefore clinical judgment must always be applied for each interaction listed.

DENTAL CONSIDERATIONS, includes general information related to dental concerns in treating a patient taking a given drug, suggestions for medical consultations, and recommendations for the patient/family in preventing dental complications or disease

Appendixes following the drug monograph section include the following:

APPENDIX A   Abbreviations
APPENDIX B   Drugs causing dry mouth
APPENDIX C   Controlled substances chart
APPENDIX D   FDA pregnancy categories
APPENDIX E   Drugs that affect taste
APPENDIX F   Combination products
APPENDIX G   Dose calculations by weight
APPENDIX H   Herbal and nonherbal remedies
APPENDIX I   Drugs affecting the cytochrome P450 isoenzymes
APPENDIX J   Prescription examples
APPENDIX K   Selected references

Located on the inside cover pages are useful tables and drugs and doses for antibiotic prophylaxis.

Tommy W. Gage
Frieda Atherton Pickett

Acknowledgments

The authors wish to express their sincere gratitude for the contributions made by members of the Editorial Review Board, who were selected on the basis of their extensive experience and knowledge. A special word of appreciation goes to Brigitte Wallaert Sims for her assistance in data entry, in the laborious task of printing the completed manuscript, and in putting up with our demands.

Tommy W. Gage
Frieda Atherton Pickett

Contents

Therapeutic/Pharmacologic Index

Drugs Classified by Usual Therapeutic/Pharmacologic Category

This section of the book features drugs classified by primary therapeutic or pharmacologic group, or both. Thus you can locate drugs by knowing their primary therapeutic use or general pharmacologic class. This arrangement makes it easy to find the matching drug monograph by using the generic name. The individual drug monographs are arranged by generic name in alphabetical order and can simply be found in the appropriate alphabet section. Colored tabs on the side of the book mark the alphabetical sections. An originator or common brand name is also listed for convenience and may help with identification. This arrangement allows the book user to see other drugs in the same classification that are included in this volume.

For example, take the case of a patient using a drug for depression and having difficulty recalling the drug name. Find the *Antidepressants* section. All of the antidepressants listed in this volume can be seen and may help the patient remember the exact drug currently used. Or if you want to know which drugs are calcium channel antagonists, go to the *Antihypertensives* section and find the subtopic of calcium channel antagonists. The calcium channel antagonists included in this volume are listed. As you identify the drug, use the generic name to quickly tab to the appropriate alphabet section.

ADRENERGIC AGONISTS
ephedrine
epinephrine (Adrenalin)
isoproterenol (Isuprel)

ALZHEIMER'S
donepezil (Aricept)
galantamine (Reminyl)
rivastigmine (Exelon)
tacrine (Cognex)

AMINOGLYCOSIDES (TOPICALS)
gentamycin ophth. (Garamycin)
neomycin (Myciguent)
polymyxin B ophth. (Aerosporin)
tobramycin ophth. (Tobrex)

AMYOTROPHIC LATERAL SCLEROSIS
riluzole (Rilutek)

ANALGESICS (NONOPIOID)
acetaminophen (Tylenol)
aspirin (Zorprim, Ascriptin)
salsalate (Anaflex)

ANALGESICS (NSAIDs)
(see nonsteroidal antiinflammatory drugs)

ANALGESICS (OPIOIDS)
codeine
fentanyl transdermal (Duragesic)
fentanyl transmucosal (Fentanyl Oralet, Actiq)
hydromorphone (Dilaudid)
meperidine (Demerol)
methadone (Dolophine)
morphine (MS Contin)
oxycodone (Roxicodone)
pentazocine (Talwin Nx)
propoxyphene hydrochloride (Darvon)
propoxyphene napsylate (Darvon-N)
tramadol (Ultram)

ANESTHETICS (LOCAL)
articaine (Septocaine)
bupivacaine (Marcaine)
etidocaine (Duranest)
lidocaine (Xylocaine)
mepivacaine (Carbocaine)
prilocaine (Citanest)

ANESTHETICS (TOPICAL)
benzocaine (Hurricaine)
dyclonine HCl (Dyclone)
lidocaine (Xylocaine)
lidocaine transoral (DentiPatch)
tetracaine (Pontocaine)

ANESTHETICS (GENERAL)
midazolam (Versed)
propofol (Diprivan)

ANOREXIANTS
diethylpropion (Tenuate)
methamphetamine (Desoxyn)
phendimetrazine (Prelu-2)
phentermine (Ionamin)
sibutramine (Merida)

ANTACIDS
magaldrate (Riopan)

ANTAGONISTS
disulfiram (Antabuse)
flumazenil (Romazicon)
levomethadyl acetate (Orlaam)
nalmefene (Revex)
naloxone (Narcan)
naltrexone (ReVia, Trexan)

ANTIANGINALS
Nitrates
isorbide dinitrate (Isordil)
isorbide mononitrate (ISMO)
nitroglycerin (Transderm-Nitro)

Beta-adrenergic antagonists
atenolol (Tenormin)
metoprolol (Lopressor)
nadolol (Corgard)
propranolol (Inderal)
Calcium channel antagonists
amlodipine (Norvasc)
bepridil (Vascor)
diltiazem (Cardizem)
felodipine (Plendil)
nicardipine (Cardene)
nifedipine (Procardia)
verapamil (Calan)

ANTIANXIETY/SEDATIVE-HYPNOTICS
Barbiturates
pentobarbital (Nembutal)
phenobarbital (Luminal)
secobarbital (Seconal)
Benzodiazepines
alprazolam (Xanax)
chlordiazepoxide (Librium)
clorazepate dipotassium
    (Tranxene)
diazepam (Valium)
estazolam (ProSom)
flurazepam (Dalmane)
lorazepam (Ativan)
midazolam (Versed)
oxazepam (Serax)
quazepam (Doral)
temazepam (Restoril)
triazolam (Halcion)
Antihistamines
diphenhydramine (Benadryl)
hydroxyzine (Atarax, Vistaril)
promethazine (Phenergan)
Others
buspirone (BuSpar)
chloral hydrate (Aquachloral)
doxepin (Sinaquan)
meprobamate (Equanil,
    Miltown)
zaleplon (Sonata)
zolpidem (Ambien)

ANTIASTHMATICS
(see bronchodilators)

ANTICARIES
sodium fluoride

ANTICHOLELITHICS
ursodiol (Actigall)

ANTICHOLINERGICS
atropine (Sal-Tropine)
benztropine (Cogentin)
biperidin (Akineton)
clidinium (Quarzan)
dicyclomine (Bentyl)
glycopyrrolate (Robinul)
hyoscyamine (Levsin)
mepenzolate (Cantil)
oxybutynin (Ditropan)
propantheline (Pro-Banthine)
scopolamine
tolterodine (Detrol)

ANTICOAGULANTS
dalteparin (Fragmin)
danaparoid (Orgaran)
enoxaparin (Lovenox)
heparin
warfarin (Coumadin)

ANTICONVULSANTS
acetazolamide (Diamox)
carbamazepine (Tegretol)
clonazepam (Klonopin)
diazepam (Valium)
divalproex (Depakote)
ethosuximide (Zarontin)
ethotoin (Peganone)
felbamate (Felbatol)
fosphenytoin (Cerebyx)
gabapentin (Neurontin)
lamotrigine (Lamictal)
levetiracetam (Keppra)
mephenytoin (Mesantoin)
mephobarbital (Mebaral)
methsuximide (Celontin)
oxcarbazepine (Trileptal)

phenobarbital (Luminal)
phensuximide (Milontin)
phenytoin (Dilantin)
primidone (Mysoline)
tiagabine (Gabitril)
topiramate (Topamax)
trimethadione (Tridione)
valproic acid (Depakene)
zonisamide (Zonegran)

ANTIDEPRESSANTS
Atypical
  bupropion (Wellbutrin)
  nefazodone (Serzone)
  trazodone (Desyrel)
  venlafaxine (Effexor)
Monoamine oxidase inhibitors
  isocarboxazid (Marplan)
  phenelzine sulfate (Nardil)
  tranylcypromine sulfate
    (Parnate)
**Serotonin-specific reuptake
inhibitors**
  citalopram (Celexa)
  fluoxetine (Prozac)
  fluvoxamine (Luvox)
  paroxetine (Paxil)
  sertraline (Zoloft)
Tetracyclics
  maprotiline (Ludiomil)
  mirtazapine (Remeron)
Tricyclics
  amitriptyline (Elavil)
  amoxapine (Asendin)
  clomipramine (Anafranil)
  desipramine (Norpramin)
  doxepin (Sinequan)
  imipramine (Tofranil)
  nortriptyline (Pamelor)
  protriptyline (Vivactil)
  trimipramine (Surmontil)

ANTIDIABETICS
  acarbose (Precose)
  acetohexamide (Dymelor)
  chlorpropamide (Diabinese)

glimepiride (Amaryl)
glipizide (Glucotrol)
glyburide (DiaBeta)
insulin
metformin (Glucophage)
miglitol (Glyset)
nateglinide (Starlix)
pioglitazone (Actos)
repaglinide (Prandin)
rosiglitazone (Avandia)
tolazamide (Tolinase)
tolbutamide (Orinase)

ANTIDIARRHEALS
bismuth subsalicylate
  (Pepto-Bismol)
camphorated opium tincture
  (Paregoric)
difenoxin/atropine (Motofen)
diphenoxylate/atropine
  (Lomotil)
loperamide (Imodium-AD)

ANTIDYSRHYTHMICS
(ANTIARRHYTHMICS)
  amiodarone (Cordarone)
  digoxin (Lanoxin)
  disopyramide (Norpace)
  dofetilide (Tikosyn)
  flecainide acetate (Tambocor)
  lidocaine (Xylocaine Cardiac)
  mexiletine (Mexitil)
  moricizine (Ethmozine)
  procainamide (Pronestyl)
  propafenone (Rythmol)
  propranolol (Inderal)
  quinidine (Quinaglute)
  sotalol (Betapace)
  tocainide (Tonocard)

ANTIEMETICS
  chlorpromazine (Thorazine)
  cyclizine (Marezine)
  dimenhydrinate (Dramamine)
  dolasetron (Anzemet)
  meclizine (Bonine)

metoclopramide (Reglan)
ondansetron (Zofran)
prochlorperazine (Compazine)
promethazine (Phenergan)
scopolamine (Transderm-Scop)
thiethylperazine (Torecan)
triflupromazine (Vesprin)
trimethobenzamide (Tigan)

ANTIFUNGALS (TOPICAL)
amphotericin B (Fungizone)
butenafine (Mentax)
butoconazole (Femstat)
ciclopirox (Loprox)
clotrimazole (Mycelex)
econazole (Spectazole)
itraconazole (Sporanox)
miconazole (Monistat, Micatin)
naftifine (Naftin)
nystatin (Mycostatin)
sulconazole (Exelderm)
terbinafine (Lamisil)
terconazole (Terazol)

ANTIFUNGALS (SYSTEMIC)
fluconazole (Diflucan)
flucytosine (Ancobon)
griseofulvin (Fulvicin)
itraconazole (Sporanox)
ketoconazole (Nizoral)
terbinafine (Lamisil)

ANTIGOUTS
allopurinol (Zyloprim)
colchicine

ANTIHISTAMINES (H$_2$) ANTAGONISTS
cimetidine (Tagamet)
famotidine (Pepcid)
nizatidine (Axid)
ranitidine (Zantac)

ANTIHISTAMINES (H$_1$) ANTAGONISTS
azatadine (Optimine)
azelastine (Astelin, Optivar)
brompheniramine (Dimetane)
buclizine (Bucladin-S)
cetirizine (Zyrtec)
chlorpheniramine (Chlor-Trimeton)
clemastine fumarate (Tavist)
cyclizine (Marezine)
cyproheptadine (Periactin)
dexchlorpheniramine (Polaramine)
dimenhydrinate (Dramamine)
diphenhydramine (Benadryl)
emedastine (Emadine)
fexofenadine (Allegra)
hydroxyzine (Atarax, Vistaril)
ketotifen (Zaditor)
levocabastine (Livostin)
loratadine (Claritin)
meclizine (Bonine)
olopatadine (Patanol)
promethazine (Phenergan)
tripelennamine (PBZ)

ANTIHYPERCALCEMICS (OSTEOPOROSIS)
alendronate (Fosamax)
etidronate (Didronel)
calcitonin (Calcimar)
raloxifene (Evista)
risedronate (Actonel)
tiludronate (Skelid)
zoledronic acid (Zometa)

ANTIHYPERLIPIDEMICS
atorvastatin (Lipitor)
cholestyramine (Questran)
clofibrate (Atromid-S)
colesevelam (Welchol)
colestipol (Colestid)

fenofibrate (Tricor)
fluvastatin (Lescol)
gemfibrozil (Lopid)
lovastatin (Mevacor)
niacin (Nia-Bid)
pravastatin (Pravachol)
simvastatin (Zocor)

ANTIHYPERTENSIVES
(also see diuretics)
Alpha-adrenergic antagonists
doxazosin (Cardura)
phentolamine (Regitine)
prazosin (Minipress)
terazosin (Hytrin)
Alpha/beta-adrenergic antagonists
carvedilol (Coreg)
labetalol (Normodyne)
Angiotensin-converting enzyme inhibitors
benazepril (Lotensin)
captopril (Capoten)
enalapril (Vasotec)
fosinopril (Monopril)
lisinopril (Prinivil, Zestril)
moexipril (Univasc)
perindopril (Aceon)
quinapril (Accupril)
ramipril (Altace)
trandolapril (Mavik)
Angiotensin II receptor antagonists
candesartan (Atacand)
eprosartan (Teveten)
irbesartan (Avapro)
losartan (Cozaar)
telmisartan (Micardis)
valsartan (Diovan)
Beta-adrenergic antagonists
Selective
atenolol (Tenormin)
betaxolol (Kerlone)
bisoprolol (Zebeta)
carteolol (Cartrol)
metoprolol (Lopressor)

nadolol (Corgard)
Nonselective
penbutolol (Levatol)
pindolol (Visken)
propranolol (Inderal)
timolol (Blocadren)
Calcium channel antagonists
amlodipine (Norvasc)
bepridil (Vascor)
diltiazem (Cardizem)
felodipine (Plendil)
isradipine (DynaCirc)
mibefradil (Posicor)
nicardipine (Cardene)
nifedipine (Procardia XL)
nislodipine (Sular)
verapamil (Calan)
Centrally acting
clonidine (Catapres)
guanabenz (Wytensin)
methyldopa (Aldomet)
Other
bosentan (Tracleer)
guanadrel (Hylorel)
guanethidine (Ismelin)
hydralazine (Apresoline)
mecamylamine (Inversine)
minoxidil (Loniten)
reserpine (Serpasil)

ANTIHYPOGLYCEMIC
glucagon (Glucagon Emergency Kit)

ANTIINFECTIVES (TOPICAL)
chlorhexidine (Peridex, PerioGard)
erythromycin (Erytroderm)
mupirocin (Bactroban)
povidone-iodine (Betadine)

ANTIINFECTIVES (MISCELLANEOUS)
atovaquone (Mepron)
clofazimine (Lamprene)
dapsone

linezolid (Zyvox)
metronidazole (Flagyl)
pentamidine (NebuPent)

ANTIINFECTIVES (SYSTEMIC)
(see specific class: penicillins,
cephalosporins, etc.)

ANTIINFLAMMATORY
ANTIARTHRITICS
allopurinol (Zyloprim)
aspirin
auranofin gold (Ridaura)
aurothioglucose (Solganal)
celecoxib (Celebrex)
choline salicylate (Arthropan)
colchicine
diflunisal (Dolobid)
etanercept (Enbrel)
etodolac (Lodine)
fenoprofen (Nalfon)
gold sodium thiomalate
   (Myochrysine)
ibuprofen (Motrin)
indomethacin (Indocin)
infliximab (Remicade)
ketoprofen (Orudis)
leflunomide (Arava)
methotrexate (Rheumatrex)
nabumetone (Relafen)
naproxen sodium (Anaprox)
naproxen (Naprosyn)
oxaprozin (Daypro)
piroxicam (Feldene)
probenecid (Benemid)
rofecoxib (Vioxx)
salsalate (Anaflex)
sulindac (Clinoril)
tolmetin (Tolectin)
valdecoxib (Bextra)

ANTIMALARIALS
chloroquine (Aralen)
hydroxychloroquine (Plaquenil)
primaquine
quinine

ANTIPARKINSONIANS
amantadine (Symmetrel)
benztropine (Cogentin)
biperiden (Akineton)
bromocriptine (Parlodel)
diphenhydramine (Benadryl)
entacapone (Comtan)
levodopa (Larodopa)
levodopa/carbidopa (Sinemet)
pergolide (Permax)
pramipexole (Mirapex)
procyclidine (Kemadrin)
ropinirole (ReQuip)
selegiline (Eldepryl)
tolcapone (Tasmar)
trihexyphenidyl (Artane)

ANTIPSYCHOTICS
Phenothiazines
chlorpromazine (Thorazine)
fluphenazine (Prolixin)
mesoridazine (Serentil)
perphenazine (Trilafon)
prochlorperazine (Compazine)
thioridazine (Mellaril)
trifluoperazine (Stelazine)
triflupromazine (Vesprin)
Butyrophenone
haloperidol (Haldol)
Thioxanthene
thiothixene (Navane)
Others
clozapine (Clozaril)
loxapine (Loxitane)
molindone (Moban)
olanzapine (Zyprexa)
pimozide (Orap)
quetiapine (Seroquel)
risperidone (Risperdal)
ziprasidone (Geodon)
Bipolar disease
lithium carbonate (Eskalith)
valproic acid (Depakene)

ANTITHYROIDS
  methimazole (Tapazole)
  propylthiouracil

ANTITUBERCULARS
  aminosalicylic acid (Paser)
  cycloserine (Seromycin)
  ethambutol (Myambutol)
  ethionamide (Trecator)
  isoniazid (Laniazid)
  pyrazinamide
  rifabutin (Mycobutin)
  rifampin (Rifadin)
  rifapentine (Priftin)

ANTITUSSIVES/ EXPECTORANTS
  benzonatate (Tessalon)
  codeine
  dextromethorphan (Robitussin)
  diphenhydramine (Benadryl)
  guaifenesin (Humibid)
  hydrocodone (Hycodan)

ANTIVIRALS (SYSTEMIC)
Herpes viruses
  acyclovir (Zovirax)
  famciclovir (Famvir)
  foscarnet (Foscavir)
  ganciclovir (Cytovene)
  valacyclovir (Valtrex)
  valganciclovir (Valcyte)
Influenza viruses
  amantadine (Symmetrel)
  oseltamivir (Tamiflu)
  rimantadine (Flumadine)
  zanamivir (Relenza)
HIV—nonnucleoside analogs
  delavirdine (Rescriptor)
  efavirenz (Sustiva)
  nevirapine (Viramune)
  tenofovir (Viread)
HIV—nucleoside analogs
  abacavir (Ziagen)
  didanosine (ddl) (Videx)

  lamivudine (3TC) (Epivir)
  stavudine (d4T) (Zerit)
  zalcitabine (Hivid)
  zidovudine (AZT) (Retrovir)
HIV—protease inhibitors
  amprenavir (Agenerase)
  indinavir (Crixivan)
  nelfinavir (Viracept)
  ritonavir (Norvir)
  saquinavir (Invirase, Fortovase)

ANTIVIRALS (TOPICAL)
  acyclovir (Zovirax)
  docosanol (Abreva)
  penciclovir (Denavir)
  vidarabine (Vira-A)

APHTHOUS STOMATITIS
  amlexanox (Aphthasol)
  chlorhexidine (Peridex)

APPETITE SUPPRESSANTS
  diethylpropion (Tenuate)
  methamphetamine (Desoxyn)
  orlistat (Xenical)
  phendimetrazine (Prelu-2)
  phentermine (Ionamin)
  sibutramine (Meridia)

ASTHMA TREATMENT
(see bronchodilators)

ASTHMA PREVENTION
  montelukast (Singulair)
  salmeterol (Serevent)
  zafirlukast (Accolate)
  zileuton (Zyflo)

BARBITURATES
  pentobarbital (Nembutal)
  phenobarbital (Luminal)
  secobarbital (Seconal)

BRONCHODILATORS
  albuterol (Proventil, Ventolin)
  aminophylline (Somophyllin)

bitolterol (Tornalate)
dyphylline (Dilor)
ephedrine
epinephrine (Adrenalin)
epinephrine inhalation
(Primatene)
formoterol (Foradil)
ipratropium (Atrovent)
isoetharine (Bronkometer)
isoproterenol (Isuprel)
levalbuterol (Xopenex)
metaproterenol (Alupent)
oxtriphylline (Choledyl)
pirbuterol (Maxair)
terbutaline (Brethine)
theophylline (Theo-Dur)

CANCER CHEMOTHERAPY
bicalutamide (Casodex)
busulfan (Myleran)
capecitabine (Xeloda)
chlorambucil (Leukeran)
cyclophosphamide (Cytoxan)
fluorouracil (Efudex)
flutamide (Eulexin)
hydroxyurea (Hydrea)
interferon alfa-2a (Roferon-A)
interferon alfa-2b (Intron-A)
imatinib (Gleevec)
letrozole (Femara)
leucovorin (Wellcovorin)
lomustine (CeeNU)
megestrol (Megace)
melphalan (Alkeran)
mercaptopurine (Purinethol)
methotrexate (Folex)
mitotane (Lysodren)
paclitaxel (Taxol)
peginterferon alfa-2b
(PEG-Intron)
procarbazine (Matulane)
tamoxifen (Novaldex)
toremifene (Fareston)

CARDIAC GLYCOSIDES
digoxin (Lanoxin)

CENTRAL NERVOUS SYSTEM STIMULANTS
dextroamphetamine (Dexedrine)
methylphenidate (Ritalin)
methamphetamine (Desoxyn)
modafinil (Provigil)
pemoline (Cylert)

CEPHALOSPORINS
cefaclor (Ceclor)
cefadroxil (Duricef)
cefazolin (Ancef)
cefdinir (Omnicef)
cefepime (Maxipime)
cefixime (Suprax)
cefpodoxime (Vantil)
cefprozil (Cefzil)
ceftibuten (Cedax)
cefuroxime (Ceftin)
cephalexin (Keflex)
cephradine (Velosef)
loracarbef (Lorabid)

CHOLESTEROL LOWERING AGENTS
atorvastatin (Lipitor)
fluvastatin (Lescol)
lovastatin (Mevacor)
pravastatin (Pravachol)

CHOLINERGIC AGONISTS
bethanechol (Urecholine)
pyridostigmine (Mestinon)

CHOLINESTRASE INHIBITORS
ambenonium (Mytelase)
neostigmine (Prostigmin)
pyridostigmine (Mestinon)

DECONGESTANTS
oxymetazoline (Afrin)
phenylephrine (Neo-Synephrine)
pseudoephedrine (Sudafed)

D

DEMENTIA/ALZHEIMER'S
donepezil (Aricept)
ergoloid mesylate (Hydergine)
galantamine (Reminyl)
rivastigmine (Exelon)
tacrine (Cognex)

DERMATOLOGICS
acitretin (Soriatane)
alitretinoin (Panretin)
azelaic acid (Azelex)
capsaicin (Zostrix)
doxepin (Zonalon)
isotretinoin (Accutane)
methotrexate (Folex)
minoxidil (Rogaine)
tacrolimus (Protopic)
tazarotene (Tazorac)
tretinoin (Retin-A)

DIURETICS
Loop diuretics
bumetanide (Bumex)
ethacrynate (Edecrin)
furosemide (Lasix)
torsemide (Demadex)
Potassium sparing
amiloride (Midamor)
spironolactone (Aldactone)
triamterene (Dyrenium)
Thiazides
chlorothiazide (Diuril)
hydrochlorothiazide
 (HydroDIURIL)
polythiazide (Renese)
Thiazide-like
chlorthalidone (Hygroton)
indapamide (Lozol)
metolazone (Zaroxolyn)
Others
acetazolamide (Diamox)
methazolamide (Neptazane)

ENDOCRINE
clomiphene (Clomid)
conjugated estrogens (Premarin)

conjugated estrogens, synthetic
 (Cenestin)
danazol (Danocrine)
desmopressin (DDAVP)
esterified estrogens (Estrab)
estradiol transdermal
 (Estraderm)
estradiol valerate (Estrace)
estropipate (Ogen)
estrogen substance conjugated
 (Premarin)
ethinyl estradiol (Estinyl)
finasteride (Proscar)
fluoxymesterone (Halotestin)
glucagon (Glucagon
 Emergency Kit)
levonorgestrel (Norplant System)
levothyroxine (Synthroid)
liothyronine (Cytomel)
liotrix (Euthroid)
medroxyprogesterone (Provera)
norethindrone (Aygestin)
norgestrel (Ovrette)
oral contraceptives (many
 brands)
oxandrolone (Oxandrin)
oxymetholone (Anadrol)
raloxifene (Evista)
stanozolol (Winstrol)
testosterone (Androderm)
thyroid (Armour Thyroid)

ERECTILE DYSFUNCTION
alprostadil (Caverject)
sildenafil (Viagra)

ERGOT ALKALOIDS
(see migraine)
ergotamine (Ergostat)

EXPECTORANT
guaifenesin (Humibid)

FLUOROQUINOLONES
alatrofloxacin (Trovan IV)
ciprofloxacin (Cipro)
enoxacin (Penetrex)

gatifloxacin (Tequin)
levofloxacin (Levaquin)
lomefloxacin (Maxaquin)
moxifloxacin (Avelox)
norfloxacin (Noroxin)
ofloxacin (Floxin)
sparfloxacin (Zagam)
trovafloxacin (Trovan)

FOLATE ANTAGONIST
trimetrexate (Neutrexin)

GASTROESOPHAGEAL REFLUX DISEASE
esomeprazole (Nexium)
lansoprazole (Prevacid)
omeprazole (Prilosec)
pantoprazole (Protonix)
rabeprazole (Aciphex)

GASTROINTESTINAL DRUGS
balsalazide (Colazal)
infliximab (Remicade)
lansoprazole (Prevacid)
mesalamine (Asacol)
metoclopramide (Reglan)
misoprostol (Cytotec)
olsalazine (Dipentum)
pancrelipase (Cotazym)
rabeprazole (Aciphex)
sucralfate (Carafate)
sulfasalazine (Azulfidine)

GLAUCOMA TREATMENT
acetazolamide (Diamox)
apraclonidine (Iopidine)
betaxolol (Betoptic)
bimatoprost (Lumigan)
brimonidine (Alphagan)
brinzolamide (Azopt)
carteolol (Ocupress)
dipivefrin (Propine C)
dorzolamide (Trusopt)
emedastine (Emadine)
latanoprost (Xalatan)
levobunolol (Betagan)

methazolamide (Neptazane)
pilocarpine (Isopto-Carpine)
timolol (Timoptic)
travoprost (Travatan)
unoprostone (Rescula)

GLUCOCORTICOIDS
Inhalant sprays
beclomethasone (Vanceril Inh)
budesonide (Rhinocort Inh)
flunisolide (Aerobid Inh)
fluticasone (Flonase)
mometasone (Nasonex)
triamcinolone (Azmacort)
Systemic
betamethasone (Celestone)
cortisone (Cortone)
dexamethasone (Dexadron)
fludrocortisone (Florinef)
hydrocortisone (Cortef)
methylprednisolone (Medrol)
prednisolone (Delta-Cortef)
prednisone (Meticorten)
triamcinolone (Aristocort)
Topical
betamethasone (Diprolene)
clobetasol (Temovate)
clobetasol foam (Olux)
clocortolone (Cloderm)
desonide (DesOwen)
desoximetasone (Topicort)
dexamethasone (Decaderm)
diflorasone (Florone)
fluocinonide (Lidex)
flurandrenolide (Cordran)
fluticasone (Cutivate)
halcinonide (Halog)
halobetasol (Ultravate)
hydrocortisone (Allercort)
hydrocortisone buteprate
  (Pandel)
loteprednol (Lotemax, Alrex)
prednicarbate (Dermatop)
rimexolone (Vexol)
triamcinolone topical (Kenalog)

HEMOSTATICS
- absorbable gelatin sponge (Gelfoam)
- aminocaproic acid (Amicar)
- oxidized cellulose (Surgicel)
- tranexamic acid (Cyklokapron)

IMMUNOMODULATORS
- imiquimod (Aldara)
- interferon alfa-2a (Roferon-A)
- interferon alfa-2b (Intron-A)
- interferon alfa-n_1 (Wellferon)
- interferon alfa-n_3 (Alferon-N)
- interferon beta-1a (Avonex)
- interferon gamma-1b (Actimmune)
- levamisole (Ergamisol)
- peginterferon alfa-2b (PEG-Intron)

IMMUNOSUPPRESSANTS
- azathioprine (Imuran)
- cyclosporine (Sandimmune)
- daclizumab (Zenapax)
- mycophenolate (CellCept)
- prednisone (Meticorten)
- tacrolimus (Prograf)
- tacrolimus (Protopic)

LEUKOTRIENE RECEPTOR ANTAGONIST
- montelukast (Singulair)
- zafirlukast (Accolate)

LEUKOTRIENE PATHWAY INHIBITOR
- zileuton (Zyflo)

LINCOSAMIDES
- clindamycin (Cleocin)
- lincomycin (Lincocin)

MACROLIDES
- azithromycin (Zithromax)
- clarithromycin (Biaxin)
- dirithromycin (DynaBac)
- erythromycin (Erythrocin)

MALE PATTERN BALDNESS
- finasteride (Propecia)
- minoxidil (Rogaine)

MAST CELL STABILIZERS
- cromolyn (Intal)
- lodoxamide (Alomide)
- nedocromil (Tilade)
- permirolast (Alamast)

MIGRAINE
(see ergot alkaloids)
- almotriptan (Axert)
- divalproex (Depakote)
- frovatriptan succinate (Frova)
- methysergide (Sansert)
- naratriptan (Amerge)
- propranolol (Inderal)
- rizatriptan (Maxalt)
- sumatriptan (Imitrex)
- timolol (Blocadren)
- zolmitripan (Zomig)

MINERALS
- ferrous gluconate
- ferrous sulfate (Feosol)
- ferrous fumarate
- potassium chloride (Micro-K)
- sodium fluoride

MUCOLYTIC
- dornase alfa (Pulmozyme)

MULTIPLE SCLEROSIS
- tizanidine (Zanaflex)

MYASTHENIA GRAVIS
- ambenonium (Mytelase)
- neostigmine (Prostigmin)
- pyridostigmine (Mestinon)

MYDRIATIC
- atropine sulfate (optic) (Isopto Atropine)

homatropine hydrobromide
(optic) (Isopto Homatropine)

NARCOTICS
(see analgesics [opioid])

NITROIMIDAZOLE
metronidazole (Flagyl)

NONSTEROIDAL ANTIINFLAMMATORY DRUGS
aspirin
celecoxib (Celebrex)
diclofenac (Voltaren)
diflunisal (Dolobid)
etodolac (Lodine)
fenoprofen (Nalfon)
flurbiprofen (Ansaid)
ibuprofen (Motrin)
indomethacin (Indocin)
ketoprofen (Orudis)
ketorolac (Toradol)
meclofenamate (Meclomen)
mefenamic acid (Ponstel)
meloxicam (Mobic)
nabumetone (Relafen)
naproxen (Naprosyn)
naproxen sodium (Anaprox)
oxaprozin (Daypro)
piroxicam (Feldene)
rofecoxib (Vioxx)
sulindac (Clinoril)
tolmetin (Tolectin)
valdecoxib (Bextra)

OPHTHALMICS
atropine sulfate (optic)
(Isopto Atropine)
azelastine (Optivar)
betaxolol (Betoptic)
bimatoprost (Lumigan)
carteolol (Occupres)
ciprofloxacin (Ciloxan)
dipivefrin (Propine)
erythromycin (Ilotycin)
flurbiprofen (Ocufen)
gentamicin (Garamycin)

homatropine hydrobromide
(optic) (Isopto Homatropine)
ketotifen (Zaditor)
levocabastine (Livostin)
loteprednol (Lotemax, Alrex)
naphazoline (Naphcon)
ofloxacin (Ocuflox)
olopatadine (Patanol)
permirolast (Alamast)
pilocarpine (Isopto Carpine)
polymyxin (Aerosporin)
sulfacetamide (Sulamyd)
timolol (Timoptic)
tobramycin (Tobrex)
travoprost (Travatan)
trifluridine (Viroptic)
unoprostone (Rescula)
vidarabine (Vira-A)

PENICILLINS
amoxicillin (Amoxil)
amoxicillin/clavulanate
(Augmentin)
ampicillin (Omnipen)
cloxacillin (Tegopen)
dicloxacillin (Dynapen)
oxacillin (Prostaphlin)
penicillin G benzathine
(Bicillin)
penicillin V potassium
(V-Cillin K)

PEPTIDE ANTIINFECTIVE
vancomycin (Vancocin)

PERIODONTAL SPECIALTY PRODUCTS
chlorhexidine (PerioChip)
doxycycline (Atridox)
doxycycline (Periostat)
minocycline (Arestin)

PERIPHERAL VASCULAR DISEASE
cilostazol (Pletal)
isoxsuprine (Vasodilan)

P

papaverine (Pavabid)
pentoxifylline (Trental)

PLATELET AGGREGATION INHIBITORS
anagrelide (Agrylin)
aspirin
clopidogrel (Plavix)
dipyridamole (Persantine)
ticlopidine (Ticlid)

PNEUMOCYSTIC PNEUMONITIS
atovaquone (Mepron)
pentamidine (Pentam 300)
sulfamethoxazole/trimethoprim
(Bactrim, Septra)
trimetrexate (Neutrexin)

PROSTAGLANDIN
alprostadil (Caverject)
bimatoprost (Lumigan)
misoprostol (Cytotec)
travoprost (Travatan)

PROSTATE HYPERPLASIA
finasteride (Proscar)
tamsulosin (Flomax)
terazosin (Hytrin)

SALIVARY STIMULANTS
amifostine (Ethyol)
cevimeline (Evoxac)
pilocarpine (Salagen)

SKELETAL MUSCLE RELAXANTS
baclofen (Lioresal)
carisoprodol (Soma)
chlorphenesin (Maolate)
chlorzoxazone (Paraflex)
cyclobenzaprine (Flexeril)
dantrolene (Dantrium)
metaxalone (Skelexan)
methocarbamol (Robaxin)
orphenadrine (Norflex)

SMOKING CESSATION
bupropion (Zyban)
nicotine polacrylex (Nicorette)
nicotine transdermal (Habitrol,
ProStep)

SULFONAMIDES
sulfacetamide sodium
(Sulamyd Sodium)
sulfamethoxazole/trimethoprim
(Septra, Bactrim)
sulfamethoxazole (Gantanol)
sulfisoxazole (Gantrisin)

TETRACYCLINES
demeclocycline (Declomycin)
doxycycline (Atridox)
doxycycline (Periostat)
doxycycline (Vibramycin)
minocycline (Minocin, Arestin)
tetracycline (Achromycin)
tetracycline fiber (Actisite)

URICOSURIC
probenecid (Benemid)
sulfinpyrazone (Anturane)

URINARY TRACT INFECTIONS
cinoxacin (Cinobac)
flavoxate (Urispas)
fosfomycin (Monurol)
methenamine (Hiprex)
nitrofurantoin (Furadantin)
phenazopyridine (Pyridium)
sulfamethoxazole (Gantanol)
sulfamethoxazole/trimethoprim
(Bactrim, Septra)

VASOCONSTRICTOR
epinephrine (Adrenalin)
phenylephrine (Neo-Synephrine)

VITAMINS
ascorbic acid
calcipotriene (Dovonex, D_3)

cyanocobalamin (Rubramin)
dihydrotachysterol (Hytakerol)
doxercalciferol (Hectorol)
folic acid (Folvite, B_9)
niacin (Nicolid)
phytonadione (Aqua
  MEPHYTON)
pyridoxine (B_6)
riboflavin (B_2)
thiamine (B_1)
vitamin A (Aquasol A)
vitamin D (Calciferol)

vitamin E (Aquasol E)

WOUND REPAIR
becaplermin (Regranex)

XANTHINES AND XANTHINE DERIVATIVES
aminophylline (Somophyllin)
dyphylline (Dilor)
oxtriphylline (Choledyl)
pentoxifylline (Trental)
theophylline (Theo-Dur)

x

Individual Drugs

abacavir sulfate

(a-bak′a-veer)

Ziagen

Drug class.: Antiviral, nucleoside analog

Action: Converted to an active metabolite, carbovir triphosphate, that inhibits reverse transcriptase enzymes in human immunodeficiency virus type 1 (HIV-1)

Uses: Used in combination with other antiviral drugs for treatment of HIV-1 infection

Dosage and routes:

• *Adult:* PO 300 mg bid in combination with other antiretroviral drugs

• *Child 3 mo-16 yr:* PO 8 mg/kg bid not to exceed adult dose; use with other antiviral drugs for HIV-1

Available forms include: Tabs 300 mg, oral sol 20 mg/ml in 240 ml vol

Side effects/adverse reactions:

▼ *ORAL:* Mucous membrane lesions

CNS: Insomnia, fatigue, headache, asthenia, lethargy

CV: Edema

*GI: Nausea, vomiting, diarrhea, anorexia, **lactic acidosis, pancreatitis***

RESP: Shortness of breath

INTEG: Rash, urticaria

META: Elevation of blood glucose, triglyceride elevation, alteration of liver enzymes

HEMA: Decreased lymphocytes

MS: Myalgia, arthralgia

*MISC: **Fatal hypersensitivity reactions,** fever*

Contraindications: Hypersensitivity

Precautions: Do not breast-feed, pregnancy category C, bone marrow depression, renal or hepatic impairment, use with other antivirals to avoid emergence of resistant viruses, avoid alcohol use

Pharmacokinetics:

PO: Bioavailability (83%), plasma protein binding (50%), hepatic metabolism (alcohol dehydrogenase), primarily renal excretion, fecal excretion (16%)

🦷 **Drug interactions of concern to dentistry:**

• None reported

DENTAL CONSIDERATIONS

General:

• Examine for oral manifestation of opportunistic infection.

• Patient on chronic drug therapy may rarely have symptoms of blood dyscrasias, which include infection, bleeding, and poor healing.

• Avoid dental light in patient's eyes; offer dark glasses for patient comfort.

• Place on frequent recall due to oral side effects.

• Consider semisupine chair position for patient comfort if GI side effects occur.

Consultations:

• In a patient with symptoms of blood dyscrasias, request a medical consult for blood studies and postpone treatment until normal values are reestablished.

• Medical consult may be required to assess disease control.

Teach patient/family:

• Importance of good oral hygiene to prevent soft tissue inflammation

• To prevent trauma when using oral hygiene aids

• To be alert for the possibility of

---

bold italic = life-threatening conditions

secondary oral infection and the need to see dentist immediately if signs of infection occur

---

absorbable gelatin sponge

Gelfoam

Drug class.: Hemostatic, purified gelatin sponge

Action: Absorbs blood, provides area for clot formation
Uses: Hemostasis adjunct in dental surgery
Dosage and routes:
Dental use
• *Adult:* TOP can be applied dry or moistened with normal saline solution; blot on sterile gauze to remove excess solution, shape to fit with light finger compression; hold pressure on dry foam for 1-2 min
Available forms include: Dental packs, size 4 (2 × 2 cm)
Side effects/adverse reactions:
• None reported
Contraindications: Hypersensitivity, frank infection
Precautions: Avoid use in presence of infection, potential nidus of infection, do not resterilize product
Pharmacokinetics:
IMPLANT: Absorbed in 4-6 wk
DENTAL CONSIDERATIONS
Teach patient/family:
• To immediately report any sign of infection to the dentist

---

acarbose

(ay´car-bose)
Precose
♣ Prandase
Drug class.: Oral antidiabetic

Action: Inhibits α-glucosidase and pancreatic α-amylase in the GI tract to delay the breakdown of carbohydrates to glucose, resulting in lower postprandial plasma glucose levels
Uses: Use as single drug or in combination with insulin or oral hypoglycemics (sulfonylureas) in type 2 diabetes (NIDDM) when diet control is ineffective in controlling blood glucose levels
Dosage and routes:
• *Adult:* PO initial dose 25 mg tid at start of each meal; after testing may be increased to 50 mg tid at start of each meal; max dose >60 kg is 100 mg tid; max dose <60 kg is 50 mg tid
Caution: Doses must be individualized for each patient
Available forms include: Tabs 50, 100 mg
Side effects/adverse reactions:
GI: Bloating, flatulence, diarrhea, abdominal pain
META: Elevations of AST/ALT
Contraindications: Hypersensitivity, diabetic ketoacidosis, cirrhosis, inflammatory or obstructive GI disease, severe renal impairment
Precautions: Use glucose for hypoglycemia, monitor blood glucose levels, pregnancy category B, avoid use in lactation, children
Pharmacokinetics:
PO: Limited oral absorption, absorbed dose excreted in urine, metabolized in the GI tract and major portion of dose excreted in feces
🦷 **Drug interactions of concern to dentistry:**
• None reported; this is a new drug and information is lacking
DENTAL CONSIDERATIONS
General:
• Ensure that patient is following

prescribed diet and takes medication regularly.

• Type 2 patients may also be using insulin. Should symptomatic hypoglycemia occur while taking this drug use dextrose rather than sucrose because of interference with sucrose metabolism.

• Place on frequent recall to evaluate healing response.

• Patients with diabetes may be more susceptible to infection and have delayed wound healing.

• Question the patient about self-monitoring the drug's antidiabetic effect.

• Consider semisupine chair position for patient comfort when GI side effects occur.

Consultations:

• Medical consult may be required to assess disease control and patient's ability to tolerate stress.

Teach patient/family:

• Importance of good oral hygiene to prevent soft tissue inflammation

---

acetaminophen

(a-seet-a-min'oh-fen)

Anacin-3, Anacin-3 Extra Strength, Apacet, Aspirin Free Anacin Maximum Strength, Aspirin Free Excedrin, Dapa, Datril Extra Strength, Excedrin Extra Strength, Liquiprin, Panadol, Tempra, Tylenol, Tylenol Arthritis Extended Relief, Valorin, and many others

♣ Abenol, Atasol, Robigesic, Rounax

Drug class.: Nonnarcotic analgesic

Action: Analgesic action not fully determined; presumed to block the initiation of pain impulses by inhibition of prostaglandin synthesis; acts mainly in the CNS and to a lesser degree in peripheral nerves; antipyretic action results from inhibition of prostaglandin synthesis in the hypothalamic heat-regulating center

Uses: Mild-to-moderate pain, fever; also used in combination with other ingredients, including opioids

Dosage and routes:

• *Adult and child >12 yr:* PO 325-650 mg q4h prn or 1 g q6h, not to exceed 4 g/day; REC: 325-650 mg q4-6h prn, not to exceed 4 g/day

• *Adult:* PO for osteoarthritis, 1300 mg tid

• *Child 0-3 mo:* PO 40 mg/dose q4h

• *Child 4-12 mo:* PO 80 mg/dose q4h

• *Child 1-2 yr:* PO 120 mg/dose q4h

• *Child 2-4 yr:* PO/REC 160 mg/dose q4h

• *Child 4-6 yr:* PO/REC 240 mg/dose q4h

• *Child 6-9 yr:* PO/REC 320 mg/dose q4h

• *Child 9-11 yr:* PO/REC 320-400 mg/dose q4h

• *Child 11-12 yr:* PO/REC 320-480 mg/dose q4h

Available forms include: Rec supp 120, 125, 325, 650 mg; chew tab 80, 160 mg; tabs 325, 500, 650 mg; caps 500 mg; elix 120, 160, 325 mg/5 ml; liq 160 mg/5 ml, 500 mg/15 ml; sol (infant drops) 100 mg/1 ml, 120 mg/2.5 ml

Side effects/adverse reactions:

CNS: Stimulation, drowsiness

GI: **Hepatotoxicity,** nausea, vomiting, abdominal pain

HEMA: **Leukopenia, neutropenia, hemolytic anemia** (long-term use), **thrombocytopenia, pancytopenia**

---

bold italic = life-threatening conditions

*INTEG: **Angioedema,*** rash, urticaria

*TOXICITY: **Cyanosis, anemia, neutropenia, jaundice, pancytopenia, CNS stimulation, delirium; then vascular collapse, convulsions, coma, death***

Contraindications: Hypersensitivity, chronic heavy alcohol use

Precautions: Anemia, hepatic disease, renal disease, chronic alcoholism, pregnancy category B

Pharmacokinetics:

PO: Onset 10-30 min, peak 0.5-2 hr, duration 4-6 hr, half-life 1-3 hr

REC: Slow, variable onset

For all routes, is metabolized in the liver, excreted by the kidneys, crosses the placenta, and found in breast milk

🦷 **Drug interactions of concern to dentistry:**

• Decreased effects: barbiturates

• Nephrotoxicity: NSAIDs, salicylates (chronic, high-dose concurrent use)

• Liver toxicity: chronic use of hydantoins, chronic alcohol use, high dose carbamazepine

• *Buffered acetaminophen:* decreased absorption of tetracycline

• *When prescribed for dental pain:* question patients about recent use of acetaminophen because acetaminophen has been shown to increase the INR to 4.0 or greater depending on the amount of acetaminophen taken. Obtain a new PT or INR value if surgical procedures are required.

• Data indicate that use of four regular strength acetaminophen tablets (325 mg) qd for 1 wk can increase the risk of INR values greater than 6.0. If acetaminophen must be used for a long duration, it is important to closely monitor INR values. *JAMA* 279:657-662.

DENTAL CONSIDERATIONS

General:

• Avoid prolonged use with aspirin-containing products.

• Determine why the patient is taking the drug.

• Patients on chronic drug therapy may rarely have symptoms of blood dyscrasias, which can include infection, bleeding, and poor healing.

Consultations:

• In a patient with symptoms of blood dyscrasias, request a medical consult for blood studies and postpone dental treatment until normal values are reestablished.

---

acetazolamide/ acetazolamide sodium

(a-set-a-zole′a-mide)

Ak-Zol, Dazamide, Diamox, Storzolamide

🍁 Acetazolam,   Apo-Acetazolamide

Drug class.: Diuretic, carbonic anhydrase inhibitor

Action: Inhibits carbonic anhydrase activity in proximal renal tubular cells to decrease reabsorption of water, sodium, potassium, bicarbonate; decreases carbonic anhydrase in CNS, increasing seizure threshold; able to decrease aqueous humor in eye, which lowers intraocular pressure

Uses: Open-angle glaucoma, narrow-angle glaucoma (preoperatively, if surgery delayed), epilepsy (petit mal, grand mal, mixed), edema in CHF, drug-induced edema, acute altitude sickness

Dosage and routes:
Narrow-angle glaucoma
• *Adult:* PO/IM/IV 250 mg q4h, or 250 mg bid, to be used for short-term therapy; ext rel 500 mg bid
Open-angle glaucoma
• *Adult:* PO/IM/IV 250 mg-1 g/day in divided doses for amounts over 250 mg
Available forms include: Tabs 125, 250 mg; sus rel caps 500 mg; inj IM/IV 500 mg
Side effects/adverse reactions:
▼ *ORAL:* Dry/burning mouth, tongue, lips; paresthesia; metallic taste; thirst
CNS: Drowsiness, paresthesia, anxiety, depression, headache, dizziness, confusion, stimulation, fatigue, seizures, sedation, nervousness
GI: Nausea, vomiting, anorexia, hepatic insufficiency, constipation, diarrhea, melena, weight loss
HEMA: Aplastic anemia, hemolytic anemia, leukopenia, agranulocytosis, thrombocytopenia, purpura, pancytopenia
GU: Frequency, hypokalemia, uremia, polyuria, glucosuria, hematuria, dysuria
EENT: Myopia, tinnitus
INTEG: Rash, Stevens-Johnson syndrome, photosensitivity, pruritus, urticaria, fever
ENDO: Hyperglycemia
Contraindications: Hypersensitivity to sulfonamides, severe renal disease, severe hepatic disease, electrolyte imbalances (hyponatremia, hypokalemia), hyperchloremic acidosis, Addison's disease, long-term use in narrow-angle glaucoma, COPD
Precautions: Hypercalciuria, pregnancy category C; chronic use of

oral sulfonylureas has been associated with increased risk of CV mortality; risk is controversial
Pharmacokinetics:
PO: Onset 1-1.5 hr, peak 1-3 hr, duration 6-12 hr
PO (SUS REL): Onset 2 hr, peak 8-12 hr, duration 18-24 hr
IV: Onset 2 min, peak 15 min, duration 4-5 hr
65% absorbed if fasting (oral), 75% absorbed if given with food; half-life 2.5-5.5 hr; excreted unchanged by kidneys (80% within 24 hr); crosses placenta
Drug interactions of concern to dentistry:
• Toxicity: salicylates (large doses)
• Hypokalemia: corticosteroids (systemic use)
• Crystalluria: ciprofloxacin
DENTAL CONSIDERATIONS:
General:
• Patients on chronic drug therapy may rarely have symptoms of blood dyscrasias, which can include infection, bleeding, and poor healing.
• Assess salivary flow as a factor in caries, periodontal disease, and candidiasis.
• Avoid drugs that may exacerbate glaucoma (e.g., anticholinergics).
Consultations:
• In a patient with symptoms of blood dyscrasias, request a medical consult for blood studies and postpone dental treatment until normal values are reestablished.
• Consult may be required to assess disease control.
Teach patient/family:
• Importance of good oral hygiene to prevent soft tissue inflammation
• Caution to prevent injury when using oral hygiene aids

---

bold italic = life-threatening conditions   *For periodic updates, visit* **www.mosby.com**

When chronic dry mouth occurs, advise patient:

• To avoid mouth rinses with high alcohol content due to drying effects
• To use daily home fluoride products for anticaries effect
• To use sugarless gum, frequent sips of water, or saliva substitutes

---

acetohexamide

(a-set-oh-hex′a-mide)
Dymelor
♣ Dimelor

Drug class.: Sulfonylurea (first generation), antidiabetic

Action: Causes functioning beta cells in pancreas to release insulin, leading to drop in blood glucose levels; may improve binding between insulin and insulin receptors or increase number of insulin receptors; not effective if patient lacks functioning beta cells
Uses: Stable adult-onset diabetes mellitus (type 2)
Dosage and routes:
• *Adult:* PO 250 mg-1.5 g/day; usually given before breakfast, unless large dose is required, then dose is divided in two
Available forms include: Tabs 250, 500 mg scored
Side effects/adverse reactions:
CNS: Headache, weakness, tinnitus, fatigue, dizziness, vertigo
GI: ***Hepatotoxicity, jaundice,*** heartburn, nausea, vomiting, diarrhea
HEMA: ***Leukopenia, thrombocytopenia, agranulocytosis, aplastic anemia, hemolytic anemia,*** increased AST/ALT, alk phosphatase
INTEG: Rash, allergic reactions, pruritus, urticaria, eczema, photosensitivity, erythema
ENDO: ***Hypoglycemia***
Contraindications: Hypersensitivity to sulfonylureas, juvenile or brittle diabetes
Precautions: Pregnancy category C, elderly, cardiac disease, renal disease, hepatic disease, thyroid disease, severe hypoglycemic reactions
Pharmacokinetics:
PO: Onset 1 hr, peak 2-4 hr, duration 12-24 hr, half-life 6-8 hr; completely absorbed by GI route; metabolized in liver; excreted in urine (active metabolites, unchanged drug)
🦷 Drug interactions of concern to dentistry:
• Increased hypoglycemic effects: salicylates (large doses), NSAIDs, ketoconazole, miconazole
• Decreased action: corticosteroids
• Disulfiram-like reaction: alcohol
DENTAL CONSIDERATIONS
General:
• Monitor vital signs every appointment due to cardiovascular effects of diabetes.
• Patients on chronic drug therapy may rarely have symptoms of blood dyscrasias, which can include infection, bleeding, and poor healing.
• Place on frequent recall to evaluate healing response.
• Ensure that patient is following prescribed diet and takes medication regularly.
• Question patient about self-monitoring of drug's antidiabetic effect, including blood glucose values (SMBG) or finger-stick records.
• Avoid prescribing aspirin-containing products.

• Early morning appointments and a stress reduction protocol may be required for anxious patients.
• Patients with diabetes may be more susceptible to infection and have delayed wound healing.

Consultations:
• In a patient with symptoms of blood dyscrasias, request a medical consult for blood studies and postpone dental treatment until normal values are reestablished.
• Medical consult may include data from patient's blood glucose monitoring, including glycosylated hemoglobin (GHb) or HbA_{1c} testing.

Teach patient/family:
• Importance of good oral hygiene to prevent soft tissue inflammation
• Caution to prevent injury when using oral hygiene aids
• To avoid mouth rinses with high alcohol content

---

acitretin
(a-si-tre′tin)
Soriatane
Drug class.: Systemic retinoid

Action: Unclear; may enhance the inflammatory response and accelerate reappearance of the stratum corneum; binds to nuclear retinoic acid receptors (RAR) and may alter gene expression
Uses: Severe psoriasis; unlabeled uses: nonpsoritic dermatoses, keratinization disorders, palmoplantar keratoses, lichen planus, Darier's disease, Sjögren-Larrson syndrome
Dosage and routes:
• *Adult:* PO initial dose 25-50 mg qd taken with the main meal, adjust dose by patient response

Available forms include: Caps 10, 25 mg
Side effects/adverse reactions:
▼ *ORAL: Xerostomia (30%), ulcerative and nonulcerative stomatitis, taste perversion, cheilitis, gingival bleeding,* gingival hyperplasia
CNS: Fatigue, headache, dizziness, dysesthesia
*CV: Flushing, **pseudotumor cerebri***
*GI: Abdominal pain, diarrhea, nausea, **hepatitis, pancreatitis***
RESP: Sinusitis
HEMA: Thrombocytosis
EENT: Rhinitis, xerophthalmia, earache, tinnitus, dry eyes, dry nose, conjunctivitis, epistaxis, blurred vision, eye pain, photophobia
INTEG: Abnormal skin color, dry skin, alopecia, bulbous eruption, dermatitis, rash, purpura, skin fissures and ulcerations, photosensitivity
META: Elevation in serum transaminase, lipid disturbances, hyperglyceridemia
MS: Arthralgia, myalgia, spinal hyperostosis
MISC: Joint pains, asthenia, chills, diaphoresis
Contraindications: Hypersensitivity, hypersensitivity to etretinate, pregnancy, ethanol use, concurrent use with vitamin A, hepatic disease, tetracyclines
Precautions: Women are advised to use effective contraception during use and for 2 yr after use, renal impairment, lactation, pregnancy category X, hyperlipidemia, cardiovascular disease

---

Pharmacokinetics:
PO: Peak serum levels 2-5 hr; food enhances bioavailability, highly plasma protein bound (99.9%), hepatic metabolism, active metabolite; excreted in urine and bile

♣ Drug interactions of concern to dentistry:
• Avoid vitamin preparations containing vitamin A
• Avoid tetracyclines and other drugs that cause photosensitivity

DENTAL CONSIDERATIONS
General:
• Determine why patient is taking the drug.
• Apply lubricant to dry lips for patient comfort before dental procedures.
• Assess salivary flow as factor in caries, periodontal disease, and candidiasis.
• Palliative medication may be required for management of oral side effects.
• Place on frequent recall due to oral side effects.
• Consider semisupine chair position for patient comfort if GI side effects occur.
• Avoid dental light in patient's eyes; offer dark glasses for patient comfort.

Consultations:
• Medical consult may be required to assess disease control.

Teach patient/family:
• Importance of good oral hygiene to prevent soft tissue inflammation
• Caution patient to prevent trauma when using oral hygiene aids
• To report oral lesions, soreness, or bleeding to dentist
When chronic dry mouth occurs, advise patient:

• To avoid mouth rinses with high alcohol content due to drying effects
• To use daily home fluoride products for anticaries effect
• To use sugarless gum, frequent sips of water, or saliva substitutes

---

acyclovir (topical)
(ay-sye′kloe-ver)
Zovirax
Drug class.: Antiviral

Action: Converted to acyclovir triphosphate by herpes simplex thymidine kinase resulting in inhibition of DNA polymerase, thereby inhibiting HSV DNA replication
Uses: Simple mucocutaneous herpes simplex, and in immunocompromised patients with initial herpes genitalis; unapproved: herpes zoster

Dosage and routes:
• *Adult and child:* TOP apply to all lesions q3h while awake, 6 × daily × 1 wk
Available forms include: TOP oint 5% (50 mg/g) in 3 g and 15 g tubes; top cream 5% (Canada)

Side effects/adverse reactions:
▼ ORAL: Stinging sensation (lip application)
INTEG: Rash, urticaria, stinging, burning, pruritus, vulvitis
Contraindications: Hypersensitivity
Precautions: Pregnancy category C, lactation; cutaneous use only

DENTAL CONSIDERATIONS
General:
• Postpone dental treatment when oral herpetic lesions are present.

Teach patient/family:
• To dispose of toothbrush or other contaminated oral hygiene devices

used during period of infection to prevent reinoculation of herpetic infection

• To apply with a finger cot or latex glove to prevent herpes infection on fingers

• To avoid mouth rinses with high alcohol content due to irritating effects

---

acyclovir sodium

(ay-sye′kloe-ver)
Zovirax
♣ Avirax
Drug class.: Antiviral

Action: Converted to acyclovir triphosphate by herpes simplex thymidine kinase resulting in inhibition of DNA polymerase, thereby inhibiting HSV DNA replication

Uses: Initial episodes of herpes genitalis (HSV-2), *herpes simplex*, neonatal *herpes simplex* in immunocompromised patients, *herpes zoster* in all patients, varicella (chickenpox); unapproved: prophylaxis of *herpes simplex* or *herpes zoster*

Dosage and routes:

Herpes simplex (mucocutaneous)

• *Adult:* PO 200-400 mg 5 × daily for 10 days in immunocompromised patients

Genital herpes

• *Adult:* PO initial dose 200 mg q4h 5 × daily while awake for 10 days; chronic suppressive therapy 400 mg bid or 200 mg 3-5 × day up to 12 mo

Herpes zoster

• 800 mg q4h, 5 × daily for 7-10 days

Chickenpox

• *Child >2 yr:* PO 20 mg/kg per dose (limit 800 mg), 4 × daily for 5 days; start at earliest sign of symptoms

• *Adult and child >40 kg:* PO 800 mg 4 × daily × 5 days

Available forms include: Caps 200 mg; tabs 400 mg and 800 mg; powder for inj IV 500 mg and 1000 mg vials; susp 200 mg/5 ml

Side effects/adverse reactions:

▼ *ORAL:* Glossitis, medication taste

*CNS: **Convulsions,** confusion, lethargy, hallucinations, dizziness, headache

CV: Peripheral edema

GI: Nausea, vomiting, diarrhea, abdominal pain

*HEMA: **Thrombocytopenia, leukopenia,** lymphadenopathy

GU: Elevated creatinine

EENT: Visual abnormalities

*INTEG: **Erythema multiforme, toxic epidermal necrolysis,** rash,* urticaria, pruritus, phlebitis at IV site

META: Increased ALT/AST

*MISC: **Anaphylaxis,** fever

Contraindications: Hypersensitivity

Precautions: Lactation, hepatic disease, renal disease, electrolyte imbalance, dehydration, pregnancy category B

Pharmacokinetics:

IV: Peak 1 hr, half-life 20 min to 3 hr (terminal); metabolized by liver; excreted by kidneys as unchanged drug (95%); crosses placenta

PO: Peak levels 1.5-2 hr, plasma half-life 2.5-3 hr; low protein binding

🦷 **Drug interactions of concern to dentistry:**

• No dental drug interactions reported

---

bold italic = life-threatening conditions   *For periodic updates, visit* **www.mosby.com**

DENTAL CONSIDERATIONS
General:
• Patients on chronic drug therapy may rarely have symptoms of blood dyscrasias, which can include infection, bleeding, and poor healing.
• Determine why the patient is taking the drug.
Consultations:
• In a patient with symptoms of blood dyscrasias, request a medical consult for blood studies and postpone dental treatment until normal values are reestablished.
• Medical consult may be required to assess disease control.
Teach patient/family:
• Importance of good oral hygiene to prevent soft tissue inflammation
• Caution to prevent injury when using oral hygiene aids
• To avoid mouth rinses with high alcohol content due to drying effects
• To dispose of toothbrush or other contaminated oral hygiene devices used during period of infection to prevent reinoculation of herpetic infection

---

albuterol and albuterol sulfate

(al-byoo′ter-ole)

Airet, Gen-Salbutamol, Proventil, Proventil HFA, Proventil Repetabs, Ventodisk, Ventolin, Ventolin Rotacaps, Volmax
♣ Apo-Salvent, Novo-Salmol, Ventolin Nebules

Drug class.: Adrenergic β_2-agonist

Action: Causes bronchodilation by agonist action on β_2-receptors by increasing levels of cAMP, which relaxes smooth muscle with very little effect on heart rate; may also inhibit the release of immediate hypersensitivity mediators

Uses: Prevention of exercise-induced asthma, bronchospasm with reversible obstructive airway disease, exercise-induced bronchospasm; unlabeled use acute, serious hyperkalemia in hemodialysis patients

Dosage and routes:
INH sulfate solution (bronchodilation):
• *Adult and child >12 yr:* INH 2.5 mg by nebulization over 5-15 min q4-6h
• *Child 2-12 yr:* INH 1.25-2.5 mg by nebulization over 5-15 min q4-6h
INH sulfate capsules (bronchodilation):
• *Adult and child >4 yr:* INH 200-400 μg q4-6h prophylaxis for exercise-induced bronchospasm
• *Adult and child >4 yr:* INH 200 μg 15 min before exercise
INH aerosol (bronchodilation):
• *Adult and child >4 yr:* INH 2 inhalations (180-200 μg) q4-6h prophylaxis for exercise-induced bronchospasm
• *Adult and child >4 yr:* INH 2 inhalations 15 min prior to exercise
Tablets (bronchodilation):
• *Adult and child >12 yr:* PO 2-4 mg tid or qid; limit 32 mg/day
• *Child 6-12 yr:* PO 2 mg tid or qid; limit 24 mg/day
Extended release tablets (bronchodilation):
• *Adult and child >12 yr:* PO 4-8 mg q12h, limit 16 mg bid
• *Child 6-12 yr:* PO 4 mg q12h; limit 12 mg bid
Syrup:
• *Adult and child >14 yr:* PO 2-4 mg tid or qid; limit 8 mg qid

• *Child 6-14 yr:* PO 2 mg tid or qid; limit 24 mg/day
• *Child 2-6 yr:* PO 0.1 mg/kg tid; limit 2 mg tid
• *Elderly and patients sensitive to β-adrenergic agonists:* PO 2 mg tid or qid

Available forms include: Aerosol 90, 100 μ/actuation; tabs 2, 4 mg; ext rel tabs 4, 8 mg; syr 2 mg/5 ml; inhal sol 0.083%, 0.5%; cap inh 200 μ

Side effects/adverse reactions:

▼ *ORAL:* Taste changes, dry mouth, teeth discoloration
CNS: Tremors, anxiety, insomnia, headache, dizziness, stimulation, restlessness, hallucinations, flushing, irritability, fatigue
CV: Palpitation, tachycardia, hypertension, angina, hypotension, dysrhythmias
GI: Heartburn, nausea, vomiting, diarrhea
RESP: Bronchospasm, bronchitis
GU: Difficulty in urination
EENT: Dry nose, irritation of nose and throat, nasal congestion, epistaxis
MS: Muscle cramps

Contraindications: Hypersensitivity to sympathomimetics, tachydysrhythmias, severe cardiac disease

Precautions: Lactation, pregnancy category C, cardiac disorders, hyperthyroidism, diabetes mellitus, hypertension, prostatic hypertrophy, narrow-angle glaucoma, seizures

Pharmacokinetics:

PO: Onset 0.5 hr, peak 2.5 hr, duration 4-6 hr, half-life 2.5 hr
INH: Onset 5-15 min, peak 0.5-2 hr, duration 3-6 hr, half-life 4 hr

Metabolized in the liver; excreted in urine; crosses placenta, breast milk, blood-brain barrier

⚕ Drug interactions of concern to dentistry:

• Increased dysrhythmias: halogenated hydrocarbon anesthetics

DENTAL CONSIDERATIONS
General:

• Monitor vital signs every appointment due to cardiovascular and respiratory side effects.
• Assess salivary flow as a factor in caries, periodontal disease, and candidiasis.
• Consider semisupine chair position for patients with respiratory disease.
• Midday appointments and a stress reduction protocol may be required for anxious patients.
• Be aware that aspirin or sulfite preservatives in vasoconstrictor-containing products can exacerbate asthma.
• Acute asthmatic episodes may be precipitated in the dental office. Sympathomimetic inhalants should be available for emergency use.

Consultations:

• Medical consult may be required to assess disease control.
• Medical consult may be required to assess patient's ability to tolerate stress.

Teach patient/family:

• For inhalation dosage forms, rinse mouth with water after each dose to prevent dryness
When chronic dry mouth occurs, advise patient:
• To avoid mouth rinses with high alcohol content due to drying effects
• To use daily home fluoride products for anticaries effect

---

bold italic = life-threatening conditions   *For periodic updates, visit* **www.mosby.com**

• To use sugarless gum, frequent sips of water, or saliva substitutes

---

alendronate sodium
(a-len'droe-nate)
Fosamax
Drug class.: Amino biphosphonate

Action: Acts as a specific inhibitor of osteoclast-mediated bone resorption

Uses: Osteoporosis treatment and prevention in men and postmenopausal women, glucocorticoid-induced osteoporosis in men and women receiving glucocorticoids at daily dose of 7.5 mg prednisone, Paget's disease of bone

Dosage and routes:
Osteoporosis-Treatment
• *Postmenopause:* PO 10 mg/day; must be taken at least 30 min before first food, beverage, or other medication of the day; take with full glass of water and avoid lying down for 30 min after dose; supplemental calcium and vitamin D required for all patients if dietary intake is inadequate; or 70 mg once weekly
• *Men:* PO 10 mg once daily, as described above

Prevention of osteoporosis in postmenopause
• *Adult:* PO 5 mg/day or 35 mg once weekly taken as described above

Glucocorticoid-induced osteoporosis:
• *Adult:* PO 5 mg/day as described above; in postmenopausal women not receiving estrogen, the dose is 10 mg/day as described above

Paget's disease
• *Adult:* PO 40 mg/day × 6 mo; take as described above; supple-mental calcium and vitamin D required for all patients if dietary intake is inadequate

Available forms include: Tabs 5, 10, 35, 40, 70 mg

Side effects/adverse reactions:
▼ *ORAL:* Taste alteration
CNS: Headache, nervousness
GI: Abdominal pain, nausea, constipation, diarrhea, acid regurgitation, gastritis, esophagitis
INTEG: Rash, erythema
MS: Pain, cramps

Contraindications: Hypersensitivity, hypocalcemia, esophageal abnormalities, inability to sit upright for 30 min

Precautions: Renal insufficiency, active upper GI disease, may see decrease in serum calcium/phosphate, pregnancy category C, lactation

Pharmacokinetics:
PO: Food, coffee, or juice reduces bioavailability; rapidly distributed to bone; not metabolized; almost complete urinary excretion

🦷 **Drug interactions of concern to dentistry:**
• Increased risk of GI side effects in doses >10 mg/day: Use NSAIDs, ASA with caution
• After administration, must wait at least 30 min before taking any other drug

DENTAL CONSIDERATIONS
General:
• Be aware of oral manifestations of Paget's disease (macrognathia, alveolar pain).
• Consider semisupine chair position for patient comfort due to pain experienced in osteoporosis and possible GI side effects of drug.
• Consider short appointments for patient comfort.

Consultations:
• Medical consult may be required to assess disease control and patient's ability to tolerate stress.

---

alitretinoin gel
(a-li-tret'-i-noyn)
Panretin
Drug class.: Topical retinoid

Action: Binds to all known intracellular retinoid receptor subtypes to function as a transcription factor in the regulation of gene expression that controls the process of cellular differentiation and proliferation in both normal and neoplastic cells

Uses: Topical treatment of cutaneous lesions in patients with AIDS-related Kaposi's sarcoma

Dosage and routes:
• *Adult:* TOP apply bid; can increase to tid or qid if application toxicity is not severe; apply enough gel to cover the lesion

Available forms include: Gel 0.1%, 60 g tube

Side effects/adverse reactions:
INTEG: Rash, pain, pruritus, erythema, edema, exfoliative dermatitis, vesiculation

Contraindications: Hypersensitivity, avoid application to mucous membranes and normal skin, hypersensitivity to retinoids

Precautions: Avoid pregnancy, pregnancy category D, discontinue breast-feeding when used, safe use in children unknown, patients >65 yr, occlusive dressings

Pharmacokinetics: No data

☙ Drug interactions of concern to dentistry:
• Risk of photosensitivity reaction: tetracyclines, fluoroquinolones, other photosensitizing drugs

DENTAL CONSIDERATIONS
General:
• Patients will be taking antiviral drugs; note which drugs are being used, because some have potential for significant drug interactions.
• Take a complete medical history, including a current drug history with doses and duration of therapy.

---

allopurinol/allopurinol sodium
(al-oh-pure'i-nole)
Lopurin, Zyloprim
❧ Alloprin, Apo-Allopurinol, Purinol, Zyloprim
Drug class.: Antigout drug

Action: Inhibits the enzyme xanthine oxidase, reducing uric acid synthesis

Uses: Chronic gout, hyperuricemia associated with malignancies, recurrent calcium oxalate calculi, uric acid nephropathy

Dosage and routes:
Gout/hyperuricemia
• *Adult:* PO 100-600 mg qd depending on severity, not to exceed 800 mg/day; maintenance dose 200-300 mg daily
• *Child 6-10 yr:* 300 mg qd or 100 mg tid
• *Child <6 yr:* 50 mg tid

Available forms include: Tabs 100, 200, 300 mg Note: Zyloprim for injection (allopurinol sodium) used only for patients with certain cancers for control of uric acid levels

Side effects/adverse reactions:
▼ *ORAL:* Metallic taste, stomatitis, lichenoid drug reaction, salivary gland swelling

---

CNS: Headache, drowsiness, neuritis, paresthesia

GI: Nausea, vomiting, anorexia, malaise, cramps, peptic ulcer, diarrhea

*HEMA: **Agranulocytosis, thrombocytopenia, aplastic anemia, pancytopenia, leukopenia, bone marrow depression, eosinophilia***

EENT: Retinopathy, cataracts, epistaxis

INTEG: Fever, chills, dermatitis, pruritus, purpura, erythema, ecchymosis, alopecia

MISC: Myopathy, arthralgia, hepatomegaly, ***cholestatic jaundice, renal failure***

Contraindications: Hypersensitivity

Precautions: Pregnancy category C, lactation, renal disease, hepatic disease, children

Pharmacokinetics:

PO: Peak 2-4 hr, half-life 1-2 hr; excreted in feces, urine

⚡ Drug interactions of concern to dentistry:

• Increased risk of rash: ampicillin, amoxicillin, bacampicillin, hetacillin

DENTAL CONSIDERATIONS

General:

• Patients on chronic drug therapy may rarely have symptoms of blood dyscrasias, which can include infection, bleeding, and poor healing.

Consultations:

• In a patient with symptoms of blood dyscrasias, request a medical consult for blood studies and postpone dental treatment until normal values are reestablished.

• Medical consult may be required to assess disease control.

Teach patient/family:

• Importance of good oral hygiene to prevent soft tissue inflammation

• To avoid mouth rinses with high alcohol content due to drying effects

---

almotriptan malate

(al-moh-trip′tan)

Axert

Drug class.: Serotonin agonist

Action: A selective serotonin agonist for 5HT-$_{1/b.1/d}$ receptors with effects on intracranial blood vessels, trigeminal sensory nerves (cranial vessel constriction) and inhibition of proinflammatory vasoactive neuropeptide release

Uses: Acute treatment of migraine with or without aura in adults

Dosage and routes:

• *Adult:* PO single dose of 6.25-12.5 mg; can repeat in 2 hr if headache reoccurs; limit 2 doses in 24 hr

Available forms include: Tab 6.25, 12.5 mg

Side effects/adverse reactions:

▼ *ORAL: Dry mouth,* taste alteration

CNS: Headache, somnolence, dizziness, asthenia, paresthesia, anxiety

CV: Slight increase in BP, palpitation

GI: Nausea, abdominal pain, dyspepsia

EENT: Pharyngitis, rhinitis, ear pain, tinnitus, dry eyes

INTEG: Pruritus, rash, dermatitis

META: Hyperglycemia

MS: Myalgia, weakness

Contraindications: Hypersensitivity, heart disease, uncontrolled hypertension, hemiplegic or basilar migraine, use of another serotonin agonist, ergotamine-type drug in last 24 hr, MAOIs

Precautions: Hypertension, diabetes, elevated cholesterol, obesity, smoking, postmenopause, male >40 yr, preexisting heart disease, elderly, pregnancy category C, lactation, safety/efficacy for pediatric patients not evaluated

Pharmacokinetics:

PO: Bioavailability 80%, peak effect 2.5 hr, half-life 3.1 hr, plasma protein binding 35%, metabolized by CYP3A4 and monoamine oxidase A, most excreted in urine (70%), feces (13%)

🦷 Drug interactions of concern to dentistry:

• Avoid concurrent use of ketoconazole, itraconazole, erythromycin

DENTAL CONSIDERATIONS

General:

• This is an acute-use drug; it is doubtful that patients will present for dental treatment during acute migraine attacks

• Be aware of patient's disease, its severity, frequency when known

Consultations:

• If treating chronic orofacial pain, consult with physician of record.

• Medical consult may be required to assess disease control and patient's ability to tolerate stress.

Teach patient/family:

• That dryness of the mouth may occur when taking this drug; avoid mouth rinses with high alcohol content due to additional drying effects

• Importance of updating health and drug history if physician makes any changes in evaluation or drug regimens

alosetron HCl

(a-loe'se-tron)

Lotronex

Drug class.: Selective serotonin antagonist, neuroenteric modulator

Action: A selective 5-HT$_3$ (serotonin) receptor antagonist; especially those 5-HT$_3$ receptors in enteric neurons of the GI tract

Uses: Treatment of women with diarrhea-predominant irritable bowel syndrome (IBS)

Dosage and routes:

• *Adult:* PO 1 mg bid

Available forms include: Tabs 1 mg

Side effects/adverse reactions:

▼ *ORAL:* Unusual taste (rare)

CNS: Sleep disorders, depression

CV: Hypertension, arrhythmias (infrequent)

*GI: Nausea, GI discomfort, abdominal pain, gas symptoms, dyspepsia, hemorrhoids, **serious complications of constipation, ischemic colitis***

EENT: Allergic rhinitis, throat pain, eye, ear and nose infections

META: Increase in ALT, abnormal bilirubin

MISC: Allergies (rare)

Contraindications: Hypersensitivity; patients with constipation, chronic or severe constipation, history of sequela from constipation, intestinal obstruction, stricture, toxic megacolon, GI perforation, adhesions, ischemic colitis, Crohn's disease, ulcerative colitis, diverticulitis

---

bold italic = life-threatening conditions   *For periodic updates, visit* **www.mosby.com**

Precautions: Food retards absorption, elderly, reduced hepatic or renal function, notify physician immediately if severe constipation or worse occurs, pregnancy category B, lactation, children

Pharmacokinetics:

PO: Rapid absorption, bioavailability 50%-60%, peak plasma levels 1 hr, widely distributed, plasma protein binding 82%, extensively metabolized (cytochrome P450 enzymes), excreted mostly in urine (73%), feces (24%)

🦷 Drug interactions of concern to dentistry:

• Does not appear to induce CYP450 enzymes; no interactions are documented

• Avoid use of drugs (opioids) which could lead to increased risk of constipation

• Use NSAIDs or acetaminophen for mild to moderate dental pain

DENTAL CONSIDERATIONS

General:

• Short appointments and a stress reduction protocol may be required for anxious patients.

• Consider semisupine chair position for patient comfort due to GI side effects of disease.

• Avoid drugs with anticholinergic activity, such as antihistamines, opioids, benzodiazepines, propantheline, atropine, and scopolamine.

• Question patient about tolerance of NSAIDS or aspirin related to GI disease.

Consultations:

• Consult with physician before prescribing drugs that can cause constipation (opioids).

• Consultation with physician may be needed if sedation or general anesthesia is required.

• Medical consult may be required to assess disease control and patient's ability to tolerate stress.

Teach patient/family:

• Importance of updating health and drug history if physician makes any changes in evaluation or drug regimens

---

alprazolam

(al-pray′zoe-lam)

Xanax

♣ Apo-Alpraz, Novo-Alprazol, Nu-Alpraz, Xanax TS

Drug class.: Benzodiazepine

Controlled Substance Schedule IV

Action: Produces CNS depression by interacting with benzodiazepine receptors to facilitate the action of the inhibitory neurotransmitter γ-aminobutyric acid (GABA)

Uses: Anxiety, panic disorders, anxiety with depressive symptoms; unapproved: agoraphobia

Dosage and routes:

• *Adult:* PO 0.25-0.5 mg tid, not to exceed 4 mg in divided doses/day

Panic disorder

• *Adult:* PO 0.5 mg tid; may increase dose by no more than 1 mg/day

• *Geriatric:* PO 0.25 mg bid-tid

Available forms include: Tab 0.25, 0.5, 1, 2 mg; oral sol 0.5 mg/5 ml; intensol sol 1 mg/ml

Side effects/adverse reactions:

▼ *ORAL:* Dry mouth

CNS: Dizziness, drowsiness, confusion, headache, anxiety, tremors, stimulation, fatigue, depression, insomnia, hallucinations

CV: *Orthostatic hypotension,* **ECG changes, tachycardia,** hypotension

GI: Constipation, nausea, vomiting, anorexia, diarrhea

EENT: *Blurred vision,* tinnitus, mydriasis

INTEG: Rash, dermatitis, itching

Contraindications: Hypersensitivity to benzodiazepines, narrow-angle glaucoma, psychosis, pregnancy category D, child <18 yr, ketoconazole, itraconazole, ritonavir, indinavir

Precautions: Elderly, debilitated, hepatic disease, renal disease

Pharmacokinetics:

PO: Onset 30 min, peak 1-2 hr, duration 4-6 hr, half-life 12-15 hr; therapeutic response 2-3 days; metabolized by liver; excreted by kidneys; crosses placenta, breast milk

🦷 Drug interactions of concern to dentistry:

• Increased CNS depression: alcohol, other CNS depressants, clarithromycin, erythromycin, fluconazole, miconazole, fluoxetine, isoniazid

• Contraindicated with ketoconazole, itraconazole, ritonavir, indinavir

DENTAL CONSIDERATIONS

General:

• Monitor vital signs every appointment due to cardiovascular side effects.

• After supine positioning, have patient sit upright for at least 2 min to avoid orthostatic hypotension.

• Assess salivary flow as a factor in caries, periodontal disease, and candidiasis.

• Psychologic and physical dependence may occur with chronic administration.

Consultations:

• Medical consult may be required to assess disease control.

Teach patient/family: *When chronic dry mouth occurs, advise patient:*

• To avoid mouth rinses with high alcohol content due to drying effects

• To use daily home fluoride products for anticaries effect

• To use sugarless gum, frequent sips of water, or saliva substitutes

---

alprostadil

(al-pros′ta-dil)

Caverject, Edex, Muse

Drug class.: Naturally occurring prostaglandin (E_1, PGE_1)

Action: Induces erection by relaxation of trabecular smooth muscle and by dilation of cavernosal arteries

Uses: Treatment of erectile dysfunction due to neurogenic, vasculogenic, psychogenic, or mixed etiology (Note: Another alprostadil-containing product, Prostin VR Pediatric, is used to maintain ductus arteriosus patency in neonates until surgery can be performed.)

Dosage and routes:

Male gender

• *Adult:* Intracavernosal–initial dose must be determined in physician's office, individualized dose for each patient; initial doses range from 1.25-2.5 µg, titrate dose in increments of 5-10 µg until erection suitable for intercourse is obtained, doses >60 µg are not recommended; administer with

---

supplied self-injection system by injecting into the corpora cavernosa; onset varies from 5-20 min, duration <60 min; use more than 3 × wk is not recommended; alternate side and site of injection

• *Adult:* Intraurethral—the dose must be individualized in the physician's office; no more than two doses in 24 hr, follow package instructions for correct administration technique

Available forms include: Vial powder with diluent and self-injection system 5, 10, 20, 40 µg/ml; pellets: 125, 250, 500, and 1000 µg; instructions for use and administration accompany package

Side effects/adverse reactions:
CNS: Headache, dizziness
CV: Hypotension
RESP: Flulike syndrome, cough
GU: Penile pain, priapism, fibrosis, hematoma, rash or edema at site of injection, prostatic disorder, penile trauma
EENT: Nasal congestion, sinusitis
MS: Pain

Contraindications: Hypersensitivity, conditions predisposing to priapism (sickle cell anemia, sickle trait, multiple myeloma, or leukemia), penile deformation, penile implants, or Peyronie's disease

Precautions: Patients on anticoagulant therapy, use of sterile technique, care of syringe, physician instruction in use required, sexually transmitted disease

Pharmacokinetics: Rapidly metabolized and cleared from body by urinary excretion

👢 **Drug interactions of concern to dentistry:**
• None reported

---

amantadine HCl
(a-man'ta-deen)
Symadine, Symmetrel
Drug class.: Antiviral, antiparkinsonian agent

Action: Prevents uncoating of nucleic acid in viral cell, preventing penetration of virus to host; causes release of dopamine and norepinephrine from neurons; may block reuptake of dopamine and norepinephrine into presynaptic neurons
Uses: Prophylaxis or treatment of respiratory tract illness caused by influenza type A; extrapyramidal reactions; parkinsonism
Dosage and routes:
Influenza type A
• *Adult and child >12 yr:* PO 200 mg/day in single dose or divided bid
• *Adult >65 yr:* PO 200 mg daily
• *Child 9-12 yr:* PO 100 mg q12h
• *Child 1-9 yr:* PO 2.2-4.4 mg/kg/day q12h, not to exceed 150 mg/day
Extrapyramidal reaction/parkinsonism
• *Adult:* PO 100 mg bid, up to 400 mg/day in EPS; give for 1 wk, then 100 mg as needed in parkinsonism
Available forms include: Caps 100 mg; syr 50 mg/5 ml
Side effects/adverse reactions:
▼ *ORAL: Dry mouth,* glossitis
CNS: Convulsions, headache, dizziness, drowsiness, fatigue, anxiety, psychosis, impaired concentration, insomnia, depression, hallucinations, tremors
CV: CHF, orthostatic hypotension
GI: Nausea, vomiting, constipation

italic = common side effects

HEMA: **Leukopenia**
GU: Frequency, retention
EENT: Blurred vision
INTEG: Photosensitivity, dermatitis
Contraindications: Hypersensitivity, lactation, child <1 yr, pregnancy category C
Precautions: Epilepsy, CHF, orthostatic hypotension, psychiatric disorders, hepatic disease, renal disease (necessitates dose adjustment)
Pharmacokinetics:
PO: Onset 48 hr, half-life 24 hr; not metabolized; excreted in urine (90%) unchanged; crosses placenta; excreted in breast milk
⚡ Drug interactions of concern to dentistry:
• Increased anticholinergic response: anticholinergic drugs
• Increased CNS depression: alcohol, other CNS depressants
DENTAL CONSIDERATIONS
General:
• Monitor vital signs every appointment due to cardiovascular side effects.
• Assess salivary flow as a factor in caries, periodontal disease, and candidiasis.
• After supine positioning, have patient sit upright for at least 2 min to avoid orthostatic hypotension.
• Avoid dental light in patient's eyes; offer dark glasses for patient comfort.
• Short appointments and stress reduction protocol may be required for anxious patients.
• Consider semisupine chair position for patients with respiratory distress.
Teach patient/family:
• To avoid mouth rinses with high alcohol content due to drying effects

• To use electric toothbrush if patient has difficulty holding conventional devices

---

ambenonium chloride
(am-be-noe′nee-um)
Mytelase
Drug class.: Cholinesterase inhibitor

Action: An acetylcholinesterase inhibitor; inhibits destruction of acetylcholine, which increases concentration at sites in which acetylcholine is released; this facilitates transmission of impulses across the myoneural junction
Uses: Myasthenia gravis, when other drugs cannot be used
Dosage and routes:
• *Adult:* PO 5 mg tid or qid, then gradually increased q1-2d; 5-75 mg/dose is usually sufficient. Caution: doses more than 200 mg per day
Available forms include: Tabs 10 mg
Side effects/adverse reactions:
▼ *ORAL: Increased salivary secretions*
*CNS: **Paralysis, loss of consciousness, convulsions,** drowsiness, dizziness, headache, weakness, incoordination*
*CV: **Cardiac arrest,** tachycardia, dysrhythmias, bradycardia, hypotension, AV block, ECG changes, syncope*
GI: Nausea, diarrhea, vomiting, cramps, gastric secretions, dysphagia, increased peristalsis
*RESP: **Respiratory depression, bronchospasm, constriction, laryngospasm, respiratory arrest,** increased secretions, dyspnea*

---

bold italic = life-threatening conditions   *For periodic updates, visit* **www.mosby.com**

GU: Frequency, incontinence, urgency

EENT: Miosis, blurred vision, lacrimation, visual changes

INTEG: Rashes, urticaria, sweating

Contraindications: Obstruction of intestine or renal system, hypersensitivity

Precautions: Seizure disorders, bronchial asthma, coronary occlusion, hyperthyroidism, dysrhythmias, peptic ulcer, megacolon, poor GI motility, pregnancy category C, bradycardia, hypotension, lactation, children

Pharmacokinetics:

PO: Onset 20-30 min, duration 3-8 hr

🦷 Drug interactions of concern to dentistry:

• Avoid drugs with anticholinergic activity and neuromuscular blocking agents

• Avoid systemic use of ester-type local anesthetics due to reduced plasma cholinesterase activity

DENTAL CONSIDERATIONS

General:

• Control excessive salivary flow with rubber dam and suction.

• Avoid drugs that reduce salivary flow, because they will antagonize this drug.

• Patient may be unable to keep mouth open for long periods due to disease; short appointments may be necessary.

• Monitor vital signs every appointment due to cardiovascular side effects. Evaluate respiration characteristics and rate.

• Consider semisupine chair position for patient comfort due to GI side effects of the drug.

• After supine positioning, have patient sit upright for at least 2 min to avoid orthostatic hypotension.

---

amifostine

(am-i-fos′teen)

Ethyol

Drug class.: Cytoprotective, radio-protective

Action: An active free-thiol metabolite that reduces cytotoxicity by binding to and detoxifying cisplatin metabolites or other alkylating agents; acts as a free-radical scavenger.

Uses: (1) Incidence reduction in moderate to severe xerostomia in patients undergoing postoperative head and neck radiation for cancer where the radiation port includes a substantial part of the parotid gland; (2) Reduction in cumulative renal toxicity associated with repeated cisplatin use in patients with advanced ovarian or non–small cell lung cancers

Dosage and routes:

Xerostomia reduction

• *Adult:* IV infusion 200 mg/m^2 given once daily in a 3 min IV infusion starting 15-30 min before standard radiation therapy (1.8-2.0 Gy)

Cisplatin toxicity reduction

• *Adult:* IV infusion 910 mg/m^2 given once daily in a 15 min IV infusion 30 min before beginning cisplatin use

Available forms include: Vial 500 mg powder

Side effects/adverse reactions:

CNS: Somnolence, dizziness

CV: Hypotension

GI: Nausea, vomiting, hiccups

INTEG: Skin rash, flushing
META: Hypocalcemia
MISC: Hypersensitivity reactions (rare)

Contraindications: Hypersensitivity to aminothiol compounds

Precautions: Patients should be well hydrated, monitor blood pressure, safety not established in CV disease; elderly, cerebrovascular disease, pregnancy category C, lactation, children

Pharmacokinetics:

IV INFUSION: Rapidly cleared from plasma ~6 min, rapidly metabolized to an active free thiol metabolite, dephosphorylated by alk phosphatase, elimination due to rapid tissue distribution and metabolism, small amounts excreted in urine

🦷 Drug interactions of concern to dentistry:

• None reported

DENTAL CONSIDERATIONS

General:

• This is an in hospital or outpatient chemotherapy administered drug. Confirm the patient's disease and treatment status. Dental treatment may be provided if necessary during treatment.

• Monitor vital signs every appointment due to cardiovascular side effects.

• Consider semisupine chair position for patient comfort if GI side effects occur.

• Patients taking opioids for acute or chronic pain should be given alternative analgesics for dental pain.

• Short appointments and a stress reduction protocol may be required for anxious patients.

• Palliative medication may be required for management of oral side effects caused by chemotherapeutic drugs.

Consultations:

• Medical consult may be required to assess immunologic status during cancer therapy and determine safety risks posed by dental treatment.

• Consultation with physician may be needed if sedation or general anesthesia is required.

Teach patient/family:

• To prevent trauma when using oral hygiene aids

• Importance of good oral hygiene to prevent soft tissue inflammation, infection

• To report oral lesions, soreness, or bleeding to dentist

When chronic dry mouth occurs advise patient:

• To avoid mouth rinses with high alcohol content due to drying effects

• To use daily home fluoride products for anticaries effect

• To use sugarless gum, frequent sips of water or saliva substitutes

• Importance of updating health and drug history, reporting changes in health status, drug regimen changes or disease/treatment status

---

amiloride HCl

(a-mil'oh-ride)

Midamor

Drug class.: Potassium-sparing diuretic

Action: Acts primarily on distal tubule and secondarily by inhibiting reabsorption of sodium and increasing potassium retention

---

Uses: Edema in CHF in combination with other diuretics, for hypertension, adjunct with other diuretics to maintain potassium

Dosage and routes:

• *Adult:* PO 5 mg qd, may be increased to 10-20 mg qd if needed

Available forms include: Tab 5 mg

Side effects/adverse reactions:

▼ *ORAL:* Dry mouth, increased thirst

CNS: Headache, dizziness, fatigue, weakness, paresthesias, tremor, depression, anxiety

CV: Orthostatic hypotension

GI: Nausea, diarrhea, vomiting, anorexia, cramps, constipation, abdominal pain, jaundice, bleeding

HEMA: Aplastic anemia, neutropenia (rare)

GU: Polyuria, dysuria, frequency, impotence

EENT: Loss of hearing, tinnitus, blurred vision, nasal congestion, increased intraocular pressure

INTEG: Rash, pruritus, alopecia, urticaria

ELECT: Acidosis, hyponatremia, *hyperkalemia,* hypochloremia

MS: Cramps, joint pain

Contraindications: Anuria, hypersensitivity, hyperkalemia, impaired renal function

Precautions: Dehydration, pregnancy category B, diabetes, acidosis, lactation

Pharmacokinetics:

PO: Onset 2 hr, peak 6-10 hr, duration 24 hr, half-life 6-9 hr; excreted in urine, feces

Drug interactions of concern to dentistry:

• Decreased effects: corticosteroids, NSAIDs, indomethacin

DENTAL CONSIDERATIONS

General:

• Monitor vital signs every appointment due to cardiovascular side effects.

• Assess salivary flow as a factor in caries, periodontal disease, and candidiasis.

• After supine positioning, have patient sit upright for at least 2 min to avoid orthostatic hypotension.

• Patients on chronic drug therapy may rarely have symptoms of blood dyscrasias, which can include infection, bleeding, and poor healing.

• Limit use of sodium-containing products such as saline IV fluids for those patients with a dietary salt restriction.

Consultations:

• Medical consult may be required to assess patient's ability to tolerate stress.

• Medical consult may be required to assess disease control.

• In a patient with symptoms of blood dyscrasias, request a medical consult for blood studies and postpone dental treatment until normal values are reestablished.

Teach patient/family:

• Importance of good oral hygiene to prevent soft tissue inflammation

• Caution to prevent injury when using oral hygiene aids

When chronic dry mouth occurs, advise patient:

• To avoid mouth rinses with high alcohol content due to drying effects

• To use daily home fluoride products for anticaries effect

• To use sugarless gum, frequent sips of water, or saliva substitutes

---

aminocaproic acid

(a-mee-noe-ka-proe'ik)

Amicar

Drug class.: Hemostatic

Action: Inhibits fibrinolysis by inhibiting plasminogen activator substances

Uses: Hemorrhage from hyperfibrinolysis; adjunctive therapy in hemophilia, postsurgical hemorrhage

Dosage and routes:

• *Adult:* PO/IV 5 g loading dose, then 1-1.25 g qh if needed, not to exceed 30 g/day

Available forms include: Inj IV 250 mg/ml; tab 500 mg; syr 250 mg/ml

Side effects/adverse reactions:

*CNS: Headache, dizziness, **convulsions,** malaise, fatigue, hallucinations, delirium, psychosis, weakness*

*CV: **Dysrhythmias,** orthostatic hypotension, bradycardia*

GI: Nausea, vomiting, abdominal cramps, diarrhea

*HEMA: **Thrombosis***

*GU: **Renal failure,** dysuria, frequency, oliguria, ejaculatory failure, menstrual irregularities*

EENT: Tinnitus, nasal congestion, conjunctival suffusion

INTEG: Rash

Contraindications: Hypersensitivity, abnormal bleeding, postpartum bleeding, DIC, upper urinary tract bleeding, new burns

Precautions: Neonates/infants, mild or moderate renal disease, hepatic disease, thrombosis, cardiac disease, pregnancy category C

Pharmacokinetics:

PO: Peak 2 hr, excreted by kidneys as unmetabolized drug, rapidly absorbed

DENTAL CONSIDERATIONS

General:

• Monitor vital signs every appointment due to cardiovascular side effects.

• After supine positioning, have patient sit upright for at least 2 min to avoid orthostatic hypotension.

• Consider additional local hemostasis measures to prevent excessive bleeding in patients with hemophilia.

• Determine why the patient is taking the drug.

• Avoid drugs such as aspirin; NSAIDs may have the potential to prolong bleeding.

Consultations:

• Medical consult may be required to assess disease control.

• Medical consult may be required to assess patient's ability to tolerate stress.

Teach patient/family:

• Importance of good oral hygiene to prevent soft tissue inflammation

• Caution to prevent injury when using oral hygiene aids

---

aminophylline (theophylline ethylenediamine)

(am-in-off'i-lin)

Phyllocontin, Truphylline

♣ Phyllocontin-350

Drug class.: Xanthine

Action: Relaxes smooth muscle of respiratory system by blocking phosphodiesterase, which increases AMP

Uses: Bronchial asthma, bronchospasm, Cheyne-Stokes respirations

Dosage and routes:

• *Adult:* PO 6 mg/kg q6h, dose titrated to need in 3-4 doses/day; usually 300 mg/day (400-600 mg daily could be used if titrated and tolerated)

• *Child:* PO 7.5 mg/kg, then 3-6 mg/kg q6-8h; IV 7.5 mg/kg, then 3-6 mg/kg q6-8h injected over 5 min, do not exceed 25 mg/min, may give loading dose of 5.6 mg/kg over 1/2 hr; CONT IV 1 mg/kg/hr (maintenance)

Available forms include: Inj IV 250 mg/10 ml; rec supp 250, 500 mg; oral liq 105 mg/5 ml; tabs 100, 200 mg; con rel tabs 225 mg

Side effects/adverse reactions:

▼ *ORAL:* Bitter taste

CNS: Anxiety, restlessness, insomnia, dizziness, convulsions, headache, light-headedness, muscle twitching

CV: Palpitation, sinus tachycardia, hypotension, flushing, dysrhythmias

GI: Nausea, vomiting, anorexia, diarrhea, dyspepsia, anal irritation (suppositories), epigastric pain

RESP: Increased rate

GU: Urinary frequency

INTEG: Flushing, urticaria

Contraindications: Hypersensitivity to xanthines, tachydysrhythmias

Precautions: Elderly, CHF, cor pulmonale, hepatic disease, active peptic ulcer disease, diabetes mellitus, hyperthyroidism, hypertension, children, pregnancy category C, glaucoma, prostatic hypertrophy

Pharmacokinetics:

IV: Peak 30 min; 16 mg of anhydrous aminophylline provides a dose equivalent to 100 mg anhydrous theophylline

⚖ Drug interactions of concern to dentistry:

• Increased action: erythromycin (macrolides), ciprofloxacin

• Cardiac dysrhythmia: CNS stimulants, hydrocarbon inhalation anesthetics

• Decreased effects: barbiturates, carbamazepine

• Decreased effects of benzodiazepines

DENTAL CONSIDERATIONS

General:

• Monitor vital signs every appointment due to cardiovascular and respiratory side effects.

• Consider semisupine chair position for patient comfort due to respiratory disease and GI side effects of the drug.

• Midday appointments and a stress reduction protocol may be required for anxious patients.

• Be aware that aspirin or sulfite preservatives in vasoconstrictor-containing products can exacerbate asthma.

• Acute asthmatic episodes may be precipitated in the dental office. Sympathomimetic inhalants should be available for emergency use.

Consultations:
• Medical consult may be required to assess disease control.

---

aminosalicylic acid

(a-mee-noe-sal-i-sil'ik)

Paser

Drug class.: Antitubercular antiinfective

Action: Bacteriostatic for *M. tuberculosis;* postulated mechanisms are related to inhibition of folic acid synthesis or inhibition of the cell wall component, mycobactin

Uses: Tuberculosis, in combination with other *M. tuberculosis* antiinfectives

Dosage and routes:
Multidrug resistant TB cases
• Adult: PO 4 g tid

Available forms include: Packets 4 g; carton of 30 packets

Side effects/adverse reactions:

CV: Pericarditis

GI: Nausea, vomiting, diarrhea, abdominal pain, jaundice, hepatitis

*HEMA: **Agranulocytosis, thrombocytopenia,*** leukopenia, anemia, reduction in prothrombin

GU: Crystalluria

EENT: Optic neuritis

*INTEG: **Exfoliative dermatitis,*** rash, eruptions

MISC: Fever, infectious mononucleosis-like and lymphoma-like symptoms

Contraindications: Hypersensitivity, severe renal impairment

Precautions: Hepatic dysfunction, refrigeration required for storage, malabsorption of vitamin B_{12}, pregnancy category C, no data on safe use in children or lactation

Pharmacokinetics:

PO: Protect granules by giving with acidic foods, mean peak serum levels 6 hr, 50%-60% protein bound; acetylated form excreted mostly in urine

⚕ Drug interactions of concern to dentistry:
• None reported

DENTAL CONSIDERATIONS

General:
• Determine that noninfectious status exists by ensuring that (1) antiTB drugs have been taken more than 3 wk, (2) culture confirmed TB susceptibility to antiinfectives, (3) patient has had three consecutive negative sputum smears, and (4) patient is not in the coughing stage.
• Determine why patient is taking drug (i.e., for prophylaxis or active therapy).
• Importance of taking medication for full length of regimen to ensure effectiveness of treatment and to prevent the emergence of resistant strains.
• Patient on chronic drug therapy may rarely present with symptoms of blood dyscrasias, which can include infection, bleeding, and poor healing.
• Consider semisupine chair position for patient comfort if GI side effects occur.

Consultations:
• Medical consult may be required to assess disease control and patient's ability to tolerate stress.
• In a patient with symptoms of blood dyscrasias, request a medical consult for blood studies and postpone treatment until normal values are reestablished.

Teach patient/family:
• Importance of updating health

---

bold italic = life-threatening conditions

and drug history if physician makes any changes in evaluation or drug regimens
• To prevent trauma when using oral hygiene aids

---

amiodarone HCl

(a-mee'oh-da-rone)

Cordarone, Cordarone IV, Pacerone

Drug class.:   Antidysrhythmic (class III)

Action: Prolongs action potential duration and effective refractory period, noncompetitive α- and β-adrenergic receptor inhibition
Uses: Documented life-threatening ventricular tachycardia; unapproved: ventricular fibrillation not controlled by first-line agents
Dosage and routes:
• *Adult:* PO loading dose 800-1600 mg/day 1-3 wk, then 600-800 mg/day 1 mo; maintenance 200-600 mg/day; also given by IV infusion, must follow package insert rates
Available forms include: Tabs 200, 400 mg; INJ 50 mg/ml
Side effects/adverse reactions:
▼ *ORAL:* Bitter taste sensation, dry mouth
CNS: Headache, dizziness, involuntary movement, tremors, peripheral neuropathy, malaise, fatigue, ataxia, paresthesias, insomnia
CV: Hypotension, bradycardia, si-nus arrest, CHF, dysrhythmias, SA node dysfunction prolonged QT interval
GI: Hepatotoxicity, nausea, vomiting, diarrhea, abdominal pain, anorexia, constipation
RESP: Pulmonary fibrosis, pulmonary inflammation

EENT: ***Corneal microdeposits,*** blurred vision, halos, photophobia, dry eyes
INTEG: Rash, photosensitivity, bluish-gray skin discoloration, rash, alopecia, spontaneous ecchymosis
ENDO: Hyperthyroidism or hypothyroidism
MS: Weakness, pain in extremities
MISC: Flushing, abnormal smell, edema, coagulation abnormalities
Precautions: Goiter, Hashimoto's thyroiditis, SN dysfunction, second- or third-degree AV block, electrolyte imbalances, pregnancy category C, bradycardia, lactation
Pharmacokinetics:
PO: Onset 1-3 wk, peak 3-7 hr, half-life 15-100 days; metabolized by liver; excreted by kidneys
⚞ Drug interactions of concern to dentistry:
• Bradycardia, hypotension: inhalation anesthetics, lidocaine, anticholinergics, vasoconstrictors
• Increased photosensitization: tetracyclines
DENTAL CONSIDERATIONS
General:
• Monitor vital signs every appointment due to cardiovascular and respiratory side effects.
• Assess salivary flow as a factor in caries, periodontal disease, and candidiasis.
• Avoid dental light in patient's eyes; offer dark glasses for patient comfort.
• After supine positioning, have patient sit upright for at least 2 min before standing to avoid orthostatic hypotension.
• Use vasoconstrictors with caution, in low doses, and with careful aspiration. Avoid gingival retraction cord with epinephrine.

• Stress from dental procedures may compromise cardiovascular function; determine patient risk.

• Delay or avoid dental treatment if patient shows signs of cardiac symptoms or respiratory distress.

Consultations:

• Medical consult may be required to assess patient's ability to tolerate stress.

• Medical consult may be required to assess disease control.

Teach patient/family: *When chronic dry mouth occurs, advise patient:*

• To avoid mouth rinses with high alcohol content due to drying effects

• To use daily home fluoride products for anticaries effect

• To use sugarless gum, frequent sips of water, or saliva substitutes

---

amitriptyline HCl

(a-mee-trip'ti-leen)
Elavil
♣ Apo-Amitriptyline, Levate, Novotriptyn

Drug class.: Antidepressant–tricyclic

Action: Inhibits both norepinephrine and serotonin (5-HT) uptake in the brain, although the precise antidepressant mechanism remains unclear

Uses: Major depression; unapproved: enuresis and neurogenic pain

Dosage and routes:

• *Adult:* PO 75 mg/day in divided doses or 50-100 mg hs, may increase to 150 mg qd; IM 20-30 mg qid or 80-120 mg hs

• *Adolescent/geriatric:* PO 30 mg/day in divided doses, may be increased to 150 mg/day

Available forms include: Tabs 10, 25, 50, 75, 100, 150 mg; inj IM 10 mg/ml; syr 10 mg/5 ml

Side effects/adverse reactions:

▼ *ORAL: Dry mouth, unpleasant taste,* stomatitis, salivary gland pain

CNS: Dizziness, drowsiness, confusion, headache, anxiety, tremors, stimulation, weakness, insomnia, nightmares, EPS (elderly), increased psychiatric symptoms, seizures, ataxia, paresthesias

CV: Orthostatic hypotension, ECG changes, tachycardia, hypertension, palpitation, syncope, prolonged QT interval

GI: Diarrhea, paralytic ileus, hepatitis, increased appetite, cramps, epigastric distress, jaundice, nausea, vomiting

HEMA: Agranulocytosis, thrombocytopenia, eosinophilia, leukopenia

GU: Retention

EENT: Blurred vision, tinnitus, mydriasis, ophthalmoplegia

INTEG: Rash, urticaria, sweating, pruritus, photosensitivity

Contraindications: Hypersensitivity to tricyclic antidepressants, recovery phase of MI

Precautions: Suicidal patients, convulsive disorders, prostatic hypertrophy, schizophrenia, psychotic disorders, severe depression, increased intraocular pressure, narrow-angle glaucoma, urinary retention, cardiac disease, hepatic disease, renal disease, hyperthyroidism, electroshock therapy, elective surgery, child <12 yr, pregnancy category C, elderly, MAO inhibitors

---

bold italic = life-threatening conditions

Pharmacokinetics:
PO/IM: Onset 45 min, peak 2-12 hr, therapeutic response 2-3 wk, half-life 10-50 hr; metabolized by liver; excreted in urine, feces, breast milk; crosses placenta

🦷 Drug interactions of concern to dentistry:
• Increased anticholinergic effects: muscarinic blockers, antihistamines, phenothiazines
• Increased effects of direct-acting sympathomimetics (epinephrine, levonordefrin)
• Possible risk of increased CNS depression: alcohol, barbiturates, benzodiazepines, CNS depressants
• Decreased antihypertensive effect: clonidine, guanadrel, guanethidine

DENTAL CONSIDERATIONS
General:
• Take vital signs every appointment due to cardiovascular side effects.
• Assess salivary flow as a factor in caries, periodontal disease, and candidiasis.
• Patients on chronic drug therapy may rarely have symptoms of blood dyscrasias, which can include infection, bleeding, and poor healing.
• After supine positioning, have patient sit upright for at least 2 min to avoid orthostatic hypotension.
• Use vasoconstrictors with caution, in low doses, and with careful aspiration. Avoid use of gingival retraction cord with epinephrine.
• Place on frequent recall due to oral side effects.
Consultations:
• In a patient with symptoms of blood dyscrasias, request a medical consult for blood studies and postpone dental treatment until normal values are reestablished.
• Medical consult may be required to assess disease control.
• Physician should be informed if significant xerostomic side effects occur (e.g., increased caries, sore tongue, problems eating or swallowing, difficulty wearing prosthesis) so a medication change can be considered.

Teach patient/family:
• Importance of good oral hygiene to prevent soft tissue inflammation
• Caution to prevent injury when using oral hygiene aids
When chronic dry mouth occurs, advise patient:
• To avoid mouth rinses with high alcohol content due to drying effects
• To use daily home fluoride products for anticaries effect
• To use sugarless gum, frequent sips of water, or saliva substitutes

---

amlexanox
(am-lex'an-ox)
Aphthasol
Drug class.: Topical antiinflammatory

Action: Mechanism of action is unknown; has antiinflammatory and antiallergic activities; accelerates the resolution of pain and healing of aphthous ulcers
Uses: Aphthous ulcers in patients with normal immune systems
Dosage and routes:
• *Adult:* TOP squeeze dab (0.5 cm) of paste onto fingertip and dab each ulcer qid, after oral hygiene, after each meal, and hs; use until ulcer heals

Available forms include: Oral paste 5%, 5 g tube

Side effects/adverse reactions:

▼ *ORAL:* Transient stinging and burning on application, contact mucositis

GI: Nausea, diarrhea

Contraindications: Hypersensitivity

Precautions: Wash hands immediately before and after each use; discontinue if mucositis appears, pregnancy category B, lactation, children

Pharmacokinetics:

TOP: Systemic absorption from GI tract if swallowed, drug and metabolites excreted in urine

🦷 **Drug interactions of concern to dentistry:**

• None reported

DENTAL CONSIDERATIONS

General:

• Recurrent aphthous ulcers may be associated with systemic conditions; evaluate as needed if healing has not occurred after 10 days.

Teach patient/family:

• To apply paste as directed and wash hands immediately before and after each use

• To report oral lesions or soreness to dentist

---

amlodipine besylate

(am-loe′di-peen)

Norvasc

Drug class.: Calcium channel blocker

Action: Inhibits calcium ion influx across cell membrane during cardiac depolarization; produces relaxation of coronary vascular smooth muscle; dilates coronary arteries; decreases SA/AV node conduction; dilates peripheral arteries

Uses: Hypertension as a single agent or in combination with other antihypertensives, chronic stable angina pectoris, vasospastic angina

Dosage and routes:

Hypertension

• *Adult:* PO 5 mg/day; max daily dose 10 mg

• *Geriatric or small, fragile adult:* PO 2.5 mg/day

Available forms include: Tabs 2.5, 5, 10 mg

Side effects/adverse reactions:

▼ *ORAL:* Dry mouth, altered taste; gingival overgrowth has been reported with other calcium channel blockers

CNS: Headache, fatigue, lethargy, somnolence, dizziness, light-headedness

CV: Peripheral edema, palpitation, syncope, CHF, tachycardia, chest pain

GI: Nausea, dyspepsia, discomfort, diarrhea, flatulence

RESP: Pulmonary edema

GU: Sexual difficulties

EENT: Diplopia, eye pain

INTEG: Petechiae, bruising, ecchymoses, purpura

MS: Muscle cramps, joint stiffness

Contraindications: Sick sinus syndrome, second- or third-degree heart block, hypotension less than 90 mm Hg systolic, cardiogenic shock, severe CHF

Precautions: Pregnancy category C, CHF, hypotension, hepatic injury, lactation, children, renal disease

Pharmacokinetics:

PO: Peak plasma levels 6-12 hr, half-life 30-50 hr; highly protein

---

bold italic = life-threatening conditions

bound; metabolized in liver; excreted in urine

👆 **Drug interactions of concern to dentistry:**

• Decreased effect: indomethacin, possibly other NSAIDs, phenobarbital

• Increased effect: parenteral and inhalational general anesthetics or other drugs with hypotensive actions

DENTAL CONSIDERATIONS

General:

• Monitor cardiac status; take vital signs at each appointment because of CV side effects. Consider a stress reduction protocol to prevent stress-induced angina during the dental appointment.

• After supine positioning, have patient sit upright for at least 2 min to avoid orthostatic hypotension.

• Limit use of sodium-containing products such as saline IV fluids for those patients with a dietary salt restriction.

• Assess salivary flow as a factor in caries, periodontal disease, and candidiasis.

Consultations:

• Medical consult may be required to assess disease control.

Teach patient/family:

• Need for frequent oral prophylaxis if gingival overgrowth should occur

When chronic dry mouth occurs, advise patient:

• To avoid mouth rinses with high alcohol content due to drying effects

• To use daily home fluoride products for anticaries effect

• To use sugarless gum, frequent sips of water, or artificial saliva

amoxapine
(a-mox′a-peen)
Asendin
Drug class.: Antidepressant–tricyclic

Action: Inhibits both norepinephrine and serotonin (5-HT) uptake in the brain, although the precise antidepressant mechanism remains unclear

Uses: Depression

Dosage and routes:

• *Adult:* PO 50 mg tid, may increase to 100 mg tid on third day of therapy, not to exceed 300 mg/day unless lower doses have been given for at least 2 wk; may be given daily dose hs, not to exceed 600 mg/day in divided doses in hospitalized patients

Available forms include: Tabs 25, 50, 100, 150 mg

Side effects/adverse reactions:

▼ *ORAL: Dry mouth,* stomatitis
CNS: Dizziness, drowsiness, confusion, headache, anxiety, tremors, tardive dyskinesia, stimulation, weakness, insomnia, nightmares, EPS (elderly), increased psychiatric symptoms, paresthesia
CV: Orthostatic hypotension, ECG changes, tachycardia, **hypertension,** palpitation
GI: Diarrhea, constipation, **paralytic ileus, hepatitis,** nausea, vomiting, increased appetite, cramps, epigastric distress, jaundice
HEMA: **Agranulocytosis, thrombocytopenia, eosinophilia, leukopenia**
GU: **Acute renal failure,** urinary retention
EENT: Blurred vision, tinnitus, mydriasis, ophthalmoplegia

INTEG: Rash, urticaria, sweating, pruritus, photosensitivity

Contraindications: Hypersensitivity to tricyclic antidepressants, recovery phase of MI, convulsive disorders, prostatic hypertrophy

Precautions: Suicidal patients, severe depression, increased intraocular pressure, narrow-angle glaucoma, urinary retention, cardiac disease, hepatic disease, hyperthyroidism, electroshock therapy, elective surgery, elderly, pregnancy category C, MAO inhibitors

Pharmacokinetics:

PO: Peak blood levels 90 min, steady state 7 days, half-life 8 hr; metabolized by liver; excreted by kidneys; crosses placenta

☙ Drug interactions of concern to dentistry:

• Increased anticholinergic effects: muscarinic blockers, antihistamines, phenothiazines

• Increased effects of direct-acting sympathomimetics (epinephrine, levonordefrin)

• Potential risk of increased CNS depression: alcohol, barbiturates, benzodiazepines, CNS depressants

• Decreased antihypertensive effect: clonidine, guanadrel, guanethidine

DENTAL CONSIDERATIONS

General:

• Take vital signs every appointment due to cardiovascular side effects.

• Assess salivary flow as a factor in caries, periodontal disease, and candidiasis.

• Patients on chronic drug therapy may rarely have symptoms of blood dyscrasias, which can include infection, bleeding, and poor healing.

• After supine positioning, have patient sit upright for at least 2 min to avoid orthostatic hypotension.

• Use vasoconstrictors with caution, in low doses, and with careful aspiration. Avoid use of gingival retraction cord with epinephrine.

• Place on frequent recall due to oral side effects.

Consultations:

• In a patient with symptoms of blood dyscrasias, request a medical consult for blood studies and postpone dental treatment until normal values are reestablished.

• Medical consult may be required to assess disease control.

• Physician should be informed if significant xerostomic side effects occur (e.g., increased caries, sore tongue, problems eating or swallowing, difficulty wearing prosthesis) so a medication change can be considered.

Teach patient/family:

• Importance of good oral hygiene to prevent soft tissue inflammation

• Caution to prevent injury when using oral hygiene aids

When chronic dry mouth occurs, advise patient:

• To avoid mouth rinses with high alcohol content due to drying effects

• To use daily home fluoride products for anticaries effect

• To use sugarless gum, frequent sips of water, or saliva substitutes

---

amoxicillin/clavulanate potassium

(a-mox-i-sil'in)/(klav'yoo-la-nate)

Augmentin, Augmentin ES-600, Augmentin SR

♣ Clavulin

Drug class.: Aminopenicillin with a β-lactamase inhibitor

Action: Interferes with cell-wall replication of susceptible organisms; the cell wall, rendered osmotically unstable, swells and bursts from osmotic pressure

Uses: Sinusitis, pneumonia, lower RTI, otitis media, skin and urinary tract infections caused by susceptible microorganisms that include β-lactamase-producing organisms

Dosage and routes:

• *Adult:* PO one 500 mg tab q12h or one 250 mg tab q8h depending on severity of infection

• *Child:* PO 20-40 mg/kg/day in divided doses q8h

*Do not use the 250/125 mg tab until child weighs at least 40 kg or more.

Severe and respiratory tract infections

• *Adult:* PO one 875 mg tab q12h or one 500 mg tab q8h

Recurrent or persistent otitis media

• *Child:* PO (amoxicillin) 90 mg/kg/day in two equal doses

Available forms include: Amoxicillin/clavulanate K amounts: Tabs 250/125, 500/125, 875/125 mg; chew tabs 125/31.25, 200/28.5, 250/62.5, 400/57 mg; powder for oral susp 125/31.25, 200/28.5, 250/62.5, 400/57 mg/5 ml when reconstituted; note that the single dose of clavulanate K should not exceed 125 mg. Augmentin 250 mg tab and Augmentin 250 mg chewable tab do not contain the same amount of clavulanic acid. They are not interchangeable; ES-600 oral suspension (amoxicillin 600 mg and clavulanic acid 42.9 mg/5 ml)

Side effects/adverse reactions:

▼ *ORAL:* Discolored tongue, glossitis, increased thirst, candidiasis, stomatitis

CNS: Headache

GI: Nausea, diarrhea, vomiting, increased AST/ALT, abdominal pain, colitis, antibiotic-associated pseudomembranous colitis

*HEMA: **Bone marrow depression, granulocytopenia, leukopenia, eosinophilia,** thrombocytopenic purpura, anemia*

*GU: Vaginitis, moniliasis, **glomerulonephritis,** oliguria, proteinuria, hematuria*

INTEG: Pemphigus-like reaction

META: Hyperkalemia, hypokalemia, alkalosis, hypernatremia

*SYST: **Anaphylaxis,** pruritus, urticaria, angioedema, bronchospasm (allergy symptoms)*

Contraindications: Hypersensitivity to penicillins; neonates, clavulanate K–associated cholestatic/hepatic dysfunction

Precautions: Pregnancy category B, hypersensitivity to cephalosporins, hepatic function impairment

Pharmacokinetics:

PO: Good oral absorption with or without food; peak 2 hr, duration 6-8 hr, half-life 1-1.33 hr; metabolized in liver; excreted in urine; crosses placenta; enters breast milk

🦷 **Drug interactions of concern to dentistry:**

• Decreased antimicrobial effectiveness: tetracyclines, erythromycins, lincomycins

• Increased amoxicillin concentrations: probenecid
• Increased risk of skin rashes: allopurinol

When used for dental infection:
• Oral contraceptives: advise patient of a potential risk for decreased contraceptive action, to maintain compliance with oral contraceptive use while using antibiotics, and to consider the use of additional nonhormonal contraception

DENTAL CONSIDERATIONS

General:
• Take precautions regarding allergy to medication.
• Determine why the patient is taking the drug.

Consultations:
• Medical consult may be required to assess disease control.

Teach patient/family:
• Importance of good oral hygiene to prevent soft tissue inflammation
• Caution to prevent injury when using oral hygiene aids

When used for dental infection, advise patient:
• To report sore throat, oral burning sensation, fever, and fatigue, any of which could indicate superinfection
• To take at prescribed intervals and complete dosage regimen
• To immediately notify the dentist if signs or symptoms of infection increase

---

amoxicillin trihydrate
(a-mox-i-sil'in)
Amoxil, Trimox, Wymox
♣ Apo-Amoxi, Nova moxin, Nu-Amox
Drug class.: Aminopenicillin

Action: Interferes with cell-wall replication of susceptible organisms; the cell wall, rendered osmotically unstable, swells and bursts from osmotic pressure

Uses: Sinus infections, pneumonia, otitis media, skin infections, urinary tract infections; effective for strains of *E. coli, P. mirabilis, H. influenzae, S. faecalis, S. pneumoniae;* unlabeled uses for chlamydia, *H. pylori*

Dosage and routes:
Systemic infections
• *Adult:* PO 250-500 mg q8h or q12h depending on severity of infection
• *Child:* PO 20-40 mg/kg/day in divided doses q8h; optional dose 200 mg q12h (in place of 125 mg q8h) or 400 mg q12h (in place of 250 mg q8h)

Bacterial endocarditis prophylaxis
• *Adult:* PO 2 g 1 hr before dental procedure
• *Child:* PO 50 mg/kg of body weight, not to exceed the adult dose, 1 hr before dental procedure

Prosthetic joint prophylaxis (when indicated)
• *Adult:* PO 2 g 1 hr before dental procedure

Available forms include: Caps 250, 500 mg; tabs 500, 875 mg; chew tabs 125, 250 mg; powder for oral susp 50 mg/ml and 125, 250 mg/5 ml

Side effects/adverse reactions:
▼ *ORAL:* Discolored tongue, glossitis, increased thirst, candidiasis, stomatitis
CNS: Headache
GI: Nausea, vomiting, diarrhea, increased AST/ALT, abdominal pain, colitis

---

bold italic = life-threatening conditions

HEMA: ***Bone marrow depression,*** ***granulocytopenia,*** anemia, increased bleeding time

INTEG: Pemphigus-like reaction

SYST: ***Anaphylaxis*** (allergy symptoms), pruritus, urticaria, angioedema, bronchospasm

Contraindications: Hypersensitivity to penicillins; neonates

Precautions: Pregnancy category B, hypersensitivity to cephalosporins

Pharmacokinetics:

PO: Peak 2 hr, duration 6-8 hr, half-life 1-1.33 hr; metabolized in liver; excreted in urine; crosses placenta; enters breast milk

Drug interactions of concern to dentistry:

• Decreased antimicrobial effectiveness: tetracyclines, erythromycins, lincomycins

• Increased amoxicillin concentrations: probenecid

• Suspected increase in methotrexate toxicity

When used for dental infection:

• Oral contraceptives: advise patient of a potential risk for decreased contraceptive action, to maintain compliance with oral contraceptive use while using antibiotics, and to consider the use of additional nonhormonal contraception

DENTAL CONSIDERATIONS

General:

• Take precautions regarding allergy to medication.

• Determine why the patient is taking the drug.

Consultations:

• Medical consult may be required to assess disease control

Teach patient/family:

• Importance of good oral hygiene to prevent soft tissue inflammation

• Caution to prevent injury when using oral hygiene aids

When used for dental infection, advise patient:

• To report sore throat, oral burning sensation, fever, and fatigue, any of which could indicate superinfection

• To take at prescribed intervals and complete dosage regimen

• To immediately notify the dentist if signs or symptoms of infection increase

---

amphotericin B (topical)

(am-foe-ter'i-sin)

Fungizone Oral Suspension

Drug class.: Polyene antifungal

Action: Increases cell membrane permeability in susceptible organisms by binding to cell membrane sterols

Uses: Oral mucocutaneous infections caused by *Candida*

Dosage and routes:

• *Adult and child:* SOL oral suspension rinse with 1 ml (100 mg) qid; shake well before using, place dose on tongue using the dropper, swish as long as reasonable, can swallow.

Available forms include: Oral suspension 100 mg/ml in 24 ml dropper bottle

Side effects/adverse reactions:

GI: Nausea, vomiting, diarrhea

INTEG: Urticaria, angioedema (rare), ***Stevens-Johnson syndrome***

Contraindications: Hypersensitivity

Precautions: Pregnancy category

C, lactation; not for systemic fungal infections

Pharmacokinetics: Topical rinse only, poorly absorbed if swallowed

Drug interactions of concern to dentistry:
• None reported

DENTAL CONSIDERATIONS

General:
• Determine why the patient is taking the drug.
• Broad-spectrum antibiotics may contribute to oral *Candida* infections.

Teach patient/family:
• That long-term therapy may be needed to clear infection; complete entire course of medication
• Not to use commercial mouthwashes for mouth infection unless prescribed by dentist
• That patient with removable dental appliance should soak appliance in antifungal agent overnight
• To prevent reinoculation of *Candida* infection by disposing of toothbrush or other contaminated oral hygiene devices used during period of infection

---

ampicillin/ampicillin sodium/ampicillin trihydrate
(am-pi-sil'in)

Ampicillin sodium (parenteral):
Omnipen-N
✤ Ampicin, Penbritin
Ampicillin: Marcillin, Omnipen, Polycillin, Principen, Totacillin
✤ Apo-Ampi, Novo-Ampicillin, Nu-Ampi

Drug class.: Aminopenicillin

Action: Interferes with cell-wall replication of susceptible organisms; the cell wall, rendered osmotically unstable, swells and bursts from osmotic pressure

Uses: Sinus infections, pneumonia, otitis media, skin infections, UTIs; effective for strains of *E. coli, P. mirabilis, H. influenzae, S. faecalis, S. pneumoniae*

Dosage and routes:

Systemic infections
• *Adult:* PO 250-500 mg q6h depending on severity of infection; IV/IM 2-8 g qd in divided doses q4-6h
• *Child:* PO 50-100 mg/kg/day in divided doses q6h; IV/IM 100-200 mg/kg/day in divided doses q6h

Bacterial endocarditis prophylaxis
• *Adult:* IV or IM for patients unable to take oral medications and who are not allergic to penicillin 2 g within 30 min of dental procedure
• *Child:* IV or IM for patients unable to take oral medications and who are not allergic to penicillin 50 mg/kg of body weight not to exceed the adult dose

Prosthetic joint prophylaxis (when indicated)
• *Adult:* IV or IM for patients unable to take oral medications and who are not allergic to penicillin 2 g 1 hr before dental procedure

Available forms include: Powder for inj IV/IM 125, 250, 500 mg and 1, 2, 10 g; IV inf 500 mg and 1, 2 g; caps 250, 500 mg; powder for oral susp 125, 250 mg/5 ml

Side effects/adverse reactions:

▼ *ORAL:* Discolored tongue, glossitis, increased thirst, candidiasis, stomatitis

---

bold italic = life-threatening conditions

*CNS: **Coma, convulsions,*** lethargy, hallucinations, anxiety, depression, twitching

GI: Nausea, vomiting, diarrhea

*HEMA: **Bone marrow depression, granulocytopenia,*** anemia, increased bleeding time

*GU: Vaginitis, moniliasis, **glomerulonephritis,*** oliguria, proteinuria, hematuria

INTEG: Rash, urticaria

*SYST: **Anaphylaxis,*** pruritus, urticaria, angioedema, bronchospasm (allergy symptoms)

Contraindications: Hypersensitivity to penicillins

Precautions: Pregnancy category B, hypersensitivity to cephalosporins, neonates

Pharmacokinetics:

PO: Peak 2 hr

IV: Peak 5 min

IM: Peak 1 hr, half-life 50-110 min; metabolized in liver; excreted in urine, bile, breast milk; crosses placenta

⚡ **Drug interactions of concern to dentistry:**

• Decreased antimicrobial effectiveness: tetracyclines, erythromycins, lincomycins

• Increased ampicillin concentrations: probenecid

When used for dental infection:

• Oral contraceptives: advise patient of a potential risk for decreased contraceptive action, to maintain compliance with oral contraceptive use while using antibiotics, and to consider the use of additional nonhormonal contraception

DENTAL CONSIDERATIONS

General:

• Take precautions regarding allergy to medication.

• Determine why the patient is taking the drug.

Consultations:

• Medical consult may be required to assess disease control.

Teach patient/family:

• Importance of good oral hygiene to prevent soft tissue inflammation

• Caution to prevent injury when using oral hygiene aids

When used for dental infection, advise patient:

• To report sore throat, oral burning sensation, fever, and fatigue, any of which could indicate superinfection

• To take at prescribed intervals and complete dosage regimen

• To immediately notify the dentist if signs or symptoms of infection increase

---

amprenavir

(am-pren′a-veer)

Agenerase

Drug class.: Antiviral

Action: Inhibits human immunodeficiency virus (HIV) protease enzymes

Uses: HIV-1 infection, in combination with other antiretroviral agents

Dosage and routes:

• *Adult:* PO 1200 mg bid in combination with other antiretroviral drugs

• *Child 13-16 yr:* PO 1200 mg bid in combination with other antiretroviral drugs

• *Child 4-12 yr or 13-16 yr weighing less than 50 kg:* PO 20 mg/kg bid or 15 mg/kg tid (max 2400 mg/day) in combination with other antiretroviral drugs

Oral solution
• *Child 4-12 yr or 13-16 yr weighing less than 50 kg:* PO 22.5 mg/kg (1.5 ml/kg) bid or 17 mg/kg (1.1 ml/kg) tid in combination with other antiretroviral drugs; max daily limit 2800 mg

Available forms include: Caps 50, 150 mg; oral sol 15 mg/ml in 240 ml

(Note: capsules and oral solution are not interchangeable on a mg per mg basis)

Side effects/adverse reactions:
▼ *ORAL: Perioral paresthesia, taste disorders*
CNS: Headache, peripheral paresthesia, depression
GI: Nausea, vomiting, diarrhea, abdominal pain
HEMA: **Acute hemolytic anemia**
INTEG: Rash, **Stevens-Johnson syndrome**
META: Hyperglycemia, hyperlipidemia, hypercholesterolemia
MISC: Fatigue

Contraindications: Concurrent use with midazolam, triazolam, bepridil, and ergotlike drugs; hypersensitivity; serious reactions could occur with lidocaine (systemic) and tricyclic antidepressants; avoid use of drugs metabolized by CYP3A4 enzymes; lactation

Precautions: Exacerbation of diabetes, hyperglycemia, use of additional vitamin E, hemophilia, viral resistance, risk of cross allergy with sulfonamides, fat redistribution, pregnancy category C, children <4 yr, hepatic disease, patients on oral contraceptives, sildenafil

Pharmacokinetics:
PO: Rapid oral absorption (except with fatty meal), bioavailability of oral solutions is less than capsules, peak plasma concentration 1-2 hr, plasma protein binding 90%, hepatic metabolism (CYP450, CYP3A4), excreted in feces (75%) and urine

🦷 Drug interactions of concern to dentistry:
• Contraindicated with midazolam, triazolam, tricyclic antidepressants
• Increased plasma levels of erythromycin, clarithromycin, itraconazole, alprazolam, chlorazepate, diazepam, carbamazepine, loratadine, flurazepam, ketoconazole; lidocaine (systemic use for cardiac arrhythmias)

DENTAL CONSIDERATIONS
General:
• Palliative medication may be required for management of oral side effects.
• Examine for oral manifestation of opportunistic infection.
• Patient on chronic drug therapy may rarely have symptoms of blood dyscrasias, which can include infection, bleeding, and poor healing.
• Consider semisupine chair position for patient comfort if GI side effects occur.

Consultations:
• In a patient with symptoms of blood dyscrasias, request a medical consult for blood studies and postpone treatment until normal values are reestablished.
• Medical consult may be required to assess disease control and patient's ability to tolerate stress.

Teach patient/family:
• Importance of good oral hygiene to prevent soft tissue inflammation
• To prevent trauma when using oral hygiene aids
• Importance of updating health

---

bold italic = life-threatening conditions   *For periodic updates, visit* **www.mosby.com**

and drug history if physician makes any changes in evaluation or drug regimens
• That secondary oral infection may occur; must see dentist immediately if infection occurs

---

anagrelide hydrochloride

(an-ag′gre-lide)
Agrylin

Drug class.: Platelet-reducing agent

Action: Unclear; may involve a reduction in megakaryocyte hypermaturation without affecting WBC count or coagulation, insignificant reduction in RBC count; platelet aggregation may be inhibited in larger doses

Uses: Treatment of essential thrombocythemia, polycythemia vera

Dosage and routes:
• *Adult:* PO (requires close medical supervision)—initial dose 0.5 mg qid or 1.0 mg bid; after 1 wk adjust dose to maintain platelet count below 600,000/µl; limit dose increases to 0.5 mg/day; dose limit 10 mg/day and 2.5 mg per single dose

Available forms include: Tabs 0.5 mg and 1.0 mg

Side effects/adverse reactions:
▼ *ORAL:* Aphthous stomatitis
CNS: Headache, dizziness, paresthesia, seizures
CV: Palpitation, edema, tachycardia
GI: Diarrhea, abdominal pain, nausea, dyspepsia, flatulence, vomiting, anorexia, **pancreatitis,** ulceration

RESP: **Pulmonary infiltrate, pulmonary hypertension**
EENT: Rash, urticaria
MS: Back pain, arthralgia
MISC: Asthenia, malaise

Precautions: Cardiac disease, renal impairment, hepatic impairment, monitor reduction in platelets, risk of thrombocytopenia especially while correct dose is being found, sudden discontinuance of use, pregnancy category C, lactation, children <16 yr

Pharmacokinetics:
PO: Extensive hepatic metabolism, urinary excretion, half-life 1.3 hr

Drug interactions of concern to dentistry:
• Possible risk of hemorrhage: NSAIDs, aspirin

DENTAL CONSIDERATIONS
General:
• Laboratory studies should include routine CBCs.
• Patients have risk of thrombohemorrhagic complications; prolonged bleeding time, anemia, or splenomegaly may occur in some patients with this disease. However, thrombosis may also occur in some patients.
• Mucosal bleeding can be a symptom of disease.
• Patients with severe symptoms may be taking chemotherapy.
• Monitor vital signs every appointment due to cardiovascular side effects.
• Consider semisupine chair position for patient comfort when GI side effects occur.

Consultations:
• Medical consult with hematologist or physician directing therapy is essential before dental treatment.

Teach patient/family:
• To inform dentist of unusual bleeding episodes following dental treatment
• Importance of updating health and drug history if physician makes any changes in evaluation or drug regimens

---

apraclonidine
(a-pra-kloe'ni-deen)
Iopidine
Drug class.: Selective α_2-adrenergic agonist

Action: Reduces elevated or normal intraocular pressure
Uses: Control or prevention of increases in intraocular pressure related to laser surgery of eye; short-term control of increased intraocular pressure as an adjunctive drug
Dosage and routes:
• *Adult:* TOP INSTILL 1 or 2 gtt (0.5% sol) tid; allow a 5 min interval between other required ophthalmic drops
• *Adult:* TOP prelaser surgery use 1 gtt (1% sol) 1 hr before surgery and 1 gtt when surgery is completed
Available forms include: Sterile ophthalmic sol 0.5% and 1.0%
Side effects/adverse reactions:
▼ *ORAL:* Dry mouth, taste alterations (both 1%)
CNS: Insomnia, paresthesia, head-ache, dizziness
CV: Bradycardia, vasovagal syncope, palpitation
GI: Abdominal pain, diarrhea, emesis, nausea
RESP: Dyspnea, asthma
EENT: Hyperemia, discomfort, edema, tearing, mydriasis, blurred vision

INTEG: Pruritus
MISC: Facial edema
Contraindications: Hypersensitivity to this drug or clonidine; concurrent use of monoamine oxidase inhibitors
Precautions: Tachyphylaxis, impaired renal or liver function, depression, pregnancy category A, lactation, children, cardiovascular disease, cardiovascular drugs
Pharmacokinetics:
TOP: Onset 1 hr, maximum effect 3-5 hr; some systemic absorption
⚡ Drug interactions of concern to dentistry:
• No drug interactions have been reported; this is a new drug and data are lacking
• Avoid using drugs that can exacerbate glaucoma: anticholinergic drugs
DENTAL CONSIDERATIONS
General:
• Protect patient's eyes from accidental spatter during dental treatment.
• Avoid dental light in patient's eyes; offer dark glasses for patient comfort.
• Determine why the patient is taking the drug.
• Assess salivary flow as a factor in caries, periodontal disease, and candidiasis.
Consultations:
• Medical consult may be required to assess disease control.
Teach patient/family: *When chronic dry mouth occurs, advise patient:*
• To avoid mouth rinses with high alcohol content due to drying effects
• Need for daily home fluoride to prevent caries

• To use sugarless gum, frequent sips of water, or saliva substitutes

---

articaine HCl (local)
(ar-te'kane)
Septocaine

Drug class.: Amide local anesthetic with vasoconstrictor (epinephrine)

Action: Inhibits ion fluxes across membranes, particularly sodium transport across cell membrane; decreases rise of depolarization phase of action potential; blocks nerve action potential

Uses: Local, infiltrative, or conductive anesthesia in both simple and complex dental and periodontal procedures

Dosage and routes:
Infiltration
• *Adult:* INJ 0.5-2.5 ml (20-100 mg)
Nerve block
• *Adult:* INJ 0.5-3.4 ml (20-136 mg)
Oral surgery
• *Adult:* INJ 1.0-5.1 ml (40-204 mg)
Maximum recommended doses should not exceed 7 mg/kg or 3.2 mg/lb. Reduce doses for pediatric, elderly and patients with cardiac or liver disease.
• *Child:* Use not recommended for child <4 yr. Do not exceed maximum recommended dose and adjust for age, body weight, and physical condition.

Example calculations illustrating amount of drug administered per dental cartridge(s)

# cartridges (1.7 ml)	mg of articaine (4%)	mg (µg) of vasoconstrictor (1:100,000)
1	68	0.017 (17)
2	136	0.034 (34)
3	204	0.051 (51)

Available forms include: Inj 4% with epinephrine 1:100,000 in 1.7 ml vol (50 per carton)

Side effects/adverse reactions:
▼ *ORAL: Facial edema, gingivitis,* glossitis, tongue edema, mouth ulcer, taste perversion, dry mouth
CNS: Headache, paresthesia, migraine
CV: Syncope, tachycardia (infrequent)
GI: Nausea, vomiting, diarrhea
RESP: Pharyngitis
HEMA: Ecchymosis
GU: Dysmenorrhea
EENT: Rhinitis, ear pain
INTEG: Pruritus, rash
META: Edema, thirst
MS: Arthralgia, myalgia
MISC: Infection, localized pain

Contraindications: Hypersensitivity to amides or sodium metabisulfite

Precautions: Accidental intravascular injections may be associated with convulsions, CNS depression or cardiorespiratory depression, reduce dose for elderly, debilitated or pediatric patients, exaggerated response to intravascular epinephrine, severe hepatic impairment, pregnancy category C, lactation

Pharmacokinetics: Onset 1-6 min; duration about 1 hr; pKa 7.8,

---

italic = common side effects

pH of sol is 5.0; peak blood levels in 25 min, plasma levels after 68 mg is 385 ng/ml, after 204 mg is 900 ng/ml, 60%-80% plasma protein bound, metabolized by plasma carboxylesterase; liver P450 enzymes metabolize 5%-10% of available articaine; urinary excretion mainly

🦷 **Drug interactions of concern to dentistry:**
• CNS depressants: increased risk of CNS depression with all CNS depressants, especially in children and when larger doses are used
• Avoid placing dental cartridges in disinfectant solutions with heavy metals or surface-active agents; may see release of metal ions into local anesthetic solutions with tissue irritation following injection
• Risk of cardiovascular side effects; rapid intravascular administration of local anesthetic containing vasoconstrictor, either alone or in patients taking tricyclic antidepressants, MAO inhibitors, digitalis drugs, cocaine, phenothiazines, β-blockers, and in presence of halogenated hydrocarbon general anesthetics; use smallest effective vasoconstrictor dose and careful aspiration technique
• Avoid use of vasoconstrictors in patients with uncontrolled hyperthyroidism, diabetes, angina, or hypertension; refer these patients for medical treatment before elective dental procedures

DENTAL CONSIDERATIONS
General:
• Monitor vital signs every appointment due to cardiovascular side effects.

• Apply lubricant to dry lips for patient comfort prior to dental procedures.
• Use vasoconstrictor with caution, in low doses and with careful aspiration.

Teach patient/family:
• To use care to prevent injury while numbness exists and to not chew gum or eat following dental anesthesia
• To report any signs of infection, muscle pain, or fever to dentist when feeling returns
• To report any unusual soft tissue reactions

---

ascorbic acid (vitamin C)
(a-skor′bic)
Cevi-Bid, Dull-C, Vita-C
♣ Apo-C

Drug class.: Vitamin C, water-soluble vitamin

Action: Needed for wound healing, collagen synthesis, antioxidant, carbohydrate metabolism, absorption of iron, and other metabolic processes
Uses: Vitamin C deficiency, scurvy, urine acidification, and supplemental use in a variety of debilitated patients with poor vitamin C intake
Dosage and routes:
Scurvy
• *Adult:* PO/SC/IM/IV 100-500 mg qd, then 50 mg or more qd
• *Child:* PO/SC/IM/IV 100-300 mg qd, then 35 mg or more qd
Wound healing/chronic disease/fracture
• *Adult:* SC/IM/IV/PO 200-500 mg qd

• *Child:* SC/IM/IV/PO 100-200 mg added doses

Urine acidification

• *Adult:* SC/IM/IV/PO 4-12 g qd in divided doses

Available forms include: Tabs 250, 500, 1000, 1500 mg; sus rel tabs 500, 1000 mg; crys 4 g/tsp; powd 4 g/tsp; sol 100 mg/ml; inj SC/IM/IV 500 mg/ml; loz 60 mg

Side effects/adverse reactions:

▼ *ORAL:* Enamel erosion, caries (chewable form, chronic use)

CNS: Headache, insomnia, dizziness, fatigue, flushing

GI: Nausea, vomiting, diarrhea, anorexia, heartburn, cramps

HEMA: Hemolytic anemia in patients with G6PD

GU: Polyuria, urine acidification, oxalate or urate renal stones

Contraindications: None significant

Precautions: Gout, pregnancy category A

Pharmacokinetics:

PO/INJ: Metabolized in liver; unused amounts excreted in urine (unchanged) and metabolites; crosses placenta and excreted in breast milk

🥄 **Drug interactions of concern to dentistry:**

• Increased urinary excretion: salicylates, barbiturates

DENTAL CONSIDERATIONS

General:

• An increased incidence of caries and soft tissue injury has been reported with excessive use of chewable ascorbic acid tablets.

aspirin (acetylsalicylic acid)

(as′pir-in)

Arthritis Foundation Pain Reliever, ASA, Ascriptin, Aspergum, Aspirin, Bayer Children's Aspirin, Ecotrin, Empirin, Genuine Bayer, Maximum Bayer, Norwich Extra-Strength, St. Joseph Adult Chewable Aspirin, Zorprim, others

Combinations: Often combined with other analgesic drugs

♣ Entrophen, Novasen, Sal-Adult, Sal-Infant, Supasa

Drug class.: Nonnarcotic analgesic salicylate

Action: Inhibits prostaglandin synthesis by interfering with cyclo-oxygenase needed for biosynthesis; possesses analgesic, antiinflammatory, antipyretic properties

Uses: Mild-to-moderate pain or fever, including arthritis, thromboembolic disorders, transient ischemic attacks in men, rheumatic fever, postmyocardial infarction

Dosage and routes:

Arthritis

• *Adult:* PO 3.2-6 g/day in divided doses q4-6h

Juvenile rheumatoid arthritis

• *Child:* PO 60-110 mg/kg/day in divided doses q6-8h

Pain/fever

• *Adult:* PO/REC 500 mg q3h, 325-650 mg q4h or 1000 mg q6h

• *Child 2-3 yr:* PO/REC 160 mg q4h

• *Child 4-5 yr:* PO/REC 240 mg q4h

• *Child 6-8 yr:* PO/REC 325 mg q4h

• *Child 9-10 yr:* PO/REC 400 mg q4h
• *Child 11 yr:* PO/REC 480 mg q4h
• *Child 12 yr:* PO/REC 650 mg q4h
Platelet aggregation inhibitor
• *Adult:* PO 80-325 mg/day
Transient ischemic attacks in men
• *Adult:* PO 325 mg-1.0 g/day
Available forms include: Tabs 81,165, 325, 500, 650, 975 mg; chew tabs 81 mg; caps 325, 500 mg; con rel tabs 800 mg; time rel tabs 650 mg; supp 120, 200, 300, 600 mg, and 1.2 g; gum 227.5 mg
Side effects/adverse reactions:
▼ *ORAL:* Increased bleeding (chronic, high doses)
CNS: ***Coma, convulsion,*** stimulation, drowsiness, dizziness, confusion, headache, flushing, hallucinations
CV: Rapid pulse, pulmonary edema
GI: Nausea, vomiting, ***GI bleeding, hepatitis,*** diarrhea, heartburn, anorexia
RESP: Wheezing, hyperpnea
HEMA: ***Thrombocytopenia, agranulocytosis, leukopenia, neutropenia, hemolytic anemia,*** increased pro-time, bleeding time
EENT: Tinnitus, hearing loss
INTEG: *Rash,* urticaria, bruising
ENDO: Hypoglycemia, hyponatremia, hypokalemia
Contraindications: Hypersensitivity to salicylates, GI bleeding, bleeding disorders, children <3 yr, children with flulike symptoms, pregnancy category C, lactation, vitamin K deficiency, peptic ulcer
Precautions: Anemia, hepatic disease, renal disease, Hodgkin's disease, preoperative, postoperative
Pharmacokinetics:
PO: Onset 15-30 min, peak 1-2 hr, duration 4-6 hr

REC: Onset slow, duration 4-6 hr, half-life 1-3.5 hr; metabolized by liver; excreted by kidneys; crosses placenta; excreted in breast milk
🦷 **Drug interactions of concern to dentistry:**
• Increased risk of GI complaints and occult blood loss: alcohol, NSAIDs, corticosteroids
• *Buffered aspirin:* Decreased absorption of tetracycline
• Recent report indicated ibuprofen may block clot-preventing effects of aspirin
Interactions when used as a dental drug:
• Increased risk of bleeding: oral anticoagulants, valproic acid, dipyridamole
• Increased risk of hypoglycemia: sulfonylureas
• Increased risk of toxicity: methotrexate, lithium, zidovudine
• Decreased effects of probenecid, sulfinpyrazone
• Avoid prolonged or concurrent use with NSAIDs, corticosteroids, acetaminophen
DENTAL CONSIDERATIONS
General:
• Patients on chronic drug therapy may rarely have symptoms of blood dyscrasias, which can include infection, bleeding, and poor healing.
• Avoid prescribing buffered aspirin-containing products if patient is on a sodium-restricted diet.
• Chewable forms of aspirin should not be used for 7 days following oral surgery because of possible soft tissue injury.
• Evaluate allergic reactions: rash, urticaria; patients with allergy to

salicylates may not be able to take NSAIDs; drug may need to be discontinued.

Consultations:

• In a patient with symptoms of blood dyscrasias, request a medical consult for blood studies and postpone dental treatment until normal values are reestablished.

• Take precautions if dental surgery is anticipated due to risk of increased bleeding; avoid prescribing aspirin before dental surgery.

• Tinnitus, ringing, roaring in ears after high-dose and long-term therapy necessitates referral for salicylism.

Teach patient/family:

• That aspirin or buffered aspirin tablets should not be placed directly on a tooth or mucosal surface due to the risk of chemical burn

• To read label on other OTC drugs; may contain aspirin

• To avoid alcohol ingestion; GI bleeding may occur

---

atenolol

(a-ten′oh-lole)
Tenormin
♣ Apo-Atenol, Novo-Atenolol

Drug class.: Antihypertensive, selective β_1-blocker

Action: This is a selective β_1-adrenergic antagonist. At higher doses selectivity may be lost with antagonism of β_2-receptors as well. The antihypertensive mechanism of action is unclear, but may include a reduction in cardiac output and inhibition of renin release by the renal juxtaglomerular apparatus. Peripheral resistance decreases with long-term use. The antianginal action (when indicated for this use) may be related to a decrease in myocardial oxygen demand and negative chronotropic and inotropic effects. The antiarrhythmic action (when indicated for this use) has been related to a reduction in spontaneous pacemaker firing and slowing of AV nodal conduction.

Uses: Mild-to-moderate hypertension, treatment and prophylaxis of angina pectoris, arrhythmia, adjunct therapy in hypertrophic cardiomyopathy, MI therapy and prophylaxis, adjunct therapy in pheochromocytoma, prophylaxis for vascular headache, adjunct therapy in thyrotoxicosis

Dosage and routes:

Hypertension

• *Adult:* PO 50 mg qd, increasing q1-2wk to 100 mg qd used alone or in combination with other antihypertensive drugs

Angina pectoris

• *Adult:* PO 50 mg/day, can increase to 100 mg/day in 1 wk; max dose 200 mg/day

Available forms include: Tabs 25, 50, 100 mg; inj 5 mg/10 ml ampules

Side effects/adverse reactions:

▼ *ORAL:* Dry mouth

CNS: Insomnia, fatigue, dizziness, mental changes, memory loss, hallucinations, depression, lethargy, drowsiness, strange dreams, catatonia

CV: Profound hypotension, bradycardia, CHF, cold extremities, postural hypotension, second- or third-degree heart block

GI: Nausea, diarrhea, mesenteric arterial thrombosis, ischemic colitis, vomiting

RESP: Bronchospasm, dyspnea, wheezing

HEMA: Agranulocytosis, thrombocytopenia, purpura
GU: Impotence
EENT: Sore throat, dry burning eyes
INTEG: Rash, fever, alopecia
ENDO: Hypoglycemia

Contraindications: Hypersensitivity to β-blockers, cardiogenic shock, second- or third-degree heart block, sinus bradycardia, CHF, cardiac failure

Precautions: Major surgery, pregnancy category D, lactation, diabetes mellitus, severe renal disease, thyroid disease, COPD, asthma, well-compensated heart failure

Pharmacokinetics:
PO: Peak 2-4 hr; half-life 6-7 hr; excreted unchanged in urine; protein binding 5%-15%; up to 50% excreted unchanged in feces as unabsorbed drug

🐝 Drug interactions of concern to dentistry:
• Decreased antihypertensive effects: NSAIDs, indomethacin
• May slow metabolism of lidocaine
• Decreased β-blocking effects (or decreased β-adrenergic effects) of epinephrine, levonordefrin, isoproterenol, and other sympathomimetics

DENTAL CONSIDERATIONS
General:
• Monitor vital signs every appointment due to cardiovascular and respiratory side effects.
• After supine positioning, have patient sit upright for at least 2 min before standing to avoid orthostatic hypotension.
• Patients on chronic drug therapy may rarely have symptoms of blood dyscrasias, which can include infection, bleeding, and poor healing.
• Assess salivary flow as a factor in caries, periodontal disease, and candidiasis.
• Stress from dental procedures may compromise cardiovascular function; determine patient risk.
• Short appointments and a stress reduction protocol may be required for anxious patients.
• Use vasoconstrictors with caution, in low doses, and with careful aspiration. Avoid use of gingival retraction cord with epinephrine.

Consultations:
• In a patient with symptoms of blood dyscrasias, request a medical consult for blood studies and postpone dental treatment until normal values are reestablished.
• Medical consult may be required to assess disease control and stress tolerance of patient.
• Use precautions if general anesthesia is required for dental surgery.

Teach patient/family:
• Importance of good oral hygiene to prevent soft tissue inflammation
• Caution to prevent injury when using oral hygiene aids
When chronic dry mouth occurs, advise patient:
• To avoid mouth rinses with high alcohol content due to drying effects
• To use daily home fluoride products for anticaries effect
• To use sugarless gum, frequent sips of water, or saliva substitutes

---

atorvastatin calcium

(a-tore′va-sta-tin)

Lipitor

Drug class.: Cholesterol-lowering agent

Action: Inhibits HMG-CoA reductase enzyme, which reduces cholesterol synthesis; reduced synthesis of VLDL; plasma triglyceride levels may also be decreased

Uses: As an adjunct in homozygous familial hypercholesterolemia, mixed lipidemia, elevated serum triglyceride levels and Ttype IV hyperproteinemia, also reduces total cholesterol, LDL-C, apo B, and triglyceride levels; patient should first be placed on cholesterol-lowering diet

Dosage and routes:

• *Adult:* PO initial 10 mg daily; dose can be modified according to lipid lab values at 2-4 wk; dose range 10-80 mg daily

Available forms include: Tabs 10, 20, 40, 80 mg

Side effects/adverse reactions:

▼ *ORAL:* Angioneurotic edema, lichenoid reaction

CNS: Headache, insomnia

CV: Chest pain

GI: Flatulence, dyspepsia, abdominal pain, nausea

RESP: Bronchitis, rhinitis

EENT: Rash, pruritus

META: Elevated liver enzymes

MS: Myalgia, arthritis

MISC: Allergy, urinary tract infection, peripheral edema

Contraindications: Hypersensitivity, active liver disease, pregnancy, lactation

Precautions: Chronic alcohol liver disease, pregnancy X, monitor liver function and lipid levels

Pharmacokinetics:

PO: First-pass metabolism, half-life 14 hr, 98% protein bound

🖢 **Drug interactions of concern to dentistry:** Severe myopathy or rhabdomyolysis: erythromycin, niacin, itraconazole Increase in plasma levels: erythromycin, itraconazole

DENTAL CONSIDERATIONS

General:

• Consider semisupine chair position for patient comfort if GI side effects occur.

atovaquone

(a-toe′va-kwone)

Mepron

Drug class.: Antipneumocystic (antiprotozoal)

Action: Mechanism of action unknown; may act through ubiquinone to inhibit synthesis of ATP and nucleic acids

Uses: Treatment and prevention of mild to moderate *P. carinii* pneumonia in patients who are intolerant to trimethoprim-sulfamethoxazole

Dosage and routes:

• *Adult and child 13-16 yr:* PO 750 mg bid with a meal × 21 days

Prevention

• *Child 13-16 yr:* PO 1500 mg/day at mealtime

Available forms include: Oral susp 750 mg/5 ml

Side effects/adverse reactions:

▼ *ORAL: Candidiasis,* taste alteration

CNS: Headache, insomnia, dizziness, anxiety

CV: Hypotension, hyponatremia

GI: Nausea, vomiting, abdominal pain, diarrhea, constipation
RESP: Cough
*HEMA: **Neutropenia,*** anemia
INTEG: Rash, sweating
MISC: Fever, hypoglycemia, asthenia
Contraindications: Hypersensitivity
Precautions: Pregnancy category C, lactation, children, elderly, GI diseases with malabsorption complications, hepatic disease; must do CBC, ALT, and AST values
Pharmacokinetics: Fatty meals enhance absorption; highly protein bound (99%); two peak plasma periods (first 1-8 hr, second 24-96 hr); metabolites excreted in urine
Drug interactions of concern to dentistry:
• Aspirin: there are no data on drug interactions related to specific dental medications; however, because of its high protein binding there is always a risk of displacement when other highly protein bound drugs are administered.

DENTAL CONSIDERATIONS
General:
• Examine patient for signs of oral manifestations of opportunistic infections.
• Place on frequent recall because of drug and disease oral side effects.
• Consider semisupine chair position due to GI side effects.
• Consider semisupine chair position for patients with respiratory disease.
• Patients on chronic drug therapy may rarely have symptoms of blood dyscrasias, which can include infection, bleeding, and poor healing.

Consultations:
• Medical consult may be required to assess disease control and stress tolerance.
• In a patient with symptoms of blood dyscrasias, request a medical consult for blood studies and postpone dental treatment until normal values are reestablished.
• Acute oral infection may require physician consult for coordination of antiinfective therapy.
Teach patient/family:
• Importance of good oral hygiene to prevent soft tissue inflammation
• Caution to prevent injury when using oral hygiene aids
• Importance of dietary suggestions to maintain oral and systemic health
• That secondary oral infections may occur; must see dentist immediately if infection occurs

---

atropine sulfate
(a'troe-peen)
Sal-Tropine
Drug class.: Anticholinergic

Action: Inhibits muscarinic actions of acetylcholine at postganglionic parasympathetic neuroeffector sites; dries secretions by antagonism of muscarinic cholinergic receptors
Uses: Reduction of salivary and bronchial secretions
Dosage and routes:
• *Adult:* PO 0.4 mg given 30-60 min before drying effect is required for dental procedure
• *Child:* PO >90 lb, 0.4 mg; 65-90 lb, 0.4 mg; 40-65 lb, 0.3 mg
Available forms include: Tabs 0.4 mg

---

bold italic = life-threatening conditions

Side effects/adverse reactions:

▼ *ORAL: Dry mouth,* burning sensation

CNS: Headache, dizziness, **coma (toxic dose),** involuntary movement, confusion, anxiety, flushing, drowsiness, insomnia

CV: Hypotension, paradoxic bradycardia, angina, PVCs, hypertension, tachycardia, ectopic ventricular beats

GI: Nausea, vomiting, abdominal pain, anorexia, constipation, *paralytic ileus,* abdominal distention

GU: Retention, hesitancy, impotence, dysuria

EENT: Blurred vision, photophobia, glaucoma, eye pain, pupil dilation, nasal congestion

INTEG: Rash, urticaria, contact dermatitis, dry skin, flushing

MISC: Suppression of lactation, decreased sweating

Contraindications: Hypersensitivity to belladonna alkaloids, angle-closure glaucoma, GI obstructions, myasthenia gravis, thyrotoxicosis, ulcerative colitis, prostatic hypertrophy, tachycardia/tachydysrhythmias, asthma

Precautions: Pregnancy category C, lactation, renal disease, CHF, hyperthyroidism, COPD, hepatic disease, child <6 yr, hypertension, geriatric

Pharmacokinetics:

PO: Onset 0.5-1 hr, moderate protein binding, duration of action 4-6 hr, renal excretion

⚡ Drug interactions of concern to dentistry:

• Increased anticholinergic effects: tricyclic antidepressants, antihistamines, opioid analgesics, antipsychotic medications, or other drugs with anticholinergic activity

• Decreased absorption of ketoconazole

DENTAL CONSIDERATIONS

General:

• Give PO dose 30-60 min before drying effects are required for dental procedures.

• Request that patient remove contact lenses before using due to possible drying effects in the eyes.

• Caution patients that they may feel a dry, burning sensation in the throat and experience blurred vision.

• This drug is intended for acute use, usually in single doses only; therefore chronic dry mouth should not be a concern.

• Avoid dental light in patient's eyes; offer dark glasses for patient comfort.

Consultations:

• Medical consult is advisable before using this drug in patients with a history of GI disease, cardiac disease, or glaucoma.

atropine sulfate (optic)

(a'troe-peen)

Atropine-1, Atropine Care, Atropisol, Isopto Atropine

♣ Mims Atropine

Drug class.: Mydriatic (anticholinergic)

Action: Blocks response of iris sphincter muscle and muscle of accommodation of ciliary body to cholinergic stimulation, resulting in dilation and paralysis of accommodation

Uses: Iritis, cycloplegic refraction

Dosage and routes:

• *Adult:* INSTILL SOL 1-2 gtt of a 1% sol qd-tid for iritis or

1 hr before refracting (cycloplegic refraction); INSTILL OINT bid-tid
• *Child:* INSTILL SOL 1-2 gtt of a 0.5% sol qd-tid for iritis or bid × 1-3 days before exam (cycloplegic refraction); INSTILL OINT qd-bid 2-3 days before exam

Uveitis

• *Adult:* INSTILL SOL 1-2 gtt into eye(s) up to 4 × daily
• *Child:* INSTILL SOL 1 or 2 gtt of 0.5% sol into eye(s) up to 3 × daily

Available forms include: Oint 1%; sol 0.5%, 1%, 2%

Side effects/adverse reactions:

▼ *ORAL:* Dry mouth
SYST: Tachycardia, confusion, fever, flushing, dry skin, abdominal discomfort (infants: bladder distention, irregular pulse, respiratory depression)

Contraindications: Hypersensitivity, infants <3 mo, open- or narrow-angle glaucoma, conjunctivitis, Down syndrome

Pharmacokinetics:

INSTILL: Peak 30-40 min (mydriasis), 60-180 min (cycloplegia); duration of dilation up to 6-12 days

DENTAL CONSIDERATIONS

General:

• Avoid dental light in patient's eyes; offer dark glasses for patient comfort.

---

auranofin

(au-rane'oh-fin)
Ridaura

Drug class.: Gold salt

Action: Specific antiinflammatory action unknown; may decrease phagocytosis, lysosomal activity, concentration of rheumatoid factor or immunoglobulins

Uses: Rheumatoid arthritis, unapproved: juvenile arthritis

Dosage and routes:

• *Adult:* PO 6 mg qd or 3 mg bid, may increase to 9 mg/day after 3 mo, if tolerated

Available forms include: Caps 3 mg

Side effects/adverse reactions:

▼ *ORAL: Stomatitis, lichenoid drug reaction,* metallic taste, glossitis, gingivitis
CNS: Dizziness, syncope
GI: Diarrhea, abdominal cramping, stomatitis, nausea, vomiting, enterocolitis, anorexia, flatulence, dyspepsia, jaundice, increased AST/ALT, melena, constipation
RESP: Interstitial pneumonitis, fibrosis, cough, dyspnea
HEMA: Thrombocytopenia, agranulocytosis, aplastic anemia, leukopenia, eosinophilia
GU: Proteinuria, hematuria, increased BUN, creatinine, vaginitis
INTEG: Rash, pruritus, dermatitis, exfoliative dermatitis, urticaria, alopecia, photosensitivity

Contraindications: Hypersensitivity to gold, necrotizing enterocolitis, bone marrow aplasia, child <6 yr, lactation, pulmonary fibrosis, exfoliative dermatitis, blood dyscrasias, recent radiation therapy

Precautions: Elderly, CHF, diabetes mellitus, allergic conditions, ulcerative colitis, renal disease, liver disease, pregnancy category C

Pharmacokinetics:

PO: Peak 2 hr; steady state 8-16 wk; 20%-25% absorbed by GI tract; excreted in urine and feces

DENTAL CONSIDERATIONS

General:

• Patients on chronic drug therapy may rarely have symptoms of blood dyscrasias, which can in-

clude infection, bleeding, and poor healing.
• Consider semisupine chair position for patients with arthritic disease.

Consultations:
• In a patient with symptoms of blood dyscrasias, request a medical consult for blood studies and postpone dental treatment until normal values are reestablished.

Teach patient/family:
• Importance of good oral hygiene to prevent soft tissue inflammation
• To avoid mouth rinses with high alcohol content due to drying and irritating effects

---

aurothioglucose/gold sodium thiomalate
(aur-oh-thye-oh-gloo'kose)
Aurolate (gold sodium thiomalate), Solganal (aurothioglucose)
Drug class.: Antiinflammatory gold compound

Action: Specific antiinflammatory action unknown; may decrease phagocytosis, lysosomal activity, prostaglandin synthesis
Uses: Rheumatoid arthritis; juvenile arthritis; unapproved: psoriatic arthritis, Felty's syndrome

Dosage and routes:
Aurothioglucose
• *Adult:* IM 10 mg, then 25 mg qwk × 2-3 wk, then 25-50 mg/wk until total of 800 mg-1 g is administered, then 25-50 mg q3-4wk if there is improvement without toxicity; limit 50 mg/wk
• *Child 6-12 yr:* IM 2.5 mg × 1 wk, 6.25 mg qwk × 2-3 wk, then 12.5 mg/wk until total dose of 200-250 mg, then 6.25-12.5 mg q2-3wk

Gold sodium thiomalate
• *Adult:* IM 10 mg, then 25 mg after 1 wk, then 25-50 mg qwk for total of 1 g, then 25-50 mg q2wk × 20 wk, then 25-50 mg q3-4wk for maintenance
• *Child:* IM 10 mg × 1 wk, 1 mg/kg 2nd wk (limit 50 mg), then maintenance dose
Available forms include: IM inj 50 mg/ml

Side effects/adverse reactions:
▼ *ORAL:* Stomatitis, metallic taste
CNS: Dizziness, **encephalitis,** EEG abnormalities, confusion, hallucinations
CV: Bradycardia, rapid pulse
GI: **Hepatitis,** vomiting, nausea, jaundice, diarrhea, cramping, flatulence
RESP: **Pulmonary fibrosis,** interstitial pneumonitis, pharyngitis
HEMA: **Thrombocytopenia, agranulocytosis, aplastic anemia, leukopenia, eosinophilia, neutropenia**
GU: Proteinuria, **nephrosis, tubular necrosis,** hematuria
EENT: Iritis, corneal ulcers
INTEG: Rash, pruritus, dermatitis, **exfoliative dermatitis, angioedema,** urticaria, alopecia, photosensitivity
MISC: **Anaphylaxis**
Contraindications: Hypersensitivity to gold, SLE, uncontrolled diabetes mellitus, marked hypertension, recent radiation therapy, CHF, lactation, renal disease, liver disease
Precautions: Decreased tolerance in elderly, children, blood dyscrasias, pregnancy category C
Pharmacokinetics:
IM: Peak 4-6 hr; half-life 3-27 days; half-life increases up to 168

---

days with eleventh dose; excreted in urine and feces

⚕ Drug interactions of concern to dentistry:
• None reported

DENTAL CONSIDERATIONS
General:
• Patients on chronic drug therapy may rarely have symptoms of blood dyscrasias, which can include infection, bleeding, and poor healing.
• Palliative medication may be required for management of oral side effects.
• Consider semisupine chair position for patient comfort due to arthritic disease.

Consultations:
• Medical consult may be required to assess disease control and patient's ability to tolerate stress.
• In a patient with symptoms of blood dyscrasias, request a medical consult for blood studies and postpone dental treatment until normal values are reestablished.

Teach patient/family:
• Importance of good oral hygiene to prevent soft tissue inflammation
• Alert the patient to the possibility of secondary oral infection and the need to see dentist immediately if infection occurs
• To report oral lesions, soreness, or bleeding to dentist
• To avoid mouth rinses with high alcohol content due to drying effects

---

azatadine maleate
(a-za'ta-deen)
Optimine
Drug class.: Antihistamine, H$_1$-receptor antagonist

Action: Acts on blood vessels, GI system, and respiratory system by competing with histamine for H$_1$-receptor site; decreases allergic response by blocking histamine

Uses: Allergy symptoms, rhinitis, chronic urticaria, pruritus

Dosage and routes:
• *Adult and child >12 yr:* PO 1-2 mg bid, not to exceed 4 mg/day
Available forms include: Tabs 1 mg

Side effects/adverse reactions:
▼ *ORAL:* Dry mouth
CNS: Dizziness, drowsiness, poor coordination, fatigue, anxiety, euphoria, confusion, paresthesia, neuritis, sweating, chills
CV: Hypotension, palpitation, tachycardia
GI: Constipation, nausea, vomiting, anorexia, diarrhea
RESP: Increased thick secretions, wheezing, chest tightness
HEMA: ***Thrombocytopenia, agranulocytosis, hemolytic anemia***
GU: Retention, dysuria, frequency, impotence
EENT: Blurred vision, dilated pupils, tinnitus, nasal stuffiness, dry nose/throat
INTEG: Rash, urticaria, photosensitivity

Contraindications: Hypersensitivity to H$_1$-receptor antagonist, acute asthma attack, lower respiratory tract disease, child <12 yr

Precautions: Increased intraocular pressure, renal disease, cardiac disease, bronchial asthma, seizure disorder, stenosed peptic ulcers, hyperthyroidism, prostatic hypertrophy, bladder neck obstruction, pregnancy category B, elderly, lactation

Pharmacokinetics:
PO: Peak 4 hr, half-life 9-12 hr;

---

minimally bound to plasma proteins; metabolized in liver; excreted by kidneys; crosses placenta, blood-brain barrier

👤 Drug interactions of concern to dentistry:
• Increased CNS depression: all CNS depressants, alcohol
• Increased anticholinergic effect: anticholinergics

DENTAL CONSIDERATIONS
General:
• Assess salivary flow as a factor in caries, periodontal disease, and candidiasis.
• Patients on chronic drug therapy may rarely have symptoms of blood dyscrasias, which can include infection, bleeding, and poor healing.
• Consider semisupine chair position for patient comfort due to respiratory disease.
• Monitor vital signs every appointment due to cardiovascular side effects.

Consultations:
• In a patient with symptoms of blood dyscrasia, request a medical consult for blood studies and postpone dental treatment until normal values are reestablished.

Teach patient/family:
• Importance of good oral hygiene to prevent soft tissue inflammation
• Caution to prevent injury when using oral hygiene aids
When chronic dry mouth occurs, advise patient:
• To avoid mouth rinses with high alcohol content due to drying effects
• To use daily home fluoride products for anticaries effect
• To use sugarless gum, frequent sips of water, or saliva substitutes

azathioprine

(ay-za-thye′oh-preen)
Imuran

Drug class.: Immunosuppressant

Action: Produces immunosuppression by inhibiting purine synthesis in cells, thereby preventing RNA and DNA synthesis

Uses: Renal transplants to prevent graft rejection, refractory rheumatoid arthritis, refractory ITP, glomerulonephritis, nephrotic syndrome, bone marrow transplant; unapproved: pemphigoid and pemphigus, chronic ulcerative colitis, Behçet's syndrome, Crohn's disease

Dosage and routes:
Prevention of rejection
• *Adult and child:* PO/IV 3-5 mg/kg/day, then maintenance of at least 1-2 mg/kg/day
Refractory rheumatoid arthritis
• *Adult:* PO 1 mg/kg/day, may increase dose after 2 mo by 0.5 mg/kg/day, not to exceed 2.5 mg/kg/day
Unlabeled use in pemphigoid, pemphigus
• *Adult:* PO 1 mg/kg of body weight per day; can titrate dose after 6-8 wk at 0.5 mg/kg of body weight per day. Max dose 2.5 mg/kg of body weight per day. Maintenance dose: determine the minimum effective dose by reducing dose at 0.5 mg/kg of body weight per day every 4-8 wk
Available forms include: Tabs 50 mg; inj IV 100 mg

Side effects/adverse reactions:
▼ *ORAL:* Stomatitis, oral ulceration

GI: **Pancreatitis, hepatotoxicity, jaundice,** nausea, vomiting, esophagitis
HEMA: **Leukopenia, thrombocytopenia, anemia, pancytopenia**
INTEG: Rash
MS: Arthralgia, muscle wasting
Contraindications: Hypersensitivity, pregnancy category D
Precautions: Severe renal disease, severe hepatic disease
Pharmacokinetics: Metabolized in liver; excreted in urine (active metabolite); crosses placenta
⚖ Drug interactions of concern to dentistry:
• Increased blood dyscrasias: NSAIDs, especially phenylbutazone, dapsone, phenothiazines
• Increased immunosuppression, risk of infection: corticosteroids
DENTAL CONSIDERATIONS
General:
• Patients on chronic drug therapy may rarely have symptoms of blood dyscrasias, which can include infection, bleeding, and poor healing.
• To prevent infection if surgery or deep scaling is planned, prophylactic antibiotics may be indicated in patients who develop neutropenia.
• Determine why the patient is taking the drug.
• Alert the patient to the possibility of secondary oral infection; must see dentist immediately if infection occurs.
Consultations:
• In a patient with symptoms of blood dyscrasias, request a medical consult for blood studies and postpone dental treatment until normal values are reestablished.
• Medical consult may be required to assess disease control.

• Medical consult may be required to assess patient's ability to tolerate stress.
Teach patient/family:
• Importance of good oral hygiene to prevent soft tissue inflammation
• Caution to prevent injury when using oral hygiene aids
• To avoid mouth rinses with high alcohol content due to drying effects and irritation of mucous membranes

azelaic acid
(a-zel′ay-ik)
Azelex
Drug class.: Antiacne

Action: Exact mechanism unknown; may inhibit synthesis of cellular protein; has antimicrobial activity against *P. acnes* and *S. epidermidis*
Uses: Topical therapy of mild-to-moderate inflammatory acne vulgaris; unapproved: melasma
Dosage and routes:
• *Adult and child <12 yr:* TOP wash skin and pat skin dry, apply thin film to affected area bid
Available forms include: Cream 20% in 30 g tube
Side effects/adverse reactions:
INTEG: Irritation, pruritus, burning, hypopigmentation
Contraindications: Hypersensitivity
Precautions: Prevent contact with eyes, pregnancy category B, child <12 yr, lactation
Pharmacokinetics:
TOP: Less than 4% systemic absorption
⚖ Drug interactions of concern to dentistry:
• None reported

DENTAL CONSIDERATIONS
General:
• Topical use rarely causes exacerbation of recurrent herpes labialis.
• Keep away from mouth and other mucous membranes; wash eyes if cream comes in contact; irritation can occur.

---

azelastine HCl (otic)
(a-zel'as-teen)
Optivar
Drug class.: Ophthalmic antihistamine

Action: Selective H$_1$-antagonist; may inhibit release of other mediators from mast cells
Uses: Temporary relief of signs and symptoms of allergic conjunctivitis
Dosage and routes:
• *Adult:* TOP 1 drop in affected eye(s) bid
Available forms include: Sol 0.5 mg/ml in 6 ml
Side effects/adverse reactions:
CNS: Headache
EENT: Transient burning, stinging
Contraindications: Hypersensitivity
Precautions: Pregnancy category C, lactation; safety/effectiveness in children <3 yr unknown, renal impairment
Pharmacokinetics:
TOP: Low systemic absorption, low plasma levels, plasma protein binding 88%; metabolized to active metabolite by CYP450 (N-desmethylazelastine); excreted primarily in feces
⚠ Drug interactions of concern to dentistry:
• None reported

DENTAL CONSIDERATIONS
General:
• Protect patient's eyes from accidental spatter during dental treatment.

---

azelastine HCl
(a-zel'as-teen)
Astelin
Drug class.: H$_1$-receptor antagonist

Action: Acts by competitive antagonism of H$_1$-receptors to antagonize the wheal and flare responses and nasal hypersecretion; may also inhibit the release of other inflammatory mediators, including kinins and leukotrienes
Uses: Control of symptoms associated with seasonal allergic rhinitis or nonallergic vasomotor rhinitis
Dosage and routes:
• *Adult and child >12 yr:* Nasal spray 2 sprays per nostril bid
• *Child 5-11 yr:* Nasal spray 1 spray per nostril bid
Available forms include: Nasal spray unit, 137 µg per actuation
Side effects/adverse reactions:
▼ *ORAL: Bitter taste, dry mouth*
CNS: Somnolence, headache
GI: Nausea
RESP: Paroxysmal sneezing
EENT: Nasal burning
MISC: Fatigue
Contraindications: Hypersensitivity
Precautions: Child <12 yr, no data on pregnancy or lactation, renal impairment
Pharmacokinetics:
INH: Low absorption, metabolism to active metabolite, desmethyla-

zelastine; excretion mostly in feces (75%), urine (25%)

👪 Drug interactions of concern to dentistry:
• Increased risk of anticholinergic effects: anticholinergics
• Possible additive sedation: alcohol, anxiolytics, opioid analgesics

DENTAL CONSIDERATIONS

General:
• Assess salivary flow as factor in caries, periodontal disease, and candidiasis.

Teach patient/family: *When chronic dry mouth occurs, advise patient:*
• To avoid mouth rinses with high alcohol content due to drying effects
• To use daily home fluoride products for anticaries effect
• To use sugarless gum, frequent sips of water, or saliva substitutes

---

azithromycin/ azithromycin dihydrate

(az-ith-roe-mye'sin)
Zithromax

Drug class.: Macrolide antibiotic

Action: Binds to 50S ribosomal subunits of susceptible bacteria and suppresses protein synthesis; similar spectrum of activity to erythromycin

Uses: Mild-to-moderate infections of the upper/lower respiratory tract; COPD exacerbations due to *H. influenza, M. catarrhalis,* or *S. pneumoniae;* gonorrhea, chancroid, uncomplicated skin and skin structure infections caused by *M. catarrhalis, S. pneumoniae, S. pyogenes, S. aureus, S. agalactiae, H. influenzae, Clostridium, L. pneumophila;* nongonococcal urethritis;

cervicitis due to *C. trachomatis;* otitis media due to *H. influenzae, S. pneumoniae, M. catarrhalis;* chlamydia; *M. avium* complex in HIV infection

Dosage and routes:
• *Adult:* PO 500 mg on day 1, then 250 mg qd on days 2-5 for a total dose of 1.5 g; do not take oral suspension with meals; take 1 hr before or 2 hr after eating

Chlamydia/chancroid/urinary infections
• *Adult:* PO 1 g in a single dose

Gonorrhea
• *Adult:* PO 2 g in a single dose

Otitis media
• *Child:* PO 10 mg/kg/day on day 1; then 5 mg/kg on days 2-5, do not exceed adult dose; (was also approved by FDA for a 1- and 3-day regimen, but details were not available at publication time)

Mycobacterium avium complex
• *Adult:* PO 1200 mg qwk

Bacterial endocarditis prophylaxis
• *Adult:* PO for patients allergic to amoxicillin, 500 mg 1 hr before dental procedure
• *Child:* PO for patients allergic to amoxicillin, 15 mg/kg of body weight not to exceed the adult dose 1 hr before dental procedure

Available forms include: Tab 250 (Z-Pak 6 tabs), 600 mg; powder for oral susp 100/5 ml (in 300 mg bottle), 200 mg/5 ml (in 600, 900, 1200 mg bottles); 1 g packet

Side effects/adverse reactions:
▼ *ORAL:* Stomatitis, candidiasis, angioedema (allergy)
CNS: Dizziness, headache, vertigo, somnolence, fatigue
CV: Palpitation, chest pain
GI: Nausea, vomiting, diarrhea,

---

bold italic = life-threatening conditions

*abdominal pain, **hepatotoxicity,*** heartburn, dyspepsia, flatulence, melena

GU: Vaginitis, nephritis

INTEG: **Cholestatic jaundice,** rash, urticaria, pruritus (allergy), photosensitivity

Contraindications: Hypersensitivity to azithromycin or erythromycin, pimozide therapy

Precautions: Pregnancy category C; lactation; hepatic, renal, cardiac disease; elderly; child <16 yr

Pharmacokinetics:
PO: Peak 12 hr, duration 24 hr, half-life 11-57 hr; excreted in bile, feces, urine primarily as unchanged drug

🦷 **Drug interactions of concern to dentistry:**
• Increased serum levels: carbamazepine, cyclosporine, pimozide
• Risk of severe myopathy, rhabdomyolysis: HMG-CoA reductase inhibitors (statins)
• Decreased action of clindamycin, penicillin, lincomycin
• Oral contraceptives: advise patient of a potential risk for decreased contraceptive action, to maintain compliance with oral contraceptive use while using antibiotics, and to consider the use of additional nonhormonal contraception

DENTAL CONSIDERATIONS
General:
• Alternative drug of choice for mild infection due to susceptible organisms in patients allergic to penicillin.
• Determine why the patient is taking the drug.
• Consider semisupine chair position for patient comfort if GI side effects occur.

Teach patient/family: *When used for dental infection, advise patient:*
• To report sore throat, oral burning sensation, fever, fatigue, any of which could indicate superinfection
• To take at prescribed intervals and complete dosage regimen
• To immediately notify the dentist if signs or symptoms of infection increase

---

baclofen
(bak'loe-fen)
Lioresal, Lioresal Intrathecal
♣ Alpha-Baclofen, PMS-Baclofen
Drug class.: Skeletal muscle relaxant, central acting

Action: Precise mechanism of action is unknown; inhibits both monosynaptic and polysynaptic reflexes in the spinal cord and may act as an agonist for GABA$_B$ receptors; also causes some CNS depression

Uses: Skeletal muscle spasticity in multiple sclerosis, spinal cord injury, children with cerebral palsy; intrathecal dose form for severe spasticity in spinal cord injury or those not responsive to oral dose form; unapproved: trigeminal neuralgia

Dosage and routes:
• *Adult:* PO 5 mg tid × 3 days, then 10 mg tid × 3 days, then 15 mg tid × 3 days, then 20 mg tid × 3 days, then titrated to response, not to exceed 80 mg/day
Trigeminal neuralgia
• *Adult:* PO 50-60 mg/day

Intrathecal doseform
• *Adult:* INJ necessitates use of implantable pumps and titration of doses for each individual

Available forms include: Tabs 10, 20 mg; intrathecal 10 mg/20 ml, 10 mg/5 ml

Side effects/adverse reactions:

▼ *ORAL:* Dry mouth, taste alteration

CNS: Dizziness, weakness, fatigue, drowsiness, headache, disorientation, insomnia, paresthesias, tremors, convulsions, anxiety

CV: Hypotension, chest pain, palpitation, edema

GI: Nausea, vomiting, constipation, increased AST, alk phosphatase, abdominal pain, anorexia

GU: Urinary frequency, incontinence

EENT: Nasal congestion, blurred vision, mydriasis, tinnitus

INTEG: Rash, pruritus, urticaria

MS: Hypotonia

META: Elevated AST, alk phosphatase, blood sugar

Contraindications: Hypersensitivity

Precautions: Peptic ulcer disease, renal disease, hepatic disease, stroke, seizure disorder, diabetes mellitus, pregnancy category C, lactation, elderly, psychotic disorders, ovarian cysts, MAO inhibitors

Pharmacokinetics:

PO: Peak 2-3 hr, duration <8 hr, half-life 2.5-4 hr; partially metabolized in liver; excreted in urine (unchanged)

🥄 **Drug interactions of concern to dentistry:**
• Increased CNS depression: alcohol, all CNS depressants

• Muscle hypertonia: tricyclic antidepressants

When used in dentistry:
• Warn patient of sedative effects while taking medication

DENTAL CONSIDERATIONS:
General:
• Monitor vital signs every appointment due to cardiovascular side effects.
• Assess salivary flow as a factor in caries, periodontal disease, and candidiasis.
• After supine positioning, have patient sit upright for at least 2 min to avoid orthostatic hypotension.

Teach patient/family: *When chronic dry mouth occurs, advise patient:*
• To avoid mouth rinses with high alcohol content due to drying effects
• To use daily home fluoride products for anticaries effect
• To use sugarless gum, frequent sips of water, or saliva substitutes

---

balsalazide disodium
(bal-sal′a-zide)
Colazal
Drug class.: Antiinflammatory

Action: Converted by colon bacteria to mesalamine, mechanism of action unknown, may act topically in bowel by blocking synthesis of arachidonic acid metabolites

Uses: Mild to moderately active ulcerative colitis

Dosage and routes:
• *Adult:* PO 2.25 g (three capsules) taken tid for total daily dose of 6.75 g × 8–12 wk

Available forms include: Cap 750 mg

Side effects/adverse reactions:

▼ *ORAL:* Dry mouth (1%)

CNS: Headache, insomnia, fatigue, anorexia, dizziness

CV: Hot flushes

GI: Abdominal pain, diarrhea, nausea, vomiting, flatulence, rectal bleeding

RESP: Respiratory infection, pharyngitis, coughing

HEMA: Anemia

EENT: Rhinitis, sinusitis

INTEG: Rash, pruritus

MS: Back pain, myalgia

MISC: Arthralgia, fever

Contraindications: Hypersensitivity, including hypersensitivity to mesalamine or salicylates

Precautions: Hepatic or renal impairment, pyloric stenosis, pregnancy category B, lactation, pediatric patients not evaluated

Pharmacokinetics:

PO: Drug reaches colon intact; bacterial azoreductases release 5-aminobenzyl-B-analine and mesalamine (active metabolite); low, variable systemic absorption; peak concentration 1-2 hr, protein binding ~99%; less than 1% renal excretion; most excreted in feces (65%)

👄 **Drug interactions of concern to dentistry:**

• None reported

DENTAL CONSIDERATIONS

General:

• Consider semisupine chair position for patient comfort due to GI side effects of disease.

Consultations:

• To reduce any potential risk of antibiotic-associated pseudomembranous colitis, a consult is recommended before selecting an antibiotic for a dental infection.

becaplermin

(bee-kap'ler-min)

Regranex Gel

Drug class.: Topical wound repair

Action: A recombinant human platelet-derived growth factor (rhPDGF-BB) that promotes chemotactic recruitment and proliferation of cells involved in wound repair and formation of granulation tissue

Uses: As an adjunct to good ulcer care practices in lower extremity diabetic, neuropathic ulcers that extend into subcutaneous tissues or beyond and have adequate blood supply

Dosage and routes:

• *Adult and child >16 yr:* TOP Calculate the amount of gel to apply by the area (l × w) of the ulcer according to manufacturer's formula in gel package insert. Apply the gel once daily in a 1/16-inch-thick layer spread evenly on the ulcerated area. As the ulcer heals, the dose must be recalculated at weekly or biweekly intervals.

Available forms include: Gel 0.01% in 2, 7.5, and 15 g tubes

Side effects/adverse reactions:

INTEG: Erythematous rashes, pain, infection

Contraindications: Hypersensitivity, neoplasms at the site of application, ulcers due to vascular insufficiency

Precautions: Nonsterile, low-bioburden product that is not for use in ulcers that heal by primary intention, external use only, do not apply with fingers, pregnancy category C, lactation, children <16 yr

🦷 **Drug interactions of concern to dentistry:**

• Unknown

DENTAL CONSIDERATIONS:

General:

• Patients requiring use of this medication will probably be limited in activities or bedridden.

• Determine why patient is taking the drug.

• Diabetes: question patient about self-monitoring of blood glucose values or finger-stick records.

• Diabetics may be more susceptible to infection and have delayed wound healing.

• Examine for oral manifestation of opportunistic infection.

• Patients with advanced diabetes should be questioned about any limitations in activities or stress tolerance. Some will also be receiving dialysis treatment if renal function is compromised. Dental treatment can usually be performed the day after dialysis.

Consultations:

• Medical consult may be required to assess disease control and patient's ability to tolerate stress.

• Medical consult may include data from patient's blood glucose monitoring, including glycosylated hemoglobin (GHb) or HbA_{1c} testing.

• Patients in dialysis may require antibiotic prophylaxis; determine need.

Teach patient/family:

• Importance of good oral hygiene to prevent soft tissue inflammation

• To prevent trauma when using oral hygiene aids

• Importance of updating health and drug history if physician makes any changes in evaluation or drug regimens

beclomethasone dipropionate/ beclomethasone dipropionate HFA

(be-kloe-meth′a-sone)

Oral inhalation: Qvar, Vanceril, Vanceril Double Strength

Nasal inhalation: Beconase, Beconase AQ Nasal, Vancenase AQ 84 mcg, Vancenase Pockethaler

Drug class.: Corticosteroid, synthetic

Action: Glucocorticoids have multiple actions that include antiinflammatory and immunosuppressant effects. They inhibit phospholipase A_2, interfering with or reducing the synthesis of prostaglandins and leukotrienes. They also bind to cytoplasmic glucocorticoid receptors (GRs) and enter the cell nucleus to bind with DNA. This results in the synthesis of various enzymes such as collagenase, elastase, and cytokines that play important roles in inflammation and immunosuppression. They also suppress the production of lymphocytes, monocytes, and eosinophils.

Uses: Chronic asthma, prevent recurrent nasal polyps, allergic and nonallergic rhinitis

Dosage and routes:

Oral inhalation:

• *Adult:* INH 2 puffs tid-qid, not to exceed 20 inhalations/day

---

bold italic = life-threatening conditions

• *Child 6-12 yr:* INH 1-2 puffs tid-qid, not to exceed 10 inhalations/day

Oral inhalation (double strength):
• *Adult:* INH 2 puffs bid, can be more frequent in severe asthma; limit 10 inhalations/day
• *Child 6-12 yr:* INH 2 puffs bid, limit 5 inhalations/day

Nasal inhalation:
• *Adult and child >12 yr:* INSTILL 1-2 sprays in each nostril bid-qid; 84 μg double strength is once daily dose
• *Child 6-12 yr:* INSTILL 1 spray in each nostril once daily, QVAR use in children <12 yr not established

Pockethaler:
• *Adult and child >12 yr:* INH 1 spray in each nostril bid-qid

Available forms include: Aerosol 42, 84 μg/actuation in canisters, and pockethaler containing 200 metered actuations; QVAR 40, 80 μg/actuations

Side effects/adverse reactions:
▼ *ORAL:* Dry mouth, candidiasis (rare)
RESP: **Bronchospasm**
EENT: Hoarseness, sore throat

Contraindications: Hypersensitivity; status asthmaticus (primary treatment); nonasthmatic bronchial disease; bacterial, fungal, or viral infections of mouth, throat, or lungs; child <3 yr

Precautions: Nasal disease/surgery, pregnancy category C

Pharmacokinetics:
INH: Onset 10 min, half-life 3-15 hr; crosses placenta; metabolized in lungs, liver, GI system; excreted in feces (metabolites)

DENTAL CONSIDERATIONS
General:
• Evaluate respiration characteristics and rate.
• Assess salivary flow as a factor in caries, periodontal disease, and candidiasis
• Place on frequent recall due to oral side effects.
• Be aware that aspirin or sulfite preservatives in vasoconstrictor-containing products can exacerbate asthma.
• Acute asthmatic episodes may be precipitated in the dental office. Sympathomimetic inhalants should be available for emergency use.
• Midday appointments and a stress reduction protocol may be required for anxious patients.
Consultations:
• Medical consult may be required to assess patient's ability to tolerate stress.
Teach patient/family:
• That gargling and rinsing with water after each dose helps prevent candidiasis
When chronic dry mouth occurs, advise patient:
• To avoid mouth rinses with high alcohol content due to drying effects
• To use daily home fluoride products for anticaries effect
• To use sugarless gum, frequent sips of water, or saliva substitutes

---

benazepril
(ben-a′ze-pril)
Lotensin
Drug class.: Angiotensin-converting enzyme (ACE) inhibitor

Action: Selectively suppresses renin-angiotensin-aldosterone system; inhibits ACE; prevents conversion of angiotensin I to angiotensin II; results in dilation of arterial, venous vessels

Uses: Hypertension, alone or in combination with thiazide diuretics

Dosage and routes:
• *Adult:* PO 10 mg qd initially, then 20-40 mg/day divided bid or qd as a single drug

Renal impairment and with diuretics: PO 5 mg qd with Ccr <30 ml/min/1.73 m^2, increase as needed to max of 40 mg/day

Available forms include: Tabs 5, 10, 20, 40 mg

Side effects/adverse reactions:

▼ *ORAL:* Angioedema, dry mouth (rare)

CNS: Anxiety, hypertonia, insomnia, paresthesia, headache, dizziness, fatigue

CV: Hypotension, postural hypotension, syncope, palpitation, angina

GI: Nausea, constipation, vomiting, gastritis, melena

RESP: Cough, asthma, bronchitis, dyspnea, sinusitis

HEMA: Neutropenia, agranulocytosis

GU: Increased BUN, creatinine, decreased libido, impotence, UTI

INTEG: Rash, flushing, sweating

MS: Arthralgia, arthritis, myalgia

META: Hyperkalemia, hyponatremia

Contraindications: Hypersensitivity to ACE inhibitors, pregnancy category D, lactation, children

Precautions: Impaired renal or liver function, dialysis patients, hypovolemia, blood dyscrasias, CHF, COPD, asthma, elderly

Pharmacokinetics:
PO: Peak 0.5-1 hr, half-life 10-11 hr; serum protein binding 97%;

metabolized by liver (metabolites); excreted in urine

🦷 **Drug interactions of concern to dentistry:**
• Increased hypotension: alcohol, phenothiazines
• Decreased hypotensive effects: indomethacin and possibly other NSAIDs, sympathomimetics

DENTAL CONSIDERATIONS:
General:
• Monitor vital signs every appointment due to cardiovascular and respiratory side effects.
• After supine positioning, have patient sit upright for at least 2 min to avoid orthostatic hypotension.
• Patients on chronic drug therapy may rarely have symptoms of blood dyscrasias, which can include infection, bleeding, and poor healing.
• Assess salivary flow as a factor in caries, periodontal disease, and candidiasis.
• Limit use of sodium-containing products such as saline IV fluids for those patients with a dietary salt restriction.
• Use vasoconstrictors with caution, in low doses, and with careful aspiration.
• Stress from dental procedures may compromise cardiovascular function; determine patient risk.
• Short appointments and a stress reduction protocol may be required for anxious patients.

Consultations:
• Medical consult may be required to assess disease control and patient's ability to tolerate stress.
• In a patient with symptoms of blood dyscrasias, request a medical consult for blood studies and postpone dental treatment until normal values are reestablished.

---

bold italic = life-threatening conditions   *For periodic updates, visit* **www.mosby.com**

• Take precautions if dental surgery is anticipated and sedation or general anesthesia is required; there is risk of a hypotensive episode.

Teach patient/family:

• Importance of good oral hygiene to prevent soft tissue inflammation

• Caution to prevent injury when using oral hygiene aids

When chronic dry mouth occurs, advise patient:

• To avoid mouth rinses with high alcohol content due to drying effects

• To use daily home fluoride products for anticaries effect

• To use sugarless gum, frequent sips of water, or saliva substitutes

---

benzocaine (topical)
(ben′zoe-kane)

Benzocaine liquid 20%: Maximum Strength Anbesol, Orajel Mouth Aid

Benzocaine gel 20%: Americaine Anesthetic Lubricant, Hurricaine, Orajel Mouth-Aid

Benzocaine gel 15%: Orabase Gel

Benzocaine cream 6%: Bicozene, Lanacaine

Benzocaine lotion 8%: Dermoplast

Benzocaine spray 20%: Americaine, Dermoplast, Hurricaine, Lanacaine, Solarcaine

Benzocaine ointment/paste 20%: Boil-Ease

Drug class.: Topical ester, local anesthetic

Action: Inhibits conduction of nerve impulses from sensory nerves

Uses: Oral irritation, toothache, cold sore, canker sore, pain, teething pain, pain caused by dental

prostheses or orthodontic appliances

Dosage and routes:

• *Adult and child >6 yr:* TOP apply to affected area according to manufacturer's labeled instructions

Available forms include: Liq 20%; gel 20%, 15%, 10%, 7.5%, 6%; spray 20%; oint 20%; paste 20%

Side effects/adverse reactions:

▼ *ORAL:* Numbness, tingling

EENT: Itching, irritation

INTEG: Rash, urticaria

Contraindications: Hypersensitivity

Precautions: Pregnancy category C

Pharmacokinetics:

TOP: Onset 1 min, duration 0.5-1 hr; esters metabolized by plasma esterases; excreted as urinary metabolites

DENTAL CONSIDERATIONS

General:

• Do not use for topical anesthesia if medical history reveals allergy to procaine, PABA, parabens, or other ester-type local anesthetics.

• Use smallest effective amount in infants and children.

• Avoid applying to large denuded areas of mucosa to prevent excessive systemic absorption and potential toxicity.

---

benzonatate
(ben-zoe′na-tate)

Tessalon

Drug class.: Antitussive, nonnarcotic

Action: Inhibits cough reflex by anesthetizing stretch receptors in respiratory system, lungs, and pleura

Uses: Nonproductive cough relief

Dosage and routes:
• *Adult and child:* PO 100 mg tid, not to exceed 600 mg/day
• *Child <10 yr:* PO 8 mg/kg in 3-6 divided doses
Available forms include: Perles 100 mg; caps 200 mg
Side effects/adverse reactions:
CNS: Dizziness, drowsiness, headache
CV: Increased BP, chest tightness, numbness
GI: Nausea, constipation, upset stomach
EENT: Nasal congestion, burning eyes
INTEG: Urticaria, rash, pruritus
Contraindications: Hypersensitivity
Precautions: Pregnancy category C, lactation
Pharmacokinetics:
PO: Onset 15-20 min, duration 3-8 hr; metabolized by liver; excreted in urine
⚕ Drug interactions of concern to dentistry:
• Increased CNS depression: slight risk of increased sedation with other CNS depressants
DENTAL CONSIDERATIONS
General:
• Elective dental treatment may not be possible with significant coughing episodes.

---

benztropine mesylate
(benz'troe-peen)
Cogentin
♣ Apo-Benzotropine, PMS Benztropine
Drug class.: Anticholinergic, antidyskinetic

Action: Blockade of central acetylcholine receptors

Uses: Parkinson symptoms, extrapyramidal symptoms associated with neuroleptic drugs
Dosage and routes:
Drug-induced extrapyramidal symptoms
• *Adult:* IM/IV 1-2 ml 1-2 × daily; give PO dose as soon as possible; PO 1-4 mg qd-bid, increase by 0.5 mg q5-6d
Parkinson symptoms
• *Adult:* PO 0.5-1 mg qd, increased 0.5 mg q5-6d titrated to patient response
Available forms include: Tabs 0.5, 1, 2 mg; inj IM/IV 1 mg/ml
Side effects/adverse reactions:
▼ *ORAL: Dry mouth,* glossitis
CNS: Confusion, anxiety, restlessness, irritability, delusions, hallucinations, headache, sedation, depression, incoherence, dizziness, memory loss
CV: Palpitation, tachycardia, hypotension, bradycardia
GI: Constipation, paralytic ileus, nausea, vomiting, abdominal distress, epigastric distress
GU: Hesitancy, retention
EENT: Blurred vision, photophobia, dilated pupils, difficulty swallowing, dry eyes, mydriasis
INTEG: Rash, urticaria, dermatosis
MS: Muscular weakness, cramping
MISC: Increased temperature, flushing, decreased sweating, hyperthermia, heatstroke, numbness of fingers
Contraindications: Hypersensitivity, narrow-angle glaucoma, myasthenia gravis, GI/GU obstruction, child <3 yr, peptic ulcer, megacolon
Precautions: Pregnancy category C, elderly, lactation, tachycardia,

---

bold italic = life-threatening conditions

prostatic hypertrophy, liver or kidney disease, drug abuse history, dysrhythmias, hypotension, hypertension, psychiatric patients

Pharmacokinetics:

IM/IV: Onset 15 min, duration 6-10 hr

PO: Onset 1 hr, duration 6-10 hr

👆 Drug interactions of concern to dentistry:

• Increased anticholinergic effect: antihistamines, anticholinergics, and meperidine

• Decreased effects of phenothiazines

DENTAL CONSIDERATIONS

General:

• Monitor vital signs every appointment due to cardiovascular side effects.

• Assess salivary flow as a factor in caries, periodontal disease, and candidiasis.

• After supine positioning, have patient sit upright for at least 2 min to avoid orthostatic hypotension.

• Avoid dental light in patient's eyes; offer dark glasses for patient comfort.

• Do not use ingestible sodium bicarbonate products, such as the air polishing system (Prophy Jet), within 1 hr of taking benztropine.

• Place on frequent recall due to oral side effects.

Consultations:

• Medical consult may be required to assess disease control.

• Medical consult may be required to assess patient's ability to tolerate stress.

Teach patient/family:

• Importance of good oral hygiene to prevent soft tissue inflammation

• Use of electric toothbrush if patient has difficulty holding conventional devices

When chronic dry mouth occurs, advise patient:

• To avoid mouth rinses with high alcohol content due to drying effects

• To use daily home fluoride products for anticaries effect

• To use sugarless gum, frequent sips of water, or saliva substitutes

---

bepridil HCl

(be′pri-dil)

Bepadin, Vascor

Drug class.: Calcium channel blockers

Action: Inhibits calcium ion influx across cell membrane during cardiac depolarization; produces relaxation of coronary vascular smooth muscle; dilates coronary arteries; decreases SA/AV node conduction; dilates peripheral arteries

Uses: Stable angina, used alone or in combination with propranolol

Dosage and routes:

Angina

• *Adult:* PO 200 mg qd, can titrate to 300 mg or 400 mg qd; usual dose 200 mg/day

Available forms include: Film-coated tabs, PO 200, 300, 400 mg

Side effects/adverse reactions:

▼ *ORAL:* Dry mouth, taste changes (gingival overgrowth has been reported with other calcium channel blockers)

CNS: Headache, fatigue, drowsiness, dizziness, anxiety, depression, weakness, insomnia, confu-

---

sion, light-headedness, nervousness

CV: Dysrhythmia, edema, CHF, bradycardia, hypotension, palpitation, AV block

GI: Nausea, vomiting, diarrhea, gastric upset, constipation, increased liver function studies

GU: Nocturia, polyuria

Contraindications: Sick sinus syndrome, second- or third-degree heart block, Wolff-Parkinson-White syndrome, hypotension <90 mm Hg (systolic), cardiogenic shock

Precautions: CHF, hypotension, hepatic injury, pregnancy category C, lactation, children, renal disease

Pharmacokinetics:

PO: Onset 60 min, peak 2-3 hr, half-life 42 hr; 99% plasma protein bound; completely metabolized in liver; excreted in urine and feces

🦷 Drug interactions of concern to dentistry:

• Decreased effect: indomethacin, possibly other NSAIDs, phenobarbital

• Increased effect: parenteral and inhalational general anesthetics or other drugs with hypotensive actions

• Increased effects of carbamazepine

DENTAL CONSIDERATIONS

General:

• Monitor cardiac status; take vital signs at each appointment because of cardiovascular side effects. Consider a stress reduction protocol to prevent stress-induced angina during the dental appointment.

• After supine positioning, have patient sit upright for at least 2 min to avoid orthostatic hypotension.

• Limit use of sodium-containing products such as saline IV fluids for those patients with a dietary salt restriction.

• Assess salivary flow as a factor in caries, periodontal disease, and candidiasis.

Consultations:

• Medical consult may be required to assess disease control and stress tolerance of patient.

Teach patient/family:

• Need for frequent oral prophylaxis if gingival overgrowth occurs

When chronic dry mouth occurs, advise patient:

• To avoid mouth rinses with high alcohol content due to drying effects

• To use daily home fluoride products for anticaries effect

• To use sugarless gum, frequent sips of water, or saliva substitutes

---

betamethasone valerate/ betamethasone benzoate/ betamethasone dipropionate

(bay-ta-meth′a-sone)

Betamethasone dipropionate augmented cream 0.05%: Diprolene, Diprolene AF

Betamethasone dipropionate augmented ointment 0.05%: Diprolene

Betamethasone dipropionate augmented gel 0.05%: Diprolene

Betamethasone dipropionate augmented lotion 0.05%: Diprolene

Betamethasone dipropionate cream 0.05%: Alphatrex, Diprosone, Maxivate, Teldar

Betamethasone dipropionate oint 0.05%: Alphatrex, Diprolene, Diprosone, Maxivate, Topilene, Topisone

Betamethasone dipropionate lotion 0.05%: Alphatrex, Diprosone, Maxivate, Topisone

Betamethasone valerate cream 0.1 or 0.01%: Betatrex, Beta-Val, Prevex B, Valisone, Valisone Reduced Strength

♣ *Betamethasone benzoate gel 0.025%:* Bepen

Betamethasone valerate cream 0.1 or 0.01%: Bentovate-1/2, Celestoderm-V/2, Ectosone Mild, Metaderm Mild, Metaderm Regular, NovoBetament

Drug class.: Topical corticosteroid

Action: Glucocorticoids have multiple actions that include anti-inflammatory and immunosuppressant effects. They inhibit phospholipase A_2, interfering with or reducing the synthesis of prostaglandins and leukotrienes. They also bind to cytoplasmic glucocorticoid receptors (GRs) and enter the cell nucleus to bind with DNA. This results in the synthesis of various enzymes such as collagenase, elastase, betamethasone, and cytokines that play important roles in inflammation and immunosuppression. They also suppress the production of lymphocytes, monocytes, and eosinophils.

Uses: Psoriasis, eczema, contact dermatitis, pruritus, oral ulcerative inflammatory lesions

Dosage and routes

• *Adult and child:* TOP apply to affected area qid

Available forms include: Oint 0.05%; cream 0.025% and 0.05%; lotion 0.1% and 0.01%; gel 0.05% (gel available in 15 and 45 g tubes)

Side effects/adverse reactions:

▼ *ORAL:* Thinning of mucosa, stinging sensation (oral application)

INTEG: Burning, dryness, itching, irritation, acne, folliculitis, hypertrichosis, perioral dermatitis, hypopigmentation, atrophy, striae, miliaria, allergic contact dermatitis, secondary infection

Contraindications: Hypersensitivity to corticosteroids, fungal infections

Precautions: Pregnancy category C, lactation, viral infections, bacterial infections

italic = common side effects

DENTAL CONSIDERATIONS
General:
• Place on frequent recall to evaluate healing response.
Teach patient/family:
• When used for oral lesions, advise patient to return for oral evaluation if response of oral tissues has not occurred in 7-14 days
• Importance of good oral hygiene to prevent soft tissue inflammation
• To apply at bedtime or after meals for maximum effect
• To apply with cotton-tipped applicator by pressing, not rubbing, paste on lesion
• That use on oral herpetic ulcerations is contraindicated

---

betamethasone/ betamethasone sodium phosphate/ betamethasone sodium phosphate and betamethasone acetate
(bay-ta-meth′a-sone)

Betamethasone oral: Celestone
Betamethasone sodium phosphate injection USP: Celestone Phosphate, Cel-U-Jec
Betamethasone sodium phosphate and betamethasone acetate USP: Celestone Soluspan
✤ *Betamethasone oral:* Betnelan, Betnesol, Celestone Extended Release

Drug class.: Glucocorticoid, long acting

Action: Glucocorticoids have multiple actions that include anti-inflammatory and immunosuppressant effects. They inhibit phospholipase A_2, interfering with or reducing the synthesis of prostaglandins and leukotrienes. They also bind to cytoplasmic glucocorticoid receptors (GRs) and enter the cell nucleus to bind with DNA. This results in the synthesis of various enzymes such as collagenase, elastase, and cytokines that play important roles in inflammation and immunosuppression. They also suppress the production of lymphocytes, monocytes, and eosinophils.
Uses: Severe inflammation, shock, adrenal insufficiency, collagen disorders

Dosage and routes:
Betamethasone tablets or syrup
• *Adult:* PO 0.6-7.2 mg/day as a single dose or in divided doses; all doses must be individualized for the patient depending on the disease and patient response
• *Child:* 62.5-250 µg/kg of body weight in 3 or 4 divided doses daily for most indications; for adrenal cortical insufficiency: 17.5 µg/kg of body weight
Betamethasone sodium phosphate injection
• *Adult:* IM or IV up to 9 mg/day; intraarticular, intralesional, or soft tissue injection up to 9 mg as needed
Betamethasone sodium phosphate and betamethasone acetate suspension
• *Adult:* IM can be mixed with paraben-free 1% or 2% lidocaine for injection, 0.5-9 mg/day; intrabursal INJ 1.0 ml/0.6 mg; intraarticular INJ 0.5-2.0 mg (1.5-12 mg) depending on joint size; intradermal or intralesional INJ 1.2 mg/cm² of affected skin up to 6 mg at weekly intervals

---

bold italic = life-threatening conditions

Available forms include: Tabs 0.6 mg, effervescent tabs 0.5 mg; syrup 0.6 mg/5 ml; inj 4 mg betamethasone phosphate/ml in 5 ml vials; 3 mg betamethasone acetate with 3 mg betamethasone sodium phosphate in 5 ml vials

Side effects/adverse reactions:

▼ *ORAL:* Candidiasis, dry mouth
CNS: Depression, flushing, sweating, headache, mood changes
CV: Hypertension, *circulatory collapse, thrombophlebitis, embolism,* tachycardia, edema
GI: Diarrhea, nausea, abdominal distention, *GI hemorrhage, pancreatitis,* increased appetite
HEMA: Thrombocytopenia
EENT: Fungal infections, increased intraocular pressure, blurred vision
INTEG: Acne, poor wound healing, ecchymosis, petechiae
MS: Fractures, osteoporosis, weakness

Contraindications: Psychosis, hypersensitivity, idiopathic thrombocytopenia, acute glomerulonephritis, amebiasis, fungal infections, nonasthmatic bronchial disease, child <2 yr, AIDS, TB

Precautions: Pregnancy category C, diabetes mellitus, glaucoma, osteoporosis, seizure disorders, ulcerative colitis, CHF, myasthenia gravis, renal disease, peptic ulcer, esophagitis

Pharmacokinetics:
PO: Peak 1-2 hr, duration 2.33 days
IM: Peak 8 hr, duration 6 days; half-life 3-4.5 hr

🐾 **Drug interactions of concern to dentistry:**
• Decreased action: barbiturates
• Increased GI side effects: alcohol, salicylates, and other NSAIDs
• Increased action: ketoconazole, macrolide antibiotics

DENTAL CONSIDERATIONS
General:
• Monitor vital signs every appointment due to cardiovascular side effects.
• Patients on chronic drug therapy may rarely have symptoms of blood dyscrasias, which can include infection, bleeding, and poor healing.
• Symptoms of oral infections may be masked.
• Determine dose and duration of steroid therapy for each patient to assess risk for stress tolerance and immunosuppression.
• Avoid prescribing aspirin-containing products.
• Place on frequent recall to evaluate healing response.
• Prophylactic antibiotics may be indicated to prevent infection if surgery or deep scaling is planned.
• Patients who have been or are currently on chronic steroid therapy (>2 wk) may require supplemental steroids for dental treatment.

Consultations:
• In a patient with symptoms of blood dyscrasias, request a medical consult for blood studies and postpone dental treatment until normal values are reestablished.
• Medical consult may be required to assess disease control.
• Consult may be required to confirm steroid dose and duration of use.

Teach patient/family:
• Importance of good oral hygiene to prevent soft tissue inflammation
• Caution to prevent injury when using oral hygiene aids

betaxolol HCl

(be-tax'oh-lol)
Kerlone

Drug class.: Antihypertensive, selective β_1-blocker

Action: This is a selective β_1-adrenergic antagonist. At higher doses selectivity may be lost with antagonism of β_2-receptors as well. The antihypertensive mechanism of action is unclear, but may include a reduction in cardiac output and inhibition of renin release by the renal juxtaglomerular apparatus. Peripheral resistance decreases with long-term use. The antianginal action (when indicated for this use) may be related to a decrease in myocardial oxygen demand and negative chronotropic and inotropic effects. The antiarrhythmic action (when indicated for this use) has been related to a reduction in spontaneous pacemaker firing and slowing of AV nodal conduction.
Uses: Hypertension, alone or in combination with other antihypertensive drugs, especially thiazide diuretics

Dosage and routes:
• *Adult:* PO 10 mg qd, increasing to 20 mg qd if response is inadequate after 14 days
Available forms include: Tabs 10, 20 mg

Side effects/adverse reactions:
▼ *ORAL:* Dry mouth (less than 2%)
CNS: Dizziness, fatigue, lethargy, depression, headache
CV: Bradycardia, hypotension, dysrhythmias
GI: Nausea, dyspepsia, diarrhea

RESP: **Bronchospasm,** dyspnea, pharyngitis
GU: Impotence
EENT: Eye irritation, conjunctivitis, keratitis
INTEG: Rash, urticaria
Contraindications: Hypersensitivity to β-blockers, cardiogenic shock, second- or third-degree heart block, sinus bradycardia, CHF, cardiac failure
Precautions: Major surgery, pregnancy category C, lactation, diabetes mellitus, renal disease, thyroid disease, COPD, asthma, well-compensated heart failure, aortic or mitral valve disease
Pharmacokinetics:
PO: Peak 3-4 hr, half-life 14-22 hr; protein binding 50%; some hepatic metabolism; excreted in urine mostly unchanged
⚡ Drug interactions of concern to dentistry:
• Decreased antihypertensive effects: NSAIDs, indomethacin
• May slow metabolism of lidocaine
• Decreased β-blocking effects (or decreased β-adrenergic effects) of epinephrine, levonordefrin, isoproterenol, and other sympathomimetics
DENTAL CONSIDERATIONS
General:
• Monitor vital signs every appointment due to cardiovascular and respiratory side effects.
• After supine positioning, have patient sit upright for at least 2 min to avoid orthostatic hypotension.
• Assess salivary flow as a factor in caries, periodontal disease, and candidiasis.

---

bold italic = life-threatening conditions   *For periodic updates, visit* **www.mosby.com**

• Stress from dental procedures may compromise cardiovascular function; determine patient risk.

• Short appointments and a stress reduction protocol may be required for anxious patients.

• Use vasoconstrictors with caution, in low doses, and with careful aspiration. Avoid use of gingival retraction cord with epinephrine.

Consultations:

• Medical consult may be required to assess disease control and stress tolerance of patient.

• Use precautions if general anesthesia is required for dental surgery.

Teach patient/family:

• Importance of good oral hygiene to prevent soft tissue inflammation

• Caution to prevent injury when using oral hygiene aids

When chronic dry mouth occurs, advise patient:

• To avoid mouth rinses with high alcohol content due to drying effects

• To use daily home fluoride products for anticaries effect

• To use sugarless gum, frequent sips of water, or saliva substitutes

---

betaxolol HCl (optic)

(be-tax'oh-lol)
Betoptic Solution, Betoptic S-Suspension
Drug class.: Selective β_1-blocker

Action: Reduces intraocular pressure by reducing production of aqueous humor

Uses: Chronic open-angle glaucoma, ocular hypertension

Dosage and routes:

• *Adult:* INSTILL 1-2 gtt bid

Available forms include: Susp 0.25%; sol 0.5%

Side effects/adverse reactions:

CNS: Insomnia, dizziness, headache, depression (all rarely occur)

CV: Bradycardia (rare)

RESP: **Bronchospasm** (rare)

EENT: Eye irritation, conjunctivitis, keratitis

Contraindications: Hypersensitivity, asthma, second- or third-degree heart block, right ventricular failure, congenital glaucoma (infants), COPD

Precautions: Pregnancy category C

Pharmacokinetics: Onset 30 min, max effect 2 hr, duration 12 hr

♣ Drug interactions of concern to dentistry:

• Avoid use of anticholinergic drugs, atropine-like drugs, propantheline, and diazepam (benzodiazepines)

DENTAL CONSIDERATIONS

General:

• Monitor vital signs every appointment due to cardiovascular side effects.

• Check compliance of patient with prescribed drug regimen for glaucoma.

• Avoid dental light in patient's eyes; offer dark glasses for patient comfort.

Consultations:

• Consultation with physician may be needed if sedation or anesthesia is required.

---

　　　italic = common side effects

bethanechol chloride
(be-than'e-kole)

Drug class.: Cholinergic stimulant

Action: Stimulates muscarinic ACh receptors directly; mimics effects of parasympathetic nervous system stimulation; stimulates gastric motility, stimulates ganglia

Uses: Urinary retention (postoperative, postpartum), neurogenic atony of bladder with retention; unapproved: gastric atony

Dosage and routes:
• *Adult:* PO 10-50 mg tid-qid

Available forms include: Tabs 5, 10, 25, 50 mg

Side effects/adverse reactions:
▼ *ORAL:* Increased salivation

CNS: **Convulsions,** dizziness, headache, confusion, weakness

CV: **Cardiac arrest, circulatory collapse,** hypotension, bradycardia, orthostatic hypotension, reflex tachycardia

GI: Nausea, bloody diarrhea, vomiting, cramps, fecal incontinence

RESP: Acute asthma, dyspnea

GU: Frequency, incontinence

EENT: Miosis, lacrimation, blurred vision

INTEG: Rash, urticaria, flushing, increased sweating, hypothermia

Contraindications: Hypersensitivity, severe bradycardia, asthma, severe hypotension, hyperthyroidism, peptic ulcer, parkinsonism, seizure disorders, CAD, coronary occlusion, mechanical obstruction

Precautions: Hypertension, pregnancy category C, lactation, child <8 yr, urinary retention

Pharmacokinetics:
PO: Onset 30-90 min, duration 6 hr
SC: Onset 5-15 min, duration 2 hr; excreted by kidneys

💊 **Drug interactions of concern to dentistry:**
• Decreased effects: anticholinergics

DENTAL CONSIDERATIONS
General:
• Monitor vital signs every appointment due to cardiovascular and respiratory side effects.
• After supine positioning, have patient sit upright for at least 2 min to avoid orthostatic hypotension.

Consultations:
• For excessive, troublesome salivation, reassure patient that treatment duration is usually limited to a few days; otherwise consult to lower bethanechol dose.

bicalutamide
(bye-ka-loo'ta-mide)
Casodex

Drug class.: Nonsteroidal antiandrogen, antineoplastic

Action: Competitively inhibits the action of androgens by binding to androgen receptors in target tissues

Uses: Combination therapy with a luteinizing hormone-releasing hormone (LHRH) analog for advanced prostate cancer

Dosage and routes:
• *Adult:* PO 50 mg daily with or without food

Available forms include: Tabs 50 mg

Side effects/adverse reactions:

▼ *ORAL:* Dry mouth (<5%)

CNS: Headache, dizziness, paresthesia, insomnia

CV: Hot flashes, hypertension, peripheral edema

GI: Diarrhea, abdominal pain, constipation, flatulence, vomiting

RESP: Dyspnea, cough

HEMA: Anemia

GU: Nocturia, hematuria, UTI, incontinence, inhibition of spermatogenesis

INTEG: Rash, sweating

ENDO: Gynecomastia, hyperglycemia

MS: Back pain, asthenia, bone pain

MISC: Breast pain, weight loss

Contraindications: Hypersensitivity, women who may become pregnant, pregnancy category X

Precautions: Hepatic impairment, lactation, children

Pharmacokinetics:

PO: Rapid absorption; 96% plasma protein binding; hepatic metabolism; excretion in feces and urine

🦷 **Drug interactions of concern to dentistry:**

• Avoid drugs that could exacerbate urinary retention, such as anticholinergics

DENTAL CONSIDERATIONS

General:

• Patients taking opioids for acute or chronic pain should be given alternative analgesics for dental pain.

• Palliative medication may be required for management of oral side effects.

• Assess salivary flow as a factor in caries, periodontal disease, and candidiasis.

• Monitor vital signs every appointment due to cardiovascular and respiratory side effects.

• Short appointments may be required for patient comfort.

• Consider semisupine chair position for patient comfort due to disease and drug side effects.

Consultations:

• Medical consult may be required to assess disease control and patient's ability to tolerate stress.

Teach patient/family:

• Place on frequent recall due to oral side effects

• Importance of updating medical/drug record if physician makes any changes in evaluations/drug regimens

When chronic dry mouth occurs, advise patient:

• To avoid mouth rinses with high alcohol content due to drying effects

• Of need for daily home fluoride to prevent caries

• To use sugarless gum, frequent sips of water, or saliva substitutes

---

bimatoprost ophthalmic solution
(bye′ma-to-prost)
Lumigan

Drug class.: A prostamide (synthetic structural analog of prostaglandin)

Action: Mimics the intraocular pressure lowering activity of natural prostamides; believed to lower intraocular pressure (IOP) by increasing outflow of aqueous humor through both the trabecular meshwork and uveoscleral routes

Uses: Reduction of elevated IOP in patients with open-angle glaucoma or ocular hypertension who are intolerant of, or insufficiently responsive to, other IOP-lowering drugs

Dosage and routes:
• *Adult:* TOP 1 drop in affected eye(s) once daily in PM

Available forms include: Sterile sol 0.03% in 2.5, 5, 7.5 ml

Side effects/adverse reactions:

CNS: Headache

RESP: URI, colds

EENT: Conjunctival hyperemia, growth of eyelashes, dryness, burning, ocular pruritus, eye pain, pigmentation, eyelash darkening, foreign body sensation, visual disturbance

META: Abnormal liver function tests

MS: Asthenia

MISC: Hirsutism

Contraindications: Hypersensitivity

Precautions: Increased pigmentation in iris and eyelid, change in eye color, changes in eyelashes (color, length, shape); uveitis, macular edema; renal or hepatic impairment, remove contact lenses to apply, pregnancy category C, lactation, pediatric use

Pharmacokinetics:

TOP: Very low absorption, no systemic accumulation, some tissue distribution, 12% of absorbed dose seen in the plasma, metabolized to multiple metabolites, excreted mostly in urine (67%), feces (25%)

Drug interactions of concern to dentistry:
• None reported

DENTAL CONSIDERATIONS
General:
• Avoid drugs with anticholinergic activity, such as antihistamines, opioids, benzodiazepines, propantheline, atropine, and scopolamine.

• Protect patient's eyes from accidental spatter during dental treatment.
• Avoid dental light in patient's eyes; offer dark glasses for patient comfort.

Consultations:
• Medical consult may be required to assess disease control.

Teach patient/family:
• Importance of updating health and drug history if physician makes any changes in evaluation or drug regimens

---

biperiden HCl/ biperiden lactate

(bye-per'i-den)
Akineton

Drug class.: Anticholinergic

Action: Centrally acting competitive anticholinergic

Uses: Parkinson symptoms, extrapyramidal symptoms secondary to neuroleptic drug therapy

Dosage and routes:

Extrapyramidal symptoms
• *Adult:* PO 2 mg tid-qid; IM/IV 2 mg q30min, if needed, not to exceed 8 mg/24 hr

Parkinson symptoms
• *Adult:* PO 2 mg tid-qid; max daily dose 16 mg/24 hr

Available forms include: Tabs 2 mg; inj IM/IV 5 mg/ml (lactate)

Side effects/adverse reactions:

▼ *ORAL: Dry mouth,* glossitis

CNS: Confusion, anxiety, restlessness, irritability, delusions, hallucinations, headache, sedation, depression, incoherence, dizziness, euphoria, tremors, memory loss

CV: Palpitation, tachycardia, postural hypotension, bradycardia

*GI: Constipation, **paralytic ileus,*** nausea, vomiting, abdominal distress

GU: Hesitancy, retention

EENT: Blurred vision, photophobia, dilated pupils, difficulty swallowing, mydriasis

INTEG: Rash, urticaria, dermatosis

MS: Weakness, cramping

MISC: Increased temperature, flushing, decreased sweating, hyperthermia, heatstroke, numbness of fingers

Contraindications: Hypersensitivity, narrow-angle glaucoma, myasthenia gravis, GI/GU obstruction, megacolon, stenosing peptic ulcers

Precautions: Pregnancy category C, elderly, lactation, tachycardia, prostatic hypertrophy, dysrhythmias, liver or kidney disease, drug abuse, hypotension, hypertension, psychiatric patients, children

Pharmacokinetics:

IM/IV: Onset 15 min, duration 6-10 hr

PO: Onset 1 hr, duration 6-10 hr

🦷 **Drug interactions of concern to dentistry:**

• Increased anticholinergic effect: antihistamines, anticholinergic-acting drugs, meperidine

• Increased CNS depression: alcohol, CNS depressants

• Decreased effects of phenothiazines

DENTAL CONSIDERATIONS

General:

• Monitor vital signs every appointment due to cardiovascular side effects.

• After supine positioning, have patient sit upright at least 2 min to avoid orthostatic hypotension.

• Assess salivary flow as a factor in caries, periodontal disease, and candidiasis.

• Avoid dental light in patient's eyes; offer dark glasses for patient comfort.

Consultations:

• Medical consult may be required to assess disease control and patient's ability to tolerate stress.

Teach patient/family:

• To use electric toothbrush if patient has difficulty holding conventional devices

• Importance of good oral hygiene to prevent soft tissue inflammation

When chronic dry mouth occurs, advise patient:

• To avoid mouth rinses with high alcohol content due to drying effects

• To use daily home fluoride products for anticaries effect

• To use sugarless gum, frequent sips of water, or saliva substitutes

---

bismuth subsalicylate

(bis'meth)

Bismatrol, Bismatrol Extra Strength, Pepto-Bismol, Pepto-Bismol Maximum Strength, Pink-Bismuth

♣ PMS-bismuth subsalicylate

Drug class.: Antidiarrheal, also used in combination with antibiotics (amoxicillin, clarithromycin, metronidazole, tetracyclines), proton pump inhibitors (omeprazole or lansoprazole), or ranitidine for *H. pylori* infection

Action: Mechanism of action is not known; may act through antisecretory, antimicrobial, or antiinflammatory effects

Uses: Diarrhea (cause undetermined), prevention of diarrhea when traveling; unapproved: gastritis, duodenal ulcer associated with *H. pylori*

Dosage and routes:

• *Adult:* PO 30 ml or 2 tabs q30-60 min, not to exceed 8 doses for >2 days

• *Child 9-12 yr:* PO 15 ml or 1 tab

• *Child 6-9 yr:* PO 10 ml or 2/3 tab

• *Child 3-6 yr:* PO 5 ml or 1/3 tab

Available forms include: Caps 262 mg; Chew tabs 262 mg; susp 262 mg/15 ml, 524 mg/15 ml

Side effects/adverse reactions:

▼ *ORAL:* Metallic taste, gray discoloration of tongue

CNS: Confusion, twitching

GI: Increased fecal impaction (high doses), dark stools

HEMA: Increased bleeding time

EENT: Hearing loss, tinnitus

Contraindications: Child <3 yr

Precautions: Anticoagulant therapy

Pharmacokinetics:

PO: Onset 1 hr, peak 2 hr, duration 4 hr

⚡ Drug interactions of concern to dentistry:

• Salicylate toxicity: other salicylates

• Decreased absorption of tetracyclines

DENTAL CONSIDERATIONS

General:

• Avoid prescribing aspirin-containing products for analgesia.

---

bisoprolol fumarate

(bis-oh′proe-lol)

Zebeta

Drug class.: Antihypertensive, selective β₁-blocker

Action: Produces fall in BP without reflex tachycardia or significant reduction in heart rate; acts to block β₁-adrenergic receptors; elevated plasma renins are reduced; blocks β₁-adrenergic receptors in bronchial and vascular smooth muscle only at high doses

Uses: Hypertension as a single agent or in combination with other antihypertensives; unapproved: angina pectoris, PVCs, supraventricular tachydysrhythmias

Dosage and routes:

• *Adult:* PO 5 mg/day, limit 20 mg/day

• *Geriatric:* PO 2.5 mg/day

Available forms include: Tabs 5, 10 mg

Side effects/adverse reactions:

▼ *ORAL:* Dry mouth

*CNS: Insomnia, dizziness, **depression,** mental changes, hallucinations, anxiety, headaches, nightmares, confusion, fatigue*

*CV: Bradycardia, palpitation, **cardiac arrest, AV block,** hypotension, dysrhythmias, CHF*

GI: Hiccups, nausea, vomiting, colitis, cramps, diarrhea, constipation, flatulence

*RESP: **Bronchospasm,** dyspnea, wheezing*

*HEMA: **Agranulocytosis, eosinophilia, thrombocytopenic purpura***

GU: Impotence

EENT: Sore throat, dry burning eyes

INTEG: Rash, purpura, alopecia, dry skin, urticaria, pruritus

Contraindications: Hypersensitivity to β-blockers, cardiogenic shock, second- or third-degree heart block, sinus bradycardia, CHF, bronchial asthma

Precautions: Pregnancy category C, major surgery, lactation, diabe-

---

bold italic* = life-threatening conditions*

tes mellitus, renal disease, thyroid disease, COPD, heart failure, CAD, nonallergic bronchospasm, hepatic disease

Pharmacokinetics:

PO: Half-life 9-12 hr; highly protein bound; 50% excreted unchanged in urine, rest as metabolites

⚡ Drug interactions of concern to dentistry:

• Decreased antihypertensive effects: NSAIDs, indomethacin, sympathomimetics

• May slow metabolism of lidocaine

• Decreased β-blocking effects (or decreased β-adrenergic effects) of epinephrine, levonordefrin, isoproterenol, and other sympathomimetics

DENTAL CONSIDERATIONS

General:

• Monitor vital signs every appointment due to cardiovascular side effects.

• After supine positioning, have patient sit upright for at least 2 min to avoid orthostatic hypotension.

• Patients on chronic drug therapy may rarely have symptoms of blood dyscrasias, which can include infection, bleeding, and poor healing.

• Assess salivary flow as a factor in caries, periodontal disease, and candidiasis.

• Stress from dental procedures may compromise cardiovascular function; determine patient risk.

• Short appointments and a stress reduction protocol may be required for anxious patients.

• Use vasoconstrictors with caution, in low doses, and with careful aspiration. Avoid use of gingival retraction cord with epinephrine.

Consultations:

• In a patient with symptoms of blood dyscrasias, request a medical consult for blood studies and postpone dental treatment until normal values are reestablished.

• Medical consult may be required to assess disease control and patient's ability to tolerate stress.

• Take precautions if general anesthesia is required for dental surgery.

Teach patient/family: *When chronic dry mouth occurs, advise patient:*

• To avoid mouth rinses with high alcohol content due to drying effects

• To use daily home fluoride products for anticaries effect

• To use sugarless gum, frequent sips of water, or saliva substitutes

---

bitolterol mesylate

(bye-tole'ter-ole)

Tornalate

Drug class.: Adrenergic β$_2$-agonist

Action: Causes bronchodilation by action on β$_2$-receptors by increasing levels of cAMP, which relaxes smooth muscle with very little effect on heart rate

Uses: Treatment or prophylaxis of asthma, bronchitis, bronchospasm

Dosage and routes:

Treatment

• *Adult and child >12 yr:* INH 2 inhalations at intervals of 1-3 min, followed by third inhalation if

---

needed; not to exceed 3 inh q6h or 2 inh q4h

Prophylaxis
• *Adult and child >12 yr:* INH 2 inhalations q8h, not to exceed 3 INH q6h or 2 INH q4h; administer sol over 10-15 min

Available forms include: Aerosol 0.37 mg/actuation in 15 ml; sol for INH 0.2% in 10, 30, 60 ml

Side effects/adverse reactions:
▼ *ORAL:* Taste change, dry mouth, discolored teeth
CNS: Tremors, anxiety, insomnia, *headache, dizziness,* stimulation, restlessness, flushing, irritability, hallucinations
CV: Palpitation, tachycardia, hypertension, angina, dysrhythmias, chest pain
GI: Heartburn, nausea, vomiting, diarrhea
RESP: **Paradoxic bronchospasm**
GU: Difficult or painful urination
EENT: Dry nose, irritation of nose and throat
MS: Muscle cramps, twitching

Contraindications: Hypersensitivity to sympathomimetics, tachydysrhythmia, severe cardiac disease

Precautions: Lactation, pregnancy category C, cardiac disorders, hyperthyroidism, diabetes mellitus, hypertension, prostatic hypertrophy, narrow-angle glaucoma, pheochromocytoma, seizures

Pharmacokinetics:
INH: Onset 3-4 min, peak 0.5-1 hr, duration 5-8 hr

🦶 Drug interactions of concern to dentistry:
• Increased dysrhythmias: halogenated hydrocarbon anesthetics

• Increased CNS stimulation: cocaine and other CNS stimulants

DENTAL CONSIDERATIONS
General:
• Monitor vital signs every appointment due to cardiovascular and respiratory side effects.
• Assess salivary flow as a factor in caries, periodontal disease, and candidiasis.
• Consider semisupine chair position for patients with respiratory disease.
• Midday appointments and a stress reduction protocol may be required for anxious patients.
• Be aware that aspirin or sulfite preservatives in vasoconstrictor-containing products can exacerbate asthma.
• Acute asthmatic episodes may be precipitated in the dental office. Sympathomimetic inhalants should be available for emergency use.

Consultations:
• Medical consult may be required to assess disease control.
• Medical consult may be required to assess patient's ability to tolerate stress.

Teach patient/family:
• For inhalation dosage forms: rinse mouth with water after each dose to prevent dryness
When chronic dry mouth occurs, advise patient:
• To avoid mouth rinses with high alcohol content due to drying effects
• Of need for daily home fluoride to prevent caries
• To use sugarless gum, frequent sips of water, or saliva substitutes

---

bosentan

(boe-sen'-tan)
Tracleer
Drug class.: Antihypertensive

Action: Acts as an antagonist for endothelin-1 receptors (endothelin A and B), thereby antagonizing the vasoconstrictor action of endothelin-1 endogenous peptide

Uses: Treatment of pulmonary arterial hypertension in patients with WHO class III and IV symptoms

Dosage and routes:
• *Adult:* PO initial dose is 62.5 mg bid × 4 wk; then increase to 125 mg bid as a maintenance dose. Low body weight patients should use the lower dose, 62.5 mg, as a maintenance dose.

Available forms include: Tabs: 62.5 and 125 mg

Side effects/adverse reactions:
CNS: Headache, fatigue
CV: Flushing, hypotension, palpitation
GI: Dyspnea
HEMA: Decrease in hemoglobin, hematocrit
EENT: Nasopharyngitis
INTEG: Pruritus
ENDO: Potential liver injury, abnormal liver function, altered liver enzymes
MISC: Lower-limb edema

Contraindications: Hypersensitivity, pregnancy, concurrent use of cyclosporine or glyburide

Precautions: Potential for serious liver injury, risk of major birth defect, hepatic impairment, pregnancy category X, use during lactation or in children has not been determined, necessitates monthly tests for pregnancy during use

Pharmacokinetics:
PO: Bioavailability 50%, highly plasma protein bound (98%), hepatic metabolism (CYP 2C9 and CYP 3A4), active metabolites, biliary excretion

Drug interactions of concern to dentistry:
• Increased plasma concentrations: ketoconazole and possible other drugs that inhibit or induce CYP 450 enzymes involved with metabolism
• See contraindications for other drugs

DENTAL CONSIDERATIONS
General:
• Acute pulmonary arterial hypertension rarely occurs and is a major medical problem. Patients are at high risk.
• Chronic pulmonary arterial hypertension also occurs. Patients may be taking a variety of antihypertensive medications. It is advisable to consult with the physician of record to determine quality of disease control, patient's ability to tolerate stress, and, with this particular drug, liver function.

Teach patient/family:
• Importance of good oral hygiene to prevent tissue inflammation and dental caries
• Importance of updating health and drug history if physician makes any changes in evaluation or drug regimens

brimonidine tartrate

(bri-moe'ni-deen)
Alphagan, Alphagan-P
Drug class.: α-adrenergic agonist

Action: Selective α₂-adrenergic

agonist that reduces aqueous humor production and increases uveoscleral outflow

Uses: Lowering of intraocular pressure in open-angle glaucoma or ocular hypertension; prevention of postoperative intraocular pressure elevation after argon laser trabeculoplasty

Dosage and routes:

• *Adult:* OPTH 1 drop in affected eye(s) tid q8h (Recently approved for children >2 yr–recommended dose not available at time of publication.)

Available forms include: Sol 0.2% and 0.5%; 5, 10 ml; (Alphagan-P) 0.15% in 10 ml, 15 ml

Side effects/adverse reactions:

▼ *ORAL: Dry mouth,* abnormal taste

CNS: Headache, drowsiness, fatigue, insomnia, depression

CV: Hypertension, palpitation, syncope

EENT: Ocular hyperemia, burning, stinging, ocular allergy, blurring, foreign body reaction, photophobia

MS: Muscular pain

Contraindications: Hypersensitivity, MAO inhibitor

Precautions: Wait 15 min after using before inserting contact lens; tricyclic antidepressants, β-blockers, CNS depressants; severe CV disease, hepatic or renal impairment, depression, cerebral or coronary insufficiency, Raynaud's phenomenon, orthostatic hypotension, thromboangiitis obliterans, pregnancy category B, lactation, children

Pharmacokinetics:

TOP: Peak plasma levels 1-4 hr;

half-life 3 hr; hepatic metabolism, urinary excretion

🦷 **Drug interactions of concern to dentistry:** *Drug interactions have not been studied; however, the following possibilities exist:*

• Increased CNS depression: opioids, sedatives, alcohol, and general anesthetics

• Possible risk of interference with lowering intraocular pressure: anticholinergic drugs or drugs with anticholinergic actions; tricyclic antidepressants

DENTAL CONSIDERATIONS

General:

• Assess salivary flow as factor in caries, periodontal disease, and candidiasis.

• Avoid dental light in patient's eyes; offer dark glasses for patient comfort.

• Question patient about compliance with prescribed drug regimen for glaucoma.

• Avoid drugs with anticholinergic activity, such as antihistamines, opioids, benzodiazepines, propantheline, atropine, and scopolamine.

• Monitor vital signs every appointment due to cardiovascular side effects.

Consultations:

• Consultation with physician may be needed if sedation or general anesthesia is required.

Teach patient/family:

• Importance of updating health and drug history if physician makes any changes in evaluation or drug regimens

When chronic dry mouth occurs, advise patient:

• To avoid mouth rinses with high alcohol content due to drying effects

---

• To use daily home fluoride products for anticaries effect
• To use sugarless gum, frequent sips of water, or saliva substitutes

---

brinzolamide (optic)
(brin-zoh′la-mide)
Azopt

Drug class.: Carbonic anhydrase inhibitor

Action: Reduces intraocular pressure through inhibition of carbonic anhydrase enzyme
Uses: Ocular hypertension, open-angle glaucoma
Dosage and routes:
• *Adult:* OPTH 1 gtt in affected eye tid
Available forms include: Ophthalmic suspension 1% in 2.5, 5, 10, 15 ml
Side effects/adverse reactions:
▼ *ORAL: Bitter taste,* dry mouth (>1%)
CNS: Headache, dizziness
GI: Diarrhea
EENT: Blurred vision, blepharitis, dry eye, ocular pain, foreign body sensation
MISC: Allergy
Contraindications: Hypersensitivity
Precautions: Pregnancy category C, lactation, no pediatric data for use
Pharmacokinetics:
TOP: Some systemic absorption, active metabolite, plasma protein binding 60%, urinary excretion
 Drug interactions of concern to dentistry:
• Avoid drugs that can exacerbate glaucoma (e.g., anticholinergics)

DENTAL CONSIDERATIONS
General:
• Avoid dental light in patient's eyes; offer dark glasses for patient comfort.
• Question patient about compliance with prescribed drug regimen for glaucoma.
Consultations:
• Medical consult may be required to assess disease control.

---

bromocriptine mesylate
(broe-moe-krip′teen)
Parlodel, Parlodel SnapTabs
♣ Alti-Bromocriptine, Apo-Bromocriptine

Drug class.: Dopamine receptor agonist, ovulation stimulant

Action: Inhibits prolactin release by activating postsynaptic dopamine receptors; activation of striatal dopamine receptors could be reason for improvement in Parkinson's disease
Uses: Female infertility, Parkinson's disease, prevention of postpartum lactation, amenorrhea caused by hyperprolactinemia, acromegaly
Dosage and routes:
Hyperprolactinemic indications
• *Adult:* PO 0.5-2.5 mg with meals; may increase by 2.5 mg q3-7d; usual range 5-7.5 mg
Acromegaly
• *Adult:* PO 1.25-2.5 mg × 3 days hs, may increase by 1.25-2.5 mg q3-7d, usual range 20-30 mg/day
Postpartum lactation
• *Adult:* PO 2.5 mg qd-tid with meal × 14 or 21 days

Parkinson's disease
• *Adult:* PO 1.25 mg bid with meals, may increase q2-4wk by 2.5 mg/day, not to exceed 100 mg qd
Available forms include: Caps 5 mg; tabs 2.5 mg
Side effects/adverse reactions:
▼ *ORAL:* Dry mouth
CNS: Headache, **convulsions,** depression, restlessness, anxiety, nervousness, confusion, hallucinations, dizziness, fatigue, drowsiness, abnormal involuntary movements, psychosis
CV: **Shock,** orthostatic hypotension, decreased BP, palpitation, extra systole, dysrhythmias, bradycardia
GI: Nausea, vomiting, anorexia, cramps, constipation, diarrhea, hemorrhage
GU: Frequency, retention, incontinence, diuresis
EENT: Blurred vision, diplopia, burning eyes, nasal congestion
INTEG: Rash on face/arms, alopecia
Contraindications: Hypersensitivity to ergot, severe ischemic disease, pregnancy category D, severe peripheral vascular disease
Precautions: Lactation, hepatic disease, renal disease, children
Pharmacokinetics:
PO: Peak 1-3 hr, duration 4-8 hr, half-life 3 hr; 90%-96% protein bound; metabolized by liver (inactive metabolites); excreted in urine, feces
🦶 **Drug interactions of concern to dentistry:**
• Decreased action: phenothiazines, loxapine, haloperidol, droperidol, amitriptyline
• Increased plasma levels: erythromycin

General:
• Monitor vital signs every appointment due to cardiovascular side effects.
• After supine positioning, have patient sit upright for at least 2 min to avoid orthostatic hypotension.
• Assess salivary flow as a factor in caries, periodontal disease, and candidiasis.
• Short appointments may be required due to disease effects on musculature.
Consultations:
• Medical consult may be required to assess disease control.
Teach patient/family:
• To avoid mouth rinses with high alcohol content due to drying effects

---

brompheniramine maleate
(brome-fen-ir′a-meen)
Bromphen, Codimal-A, Conjec-B, Cophene-B, Dehist, Diamine TD, Dimetane, Dimetane Extentabs, Dimetapp Allergy, Histaject Modified, Oraminic II, Veltane
♣ Chlorphed, Nasahist-B, ND-Stat Revised

Drug class.: Antihistamine, H_1-receptor antagonist

Action: Acts on blood vessels, GI system, respiratory system by competing with histamine for H_1-receptor sites; decreases allergic response by blocking histamine
Uses: Allergy symptoms, rhinitis
Dosage and routes:
• *Adult:* PO 4-8 mg tid-qid, not to exceed 36 mg/day; TIME REL 8-12 mg bid-tid, not to exceed 24

---

mg/day; IM/IV/SC 5-20 mg q6-12h, not to exceed 40 mg/day
• *Child >6 yr:* PO 2 mg tid-qid, not to exceed 12 mg/day; IM/IV/SC 0.5 mg/kg/day divided tid or qid
• *Child <6 yr:* Only as directed by physician
Available forms include: Tabs 4 mg; time rel tabs 8, 12 mg; elix 2 mg/5 ml; inj IM/SC/IV 10, 100 mg/ml
Side effects/adverse reactions:
▼ *ORAL:* Dry mouth
CNS: Dizziness, drowsiness, poor coordination, fatigue, anxiety, euphoria, confusion, paresthesia, neuritis
CV: Hypotension, palpitation, tachycardia
GI: Nausea, vomiting, anorexia, constipation, diarrhea
RESP: Increased thick secretions, wheezing, chest tightness
HEMA: ***Thrombocytopenia, agranulocytosis, hemolytic anemia***
GU: Retention, dysuria, frequency, impotence
EENT: Blurred vision, dilated pupils, tinnitus, nasal stuffiness, dry nose/throat
INTEG: Photosensitivity
Contraindications: Hypersensitivity to H_1-receptor antagonists, acute asthma attack, lower respiratory tract disease, child <6 yr
Precautions: Increased intraocular pressure, renal disease, cardiac disease, hypertension, bronchial asthma, seizure disorder, stenosed peptic ulcers, hyperthyroidism, prostatic hypertrophy, bladder neck obstruction, pregnancy category C
Pharmacokinetics:
PO: Peak 2-5 hr, duration to 48 hr, half-life 12-34 hr; metabolized in liver; excreted by kidneys

🦷 **Drug interactions of concern to dentistry:**
• Increased CNS depression: alcohol, all CNS depressants
• Additive photosensitization: tetracyclines
• Increased drying effect: anticholinergics
• Hypotension: general anesthetics
DENTAL CONSIDERATIONS
General:
• Assess salivary flow as a factor in caries, periodontal disease, and candidiasis.
• Consider semisupine chair position for patients with respiratory disease.
• Determine why the patient is taking the drug.
Teach patient/family:
• Importance of good oral hygiene to prevent soft tissue inflammation
• To avoid mouth rinses with high alcohol content due to drying effects

---

budesonide

(byoo-des'oh-nide)
Pulmacort Turbuhaler, Pulmicort Respules, Rhinocort Aqua, Rhinocort Nasal Inhaler

Drug class.: Corticosteroid, synthetic

Action: Glucocorticoids have multiple actions that include antiinflammatory and immunosuppressant effects. They inhibit phospholipase A_2, interfering with or reducing the synthesis of prostaglandins and leukotrienes. They also bind to cytoplasmic glucocorticoid receptors (GRs) and enter the cell nucleus to bind with DNA. This results in the synthesis of various enzymes such as collagenase, elastase, and cytokines that play important roles in inflammation and immunosuppression. They also suppress the production of lymphocytes, monocytes, and eosinophils.

Uses: Management of symptoms of perennial allergic rhinitis in adults and children, perennial nonallergic rhinitis in adults

Dosage and routes:

For intranasal use only

• *Adult and child >6 yr:* INH 1 spray in each nostril AM and PM, up to 4 sprays in each nostril in AM, then reduce to smallest amount required for symptom control

• *Child >12 mo:* INH NEB 0.5 mg either qd or bid in divided doses

For respules

• *Child 12 mo-8 yr:* INH used only for maintenance therapy in chronic asthma

Available forms include: Metered inhaler: 7 g canister (contains 200 doses); each actuation provides 32 µg; nebulizer 0.25, 0.5 mg in 2 ml plastic amps; turbihaler 200 µg in each actuation (200 doses); INH susp 0.25 mg/2 ml

Side effects/adverse reactions:

▼ *ORAL: Dry mouth, alteration of taste*

CNS: Nervousness

GI: Nausea

RESP: Wheezing, dyspnea

EENT: Irritation of nasal membranes, sneezing, coughing, epistaxis, candidosis, altered smell, nasal septum injury

INTEG: Rash, pruritus, facial edema

MS: Myalgia, arthralgia

Contraindications: Hypersensitivity; bacterial, viral, or fungal infections of mouth, throat, or lungs

Precautions: Pregnancy category B, lactation, child age <6 yr with nonallergic rhinitis; larger doses may cause symptoms of hypercorticism and suppress HPA function

Pharmacokinetics: INH approximately 20% of inhaled dose is absorbed; highly protein bound; liver metabolism; urinary excretion

Drug interactions of concern to dentistry:

• None reported

DENTAL CONSIDERATIONS

General:

• Evaluate respiration characteristics and rate.

• Assess salivary flow as a factor in caries, periodontal disease, and candidiasis.

• Midday appointments suggested with stress reduction protocol for anxious patients.

• Place on frequent recall due to oral side effects.

• Acute asthmatic episodes may be precipitated in the dental office. Rapid-acting sympathomimetic inhalants should be available for emergency use. Budesonide is not a rapid-acting drug and is not intended for use in acute asthmatic attacks.

Consultations:

• Medical consult may be required to assess disease control.

Teach patient/family:

• Importance of good oral hygiene to prevent soft tissue inflammation

• That gargling and rinsing with water after each dose helps prevent fungal infection

When chronic dry mouth occurs, advise patient:

• To avoid mouth rinses with high alcohol content due to drying effects

---

bold italic = life-threatening conditions   *For periodic updates, visit* **www.mosby.com**

- To use daily home fluoride products for anticaries effect
- To use sugarless gum, frequent sips of water, or artificial saliva substitutes

---

bumetanide

(byoo-met′a-nide)
Bumex
Drug class.: Loop diuretic

Action: Acts on loop of Henle to decrease the reabsorption of chloride and sodium with resultant diuresis

Uses: Edema in CHF, liver disease, renal disease (nephrotic syndrome), pulmonary edema, ascites (nephrotic syndrome), hypertension

Dosage and routes:
- *Adult:* PO 0.5-2.0 mg qd, may give second or third dose at 4-5 hr intervals, not to exceed 10 mg/day, may be given on alternate days or intermittently; IV/IM 0.5-1.0 mg/day, may give second or third dose at 2-3 hr intervals, not to exceed 10 mg/day

Available forms include: Tabs 0.5, 1, 2 mg; inj IV/IM 0.25 mg/ml

Side effects/adverse reactions:

▼ *ORAL:* Dry mouth, increased thirst
CNS: Headache, fatigue, weakness, vertigo
CV: Circulatory collapse, chest pain, hypotension, ECG changes
GI: Nausea, *acute pancreatitis, jaundice,* diarrhea, vomiting, anorexia, cramps, upset stomach, abdominal pain
HEMA: Thrombocytopenia, agranulocytosis, neutropenia
GU: Polyuria, *renal failure,* glycosuria

EENT: Loss of hearing, ear pain, tinnitus, blurred vision
*INTEG: Rash, pruritus, **Stevens-Johnson syndrome,*** purpura, sweating, photosensitivity
ENDO: Hyperglycemia
ELECT: Hypokalemia, hypochloremic alkalosis, hypomagnesemia, hyperuricemia, hypocalcemia, hyponatremia
MS: Cramps, arthritis, stiffness
Contraindications: Hypersensitivity to sulfonamides, anuria, hepatic coma, hypovolemia, lactation
Precautions: Dehydration, ascites, severe renal disease, pregnancy category C
Pharmacokinetics:
PO: Onset 0.5-1 hr, duration 4 hr
IM: Onset 40 min, duration 4 hr
IV: Onset 5 min, duration 2-3 hr; excreted by kidneys; crosses placenta; excreted by breast milk
🦷 **Drug interactions of concern to dentistry:**
- Decreased diuretic effect: NSAIDs, indomethacin
- Masked ototoxicity: phenothiazines
- Increased electrolyte imbalance: nondepolarizing skeletal muscle relaxants, corticosteroids

DENTAL CONSIDERATIONS
General:
- Monitor vital signs every appointment due to cardiovascular side effects.
- Patients on chronic drug therapy may rarely have symptoms of blood dyscrasias, which can include infection, bleeding, and poor healing.
- After supine positioning, have patient sit upright for at least 2 min to avoid orthostatic hypotension.
- Assess salivary flow as a factor in

caries, periodontal disease, and candidiasis.

• Limit use of sodium-containing products such as saline IV fluids for patients with a dietary salt restriction.

• Patients on high-potency diuretics should be monitored for serum K^+ levels.

Consultations:

• In a patient with symptoms of blood dyscrasias, request a medical consult for blood studies and postpone dental treatment until normal values are reestablished.

• Medical consult may be required to assess disease control.

Teach patient/family:

• Importance of good oral hygiene to prevent soft tissue inflammation

• Caution to prevent injury when using oral hygiene aids

When chronic dry mouth occurs, advise patient:

• To avoid mouth rinses with high alcohol content due to drying effects

• To use daily home fluoride products for anticaries effect

• To use sugarless gum, frequent sips of water, or saliva substitutes

---

bupivacaine HCl (local)
(byoo-piv′a-kane)

Marcaine, Sensorcaine, Sensorcaine-MPF

With vasoconstrictor: Marcaine Hydrochloride with Epinephrine, Sensorcaine with Epinephrine, Sensorcaine-MPF with Epinephrine

Drug class.: Amide local anesthetic

Action: Inhibits ion fluxes across membranes, particularly sodium transport across cell membrane; decreases rise of depolarization phase of action potential; blocks nerve action potential

Uses: Local dental anesthesia, epidural anesthesia, peripheral nerve block, caudal anesthesia

Dosage and routes:

Dental injection: infiltration or conduction block

• *Bupivacaine 0.5% with epinephrine 1:200,000:* Max dose 1.3 mg/kg or 0.6 mg/lb; limit 90 mg* per dental appointment for healthy patients; doses must be adjusted downward for medically compromised, debilitated, or elderly and for each individual patient. **Always use the lowest effective dose, a slow injection rate, and careful aspiration technique.**

Example calculations illustrating amount of drug administered per dental cartridge

# of cartridges (1.8 ml)	mg of bupivacaine (0.5%)	mg (µg) of vasoconstrictor (1:200,000)
1	9	0.009 (9)
2	18	0.018 (18)
4	36	0.036 (36)
6	54	0.054 (54)
10	90	0.090 (90 g)

*Maximum dose is cited from the *USP-DI*, ed 16, 1996, US Pharmacopeial Convention, Inc. Doses may differ in other published reference resources.

• Package insert does not recommend bupivacaine for children <12 yr.

Available forms include: Inj 0.25%, 0.5%, 0.75%; inj with epinephrine 1:200,000 in 0.25%, 0.5%, 0.75%

Side effects/adverse reactions:

▼ *ORAL:* Numbness, tingling, trismus

CNS: **Convulsions, loss of consciousness,** drowsiness, disorientation, tremors, shivering, anxiety, restlessness

CV: **Myocardial depression, cardiac arrest, dysrhythmias,** bradycardia, hypotension, hypertension, fetal bradycardia

GI: Nausea, vomiting

RESP: **Status asthmaticus, respiratory arrest, anaphylaxis**

EENT: Blurred vision, tinnitus, pupil constriction

INTEG: Rash, urticaria, allergic reactions, edema, burning, skin discoloration at injection site, tissue necrosis

Contraindications: Hypersensitivity, cross sensitivity between amides (rare), severe liver disease, 0.75% sol in dentistry

Precautions: Elderly, severe drug allergies, pregnancy category C, use in children (risk of local injury due to long duration of anesthesia)

Pharmacokinetics: INJ onset 4-17 min, duration 4-12 hr; excreted in urine (metabolites); metabolized by liver

Drug interactions of concern to dentistry:

• CNS depressants: may see increased risk of CNS depression with all CNS depressants, especially in children and when larger doses are used

• Avoid placing dental cartridges in disinfectant solutions with heavy metals or surface-active agents; may see release of metal ions into local anesthetic solutions, with tissue irritation following injection

• Avoid excessive exposure of dental cartridges to light or heat; it hastens deterioration of vasoconstrictor; color change in local anesthetic solution indicates breakdown of vasoconstrictor

• Risk of cardiovascular side effects: rapid intravascular administration of local anesthetic containing vasoconstrictor, either alone or in patients taking tricyclic antidepressants, MAO inhibitors, digitalis drugs, cocaine, phenothiazines, β-blockers, and in the presence of halogenated hydrocarbon general anesthetics; always use the smallest effective vasoconstrictor dose and careful aspiration technique

• Avoid use of vasoconstrictors in patients with uncontrolled hyperthyroidism, diabetes, angina, or hypertension; refer these patients for medical treatment before elective dental procedures

DENTAL CONSIDERATIONS

General:

• Monitor vital signs every appointment due to cardiovascular and respiratory side effects.

• Lubricate dry lips before injection or dental treatment as required.

Teach patient/family:

• To use care to prevent injury while numbness exists; do not chew gum or eat following dental anesthesia

• That numbness with this drug is expected to last for a considerable period

• To report any signs of infection, muscle pain, or fever to dentist when oral sensations return

• To report any unusual soft tissue reactions

bupropion hydrochloride

(byoo-proe'pee-on)

Wellbutrin, Wellbutrin SR, Zyban

Drug class.: Antidepressant

Action: Weak uptake inhibitor of dopamine, serotonin, norepinephrine; antidepressant and smoking cessation mechanism unknown

Uses: Depression; smoking cessation treatment (Zyban)

Dosage and routes:

Depression

• *Adult:* PO 100 mg bid initially, then increase after third day to 100 mg tid if needed; may increase after 1 mo to 150 mg tid. Usual dose 300 mg/day in three equally divided doses; limit use of higher doses to 450 mg/day

Smoking cessation

• *Adult:* PO initial dose 150 mg/day × 3 days, can increase to 150 mg bid if required; max daily dose 300 mg; initiate dose while patient is still smoking to allow for achievement of steady-state blood levels; set stop smoking date within 2 wk of administration; continue doses for 7 wk; if progress is not made by week 7 it is unlikely patient will stop smoking during the session; maintenance doses may be required through week 12; may be used in combination with nicotine transdermal system

Available forms include: Tabs 75, 100 mg; sus rel tabs 50, 100, 150 mg; Zyban sus rel tabs 100 and 150 mg

Side effects/adverse reactions:

▼ *ORAL: Dry mouth*

CNS: Headache, agitation, confu-sion, *seizures,* akathisia, delusions, insomnia, sedation, tremors

CV: Dysrhythmias, hypertension, palpitation, tachycardia, hypotension

GI: Nausea, vomiting, increased appetite, constipation

GU: Impotence, frequency, retention

EENT: Blurred vision, auditory disturbance

INTEG: Rash, pruritus, sweating

Contraindications: Hypersensitivity, seizure disorder, eating disorders (bulimia, anorexia), ritonavir, MAO inhibitors

Precautions: Renal and hepatic disease, recent MI, cranial trauma, pregnancy category B, lactation, children, low abuse potential

Pharmacokinetics:

PO: Onset 2-4 wk, half-life 12-14 hr, metabolized by liver

🥄 Drug interactions of concern to dentistry:

• Increased adverse reactions (seizures): tricyclic antidepressants, phenothiazines, benzodiazepines, alcohol, haloperidol, and trazodone

DENTAL CONSIDERATIONS

General:

• Assess salivary flow as a factor in caries, periodontal disease, and candidiasis.

• Short appointments and a stress reduction protocol may be required for anxious patients.

• See nicotine transdermal systems for additional smoking cessation considerations.

Consultations:

• Medical consult may be required to assess disease control and patient's ability to tolerate stress.

• Physician should be informed if significant xerostomic side effects occur (e.g., increased caries, sore tongue, problems eating or swallowing, difficulty wearing prosthesis) so a medication change can be considered.

Teach patient/family: *When chronic dry mouth occurs, advise patient:*

• To avoid mouth rinses with high alcohol content due to drying effects

• To use daily home fluoride products for anticaries effect

• To use sugarless gum, frequent sips of water, or saliva substitutes

---

buspirone HCl
(byoo-spye'rone)
BuSpar
Drug class.: Antianxiety agent

Action: Unknown; may act by inhibiting 5-HT receptors or dopamine receptors

Uses: Management and short-term relief of anxiety disorders; unapproved: PMS

Dosage and routes:

• *Adult:* PO 5 mg tid, may increase by 5 mg/day q2-3d, not to exceed 60 mg/day

Available forms include: Tabs 5, 10, 30 mg

Side effects/adverse reactions:

▼ *ORAL:* Dry mouth

CNS: Dizziness, headache, depression, stimulation, insomnia, nervousness, light-headedness, numbness, paresthesia, incoordination, tremors, excitement, involuntary movements, confusion, akathisia

CV: Tachycardia, palpitation, CVA, CHF, MI, hypotension, hypertension

GI: Nausea, diarrhea, constipation, flatulence, increased appetite, rectal bleeding

RESP: Hyperventilation, chest congestion, shortness of breath

GU: Frequency, hesitancy, menstrual irregularity, change in libido

EENT: Sore throat, tinnitus, blurred vision, nasal congestion, red/itching eyes, change in smell

INTEG: Rash, edema, pruritus, alopecia, dry skin

MS: Pain, weakness, muscle cramps, spasms

MISC: Sweating, fatigue, weight gain, fever

Contraindications: Hypersensitivity, child <18 yr

Precautions: Pregnancy category B, lactation, elderly, impaired hepatic/renal function

Pharmacokinetics:

PO: Peak plasma levels 30-60 min, highly protein bound; metabolized in liver; mainly renal excretion of metabolites, some fecal excretion; full antianxiety effects may not be seen until after 2 wk

🦷 **Drug interactions of concern to dentistry:**

• Increased sedation: alcohol, all CNS depressants

• Increased plasma levels: fluconazole, ketoconazole, itraconazole, miconazole, erythromycin, clarithromycin, troleandomycin

DENTAL CONSIDERATIONS

General:

• Monitor vital signs every appointment due to cardiovascular side effects.

• Assess salivary flow as a factor in caries, periodontal disease, and candidiasis.

• Short appointments and a stress reduction protocol may be required for anxious patients.

• Determine why the patient is taking the drug.

Consultations:

• Medical consult may be required to assess disease control.

Teach patient/family: *When chronic dry mouth occurs, advise patient:*

• To avoid mouth rinses with high alcohol content due to drying effects

• To use daily home fluoride products for anticaries effect

• To use sugarless gum, frequent sips of water, or saliva substitutes

---

busulfan

(byoo-sul′fan)
Busulfex, Myleran
Drug class.: Antineoplastic

Action: Changes essential cellular ions to covalent bonding with resultant alkylation, which interferes with biologic function of DNA; activity is not phase specific; effect is due to myelosuppression

Uses: Chronic myelogenous leukemia, orphan drug in preparative therapy for malignancies treated with bone marrow transplant

Dosage and routes:

• *Adult:* PO 1.8 mg/m^2/day initially until WBC levels fall to 15,000/mm^3, then drug is stopped until WBC levels rise over 50,000/mm^3, then 1-12 mg/day

• *Child:* PO 0.06-0.12 mg/kg or 1.8-4.6 mg/m^2 day; dose is titrated to maintain WBC levels at 20,000/mm^3

Available forms include: Tabs 2 mg

Side effects/adverse reactions:

▼ *ORAL:* Dry mouth, cheilosis, stomatitis

*CV: **Endocardial fibrosis***

GI: Diarrhea, weight loss, nausea, vomiting, anorexia

*RESP: **Irreversible pulmonary fibrosis,*** pneumonitis

*HEMA: **Thrombocytopenia, leukopenia, pancytopenia, severe bone marrow depression,*** anemia

*GU: **Renal toxicity,*** impotence, sterility, amenorrhea, gynecomastia, hyperuricemia, adrenal insufficiency–like syndrome

EENT: Cataracts

INTEG: Hyperpigmentation, dermatitis, alopecia

*MISC: **Chromosomal aberrations,*** weakness, fatigue

Contraindications: Radiation, chemotherapy, lactation, pregnancy category D, blastic phase of chronic myelocytic leukemia, hypersensitivity

Precautions: Childbearing-age men and women, leukopenia, thrombocytopenia, anemia, hepatotoxicity, renal toxicity

Pharmacokinetics:

PO: Well absorbed orally; hepatic metabolism, excreted in urine; crosses placenta; excreted in breast milk; long retention of metabolites in body

🦷 **Drug interactions of concern to dentistry:**

• May be an increased risk of bleeding with aspirin

DENTAL CONSIDERATIONS
General:
• Patients taking opioids for acute or chronic pain should be given alternative analgesics for dental pain.
• Consider semisupine chair position for patient comfort if GI side effects occur.
• Chlorhexidine mouth rinse (nonalcoholic) before and during chemotherapy may reduce severity of mucositis.
• Patients on chronic drug therapy may rarely have symptoms of blood dyscrasias, which can include infection, bleeding, and poor healing.
• Palliative medication may be required for management of oral side effects.
• Apply lubricant to dry lips for patient comfort before dental procedures.
• Assess salivary flow as factor in caries, periodontal disease, and candidiasis.
• Patients in active chemotherapy treatment should have adequate WBC count before completing dental procedures that may produce a wound. Consultation with the oncologist may be required to determine WBC values before treatment.
Consultations:
• Medical consult may be required to assess disease control and patient's ability to tolerate stress.
• In a patient with symptoms of blood dyscrasias, request a medical consult for blood studies and postpone dental treatment until normal values are reestablished.

• Consult oncologist; prophylactic or therapeutic antibiotics may be indicated to prevent/treat infection if surgery or deep scaling is planned.
Teach patient/family:
• Importance of good oral hygiene to prevent soft tissue inflammation
• To prevent trauma when using oral hygiene aids
• To report oral lesions, soreness, or bleeding to dentist
• That secondary oral infection may occur; must see dentist immediately if infection occurs
• Importance of updating medical/drug record if physician makes any changes in evaluation or drug regimen
When chronic dry mouth occurs, advise patient:
• To avoid mouth rinses with high alcohol content due to drying effects
• To use daily home fluoride products for anticaries effect
• To use sugarless gum, frequent sips of water, or artificial saliva substitutes

---

butenafine
(byoo'ten-a-feen)
Lotrimin Ultra (OTC), Mentax
Drug class.: Antifungal

Action: Inhibits epoxidation of squalene, thereby interfering with the synthesis of fungal cell membranes
Uses: Tinea pedis caused by *E. floccosum, T. mentagrophytes,* or *T. rubrum;* and Tinea versicolor caused by *Malassezia furfur*

Dosage and routes:
• *Adult:* TOP apply to affected area and adjacent skin once daily for 4 wk
Available forms include: Cream 1% in 2, 15, and 30 g sizes
Side effects/adverse reactions:
INTEG: Dermatitis, burning, stinging, erythema, itching
Contraindications: Hypersensitivity
Precautions: External use only, pregnancy category B, lactation, children <12 yr, not for oral use
Pharmacokinetics:
TOP: Some systemic absorption, hepatic metabolism
DENTAL CONSIDERATIONS
General:
• There are no dental drug interactions or relevant considerations to dentistry for this drug.

---

butoconazole nitrate
(byoo-toe-koe′na-zole)
Femstat, FemStat One, Femstat 3, Gynazole-1, Mycelex-3
Drug class.: Antifungal

Action: Binds sterols in fungal cell membrane, which increases permeability
Uses: Vulvovaginal infections caused by *Candida*
Dosage and routes:
• *Adult:* INTRA VAG 1 applicator × 6 days (second/third trimester pregnancy)
• *Three day treatment:* INTRAVAG insert 1 applicator for 3 days
Available forms include: Vaginal cream 2%

Side effects/adverse reactions:
GU: Rash, stinging, burning, vulvovaginal itching, soreness, swelling, discharge
Contraindications: Hypersensitivity
Precautions: Pregnancy category C, lactation
DENTAL CONSIDERATIONS
General:
• Examine oral mucous membranes for signs of yeast infection.
• Broad-spectrum antibiotics for dental infections may cause vaginal yeast infection.

---

calcipotriene
(kal-si-poe′try-een)
Dovonex
Drug class.: Vitamin D_3 analog (synthetic)

Action: Regulation of skin cell production and development
Uses: Chronic, mild-to-moderate plaque psoriasis
Dosage and routes:
• *Adult:* TOP: Apply small amount to skin bid, rub in gently; do not exceed 100 g cream/ointment per wk
Available forms include: Ointment, cream 0.005%; 30, 60, 100 g
Side effects/adverse reactions:
INTEG: Local irritation, itching, burning, dry skin, dermatitis
Contraindications: Hypersensitivity
Precautions: Pregnancy category C, external use only, elderly >65 yr, lactation, children, hypercalcemia

---

Drug interactions of concern to dentistry:
• None reported

DENTAL CONSIDERATIONS

General:
• Be aware that psoriasis may have oral manifestations.

---

calcitonin (salmon)

(kal-si-toe'nin)

Calcimar, Micalcin Nasal Spray, Osteocalcin, Salmonine

Drug class.: Synthetic polypeptide calcitonins

Action: Inhibits bone resorption; reduces osteoclast function; reduces serum calcium levels in hypercalcemia

Uses: Paget's disease, postmenopausal osteoporosis, hypercalcemia, unlabeled use in intractable bone pain

Dosage and routes:

Paget's disease
• *Adult:* SC/IM 50-100 IU daily; monitor disease symptoms, serum alk phosphatase, and urinary hydroxyproline; maintenance dose of 50 IU qd-qid may be sufficient

Postmenopausal osteoporosis
• *Adult:* SC/IM 100 IU daily with supplemental calcium and vitamin D; NASAL spray 200 IU daily

Hypercalcemia
• *Adult:* SC/IM 4 IU q12h for 1-2 days, increasing if required to 8 IU q12h; maximum dose 8 IU q6-12h

Available forms include: Inj 100, 200 IU/ml; nasal spray 200 IU in 2 ml

Side effects/adverse reactions:

▼ *ORAL:* Dry mouth, metallic taste (all infrequent)

CNS: Headache, dizziness, insomnia, anorexia, anxiety, depression
CV: Hypertension, angina pectoris, tachycardia, palpitation
GI: Nausea, vomiting, diarrhea, abdominal pain
RESP: URI, coughing, dyspnea, bronchospasm
HEMA: Lymphadenopathy, anemia
GU: Frequency of urination, cystitis, hematuria, renal calculus
EENT (NASAL SPRAY): Epistaxis, rhinitis, nasal irritation, dryness, sores, crusting, tinnitus
INTEG: Erythematous skin rashes, flushing face and hands, inflammation at injection site, pruritus
ENDO: Goiter, hyperthyroidism
MS: Myalgia, arthrosis
MISC: Fatigue, flulike symptoms, severe allergic reactions

Contraindications: Hypersensitivity (skin test before use)

Precautions: Allergy, hypocalcemic tetany, routine monitoring of urine sediment, osteogenic sarcoma in Paget's disease, pregnancy category C, lactation, children

Pharmacokinetics:

NASAL: Low bioavailability
IM/SC: Therapeutic response; see decrease in serum calcium in 2 hr, duration 6-8 hr; pain relief in bone may take 8-10 days; Paget's disease response may take several months; rapidly metabolized in kidney and other tissues; renal excretion

Drug interactions of concern to dentistry:
• Supplemental calcium and vitamin D may already be used; not to use additional amounts

DENTAL CONSIDERATIONS:

General:
• Consider semisupine chair posi-

---

italic = common side effects

tion for patient comfort due to effects of disease.
• Consider semisupine chair position for patient comfort if GI side effects occur.
• Assess salivary flow as factor in caries, periodontal disease, and candidiasis.

Teach patient/family:
• Importance of good oral hygiene to prevent soft tissue inflammation
When chronic dry mouth occurs, advise patient:
• To avoid mouth rinses with high alcohol content due to drying effects
• To use daily home fluoride products for anticaries effect
• To use sugarless gum, frequent sips of water, or saliva substitutes

---

camphorated opium tincture

(oh'pee-um)
Paregoric
Drug class.: Antidiarrheal

Controlled Substance Schedule III, Canada N
Action: Antiperistaltic and analgesic with activity related to morphine content
Uses: Diarrhea
Dosage and routes:
• *Adult:* PO 5-10 ml qd-qid
• *Child:* PO 0.25-0.5 ml/kg qd-qid
Available forms include: Liq 2 mg morphine equivalent per 5 ml
Side effects/adverse reactions:
▼ *ORAL:* Dry mouth
CNS: **CNS depression,** dizziness, drowsiness, fainting, flushing, physical dependency
GI: Nausea, vomiting, constipation, abdominal pain

Contraindications: Hypersensitivity, severe ulcerative colitis, pseudomembranous colitis
Precautions: Liver disease, addiction-prone individuals, prostatic hypertrophy (severe), pregnancy category B
Pharmacokinetics:
PO: Duration 4 hr, half-life 2-3 hr; metabolized in liver; excreted in urine

🥄 Drug interactions of concern to dentistry:
• Increased action of both drugs: alcohol, all other CNS depressants
• Decreased peristalsis: anticholinergic drugs
DENTAL CONSIDERATIONS
General:
• Psychologic and physical dependence may occur with chronic administration.
• Determine why the patient is taking the drug.
Teach patient/family:
• To avoid mouth rinses with high alcohol content due to drying effects

---

candesartan cilexetil

(kan-de-sar'tan)
Atacand
Drug class.: Angiotensin II (AT$_1$) receptor antagonist

Action: Blocks the vasoconstrictor and aldosterone-releasing effects of angiotensin II
Uses: Hypertension, as a single drug or in combination with other antihypertensives
Dosage and routes:
• *Adult:* Usual starting dose 16 mg once a day when use as mono-

---

bold italic = life-threatening conditions

therapy if not volume depleted; can be given qd or bid with total daily dose range 8-32 mg

Available forms include: Tabs 4, 8, 16, 32 mg

Side effects/adverse reactions:

CNS: Headache, dizziness, fatigue, anxiety

CV: Peripheral edema, chest pain, tachycardia, palpitation

GI: Dyspepsia

RESP: URI, bronchitis, cough

GU: Hematuria

EENT: Pharyngitis, rhinitis, sinusitis

INTEG: Rash, sweating

MS: Back pain, myalgia

Contraindications: Hypersensitivity

Precautions: Discontinue drug if pregnancy occurs, risk of fetal and neonatal injury, correct volume depletion if present, renal impairment, pregnancy category C (first trimester) and D (second and third trimesters), lactation

Pharmacokinetics:

PO: Pro-drug rapidly converted to candesartan on absorption, bioavailability 15%, peak serum levels 3-4 hr, highly plasma protein bound (99%), minor hepatic metabolism, 67% excreted in feces, 33% in urine

Drug interactions of concern to dentistry:

• Potential for increased hypotensive effects with other hypotensive and sedative drugs

DENTAL CONSIDERATIONS
General:

• Monitor vital signs at every appointment in patients with history of hypertension.

• Evaluate respiration characteristics and rate due to respiratory side effects.

• Consider semisupine chair position for patient comfort if GI side effects occur.

• Limit use of sodium-containing products such as saline IV fluids for those patients with a dietary salt restriction.

• Stress from dental procedures may compromise cardiovascular function; determine patient risk.

• Short appointments and a stress reduction protocol may be required for anxious patients.

• Use precaution if sedation or general anesthesia is required; risk of hypotensive episode.

Consultations:

• Medical consult may be required to assess disease control and patient's ability to tolerate stress.

Teach patient/family:

• Importance of updating health and drug history if physician makes any changes in evaluation or drug regimens

---

capecitabine

(ka-pe-site'a-been)

Xeloda

Drug class.: Antineoplastic

Action: A pro-drug that is enzymatically converted to 5-fluorouracil (5-FU). 5-FU is metabolized by both normal and tumor cells to other metabolites that prevent the synthesis of thymidylate (essential for DNA synthesis), thus inhibiting cell division, or by action as an antimetabolite that can interfere with RNA processing and protein synthesis

Uses: First-line treatment of patients with metastatic colorectal cancer and metastatic breast cancer resistant to both paclitaxel or an anthracycline-containing chemotherapy regimen; colorectal cancer when treatment with a fluoropyrimidine alone is preferred

Dosage and routes:

• *Adult:* PO 2500 mg/m^2/day in two divided doses AM and PM for 2 wk followed by a 1-wk rest period given in 3-wk cycles; take within 30 min of the end of a meal

Available forms include: Tabs 150, 500 mg

Side effects/adverse reactions:

▼ *ORAL: Stomatitis,* taste alteration, candidiasis

CNS: Fatigue, weakness, fever, headache, dizziness

CV: Edema, chest pain, ***cardiotoxicity, MI, dysrhythmias***

GI: Severe diarrhea, nausea, vomiting, abdominal pain, constipation, GI bleeding, ileus

RESP: Dyspnea, cough, URI

HEMA: ***Neutropenia, thrombocytopenia, lymphopenia,*** anemia

EENT: Eye irritation, abnormal vision, sore throat, epistaxis

INTEG: Dermatitis, hand and foot syndrome (tingling, swelling, desquamation, pain), alopecia, skin discoloration, photosensitivity, sweating

META: Hyperbilirubinemia, decreased appetite

MS: Back pain, arthralgia, pain in limbs, paresthesia

MISC: Peripheral neuropathy, viral infections

Contraindications: Hypersensitivity to 5-FU, pregnancy, severe renal impairment

Precautions: Food reduces absorption, renal insufficiency, altered coagulation when taken with Coumadin, patients >80 yr, pregnancy category D, hepatic dysfunction due to liver metastases, lactation, children <18 yr, avoid use of folic acid

Pharmacokinetics:

PO: Readily absorbed, peak blood levels 1.5 hr, plasma protein binding <60%, extensively metabolized in liver to 5-FU (fluorouracil), renal excretion (95.5%)

Drug interactions of concern to dentistry:

• Dental drug interactions not reported; however, patients taking this drug with coumarin oral anticoagulants have altered coagulation parameters and/or bleeding

DENTAL CONSIDERATIONS

General:

• Monitor vital signs every appointment due to cardiovascular side effects.

• Patient on chronic drug therapy may present with symptoms of blood dyscrasias, which can include infection, bleeding, and poor healing.

• Patients taking opioids for acute or chronic pain should be given alternative analgesics for dental pain.

• Short appointments and a stress reduction protocol may be required for anxious patients.

• Consider semisupine chair position for patient comfort if GI side effects occur.

• Question patient about tolerance of NSAIDs or aspirin related to GI effects of drug.

• Consider local hemostasis measures to control and prevent excessive bleeding.

• Examine for oral manifestation of opportunistic infection.

---

bold italic = life-threatening conditions   *For periodic updates, visit* **www.mosby.com**

• Be aware of oral side effects and potential sequela.
• Palliative medication may be required for management of oral side effects.
• Avoid dental light in patient's eyes; offer dark glasses for patient comfort.
• Prophylactic or therapeutic antibiotics may be indicated to prevent or treat infection if surgery or periodontal débridement is required.

Consultations:
• In a patient with symptoms of blood dyscrasias, request a medical consult for blood studies and postpone treatment until normal values are reestablished.
• Medical consult may be required to assess disease control and patient's ability to receive dental treatment.
• Consultation with physician may be needed if sedation or general anesthesia is required.

Teach patient/family:
• To prevent trauma when using oral hygiene aids
• That secondary oral infection may occur; need to see dentist immediately if infection occurs
• Importance of good oral hygiene to prevent soft tissue inflammation
• To report oral lesions, soreness, or bleeding to dentist
• Importance of updating health and drug history if physician makes any changes in evaluation or drug regimens

capsaicin

(kap'say-sin)

Capsin, Capzasin-P, No Pain-HP, Pain Doctor, Pain X, R-Gel, Zostrix, Zostrix-HP

Drug class.: Topical analgesic for selected pain syndromes

Action: Exact mechanism unknown; depletes and prevents reaccumulation of substance P in peripheral sensory neurons

Uses: Neuralgia associated with herpes zoster or diabetic neuropathy; pain of osteoarthritis and rheumatoid arthritis; unapproved: postmastectomy pain, causalgia, and TMD pain

Dosage and routes:
• *Adult and child >2 yr:* TOP apply sparingly to affected area tid or qid; transient burning may occur

Available forms include: Cream 0.025% in 45, 90 g tubes; cream 0.075% in 30, 60 g tubes; lotion 0.025%, 0.075%; gel 0.025%, 0.05%; roll-on 0.075%

Side effects/adverse reactions:
EENT: Coughing if inhaled
INTEG: Local burning sensation, stinging

Contraindications: Hypersensitivity, persons especially sensitive to hot peppers, children <2 yr

Precautions: Pregnancy category not reported, lactation, avoid use on broken skin

🔥 Drug interactions of concern to dentistry:
• None reported

DENTAL CONSIDERATIONS
General:
• Determine why the patient is taking the drug.

• Consider location of lesions and alter dental procedures accordingly.

Teach patient/family:

• To wash hands thoroughly after use and avoid contact with mouth or eyes

---

captopril

(kap'toe-pril)

Capoten

Drug class.: Angiotensin-converting enzyme (ACE) inhibitor

Action: Selectively suppresses renin-angiotensin-aldosterone system; inhibits ACE; prevents conversion of angiotensin I to angiotensin II; results in dilation of arterial, venous vessels

Uses: Hypertension, heart failure not responsive to conventional therapy, left ventricular dysfunction (LVD) after MI, diabetic nephropathy; unapproved: hypertension of scleroderma

Dosage and routes:

Hypertension (alone or with other antihypertensives, esp. thiazide diuretics)

• *Initial dose–Adult:* PO 25 mg bid/tid; may increase to 50 mg bid-tid at 1-2 wk intervals; usual range 25-150 mg bid-tid; max 450 mg

CHF

• *Adult:* PO 6.25-12.5 mg tid, given with a diuretic, digitalis; may increase to 50 mg bid-tid, after 14 days; may increase to 150 mg tid if needed

LVD post MI

• *Adult:* PO single dose of 6.25 mg; then 12.5 mg tid increasing to 25 mg tid over several days, then to 50 mg tid over several wk

Diabetic nephropathy

• *Adult:* PO 25 mg tid

Available forms include: Tabs 12.5, 25, 50, 100 mg

Side effects/adverse reactions:

▼ *ORAL:* Dry mouth, glossitis, oral ulceration (Stevens-Johnson syndrome), angioedema, bleeding, lichenoid drug reaction

CNS: Fever, chills

CV: Hypotension

RESP: **Bronchospasm,** dyspnea, cough

HEMA: **Neutropenia**

GU: **Nephrotic syndrome, acute reversible renal failure,** polyuria, oliguria, frequency, impotence, dysuria, nocturia, proteinuria

INTEG: Angioedema, rash, pemphigus-like reaction

META: Hyperkalemia

Contraindications: Hypersensitivity, pregnancy category D, lactation, heart block, children, K-sparing diuretics

Precautions: Dialysis patients, hypovolemia, leukemia, scleroderma, lupus erythematosus, blood dyscrasias, CHF, diabetes mellitus, renal disease, thyroid disease, COPD, asthma

Pharmacokinetics:

PO: Peak 1-1.5 hr, duration 2-6 hr, half-life 3 hr; metabolized by liver (metabolites); excreted in urine; crosses placenta; excreted in breast milk

☙ **Drug interactions of concern to dentistry:**

• Increased hypotension: alcohol, phenothiazines

• Decreased hypotensive effects: indomethacin and possibly other NSAIDs, sympathomimetics

DENTAL CONSIDERATIONS

General:

• Monitor vital signs every ap-

---

bold italic = life-threatening conditions

pointment due to cardiovascular side effects.

• After supine positioning, have patient sit upright at least 2 min before standing to avoid orthostatic hypotension.

• Patients on chronic drug therapy may rarely have symptoms of blood dyscrasias, which can include infection, bleeding, and poor healing.

• Assess salivary flow as a factor in caries, periodontal disease, and candidiasis.

• Limit use of sodium-containing products such as saline IV fluids for patients with a dietary salt restriction.

• Stress from dental procedures may compromise cardiovascular function; determine patient risk.

• Short appointments and a stress reduction protocol may be required for anxious patients.

Consultations:

• Medical consult may be required to assess patient's ability to tolerate stress.

• In a patient with symptoms of blood dyscrasias, request a medical consult for blood studies and postpone dental treatment until normal values are reestablished.

• Take precautions if dental surgery is anticipated and sedation or general anesthesia is required; there is risk of a hypotensive episode.

Teach patient/family:

• Importance of good oral hygiene to prevent soft tissue inflammation

• Caution to prevent injury when using oral hygiene aids

When chronic dry mouth occurs, advise patient:

• To avoid mouth rinses with high alcohol content due to drying effects

• To use daily home fluoride products for anticaries effect

• To use sugarless gum, frequent sips of water, or saliva substitutes

---

carbamazepine

(kar-ba-maz'e-peen)

Atretol, Carbatrol, Epitol, Tegretol, Tegretol Chewtabs, Tegretol CR, Tegretol XR

♣ Apo-Carbamazepine, Novo-Carbamaz, Nu-Carbamazepine, Taro-Carbamazepine

Drug class.: Anticonvulsant

Action: Exact mechanism unknown, inhibits nerve impulses by limiting influx of sodium ions across cell membrane in motor cortex, may also decrease synaptic transmission

Uses: Tonic-clonic, complex-partial, mixed seizures; trigeminal neuralgia; unapproved: neurogenic pain, some psychotic disorders, diabetes insipidus, alcohol withdrawal

Dosage and routes:

Seizures

• *Adult and child >12 yr:* PO 200 mg bid, may be increased at weekly intervals by 200 mg/day in divided doses q6-8h or 2 × daily with extended release tab; adjustment is needed to minimum dose to control seizures; up to 1.6 g/day; maintenance dose 800-1200 mg/day

• *Child 6-12 yr:* PO 100 mg bid, can increase at weekly intervals by 100 mg/day q6-8h or 2 × daily for extended release tab; maximum doses 1000 mg/day

Trigeminal neuralgia

• *Adult:* PO 100 mg bid, may increase 100 mg q12h until pain subsides, not to exceed 1.2 g/day; maintenance is 200-400 mg bid

Available forms include: Chew tabs 100 mg; tabs 200 mg; ext rel tabs 100, 200, 400 mg; ext rel caps 200, 300 mg; oral susp 100 mg/5 ml

Side effects/adverse reactions:

▼ *ORAL:* Dry mouth, oral ulceration, glossitis, lichenoid reaction

CNS: Drowsiness, *paralysis,* dizziness, confusion, fatigue, headache, hallucinations

CV: **Hypertension, CHF,** hypotension, aggravation of CAD

GI: Nausea, constipation, diarrhea, **hepatitis,** anorexia, vomiting, abdominal pain, increased liver enzymes

RESP: Pulmonary hypersensitivity (fever, dyspnea, pneumonitis)

HEMA: **Thrombocytopenia, agranulocytosis, leukocytosis, neutropenia, aplastic anemia, eosinophilia,** increased pro-time

GU: Frequency, retention, albuminuria, glycosuria, impotence

EENT: Tinnitus, blurred vision, diplopia, nystagmus, conjunctivitis

INTEG: Rash, **Stevens-Johnson syndrome,** urticaria

Contraindications: Hypersensitivity to carbamazepine or tricyclic antidepressants, bone marrow depression, concomitant use of MAO inhibitors

Precautions: Glaucoma, hepatic disease, renal disease, cardiac disease, psychosis, pregnancy category C, lactation, child <6 yr

Pharmacokinetics:

PO: Onset slow, peak 4-8 hr, half-life 14-16 hr; metabolized in liver by cytochrome P450 3A4 isoenzymes; excreted in urine, feces; crosses placenta; excreted in breast milk; trigeminal neuralgia pain relief 8-72 hr

🦷 **Drug interactions of concern to dentistry:**

• Decreased metabolism, risk of toxicity: erythromycin, clarithromycin, propoxyphene, troleandomycin, metronidazole, ketoconazole, fluconazole, itraconazole or any drug that inhibits CYP450 3A4 enzymes

• Increased serum levels: tricyclic antidepressants, fluoxetine, fluvoxamine, nefazodone, ketoconazole, itraconazole

• Increased CNS depression: haloperidol, phenothiazines

• Decreased half-life: doxycycline

• Potential hepatotoxicity: chronic high doses carbamazepine with acetaminophen

• Decreased effects of phenobarbital, corticosteroids, benzodiazepines, doxycycline, sertraline

DENTAL CONSIDERATIONS

General:

• Monitor vital signs every appointment due to cardiovascular side effects.

• Patients on chronic drug therapy may rarely have symptoms of blood dyscrasias, which can include infection, bleeding, and poor healing.

• Assess salivary flow as a factor in caries, periodontal disease, and candidiasis.

• Short appointments and a stress reduction protocol may be required for anxious patients.

• Talk with patient about type of epilepsy, seizure frequency, and quality of seizure control.

Consultations:

• In a patient with symptoms of blood dyscrasias, request a medical

---

bold italic = life-threatening conditions

consult for blood studies and postpone dental treatment until normal values are reestablished.

• Medical consult may be required to assess disease control and patient's ability to tolerate stress.

Teach patient/family:

• Importance of good oral hygiene to prevent soft tissue inflammation

• Caution to prevent injury when using oral hygiene aids

When chronic dry mouth occurs, advise patient:

• To avoid mouth rinses with high alcohol content due to drying effects

• To use daily home fluoride products for anticaries effect

• To use sugarless gum, frequent sips of water, or saliva substitutes

---

carisoprodol

(kar-eye-soe-proe'dole)

Soma

Drug class.: Skeletal muscle relaxant, central acting

Action: Mechanism unknown, may act by blocking interneuronal activity in spinal cord, produces nonspecific CNS sedation

Uses: Adjunct for relief of acute, painful musculoskeletal conditions

Dosage and routes:

• *Adult and child >12 yr:* PO 350 mg tid and hs

Available forms include: Tabs 350 mg

Side effects/adverse reactions:

▼ *ORAL:* Glossitis, swelling of lips

CNS: Dizziness, weakness, drowsiness, headache, tremor, depression, insomnia, ataxia, irritability

CV: Postural hypotension, tachycardia

GI: Nausea, vomiting, hiccups, epigastric discomfort

EENT: Diplopia, temporary loss of vision

INTEG: Rash, pruritus, fever, facial flushing

Contraindications: Hypersensitivity, intermittent porphyria

Precautions: Renal disease, hepatic disease, addictive personalities, pregnancy category C, elderly, children <12 yr

Pharmacokinetics:

PO: Onset 0.5 hr, duration 4-6 hr, half-life 8 hr; metabolized by liver; excreted in urine; crosses placenta; excreted in breast milk (large amounts)

🦷 Drug interactions of concern to dentistry:

• Increased CNS depression: alcohol, all CNS depressants

DENTAL CONSIDERATIONS

General:

• When used in dentistry, may be more effective when used in combination with aspirin or NSAIDs.

Teach patient/family:

• To use electric toothbrush if patient has difficulty holding conventional devices

---

carteolol

(kar-tee'oh-lole)

Cartrol

Drug class.: Nonselective β-adrenergic blocker

Action: This is a nonselective β_1- and β_2-adrenergic antagonist. The antihypertensive mechanism of action is unclear but may include a reduction in cardiac output and inhibition of renin release by the renal juxtaglomerular apparatus. Peripheral resistance decreases with long-term use. The antianginal action (when indicated for this use) may be related to a decrease in myocardial oxygen demand and negative chronotropic and inotropic effects. The antiarrhythmic action (when indicated for this use) has been related to a reduction in spontaneous pacemaker firing and slowing of AV nodal conduction.

Uses: Mild-to-moderate hypertension, alone or with other antihypertensive drugs; unapproved: angina pectoris

Dosage and routes:
• *Adult:* PO 2.5 mg tid initially, may gradually increase to desired response up to 10 mg/day
Available forms include: Tabs 2.5, 5 mg

Side effects/adverse reactions:
▼ *ORAL:* Dry mouth
CNS: Dizziness, mental changes, drowsiness, fatigue, headache, catatonia, depression, anxiety, nightmares, paresthesia, lethargy, insomnia, decreased concentration
CV: Bradycardia, CHF, ventricular dysrhythmias, AV block, peripheral vascular insufficiency, palpitation, orthostatic hypotension
GI: Nausea, vomiting, diarrhea, flatulence, constipation, anorexia
RESP: Bronchospasm, dyspnea, wheezing, nasal stuffiness, pharyngitis
HEMA: Agranulocytosis, thrombocytopenic purpura (rare)
GU: Impotence, dysuria, ejaculatory failure, urinary retention
EENT: Tinnitus, visual changes, sore throat, double vision, dry/burning eyes
INTEG: Rash, alopecia, urticaria, pruritus, fever
MS: Joint pain, arthralgia, muscle cramps, pain

MISC: Facial swelling, decreased exercise tolerance, weight change, Raynaud's disease

Contraindications: Hypersensitivity to β-blockers, cardiogenic shock, second- or third-degree heart block, sinus bradycardia, CHF, bronchial asthma

Precautions: Major surgery, pregnancy category C, lactation, diabetes mellitus, renal disease, thyroid disease, COPD, well-compensated heart failure, CAD, nonallergic bronchospasm

Pharmacokinetics:
PO: Onset 1-2 hr, peak 2-4 hr, duration 8-12 hr, half-life 6-8 hr; metabolized by liver (metabolites inactive); crosses placenta; excreted in breast milk, urine, bile

⚖ Drug interactions of concern to dentistry:
• Hypertension, bradycardia: sympathomimetics (epinephrine, ephedrine)
• Slow metabolism of drug: lidocaine
• Increased hypotension, myocardial depression: fentanyl derivatives, hydrocarbon inhalation anesthetics
• Decreased hypotensive effect: indomethacin and other NSAIDs

DENTAL CONSIDERATIONS
General:
• Monitor vital signs every appointment due to cardiovascular side effects.
• Patients on chronic drug therapy may rarely have symptoms of blood dyscrasias, which can include infection, bleeding, and poor healing.
• After supine positioning, have patient sit upright for at least 2 min before standing to avoid orthostatic hypotension.

---

bold italic = life-threatening conditions   *For periodic updates, visit* **www.mosby.com**

• Limit use of sodium-containing products such as saline IV fluids for patients with a dietary salt restriction.

• Assess salivary flow as a factor in caries, periodontal disease, and candidiasis.

• Stress from dental procedures may compromise cardiovascular function; determine patient risk.

• Short appointments and a stress reduction protocol may be required for anxious patients.

Consultations:

• In a patient with symptoms of blood dyscrasias, request a medical consult for blood studies and postpone dental treatment until normal values are reestablished.

• Take precautions if dental surgery is anticipated and anesthesia is required.

• Medical consult may be required to assess disease control and patient's ability to tolerate stress.

Teach patient/family:

• Importance of good oral hygiene to prevent soft tissue inflammation

• Caution to prevent injury when using oral hygiene aids

When chronic dry mouth occurs, advise patient:

• To avoid mouth rinses with high alcohol content due to drying effects

• To use daily home fluoride products for anticaries effect

• To use sugarless gum, frequent sips of water, or saliva substitutes

---

carteolol HCl

(kar-tee'oe-lole)

Ocupress

Drug class.: β-adrenergic blocker

Action: Nonselective β-adrenergic

blocking agent, reduces production of aqueous humor by unknown mechanisms

Uses: Chronic open-angle glaucoma, ocular hypertension

Dosage and routes:

• *Adult:* INSTILL 1 gtt in affected eye bid

Available forms include: Sol 1%

Side effects/adverse reactions:

CNS: Ataxia, dizziness, lethargy

CV: Bradycardia, hypotension, dysrhythmias

GI: Nausea

RESP: **Bronchospasm**

EENT: Eye irritation, conjunctivitis

Contraindications: Hypersensitivity, asthma, second- and third-degree heart block, right ventricular failure, congenital glaucoma (infants), COPD

Precautions: Pregnancy category C, lactation, elderly, children

Pharmacokinetics: INSTILL: Onset 1 hr, peak effects 2 hr, duration of action 6-8 hr

⚕ Drug interactions of concern to dentistry:

• Avoid use of anticholinergic drugs, including atropine-like drugs, propantheline, and diazepam (benzodiazepine)

DENTAL CONSIDERATIONS

General:

• Check compliance of patient with prescribed drug regimen for glaucoma.

• Avoid dental light in patient's eyes; offer dark glasses for comfort.

Consultations:

• Consultation with physician may be needed if sedation or anesthesia is required.

C

carvedilol

(kar've-di-lole)
Coreg

Drug class.: Nonselective β-adrenergic blocking agent with α₁-blocking activity

Action: Produces fall in BP without reflex tachycardia or significant reduction in heart rate through mixture of α-blocking, β-blocking effects; elevated plasma renin reduced

Uses: Essential hypertension, alone or with other antihypertensives, CHF; unlabeled use in angina

Dosage and routes:

Essential hypertension

• *Adult:* PO initially 6.25 mg bid for 7-14 days, then 12.5 mg bid if required for 7-14 days, then 25 mg bid; take with food to minimize risk of orthostatic hypotension

CHF

• *Adult:* PO 3.125 mg bid for 2 wk, patients must be closely monitored by physician

Available forms include: Tabs 3.125, 6.25, 12.5, 25 mg

Side effects/adverse reactions:

▼ *ORAL:* Dry mouth (<1%)

CNS: Dizziness, insomnia, somnolence

*CV: **Heart block,** orthostatic hypotension, syncope, bradycardia,* peripheral edema, fatigue

GI: Diarrhea, hepatocellular injury, abdominal pain

*RESP: **Status asthmaticus,** rhinitis,* pharyngitis, dyspnea

*HEMA: **Thrombocytopenia***

GU: UTI, impotence

INTEG: Pruritus, rash

MS: Back pain

MISC: Hypertriglyceridemia

Contraindications: Class IV heart failure, bronchial asthma, bronchospastic diseases, second- or third-degree AV block, cardiogenic shock or severe bradycardia, hypersensitivity

Precautions: Elderly, hepatic impairment, renal impairment, pregnancy category C, lactation, child <18 yr

Pharmacokinetics:

PO: Rapid oral absorption, hepatic metabolism, metabolites excreted in feces, 98% plasma protein binding

🦷 **Drug interactions of concern to dentistry:**

• Decreased hypotensive effect: indomethacin, NSAIDs

• Increased hypotension, myocardial depression: hydrocarbon inhalation anesthetics

• Hypertension, bradycardia: sympathomimetics (epinephrine, ephedrine)

DENTAL CONSIDERATIONS

General:

• Monitor vital signs every appointment due to cardiovascular side effects.

• After supine positioning, have patient sit upright for at least 2 min before standing to avoid orthostatic hypotension.

• Assess salivary flow as a factor in caries, periodontal disease, and candidiasis.

• Patients on chronic drug therapy may rarely have symptoms of blood dyscrasias, which can include infection, bleeding, and poor healing.

• Limit use of sodium-containing products, such as saline IV fluids, for those patients with a dietary salt restriction.

• Stress from dental procedures

---

bold italic = life-threatening conditions

may compromise cardiovascular function; determine patient risk.

• Short appointments and a stress reduction protocol may be required for anxious patients.

Consultations:

• In a patient with symptoms of blood dyscrasias, request a medical consult for blood studies and postpone dental treatment until normal values are reestablished.

• Medical consult may be required to assess disease control and patient's ability to tolerate stress.

Teach patient/family:

• To report oral lesions, soreness, or bleeding to dentist

When chronic dry mouth occurs, advise patient:

• To avoid mouth rinses with high alcohol content due to drying effects

• Of need for daily home fluoride to prevent caries

• To use sugarless gum, frequent sips of water, or saliva substitutes

---

cefaclor

(sef′a-klor)

Ceclor, Ceclor CD

♣ Apo-Cefaclor

Drug class.: Antibiotic, cephalosporin (second generation)

Action: Inhibits bacterial cell wall synthesis, rendering cell wall osmotically unstable

Uses: For use in the treatment of the following infections when caused by susceptible strains of named microorganisms: otitis media caused by *S. pneumoniae, H. influenza,* staphylococci, and *S. pyogenes;* lower respiratory tract infections caused by *S. pneumoniae, H. influenza,* and *S. pyo-*

genes; pharyngitis and tonsillitis caused by *S. pyogenes;* urinary tract infections caused by *E. coli, P. mirabilis,* Klebsiella species, and coagulase-negative staphylococci; skin and skin structure infections caused by *S. aureus* and *S. pyogenes;* and in vitro activity against *Peptococcus, Peptostreptococcus,* and *Propionibacterium* (clinical significance unknown)

Dosage and routes:

• *Adult:* PO 250-500 mg q8h, not to exceed 4 g/day

• *Child >1 mo:* PO 20-40 mg/kg/qd in divided doses q8h, not to exceed 1 g/day

Available forms include: Caps 250, 500 mg; powder for oral susp 125, 187, 250, 375 mg/5 ml; ext rel tabs 375, 500 mg

Side effects/adverse reactions:

▼ *ORAL:* Candidiasis, glossitis

CNS: Headache, dizziness, weakness, paresthesia, fever, chills

GI: Diarrhea, anorexia, nausea, vomiting, pain, bleeding, increased AST/ALT, bilirubin, LDH, alk phosphatase, abdominal pain

RESP: Dyspnea

HEMA: Leukopenia, thrombocytopenia, agranulocytosis, neutropenia, lymphocytosis, eosinophilia, pancytopenia, hemolytic anemia, anemia

GU: Nephrotoxicity, renal failure, proteinuria, vaginitis, pruritus, candidiasis, increased BUN

INTEG: Anaphylaxis, rash, urticaria, dermatitis

Contraindications: Hypersensitivity to cephalosporins, infants <1 mo

Precautions: Hypersensitivity to penicillins, pregnancy category B, lactation, renal disease

---

italic = common side effects

Pharmacokinetics:

PO: Peak 0.5-1 hr, half-life 36-54 min; 25% bound by plasma proteins; 60%-85% eliminated unchanged in urine in 8 hr; crosses placenta; excreted in breast milk

⚗ Drug interactions of concern to dentistry:

• Decreased bactericidal effects: tetracyclines, erythromycins
• Increased and prolonged serum levels: probenecid
• Oral contraceptives: advise patient of a potential risk for decreased contraceptive action, to maintain compliance with oral contraceptive use while using antibiotics, and to consider the use of additional nonhormonal contraception

DENTAL CONSIDERATIONS
General:

• Take precautions regarding allergy to medication.
• Determine why the patient is taking the drug.

Consultations:

• Medical consult may be required to assess disease control.

Teach patient/family:

• Importance of good oral hygiene to prevent soft tissue inflammation
• To avoid mouth rinses with high alcohol content due to drying effects and possible drug-drug reaction

When used for dental infection, advise patient:

• To report sore throat, oral burning sensation, fever, fatigue, any of which could indicate superinfection
• To take at prescribed intervals and complete dosage regimen

• To immediately notify the dentist if signs or symptoms of infection increase

---

cefadroxil

(sef-a-drox'il)
Duricef

Drug class.: Cephalosporin (first generation)

Action: Inhibits bacterial cell wall synthesis, rendering cell wall osmotically unstable

Uses: Gram-negative bacilli: *E. coli, P. mirabilis, Klebsiella* (UTI only); gram-positive organisms: *S. pneumoniae, S. pyogenes, S. aureus;* upper/lower respiratory tract, urinary tract, skin infections; otitis media; tonsillitis; particularly for UTI

Dosage and routes:

• *Adult:* PO 500 mg-1 g q12h; dosage reduction indicated in renal impairment (CrCl <50 ml/min); limit 4 g/day
• *Child:* PO 30 mg/kg/day or 15 mg/kg q12h

Bacterial endocarditis prophylaxis

• *Adult:* PO 2 g 1 hr before dental procedure
• *Child:* PO 50 mg/kg 1 hr before dental procedure, not to exceed the adult dose

Available forms include: Caps 500 mg; tabs 1 g; oral susp 125, 250, 500 mg/5 ml

Side effects/adverse reactions:

▼ *ORAL:* Candidiasis, glossitis
CNS: Headache, dizziness, weakness, paresthesia, fever, chills
GI: Diarrhea, anorexia, **pseudomembranous colitis,** nausea, vomiting, pain, bleeding, increased AST/ALT, bilirubin, LDH, alk phosphatase, abdominal pain

---

bold italic = life-threatening conditions *For periodic updates, visit* **www.mosby.com**

RESP: Dyspnea
*HEMA: **Leukopenia, thrombocytopenia, agranulocytosis, neutropenia, lymphocytosis, eosinophilia, pancytopenia, hemolytic anemia***
*GU: **Nephrotoxicity, renal failure,*** proteinuria, vaginitis, pruritus, candidiasis, increased BUN
*INTEG: **Anaphylaxis,*** rash, urticaria, dermatitis

Contraindications: Hypersensitivity to cephalosporins, infants <1 mo

Precautions: Hypersensitivity to penicillins, pregnancy category B, lactation, renal disease

Pharmacokinetics:
PO: Peak 1-1.5 hr, half-life 1-2 hr; 20% bound by plasma proteins; crosses placenta; excreted in breast milk

⚘ Drug interactions of concern to dentistry:
• Decreased bactericidal effects: tetracyclines, erythromycins
• Increased and prolonged serum levels: probenecid
• Oral contraceptives: advise patient of a potential risk for decreased contraceptive action, to maintain compliance with oral contraceptive use while using antibiotics, and to consider the use of additional nonhormonal contraception

DENTAL CONSIDERATIONS
General:
• Take precautions regarding allergy to medication.
• Determine why the patient is taking the drug.
Consultations:
• Medical consult may be required to assess disease control.
Teach patient/family:
• Importance of good oral hygiene to prevent soft tissue inflammation

• To avoid mouth rinses with high alcohol content due to drying effects and possible drug-drug reaction
When used for dental infection, advise patient:
• To report sore throat, oral burning sensation, fever, fatigue, any of which could indicate superinfection
• To take at prescribed intervals and complete dosage regimen
• To immediately notify the dentist if signs or symptoms of infection increase

cefazolin sodium
(sef-a′zoe-lin)
Ancef, Kefzol, Zolicef

Drug class.: Cephalosporin (first generation)

Action: Inhibits bacterial cell wall synthesis, rendering cell wall osmotically unstable
Uses: Indicated for use when caused by susceptible microorganisms: respiratory tract infections caused by *S. pneumoniae,* Klebsiella species, *H. influenza, S. aureus* and group A β-hemolytic streptococci; UTI infections caused by *E. coli, P. mirabilis,* Klebsiella species, and some enterobacter and enterococci; skin and skin structure infections caused by *S. aureus,* group A β-hemolytic streptococci; biliary tract infections caused by *E. coli, P. mirabilis, S. aureus,* Klebsiella species, and various strains of streptococci; bone and joint infections caused by *S. aureus;* genital infections caused by *E. coli, P. mirabilis,* Klebsiella species, and some enterococci; septicemia caused by *S. pneumoniae, S. au-*

reus, P. mirabilis, E. coli, and Klebsiella species; endocarditis caused by *S. aureus* and group A β-hemolytic streptococci

Dosage and routes:

Life-threatening infections
- *Adult:* IM/IV 1-1.5 g q6h
- *Child >1 mo:* IM/IV 100 mg/kg in 3-4 equal doses

Mild-to-moderate infections
- *Adult:* IM/IV 250-500 mg q8h
- *Child >1 mo:* IM/IV 25-50 mg/kg in 3-4 equal doses

Dosage reduction indicated in renal impairment (CrCl <54 ml/min)

Bacterial endocarditis prophylaxis
- *Adult:* IM or IV patients unable to take oral medications (caution allergy to amoxicillin) 1 g 30 min before dental procedure
- *Child:* IM or IV 25 mg/kg of body weight not to exceed the adult dose 30 min before dental procedure

Prosthetic joint prophylaxis (when indicated)
- *Adult:* IM or IV 1 g 1 hr before dental procedure

Available forms include: Inj IM/IV 250, 500 mg; 1, 5, 10 g

Side effects/adverse reactions:

▼ *ORAL:* Candidiasis

CNS: Headache, dizziness, weakness, paresthesia, fever, chills

GI: Diarrhea, anorexia, nausea, vomiting, pain, glossitis, bleeding, increased AST/ALT, bilirubin, LDH, alk phosphatase, abdominal pain

HEMA: Leukopenia, thrombocytopenia, agranulocytosis, anemia, neutropenia, lymphocytosis, eosinophilia, pancytopenia, hemolytic anemia

GU: Nephrotoxicity, renal failure, proteinuria, vaginitis, pruritus, increased BUN

INTEG: Anaphylaxis, rash, urticaria, dermatitis

Contraindications: Hypersensitivity to cephalosporins, infants <1 mo

Precautions: Hypersensitivity to penicillins, pregnancy category B, lactation, renal disease

Pharmacokinetics:
IM: Peak 0.5-2 hr, half-life 1.5-2.25 hr
IV: Peak 10 min, eliminated unchanged in urine 70%-86% protein bound

⚡ Drug interactions of concern to dentistry:
- Decreased bactericidal effects: tetracyclines, erythromycins
- Increased and prolonged serum levels: probenecid
- Oral contraceptives: advise patient of a potential risk for decreased contraceptive action, to maintain compliance with oral contraceptive use while using antibiotics, and to consider the use of additional nonhormonal contraception

DENTAL CONSIDERATIONS
General:
- Take precautions regarding allergy to medication.
- Determine why the patient is taking the drug.

Consultations:
- Medical consult may be required to assess disease control.

Teach patient/family:
- Importance of good oral hygiene to prevent soft tissue inflammation
- To avoid mouth rinses with high alcohol content due to drying effects and possible drug-drug reaction

When used for dental infection, advise patient:
- To report sore throat, oral burning

sensation, fever, fatigue, any of which could indicate superinfection

• To take at prescribed intervals and complete dosage regimen

• To immediately notify the dentist if signs or symptoms of infection increase

---

cefdinir

(sef'di-ner)

Omnicef

Drug class.: Cephalosporin (third generation)

Action: Inhibits bacterial cell wall synthesis, rendering cell wall osmotically unstable

Uses: Infections caused by susceptible strains of organisms that cause community-acquired pneumonia, acute exacerbation of chronic bronchitis, pharyngitis, tonsillitis, uncomplicated skin and skin structure infections, acute maxillary sinusitis, and acute bacterial otitis media

Dosage and routes:

• *Adult and child <13 yr:* PO dose depends on type of infection and patient; range is from 300 mg every 12 hr to 600 mg every 24 hr for 5-10 days taken with or without food

• *Child <6 mo-12 yr:* PO dose depends on type of infection and patient: range is from 7 mg/kg of body weight every 12 hr to 14 mg/kg of body weight every 24 hr for 5-10 days with or without food

Available forms include: Caps 300 mg; powder for oral suspension 125 mg/5 ml

Side effects/adverse reactions:

▼ *ORAL:* None reported, but most antiinfectives carry a risk of opportunistic candidiasis

CNS: Dizziness, insomnia, somnolence

*GI: Diarrhea, nausea, abdominal pain, **antibiotic-associated pseudomembranous colitis***

RESP: Dyspnea

HEMA: Eosinophilia

GU: Vaginal candidiasis

INTEG: Rash, cutaneous candidiasis

META: Abnormal liver function tests, elevated AST/ALT, bilirubin, potassium, and urinary pH

MS: Asthenia, ***anaphylaxis***

Contraindications: Hypersensitivity

Precautions: Hypersensitivity to other cephalosporins, penicillins, or penicillamine; renal impairment (need dose reduction); ulcerative colitis, pseudomembranous colitis, bleeding disorders, renal impairment, hemodialysis, β-lactamase-resistant organisms, pregnancy category B, not detected in breast milk, child <6 mo

Pharmacokinetics:

PO: Slow absorption, peak serum levels 2-4 hr, bioavailability ranges from 16%-25%, depending on dose and dose form, plasma protein binding 60%-70%, little to no metabolism, renal excretion

🍃 **Drug interactions of concern to dentistry:**

• Absorption retarded by iron salts, magnesium, or aluminum antacids: take antiinfective dose at least 2 hr before antacids or iron preparations

• Increased plasma levels: probenecid

• Oral contraceptives: advise patient of a potential risk for decreased contraceptive action, to maintain compliance with oral contraceptive use while using antibiotics, and to consider the use of additional nonhormonal contraception

DENTAL CONSIDERATIONS
General:
• Use precaution regarding allergy to medication.
• Determine why patient is taking the drug.
• Examine for oral manifestation of opportunistic infection.
Consultations:
• Medical consult may be required to assess disease control.
Teach patient/family:
• Importance of good oral hygiene to prevent soft tissue inflammation

---

cefepime

(sef'e-pim)
Maxipime

Drug class.: Cephalosporin (fourth generation)

Action: Inhibits bacterial cell wall synthesis
Uses: Urinary tract infections (uncomplicated and complicated), skin and soft tissue infections, complicated intraabdominal infections (in combination with metronidazole) and pneumonia caused by susceptible strains of microorganisms, including *E. coli, K. pneumonia, P. mirabilis, S. aureus* (methicillin susceptible), *S. pneumoniae* and *S. pyogenes;* febrile neutropenia
Dosage and routes:
Mild to moderate infections
• *Adult:* IV/IM 0.5-1.0 g q12h depending on severity of the infection for 7-10 days; IM doses for mild infections only

Moderate to severe infections
• *Adult:* IV 1.0-2.0 g q12h for 10 days depending on severity of the infection; adjust all doses in patients with renal impairment
Available forms include: Powder for injection vials 500 mg, 1, 2 g
Side effects/adverse reactions:
▼ *ORAL:* Candidiasis
CNS: Headache, light-headedness
CV: Phlebitis
GI: Diarrhea, pseudomembranous colitis, vomiting, dyspepsia
GU: Vaginitis
EENT: Blurred vision
INTEG: Urticaria, pruritus, rash
META: Elevation of liver function tests
MISC: Local reactions, fever
Contraindications: Hypersensitivity to cephalosporins or penicillins
Precautions: Renal impairment, overgrowth of resistant organisms, colitis, monitor prothrombin, pregnancy category B, lactation, child <12 yr
Pharmacokinetics:
IV: Peak levels vary with dose and occur within 0.5-1 hr, protein binding 20%, urinary excretion (85% of dose), therapeutic serum levels up to 8 hr
IM: Peak levels 0.5-1.5 hr
🍃 Drug interactions of concern to dentistry:
• Increased risk of nephrotoxicity, ototoxicity: aminoglycosides in high doses, furosemide
DENTAL CONSIDERATIONS
General:
• Precaution regarding allergy to medication.
• Determine why patient is taking the drug.
• Oral contraceptives: advise patient of a potential risk for de-

---

creased contraceptive action, to maintain compliance with oral contraceptive use while using antibiotics, and to consider the use of additional nonhormonal contraception

Consultation: Medical consult may be required to assess disease control.

Teach patient/family:
• Importance of good oral hygiene to prevent soft tissue inflammation
• To report sore throat, oral burning sensation, fever, fatigue, any of which could indicate presence of a superinfection

---

cefixime

(sef-ix′eem)

Suprax

Drug class.: Cephalosporin (third generation)

Action: Inhibits bacterial cell wall synthesis, rendering cell wall osmotically unstable

Uses: Uncomplicated UTI *(E. coli, P. mirabilis)*, pharyngitis and tonsillitis *(S. pyogenes)*, otitis media *(H. influenzae, M. catarrhalis)*, acute bronchitis, and acute exacerbations of chronic bronchitis *(S. pneumoniae, H. influenzae)*

Dosage and routes:
• *Adult:* PO 400 mg qd as a single dose or 200 mg q12h
• *Child >50 kg or >12 yr:* PO use adult dosage
• *Child <50 kg or <12 yr:* PO 8 mg/kg/day as a single dose or 4 mg/kg q12h

Available forms include: Tabs 200, 400 g; powder for oral susp 100 mg/5 ml

Side effects/adverse reactions:

▼ *ORAL:* Candidiasis, glossitis

CNS: Headache, dizziness, paresthesia, fever, chills, lethargy, fatigue, confusion

GI: Nausea, vomiting, diarrhea, anorexia, pain, bleeding, increased AST/ALT, bilirubin, LDH, alk phosphatase, heartburn, dysgeusia, flatulence

RESP: **Bronchospasm,** dyspnea, tight chest

HEMA: **Leukopenia, thrombocytopenia, agranulocytosis, neutropenia, lymphocytosis, eosinophilia, pancytopenia, hemolytic anemia**

GU: **Proteinuria, nephrotoxicity, renal failure,** pyuria, dysuria, vaginitis, pruritus, increased BUN

INTEG: **Exfoliative dermatitis, anaphylaxis,** rash, urticaria

Contraindications: Hypersensitivity to cephalosporins, infants <6 mo

Precautions: Hypersensitivity to penicillins, pregnancy category B, lactation, renal disease

Pharmacokinetics:

PO: Peak 1 hr, half-life 3-4 hr; 65% bound by plasma proteins, 50% eliminated unchanged in urine; crosses placenta; excreted in breast milk

Drug interactions of concern to dentistry:
• Decreased bactericidal effects: tetracyclines, erythromycins
• Increased and prolonged serum levels: probenecid
• Oral contraceptives: advise patient of a potential risk for decreased contraceptive action, to maintain compliance with oral contraceptive use while using antibiotics, and to consider the use of additional nonhormonal contraception

---

DENTAL CONSIDERATIONS
General:
• Take precautions regarding allergy to medication.
• Determine why the patient is taking the drug.
Consultations:
• Medical consult may be required to assess disease control.
Teach patient/family:
• Importance of good oral hygiene to prevent soft tissue inflammation
• To avoid mouth rinses with high alcohol content due to drying effects and possible drug-drug reaction
When used for dental infection, advise patient:
• To report sore throat, oral burning sensation, fever, fatigue, any of which could indicate superinfection
• To take at prescribed intervals and complete dosage regimen
• To immediately notify the dentist if signs or symptoms of infection increase

---

cefpodoxime proxetil
(cef-pode-ox′eem)
Vantin

Drug class.: Cephalosporin (third generation)

Action: Inhibits bacterial cell wall synthesis, rendering cell wall osmotically unstable
Uses: Upper/lower respiratory tract infections, pharyngitis (tonsillitis), gonorrhea, UTI, uncomplicated skin and skin structure infections caused by susceptible organisms, otitis media

Dosage and routes:
• *Adult:* PO 100-200 mg q12h for 5 days; more severe infections 400 mg q12h
Otitis media
• *Child 2 mo-12 yr:* PO 10 mg/kg/day in one dose (max daily dose 400 mg) or 5 mg/kg (max 200 mg/dose) bid for 5 days
Available forms include: Tabs 100, 200 mg; oral susp 50, 100 mg/5 ml
Side effects/adverse reactions:
▼ *ORAL:* Candidiasis, glossitis
CNS: Headache, dizziness, weakness, paresthesia, fever, chills
GI: Diarrhea, anorexia, nausea, vomiting, abdominal pain, bleeding, increased AST/ALT, bilirubin, LDH, alk phosphatase
RESP: Dyspnea
HEMA: Leukopenia, thrombocytopenia, agranulocytosis, neutropenia, lymphocytosis, eosinophilia, pancytopenia, hemolytic anemia
GU: Nephrotoxicity, renal failure, proteinuria, vaginitis, pruritus, candidiasis, increased BUN
INTEG: Anaphylaxis, rash, urticaria, dermatitis
Contraindications: Hypersensitivity to cephalosporins, infants <1 mo
Precautions: Hypersensitivity to penicillins, lactation, renal disease, pregnancy category not listed
Pharmacokinetics:
PO: Half-life 2-3 hr; excreted unchanged in urine; alter dose with renal impairment
♣ Drug interactions of concern to dentistry:
• Decreased bactericidal effects: tetracyclines, erythromycins
• Increased and prolonged serum levels: probenecid
• Oral contraceptives: advise patient of a potential risk for de-

---

bold italic = life-threatening conditions

creased contraceptive action, to maintain compliance with oral contraceptive use while using antibiotics, and to consider the use of additional nonhormonal contraception

DENTAL CONSIDERATIONS
General:
• Take precautions regarding allergy to medication.
• Determine why the patient is taking the drug.
Consultations:
• Medical consult may be required to assess disease control.
Teach patient/family:
• Importance of good oral hygiene to prevent soft tissue inflammation
• To avoid mouth rinses with high alcohol content due to drying effects and possible drug-drug reaction
When used for dental infection, advise patient:
• To report sore throat, oral burning sensation, fever, fatigue, any of which could indicate superinfection
• To take at prescribed intervals and complete dosage regimen
• To immediately notify the dentist if signs or symptoms of infection increase

---

cefprozil monohydrate
(sef-pro′zil)
Cefzil

Drug class.: Cephalosporin (second generation)

Action: Inhibits bacterial cell wall synthesis, rendering cell wall osmotically unstable
Uses: Pharyngitis/tonsillitis, otitis media, secondary bacterial infection of acute bronchitis, sinusitis; acute bacterial sinusitis; acute bacterial exacerbation of chronic bronchitis and uncomplicated skin and skin structure infections
Dosage and routes:
Upper respiratory infections
• *Adult:* PO 500 mg qd × 10 days
Otitis media
• *Child 6 mo-12 yr:* PO 15 mg/kg q12h × 10 days
Lower respiratory infections
• *Adult:* PO 500 mg bid × 10 days
Skin/skin structure infections
• *Adult:* PO 250-500 mg q12h × 10 days
Available forms include: Tabs 250, 500 mg; susp 125, 250 mg/5 ml
Side effects/adverse reactions:
▼ *ORAL:* Candidiasis, glossitis
CNS: Dizziness, headache, weakness, paresthesia, fever, chills
*GI: **Pseudomembranous colitis,** diarrhea, nausea, vomiting, pain, anorexia, bleeding, increased AST/ALT, bilirubin, LDH, alk phosphatase, abdominal pain, flatulence
*RESP: **Anaphylaxis,** dyspnea
*HEMA: **Leukopenia, thrombocytopenia, agranulocytosis, anemia, neutropenia, lymphocytosis, eosinophilia, pancytopenia, hemolytic anemia***
*GU: **Nephrotoxicity, proteinuria, increased BUN, renal failure, hematuria,** vaginitis, genitoanal pruritus, candidiasis
INTEG: Rash, urticaria, dermatitis
Contraindications: Hypersensitivity to cephalosporins
Precautions: Pregnancy category B, lactation, elderly, hypersensitivity to penicillins, renal disease
Pharmacokinetics:
PO: Peak 6-10 hr, elimination half-life 25 hr; plasma protein binding

99%; extensively metabolized to an active metabolite

🔋 **Drug interactions of concern to dentistry:**
• Decreased bactericidal effects: tetracyclines, erythromycins
• Increased and prolonged serum levels: probenecid
• Oral contraceptives: advise patient of a potential risk for decreased contraceptive action, to maintain compliance with oral contraceptive use while using antibiotics, and to consider the use of additional nonhormonal contraception

DENTAL CONSIDERATIONS
General:
• Take precautions regarding allergy to medication.
• Determine why the patient is taking the drug.
• Examine for evidence of oral manifestations of blood dyscrasia (infection, bleeding, poor healing) and superinfection.

Consultations:
• Medical consult may be required to assess disease control.

Teach patient/family:
• Importance of good oral hygiene to prevent soft tissue inflammation
• To avoid mouth rinses with high alcohol content due to drying effects and possible drug-drug reaction

When used for dental infection, advise patient:
• To report sore throat, oral burning sensation, fever, fatigue, any of which could indicate superinfection
• To take at prescribed intervals and complete dosage regimen
• To immediately notify the dentist if signs or symptoms of infection increase

ceftibuten
(sef-tye′byoo-ten)
Cedax
Drug class.: Cephalosporin (third generation)

Action: Inhibits bacterial cell wall synthesis, rendering cell wall osmotically unstable

Uses: Acute exacerbations of chronic bronchitis due to susceptible strains of *H. influenzae, M. catarrhalis, S. pneumoniae;* acute otitis media due to susceptible strains of *H. influenzae, M. catarrhalis, S. pyogenes;* pharyngitis and tonsillitis due to *S. pyogenes*

Dosage and routes:
• *Adult and child >12 yr:* PO 400 mg qd × 10 days
• *Child:* SUSP 9 mg/kg qd × 10 days, susp administered 2 hr before or 1 hr after a meal

Available forms include: Caps 400 mg; susp 90, 180 mg/5 ml in 30, 60, 120 ml volumes

Side effects/adverse reactions:

▼ *ORAL:* Candidiasis, dry mouth (<1%)

CNS: Headache, dizziness, weakness, paresthesia, fever, chills

GI: Diarrhea, dyspepsia, nausea, vomiting, abdominal pain, bleeding, anorexia, increased AST/ALT, bilirubin, LDH, alk phosphatase, antibiotic-associated pseudomembranous colitis

RESP: Dyspnea

HEMA: **Leukopenia, thrombocytopenia, agranulocytosis, neutropenia, lymphocytosis, eosinophilia, pancytopenia, hemolytic anemia**

GU: **Nephrotoxicity, renal failure,** proteinuria, vaginitis, pruritus, candidiasis, increased BUN

---

bold italic = life-threatening conditions

*INTEG: Rash, pruritus, **anaphylaxis,** urticaria, dermatitis*
Contraindications: Hypersensitivity to cephalosporins
Precautions: Hypersensitivity to penicillins, lactation, renal impairment, pregnancy category B, lactation, infants <6 mo, pseudomembranous colitis, oral suspension contains 1 g sucrose/5 ml
Pharmacokinetics:
PO: Half-life 2-3 hr; protein binding 6%, excreted mostly unchanged in urine; alter dose with renal impairment

☘ Drug interactions of concern to dentistry:
• Decreased bactericidal effects: tetracyclines, erythromycins
• Increased and prolonged serum levels: probenecid
• Aminoglycosides increase nephrotoxic potential
• Oral contraceptives: advise patient of a potential risk for decreased contraceptive action, to maintain compliance with oral contraceptive use while using antibiotics, and to consider the use of additional nonhormonal contraception

DENTAL CONSIDERATIONS
General:
• Take precautions regarding allergy to medication.
• Assess salivary flow as factor in caries, periodontal disease, and candidiasis.
• Oral suspension contains sucrose; patient should rinse mouth after use.
• Determine why the patient is taking the drug.
Consultations:
• Medical consult may be required to assess disease control.

Teach patient/family:
• Importance of good oral hygiene to prevent soft tissue inflammation
When used for dental infection, advise patient:
• To report sore throat, oral burning sensation, fever, fatigue, any of which could indicate superinfection
• To take at prescribed intervals and complete dosage regimen
• To immediately notify the dentist if signs or symptoms of infection increase

---

cefuroxime axetil
(sef-fyoor-ox´eem)
Ceftin, Kefurox, zinacef
Drug class.: Cephalosporin (second generation)

Action: Inhibits bacterial cell wall synthesis, rendering cell wall osmotically unstable
Uses: Gram-negative bacilli *(H. influenzae, E. coli, Neisseria, P. mirabilis, Klebsiella);* gram-positive organisms *(S. pneumoniae, S. pyogenes, S. aureus);* serious lower respiratory tract, urinary tract, skin, gonococcal infections; septicemia; meningitis; early Lyme disease; acute bronchitis, acute bacterial maxillary sinusitis, pharyngitis, tonsillitis, impetigo, bone and joint infections
Dosage and routes:
• *Adult and child:* PO 250 mg q12h, may increase to 500 mg q12h in serious infections; for severe infections give IV/IM according to package insert directions
Urinary tract infections
• *Adult:* PO 125 mg q12h, may increase to 250 q12h if needed

---

Otitis media
- *Child <2 yr:* PO 125 mg bid
- *Child >2 yr:* PO 250 mg bid

Available forms include: Tabs 125, 250, 500 mg; powder for inj 750 mg and 1.5, 7.5 g; oral susp 125 mg/5 ml, 250 mg/5 ml in 50 ml and 100 ml

Side effects/adverse reactions:

▼ *ORAL:* Candidiasis, glossitis

CNS: Headache, dizziness, weakness, paresthesia, fever, chills

GI: Nausea, vomiting, diarrhea, anorexia, pseudomembranous colitis, bleeding, increased AST/ALT, bilirubin, LDH, alk phosphatase, abdominal pain

RESP: Anaphylaxis

HEMA: Leukopenia, thrombocytopenia, agranulocytosis, neutropenia, lymphocytosis, eosinophilia, pancytopenia, hemolytic anemia

GU: Nephrotoxicity, renal failure, proteinuria, vaginitis, pruritus, candidiasis, increased BUN

INTEG: Rash, urticaria, dermatitis

Contraindications: Hypersensitivity to cephalosporins, infants <1 mo

Precautions: Hypersensitivity to penicillins, pregnancy category B, lactation, renal disease

Pharmacokinetics:

PO: Half-life 1-2 hr in normal renal function, 65% excreted unchanged in urine

🐝 **Drug interactions of concern to dentistry:**

- Decreased bactericidal effects: tetracyclines, erythromycins
- Increased and prolonged serum levels: probenecid
- Oral contraceptives: advise patient of a potential risk for decreased contraceptive action, to maintain compliance with oral contraceptive use while using antibiotics, and to consider the use of additional nonhormonal contraception

DENTAL CONSIDERATIONS

General:
- Take precautions regarding allergy to medication.
- Determine why the patient is taking the drug.

Consultations:
- Medical consult may be required to assess disease control.

Teach patient/family:
- Importance of good oral hygiene to prevent soft tissue inflammation
- To avoid mouth rinses with high alcohol content due to drying effects and possible drug-drug reaction

When used for dental infection, advise patient:
- To report sore throat, oral burning sensation, fever, fatigue, any of which could indicate superinfection
- To take at prescribed intervals and complete dosage regimen
- To immediately notify the dentist if signs or symptoms of infection increase

---

celecoxib

(sel-e-cox′ib)

Celebrex

Drug class.: Nonsteroidal antiinflammatory

Action: May be related to a selective inhibition of inducible cyclooxygenase 2 (COX 2) enzymes preventing the synthesis of prostaglandins

Uses: Relief of signs and symptoms of osteoarthritis and relief of signs and symptoms of rheumatoid

---

arthritis in adults; also approved for reducing the number of intestinal polyps in patients with familial adenomatous polyposis; acute pain and primary dysmenorrhea

Dosage and routes:

Osteoarthritis
• *Adult:* PO 200 mg/day as a single dose or 100 mg bid

Rheumatoid arthritis
• *Adult:* PO 100-200 mg bid

Familial adenomatosis polyposis
• *Adult:* PO 400 mg bid with food

Available forms include: Caps 100, 200 mg

Side effects/adverse reactions:

▼ *ORAL:* Dry mouth, stomatitis, taste alteration

CNS: Headache, dizziness, insomnia, anxiety

CV: May aggravate hypertension, palpitation, syncope, ***CHF***

GI: Abdominal pain, diarrhea, dyspepsia, flatulence, nausea, **severe GI bleeding**

RESP: Pharyngitis, URI, aggravates bronchospasm

HEMA: Anemia, ecchymosis, ***thrombocytopenia***

GU: UTI, ***acute renal failure***

EENT: Rhinitis, sinusitis, tinnitus, deafness, blurred vision

INTEG: Skin rash, pruritus, urticaria, Sweet's syndrome (acute febrile neutrophilic dermatosis)

META: Hyperchloremia, hypophosphatemia, elevated BUN, elevated liver enzymes (SGOT, SGPT)

MS: Myalgia, arthralgia

MISC: ***Anaphylaxis,*** back pain

Contraindications: Hypersensitivity, allergy to sulfonamides, patients who have experienced asthma, urticaria, or allergic-type reactions to ASA or NSAIDs

Precautions: Geriatric patients weighing <50 kg use lowest dose,

children <18 yr, severe hepatic or renal impairment, upper active GI disease, GI bleeding, avoid in late pregnancy (category D after 34 wk), pregnancy category C, lactation, dehydrated patients, heart failure, hypertension, asthma

Pharmacokinetics:

PO: Fatty meal delays absorption, peak plasma levels 3 hr, half-life 11 hr, metabolism (CYP450 2C9), metabolites excreted in feces (57%) and urine (27%)

🦷 Drug interactions of concern to dentistry:

• Increased plasma levels: fluconazole
• Increased risk of GI bleeding: long-duration NSAIDs, aspirin (except low doses), oral glucocorticoids, alcoholism, smoking, older age, and generally poor health
• Increased plasma levels of lithium
• Possible risk of increased INR in elderly patients taking warfarin

DENTAL CONSIDERATIONS

General:

• Patients on chronic drug therapy may rarely have symptoms of blood dyscrasias, which can include infection, bleeding, and poor healing.
• Assess salivary flow as a factor in caries, periodontal disease, and candidiasis.
• Consider semisupine chair position for patient comfort due to disease and GI side effects of drug.

Teach patient/family:

• Importance of good oral hygiene to prevent soft tissue inflammation
• Importance of updating health and drug history if physician makes any changes in evaluation or drug regimens

• Use of electric toothbrush if patient has difficulty holding conventional devices

When chronic dry mouth occurs, advise patient:

• To avoid mouth rinses with high alcohol content due to drying effects

• To use daily home fluoride products for anticaries effect

• To use sugarless gum, frequent sips of water, or saliva substitutes

---

cephalexin/cephalexin HCl monohydrate

(sef-a-lex′in)

Cephalexin: Biocef, Keflex

✚ Apo-Cephalex,   Novo-Lexin, Nu-Cephalex, PMS-Cephalexin

Cephalexin HCl monohydrate: Keftab

Drug class.: Cephalosporin (first generation)

Action: Inhibits bacterial cell wall synthesis, rendering cell wall osmotically unstable

Uses: Use for the following infections when caused by susceptible microorganisms: respiratory tract infections caused by *S. pneumoniae, S. pyogenes;* otitis media caused by *S. pneumoniae, H. influenza, M. catarrhalis,* staphylococci, streptococci; skin and skin structure infections caused by staphylococci and streptococci; bone infections caused by staphylococci, *P. mirabilis;* genitourinary tract infections caused by *E. coli, P. mirabilis, K. pneumoniae*

Dosage and routes:

• *Adult:* PO 250-500 mg q6h, up to 4 g/day

• *Child:* PO 6.25-50 mg/kg/day in 4 equal doses

Moderate skin infections

• 500 mg q12h

Severe infections

• *Adult:* PO 500 mg-1 g q6h

• *Child:* PO 50-100 mg/kg/day in 4 equal doses

Dosage reduction indicated in renal impairment (CrCl <50 ml/min)

Bacterial endocarditis prophylaxis:

• *Adult:* PO 2 g 1 hr before dental procedure for those patients unable to take amoxicillin

• *Child:* PO 50 mg/kg of body weight 1 hr before dental procedure, not to exceed the adult dose for those patients unable to take amoxicillin

Available forms include: Caps 250, 500 mg; tabs 250, 500; oral susp 125, 250 mg/5 ml; pediatric susp 100 mg/ml; monohydrate tabs 500 mg

Side effects/adverse reactions:

▼ *ORAL:* Candidiasis, glossitis

CNS: Headache, dizziness, weakness, paresthesia, fever, chills

*GI: Nausea, vomiting, diarrhea, anorexia, **pseudomembranous colitis,** bleeding, increased AST/ALT, bilirubin, LDH, alk phosphatase, abdominal pain

*RESP: **Anaphylaxis,** dyspnea

*HEMA: **Leukopenia, thrombocytopenia, agranulocytosis, neutropenia, lymphocytosis, eosinophilia, pancytopenia, hemolytic anemia**

*GU: **Nephrotoxicity, renal failure,** proteinuria, vaginitis, pruritus, candidiasis, increased BUN

INTEG: Rash, urticaria, dermatitis

Contraindications: Hypersensitivity to cephalosporins, infants <1 mo

Precautions: Hypersensitivity to penicillins, pregnancy category B, lactation, renal disease

---

bold italic = life-threatening conditions

Pharmacokinetics:

PO: Peak 1 hr, duration 6-8 hr, half-life 30-72 min; 5%-15% bound by plasma proteins, 90%-100% eliminated unchanged in urine; crosses placenta; excreted in breast milk

🦷 **Drug interactions of concern to dentistry:**

• Decreased bactericidal effects: tetracyclines, erythromycins
• Increased and prolonged serum levels: probenecid
• Oral contraceptives: advise patient of a potential risk for decreased contraceptive action, to maintain compliance with oral contraceptive use while using antibiotics, and to consider the use of additional nonhormonal contraception

DENTAL CONSIDERATIONS

General:

• Take precautions regarding allergy to medication.
• Determine why the patient is taking the drug.

Consultations:

• Medical consult may be required to assess disease control.

Teach patient/family:

• Importance of good oral hygiene to prevent soft tissue inflammation
• To avoid mouth rinses with high alcohol content due to drying effects and possible drug-drug reaction

When used for dental infection, advise patient:

• To report sore throat, oral burning sensation, fever, fatigue, any of which could indicate superinfection
• To take at prescribed intervals and complete dosage regimen
• To immediately notify the dentist if signs or symptoms of infection increase

---

cephradine

(sef'ra-deen)

Velosef

Drug class.: Cephalosporin (first generation)

Action: Inhibits bacterial cell wall synthesis, rendering cell wall osmotically unstable

Uses: Gram-negative bacilli: *H. influenzae, E. coli, P. mirabilis, Klebsiella;* gram-positive organisms: *S. pneumoniae, S. pyogenes, S. aureus;* serious respiratory tract, urinary tract, and skin infections; otitis media

Dosage and routes:

• *Adult:* IM/IV 500 mg-1 g q4-6h, not to exceed 8 g/day; PO 250 mg-1 g q6-12h; limit PO dose to 4 g/day
• *Child >1 yr:* IM/IV 12-25 mg/kg q6h; PO 6-25 mg/kg q6h

Available forms include: Powder for inj IM/IV 250, 500 mg and 1, 2 g; caps 250, 500 mg; oral susp 125, 250 mg/5 ml in 100 ml and 200 ml

Side effects/adverse reactions:

▼ *ORAL:* Candidiasis, glossitis

CNS: Headache, dizziness, weakness, paresthesia, fever, chills

GI: Nausea, vomiting, diarrhea, anorexia, pseudomembranous colitis, bleeding, increased AST/ALT, bilirubin, LDH, alk phosphatase, abdominal pain

RESP: Anaphylaxis, dyspnea

HEMA: Leukopenia, thrombocytopenia, agranulocytosis, neutropenia, lymphocytosis, eosinophilia, pancytopenia, hemolytic anemia

GU: ***Nephrotoxicity, renal failure,*** proteinuria, vaginitis, pruritus, candidiasis, increased BUN

INTEG: Rash, urticaria, dermatitis

Contraindications: Hypersensitivity to cephalosporins, infants <1 mo

Precautions: Hypersensitivity to penicillins, pregnancy category B, lactation, renal disease

Pharmacokinetics:

PO: Peak 1 hr

IV: Peak 5 min

IM: Peak 1 hr Half-life 0.75-1.5 hr; 20% bound by plasma proteins, 80%-90% eliminated unchanged in urine; crosses placenta; excreted in breast milk

⚕ Drug interactions of concern to dentistry:

• Decreased bactericidal effects: tetracyclines, erythromycins

• Increased and prolonged serum levels: probenecid

• Oral contraceptives: advise patient of a potential risk for decreased contraceptive action, to maintain compliance with oral contraceptive use while using antibiotics, and to consider the use of additional nonhormonal contraception

DENTAL CONSIDERATIONS

General:

• Take precautions regarding allergy to medication.

• Determine why the patient is taking the drug.

Consultations:

• Medical consult may be required to assess disease control.

Teach patient/family:

• Importance of good oral hygiene to prevent soft tissue inflammation

• To avoid mouth rinses with high alcohol content due to drying effects and possible drug-drug reaction

When used for dental infection, advise patient:

• To report sore throat, oral burning sensation, fever, fatigue, any of which could indicate superinfection

• To take at prescribed intervals and complete dosage regimen

• To immediately notify the dentist if signs or symptoms of infection increase

---

cetirizine hydrochloride

(se-ti′ra-zeen)

Zyrtec

♣ Reactine

Drug class.: Antihistamine

Action: Competitive antagonist for peripheral H_1-receptors

Uses: Treatment of symptoms of seasonal allergic rhinitis, perennial allergic rhinitis, chronic urticaria

Dosage and routes:

• *Adult and child >12 yr:* PO 5-10 mg bid, limit 10 mg/day

• *Child 6-11 yr:* PO 5-10 mg once daily

• *Child 2-6 yr:* PO 2.5 mg once daily, can be increased to 5 mg once day or 2.5 mg bid if required

Available forms include: Tabs 5, 10 mg; syrup 5 mg/5 ml

Side effects/adverse reactions:

▼ *ORAL: Dry mouth (5%),* taste alteration, tongue edema, orofacial dyskinesia (all rare)

CNS: Sedation, drowsiness, dizziness, headache, somnolence, depression

CV: Palpitation, tachycardia, hypertension, cardiac failure

GI: Constipation, diarrhea

---

bold italic = life-threatening conditions

HEMA: **Hemolytic anemia, thrombocytopenia**
GU: Difficult urination, urinary retention, dysmenorrhea
EENT: Pharyngitis, dry nose or throat, tinnitus, earache
INTEG: Pruritus, rash, dry skin
MS: Myalgia, arthralgia
MISC: Photosensitivity
Contraindications: Hypersensitivity to cetirizine or hypersensitivity to hydroxyzine
Precautions: Renal impairment (requires dose reduction), elderly, glaucoma, urinary obstruction, pregnancy category not listed, lactation
Pharmacokinetics:
PO: Peak plasma levels 1 hr, duration up to 24 hr, half-life 8-11 hr; highly protein bound; rapid oral absorption, minimal metabolism; excreted mostly unchanged in urine
🦷 **Drug interactions of concern to dentistry:**
• No drug interactions reported, but should be similar to other antihistamines; anticipate increased sedation with other CNS depressants and increased anticholinergic effects with anticholinergic drugs
DENTAL CONSIDERATIONS
General:
• Assess salivary flow as factor in caries, periodontal disease, and candidiasis.
Teach patient/family: *When chronic dry mouth occurs, advise patient:*
• To avoid mouth rinses with high alcohol content due to drying effects
• To use daily home fluoride products for anticaries effect
• To use sugarless gum, frequent sips of water, or saliva substitutes

cevimeline
(ce-vi-me′leen)
Evoxac
Drug class.: Cholinergic (muscarinic) agonist

Action: Acts directly on cholinergic (muscarinic) receptor sites in the CNS and in exocrine glands (i.e., salivary glands); also binds to cholinergic receptors in the GI and GU tracts; derivative of acetylcholine; peripheral effects may resemble pilocarpine
Uses: Treatment of symptoms of dry mouth associated with Sjögren's syndrome
Dosage and routes:
• *Adult:* PO 30 mg tid (higher doses have not been demonstrated to provide greater effects)
Available forms include: Caps 30 mg
Side effects/adverse reactions:
▼ *ORAL: Salivation,* facial edema (rare), salivary gland enlargement, ulcerative stomatitis
CNS: Confusion, headache, dizziness, fatigue, insomnia
CV: Palpitation, chest pain
GI: Diarrhea, nausea, abdominal pain, vomiting
GU: Urinary frequency, sinusitis, UTI, polyuria
RESP: Rhinitis, URI, *coughing*
EENT: Pharyngitis, conjunctivitis, bronchitis, abnormal vision, eye pain, ear pain, visual blurring, lacrimation
INTEG: Diaphoresis, rash, allergy, erythematous rash
MS: Back pain*,* arthralgia
MISC: Asthenia, pain, skeletal pain
Contraindications: Hypersensi-

tivity, uncontrolled asthma, acute iritis, narrow-angle glaucoma

Precautions: Has the potential to alter heart rate or cardiac conduction; use with care in cardiovascular disease, asthma, bronchitis, COPD, seizure disorders, Parkinson's disease, urinary tract/bladder obstruction, cholecystitis, cholangitis, biliary obstruction, GI ulcers, pregnancy category C, lactation, children (no data), history of adverse effects to other cholinergic agonists

Pharmacokinetics:

PO: Good oral absorption, peak concentration in 1.5-2 hr, <20% bound to plasma proteins, half-life 4-6 hr, hepatic metabolism by cytochrome P-450 (CYP2D6 and CYP3A3/4), renal excretion (97%)

🦷 Drug interactions of concern to dentistry:

• Use with caution in patients taking β-adrenergic blockers: possible conduction disturbances.

• There are no specific data on dental drug interactions; however, use caution with other cholinergic agonist.

• There is always the possibility that a cholinergic antagonist could interfere with this drug's action.

• Although there are no supporting data, use with caution in patients taking drugs that inhibit cytochrome P-450 (CYP3A3/4 and CYP2D6).

DENTAL CONSIDERATIONS

General:

• Assess salivary flow as a factor in caries, periodontal disease, and candidiasis.

• Monitor vital signs every appointment due to possible cardiovascular side effects.

• Place on frequent recall to assess effectiveness.

Consultations:

• Medical consult may be required to assess disease control.

• Medical consult may be necessary before prescribing for those patients with cardiovascular or respiratory disease.

Teach patient/family:

• That this drug may cause visual disturbances, especially with night driving, which may impair driving safety

• That the patient should drink extra fluids (water) to compensate for excessive sweating

When chronic dry mouth occurs, advise patient:

• To avoid mouth rinses with high alcohol content due to drying effects

• Of need for daily home fluoride to prevent caries

• To use sugarless gum, frequent sips of water, or saliva substitutes

---

chloral hydrate

(klor-al hye'drate)

Aquachloral Supprettes

♣ Novo-Chlorhydrate,   PMS-Chloral Hydrate

Drug class.: Sedative-hypnotic, chloral derivative

Controlled Substance Schedule IV, Schedule F

Action: Active metabolite, trichloroethanol, produces mild CNS depression

Uses: Sedation, insomnia

Dosage and routes:

Sedative-hypnotic

• *Adult:* PO/REC 250 mg tid pc; preoperative 500 mg-1 g 30 min before surgery or bedtime

---

bold italic = life-threatening conditions

• *Child:* PO 25-50 mg/kg of body weight/day not to exceed 1 g/dose
Insomnia-hypnotic dose
• *Adult:* PO/REC 500 mg-1g 0.5 hr hs
Available forms include: Caps 500 mg; syr 250, 500 mg/5 ml; supp 325, 500, 648 mg
Side effects/adverse reactions:
▼ *ORAL:* Unpleasant taste, mucosal irritation
CNS: Drowsiness, dizziness, stimulation, nightmares, ataxia, hangover (rare), light-headedness, headache, paranoia
CV: Hypotension, dysrhythmias
GI: Nausea, vomiting, flatulence, diarrhea, **gastric necrosis**
RESP: Depression
HEMA: Eosinophilia, leukopenia
INTEG: Rash, urticaria, angioedema, fever, purpura, eczema
Contraindications: Hypersensitivity to this drug, severe renal disease, severe hepatic disease, GI disorders (oral forms), gastritis
Precautions: Severe cardiac disease, depression, suicidal individuals, asthma, intermittent porphyria, pregnancy category C, lactation, elderly; no specific reversal agent available, use extreme caution in dose calculation when used in pediatric patients for sedation
Pharmacokinetics:
PO: Onset 0.5-1 hr, duration 4-8 hr
REC: Onset slow, duration 4-6 hr; metabolized by liver; excreted by kidneys (inactive metabolite) and in feces; crosses placenta; excreted in breast milk; metabolite is highly protein bound
🥄 **Drug interactions of concern to dentistry:**
• Increased action of both drugs: alcohol, all CNS depressants, including nitrous oxide

DENTAL CONSIDERATIONS
General:
• Consider semisupine chair position for patient comfort due to GI effects of drug.
• Administer syrup in juice or beverage to mask taste and reduce GI upset.
• Contraindicated for use in patients with GI ulcerative disease.
• Have someone drive patient to and from dental office when used for conscious sedation.
• Geriatric patients are more susceptible to drug effects; use lower dose.
• Psychologic and physical dependence may occur with chronic administration.

---

chlorambucil
(klor-am'byoo-sil)
Leukeran
Drug class.: Antineoplastic alkylating agent

Action: Alkylates DNA, RNA; inhibits enzymes that allow synthesis of amino acids in proteins
Uses: Chronic lymphocytic leukemia, Hodgkin's disease, other lymphomas, macroglobulinemia, nephrotic syndrome, breast carcinoma, choriocarcinoma, ovarian carcinoma
Dosage and routes:
• *Adult:* PO 0.1-0.2 mg/kg/day for 3-6 wk initially, then 2-6 mg/day; maintenance 0.2 mg/kg for 2-4 wk; course may be repeated at 2-4 wk intervals
• *Child:* PO 0.1-0.2 mg/kg/day in divided doses or 4.5 mg/m^2/day as 1 dose or in divided doses
Available forms include: Tabs 2 mg

Side effects/adverse reactions:

▼ *ORAL: Stomatitis, sore mouth, lips*

CNS: **Convulsions in children**

GI: Nausea, vomiting, diarrhea, weight loss

RESP: **Fibrosis, pneumonitis**

HEMA: **Thrombocytopenia, leukopenia, pancytopenia** (prolonged use), **permanent bone marrow depression**

GU: Hyperuremia

INTEG: Alopecia (rare), dermatitis, rash

Contraindications: Radiation therapy within 1 mo, chemotherapy within 1 mo, thrombocytopenia, smallpox vaccination, pregnancy category D (first trimester)

Precautions: *Pneumococcus* vaccination

Pharmacokinetics:

PO: Half-life 2 hr; well absorbed orally; metabolized in liver; excreted in urine

🦷 **Drug interactions of concern to dentistry:**

• Increased seizures: haloperidol, loxapine, phenothiazines, thioxanthenes

• Increased blood dyscrasia: NSAIDs, dapsone, phenothiazines

• Increased infection: corticosteroids

DENTAL CONSIDERATIONS

General:

• Patients on chronic drug therapy may rarely have symptoms of blood dyscrasias, which can include infection, bleeding, and poor healing.

• Prophylactic antibiotics may be indicated to prevent infection if surgery or deep scaling is planned.

• Caution in prescribing NSAIDs or aspirin-containing products due to risk of GI bleeding.

• Determine why the patient is taking the drug.

• Patients receiving chemotherapy may require palliative treatment for stomatitis.

Consultations:

• In a patient with symptoms of blood dyscrasias, request a medical consult for blood studies and postpone dental treatment until normal values are reestablished.

• Medical consult may be required to assess disease control.

Teach patient/family:

• Importance of good oral hygiene to prevent soft tissue inflammation

• Caution against injury when using oral hygiene aids

• To avoid mouth rinses with high alcohol content due to drying effects

---

chlordiazepoxide HCl

(klor-dye-az-e-pox'ide)

Libritabs, Librium, Mitran, Reposans-10

♣ Apo-Chlordiazepoxide, Novo-Poxide

Drug class.: Benzodiazepine antianxiety

Controlled Substance Schedule IV

Action: Produces CNS depression by interacting with a benzodiazepine receptor to facilitate the action of the inhibitory neurotransmitter γ-aminobutyric acid (GABA)

Uses: Short-term management of anxiety, acute alcohol withdrawal, preoperatively for relaxation

Dosage and routes:

Mild anxiety

• *Adult:* PO 5-10 mg tid-qid

• *Child >6 yr:* PO 5 mg bid-qid, not to exceed 10 mg bid-tid

---

Severe anxiety
• *Adult:* PO 20-25 mg tid-qid
Preoperatively
• *Adult:* PO 5-10 mg tid-qid on day before surgery; IM 50-100 mg 1 hr before surgery
Alcohol withdrawal
• *Adult:* PO/IM/IV 50-100 mg, not to exceed 300 mg/day
Available forms include: Caps 5, 10, 25 mg; tabs 10, 25 mg; powder for IM inj 100 mg

Side effects/adverse reactions:
▼ *ORAL:* Dry mouth
CNS: Dizziness, drowsiness, confusion, headache, anxiety, tremors, stimulation, fatigue, depression, insomnia, hallucinations
CV: Orthostatic hypotension, ECG changes, tachycardia, hypotension
GI: Constipation, nausea, vomiting, anorexia, diarrhea
EENT: Blurred vision, tinnitus, mydriasis
INTEG: Rash, dermatitis, itching

Contraindications: Hypersensitivity to benzodiazepines, narrow-angle glaucoma, psychosis, pregnancy category D, child <18 yr; ritonavir, indinavir

Precautions: Elderly, debilitated, hepatic disease, renal disease

Pharmacokinetics:
PO: Onset 30 min, peak 30 min, duration 4-6 hr, half-life 5-30 hr; metabolized by liver; excreted by kidneys; crosses placenta, breast milk

⚕ Drug interactions of concern to dentistry:
• Delayed elimination: erythromycin
• Increased CNS depression: CNS depressants, alcohol
• Increased serum levels and prolonged effects of benzodiazepines:

ketoconazole, itraconazole, fluconazole, miconazole (systemic)
• Contraindicated with ritonavir, indinavir

DENTAL CONSIDERATIONS
General:
• After supine positioning, have patient sit upright for at least 2 min to avoid orthostatic hypotension.
• Assess salivary flow as a factor in caries, periodontal disease, and candidiasis.
• Psychologic and physical dependence may occur with chronic administration.
• Geriatric patients are more susceptible to drug effects; use lower dose.
• Have someone drive patient to and from dental office if used for conscious sedation.

Consultations:
• Medical consult may be required to assess disease control.

Teach patient/family:
• Importance of good oral hygiene to prevent soft tissue inflammation
• To avoid mouth rinses with high alcohol content due to drying effects

---

chlorhexidine gluconate

(klor-hex'i-deen)
Peridex, PerioGard

Drug class.: Antiinfective—oral rinse

Action: Adsorbed on tooth surfaces, dental plaque, and oral mucosa; a sustained reduction of plaque organisms occurs
Uses: Treatment of gingivitis; unlabeled use: acute aphthous ulcers and denture stomatitis

---

Dosage and routes:
Gingivitis
• *Adult:* Rinse 15 ml for 30 sec bid after brushing and flossing teeth; expectorate after rinsing
Denture stomatitis
• Soak dentures for 1-2 min bid, with patient following oral rinse instructions
Available forms include: Oral rinse, 0.12% in 16-oz bottles
Side effects/adverse reactions:
▼ *ORAL: Staining of teeth, tongue, and restorations; increased calculus formation; taste alteration;* mucosal desquamation and irritation; transient parotitis
Contraindications: Hypersensitivity
Precautions: Pregnancy category B, lactation, efficacy not established for children <18 yr, not intended for periodontitis
Pharmacokinetics: Approximately 30% of chlorhexidine is retained in the oral cavity and slowly released; poorly absorbed orally

👍 **Drug interactions of concern to dentistry:**
• Disulfiram-like effects due to alcohol content: antabuse, metronidazole
DENTAL CONSIDERATIONS
General:
• Perform dental examination and prophylaxis/scaling/root planing before starting rinse.
• Place on frequent recall due to oral side effects.
• Use discretion when prescribing to patients with anterior facial restorations with rough surfaces or margins.
Teach patient/family:
• Instruct patient to eat, brush, and floss before using rinse

• Do not rinse with water after using chlorhexidine
• Inform patient of oral side effects

---

chlorhexidine gluconate chip
(klor-hex'i-deen)
PerioChip
Drug class.: Antiinfective

Action: Interferes with the integrity of the bacterial cell membrane, causing leakage of the intracellular components; penetrates into the cell, precipitates the cytoplasm, and the cell dies; effective against numerous supragingival and subgingival bacteria
Uses: Adjunct to scaling and root planing for reduction of the subgingival bacterial flora
Dosage and routes:
• *Adult:* Insert chip into a periodontal pocket with probing depth ≥5 mm. Up to eight chips may be inserted per single visit. Treatment recommended once every 3 mo in pockets ≥5 mm in depth. If chip dislodges within 48 hr of placement, replace with new chip. Do not replace chips lost after 48 hr, but reevaluate in 3 mo. If chip is dislodged 7 days or more after placement, consider this a full course of treatment.
Available forms include: CHIP 2.5 mg
Side effects/adverse reactions:
▼ *ORAL: Localized pain, tenderness, aching, throbbing, toothache* Note: All other side effects reported did not differ from placebo chip
Contraindications: Hypersensitivity
Precautions: Not recommended

for acutely abscessed periodontal pocket, pregnancy category C, use in children not established

Pharmacokinetics:

TOP: 40% of chlorhexidine released in first 24 hr, remainder released over 7-10 days; no detectable plasma levels

Drug interactions of concern to dentistry:
• None reported

DENTAL CONSIDERATIONS
General:
• Avoid brushing or use of dental floss at site of chip placement.

Teach patient/family:
• Notify dentist immediately if chip is dislodged or if pain, swelling, or other symptoms occur

---

chloroquine HCl/ chloroquine phosphate
(klor'oh-kwin)
Aralen HCl, Aralen Phosphate
Drug class.: Antimalarial

Action: Inhibits parasite replications, transcription of DNA to RNA by forming complexes with DNA of parasite; unapproved: juvenile arthritis, rheumatoid arthritis, discoid or systemic lupus erythematosus, solar urticaria

Uses: Malaria caused by *P. vivax, P. malariae, P. ovale, P. falciparum* (some strains); rheumatoid arthritis; amebiasis

Dosage and routes:
Malaria suppression
• *Adult:* 500 mg on exactly the same day each week (500 mg phosphate = 300 mg base)
• *Child:* 5 mg/kg weekly, calculated as base, on same day each week; not to exceed adult dose

Rheumatoid arthritis
• *Adult:* PO up to 4 mg/kg/day

Available forms include: Tabs 250, 500 mg; inj IM 50 mg/ml

Side effects/adverse reactions:

▼ *ORAL:* Stomatitis, discolored mucosa, lichenoid drug reaction

CNS: **Convulsion,** headache, stimulation, fatigue, irritability, bad dreams, dizziness, confusion, psychosis, decreased reflexes

CV: Hypotension, heart block, asystole with syncope, ECG changes

GI: Nausea, vomiting, anorexia, diarrhea, cramps, weight loss

HEMA: **Thrombocytopenia, agranulocytosis, hemolytic anemia, leukopenia**

EENT: Blurred vision, corneal changes, retinal changes, difficulty focusing, tinnitus, vertigo, deafness, photophobia, corneal edema

INTEG: **Exfoliative dermatitis,** alopecia, pruritus, pigmentary changes, skin eruptions, lichenoid eruptions, eczema

Contraindications: Hypersensitivity, retinal field changes, porphyria, children (long-term use)

Precautions: Pregnancy category C, children, blood dyscrasias, severe GI disease, neurologic disease, alcoholism, hepatic disease, G6PD deficiency, psoriasis, eczema

Pharmacokinetics:
PO: Peak 1-2 hr, half-life 3-5 days; metabolized in the liver; excreted in urine, feces, breast milk; crosses placenta

Drug interactions of concern to dentistry:
• Hepatotoxicity: alcohol, hepatotoxic drugs

DENTAL CONSIDERATIONS
General:
• Patients on chronic drug therapy may rarely have symptoms of blood dyscrasias, which can include infection, bleeding, and poor healing.
• Avoid dental light in patient's eyes; offer dark glasses for patient comfort.
• Determine why the patient is taking the drug.
Consultations:
• In a patient with symptoms of blood dyscrasias, request a medical consult for blood studies and postpone dental treatment until normal values are reestablished.
Teach patient/family:
• Importance of good oral hygiene to prevent soft tissue inflammation
• To avoid mouth rinses with high alcohol content due to drying effects

---

chlorothiazide
(klor-oh-thye'a-zide)
Diurigen, Diuril
Drug class.: Thiazide diuretic

Action: Acts on distal tubule by increasing excretion of water, sodium, chloride, potassium
Uses: Edema, hypertension, diuresis
Dosage and routes:
Edema, hypertension
• *Adult:* PO/IV 500 mg-1 g qd in 2 divided doses
Diuresis
• *Child >6 mo:* PO 22 mg/kg/day in 2 divided doses
• *Child <6 mo:* PO up to 33 mg/kg/day in 2 divided doses

Available forms include: Tabs 250, 500 mg; oral susp 250 mg/5 ml; inj 500 mg
Side effects/adverse reactions:
▼ *ORAL: Dry mouth, increased thirst,* lichenoid drug reaction
CNS: Dizziness, fatigue, weakness, drowsiness, paresthesia, anxiety, depression, headache
CV: Irregular pulse, orthostatic hypotension, palpitation, volume depletion
GI: Nausea, vomiting, anorexia, hepatitis, constipation, diarrhea, cramps, pancreatitis, GI irritation
HEMA: Aplastic anemia, hemolytic anemia, leukopenia, agranulocytosis, thrombocytopenia, neutropenia
GU: Frequency, uremia, polyuria, glucosuria
EENT: Blurred vision
INTEG: Rash, urticaria, purpura, photosensitivity, fever
META: Hyperglycemia, hyperuricemia, hypomagnesemia, increased creatinine, BUN
ELECT: Hypokalemia, hypercalcemia, hyponatremia, hypochloremia
Contraindications: Hypersensitivity to thiazides or sulfonamides, anuria, renal decompensation, pregnancy category D
Precautions: Hypokalemia, renal disease, hepatic disease, gout, COPD, lupus erythematosus, diabetes mellitus, elderly
Pharmacokinetics:
PO: Onset 2 hr, peak 4 hr, duration 6-12 hr; crosses placenta; excreted in breast milk
🦷 Drug interactions of concern to dentistry:
• Increased photosensitization: tetracyclines

---

bold italic = life-threatening conditions

• Decreased hypotensive response, nephrotoxicity: indomethacin and other NSAIDs

DENTAL CONSIDERATIONS

General:
• Monitor vital signs every appointment due to cardiovascular side effects.
• After supine positioning, have patient sit upright for at least 2 min before standing to avoid orthostatic hypotension.
• Patients on chronic drug therapy may rarely have symptoms of blood dyscrasias, which can include infection, bleeding, and poor healing.
• Assess salivary flow as a factor in caries, periodontal disease, and candidiasis.
• Limit use of sodium-containing products such as saline IV fluids for patients with a dietary salt restriction.
• Stress from dental procedures may compromise cardiovascular function; determine patient risk.
• Short appointments and a stress reduction protocol may be required for anxious patients.
• Patients taking diuretics should be monitored for serum K^+ levels.

Consultations:
• In a patient with symptoms of blood dyscrasias, request a medical consult for blood studies and postpone dental treatment until normal values are reestablished.
• Medical consult may be required to assess disease control and patient's ability to tolerate stress.
• Physician should be informed if significant xerostomic side effects occur (increased caries, sore tongue, problems eating or swallowing, difficulty wearing prosthe-

sis) so a medication change can be considered.

Teach patient/family:
• Importance of good oral hygiene to prevent soft tissue inflammation
• Caution to prevent injury when using oral hygiene aids
When chronic dry mouth occurs, advise patient:
• To avoid mouth rinses with high alcohol content due to drying effects
• To use daily home fluoride products for anticaries effect
• To use sugarless gum, frequent sips of water, or saliva substitutes

---

chlorphenesin carbamate
(klor-fen′e-sin)
Maolate

Drug class.: Skeletal muscle relaxant, central acting

Action: Unknown; may be related to sedative properties; does not directly relax muscle or depress nerve conduction
Uses: Adjunct for relieving pain in acute, painful musculoskeletal conditions

Dosage and routes:
• *Adult:* PO 800 mg tid, maintenance 400 mg qid, not to exceed 8 wk
Available forms include: Tabs 400 mg

Side effects/adverse reactions:
CNS: Dizziness, weakness, drowsiness, headache, tremor, depression, insomnia, confusion
CV: Postural hypotension, tachycardia
GI: Nausea, vomiting, hiccups

HEMA: **Blood dyscrasias, leukopenia, thrombocytopenia, agranulocytosis**

EENT: Diplopia, temporary loss of vision

INTEG: Rash, pruritus, fever, facial flushing

SYST: **Anaphylaxis,** drug fever

Contraindications: Hypersensitivity, child <12 yr, intermittent porphyria, carbamate derivatives

Precautions: Renal disease, hepatic disease, addictive personality, pregnancy category unknown, elderly, lactation, using for >8 wk, impairment of mental alertness

Pharmacokinetics:

PO: Onset 0.5 hr, peak 1-2 hr, duration 4-6 hr, half-life 4 hr; metabolized by liver; excreted in urine; crosses placenta; excreted in breast milk (large amounts)

Drug interactions of concern to dentistry:

• Increased CNS depression: alcohol, tricyclic antidepressants, narcotics, barbiturates, sedatives, hypnotics

DENTAL CONSIDERATIONS

General:

• Patients on chronic drug therapy may rarely have symptoms of blood dyscrasias, which can include infection, bleeding, and poor healing.

• After supine positioning, have patient sit upright for at least 2 min to avoid orthostatic hypotension.

• Consider semisupine chair position for patient comfort if GI side effects occur.

Consultations:

• In a patient with symptoms of blood dyscrasias, request a medical consult for blood studies and postpone dental treatment until normal values are reestablished.

Teach patient/family:

• Importance of good oral hygiene to prevent soft tissue inflammation

• Caution to prevent trauma when using oral hygiene aids

• To report oral lesions, soreness, or bleeding to dentist

chlorpheniramine maleate

(klor-fen-eer′a-meen)

Aller-Chlor, Chlo-Amine, Chlor-Trimeton

♣ Chlor-Tripolon, Novo-Pheniram

Drug class.: Antihistamine, H_1-receptor antagonist

Action: Acts on blood vessels, GI system, respiratory system by competing with histamine for H_1-receptor site; decreases allergic response by blocking histamine

Uses: Allergy symptoms, rhinitis

Dosage and routes:

• *Adult and child >12 yr:* PO 2 mg tid-qid, not to exceed 36 mg/day; time rel 8-12 mg bid-tid, not to exceed 36 mg/day; IM/IV/SC 5-40 mg/day

• *Child 6-11 yr:* PO 1 mg q4-6h, not to exceed 12 mg/day

• *Child 2-5 yr:* PO 0.5 mg q4-6h, not to exceed 4 mg/day

Available forms include: Chew tabs 2 mg; tabs 4 mg; time rel tabs 8, 12 mg; time rel caps 8, 12 mg; syr 2 mg/5 ml; inj IM/SC/IV 10, 100 mg/ml

Side effects/adverse reactions:

▼ *ORAL:* Dry mouth

CNS: Dizziness, drowsiness, poor

coordination, fatigue, anxiety, euphoria, confusion, paresthesia, neuritis

GI: Nausea, anorexia, diarrhea

RESP: Increased thick secretions, wheezing, chest tightness

HEMA: **Thrombocytopenia, agranulocytosis, hemolytic anemia**

GU: Retention, dysuria, frequency

EENT: Blurred vision, dilated pupils, tinnitus, nasal stuffiness, dry nose, throat

INTEG: Photosensitivity

Contraindications: Hypersensitivity to H_1-receptor antagonists, acute asthma attack, lower respiratory tract disease

Precautions: Increased intraocular pressure, renal disease, cardiac disease, hypertension, bronchial asthma, seizure disorder, stenosed peptic ulcers, hyperthyroidism, prostatic hypertrophy, bladder neck obstruction, pregnancy category B, elderly

Pharmacokinetics:

PO: Onset 20-60 min, duration 8-12 hr, half-life 20-24 hr; detoxified in liver; excreted by kidneys (metabolites/free drug)

Drug interactions of concern to dentistry:

• Increased CNS depression: alcohol, all CNS depressants

• Increased anticholinergic effect: other anticholinergics, phenothiazines, tricyclic antidepressants

DENTAL CONSIDERATIONS

General:

• Assess salivary flow as a factor in caries, periodontal disease, and candidiasis.

• Consider semisupine chair position for patients with respiratory disease.

• Determine why the patient is taking the drug.

Teach patient/family:

• Importance of good oral hygiene to prevent soft tissue inflammation

• Caution to prevent injury when using oral hygiene aids

When chronic dry mouth occurs, advise patient:

• To avoid mouth rinses with high alcohol content due to drying effects

• To use daily home fluoride products for anticaries effect

• To use sugarless gum, frequent sips of water, or saliva substitutes

---

chlorpromazine HCl

(klor-proe'ma-zeen)

Thorazine

♣ Chlorpromanyl, Novo-Chlorpromazine

Drug class.: Phenothiazine antipsychotic

Action: Blocks neurotransmission at dopaminergic synapses in the cerebral cortex, hypothalamus, and limbic system; exhibits strong peripheral α-adrenergic, anticholinergic blocking action; mechanism for antipsychotic effects is unclear

Uses: Psychotic disorders, mania, schizophrenia, anxiety, intractable hiccups, nausea, vomiting, preoperatively for relaxation, acute intermittent porphyria, behavioral problems in children

Dosage and routes:

Psychiatry

• *Adult:* PO 10-50 mg q1-4h initially, then increase up to 2000 mg/day if necessary; IM 10-50 mg q1-4h

• *Child:* PO 0.25 mg/lb q4-6h or 0.5 mg/kg; IM 0.25 mg/lb q6-8h or

0.5 mg/kg; REC 0.5 mg/lb q6-8h or 1 mg/kg

Nausea and vomiting

• *Adult:* PO 10-25 mg q4-6h prn; IM 25-50 mg q3h prn; REC 50-100 mg q6-8h prn, not to exceed 400 mg/day; IV 25-50 mg qd-qid

• *Child:* PO 0.25 mg/lb q4-6h prn; IM 0.25 mg/lb q6-8h prn not to exceed 40 mg/day (<5 yr) or 75 mg/day (5-12 yr); REC 0.5 mg/lb q6-8h prn; IV 0.55 mg/kg q6-8h

Intractable hiccups

• *Adult:* PO 25-50 mg tid-qid; IM 25-50 mg (used only if PO dose does not work); IV 25-50 mg in 500-1000 ml saline (only for severe hiccups)

Available forms include: Tabs 10, 25, 50, 100, 200 mg; sus rel caps 30, 75, 150, 200, 300 mg; syr 10 mg/5 ml; conc 30, 100 mg/ml; supp 25, 100 mg; inj IM/IV 25 mg/ml

Side effects/adverse reactions:

▼ *ORAL: Dry mouth,* lichenoid reaction

CNS: Extrapyramidal symptoms: pseudoparkinsonism, akathisia, dystonia, tardive dyskinesia, seizures, headache

*CV: Orthostatic hypotension, **cardiac arrest, tachycardia,** hypertension, ECG changes*

GI: Nausea, vomiting, anorexia, constipation, diarrhea, jaundice, weight gain

*RESP: **Laryngospasm, respiratory depression,** dyspnea*

*HEMA: **Leukopenia, leukocytosis, agranulocytosis,** anemia*

GU: Urinary retention, urinary frequency, enuresis, impotence, amenorrhea, gynecomastia, breast engorgement

EENT: Blurred vision, glaucoma, dry eyes

INTEG: Rash, photosensitivity, dermatitis

Contraindications: Hypersensitivity, circulatory collapse, liver damage, cerebral arteriosclerosis, coronary disease, severe hypertension/hypotension, blood dyscrasias, coma, child <2 yr, brain damage, bone marrow depression, alcohol and barbiturate withdrawal states

Precautions: Pregnancy category C, lactation, seizure disorders, hypertension, hepatic disease, cardiac disease, elderly

Pharmacokinetics:

PO: Onset erratic, peak 2-4 hr, duration may be detected for up to 6 mo after last dose

IM: Onset 15-30 min, peak 15-20 min, duration may be detected for up to 6 mo after last dose

IV: Onset 5 min, peak 10 min, duration may be detected for up to 6 mo after last dose

REC: Onset erratic, peak 3 hr, elimination half-life 10-30 hr; 95% bound to plasma proteins; metabolized by liver; excreted in urine (metabolites); crosses placenta; enters breast milk

🦷 **Drug interactions of concern to dentistry:**

• Increased sedation: other CNS depressants, alcohol, barbiturate anesthetics, opioid analgesics

• Hypotension, tachycardia: epinephrine (systemic)

• Increased extrapyramidal effects: related drugs such as haloperidol, droperidol, and metoclopramide

• Additive photosensitization: tetracyclines

• Increased anticholinergic effects: anticholinergics

---

bold italic = life-threatening conditions

DENTAL CONSIDERATIONS
General:
• Monitor vital signs every appointment due to cardiovascular side effects.
• Patients on chronic drug therapy may rarely have symptoms of blood dyscrasias, which can include infection, bleeding, and poor healing.
• After supine positioning, have patient sit upright for at least 2 min before standing to avoid orthostatic hypotension.
• Assess salivary flow as a factor in caries, periodontal disease, and candidiasis.
• Avoid dental light in patient's eyes; offer dark glasses for patient comfort.
• Assess for presence of extrapyramidal motor symptoms, such as tardive dyskinesia and akathisia. Extrapyramidal motor activity may complicate dental treatment.
• Geriatric patients are more susceptible to drug effects; use a lower dose.

Consultations:
• In a patient with symptoms of blood dyscrasias, request a medical consult for blood studies and postpone dental treatment until normal values are reestablished.
• Take precautions if dental surgery is anticipated, anesthesia required.
• If signs of tardive dyskinesia or akathisia are present, refer to physician.
• Physician should be informed if significant xerostomic side effects occur (increased caries, sore tongue, problems eating or swallowing, difficulty wearing prosthesis) so a medication change can be considered.

Teach patient/family:
• Importance of good oral hygiene to prevent soft tissue inflammation
• Caution to prevent injury when using oral hygiene aids
• To use electric toothbrush if patient has difficulty holding conventional devices
When chronic dry mouth occurs, advise patient:
• To avoid mouth rinses with high alcohol content due to drying effects
• To use daily home fluoride products for anticaries effect
• To use sugarless gum, frequent sips of water, or saliva substitutes

---

chlorpropamide
(klor-proe′pa-mide)
Diabinese
♣ Apo-Chlorpromaide,   Novo-propamide
Drug class.: Antidiabetic, sulfonylurea (first generation)

Action: Causes functioning β-cells in pancreas to release insulin, leading to drop in blood glucose levels; may improve insulin binding to insulin receptors or increase the number of insulin receptors; not effective if patient lacks functioning β-cells
Uses: Stable adult-onset diabetes mellitus (type 2)
Dosage and routes:
• *Adult:* PO 100-250 mg qd, initially, then 100-500 mg maintenance according to response; not to exceed 750 mg/day
Available forms include: Tabs 100, 250 mg
Side effects/adverse reactions:
▼ *ORAL:* Lichenoid drug reaction
CNS: Headache, weakness, dizzi-

ness, drowsiness, tinnitus, fatigue, vertigo

GI: ***Hepatotoxicity, cholestatic jaundice,*** nausea, vomiting, diarrhea, heartburn

HEMA: ***Leukopenia, thrombocytopenia, agranulocytosis, aplastic anemia, pancytopenia, hemolytic anemia***

INTEG: Rash, allergic reactions, pruritus, urticaria, eczema, photosensitivity, erythema

ENDO: ***Hypoglycemia***

Contraindications: Hypersensitivity to sulfonylureas, juvenile or brittle diabetes, pregnancy category D

Precautions: Elderly, cardiac disease, thyroid disease, renal disease, hepatic disease, severe hypoglycemic reactions

Pharmacokinetics:

PO: Completely absorbed by GI route, onset 1 hr, peak 3-6 hr, duration 60 hr, half-life 36 hr; 90%-95% is plasma protein bound; metabolized in liver; excreted in urine (metabolites and unchanged drug), breast milk

🦷 Drug interactions of concern to dentistry:

• Increased hypoglycemic effects: salicylates, NSAIDs, ketoconazole, miconazole

• Decreased action: corticosteroids, sympathomimetics

DENTAL CONSIDERATIONS

General:

• Patients on chronic drug therapy may rarely have symptoms of blood dyscrasias, which can include infection, bleeding, and poor healing.

• Short appointments and a stress reduction protocol may be required for anxious patients.

• Question patient about self-mon-

itoring of drug's antidiabetic effect, including blood glucose values or finger-stick records.

• Ensure that patient is following prescribed diet and regularly takes medication.

• Determine if medication controls disease. Patients with diabetes may be more susceptible to infection and have delayed wound healing.

• Question patient about self-monitoring of drug's antidiabetic effect.

• Avoid prescribing aspirin-containing products.

Consultations:

• In a patient with symptoms of blood dyscrasias, request a medical consult for blood studies and postpone dental treatment until normal values are reestablished.

• Medical consult may be required to assess disease control.

• Medical consult may include data from patient's blood glucose monitoring, including glycosylated hemoglobin or HbA_{1c} testing.

Teach patient/family:

• Importance of good oral hygiene to prevent soft tissue inflammation

• Caution to prevent injury when using oral hygiene aids

• To avoid mouth rinses with high alcohol content due to drying effects

---

chlorthalidone

(klor-thal′i-done)

Hygroton, Thalitone

🍁 Apo-Chlorthalidone, Novo-Thalidone, Uridon

Drug class.: Diuretic with thiazide-like effects

Action: Acts on distal tubule by increasing excretion of water, sodium, chloride, potassium

---

Uses: Edema, hypertension, diuresis, CHF

Dosage and routes:
• *Adult:* PO 25-100 mg/day or 100-200 mg qid; adjust dose to response
• *Child:* PO 2 mg/kg 3 × weekly

Available forms include: Tabs 15, 25, 50, 100 mg

Side effects/adverse reactions:

▼ *ORAL: Dry mouth, increased thirst*

CNS: Dizziness, fatigue, weakness, drowsiness, paresthesia, anxiety, depression, headache

CV: Irregular pulse, orthostatic hypotension, palpitation, volume depletion

GI: Nausea, vomiting, anorexia, **hepatitis,** constipation, diarrhea, cramps, pancreatitis, GI irritation

HEMA: **Aplastic anemia, hemolytic anemia, leukopenia, agranulocytosis, thrombocytopenia, neutropenia**

GU: Frequency, **uremia,** glucosuria, polyuria

EENT: Blurred vision

INTEG: Rash, urticaria, purpura, photosensitivity, fever

META: Hyperglycemia, hyperuremia, increased creatinine, BUN

ELECT: Hypokalemia, hypomagnesemia, hypercalcemia, hyponatremia, hypochloremia

Contraindications: Hypersensitivity to thiazides or sulfonamides, anuria, renal decompensation

Precautions: Hypokalemia, renal disease, pregnancy category C, hepatic disease, gout, diabetes mellitus, elderly

Pharmacokinetics:

PO: Onset 2 hr, peak 6 hr, duration 24-72 hr, half-life 40 hr; excreted unchanged by kidneys; crosses placenta; enters breast milk

🦷 **Drug interactions of concern to dentistry:**
• Increased photosensitization: tetracyclines
• Decreased hypotensive response, nephrotoxicity: NSAIDs, indomethacin

DENTAL CONSIDERATIONS

General:
• Monitor vital signs every appointment due to cardiovascular side effects.
• After supine positioning, have patient sit upright for at least 2 min before standing to avoid orthostatic hypotension.
• Patients on chronic drug therapy may rarely have symptoms of blood dyscrasias, which can include infection, bleeding, and poor healing.
• Assess salivary flow as a factor in caries, periodontal disease, and candidiasis.
• Limit use of sodium-containing products such as saline IV fluids for those patients with a dietary salt restriction.
• Short appointments and a stress reduction protocol may be required for anxious patients.
• Stress from dental procedures may compromise cardiovascular function; determine patient risk.

Consultations:
• In a patient with symptoms of blood dyscrasias, request a medical consult for blood studies and postpone dental treatment until normal values are reestablished.
• Medical consult may be required to assess disease control and patient's ability to tolerate stress.

Teach patient/family:
• Importance of good oral hygiene to prevent soft tissue inflammation

• Caution to prevent injury when using oral hygiene aids

When chronic dry mouth occurs, advise patient:

• To avoid mouth rinses with high alcohol content due to drying effects

• To use daily home fluoride products for anticaries effect

• To use sugarless gum, frequent sips of water, or saliva substitutes

---

chlorzoxazone

(klor-zox′a-zone)

Paraflex, Parafon Forte DSC, Remular-S

Drug class.: Skeletal muscle relaxant, centrally acting

Action: Depresses multisynaptic pathways in the spinal cord

Uses: Adjunct for relief of muscle spasm in musculoskeletal conditions

Dosage and routes:

• *Adult:* PO 250-750 mg tid-qid

• *Child:* PO 20 mg/kg/day in divided doses tid-qid

Available forms include: Tabs 250, 500 mg; caplets 250, 500 mg (DSC)

Side effects/adverse reactions:

CNS: Dizziness, drowsiness, headache, insomnia, stimulation, malaise

*GI: Nausea, **hepatotoxicity, jaundice,*** vomiting, anorexia, diarrhea, constipation

*HEMA: **Granulocytopenia, anemia***

GU: Urine discoloration

*INTEG: **Angioedema,*** rash, pruritus, petechiae, ecchymoses

*SYST: **Anaphylaxis***

Contraindications: Hypersensitivity, impaired hepatic function

Precautions: Pregnancy category C, lactation, hepatic disease, elderly

Pharmacokinetics:

PO: Onset 1 hr, peak 3-4 hr, duration 6 hr, half-life 1 hr; metabolized in liver; excreted in urine (metabolites)

🦷 Drug interactions of concern to dentistry:

• Increased CNS depression: alcohol, narcotics, barbiturates, sedatives, hypnotics

DENTAL CONSIDERATIONS

General:

• Determine why the patient is taking the drug.

• Consider semisupine chair position if back is involved.

• When used for dental-related problems, consider aspirin or NSAIDs to improve response.

---

cholestyramine

(koe-less-teer′a-meen)

LoCholest Light, Prevalite, Questran, Questran Lite

Drug class.: Antihyperlipidemic

Action: Absorbs, combines with bile acids to form insoluble complex that is excreted through feces; loss of bile acids lowers cholesterol levels

Uses: Primary hypercholesterolemia, pruritus associated with biliary obstruction, diarrhea caused by excess bile acid, digitalis toxicity, xanthomas

Dosage and routes:

• *Adult:* PO 4 g qd or bid ac; maintenance dose 8-24 g in 2-6 divided doses

• *Child:* PO 4 g/day in 2 divided doses; administer with food or drink

---

bold italic = life-threatening conditions

Available forms include: 4 g cholestyramine in 5, 5.5, 5.7, 6.4, 9 g powder

Side effects/adverse reactions:

CNS: Headache, dizziness, drowsiness, vertigo, tinnitus

GI: Constipation, abdominal pain, nausea, fecal impaction, hemorrhoids, flatulence, vomiting, steatorrhea, peptic ulcer

HEMA: **Hyperchloremic acidosis; bleeding;** decreased pro-time, decreased vitamin A, D, K; red cell folate content

INTEG: Rash; irritation of perianal area, tongue, skin

MS: Muscle, joint pain

Contraindications: Hypersensitivity, biliary obstruction

Precautions: Pregnancy category C, lactation, children

Pharmacokinetics:

PO: Excreted in feces, max effect in 2 wk

🦷 **Drug interactions of concern to dentistry:**

• Decreased absorption of tetracyclines, cephalexin, phenobarbital, corticosteroids, clindamycin, penicillins; administer doses several hours apart

DENTAL CONSIDERATIONS

General:

• Consider semisupine chair position for patient comfort due to GI effects of disease.

---

choline salicylate

(koe′leen)

Arthropan

Drug class.: Salicylate analgesic

Action: Inhibits prostaglandin synthesis by interfering with cyclooxygenase need for biosynthesis; possesses analgesic, antipyretic, and antiinflammatory properties

Uses: Mild-to-moderate pain or fever, arthritis, juvenile rheumatoid arthritis

Dosage and routes:

Arthritis

• *Adult:* PO 870-1740 mg qid

Pain/fever

• *Adult and child >12 yr:* PO 870 mg q3-4h prn; maximum 6 doses/day

Available forms include: Liq 870 mg/5 ml (salicylate equivalent to 650 mg aspirin)

Side effects/adverse reactions:

CNS: **Coma, convulsions,** stimulation, drowsiness, dizziness, confusion, headache, flushing, hallucinations

CV: Rapid pulse, pulmonary edema

GI: Nausea, vomiting, GI bleeding, diarrhea, heartburn, **hepatitis,** anorexia

RESP: Wheezing, hyperpnea

HEMA: **Thrombocytopenia, agranulocytosis, leukopenia, neutropenia, hemolytic anemia,** increased pro-time

EENT: Tinnitus, hearing loss

INTEG: Rash, urticaria, bruising

ENDO: Hypoglycemia, hyponatremia, hypokalemia

Contraindications: Hypersensitivity to salicylates, GI bleeding, bleeding disorders, child <3 yr, vitamin K deficiency, child with flulike symptoms

Precautions: Anemia, hepatic disease, renal disease, Hodgkin's disease, pregnancy category C, lactation, geriatric patients

Pharmacokinetics:

PO: Onset 15-30 min; metabolized by liver; excreted by kidneys;

crosses placenta; excreted in breast milk

Drug interactions of concern to dentistry:
• Increased risk of hypoglycemia: oral hypoglycemics
• Increased risk of GI complaints: alcohol, NSAIDs, steroids
• Avoid prolonged or concurrent use with ASA, NSAIDs, corticosteroids, acetaminophen
• Increased effects of anticoagulants, valproic acid, methotrexate, dipyridamole
• Decreased effects of probenecid, sulfinpyrazone

DENTAL CONSIDERATIONS
General:
• Patients on chronic drug therapy may rarely have symptoms of blood dyscrasias, which can include infection, bleeding, and poor healing.
• Consider semisupine chair position for patient comfort if GI side effects occur.
• Determine why the patient is taking the drug.
• Evaluate allergic reactions: rash, urticaria; patients with allergy to salicylates may not be able to take NSAIDs. Drug may need to be discontinued.
• Consider semisupine chair position for patient comfort due to arthritic disease.

Consultations:
• In a patient with symptoms of blood dyscrasias, request a medical consult for blood studies and postpone dental treatment until normal values are reestablished.
• Medical consult may be required to assess disease control and patient's ability to tolerate stress.
• Tinnitus, ringing, roaring in ears

after high dose and long-term therapy requires referral for evaluation for salicylism.

Teach patient/family:
• Importance of good oral hygiene to prevent soft tissue inflammation
• Caution to prevent trauma when using oral hygiene aids
• To read label on other OTC drugs; many contain aspirin
• To report oral lesions, soreness, or bleeding to dentist
• To avoid alcohol ingestion; GI bleeding may occur

ciclopirox olamine (topical)

(sye-kloe-peer′ox)
Loprox, Penlac Nail Lacquer
Drug class.: Topical antifungal

Action: Interferes with fungal cell membrane, increasing its permeability and causing leaking of cell nutrients
Uses: Tinea cruris, tinea corporis, tinea pedis, tinea versicolor, cutaneous candidiasis, nail solution for immunocompetent patients with mild to moderate onychomycosis of nails without lunula involvement; caused by *T. rubrum*
Dosage and routes:
• *Adult and child >10 yr:* TOP rub into affected area bid; nail polish apply at bedtime; nail SOL apply solution once daily to all affected nails, used in a comprehensive care program for nails
Available forms include: Cream 1%, lotion 1%, nail polish 8%
Side effects/adverse reactions:
INTEG: Rash, urticaria, stinging, burning, pruritus, pain

---

bold italic = life-threatening conditions   *For periodic updates, visit* **www.mosby.com**

Contraindications: Hypersensitivity, systemic antifungal treatment

Precautions: Pregnancy category B, lactation, child <10 yr

DENTAL CONSIDERATIONS
General:
• There are neither dental drug interactions nor relevant considerations to dentistry for this drug.

---

cilostazol
(sil-oh'-sta-zol)
Pletal

Drug class.: Phosphodiesterase inhibitor

Action: Inhibits phosphodiesterase III enzymes, decreasing cAMP degradation to increase cAMP in platelets and blood vessels; inhibits platelet aggregation and causes vasodilation in vascular beds

Uses: Reduction of symptoms of intermittent claudication (leg pain on walking)

Dosage and routes:
• *Adult:* PO 100 mg bid at least 30 min before or 2 hr after breakfast and dinner
Note: with inhibitors of CYP3A4, give 50 mg bid

Available forms include: Tabs 50, 100 mg

Side effects/adverse reactions:
▼ *ORAL:* Glossitis, gingival bleeding
CNS: Headache, palpitation, dizziness, vertigo, tachycardia
CV: Peripheral edema
GI: Diarrhea, abdominal pain, dyspepsia, nausea, flatulence, vomiting
RESP: Bronchitis
HEMA: Anemia, purpura, ecchymosis

GU: UTI
EENT: Pharyngitis, rhinitis
INTEG: Dry skin, urticaria
META: Increased creatinine, hyperlipidemia, hyperuricemia
MS: Arthralgia, leg cramps
MISC: Infection, malaise, asthenia

Contraindications: Hypersensitivity, CHF

Precautions: Pregnancy category C, lactation, children

Pharmacokinetics:
PO: High-fat meal enhances absorption; metabolized by cytochrome P-450 enzymes (3A4); active metabolites, peak plasma levels 2-3 hr; highly protein bound (95%-98%)

⚡ Drug interactions of concern to dentistry:
• Risk of interaction with other platelet aggregation inhibitors possible, not established
• Risk of drug interaction with cytochrome P-450 3A4 inhibitors: erythromycin, ketoconazole, itraconazole, diltiazem, clarithromycin, grapefruit juice

DENTAL CONSIDERATIONS
General:
• Determine why patient is taking the drug.
• Avoid products that affect platelet function, such as aspirin and NSAIDs.

Consultations:
• Consultation with physician may be needed if excessive bleeding occurs during dental treatment.
• Consult should include data on bleeding time.

Teach patient/family:
• Importance of updating health and drug history if physician makes any changes in evaluation or drug regimens

---

• To inform dentist of unusual bleeding episodes following dental treatment
• To prevent trauma when using oral hygiene aids
• Importance of good oral hygiene to prevent soft tissue inflammation

---

cimetidine
(sye-met'i-deen)
Tagamet, Tagamet HB (OTC)
♣ Apo-Cimetidine, Gen-Cimetidine, Novo-Cimetidine, PMS-Cimetidine
Drug class.: H$_2$ histamine receptor antagonist

Action: Inhibits histamine at H$_2$-receptor site in parietal cells, which inhibits gastric acid secretion
Uses: Short-term treatment of duodenal and gastric ulcers and maintenance
Dosage and routes:
Duodenal ulcer
• *Adult:* PO preferred dose 800 mg hs for 4-8 wk, heavy smokers and conditions involving larger ulcers may require 1600 mg hs. Other regimens are 300 mg qid at meals and hs; or 400 mg bid (AM and hs); treatment should continue 4-8 wk; maintenance dose is 400 mg hs; IV bol 300 mg/20 ml 0.9% NaCl over 1-2 min q6h; IV inf 300 mg/50 ml D$_5$W over 15-20 min; IM 300 mg q6h, not to exceed 2400 mg
Heartburn/acid indigestion (OTC dose): PO 200 mg qd up to bid
GERD
• *Adult:* PO 800 mg bid or 400 mg qd × 12 wk

Available forms include: Tabs (100 mg OTC) 200, 300, 400, 800 mg; liq 300 mg/5 ml; inj 150 mg/ml, 300 mg/2 ml, 300 mg/50 ml 0.9% NaCl
Side effects/adverse reactions:
▼ *ORAL:* Lichenoid reaction
CNS: Confusion, headache, convulsions, depression, dizziness, anxiety, weakness, psychosis, tremors
CV: Bradycardia, tachycardia
GI: Diarrhea, paralytic ileus, jaundice, abdominal cramps
HEMA: Agranulocytosis, thrombocytopenia, neutropenia, aplastic anemia, increase in pro-time
GU: Gynecomastia, galactorrhea, impotence, increase in BUN, creatinine
INTEG: Exfoliative dermatitis, urticaria, rash, alopecia, sweating, flushing
Contraindications: Hypersensitivity, concurrent use with dofetilide
Precautions: Pregnancy category B, lactation, child <12 yr, organic brain syndrome, hepatic disease, renal disease
Pharmacokinetics:
PO: Peak 1-1.5 hr, half-life 1.5 hr; metabolized by liver; excreted in urine (unchanged); crosses placenta; enters breast milk
Drug interactions of concern to dentistry:
• GI ulceration, bleeding: aspirin, NSAIDs
• Decreased absorption: sodium bicarbonate
• Decreased absorption of fluconazole, ketoconazole, tetracycline (take doses 2 hr apart)
• Increased blood levels of metronidazole, alcohol, lidocaine, narcotic analgesics

---

bold italic = life-threatening conditions

DENTAL CONSIDERATIONS
General:
• Monitor vital signs every appointment due to cardiovascular side effects.
• Consider semisupine chair position for patient comfort due to GI effects of disease.
• Avoid prescribing aspirin or NSAID-containing products in patients with active upper GI disease; there is a risk of irritation and ulceration.
• Sodium bicarbonate products can be used 1 hr before or 1 hr after cimetidine dose.

Teach patient/family:
• Importance of good oral hygiene to prevent soft tissue inflammation
• Caution to prevent injury when using oral hygiene aids

---

cinoxacin
(sin-ox'a-sin)
Cinobac

Drug class.: Urinary tract antibacterial

Action: Interferes with DNA replication

Uses: UTIs caused by *E. coli, Klebsiella, Enterobacter, P. mirabilis, P. vulgaris, P. morganii, Serratia, Citrobacter*

Dosage and routes:
• *Adult:* PO 1 g/day in 2-4 divided doses × 1-2 wk

Available forms include: Caps 250, 500 mg

Side effects/adverse reactions:
CNS: Dizziness, headache, agitation, insomnia, confusion
GI: Nausea, vomiting, anorexia, abdominal cramps, diarrhea

EENT: Sensitivity to light, visual disturbances, blurred vision, tinnitus
INTEG: Pruritus, rash, urticaria, photosensitivity, edema

Contraindications: Hypersensitivity to this drug, anuria, CNS damage

Precautions: Renal disease, hepatic disease, pregnancy category C, lactation

Pharmacokinetics:
PO: Duration 6-8 hr, half-life 1.5 hr; excreted in urine (unchanged/inactive metabolites)

DENTAL CONSIDERATIONS
General:
• Be aware that the patient has a UTI.

Consultations:
• May need to consult with physician when it is necessary to prescribe antiinfectives for a dental infection.

---

ciprofloxacin
(sip-roe-flox'a-sin)
Cipro, Cipro IV

Drug class.: Fluoroquinolone antiinfective

Action: A broad spectrum bactericidal agent that inhibits the enzymes topoisomerase II (DNA gyrase) and topoisomerase IV, which are required for bacterial DNA replication, transcription, repair, and recombination

Uses: Adult UTIs (including complicated) caused by *E. coli, E. cloacae, P. mirabilis, K. pneumoniae, C. freundi, S. epidermidis,* and others; lower respiratory tract infections caused by *H. parainfluenzae, H. influenzae, K. pneumoniae, E. coli, E. cloacae;* chronic bacterial prostatitis; skin and skin structure infections, bone/joint infections caused by *E. cloacae, S. marcescens, P. aeruginosa,* infectious diarrhea, typhoid fever, STDs, and acute uncomplicated cystitis in females; postexposure inhalational anthrax

Dosage and routes:
Uncomplicated UTIs
• *Adult:* PO 250 mg q12h; IV 200 mg q12h for 7-14 days; 3-day regimen: PO 100 mg bid q3d

Complicated/severe UTIs/nosocomial pneumonia
• *Adult:* PO 500 mg q12h for 7-14 days; IV 400 mg q12h

Lower respiratory tract infections (mild to moderate)
• *Adult:* PO 500 mg q12h, IV 400 mg q12h

Bone and joint infections
• *Adult:* PO 500-750 mg q12h for 4-6 wk

Postexposure inhalational anthrax
• *Adult:* PO 500 mg bid up to 60 days

Available forms include: Tabs 100, 250, 500, 750 mg; IV 200 mg/100 ml D₅W, 400 mg/200 ml D₅W; 200, 400 mg vial

Side effects/adverse reactions:
▼ *ORAL:* Candidiasis, unpleasant taste
CNS: Headache, dizziness, fatigue, insomnia, depression, restlessness, tremors, confusion, hallucinations
GI: Nausea, vomiting, diarrhea, abdominal pain, constipation, increased ALT/AST, flatulence, insomnia, heartburn, dysphagia, pseudomembranous colitis
INTEG: Rash, pruritus, urticaria, photosensitivity, flushing, fever, chills
GU: Vaginitis

EENT: Blurred vision, diplopia, tinnitus, phototoxicity
MS: Tendinitis, tendon rupture, arthralgia
META: Elevation of liver enzymes ALT, AST
MISC: Anaphylaxis
Contraindications: Hypersensitivity to quinolines
Precautions: Pregnancy category C, lactation, children, renal disease, tendon ruptures of shoulder, hand, and Achilles tendons, epilepsy, severe cerebral arteriosclerosis

Pharmacokinetics:
PO: Peak 1 hr, half-life 3-4 hr; steady state 2 days; excreted in urine as active drug, metabolites

☙ **Drug interactions of concern to dentistry:**
• Decreased absorption: divalent, trivalent antacids, iron and zinc salts
• Increased serum levels: probenecid
• Increased risk of bleeding with warfarin (monitor)
• Serious adverse effects with theophylline

DENTAL CONSIDERATIONS
General:
• Determine why the patient is taking the drug.
• Avoid dental light in patient's eyes; offer dark glasses for patient comfort.
• Minimize exposure to sunlight and wear sunscreen if sun exposure is planned.
• Ruptures of the shoulder, hand, and Achilles' tendon that required surgical repair or resulted in prolonged disability have been reported with this drug.
Consultations:
• Consult with patient's physician

if an acute dental infection occurs and another antiinfective is required.

Teach patient/family:

• To discontinue treatment and inform dentist immediately if patient experiences pain or inflammation of a tendon, and to rest and refrain from exercise

---

ciprofloxacin HCl
(sip-roe-flox′a-sin)
Ciloxan

Drug class.: Topical fluoroquinolone antiinfective

Action: A broad-spectrum bactericidal agent that inhibits the enzyme DNA gyrase needed for bacterial DNA replication
Uses: Infections caused by susceptible strains of microorganisms in conjunctivitis or corneal ulcers
Dosage and routes:
Bacterial conjunctivitis
• *Adult:* TOP solution 1-2 gtt q2h while awake × 2 days; then 1-2 gtt q4h while awake for 5 days; ointment: apply ½-inch ribbon of ointment tid × 2 days; then ½-inch ribbon bid for 5 days
Corneal ulcers:
• *Adult:* TOP solution 2 gtt in affected eye q15min × 6 hr, then 2 gtt q30min for rest of the day; on day two, 2 gtt hourly; on days 3 through 14, 2 gtt q4h
Available forms include: Sol 3.5 mg/ml in 2.5, 5 ml; oint 3.5 mg
Side effects/adverse reactions:
▼ *ORAL:* Bad taste
GI: Nausea
EENT: Burning, discomfort, eyelid

crusting, scale, white crystalline deposits, itching, foreign body sensation, blurred vision, eye pain
INTEG: Dermatitis
MISC: Allergic reactions
Contraindications: Hypersensitivity to fluoroquinolones or any ingredient in these preparations
Precautions: Prolonged use and risk of resistant microorganisms, do not contaminate sterile product
Pharmacokinetics:
TOP: Minimal systemic absorption with oral solution; no other data available
🦷 **Drug interactions of concern to dentistry:**
• Specific studies have not been conducted with topical ciprofloxacin. See systemic drug for interactions.
DENTAL CONSIDERATIONS
General:
• Protect patient's eyes from accidental spatter during dental treatment.
• Avoid dental light in patient's eyes; offer dark glasses for patient comfort.

---

citalopram hydrobromide
(ce′tal-o-pram)
Celexa

Drug class.: Antidepressant

Action: Selectively inhibits the reuptake of serotonin
Uses: Major depression
Dosage and routes:
• *Adult:* PO initial 20 mg once daily; can increase dose in 20 mg increments at intervals of at least 1 wk; doses >40 mg once daily generally not recommended

Elderly or hepatic impairment
• *Elderly:* PO 20 mg qd/daily limit
Available forms include: Tabs 20, 40 mg; oral sol 10 mg/5 ml
Side effects/adverse reactions:
▼ *ORAL: Dry mouth,* unspecified dysphagia, teeth grinding, gingivitis
CNS: Dizziness, insomnia, somnolence, agitation, fatigue, anxiety, decreased libido
CV: Tachycardia, postural hypotension, hypotension
GI: Nausea, vomiting, dyspepsia, abdominal pain
RESP: URI, cough
HEMA: Purpura, anemia
GU: Ejaculation disorder, impotence
EENT: Rhinitis, sinusitis
INTEG: Rash, pruritus
MS: Asthenia, tremor, arthralgia, myalgia
MISC: Sweating, fever, alcohol intolerance
Contraindications: Hypersensitivity, concurrent use of MAO inhibitor
Precautions: Activation of mania, hypomania, seizure disorders, hepatic impairment, pregnancy category C, lactation, safe use in children unknown, reduce doses in elderly
Pharmacokinetics:
PO: Peak blood levels approximately 4 hr, bioavailability 80%, hepatic metabolism, three active metabolites, enterohepatic circulation, fecal and renal excretion
🍃 **Drug interactions of concern to dentistry:**
• Possibly increased CNS depression: all CNS depressants, alcohol
• Decrease in plasma levels: carbamazepine

• Increase in plasma levels: macrolide antibiotics, ketoconazole, itraconazole, omeprazole

DENTAL CONSIDERATIONS
General:
• Evaluate for TMJ therapy if bruxism causes symptoms of pain.
• Assess salivary flow as a factor in caries, periodontal disease, and candidiasis.
• Monitor vital signs every appointment due to cardiovascular and respiratory side effects.
• After supine positioning, have patient sit upright for 2 min or more to avoid orthostatic hypotension.
• Consider semisupine chair position for patient comfort due to GI side effects of drug.
• Short appointments and a stress reduction protocol may be required for anxious patients.
Consultations:
• Medical consult may be required to assess disease control and patient's ability to tolerate stress.
• Physician should be informed if significant xerostomic side effects occur (e.g., increased caries, sore tongue, problems eating or swallowing, difficulty wearing prosthesis) so a medication change can be considered.
Teach patient/family:
• Importance of good oral hygiene to prevent soft tissue inflammation
• Use of electric toothbrush if patient has difficulty holding conventional devices
When chronic dry mouth occurs, advise patient:
• To avoid mouth rinses with high alcohol content due to drying effects
• To use daily home fluoride products for anticaries effect

• To use sugarless gum, frequent sips of water, or saliva substitutes

---

clarithromycin

(kla-rith'roe-mye-sin)

Biaxin, Biaxin Filmtab, Biaxin XL

Drug class.: Macrolide antibiotic

Action: Binds to 50S ribosomal subunits of susceptible bacteria and suppresses protein synthesis

Uses: Mild-to-moderate infections of the upper/lower respiratory tract; community-acquired pneumonia caused by *H. influenzae;* uncomplicated skin and skin structure infections caused by *S. pneumoniae, M. pneumoniae, C. diphtheriae, B. pertussis, L. monocytogenes, H. influenzae, S. pyogenes, S. aureus;* otitis media; maxillary sinusitis, bronchitis (XL dose form); middle ear infection; disseminated MAC (mycobacterium avium complex); unlabeled use with omeprazole or ranitidine for *H. pylori* duodenal ulcer

Dosage and routes:

• *Adult:* PO 250-500 mg bid for 7-14 days; ext rel tab 1000 mg once daily × 7 days (bronchitis) or 14 days (sinusitis), to be taken with food

Bacterial endocarditis prophylaxis

• *Adult:* PO for patients allergic to amoxicillin, 500 mg 1 hr before dental procedure

• *Child:* PO for patients allergic to amoxicillin, 15 mg/kg of body weight not to exceed the adult dose 1 hr before dental procedure

Eradicating H. pylori (double therapy)

• *Adult:* PO (days 1-14) 500 mg clarithromycin tid plus omeprazole 20 mg bid qAM; days 15-28 omeprazole 20 mg every morning

Eradicating H. pylori (triple therapy)

• *Adult:* PO 500 mg clarithromycin plus 30 mg lansoprazole plus 1 g amoxicillin q12h for 14 days

Available forms include: Tabs 250, 500 mg; ext rel 500 mg; susp 125 mg/5 ml and 250 mg/ml in 50, 100 ml

Side effects/adverse reactions:

▼ *ORAL: Abnormal taste,* candidiasis, stomatitis

*GI: Nausea, abdominal pain, diarrhea, **hepatotoxicity,** heartburn, anorexia, vomiting*

GU: Vaginitis, moniliasis

INTEG: Rash, urticaria, pruritus

MISC: Headache

Contraindications: Hypersensitivity, indinavir

Precautions: Pregnancy category C, lactation, hepatic and renal disease

Pharmacokinetics:

PO: Peak 2 hr, duration 12 hr, half-life 4-6 hr; metabolized by the liver; excreted in bile, feces

🦷 **Drug interactions of concern to dentistry:**

• Decreased effect: anticholinergic drugs

• Increased effects of cyclosporine, warfarin, cilostazol, tacrolimus, pimozide, methylprednisolone

• Decreased action of clindamycin, penicillins, lincomycin, rifabutin, rifampin, zidovudine

• Increased serum levels of carbamazepine, theophylline, digoxin

• Contraindicated with indinavir

• Suspected risk of increased CNS depression with alprazolam, diazepam, midazolam, triazolam

• Oral contraceptives: advise patient of a potential risk for de-

creased contraceptive action, to maintain compliance with oral contraceptive use while using antibiotics, and to consider the use of additional nonhormonal contraception

DENTAL CONSIDERATIONS
General:
• Determine why the patient is taking the drug.
• May prove to be an alternative drug of choice for mild infections due to a susceptible organism in patients who are allergic to penicillin.

Teach patient/family:
• Importance of good oral hygiene to prevent soft tissue inflammation
When used for dental infection, advise patient:
• To report sore throat, oral burning sensation, fever, fatigue, any of which could indicate superinfection
• To take at prescribed intervals and complete dosage regimen
• To immediately notify the dentist if signs or symptoms of infection increase

---

clemastine fumarate
(klem′as-teen)
Antihist-1, Tavist-1
♣ Tavist
Drug class.: Antihistamine, H$_1$-receptor antagonist

Action: Acts on blood vessels, GI, respiratory system by competing with histamine for H$_1$-receptor site; decreases allergic response by blocking histamine
Uses: Allergy symptoms, rhinitis, angioedema, urticaria, common cold

Dosage and routes:
• *Adult and child >12 yr:* PO 1.34-2.68 mg bid-tid, not to exceed 8.04 mg/day
Available forms include: Tabs 1.34, 2.68 mg; syr 0.67 mg/5 ml
Side effects/adverse reactions:
▼ *ORAL:* Dry mouth
CNS: Dizziness, drowsiness, poor coordination, fatigue, anxiety, euphoria, confusion, paresthesia, neuritis
CV: Hypotension, palpitation, tachycardia
GI: Constipation, nausea, vomiting, anorexia, diarrhea
RESP: Increased thick secretions, wheezing, chest tightness
HEMA: ***Thrombocytopenia, agranulocytosis, hemolytic anemia***
GU: Retention, dysuria, frequency
EENT: Blurred vision, dilated pupils, tinnitus, nasal stuffiness, dry nose/throat
INTEG: Rash, urticaria, photosensitivity
Contraindications: Hypersensitivity to H$_1$-receptor antagonists, acute asthma attack, lower respiratory tract disease
Precautions: Increased intraocular pressure, renal disease, cardiac disease, hypertension, bronchial asthma, seizure disorder, stenosed peptic ulcers, hyperthyroidism, prostatic hypertrophy, bladder neck obstruction, pregnancy category B, elderly
Pharmacokinetics:
PO: Peak 5-7 hr, duration 10-12 hr or more; metabolized in liver; excreted by kidneys
🦷 **Drug interactions of concern to dentistry:**
• Increased CNS depression: all CNS depressants, alcohol

• Increased anticholinergic effect of anticholinergics, phenothiazines, tricyclic antidepressants

DENTAL CONSIDERATIONS
General:
• Assess salivary flow as a factor in caries, periodontal disease, and candidiasis.
• Determine why the patient is taking the drug.

Teach patient/family:
• Importance of good oral hygiene to prevent soft tissue inflammation
• Caution to prevent injury when using oral hygiene aids

When chronic dry mouth occurs, advise patient:
• To avoid mouth rinses with high alcohol content due to drying effects
• To use daily home fluoride products for anticaries effect
• To use sugarless gum, frequent sips of water, or saliva substitutes

---

clidinium bromide
(kli-di'nee-um)
Quarzan
Drug class.: GI anticholinergic

Action: Inhibits muscarinic actions of acetylcholine at postganglionic parasympathetic neuroeffector sites
Uses: Treatment of peptic ulcer disease in combination with other drugs

Dosage and routes:
• *Adult:* PO 2.5-5 mg tid-qid ac, hs
• *Elderly:* PO 2.5 mg tid ac
Available forms include: Caps 2.5, 5 mg

Side effects/adverse reactions:
▼ *ORAL: Dry mouth,* taste alteration
CNS: Confusion, stimulation in el-

derly, headache, insomnia, dizziness, drowsiness, anxiety, weakness, hallucinations
CV: Palpitation, tachycardia
*GI: Constipation, **paralytic ileus,*** heartburn, nausea, vomiting, dysphagia
GU: Hesitancy, retention, impotence
EENT: Blurred vision, photophobia, mydriasis, cycloplegia, increased ocular tension
INTEG: Urticaria, rash, pruritus, anhidrosis, fever, allergic reactions
Contraindications: Hypersensitivity to anticholinergics, narrow-angle glaucoma, GI obstruction, myasthenia gravis, paralytic ileus, GI atony, toxic megacolon
Precautions: Hyperthyroidism, coronary artery disease, dysrhythmias, CHF, ulcerative colitis, hypertension, hiatal hernia, hepatic disease, renal disease, pregnancy category C, urinary retention, prostatic hypertrophy, elderly

Pharmacokinetics:
PO: Onset 1 hr, duration 3 hr; excreted in urine

⚡ Drug interactions of concern to dentistry:
• Increased anticholinergic effect: atropine, scopolamine, tricyclic antidepressants, antihistamines, opioid analgesics, and other drugs with anticholinergic actions
• Decreased effects of: ketoconazole

DENTAL CONSIDERATIONS
General:
• Assess salivary flow as a factor in caries, periodontal disease, and candidiasis.
• Avoid dental light in patient's eyes; offer dark glasses for patient comfort.

Consultations:
• Physician should be informed if significant xerostomic side effects occur (increased caries, sore tongue, problems eating or swallowing, difficulty wearing prosthesis) so a medication change can be considered.
Teach patient/family:
• Importance of good oral hygiene to prevent soft tissue inflammation *When chronic dry mouth occurs, advise patient:*
• To avoid mouth rinses with high alcohol content due to drying effects
• Of need for daily home fluoride to prevent caries
• To use sugarless gum, frequent sips of water, or saliva substitutes

---

clindamycin HCl/ clindamycin palmitate HCl/clindamycin phosphate
(klin-da-mye′sin)
Cleocin, Cleocin Pediatric
♣ Dalacin C Flavored Granules
Drug class.: Lincomycin derivative antiinfective

Action: Binds to 50S subunit of bacterial ribosomes, suppresses protein synthesis
Uses: Indications for use include serious infections caused by susceptible anaerobic bacteria and the treatment of serious infections due to susceptible strains of pneumococci and streptococci. This includes infections of the respiratory tract, serious skin and soft tissue infections, intraabdominal abscess, and infections of the female GU tracts.

Dosage and routes:
• *Adult:* PO 150-450 mg q6h; IM/IV 300 mg q6-12h, not to exceed 4800 mg/day; dose and duration determined by seriousness of the infection
• *Child >1 mo:* PO 8-25 mg/kg/day in divided doses q6-8h; IM/IV 15-40 mg/kg/day in divided doses q6-8h 3-4 equal doses; dose and duration determined by seriousness of the infection
PID
• *Adult:* IV 600 mg qid plus gentamicin
Bacterial endocarditis prophylaxis
• *Adult:* PO in patients allergic to amoxicillin, 600 mg 1 hr before dental procedure; IV for patients unable to take oral medications, 600 mg 1 hr before dental procedure
• *Child:* PO in patients allergic to amoxicillin, 20 mg/kg of body weight, not to exceed the adult dose, 1 hr before dental procedure; IV for patients unable to take oral medications, 20 mg/kg of body weight, not to exceed the adult dose, 1 hr before dental procedure
Prosthetic joint prophylaxis (when indicated)
• *Adult:* PO 600 mg 1 hr before dental procedure; IV for patients unable to take oral medications, 600 mg 1 hr before dental procedure
Available forms include: Inj 300 mg/ml, 2, 4, 6 ml; caps 75, 150, 300 mg; oral sol 75 mg/ml
Side effects/adverse reactions:
▼ *ORAL:* Candidiasis
*GI: Nausea, vomiting, abdominal pain, diarrhea, **pseudomembranous colitis,** anorexia, weight loss*

---

bold italic = life-threatening conditions

*HEMA: **Leukopenia, eosinophilia, agranulocytosis, thrombocytopenia***
GU: Vaginitis, increased AST/ALT, bilirubin, alk phosphatase, jaundice, urinary frequency
EENT: Rash, urticaria, pruritus, erythema, pain, abscess at injection site
Contraindications: Hypersensitivity to this drug or lincomycin, ulcerative colitis/enteritis, infants <1 mo
Precautions: Renal disease, liver disease, GI disease, elderly, pregnancy category B, lactation, tartrazine sensitivity
Pharmacokinetics:
PO: Peak 45 min, duration 6 hr
IM: Peak 3 hr, duration 8-12 hr, half-life 2.5 hr; metabolized in liver; excreted in urine, bile, feces as active/inactive metabolites; crosses placenta; excreted in breast milk
🥄 **Drug interactions of concern to dentistry:**
• Decreased action: erythromycin
• Increased effects of nondepolarizing muscle relaxants, hydrocarbon inhalation anesthetics
• Avoid antiperistaltic drugs if diarrhea occurs
• Possible reduced blood levels of cyclosporine
• Oral contraceptives: advise patient of a potential risk for decreased contraceptive action, to maintain compliance with oral contraceptive use while using antibiotics, and to consider the use of additional nonhormonal contraception
DENTAL CONSIDERATIONS
General:
• Determine why the patient is taking the drug.

Consultations:
• Medical consult may be required to assess disease control.
Teach patient/family:
• Importance of good oral hygiene to prevent soft tissue inflammation
• Caution to prevent injury when using oral hygiene aids
When used for dental infection, advise patient:
• To report sore throat, oral burning sensation, fever, fatigue, any of which could indicate superinfection
• To take at prescribed intervals and complete dosage regimen
• To immediately notify the dentist if signs or symptoms of infection increase

---

clobetasol propionate (topical)
(kloe-bay′ta-sol)
Olux

Drug class.: Topical corticosteroid, very high potency

Action: Glucocorticoids have multiple actions that include antiinflammatory and immunosuppressant effects. They inhibit phospholipase A_2, interfering with or reducing the synthesis of prostaglandins and leukotrienes. They also bind to cytoplasmic glucocorticoid receptors (GR) and enter the cell nucleus to bind with DNA. This results in the synthesis of various enzymes such as collagenase, elastase, and cytokines that play important roles in inflammation and immunosuppression. They also suppress the production of lymphocytes, monocytes, and eosinophils.

Uses: Treatment of inflammatory and pruritic manifestations of moderate to severe corticosteroid-responsive dermatitis of the scalp; other uses include eczema and psoriasis (ointment or cream)

Dosage and routes:
• *Adult:* TOP apply small amount of foam to affected scalp area bid (AM and PM)

Available forms include: Foam 0.05% in 100 g container

Side effects/adverse reactions:
INTEG: Burning, stinging, irritation, pruritus, contact allergy
ENDO: Possible hypothalamic-pituitary-adrenal cortex suppression

Contraindications: Hypersensitivity

Precautions: Occlusive dressings, lactation, adrenal cortical suppression, avoid use in infection, not for use in rosacea or perioral dermatitis, pregnancy category C, lactation, children more susceptible to systemic absorption

Pharmacokinetics:
TOP: Absorbed through skin, especially if abraded

⚕ Drug interactions of concern to dentistry:
• None reported. This is a new product thus limited information was available at time of publication.

DENTAL CONSIDERATIONS
General:
• Determine why patient is taking the drug.
• Avoid use of systemic corticosteroids unless a consultation is made.

clobetasol propionate
(klo-bay'ta-sol)
Embeline-E, Temovate, Temovate Emollient Cream, Temovate Gel
Drug class.: Topical corticosteroid, group I very high potency

Action: Glucocorticoids have multiple actions that include antiinflammatory and immunosuppressant effects. They inhibit phospholipase A_2, interfering with or reducing the synthesis of prostaglandins and leukotrienes. They also bind to cytoplasmic glucocorticoid receptors (GRs) and enter the cell nucleus to bind with DNA. This results in the synthesis of various enzymes such as collagenase, elastase, and cytokines that play important roles in inflammation and immunosuppression. They also suppress the production of lymphocytes, monocytes, and eosinophils.

Uses: Psoriasis, eczema, contact dermatitis, pruritus, symptomatic relief of ulcerative inflammatory lesions; usually reserved for severe dermatoses that have not responded to less potent formulations

Dosage and routes:
• *Adult and child:* TOP apply to affected area bid

Available forms include: Oint 0.05%; cream 0.05% in 15, 30, 45 g; gel 0.05% in 15, 30, 60 g; scalp application 0.05% in 25, 50 ml

Side effects/adverse reactions:
INTEG: Burning, dryness, itching, irritation, acne, folliculitis, hypertrichosis, perioral dermatitis, hypopigmentation, atrophy, striae, mili-

aria, allergic contact dermatitis, secondary infection

Contraindications: Hypersensitivity to corticosteroids, fungal infections, viral infections

Precautions: Pregnancy category C, lactation, bacterial infections

DENTAL CONSIDERATIONS

General:

• Place on frequent recall to evaluate healing response.

• Topical adrenocorticosteroids are not indicated for treating plaque-related gingivitis, which should be treated by removal of local irritants and improved oral hygiene.

Teach patient/family:

• Importance of good oral hygiene to prevent soft tissue inflammation

• That use on oral herpetic ulcerations is contraindicated

• To apply at bedtime or after meals for maximum effect

• To apply with cotton-tipped applicator by pressing, not rubbing, paste on lesion

• When used for oral lesions, advise patient to return for oral evaluation if response of oral tissues has not occurred in 7-14 days

---

clocortolone pivalate

(klo-kort'o-lone)
Cloderm

Drug class.: Topical corticosteroid, group III medium potency

---

Action: Glucocorticoids have multiple actions that include antiinflammatory and immunosuppressant effects. They inhibit phospholipase A_2, interfering with or reducing the synthesis of prostaglandins and leukotrienes. They also bind to cytoplasmic glucocorticoid receptors (GRs) and enter the cell nucleus to bind with DNA. This results in the synthesis of various enzymes such as collagenase, elastase, and cytokines that play important roles in inflammation and immunosuppression. They also suppress the production of lymphocytes, monocytes, and eosinophils.

Uses: Psoriasis, eczema, contact dermatitis, pruritus

Dosage and routes:

• *Adult and child:* Apply to affected area tid or qid

Available forms include: Cream 0.1%

Side effects/adverse reactions:

▼ *ORAL:* Perioral dermatitis

INTEG: Burning, dryness, itching, irritation, acne, folliculitis, hypertrichosis, hypopigmentation, atrophy, striae, miliaria, allergic contact dermatitis, secondary infection

Contraindications: Hypersensitivity to corticosteroids, fungal infections

Precautions: Pregnancy category C, lactation, viral infections, bacterial infections

DENTAL CONSIDERATIONS

General:

• Determine why the patient is taking the drug.

• Place on frequent recall to evaluate healing response if used on a chronic basis.

• Apply lubricant to dry lips for patient comfort before dental procedures.

---

clofazimine

(kloe-fa'zi-meen)
Lamprene

Drug class.: Leprostatic

Action: Inhibits mycobacterial

growth, binds to mycobacterial DNA

Uses: Lepromatous leprosy, dapsone-resistant leprosy, lepromatous leprosy complicated by erythema nodosum leprosum

Dosage and routes:

Erythema nodosum leprosum
• *Adult:* PO 100-200 mg qd × 3 mo, then taper dosage to 100 mg when disease is controlled, do not exceed 300 mg/day

Dapsone-related leprosy
• *Adult:* PO 100 mg/day in combination with at least one other antileprosy drug × 3 yr, then 100 mg qd clofazimine (only)

Available forms include: Caps 50 mg

Side effects/adverse reactions:

▼ *ORAL:* Stomatitis (rarely)

CNS: Dizziness, headache, fatigue, drowsiness

GI: Diarrhea, nausea, vomiting, abdominal pain, intolerance, **GI bleeding, obstruction, hepatitis,** anorexia, constipation, jaundice

EENT: Pigmentation of cornea, conjunctiva, drying, burning, itching, irritation

INTEG: Pink or brown discoloration, dryness, pruritus, rash, photosensitivity, acne, monilial cheilosis

MISC: Discolored urine, feces, sputum, sweat

Precautions: Pregnancy category C, lactation, children, abdominal pain, diarrhea, depression

Pharmacokinetics:

PO: Half-life 70 days; deposited in fatty tissue, reticuloendothelial system; small amount excreted in feces, sputum, sweat

🦷 **Drug interactions of concern to dentistry:**
• None reported

DENTAL CONSIDERATIONS

General:
• Develop awareness of the patient's disease.

Teach patient/family:
• Importance of good oral hygiene to prevent soft tissue inflammation
• To avoid mouth rinses with high alcohol content due to drying effects

---

clofibrate

(kloe-fye'brate)

Abitrate, Atromid-S
🍁 Claripex, Novofibrate

Drug class.: Antihyperlipidemic

Action: Inhibits biosynthesis of VLDL and LDL, which are responsible for triglyceride development; mobilizes triglycerides from tissue; increases excretion of neutral sterols

Uses: Hyperlipidemia (types III, IV, V)

Dosage and routes:
• *Adult:* PO 1.5-2 g/day in 2-4 divided doses

Available forms include: Caps 500 mg, 1 g

Side effects/adverse reactions:

▼ *ORAL:* Stomatitis

CNS: Fatigue, weakness, drowsiness, dizziness

CV: **Pulmonary emboli,** angina, dysrhythmias, thrombophlebitis

GI: Nausea, vomiting, dyspepsia, increased liver enzymes, flatulence

HEMA: **Leukopenia, eosinophilia,** anemia, bleeding

GU: **Hematuria,** decreased libido, impotence, dysuria, proteinuria, oliguria

INTEG: Rash, urticaria, pruritus, dry hair and skin, alopecia

---

bold italic = life-threatening conditions

MS: Myalgias, arthralgias
MISC: Polyphagia, weight gain
Contraindications: Severe hepatic disease, severe renal disease, primary biliary cirrhosis, pregnancy, lactation, children
Precautions: Peptic ulcer, pregnancy category C
Pharmacokinetics:
PO: Peak 2-6 hr, half-life 6-25 hr; plasma protein binding >90%; metabolized in liver; excreted in urine
DENTAL CONSIDERATIONS
General:
• Consider semisupine chair position for patient comfort if GI side effects occur.
• Patients on chronic drug therapy may rarely have symptoms of blood dyscrasias, which can include infection, bleeding, and poor healing.
• No dental drug interactions have been reported.
Consultations:
• In a patient with symptoms of blood dyscrasias, request a medical consult for blood studies and postpone treatment until normal values are reestablished.
Teach patient/family:
• Importance of good oral hygiene to prevent soft tissue inflammation

---

clomiphene citrate
(kloe′mi-feen)
Clomid, Milophene, Serophene
Drug class.: Nonsteroidal ovulatory stimulant

Action: Binds to estrogen receptors, resulting in increase of LH and FSH release from the pituitary, which increases maturation of ovarian follicle, ovulation, and development of corpus luteum

Uses: Female infertility
Dosage and routes:
• *Initial adult:* PO 50 mg qd × 5 days; may be repeated until conception occurs or 3-4 cycles of therapy have been completed
• *Second trial adult:* PO 100 mg/day × 5 days, can repeat third time
Available forms include: Tabs 50 mg
Side effects/adverse reactions:
CNS: Headache, depression, restlessness, anxiety, nervousness, fatigue, insomnia, dizziness, flushing
CV: Vasomotor flushing, phlebitis, deep vein thrombosis
GI: Nausea, vomiting, constipation, abdominal pain, bloating
GU: Polyuria, frequency, birth defects, spontaneous abortions, multiple ovulation, breast pain, oliguria, abnormal uterine bleeding
EENT: Blurred vision, diplopia, photophobia
INTEG: Rash, dermatitis, urticaria, alopecia
Contraindications: Hypersensitivity, pregnancy category X, hepatic disease, undiagnosed vaginal bleeding
Precautions: Hypertension, depression, convulsions, diabetes mellitus
Pharmacokinetics:
PO: Metabolized in liver, excreted in feces
DENTAL CONSIDERATIONS
General:
• Consider semisupine chair position for patient comfort due to GI effects of drug.
• Avoid dental light in patient's eyes; offer dark glasses for patient comfort.
• Be aware that patient may be in early stage of pregnancy.

---

clomipramine

(kloe-mi′pra-meen)

Anafranil

Drug class.: Tricyclic antidepressant

Action: Inhibits both norepinephrine and serotonin (5-HT) uptake in the brain, although the precise antidepressant mechanism remains unclear

Uses: Obsessive-compulsive disorder; unapproved: depression, panic disorder, narcolepsy, and neurogenic pain

Dosage and routes:

Obsessive-compulsive disorder

• *Adult:* PO 25 mg hs; increase gradually over 4 wk to a dose of 75-300 mg/day in divided doses
• *Child 10-18 yr:* PO 50 mg/day gradually increased; not to exceed 200 mg/day

Depression

• *Adult:* PO 50-150 mg/day in a single or divided dose

Anxiety/agoraphobia

• *Adult:* PO 25-75 mg/day

Available forms include: Caps 25, 50, 75 mg; tabs 10, 25, 50 mg

Side effects/adverse reactions:

▼ *ORAL: Dry mouth, unpleasant taste,* bleeding
CNS: Dizziness, tremors, mania, seizures, aggressiveness
*CV: **Cardiac arrest,*** hypotension, tachycardia, prolonged QT interval
GI: Constipation
*HEMA: **Agranulocytosis, neutropenia, pancytopenia***
GU: Delayed ejaculation, anorgasmy, retention
INTEG: Diaphoresis
ENDO: Galactorrhea, hyperprolactinemia
META: Hyponatremia

Contraindications: Pregnancy category C, hypersensitivity

Precautions: Seizures, suicidal patients, elderly, MAO inhibitors

Pharmacokinetics:

PO: Half-life: 21-hr parent compound, 36-hr metabolite; extensively bound to tissue and plasma proteins; demethylated in liver (active metabolites); excreted in urine (metabolites)

🐾 **Drug interactions of concern to dentistry:**

• Increased anticholinergic effects: muscarinic blockers, antihistamines, phenothiazines
• Increased effects of direct-acting sympathomimetics (epinephrine, levonordefrin)
• Potential risk of CNS depression: alcohol, barbiturates, benzodiazepines, and other CNS depressants
• Decreased antihypertensive effects: clonidine, guanadrel, guanethidine

DENTAL CONSIDERATIONS

General:

• Take vital signs every appointment due to cardiovascular side effects.
• Assess salivary flow as a factor in caries, periodontal disease, and candidiasis.
• Patients on chronic drug therapy may rarely have symptoms of blood dyscrasias, which can include infection, bleeding, and poor healing.
• After supine positioning, have patient sit upright for at least 2 min before standing to avoid orthostatic hypotension.
• Use vasoconstrictor with caution, in low doses, and with careful aspiration. Avoid use of gingival retraction cord with epinephrine.

---

bold italic = life-threatening conditions   *For periodic updates, visit* **www.mosby.com**

- Place on frequent recall due to oral side effects.
- A stress reduction protocol may be required.

Consultations:
- In a patient with symptoms of blood dyscrasias, request a medical consult for blood studies and postpone dental treatment until normal values are reestablished.
- Physician should be informed if significant xerostomic side effects occur (increased caries, sore tongue, problems eating or swallowing, difficulty wearing prosthesis) so a medication change can be considered.
- Medical consult may be required to assess disease control.

Teach patient/family:
- Importance of good oral hygiene to prevent soft tissue inflammation
- Caution to prevent injury when using oral hygiene aids

When chronic dry mouth occurs, advise patient:
- To avoid mouth rinses with high alcohol content due to drying effects
- To use daily home fluoride products for anticaries effect
- To use sugarless gum, frequent sips of water, or saliva substitutes

---

clonazepam

(kloe-na′zi-pam)

Klonopin

♣ Alti-Clonazepam, Apo-Clonazepam, Clonapam, Gen-Clonazepam, PMS-Clonazepam, Rivotril

Drug class.: Anticonvulsant, benzodiazepine derivative

Controlled Substance Schedule IV

Action: Inhibits spike and wave formation in absence seizures (petit mal); decreases amplitude, frequency, duration, spread of discharge in minor motor seizures; acts on benzodiazepine receptors in the CNS

Uses: Absence, atypical absence, akinetic, myoclonic seizures; panic disorder

Dosage and routes:

Seizures
- *Adult:* PO not to exceed 1.5 mg/day in 3 divided doses; may be increased 0.5-1 mg q3d until desired response; not to exceed 20 mg/day
- *Child <10 yr or 30 kg:* PO 0.01-0.03 mg/kg/day in divided doses q8h, not to exceed 0.05 mg/kg/day; may be increased 0.25-0.5 mg q3d until desired response, not to exceed 0.1-0.2 mg/kg/day

Panic disorder
- *Adult:* PO 1-2 mg/day to a maximum of 4 mg

Available forms include: Tabs 0.5, 1, 2 mg

Side effects/adverse reactions:

▼ *ORAL:* Dry mouth or increased salivation, bleeding

CNS: Drowsiness, dizziness, confusion, behavioral changes, tremors, insomnia, headache, suicidal tendencies, slurred speech

CV: Palpitation, bradycardia

GI: Nausea, constipation, polyphagia, anorexia, xerostomia, diarrhea, gastritis

RESP: **Respiratory depression,** dyspnea, congestion

HEMA: **Thrombocytopenia, leukocytosis, eosinophilia**

GU: Dysuria, enuresis, nocturia, retention

EENT: Nystagmus, diplopia, abnormal eye movements
INTEG: Rash, alopecia, hirsutism
Contraindications: Hypersensitivity to benzodiazepines, acute narrow-angle glaucoma, ritonavir
Precautions: Open-angle glaucoma, chronic respiratory disease, pregnancy category C, renal, hepatic disease, elderly
Pharmacokinetics:
PO: Peak 1-2 hr, half-life 18-50 hr; metabolized by liver; excreted in urine

🦷 **Drug interactions of concern to dentistry:**
• Increased sedation: alcohol, all CNS depressants, indinavir

DENTAL CONSIDERATIONS
General:
• Patients on chronic drug therapy may rarely have symptoms of blood dyscrasias, which can include infection, bleeding, and poor healing.
• Assess salivary flow as a factor in caries, periodontal disease, and candidiasis.
• Psychologic and physical dependence may occur with chronic administration.
• Geriatric patients are more susceptible to drug effects; use lower dose.
• Ask about type of epilepsy, seizure frequency, and quality of seizure control.
Consultations:
• Medical consult may be required to assess disease control.
• In a patient with symptoms of blood dyscrasias, request a medical consult for blood studies and postpone dental treatment until normal values are reestablished.

Teach patient/family:
• Importance of good oral hygiene to prevent soft tissue inflammation
• Caution to prevent injury when using oral hygiene aids
When chronic dry mouth occurs, advise patient:
• To avoid mouth rinses with high alcohol content due to drying effects
• To use daily home fluoride products for anticaries effect
• To use sugarless gum, frequent sips of water, or saliva substitutes

---

clonidine HCl/clonidine transdermal

(kloe'ni-deen)
Catapres, Catapres-TTS, Duraclon
♣ Dixarit

Drug class.: Antihypertensive, central α-adrenergic agonist

Action: Inhibits sympathetic vasomotor center in CNS, thus reducing impulses in sympathetic nervous system; decreases blood pressure, pulse rate, and cardiac output; analgesic action associated with α_2-adrenergic receptors in the spinal cord preventing pain signal transmission to higher centers
Uses: Hypertension, severe pain in combination with opioids for cancer patients; unapproved: opioid abstinence syndrome, nicotine withdrawal, vascular headache
Dosage and routes:
Hypertension
• *Adult:* PO/TRANS 0.1 mg bid, then increase by 0.1 mg/day or 0.2 mg/day until desired response; range 0.2-0.8 mg/day in divided doses

---

bold italic = life-threatening conditions

Severe pain
• *Adult:* INF continuous epidural infusion 30 μg/hr
Available forms include: Tabs 0.1, 0.2, 0.3 mg; transderm sys 2.5, 5, 7.5 mg delivering 0.1, 0.2, 0.3 mg/24 hr, respectively; (Duralon) 100 μg/ml in 10 ml vials

Side effects/adverse reactions:
▼ *ORAL:* Dry mouth, taste changes, salivary pain or swelling
CNS: Drowsiness, sedation, headache, fatigue, nightmares, insomnia, mental changes, anxiety, depression, hallucinations, delirium
CV: Orthostatic hypotension, palpitation, **CHF,** ECG abnormalities
GI: Nausea, vomiting, malaise, constipation
GU: Impotence, nocturia, dysuria, gynecomastia
EENT: Parotid pain
INTEG: Rash, alopecia, facial pallor, pruritus, hives, edema, burning papules, excoriation (transdermal patches)
ENDO: Hyperglycemia
MS: Muscle/joint pain, leg cramps

Contraindications: Hypersensitivity

Precautions: MI (recent), diabetes mellitus, chronic renal failure, Raynaud's disease, thyroid disease, depression, COPD, child <12 yr (patches), asthma, pregnancy category C, lactation, elderly

Pharmacokinetics:
PO: Peak 3-5 hr, half-life 12-16 hr; metabolized by liver (metabolites); excreted in urine (unchanged, inactive metabolites), feces; crosses blood-brain barrier; excreted in breast milk

🥄 **Drug interactions of concern to dentistry:**
• Increased CNS depression: alcohol, all CNS depressants
• Decreased hypotensive effects: NSAIDs, especially indomethacin, sympathomimetics, tricyclic antidepressants

DENTAL CONSIDERATIONS
General:
• Monitor vital signs every appointment due to cardiovascular side effects.
• After supine positioning, have patient sit upright for at least 2 min before standing to avoid orthostatic hypotension.
• Limit use of sodium-containing products such as saline IV fluids for patients with a dietary salt restriction.
• Assess salivary flow as a factor in caries, periodontal disease, and candidiasis.
• Stress from dental procedures may compromise cardiovascular function; determine patient risk.
• Short appointments and a stress reduction protocol may be required for anxious patients.
• Consider drug in diagnosis of taste alterations.

Consultations:
• Medical consult may be required to assess disease control.

Teach patient/family: *When chronic dry mouth occurs, advise patient:*
• To avoid mouth rinses with high alcohol content due to drying effects
• To use daily home fluoride products for anticaries effect
• To use sugarless gum, frequent sips of water, or saliva substitutes

clopidogrel bisulfate

(kloe-pid-o'grel)

Plavix

Drug class.: Platelet aggregation inhibitor

Action: Irreversibly inhibits adenosine diphosphate–induced platelet aggregation

Uses: Adjunctive treatment in MI, ischemic stroke, and peripheral vascular disease in patients with atherosclerosis

Dosage and routes:

• *Adult:* PO 75 mg qd with or without food

Available forms include: Tabs 75 mg

Side effects/adverse reactions:

GI: **Diarrhea, abdominal pain,** nausea, gastritis with bleeding, dyspepsia

RESP: RTI, bronchitis, coughing

EENT: Epistaxis, rhinitis

HEMA: Bleeding, neutropenia (rare)

INTEG: Rash, urticaria, purpura, pruritus

META: Liver function abnormalities, hepatotoxicity, hypercholesterolemia

MS: Arthralgia, back pain

Contraindications: Hypersensitivity, active bleeding, bleeding disorders, anticoagulants, antiplatelet agents

Precautions: Hepatic impairment, renal impairment, hypertension, history of bleeding disorders, major surgery, pregnancy category B

Pharmacokinetics:

PO: Well absorbed, peak levels <1 hr, hepatic metabolism, active metabolite, plasma protein binding 94%-98%, excreted in both urine and feces, maximal effect on bleeding time 5-7 days

🦷 **Drug interactions of concern to dentistry:**

• Avoid prescribing aspirin; caution in use with NSAIDs

DENTAL CONSIDERATIONS

General:

• Effects on platelet aggregation return to normal in 5-7 days.

• Patient on chronic drug therapy may rarely have symptoms of blood dyscrasias, which can include infection, bleeding, and poor healing.

• Consider local hemostasis measures to prevent excessive bleeding.

Consultations:

• Medical consult may be required to assess disease control and patient's ability to tolerate stress.

• Consult should include data on bleeding time.

• In a patient with symptoms of blood dyscrasias, request a medical consult for blood studies and postpone treatment until normal values are reestablished.

Teach patient/family:

• Importance of updating health and drug history if physician makes any changes in evaluation or drug regimens

• Caution to prevent trauma when using oral hygiene aids

• To report any unusual or prolonged bleeding episodes after dental treatment

---

bold italic = life-threatening conditions

clorazepate dipotassium

(klor-az'e-pate)

Gen-Xene, Tranxene-SD, Tranxene-SD Half Strength, Traxene T-Tab

♣ Apo-Chlorazepate, Novo-Clopate, Tranxene

Drug class.: Benzodiazepine

Controlled Substance Schedule IV

Action: Produces CNS depression by interacting with a benzodiazepine receptor to facilitate the action of the inhibitory neurotransmitter γ-aminobutyric acid (GABA)

Uses: Anxiety, acute alcohol withdrawal, adjunctive treatment of partial seizures

Dosage and routes:

Anxiety

• *Adult:* PO 15-60 mg/day in divided doses

Alcohol withdrawal

• *Adult:* PO 30 mg initially, then 30-60 mg in divided doses; day 2, 45-90 mg in divided doses; day 3, 22.5-45 mg in divided doses; day 4, 15-30 mg in divided doses; then reduce daily dose to 7.5-15 mg

Partial seizures

• *Adult and child >12 yr:* PO initial dose 7.5 mg tid; can increase by 7.5 mg qwk, limit 90 mg/day

• *Child 9-12 yr:* PO initial dose 7.5 mg bid; can increase by 7.5 mg qwk, limit 60 mg/day

Available forms include: Caps 3.75, 7.5, 15 mg; tabs 3.75, 7.5, 15 mg, single-dose tab 11.25, 22.5 mg

Side effects/adverse reactions:

▼ *ORAL:* Dry mouth

CNS: Dizziness, drowsiness, confusion, headache, anxiety, tremors, stimulation, fatigue, depression, insomnia, hallucinations

*CV: Orthostatic hypotension, **ECG changes, tachycardia,** hypotension

GI: Constipation, nausea, vomiting, anorexia, diarrhea

EENT: Blurred vision, tinnitus, mydriasis

INTEG: Rash, dermatitis, itching

Contraindications: Hypersensitivity to benzodiazepines, narrow-angle glaucoma, psychosis, pregnancy category D, child <18 yr; ritonavir

Precautions: Elderly, debilitated, hepatic disease, renal disease

Pharmacokinetics:

PO: Onset 15 min, peak 1-2 hr, duration 4-6 hr, half-life 30-100 hr; metabolized by liver; excreted by kidneys; crosses placenta, excreted in breast milk

🦷 **Drug interactions of concern to dentistry:**

• Increased effects: CNS depressants, alcohol, opioid analgesics, general anesthetics, indinavir

• Increased serum levels and prolonged effect of benzodiazepines: fluconazole, ketoconazole, itraconazole, miconazole (systemic)

DENTAL CONSIDERATIONS

General:

• Monitor vital signs every appointment due to cardiovascular side effects.

• Assess salivary flow as a factor in caries, periodontal disease, and candidiasis.

• After supine positioning, have patient sit upright for at least 2 min to avoid orthostatic hypotension.

• Psychologic and physical dependence may occur with chronic administration.

• Geriatric patients are more susceptible to drug effects; use a lower dose.
• Short appointments and a stress reduction protocol may be required for anxious patients
• Seizure: ask about type of epilepsy, seizure frequency and quality of seizure control

Consultations:
• Medical consult may be required to assess disease control and the patient's ability to tolerate stress patient.

Teach patient/family: *When chronic dry mouth occurs, advise patient:*
• To avoid mouth rinses with high alcohol content due to drying effects
• To use daily home fluoride products for anticaries effect
• To use sugarless gum, frequent sips of water, or saliva substitutes

---

clotrimazole
(kloe-trim′a-zole)

Vaginal products: Gyne-Lotrimin 3, Gyne-Lotrimin 7, Gye-Lotrimin 3 Combination Pack, Mycelex-7, Mycelex-7 Combination Pack
Topical products: Cruex, Desenex, Fungoid, Lotrimin, Lotrimin AF
Oral products: Mycelex Lozenges
♣ Canesten, Myclo-Gyne, Neo-Zol

Drug class.: Imidazole antifungal

Action: Interferes with fungal DNA replication; binds sterols in fungal cell membrane, which increases permeability, leaking of cell nutrients; fungicidal
Uses: Tinea pedis; tinea cruris; tinea corporis; tinea versicolor; *C. albicans* infection of the vagina, vulva, throat, mouth

Dosage and routes:
• *Adult and child:* TOP use OTC products daily for 4 wk; prescription products use bid AM and PM up to 4 wk VAG SUPP one intravaginally at hs for 3 consecutive days VAG CREAM one full applicator daily at hs for 3-7 consecutive days
• *Adult and child:* ORAL LOZ dissolve 1 oral troche in mouth 5 × day for 14 days

Available forms include: Cream, sol, lotion 1%; vag supp 200 mg; vag cream 1%; troche 10 mg; combo products include cream 1% with 100, 200 mg suppository

Side effects/adverse reactions:
INTEG: Rash, urticaria, stinging, burning, peeling, blistering
MISC: Abdominal cramps, bloating, urinary frequency, dyspareunia

Contraindications: Hypersensitivity

Precautions: Pregnancy category B, lactation

♣ **Drug interactions of concern to dentistry:**
• None reported

DENTAL CONSIDERATIONS
General:
• Determine why the patient is taking the drug.
• Examine oral mucous membranes for signs of fungal infection.

Teach patient/family:
• If used for oral infection: to soak full or partial dentures in an antifungal solution overnight until lesions are absent; prolonged infections may require fabrication of new prosthesis
• To dispose of toothbrush used

---

bold italic = life-threatening conditions

during oral infection after oral lesions are absent to prevent reinoculation
• That long-term therapy may be needed to clear infection; to complete entire course of medication

---

cloxacillin sodium

(klox-a-sil'in)

Cloxapen

✦ Apo Cloxi, Novo-Cloxin, Nu-Cloxi, Orbenin

Drug class.: Penicillinase-resistant penicillin

Action: Interferes with cell wall replication of susceptible organisms; the cell wall, rendered osmotically unstable, swells and bursts from osmotic pressure

Uses: Effective for gram-positive cocci *(S. aureus, S. pyogenes, E. pyogenes, S. pneumoniae),* when penicillinase-producing organisms are confirmed pathogens

Dosage and routes:
• *Adult:* PO 1-4 g/day in divided doses q6h
• *Child <40 kg:* PO 50-100 mg/kg in divided doses q6h

Available forms include: Caps 250, 500 mg; powder for oral susp 125 mg/5 ml in 100, 200 ml

Side effects/adverse reactions:

▼ *ORAL:* Discolored tongue, candidiasis, glossitis

CNS: **Coma, convulsions,** lethargy, hallucinations, anxiety, depression, twitching

GI: Nausea, vomiting, diarrhea, increased AST/ALT, abdominal pain, colitis

HEMA: **Bone marrow depression, granulocytopenia,** anemia, increased bleeding time

GU: Vaginitis, moniliasis, **glomerulonephritis,** oliguria, proteinuria, hematuria

META: Pruritus, urticaria, angioedema, bronchospasm, anaphylaxis (allergy symptoms)

Contraindications: Hypersensitivity to penicillins; neonates

Precautions: Pregnancy category B, hypersensitivity to cephalosporins

Pharmacokinetics:

PO: Peak 1 hr, duration 6 hr, half-life 0.5-1 hr; metabolized in liver; excreted in urine, bile, breast milk; crosses placenta

🦷 **Drug interactions of concern to dentistry:**
• Decreased antimicrobial effectiveness: tetracyclines, erythromycins
• Increased cloxacillin concentrations: probenecid
• Oral contraceptives: advise patient of a potential risk for decreased contraceptive action, to maintain compliance with oral contraceptive use while using antibiotics, and to consider the use of additional nonhormonal contraception

DENTAL CONSIDERATIONS

General:
• Use precautions regarding allergy to medication.
• Determine why the patient is taking the drug.

Consultations:
• Medical consult may be required to assess disease control.

Teach patient/family:
• Importance of good oral hygiene to prevent soft tissue inflammation
• Caution to prevent injury when using oral hygiene aids

When used for dental infection, advise patient:
• To report sore throat, oral burning sensation, fever, fatigue, any of which could indicate superinfection
• To take at prescribed intervals and complete dosage regimen
• To immediately notify the dentist if signs or symptoms of infection increase

clozapine
(kloʹza-pin)
Clozaril
Drug class.: Antipsychotic, atypical

Action: Interferes with binding of dopamine at D_1 and D_2 receptors with lack of extrapyramidal symptoms; also acts as an adrenergic, cholinergic, histaminergic, and serotonergic antagonist
Uses: Management of psychotic symptoms in schizophrenic patients for whom other antipsychotics have failed
Dosage and routes:
• *Adult:* PO 25 mg qd or bid, may increase by 25-50 mg/day; normal range 300-450 mg/day after 2 wk; do not increase dose more than 2 × weekly; do not exceed 900 mg/day; use lowest dose to control symptoms
Available forms include: Tabs 25, 100 mg
Side effects/adverse reactions:
▼ *ORAL: Dry mouth, increased salivation,* glossitis
CNS: Sedation, dizziness, headache, tremors, sleep problems, akinesia, fever, ***seizures,*** sweating, akathisia, confusion, fatigue, insomnia, depression, slurred speech, anxiety
CV: Tachycardia, hypotension, hypertension, chest pain, ECG changes
GI: Constipation, nausea, abdominal discomfort, vomiting, diarrhea, anorexia
RESP: Dyspnea, nasal congestion, throat discomfort
*HEMA: **Leukopenia, neutropenia, agranulocytosis, eosinophilia***
GU: Urinary abnormalities, incontinence, ejaculation dysfunction, frequency, urgency, retention
MS: Weakness; pain in back, neck, legs; spasm
Contraindications: Hypersensitivity, myeloproliferative disorders, severe granulocytopenia, CNS depression, coma, narrow-angle glaucoma
Precautions: Pregnancy category B; lactation; children <16 yr; hepatic, renal, cardiac disease; seizures; prostatic enlargement; elderly
Pharmacokinetics:
PO: Steady state 2.5 hr, half-life 8-12 hr; 95% protein bound; completely metabolized by the liver; excreted in urine and feces (metabolites)
🥄 **Drug interactions of concern to dentistry:**
• Increased anticholinergic effects: anticholinergics
• Increased CNS depression: alcohol, all CNS depressant drugs
• Increased serum concentration, leukocytosis: erythromycin base
DENTAL CONSIDERATIONS
General:
• Monitor vital signs every appointment due to cardiovascular and respiratory side effects.

---

bold italic = life-threatening conditions

• Patients on chronic drug therapy may rarely have symptoms of blood dyscrasias, which can include infection, bleeding, and poor healing.

• After supine positioning, have patient sit upright for at least 2 min before standing to avoid orthostatic hypotension.

• Assess salivary flow as a factor in caries, periodontal disease, and candidiasis.

• Determine why the patient is taking the drug.

• Place on frequent recall due to oral side effects.

Consultations:

• In a patient with symptoms of blood dyscrasias, request a medical consult for blood studies and postpone dental treatment until normal values are reestablished.

• Medical consult may be required to assess disease control and stress tolerance of patient.

• Physician should be informed if significant xerostomic side effects occur (increased caries, sore tongue, problems eating or swallowing, difficulty wearing prosthesis) so a medication change can be considered.

Teach patient/family:

• Importance of good oral hygiene to prevent soft tissue inflammation

• Caution to prevent injury when using oral hygiene aids

• To use electric toothbrush if patient has difficulty holding conventional devices

When chronic dry mouth occurs, advise patient:

• To avoid mouth rinses with high alcohol content due to drying effects

• To use daily home fluoride products for anticaries effect

• To use sugarless gum, frequent sips of water, or saliva substitutes

---

codeine sulfate/ codeine phosphate
(koe'deen)
generic codeine
Drug class.: Narcotic analgesic

Controlled Substance Schedule II, Canada N

Action: Depresses pain impulse transmission in CNS by interacting with opioid receptors

Uses: Mild-to-moderate pain, nonproductive cough

Dosage and routes:

Pain

• *Adult:* PO 15-60 mg q4h prn; IM/SC 15-60 mg q4h prn

• *Child:* PO 3 mg/kg/day in divided doses q4h prn

Cough

• *Adult:* PO 10-20 mg q4-6h, not to exceed 120 mg/day

• *Child:* PO 1-1.5 mg/kg/day in 4 divided doses, not to exceed 60 mg/day

Available forms include: Inj IM/SC 15, 30, 60 mg/ml; tabs 15, 30, 60 mg

Side effects/adverse reactions:

▼ *ORAL:* Dry mouth, lichenoid reaction

CNS: Drowsiness, sedation, dizziness, agitation, dependency, lethargy, restlessness

CV: Bradycardia, palpitation, orthostatic hypotension, tachycardia

GI: Nausea, vomiting, anorexia, constipation

*RESP: **Respiratory depression, respiratory paralysis***

GU: Urinary retention

INTEG: Flushing, rash, urticaria

Contraindications: Hypersensitivity to opiates, respiratory depression, increased intracranial pressure, seizure disorders, severe respiratory disorders

Precautions: Elderly, cardiac dysrhythmias, pregnancy category C

Pharmacokinetics:

PO: Onset 15-30 min, peak 1-2 hr, duration 4-6 hr, half-life 2.5-4 hr; metabolized by liver; excreted by kidneys; crosses placenta; excreted in breast milk

🦷 **Drug interactions of concern to dentistry:**

• Increased sedation with other CNS depressants and alcohol

• Increased effects of anticholinergics

DENTAL CONSIDERATIONS

General:

• Monitor vital signs every appointment due to cardiovascular and respiratory side effects.

• After supine positioning, have patient sit upright for at least 2 min to avoid orthostatic hypotension.

• Assess salivary flow as a factor in caries, periodontal disease, and candidiasis.

• Psychologic and physical dependence may occur with chronic administration.

Teach patient/family: *When chronic dry mouth occurs, advise patient:*

• To avoid mouth rinses with high alcohol content due to drying effects

• To use daily home fluoride products for anticaries effect

• To use sugarless gum, frequent sips of water, or saliva substitutes

colchicine

(kol'chi-seen)

generic colchicine

Drug class.: Antigout agent

Action: Inhibits deposition of uric acid crystals in soft tissues; mechanism unclear

Uses: Gout, gouty arthritis (prevention, treatment), to arrest progression of neurologic disability in multiple sclerosis

Dosage and routes:

Prevention

• *Adult:* PO 0.5-1.8 mg qd depending on severity

Treatment

• *Adult:* PO 0.5-1.2 mg, then 0.5-1.2 mg q1h until pain decreases or side effects occur

Available forms include: Tabs 0.5, 0.6 mg

Side effects/adverse reactions:

▼ *ORAL:* Metallic taste, lichenoid reaction

GI: Nausea, vomiting, anorexia, malaise, cramps, peptic ulcer, diarrhea

HEMA: Agranulocytosis, thrombocytopenia, aplastic anemia, pancytopenia

GU: Hematuria, oliguria, renal damage

INTEG: Chills, dermatitis, pruritus, purpura, erythema

MISC: Myopathy, alopecia, reversible azoospermia, peripheral neuritis

Contraindications: Hypersensitivity; serious GI, renal, hepatic, cardiac disorders; blood dyscrasias

Precautions: Severe renal disease, blood dyscrasias, pregnancy category C, hepatic disease, elderly, lactation, children, retards B_{12} absorption

---

bold italic = life-threatening conditions

Pharmacokinetics:

PO: Peak 0.5-2 hr, half-life 20 min; deacetylates in liver; excreted in feces (metabolites/active drug)

⚡ Drug interactions of concern to dentistry:

• Increased risk of GI side effects: NSAIDs, aspirin

DENTAL CONSIDERATIONS

General:

• Consider drug in diagnosis of taste alteration.

• Patients on chronic drug therapy may rarely have symptoms of blood dyscrasias, which can include infection, bleeding, and poor healing.

• Avoid prescribing aspirin-containing products.

Consultations:

• Medical consult may be required to assess disease control.

• In a patient with symptoms of blood dyscrasias, request a medical consult for blood studies and postpone dental treatment until normal values are reestablished.

Teach patient/family:

• Importance of good oral hygiene to prevent soft tissue inflammation

• Caution to prevent injury when using oral hygiene aids

• To avoid mouth rinses with high alcohol content due to drying effects

---

colesevelam HCl

(koh-le-sev´-e-lam)

Welchol

Drug class.: Antihyperlipidemic

Action: Absorbs, combines with bile acids to form insoluble complexes that are excreted through the feces; loss of bile acids lowers cholesterol levels

Uses: Adjunctive therapy to diet and exercise, alone or in combination with an HMG-CoA reductase inhibitor (statin) in patients with primary hypercholesterolemia (Type IIa) to reduce elevated LDL cholesterol

Dosage and routes:

• *Adult:* PO initial dose 3 tabs (187 mg) bid with meals and a full glass of water; or 6 tabs once/day with meals. Dose may be increased to 7 tabs depending on need.

Combination therapy with HMG-CoA reductase inhibitor

• *Adult:* PO 3 tabs (1875 mg) bid with meals or 6 tabs once/day taken with a meal

Available forms include: Tabs 625 mg

Side effects/adverse reactions:

GI: Constipation, dyspepsia

MS: Myalgia

Contraindications: Hypersensitivity, bowel obstruction

Precautions: Preexisting GI diseases, primary biliary cirrhosis, biliary obstruction, hypertriglyceridemia

Pharmacokinetics: Human data lacking, drug is not absorbed from GI tract

⚡ Drug interactions of concern to dentistry:

• None reported, but monitor if drugs with narrow therapeutic index drugs are prescribed for dental conditions

DENTAL CONSIDERATIONS

General:

• Consider semisupine chair position for patient comfort due to GI side effects of drug.

colestipol HCl
(koe-les'ti-pole)
Colestid

Drug class.: Antihyperlipidemic

Action: Absorbs, combines with bile acids to form insoluble complex that is excreted through feces; loss of bile acids lowers cholesterol levels

Uses: Primary hypercholesterolemia, xanthomas, digitalis toxicity, pruritus due to biliary obstruction, diarrhea due to bile acids

Dosage and routes:
• *Adult:* PO 5-30 g/day in 2-4 divided doses

Available forms include: Tabs 1 g, granules for oral suspension 5 g/7.5 g powder

Side effects/adverse reactions:

▼ *ORAL:* Glossitis

GI: Constipation, abdominal pain, nausea, fecal impaction, hemorrhoids, flatulence, vomiting, steatorrhea, peptic ulcer

*HEMA: Decreased vitamins A, D, K red folate content; **hyperchloremic acidosis;** bleeding; decreased protime*

INTEG: Rash, irritation of perianal area, skin

Contraindications: Hypersensitivity, biliary obstruction

Precautions: Pregnancy category B, lactation, children, bleeding disorders

Pharmacokinetics:
PO: Excreted in feces

🥄 **Drug interactions of concern to dentistry:**
• Decreased absorption of tetracyclines, cephalexin, phenobarbital, corticosteroids, clindamycin, penicillins; administer doses several hours apart

DENTAL CONSIDERATIONS
General:
• Consider semisupine chair position for patient comfort due to GI effects of disease.

cortisone acetate
(kor'ti-sone)
Cortone

Drug class.: Glucocorticoid, short-acting

Action: Glucocorticoids have multiple actions that include antiinflammatory and immunosuppressant effects. They inhibit phospholipase A_2, interfering with or reducing the synthesis of prostaglandins and leukotrienes. They also bind to cytoplasmic glucocorticoid receptors (GRs) and enter the cell nucleus to bind with DNA. This results in the synthesis of various enzymes such as collagenase, elastase, and cytokines that play important roles in inflammation and immunosuppression. They also suppress the production of lymphocytes, monocytes, and eosinophils.

Uses: Inflammation, severe allergy, adrenal insufficiency, collagen disorders, respiratory, dermatologic disorders

Dosage and routes:
• *Adult:* PO 25-300 mg qd or q2d, titrated to patient response

Available forms include: Tabs 5, 10, 25 mg; inj 50 mg/ml in 10 ml

Side effects/adverse reactions:

▼ *ORAL:* Dry mouth, poor wound healing, petechiae, candidiasis

CNS: Depression, flushing, sweating, headache, mood changes

---

bold italic = life-threatening conditions

CV: Hypertension, **circulatory collapse, thrombophlebitis, embolism, necrotizing angiitis, CHF,** tachycardia, edema

GI: Diarrhea, nausea, abdominal distention, **GI hemorrhage, pancreatitis,** increased appetite

HEMA: **Thrombocytopenia**

EENT: Fungal infections, increased intraocular pressure, blurred vision

INTEG: Acne, poor wound healing, ecchymosis, bruising, petechiae

MS: Fractures, osteoporosis, weakness

Contraindications: Psychosis, hypersensitivity, idiopathic thrombocytopenia, acute glomerulonephritis, amebiasis, fungal infections, nonasthmatic bronchial disease, child <2 yr, AIDS, TB

Precautions: Pregnancy category C, diabetes mellitus, glaucoma, osteoporosis, seizure disorders, ulcerative colitis, CHF, myasthenia gravis, renal disease, esophagitis, peptic ulcer, rifampin

Pharmacokinetics:

PO: Peak 2 hr, duration 1.5 days

IM: Peak 20-48 hr, duration 1.5 days

🦷 Drug interactions of concern to dentistry:

• Decreased action: barbiturates, rifabutin, rifampin

• Increased GI side effects: alcohol, salicylates, NSAIDs

• Increased action: ketoconazole, macrolide antibiotics

• Hepatotoxicity: acetaminophen (chronic, high doses)

DENTAL CONSIDERATIONS

General:

• Monitor vital signs every appointment due to cardiovascular side effects.

• Patients on chronic drug therapy may rarely have symptoms of blood dyscrasias, which can include infection, bleeding, and poor healing.

• Assess salivary flow as a factor in caries, periodontal disease, and candidiasis.

• Avoid prescribing aspirin-containing products.

• Symptoms of oral infections may be masked.

• Place on frequent recall to evaluate healing response.

• Prophylactic antibiotics may be indicated to prevent infection if surgery or deep scaling is planned.

• Determine dose and duration of steroid therapy for each patient to assess risk for stress tolerance and immunosuppression.

• Patients who have been or are currently on chronic steroid therapy (>2 wk) may require supplemental steroids for dental treatment.

• Determine why the patient is taking the drug.

Consultations:

• In a patient with symptoms of blood dyscrasias, request a medical consult for blood studies and postpone dental treatment until normal values are reestablished.

• Medical consult may be required to assess disease control and stress tolerance of patient.

• Consult may be required to confirm steroid dose and duration of use.

Teach patient/family:

• Importance of good oral hygiene to prevent soft tissue inflammation

• Caution to prevent injury when using oral hygiene aids

When chronic dry mouth occurs, advise patient:

• To avoid mouth rinses with high alcohol content due to drying effects

• To use daily home fluoride products for anticaries effect

• To use sugarless gum, frequent sips of water, or saliva substitutes

---

cromolyn sodium (disodium cromoglycate)

(kroe'moe-lin)

Gastrocrom, Intal, Nasalcrom

✤ Novo-Cromolyn, PMS-Sodium Chromglycate, Rynacrom

Drug class.: Antiasthmatic, mast cell stabilizer

Action: Stabilizes the membrane of the sensitized mast cell, preventing release of chemical mediators after an antigen-IgE interaction

Uses: Allergic rhinitis, severe perennial bronchial asthma, exercise-induced bronchospasm (prevention), prevention of acute bronchospasm induced by environmental pollutants, mastocytosis

Dosage and routes:

Allergic rhinitis

• *Adult and child >6 yr:* NASAL SOL 1 spray in each nostril tid-qid, not to exceed 6 doses/day

Bronchospasm

• *Adult and child >5 yr:* INH 20 mg <1 hr before exercise

Bronchial asthma

• *Adult and child >5 yr:* INH 20 mg qid; NEBULIZ 20 mg qid by nebulization

Mastocytosis

• *Adult:* PO 200 mg qid 30 min ac and hs

• *Child 2-12 yr:* PO 100 mg qid 30 min ac and hs

• *Child <2 yr:* PO 20 mg/kg of body weight per day in 4 divided doses

Available forms include: Sol 40 mg/ml; caps for inh 20 mg/2 ml; neb sol 20 mg; aerosol 800 µ/actuation; oral conc 5 ml/100 mg

Side effects/adverse reactions:

▼ *ORAL:* Dry, burning mouth, bitter taste (aerosol)

GI: Nausea, vomiting, anorexia

GU: Frequency, dysuria

INTEG: Rash, urticaria, angioedema

MS: Joint pain/swelling

Contraindications: Hypersensitivity to this drug or lactose, status asthmaticus

Precautions: Pregnancy category B, lactation, renal disease, hepatic disease, child <5 yr

Pharmacokinetics:

INH: Peak 15 min, duration 4-6 hr, half-life 80 min; excreted unchanged in feces

DENTAL CONSIDERATIONS

General:

• Assess salivary flow as a factor in caries, periodontal disease, and candidiasis.

• Consider semisupine chair position for patients with respiratory disease.

• A stress reduction protocol may be required.

• Midday appointments and a stress reduction protocol may be required for anxious patients.

• Be aware that aspirin or sulfite preservatives in vasoconstrictor-containing products can exacerbate asthma.

Consultations:

• Consider drug in diagnosis of

---

taste alteration and burning mouth syndrome.
• Medical consult may be required to assess disease control and stress tolerance of patient.

Teach patient/family:
• For inhalation dosage forms, rinse mouth with water after each dose to prevent dryness
When chronic dry mouth occurs, advise patient:
• To avoid mouth rinses with high alcohol content due to drying effects
• To use daily home fluoride products for anticaries effect
• To use sugarless gum, frequent sips of water, or saliva substitutes

---

cyanocobalamin (vitamin B$_{12}$)/ hydroxocobalamin (vitamin B$_{12}$a)

(sye-an-oh-koe-bal'a-min)
Big Shot B12, Crystamine, Crysti-1000, Cyanoject, Cyomin, HydroCobex, Hydro-Crysti-12, LA-12, Nascobal, Rubesol-1000 ♣ Anacobin, Bedoz

Drug class.: Vitamin B$_{12}$, water-soluble vitamin

Action: Needed for adequate nerve functioning, protein and carbohydrate metabolism, normal growth, RBC development, cell reproduction
Uses: Vitamin B$_{12}$ deficiency, pernicious anemia, vitamin B$_{12}$ malabsorption syndrome, Schilling test, increased requirements with pregnancy thyrotoxicosis, hemolytic anemia, hemorrhage, renal and hepatic disease

Dosage and routes:
• *Adult:* PO 25 µg qd × 5-10 days, maintenance 100-200 mg IM qmo; IM/SC 30-100 µg qd × 5-10 days, maintenance 100-200 µg IM qmo
• *Child:* PO 1 µg qd × 5-10 days, maintenance 60 µg IM qmo or more; IM/SC 1-30 µg qd × 5-10 days, maintenance 60 µg IM qmo or more
Pernicious anemia/malabsorption syndrome
• *Adult:* IM 100-1000 µg qd × 2 wk, then 100-1000 µg IM qmo
• *Child:* IM 100-500 µg over 2 wk or more given in 100-500 µg doses, then 60 µg IM/SC qmo
Schilling test
• *Adult and child:* IM 1000 µg in one dose
Available forms include: Tabs 25, 50, 100, 250, 500, 1000 µg; inj IM 100, 120, 1000 µg/ml; intranasal gel 500 µg/0.1 ml in 5 ml
Side effects/adverse reactions:
CNS: Flushing, optic nerve atrophy
CV: **CHF, pulmonary edema,** peripheral vascular thrombosis
GI: Diarrhea
INTEG: Itching, rash, pain at site
META: Hypokalemia
Contraindications: Hypersensitivity, optic nerve atrophy
Precautions: Pregnancy category A, lactation, children
Pharmacokinetics:
PO: Stored in liver, kidneys, stomach; 50%-90% excreted in urine; crosses placenta, excreted in breast milk
🥄 **Drug interactions of concern to dentistry:**
• Increased absorption: prednisone
DENTAL CONSIDERATIONS
General:
• Deficiency in B$_{12}$ and other B-

complex vitamins may cause oral symptomatology.

---

cyclizine HCl/cyclizine lactate
(sye′kli-zeen)
Marezine

Drug class.: Antiemetic, antihistaminic, anticholinergic

Action: May act centrally by blocking chemoreceptor trigger zone, which in turn acts on vomiting center; also antagonizes histamine peripherally

Uses: Motion sickness, prevention of postoperative vomiting

Dosage and routes:

Vomiting

• *Adult:* IM 50 mg 0.5 hr before termination of surgery, then q4-6h prn (lactate)

• *Child:* IM 3 mg/kg divided in 3 equal doses (lactate)

Motion sickness

• *Adult:* PO 50 mg, then q4-6h prn, not to exceed 200 mg/day (HCl)

• *Child:* PO 25 mg q4-6h prn

Available forms include: Tabs 50 mg; inj 50 mg/ml

Side effects/adverse reactions:

▼ *ORAL:* Dry mouth

CNS: Drowsiness, dizziness, convulsions in children, vertigo, fatigue, restlessness, headache, insomnia, hallucinations (auditory/visual)

GI: Nausea, anorexia

EENT: Blurred vision, tinnitus

Contraindications: Hypersensitivity to cyclizines, shock

Precautions: Children, narrow-angle glaucoma, urinary retention, lactation, prostatic hypertrophy, elderly, pregnancy category B, lactation

Pharmacokinetics:
PO: Duration 4-6 hr, other pharmacokinetics not known

🦷 **Drug interactions of concern to dentistry:**
• Increased CNS depression: alcohol, all CNS depressants
• May increase effect of anticholinergic drugs

DENTAL CONSIDERATIONS
General:
• Monitor vital signs every appointment due to cardiovascular side effects.
• Assess salivary flow as a factor in caries, periodontal disease, and candidiasis.

Teach patient/family: *When chronic dry mouth occurs, advise patient:*
• To avoid mouth rinses with high alcohol content due to drying effects
• To use daily home fluoride products for anticaries effect
• To use sugarless gum, frequent sips of water, or saliva substitutes

---

cyclobenzaprine HCl
(sye-kloe-ben′za-preen)
Flexeril

Drug class.: Skeletal muscle relaxant, centrally acting tricyclic

---

Action: Unknown; may be related to antidepressant effects, has actions similar to those of tricyclic antidepressants

Uses: Adjunct for relief of muscle spasm and pain in musculoskeletal conditions

Dosage and routes:
• *Adult:* PO 10 mg tid × 1 wk, not to exceed 60 mg/day × 3 wk

Available forms include: Tabs 10 mg

---

bold italic = life-threatening conditions

Side effects/adverse reactions:

▼ *ORAL:* Dry mouth, unpleasant taste

CNS: Dizziness, weakness, drowsiness, headache, tremor, depression, insomnia, confusion, paresthesia

CV: Postural hypotension, tachycardia, dysrhythmias

GI: Nausea, vomiting, hiccups

GU: Urinary retention, frequency, change in libido

EENT: Diplopia, temporary loss of vision

INTEG: Rash, pruritus, fever, facial flushing, sweating

Contraindications: Acute recovery phase of MI, dysrhythmias, heart block, CHF, hypersensitivity, child <12 yr, intermittent porphyria, thyroid disease

Precautions: Renal disease, hepatic disease, addictive personalities, pregnancy category B, elderly

Pharmacokinetics:

PO: Onset 1 hr, peak 3-8 hr, duration 12-24 hr, half-life 1-3 days; metabolized by liver; excreted in urine; crosses placenta; excreted in breast milk

⚖ Drug interactions of concern to dentistry:

• Increased CNS depression: alcohol, narcotics, barbiturates, sedatives, hypnotics

• Increased effects of anticholinergic drugs

• Increased effects of direct-acting sympathomimetics (epinephrine, levonordefrin)

DENTAL CONSIDERATIONS

General:

• Monitor vital signs every appointment due to cardiovascular side effects.

• Assess salivary flow as a factor in caries, periodontal disease, and candidiasis.

• After supine positioning, have patient sit upright for at least 2 min to avoid orthostatic hypotension.

• Use vasoconstrictors with caution, in low doses, and with careful aspiration. Avoid use of gingival retraction cord with epinephrine.

• Place on frequent recall due to oral side effects.

• Consider drug in diagnosis of taste alterations.

Consultations:

• Medical consult may be required to assess disease control.

Teach patient/family: *When chronic dry mouth occurs, advise patient:*

• To avoid mouth rinses with high alcohol content due to drying effects

• To use daily home fluoride products for anticaries effect

• To use sugarless gum, frequent sips of water, or saliva substitutes

---

cyclophosphamide

(sye-kloe-foss′fa-mide)

Cytoxan, Neosar

♣ Procytox

Drug class.: Antineoplastic alkylating agent

Action: Alkylates DNA, RNA; inhibits enzymes that allow synthesis of amino acids in proteins; is also responsible for cross-linking DNA strands

Uses: Hodgkin's disease; lymphomas; leukemia; cancer of female reproductive tract, lung, prostate; multiple myeloma; neuroblastoma, retinoblastoma; Ewing's sarcoma

Dosage and routes:

• *Adult:* PO initially 1-5 mg/kg over 2-5 days, maintenance 1-5 mg/kg; IV initially 40-50 mg/kg in

C

divided doses over 2-5 days, maintenance 10-15 mg/kg q7-10d or 3-5 mg/kg q3d
• *Child:* PO/IV 2-8 mg/kg or 60-250 mg/m² in divided doses for at least 6 days; maintenance 10-15 mg/kg q7-10d or 30 mg/kg q3-4wk; dose should be reduced by half when bone marrow depression occurs

Available forms include: Powder for inj IV 100, 200, 500 mg and 1, 2 g; tabs 25, 50 mg

Side effects/adverse reactions:
▼ *ORAL:* Stomatitis, swelling of lips, tongue
CNS: Headache, dizziness
CV: Cardiotoxicity (high doses)
GI: Nausea, vomiting, diarrhea, weight loss, hepatotoxicity, colitis
RESP: Fibrosis
HEMA: Thrombocytopenia, leukopenia, pancytopenia, myelosuppression
GU: Hemorrhagic cystitis, hematuria, neoplasms, amenorrhea, azoospermia, impotence, sterility, ovarian fibrosis
INTEG: Alopecia, dermatitis
ENDO: Syndrome of inappropriate antidiuretic hormone (SIADH)

Contraindications: Lactation, pregnancy category D
Precautions: Radiation therapy
Pharmacokinetics:
PO: Half-life 4-6.5 hr; 50% bound to plasma proteins; metabolized by liver; excreted in urine

🦷 **Drug interactions of concern to dentistry:**
• Increased blood dyscrasia: NSAIDs, dapsone, phenothiazines, corticosteroids
• Increased metabolism: phenobarbital

DENTAL CONSIDERATIONS
General:
• Monitor vital signs every appointment due to cardiovascular and respiratory side effects.
• Patients on chronic drug therapy may rarely have symptoms of blood dyscrasias, which can include infection, bleeding, and poor healing.
• Avoid prescribing aspirin-containing products.
• Prophylactic antibiotics may be indicated to prevent infection if surgery or deep scaling is planned due to leukopenic drug side effects.
• Patients receiving chemotherapy may require palliative treatment for stomatitis.
Consultations:
• In a patient with symptoms of blood dyscrasias, request a medical consult for blood studies and postpone dental treatment until normal values are reestablished.
• Take precautions if dental surgery is anticipated and anesthesia is required.
Teach patient/family:
• Importance of good oral hygiene to prevent soft tissue inflammation
• Caution to prevent injury when using oral hygiene aids

---

cycloserine
(sye-kloe-ser′een)
Seromycin Pulvules
Drug class.: Antitubercular

Action: Inhibits cell wall synthesis, analog of D-alanine
Uses: Pulmonary TB, extrapulmonary as adjunctive
Dosage and routes:
• *Adult:* PO 250 mg q12h × 14 days, then 250 mg q8h × 2 wk if

---

bold italic = life-threatening conditions

there are no signs of toxicity, then 250 mg q6h if there are no signs of toxicity, not to exceed 1 g/day
• *Child:* PO 10-20 mg/kg/day (max 0.75-1 g) individual doses
Available forms include: Caps 250 mg

Side effects/adverse reactions:

CNS: **Convulsions,** headache, anxiety, drowsiness, tremors, lethargy, depression, confusion, psychosis, aggression

CV: **CHF**

HEMA: **Megaloblastic anemia,** vitamin B_{12} deficiency, folic acid deficiency, leukocytosis

INTEG: Dermatitis, photosensitivity

Contraindications: Hypersensitivity, seizure disorders, renal disease, alcoholism (chronic), depression, severe anxiety, lactation, anemia

Precautions: Pregnancy category C, children

Pharmacokinetics:

PO: Peak 3-8 hr; excreted unchanged in urine; crosses placenta; excreted in breast milk

Drug interactions of concern to dentistry:
• Seizures: alcohol
• Drowsiness is a common side effect; although no drug interactions with sedatives are reported, increased drowsiness might be possible

DENTAL CONSIDERATIONS
General:
• Patients on chronic drug therapy may rarely have symptoms of blood dyscrasias, which can include infection, bleeding, and poor healing.
• Examine for evidence of oral signs of disease.

• Determine why the patient is taking the drug (i.e., for preventive or therapeutic therapy).

Consultation:
• Medical consult may be required to assess patient's ability to tolerate stress.
• In a patient with symptoms of blood dyscrasias, request a medical consult for blood studies and postpone dental treatment until normal values are reestablished.

Determine that noninfectious status exists by ensuring that:
• Anti-TB drugs have been taken more than 3 wk
• Culture confirms antibiotic susceptibility to TB microorganism
• Patient has had three consecutive negative sputum smears
• Patient is not in the coughing stage

Teach patient/family:
• To avoid mouth rinses with high alcohol content
• Caution to prevent injury when using oral hygiene aids
• Importance of good oral hygiene to prevent soft tissue inflammation
• Importance of taking medication for full length of prescribed therapy to ensure effectiveness of treatment and prevent the emergence of resistant forms of microbe

---

cyclosporine

(sye'kloe-spor-een)
Neoral, Sandimmune, SangCya
Drug class.: Immunosuppressant

Action: Produces immunosuppression by inhibiting lymphocytes (T)
Uses: To prevent rejection of tissues/organ transplants; severe re-

calcitrant psoriasis; rheumatoid arthritis (Neoral only)

Dosage and routes:

• *Adult and child:* PO 15 mg/kg several hours before surgery, daily for 2 wk, reduce dosage by 2.5 mg/kg/wk to 5-10 mg/kg/day; IV 5-6 mg/kg several hours before surgery, daily, switch to PO form as soon as possible

Rheumatoid arthritis (Neoral only)

• *Adult:* PO initial dose 2.5 mg/kg/day bid, after 8-wk dose may be increased by 0.5-0.75 mg/kg/day and again at 12 wk, max dose 4 mg/kg/day

Psoriasis (Neoral only)

• *Adult:* PO initial dose 2.5 mg/kg/day in a twice daily dose; if no progress is seen in 4 wk can increase dose in 2-wk intervals, 0.5 mg/kg/day, to a max of 4 mg/kg/day

Available forms include: Oral sol 100 mg/ml; inj IV 50 mg/ml; caps 25, 50, 100 mg; oral sol for microemulsion 100 µg/ml in 50 ml

Side effects/adverse reactions:

▼ *ORAL: Candidiasis, gingival overgrowth*

CNS: Tremors, headache

CV: Hypertension

GI: **Hepatotoxicity,** nausea, vomiting, diarrhea, pancreatitis

GU: **Albuminuria, hematuria, proteinuria, renal failure**

INTEG: Hirsutism, rash, acne

Contraindications: Hypersensitivity

Precautions: Severe renal disease, severe hepatic disease, pregnancy category C

Pharmacokinetics:

PO: Peak 4 hr, half-life (biphasic) 1.2 hr, 25 hr; highly protein bound; metabolized in liver; crosses placenta; excreted in feces, breast milk

🦷 **Drug interactions of concern to dentistry:**

• Hepatotoxicity/nephrotoxicity: erythromycin, miconazole, ketoconazole, NSAIDs

• Decreased action: barbiturates

• Possibly reduced blood levels: clindamycin

• Increased infection and immunosuppression: corticosteroids

• A single case reported elevated cyclosporine levels: ketoconazole

DENTAL CONSIDERATIONS

General:

• Monitor vital signs every appointment due to cardiovascular side effects.

• Patients on chronic drug therapy may rarely have symptoms of blood dyscrasias, which can include infection, bleeding, and poor healing.

• Place on frequent recall to evaluate gingival condition and healing response.

• Monitor time since organ/tissue transplant.

Consultations:

• Antibiotic prophylaxis is usually recommended in patients with organ transplants and immunosuppression.

• In a patient with symptoms of blood dyscrasias, request a medical consult for blood studies and postpone dental treatment until normal values are reestablished.

• Request baseline blood pressure in renal transplant patients for patient evaluation before dental treatment.

Teach patient/family:
• Importance of good oral hygiene to prevent soft tissue inflammation
• Caution to prevent injury when using oral hygiene aids

---

cyproheptadine HCl
(si-proe-hep′ta-deen)
Periactin
♣ PMS-Cyproheptadine
Drug class.: Antihistamine, H_1-receptor antagonist

Action: Acts on blood vessels, GI, respiratory system by competing with histamine for H_1 receptor site; decreases allergic response by blocking histamine

Uses: Allergy symptoms, rhinitis, pruritus, cold urticaria

Dosage and routes:
• *Adult:* PO 4 mg tid-qid, not to exceed 0.5 mg/kg/day
• *Child 7-14 yr:* PO 4 mg bid-tid, not to exceed 16 mg/day
• *Child 2-6 yr:* PO 2 mg bid-tid, not to exceed 12 mg/day

Available forms include: Tabs 4 mg; syr 2 mg/5 ml

Side effects/adverse reactions:
▼ *ORAL:* Dry mouth
CNS: Dizziness, drowsiness, poor coordination, fatigue, anxiety, euphoria, confusion, paresthesia, neuritis
CV: Hypotension, palpitation, tachycardia
GI: Constipation, nausea, vomiting, anorexia, diarrhea, weight gain
RESP: Increased thick secretions, wheezing, chest tightness

GU: Retention, dysuria, frequency, increased appetite
EENT: Blurred vision, dilated pupils, tinnitus, nasal stuffiness, dry nose/throat
INTEG: Rash, urticaria, photosensitivity

Contraindications: Hypersensitivity to H_1-receptor antagonist, acute asthma attack, lower respiratory tract disease

Precautions: Increased intraocular pressure, renal disease, cardiac disease, hypertension, bronchial asthma, seizure disorder, stenosed peptic ulcers, hyperthyroidism, prostatic hypertrophy, bladder neck obstruction, pregnancy category B, elderly

Pharmacokinetics:
PO: Duration 4-6 hr; metabolized in liver; excreted by kidneys; excreted in breast milk

🦷 **Drug interactions of concern to dentistry:**
• Increased CNS depression: alcohol, CNS depressants
• Increased effect of anticholinergic drugs

DENTAL CONSIDERATIONS
General:
• Assess salivary flow as a factor in caries, periodontal disease, and candidiasis.
• Determine why the patient is taking the drug.

Teach patient/family: *When chronic dry mouth occurs, advise patient:*
• To avoid mouth rinses with high alcohol content due to drying effects
• To use daily home fluoride products for anticaries effect
• To use sugarless gum, frequent sips of water, or saliva substitutes

daclizumab

(da-kli'si-mab)
Zenapax

Drug class.: Immunosuppressive IgG1 monoclonal antibody

Action: Saturates the Tac subunit of interleukin-2 (IL-2) receptor; acts as an IL-2 receptor antagonist

Uses: Prophylaxis of acute organ rejection in patients with renal transplants; use in combination with cyclosporine and glucocorticoids

Dosage and routes:
• *Adult:* IV infusion; 1 mg/kg of body weight as an initial dose no more than 24 hr before transplant surgery and an additional 4 doses given at intervals of 14 days

Available forms include: Vials 25 mg/5 ml

Side effects/adverse effects:
CNS: Tremor, headache, dizziness, insomnia
CV: Peripheral edema, aggravated hypertension
GI: Diarrhea, vomiting, constipation, abdominal pain
RESP: Cough, dyspnea, pulmonary edema
HEMA: Bleeding, lymphocele
GU: Oliguria, dysuria, urinary tract bleeding
EENT: Blurred vision
INTEG: Impaired wound healing, acne, pruritus, rash
MS: Myalgia, back pain
MISC: Fever, pain, fatigue

Contraindications: Hypersensitivity

Precautions: Risk of lymphoproliferative disease and opportunistic infections, anaphylaxis risk unknown, long-term effects unknown, pregnancy category C, lactation, children, geriatric patients

Pharmacokinetics:
IV: Required serum levels for Tac saturation 5-10 µg/ml, terminal elimination half-life 20 days with a range of 11-38 days, renal clearance

⚡ Drug interactions of concern to dentistry:
• None reported

DENTAL CONSIDERATIONS:
General:
• This is a hospital-type drug, but because some dosing is continued, patients may appear in the dental office while receiving this drug.
• Transplant patients may also be taking cyclosporine and glucocorticoids; review each transplant patient's medications.
• Short appointments and a stress reduction protocol may be required for anxious patients.

Consultations:
• Antibiotic prophylaxis is usually recommended in patients with organ transplants and immunosuppression.
• Medical consult may be required to assess disease control and patient's ability to tolerate stress.

Teach patient/family:
• Importance of good oral hygiene to prevent soft tissue inflammation
• To prevent trauma when using oral hygiene aids
• Importance of updating health and drug history if physician makes any changes in evaluation or drug regimens

---

bold italic = life-threatening conditions   *For periodic updates, visit* **www.mosby.com**

dalteparin sodium

(dal-te'pa-rin)
Fragmin
Drug class.: Heparin-type anticoagulant

Action: Low-molecular-weight heparin having antithrombotic actions with higher anti-Factor X_a activity compared with anti-Factor II_a

Uses: Prevention of deep vein thrombosis following abdominal surgery, treatment of life-threatening conditions such as unstable angina, non–q-wave MI; prevention of ischemia complications due to blood clot formation in patients on aspirin therapy; in combination with warfarin in deep vein thrombosis with or without pulmonary embolism

Dosage and routes:
Deep vein thrombosis prophylaxis
• *Adult:* SC 2500 IU each day starting 1-2 hr before surgery and repeated once daily for 5-10 days postoperatively
Unstable angina; non–q-wave angina
• *Adult:* SC 120 IU/kg q 12 hr with 75-165 mg oral aspirin per day for 5-8 days
Available forms include: Prefilled syringe 2500 IU, 5000 IU in 0.2 ml; vial 10,000 IU in 9.5 ml

Side effects/adverse reactions:
HEMA: Bleeding after surgery, thrombocytopenia
INTEG: Skin necrosis
MISC: Local pain, irritation, **anaphylaxis** (rare)

Contraindications: Hypersensitivity, active major bleeding, thrombocytopenia, IM administration

Precautions: Hemorrhage, cannot be used interchangeably with other forms of heparin, pregnancy category B, lactation, children, requires monitoring, GI bleeding

Pharmacokinetics:
SC INJ ONLY: Good absorption, peak levels of anti-Factor X_a activity 4 hr, renal excretion

♣ Drug interactions of concern to dentistry: Avoid concurrent use of aspirin (except as noted), NSAIDs, dipyridamole, and sulfinpyrazone

DENTAL CONSIDERATIONS:
General:
• Product may be used in outpatient therapy. Delay elective dental treatment until patient completes anticoagulant therapy.
• Determine why patient is taking the drug.
• Consider local hemostasis measures to prevent excessive bleeding.
• Avoid prescribing aspirin-containing products.

Consultations:
• Medical consult should include routine blood counts, including platelet counts and bleeding time.

Teach patient/family:
• Importance of good oral hygiene to prevent soft tissue inflammation
• To prevent trauma when using oral hygiene aids
• To report oral lesions, soreness, or bleeding to dentist

danaparoid

(da-nap'a-roid)
Orgaran
Drug class.: Heparin-type anticoagulant

Action: Low-molecular-weight

heparin having antithrombotic actions with higher anti-Factor X_a activity compared with anti-Factor II_a

Uses: Prevention of deep vein thrombosis following hip or knee replacement surgery; unapproved: thromboembolism, hemodialysis, and cardiovascular surgery

Dosage and routes:
• *Adult:* SC 750 anti-Factor X_a units bid; 1-4 hr preoperatively and not sooner than 2 hr after surgery; may be used for 7-12 days

Available forms include: Inj 750 anti-Factor X_a U/0.6 ml, amps and prefilled syringes

Side effects/adverse reactions:
CNS: Insomnia, headache, dizziness
CV: Peripheral edema
GI: Nausea, vomiting, constipation
HEMA: Bleeding after surgery, anemia
GU: UTI, urinary retention
INTEG: Rash, pruritus
MS: Asthenia
MISC: Fever, injection site pain, joint disorder

Contraindications: Hypersensitivity, severe bleeding disorders, type II thrombocytopenia, IM administration

Precautions: Cannot interchange with heparin, hemorrhage, thrombocytopenia, renal or hepatic impairment, pregnancy category B, lactation, children, antidotes not available, GI bleeding

Pharmacokinetics:
SC INJ ONLY: Bioavailability 100%, maximum activity 2-5 hr; renal excretion; half-life based on plasma anti-X_a activity is 18-28 hr

⚕ Drug interactions of concern to dentistry:
• Avoid concurrent use of platelet aggregation antagonist such as aspirin, NSAIDs, dipyridamole

DENTAL CONSIDERATIONS
General:
• Determine why patient is taking the drug.
• Consider local hemostasis measures to prevent excessive bleeding if dental treatment must be performed.
• Antibiotic prophylaxis before dental treatment may be required for joint prosthesis. See 1997 ADA guidelines.
• Delay elective dental treatment until patient completes danaparoid therapy.

Consultations:
• Medical consult should include routine blood counts, including platelet counts and bleeding time.

Teach patient/family:
• Importance of good oral hygiene to prevent soft tissue inflammation
• Caution to prevent trauma when using oral hygiene aids
• To report oral lesions, soreness, or bleeding to dentist

danazol
(da′na-zole)
Danocrine
♣ Cyclomen

Drug class.: Androgen, α-ethinyl testosterone derivative

Action: Decreases FSH and LH output and inhibits output of pituitary gonadotropins, leading to amenorrhea/anovulation

Uses: Endometriosis, prevention of hereditary angioedema, fibrocystic breast disease

Dosage and routes:

Endometriosis

• *Adult:* PO initial dose 800 mg bid, then decreased to 200-400 mg bid × 3-9 mo

Fibrocystic breast disease

• *Adult:* PO 100-400 mg qd in 2 divided doses × 2-6 mo

Hereditary angioedema

• *Adult:* PO 200 mg bid-tid until desired response, then decrease dose to 100 mg at 1-3 mo intervals

Available forms include: Caps 50, 100, 200 mg

Side effects/adverse reactions:

▼ *ORAL:* Gingival bleeding (rare), stomatitis, Stevens-Johnson syndrome (rare)

CNS: Dizziness, headache, fatigue, tremors, paresthesia, flushing, sweating, anxiety, lability, insomnia

CV: Increased BP

GI: Cholestatic jaundice, nausea, vomiting, constipation, weight gain

GU: Hematuria, amenorrhea, atrophic vaginitis, decreased libido, decreased breast size, clitoral hypertrophy, testicular atrophy

EENT: Carpal tunnel syndrome, conjunctival edema, nasal congestion

INTEG: Rash, acneiform lesions, oily hair/skin, flushing, sweating, acne vulgaris, alopecia, hirsutism

ENDO: Abnormal GTT

MS: Cramps, spasms

Contraindications: Severe renal disease, severe cardiac disease, severe hepatic disease, hypersensitivity, genital bleeding (abnormal), pregnancy

Precautions: Migraine headaches, seizure disorders, pregnancy category X

Pharmacokinetics: Limited data available; oral absorption variable; metabolized in the liver

🦷 **Drug interactions of concern to dentistry:**

• Increased serum concentration of carbamazepine; consider avoiding use of concurrent administration

DENTAL CONSIDERATIONS

General:

• Patients on chronic drug therapy may rarely have symptoms of blood dyscrasias, which can include infection, bleeding, and poor healing.

Consultations:

• In a patient with symptoms of blood dyscrasias, request a medical consult for blood studies and postpone dental treatment until normal values are reestablished.

Teach patient/family:

• Importance of good oral hygiene to prevent soft tissue inflammation

• To avoid mouth rinses with high alcohol content due to drying and irritating effects

---

dantrolene sodium

(dan′troe-leen)

Dantrium, Dantrium Intravenous

Drug class.: Skeletal muscle relaxant, direct acting

Action: Interferes with intracellular release of the calcium necessary to initiate contraction

Uses: Spasticity in multiple sclerosis, stroke, spinal cord injury, cerebral palsy, malignant hyperthermia

Dosage and routes:

Spasticity

• *Adult:* PO 25 mg/day; may in-

crease by 25-100 mg bid-qid, not to exceed 400 mg/day × 1 wk
• *Child:* PO 1 mg/kg/day given in divided doses bid-tid; may increase gradually, not to exceed 100 mg qid

Malignant hyperthermia
• *Adult and child:* IV 1 mg/kg, may repeat to total dose of 10 mg/kg; PO 4-8 mg/kg/day in 4 divided doses × 3 days to prevent further hyperthermia

Available forms include: Caps 25, 50, 100 mg; powder for inj IV 20 mg/vial

Side effects/adverse reactions:
▼ *ORAL:* Alteration of taste
CNS: Dizziness, weakness, fatigue, drowsiness, headache, disorientation, insomnia, paresthesia, tremors
CV: Hypotension, chest pain, palpitation, tachycardia
*GI: Nausea, **hepatotoxicity,*** constipation, vomiting, abdominal pain, diarrhea, anorexia; increased AST, alk phosphatase
*HEMA: **Eosinophilia***
GU: Urinary frequency, nocturia, impotence, crystalluria
EENT: Nasal congestion, blurred vision, mydriasis
INTEG: Rash, pruritus, photosensitivity
MS: Myalgia, backache

Contraindications: Hypersensitivity, compromised pulmonary function, active hepatic disease, impaired myocardial function

Precautions: Peptic ulcer disease, renal disease, hepatic disease, stroke, seizure disorder, diabetes mellitus, pregnancy category C, elderly; monitor liver enzymes

Pharmacokinetics:
PO: Peak 5 hr, half-life 8 hr; highly protein bound; metabolized in liver; excreted in urine (metabolites)

🐂 Drug interactions of concern to dentistry:
• Increased CNS depression: alcohol, other CNS depressants

DENTAL CONSIDERATIONS
General:
• Monitor vital signs every appointment due to cardiovascular and respiratory side effects.
• Patients on chronic drug therapy may rarely have symptoms of blood dyscrasias, which can include infection, bleeding, and poor healing.
• Requires proficiency in IV administration technique when used for emergency treatment of malignant hyperthermia.

Consultations:
• In a patient with symptoms of blood dyscrasias, request a medical consult for blood studies and postpone dental treatment until normal values are reestablished.

Teach patient/family:
• Importance of good oral hygiene to prevent soft tissue inflammation
• To avoid mouth rinses with high alcohol content due to drying effects

---

dapsone (DDS)
(dap′sone)
Avlosulfon

Drug class.: Leprostatic, antibacterial

Action: Bactericidal and bacteriostatic against *M. leprae;* may also be immunosuppressant
Uses: Leprosy (Hansen's disease); dermatitis herpetiformis; unapproved: cicatricial pemphigoid, LE, pemphigoid, malaria, *P. carinii*

---

bold italic = life-threatening conditions   *For periodic updates, visit* **www.mosby.com**

Dosage and routes:
Leprosy
• *Adult:* PO 50-100 mg qd with rifampin 600 mg qd × 6 mo
• *Child:* PO 1-2 mg/kg/day for minimum of 3 yr; not to exceed adult dose
Dermatitis herptiformis
• *Adult:* PO initial dose 50 mg/day; can increase by 50 mg every 1-2 wk until remission; dose limit 500 mg/day; gradually reduce dose to lowest effective maintenance dose
Available forms include: Tabs 25, 100 mg
Side effects/adverse reactions:
▼ *ORAL:* Oral ulceration (erythema multiforme), lichenoid drug reaction
CNS: Convulsions, peripheral neuropathy, headache, anxiety, drowsiness, tremors, lethargy, depression, confusion, psychosis, aggression
GI: Nausea, vomiting, abdominal pain, anorexia
HEMA: Megaloblastic anemia
GU: Proteinuria, nephrotic syndrome, renal papillary necrosis
EENT: Blurred vision, optic neuritis, photophobia
INTEG: Exfoliative dermatitis, photosensitivity
Contraindications: Hypersensitivity to sulfones, severe anemia
Precautions: Renal disease, hepatic disease, G6PD deficiency, pregnancy category C, lactation
Pharmacokinetics:
PO: Half-life 10-50 hr; rapid complete absorption; highly bound to plasma protein; metabolized in liver; excreted in urine
DENTAL CONSIDERATIONS
General:
• Patients on chronic drug therapy may rarely have symptoms of blood dyscrasias, which can include infection, bleeding, and poor healing.
• Avoid dental light in patient's eyes; offer dark glasses for patient comfort.
Consultations:
• In a patient with symptoms of blood dyscrasias, request a medical consult for blood studies and postpone dental treatment until normal values are reestablished.
Teach patient/family:
• Importance of good oral hygiene to prevent soft tissue inflammation
• Caution to prevent injury when using oral hygiene aids

---

darbepoetin alfa
(dar-be-poe′e-tin)
Aranesp
Drug class.: Hematopoietic agent

Action: An erythropoiesis stimulating protein; stimulates the division and differentiation of erythroid progenitors in bone marrow
Uses: Anemia associated with chronic renal failure
Dosage and routes:
• *Adult:* IV or SC start with low dose and slowly adjust upward depending on hemoglobin levels, give once weekly; to correct anemia the starting dose is 0.45 µg/kg; titrate dose to target of 12 g/l of hemoglobin
Available forms include: 25, 40, 60, 100, 200 µg/ml in 1 ml single-use vials
Side effects/adverse reactions:
CNS: Headache, fatigue, dizziness
CV: Hypertension, hypotension, CHF, acute MI, stroke, TIA, peripheral edema, arrhythmias, angina pain

GI: Diarrhea, nausea, vomiting, abdominal pain, constipation
RESP: URI, dyspnea, cough, bronchitis
*HEMA: **Thrombosis***
MS: Myalgia, chest pain, asthenia, limb pain
MISC: Infection, fever, flulike syndrome
Contraindications: Uncontrolled hypertension, hypersensitivity
Precautions: Increased risk of serious cardiovascular events, seizures in CRF, albumin formula has risk of viral diseases, pregnancy category C, safety in lactation or pediatric patients not established
Pharmacokinetics: Information unavailable
🦷 **Drug interactions of concern to dentistry:**
• No studies reported
DENTAL CONSIDERATIONS
General:
• Monitor vital signs every appointment due to cardiovascular side effects.
• Consider semisupine chair position for patient comfort if GI side effects occur.
• Monitor disease control and date of last dialysis.
• Prophylactic antibiotics may be indicated to prevent infection if surgery or deep scaling is planned.
Consultations:
• Medical consult may be required to assess disease control and patient's ability to tolerate stress.
Teach patient/family:
• Importance of good oral hygiene to prevent soft tissue inflammation/infection
• Importance of updating health and drug history if physician makes any changes in evaluation or drug regimens

delavirdine mesylate
(de-la-vir′deen)
Rescriptor
Drug class.: Antiviral, nonnucleoside

Action: Inhibits HIV-I reverse transcriptase enzymes; inhibits both DNA- and RNA-directed polymerase activity
Uses: HIV infection in combination with appropriate antiretroviral agents when therapy is warranted
Dosage and routes:
• *Adult:* PO 400 mg tid; may be given with or without food
Available forms include: Tabs 100, 200 mg
Side effects/adverse reactions:
▼ *ORAL:* Dry mouth (<2%), stomatitis, mouth ulcers, taste perversion
CNS: Headache, fatigue, agitation, confusion
CV: Bradycardia, palpitation, orthostatic hypotension, syncope
GI: Nausea, vomiting, abdominal pain, dyspepsia, diarrhea
RESP: Cough, congestion
HEMA: Neutropenia, leukopenia, thrombocytopenia, anemia, granulocytopenia
GU: Proteinuria
EENT: Dry eyes, conjunctivitis, diplopia
INTEG: Skin rash, pruritus
META: Altered liver function tests, elevated serum creatinine, alcohol intolerance
MS: Myalgia, cramps
Contraindications: Hypersensitivity
Precautions: Modify dose in liver disease; children <16 yr, pregnancy category C, lactation

---

bold italic = life-threatening conditions

Pharmacokinetics:
PO: Peak plasma levels 1.0 hr, highly protein bound (98%), hepatic metabolism, excreted in both urine and feces, plasma half-life 2-11 hr

🦷 **Drug interactions of concern to dentistry:**
• Reduced absorption: antacids, cimetidine
• Increased plasma levels of both delavirdine and clarithromycin
• Increased plasma levels of alprazolam, triazolam, midazolam
• Avoid coadministration with carbamazepine, phenobarbital, ketoconazole

DENTAL CONSIDERATIONS
General:
• Examine for oral manifestation of opportunistic infection.
• Patient on chronic drug therapy may rarely have symptoms of blood dyscrasias, which can include infection, bleeding, and poor healing.
• Assess salivary flow as factor in caries, periodontal disease, and candidiasis.
• After supine positioning, have patient sit upright for at least 2 min before standing to avoid orthostatic hypotension.
• Do not use ingestible sodium bicarbonate products, such as the air polishing system (ProphyJet), within 2 hr of drug use.

Consultations:
• In a patient with symptoms of blood dyscrasias, request a medical consult for blood studies and postpone treatment until normal values are reestablished.
• Medical consult may be required to assess disease control and patient's ability to tolerate stress.

Teach patient/family:
• Importance of good oral hygiene to prevent soft tissue inflammation
• Caution to prevent trauma when using oral hygiene aids
• That secondary oral infection may occur; must see dentist immediately if infection occurs
When chronic dry mouth occurs advise patient:
• To avoid mouth rinses with high alcohol content due to drying effects
• To use daily home fluoride products for anticaries effect
• To use sugarless gum, frequent sips of water, or saliva substitutes

---

demeclocycline HCl
(dem-e-kloe-sye'kleen)
Declomycin
Drug class.: Tetracycline

Action: Inhibits protein synthesis and phosphorylation in microorganisms by binding to 30S ribosomal subunits, reversibly binding to 50S ribosomal subunits; bacteriostatic

Uses: A wide variety of grampositive/gram-negative bacteria, protozoa, *Rickettsia, Mycoplasma,* agents of psittacosis and ornithosis, actinomyces species

Dosage and routes:
• *Adult:* PO 150 mg q6h or 300 mg q12h
• *Child >8 yr:* PO 3-6 mg/kg/day in divided doses q6-12h
Gonorrhea
• *Adult:* PO 600 mg, then 300 mg q12h × 4 days, total 3 g
Syndrome of inappropriate antidiuretic hormone
• *Adult:* PO 600-1200 mg/day in divided doses

Available forms include: Tabs 150, 300 mg

Side effects/adverse reactions:

▼ *ORAL:* Candidiasis, tooth discoloration, increased thirst, discolored tongue, lichenoid reaction

CNS: Fever, headache, paresthesia

CV: Pericarditis

GI: Nausea, vomiting, diarrhea, ***hepatotoxicity, pseudomembranous colitis,*** anorexia, enterocolitis, flatulence, abdominal cramps, epigastric burning

*HEMA: **Eosinophilia, neutropenia, thrombocytopenia, leukocytosis, hemolytic anemia***

*GU: Increased BUN, **renal failure, nephrotoxicity,*** polyuria, polydipsia

EENT: Dysphagia, abdominal pain

INTEG: Rash, urticaria, photosensitivity, increased pigmentation, ***exfoliative dermatitis,*** pruritus, angioedema

Contraindications: Hypersensitivity to tetracyclines, children <8 yr, pregnancy category D

Precautions: Renal disease, hepatic disease, lactation, nephrogenic diabetes insipidus

Pharmacokinetics:

PO: Peak 3-6 hr, duration 48-72 hr, half-life 10-17 hr; 36%-91% bound to serum protein; crosses placenta; excreted in urine, breast milk

🦷 **Drug interactions of concern to dentistry:**

• Decreased effect of penicillins, cephalosporins, oral contraceptives

• Oral contraceptives: advise patient of a potential risk for decreased contraceptive action, to maintain compliance with oral contraceptive use while using antibiotics, and to consider the use of additional nonhormonal contraception

DENTAL CONSIDERATIONS

General:

• Examine oral cavity for side effects if on long-term drug therapy.

• Determine why the patient is taking the drug.

• Do not prescribe during pregnancy or before age 8 yr due to tooth discoloration.

• Absorption is reduced by dairy products, metals, and antacids.

Consultations:

• Medical consult may be required to assess disease control.

Teach patient/family:

• Importance of good oral hygiene to prevent soft tissue inflammation

• Caution to prevent injury when using oral hygiene aids

When used for dental infection, advise patient:

• To report sore throat, oral burning sensation, fever, fatigue, any of which could indicate superinfection

• To take at prescribed intervals and complete dosage regimen

• To immediately notify the dentist if signs or symptoms of infection increase

---

desipramine HCl

(des-ip′ra-meen)

Norpramin, Pertofrane

Drug class.: Antidepressant, tricyclic

Action: Inhibits both norepinephrine and serotonin (5-HT) uptake in the brain, although the precise antidepressant mechanism remains unclear

Uses: Depression; unapproved: neurogenic pain

---

bold italic = life-threatening conditions

Dosage and routes:
• *Adult:* PO 100-200 mg/day in divided doses, may increase to 300 mg/day or may give daily dose hs
• *Adolescent/geriatric:* PO 25-50 mg/day, may increase to 100 mg/day

Available forms include: Tabs 10, 25, 50, 75, 100, 150 mg

Side effects/adverse reactions:

▼ *ORAL: Dry mouth, unpleasant taste,* bleeding, stomatitis

CNS: Dizziness, drowsiness, confusion, headache, anxiety, tremors, stimulation, weakness, insomnia, nightmares, EPS (elderly), increased psychiatric symptoms, paresthesia

CV: Orthostatic hypotension, ECG changes, tachycardia, **hypertension,** palpitation, prolonged QT interval

GI: Diarrhea, **paralytic ileus, hepatitis,** increased appetite, cramps, epigastric distress, jaundice, nausea, vomiting

HEMA: **Agranulocytosis, thrombocytopenia, eosinophilia, leukopenia**

GU: Retention, **acute renal failure**

EENT: Blurred vision, tinnitus, mydriasis, ophthalmoplegia

INTEG: Rash, urticaria, sweating, pruritus, photosensitivity

Contraindications: Hypersensitivity to tricyclic antidepressants, recovery phase of MI, narrow-angle glaucoma, convulsive disorders, prostatic hypertrophy, child <12 yr

Precautions: Suicidal patients, severe depression, increased intraocular pressure, narrow-angle glaucoma, elderly, pregnancy category C, MAO inhibitors

Pharmacokinetics:
PO: Steady state 2-11 days, half-life 14-62 hr; metabolized by liver; excreted by kidneys; crosses placenta

🐾 **Drug interactions of concern to dentistry:**
• Increased anticholinergic effects: muscarinic blockers, antihistamines, phenothiazines
• Increased effects of direct-acting sympathomimetics: epinephrine, levonordefrin
• Potential risk for increased CNS depression: alcohol, barbiturates, benzodiazepines, and other CNS depressants
• Decreased antihypertensive effects: clonidine, guanadrel, guanethidine
• At higher tricyclic doses, serum levels of fluconazole and ketoconazole may be elevated

DENTAL CONSIDERATIONS
General:
• Take vital signs every appointment due to cardiovascular side effects.
• Assess salivary flow as a factor in caries, periodontal disease, and candidiasis.
• Patients on chronic drug therapy may rarely have symptoms of blood dyscrasias, which can include infection, bleeding, and poor healing.
• After supine positioning, have patient sit upright for at least 2 min to avoid orthostatic hypotension.
• Use vasoconstrictors with caution, in low doses, and with careful aspiration. Avoid use of gingival retraction cord with epinephrine.
• Place on frequent recall due to oral side effects.
Consultations:
• In a patient with symptoms of

blood dyscrasias, request a medical consult for blood studies and postpone dental treatment until normal values are reestablished.

• Medical consult may be required to assess disease control.

• Physician should be informed if significant xerostomic side effects occur (increased caries, sore tongue, problems eating or swallowing, difficulty wearing prosthesis) so a medication change can be considered.

Teach patient/family:

• Importance of good oral hygiene to prevent soft tissue inflammation

• Caution to prevent injury when using oral hygiene aids

When chronic dry mouth occurs, advise patient:

• To avoid mouth rinses with high alcohol content due to drying effects

• To use daily home fluoride products for anticaries effect

• To use sugarless gum, frequent sips of water, or saliva substitutes

---

desloratadine

(des-lor-at′-a-deen)

Clarinex

Drug class: Antihistamine, histamine H_1 antagonist

Action: Antagonism of H_1 receptors, blocking typical allergic manifestations of histamine release
Use: Seasonal allergic rhinitis; chronic idiopathic urticaria
Dose and routes:
• *Adult and child >12 yr:* PO 5 mg once daily
Available forms include: Tab 5 mg
Side effects/adverse reactions:
▼ *ORAL:* Dry mouth

CNS: Somnolence, fatigue, headache, dizziness
CV: Tachycardia
GI: Nausea, dyspepsia
METAB: Elevated liver enzymes, elevated bilirubin
EENT: Pharyngitis
INTEG: Rash, pruritus, urticaria
MS: Myalgia
MISC: Rarely edema, anaphylaxis, dyspnea
Contraindications: Hypersensitivity to this drug or loratadine
Precautions: Pregnancy category C, distributed to breast milk (caution in nursing), incomplete dosing studies in the elderly, safety has not been established in children <12 yr, dosage adjustment required in hepatic impairment
Pharmacokinetics:
PO: Good oral absorption; peak levels 3 hr; metabolized to 3-hydroxydesloratadine (active metabolite), highly plasma protein bound (desloratadine—82% to 87%; 3-hydroxydesloratadine—85% to 87%); glucuronidated metabolites excreted in urine
🦷 **Drug interactions of concern to dentistry:**
• Limited studies with concurrent doses of erythromycin; ketoconazole and azithromycin show slight elevations of plasma levels, but no clinically relevant changes in electrocardiographic parameters
• One report indicated a potential for increased anticholinergic effects with other anticholinergic drugs and increased somnolence with CNS depressants; however, data are lacking
DENTAL CONSIDERATIONS
General:
• Assess salivary flow as a factor in

---

bold italic = life-threatening conditions

caries, periodontal disease, and candidiasis

Teach patient/family:

• Importance of good oral hygiene to prevent soft tissue inflammation

When chronic dry mouth occurs advise patient:

• To avoid mouth rinses with high alcohol content due to drying effects

• To use sugarless gum, frequent sips of water, or saliva substitutes

• To use daily home fluoride products for anticaries effect

---

desmopressin acetate

(des-moe-press'in)

DDAVP, DDAVP Nasal Solution, Stimate Nasal Solution
♣ DDAVP Rhinal Tube, DDAVP Rhinyl Nasal Solution, DDAVP Spray, Octosim

Drug class.: Synthetic antidiuretic hormone (a synthetic analog of vasopressin)

Action: Promotes reabsorption of water by action on renal tubular epithelium; also causes an increase in Factor VIII levels

Uses: Primary nocturnal enuresis, hemophilia A with Factor VIII levels >5%, von Willebrand's disease, neurogenic diabetes insipidus, renal concentration capacity

Dosage and routes:

Diabetes insipidus

• *Adult:* INTRANASAL 0.1-0.4 ml qd in divided doses; IV/SC 0.5-1 ml qd in divided doses

• *Adult:* PO initial dose 0.05 mg bid, increase to 0.1-1.2 mg in divided doses as required

• *Child 3 mo-12 yr:* INTRANASAL 0.05-0.3 ml qd in divided doses

Hemophilia/von Willebrand's disease

• *Adult and child:* IV 0.3 µg/kg in NaCl over 15-30 min; may repeat if needed

Available forms include: Nasal sol 1.5 mg/ml; nasal spray pump 0.1 mg/ml; intranasal test 0.1 mg/ml; inj IV/SC 4, 15 µg/ml; tab 0.1 and 0.2 mg

Side effects/adverse reactions:

CNS: Headache, drowsiness, lethargy, flushing

CV: Increased BP

GI: Nausea, *mild abdominal cramps,* heartburn

GU: Vulval pain

EENT: Nasal irritation, congestion, rhinitis

Contraindications: Hypersensitivity, nephrogenic diabetes insipidus

Precautions: Pregnancy category B, CAD, lactation, hypertension

Pharmacokinetics:

NASAL: Onset 1 hr, peak 1-2 hr, duration 8-20 hr, half-life 8 min, 76 min (terminal)

🦷 Drug interactions of concern to dentistry:

• Decreased antidiuretic effects: demeclocycline

• Increased antidiuretic effects: carbamazepine

DENTAL CONSIDERATIONS

General:

• Monitor vital signs every appointment due to cardiovascular side effects.

• Avoid prescribing aspirin-containing products if treatment is for bleeding disorder.

• Consider local hemostasis measures to prevent excessive bleeding.

• Determine why the patient is taking the drug.

• Consider semisupine chair position for patient comfort due to GI effects of disease.

Consultations:

• Medical consult may be required to assess disease control; definite consult for patients with chronic bleeding disorders.

• Medical consult should include partial prothrombin or prothrombin times.

Teach patient/family:

• To advise dentist if excessive bleeding occurs or continues after dental treatment

---

desonide

(dess'oh-nide)

DesOwen, Tridesilon

Drug class.: Topical corticosteroid, group IV low potency

Action: Glucocorticoids have multiple actions that include antiinflammatory and immunosuppressant effects. They inhibit phospholipase A_2, interfering with or reducing the synthesis of prostaglandins and leukotrienes. They also bind to cytoplasmic glucocorticoid receptors (GRs) and enter the cell nucleus to bind with DNA. This results in the synthesis of various enzymes such as collagenase, elastase, and cytokines that play important roles in inflammation and immunosuppression. They also suppress the production of lymphocytes, monocytes, and eosinophils.

Uses: Psoriasis, eczema, contact dermatitis, pruritus

Dosage and routes:

• *Adult and child:* TOP apply to affected area bid-tid

Available forms include: Cream 0.05%; oint 0.05%; lotion 0.05%

Side effects/adverse reactions:

▼ *ORAL:* Perioral dermatitis

INTEG: Burning, dryness, itching, irritation, acne, folliculitis, hypertrichosis, hypopigmentation, atrophy, striae, miliaria, allergic contact dermatitis, secondary infection

Contraindications: Hypersensitivity to corticosteroids, fungal infections

Precautions: Pregnancy category C, lactation, viral infections, bacterial infections

DENTAL CONSIDERATIONS

General:

• Determine why the patient is taking the drug.

• Place on frequent recall to evaluate healing response if used on chronic basis.

• Apply lubricant to dry lips for patient comfort before dental procedures.

---

desoximetasone

(des-ox-i-met'a-sone)

Topicort, Topicort LP

♣ Topicort Mild

Drug class.: Topical corticosteroid, group II potency (0.25%), group III potency (0.05%)

Action: Glucocorticoids have multiple actions that include antiinflammatory and immunosuppressant effects. They inhibit phospholipase A_2, interfering with or reducing the synthesis of prostaglandins and leukotrienes. They also bind to cytoplasmic glucocorticoid receptors (GRs) and enter the cell nucleus to bind with DNA. This results in the synthesis of various enzymes such as collagenase, elastase, and cytokines that play important roles in inflammation and immunosuppression. They also suppress the production of lymphocytes, monocytes, and eosinophils.

Uses: Psoriasis, eczema, contact dermatitis, pruritus

Dosage and routes:
• *Adult and child:* TOP apply to affected area bid-tid

Available forms include: Cream 0.05%, 0.25%; oint 0.25%; gel 0.05% in 15 and 60 g tubes

Side effects/adverse reactions:
▼ *ORAL:* Thinning of mucosa, stinging sensation (oral application)

INTEG: Burning, dryness, itching, irritation, acne, folliculitis, hypertrichosis, perioral dermatitis, hypopigmentation, atrophy, striae, miliaria, allergic contact dermatitis, secondary infection

Contraindications: Hypersensitivity to corticosteroids, fungal infections

Precautions: Pregnancy category C, lactation, viral infections, bacterial infections

DENTAL CONSIDERATIONS
General:
• Gel formulations are used in the treatment of oral lichen planus lesions when the diagnosis has been confirmed by immunofluorescent biopsy testing.
• Place on frequent recall to evaluate healing response.

Teach patient/family:
• When used for oral lesions, to return for oral evaluation if response of oral tissues has not occurred in 7-14 days
• Importance of good oral hygiene to prevent soft tissue inflammation
• That use on oral herpetic ulcerations is contraindicated

• To apply at bedtime or after meals for maximum effect
• To apply with cotton-tipped applicator, dabbing gently, not rubbing medication on lesion

---

dexamethasone/ dexamethasone sodium phosphate

(dex-a-meth′a-sone)

Aeroseb-Dex, Decaderm, Decadron Phosphate, Decaspray

Drug class.: Synthetic topical corticosteroid

Action: Glucocorticoids have multiple actions that include antiinflammatory and immunosuppressant effects. They inhibit phospholipase A_2, interfering with or reducing the synthesis of prostaglandins and leukotrienes. They also bind to cytoplasmic glucocorticoid receptors (GRs) and enter the cell nucleus to bind with DNA. This results in the synthesis of various enzymes such as collagenase, elastase, and cytokines that play important roles in inflammation and immunosuppression. They also suppress the production of lymphocytes, monocytes, and eosinophils.

Uses: Corticosteroid-responsive dermatoses, oral ulcerative inflammatory lesions

Dosage and routes:
• *Adult and child:* TOP apply to affected area bid-qid

Available forms include: Gel 0.1%; aerosol 0.01%, 0.04%; cream 0.1%

Side effects/adverse reactions:
▼ *ORAL:* Thinning of mucosa, stinging sensation (oral application)

INTEG: Burning, dryness, itching, irritation, acne, folliculitis, hypertrichosis, perioral dermatitis, hypopigmentation, atrophy, striae, miliaria, allergic contact dermatitis, secondary infection

Contraindications: Hypersensitivity to corticosteroids, fungal infections, viral infections

Precautions: Pregnancy category C, lactation, viral infections, bacterial infections

DENTAL CONSIDERATIONS
General:
• Place on frequent recall to evaluate healing response.

Teach patient/family:
• When used for oral lesions, to return for oral evaluation if response of oral tissues has not occurred in 7-14 days
• Importance of good oral hygiene to prevent soft tissue inflammation
• To apply approximately 0.25 inch; measure and apply with cotton-tipped applicator by gently dabbing, not rubbing, medication on lesion
• To apply at bedtime or after meals for maximum effect
• That use on oral herpetic ulcerations is contraindicated dexamethasone/dexamethasone acetate

dexamethasone/ dexamethasone acetate/ dexamethasone sodium phosphate
(dex-a-meth′a-sone)

Dexamethasone oral tab: Decadron, Decadron DosePak, Dexameth, Dexaone, Hexadrol, Hexadrol Therapeutic Pack
♣ Deronil, Dexasone, Oradexan
Dexamethasone elixir: Decadron, Hexadrol
Dexamethasone oral solution: Intensol
Dexamethasone acetate (long-lasting injection NOT FOR IV USE): Dalalaone DP, Dalalone LA, Decadron LA, Decaject-LA, Dexasone-LA, Dexone LA, Solurex-LA
Dexamethasone sodium phosphate (inj): Cortastat, Dalaone, Decadron Phosphate, Decaject, Dexone, Hexadrol Phosphate, Solurex

Drug class.: Glucocorticoid, long acting

Action: Glucocorticoids have multiple actions that include antiinflammatory and immunosuppressant effects. They inhibit phospholipase A_2, interfering with or reducing the synthesis of prostaglandins and leukotrienes. They also bind to cytoplasmic glucocorticoid receptors (GRs) and enter the cell nucleus to bind with DNA. This results in the synthesis of various enzymes such as collagenase, elastase, and cytokines that play important roles in inflammation and immunosuppression. They also suppress the production of lymphocytes, monocytes, and eosinophils.

Uses: Inflammation, allergies, neoplasms, cerebral edema, shock, collagen disorders

Dosage and routes:

Inflammation
• *Adult:* PO 0.25-4 mg bid-qid; IM 4-16 mg q1-3wk (acetate)

Shock
• *Adult:* IV 1-6 mg/kg or 40 mg q2-6h (phosphate)

Cerebral edema
• *Adult:* IV 10 mg, then 4-6 mg q6h × 2-4 days, then taper over 1 wk
• *Child:* PO 0.2 mg/kg/day in divided doses

Available forms include: Tabs 0.25, 0.5, 0.75, 1, 1.5, 2, 4, 6 mg; inj IM acetate 8, 16 mg/ml; inj IV phosphate 4, 10, 20, 24 mg/ml; elix 0.5 mg/5 ml; oral sol 0.5 mg/5 ml, 0.5 mg/0.5 ml

Side effects/adverse reactions:

▼ *ORAL: Candidiasis,* dry mouth
CNS: Depression, flushing, sweating, headache, mood changes
*CV: Hypertension, **circulatory collapse, thrombophlebitis, embolism,** tachycardia, edema*
*GI: Diarrhea, nausea, abdominal distention, **GI hemorrhage, pancreatitis,** increased appetite*
*HEMA: **Thrombocytopenia***
EENT: Fungal infections, increased intraocular pressure, blurred vision
INTEG: Acne, poor wound healing, ecchymosis, petechiae
MS: Fractures, osteoporosis, weakness

Contraindications: Psychosis, hypersensitivity, idiopathic thrombocytopenia, acute glomerulonephritis, amebiasis, fungal infections, nonasthmatic bronchial disease, child <2 yr, AIDS, TB

Precautions: Pregnancy category C, diabetes mellitus, glaucoma, osteoporosis, seizure disorders, ulcerative colitis, CHF, myasthenia gravis, renal disease, peptic ulcer, esophagitis

Pharmacokinetics:
PO: Peak 1-2 hr, duration 2.33 days
IM: Peak 8 hr, duration 6 days
Half-life 3-4.5 hr

⚕ Drug interactions of concern to dentistry:
• Decreased action: barbiturates
• Increased side effects: alcohol, salicylates, and other NSAIDs
• Increased action: ketoconazole, macrolide antibiotics

DENTAL CONSIDERATIONS

General:
• Monitor vital signs every appointment due to cardiovascular side effects.
• Patients on chronic drug therapy may rarely have symptoms of blood dyscrasias, which can include infection, bleeding, and poor healing.
• Symptoms of oral infections may be masked.
• Patients who have been or are currently on chronic steroid therapy (>2 wk) may require supplemental steroids for dental treatment.
• Avoid prescribing aspirin-containing products.
• Place on frequent recall to evaluate healing response.
• Prophylactic antibiotics may be indicated to prevent infection if surgery or deep scaling is planned.

Consultations:
• In a patient with symptoms of blood dyscrasias, request a medical consult for blood studies and postpone dental treatment until normal values are reestablished.
• Medical consult may be required to assess disease control.
• Consult may be required to con-

firm steroid dose and duration of use.

Teach patient/family:
• Importance of good oral hygiene to prevent soft tissue inflammation
• Caution to prevent injury when using oral hygiene aids
• To avoid mouth rinses with high alcohol content due to drug interaction

---

dexchlorpheniramine maleate

(dex-klor-fen-eer′a-meen)
Polaramine, Polaramine Repetabs

Drug class.: Antihistamine

Action: Acts on blood vessels, GI system, respiratory system by competing with histamine for H_1-receptor site; decreases allergic response by blocking histamine
Uses: Allergy symptoms, rhinitis, pruritus, contact dermatitis
Dosage and routes:
• *Adult:* PO 1-2 mg tid-qid; repeat action 4-6 mg tid
• *Child 6-11 yr:* PO 1 mg q4-6h; time rel 4 mg hs
• *Child 2-5 yr:* PO 0.5 mg q4-6h; do not use repeat-action form
Available forms include: Tabs 2 mg; timed release tab 4, 6 mg; syr 2 mg/5 ml
Side effects/adverse reactions:
▼ *ORAL:* Dry mouth
CNS: Dizziness, drowsiness, poor coordination, fatigue, anxiety, euphoria, confusion, paresthesia, neuritis
CV: Hypotension, palpitations, tachycardia
GI: Constipation, nausea, vomiting, anorexia, diarrhea

RESP: Increased thick secretions, wheezing, chest tightness
GU: Retention, dysuria, frequency
EENT: Blurred vision, dilated pupils, tinnitus, nasal stuffiness, dry nose/throat
INTEG: Rash, urticaria, photosensitivity
Contraindications: Hypersensitivity to H_1-receptor antagonist; acute asthma attack, lower respiratory tract disease
Precautions: Increased intraocular pressure, renal disease, cardiac disease, hypertension, bronchial asthma, seizure disorder, stenosed peptic ulcers, hyperthyroidism, prostatic hypertrophy, bladder neck obstruction, pregnancy category B, elderly
Pharmacokinetics:
PO (EXCEPT EXTENDED-ACTION DOSE FORMS): Onset 15 min, peak 3 hr, duration 3-6 hr; metabolized in liver; excreted by kidneys (inactive metabolites); excreted in breast milk (small amounts)
⚖ Drug interactions of concern to dentistry:
• Increased CNS depression: barbiturates, narcotics, hypnotics, tricyclic antidepressants, alcohol
• Increased anticholinergic effect: anticholinergic drugs
DENTAL CONSIDERATIONS
General:
• Assess salivary flow as a factor in caries, periodontal disease, and candidiasis.
• Consider semisupine chair position for patient comfort due to respiratory effects of disease.
Teach patient/family: *When chronic dry mouth occurs, advise patient:*
• To avoid mouth rinses with high

---

alcohol content due to drying effects

• To use sugarless gum, frequent sips of water, or saliva substitutes

• To use daily home fluoride products for anticaries effect

dextroamphetamine sulfate

(dex-troe-am-fet′a-meen)

Dexedrine, Dexedrine Spansules, DextroStat

Drug class.: Amphetamine

Controlled Substance Schedule II, Canada G

Action: Increases release of norepinephrine, dopamine in cerebral cortex to reticular activating system

Uses: Narcolepsy, attention deficit disorder with hyperactivity

Dosage and routes:

Narcolepsy

• *Adult:* PO 5-60 mg qd in divided doses

• *Child >12 yr:* PO 10 mg qd, increasing by 10 mg/day at weekly intervals, limit usually 40 mg/day

• *Child 6-12 yr:* PO 5 mg qd increasing by 5 mg/wk

Attention deficit disorder

• *Child >6 yr:* PO 5 mg qd-bid increasing by 5 mg/day at weekly intervals

• *Child 3-6 yr:* PO 2.5 mg qd increasing by 2.5 mg/day at weekly intervals

Available forms include: Tabs 5, 10 mg; sus rel caps 5, 10, 15 mg

Side effects/adverse reactions:

▼ *ORAL:* Dry mouth, metallic taste

CNS: Hyperactivity, insomnia, restlessness, talkativeness, dizziness,

headache, chills, stimulation, dysphoria, irritability, aggressiveness, tremor

CV: Palpitation, tachycardia, hypertension, decrease in heart rate, dysrhythmias

GI: Anorexia, diarrhea, constipation, weight loss

GU: Impotence, change in libido

INTEG: Urticaria

Contraindications: Hypersensitivity to sympathomimetic amines, hyperthyroidism, hypertension, glaucoma hypertrophy, severe arteriosclerosis, drug abuse, cardiovascular disease, anxiety, MAO inhibitors or within 14 days of MAO inhibitor use

Precautions: Gilles de la Tourette's syndrome, pregnancy category C, lactation, child <3 yr

Pharmacokinetics:

PO: Onset 30 min, peak 1-3 hr, duration 4-20 hr, half-life 10-30 hr; metabolized by liver; urine excretion pH dependent; crosses placenta, excreted in breast milk

🦷 **Drug interactions of concern to dentistry:**

• Increased risk of serious side effects: meperidine, propoxyphene, tricyclic antidepressants

DENTAL CONSIDERATIONS

General:

• Monitor vital signs every appointment due to cardiovascular side effects.

• Assess salivary flow as a factor in caries, periodontal disease, and candidiasis.

• Psychologic and physical dependence may occur with chronic administration.

Consultations:

• Medical consult may be required to assess disease control.

Teach patient/family: *When*

chronic dry mouth occurs, advise patient:
• To avoid mouth rinses with high alcohol content due to drying effects
• To use daily home fluoride products for anticaries effect
• To use sugarless gum, frequent sips of water, or saliva substitutes

---

dextromethorphan hydrobromide

(dex-troe-meth-or′fan)
Benylin Adult, Benylin Pediatric, Children's Hold, Drixoral Cough, Hold DM, Pertussin CS and ES, Robitussin Pediatric, Scot-Tussin DM, and many other brands
♣ DM Syrup, Robidex, Sedatuss
Drug class.: Antitussive, nonnarcotic

Action: Depresses cough center in medulla
Uses: Nonproductive cough
Dosage and routes:
• *Adult:* PO 10-20 mg q4h or 30 mg q6-8h, not to exceed 120 mg/day; con rel liq 60 mg bid, not to exceed 120 mg/day
• *Child 6-12 yr:* PO 5-10 mg q4h; con rel liq 30 mg bid, not to exceed 60 mg/day
• *Child 2-6 yr:* PO 2.5-5 mg q4h or 7.5 mg q6-8h, not to exceed 30 mg/day
Available forms include: Loz 5 mg; sol 5, 7.5, 10, 15 mg/5 ml
Side effects/adverse reactions:
CNS: Dizziness
GI: Nausea
Contraindications: Hypersensitivity, asthma/emphysema, productive cough, MAO inhibitor
Precautions: Nausea, vomiting, increased temperature, persistent headache, pregnancy category C, drug abuse
Pharmacokinetics:
PO: Onset 15-30 min, duration 3-6 hr
🦷 **Drug interactions of concern to dentistry:**
• Inhibition of metabolism: terbinafine
DENTAL CONSIDERATIONS
General:
• Consider semisupine chair position for patients with respiratory disease.

---

diazepam

(dye-az′e-pam)
Diastat, Diazc, Diazemuls, Diazepam Intensol, Valium
♣ Apo-Diazepam, Novo-Dipam, PMS Diazepam, Vivol
Drug class.: Benzodiazepine, anxiolytic

Controlled Substance
Schedule IV
Action: Produces CNS depression by interacting with a benzodiazepine receptor to facilitate the action of the inhibitory neurotransmitter γ-aminobutyric acid (GABA)
Uses: Anxiety, acute alcohol withdrawal, adjunct in seizure disorders, skeletal muscle spasm; unapproved: conscious sedation
Dosage and routes:
Anxiety/convulsive disorders/sedation
• *Adult:* PO 2-10 mg tid-qid
• *Child >6 mo:* PO 1-2.5 mg tid-qid
Tetanic muscle spasms
• *Child >5 yr:* IM/IV 5-10 mg q3-4h prn
• *Infant >30 days:* IM/IV 1-2 mg q3-4h prn

---

bold italic = life-threatening conditions

Status epilepticus
• *Adult:* IV BOLUS 5-20 mg, 2 mg/min; may repeat q5-10min, not to exceed 60 mg; may repeat in 30 min if seizures reappear
• *Child:* IV BOLUS 0.1-0.3 mg/kg (1 mg/min over 3 min); may repeat q15min × 2 doses
Adjunct in skeletal muscle spasm
• *Adult:* PO 2-10 mg tid-qid
Available forms include: Tabs 2, 5, 10 mg; IM/IV inj 5 mg/ml; oral sol 5 mg/ml

Side effects/adverse reactions:
▼ *ORAL:* Dry mouth, ulcerations
CNS: Dizziness, drowsiness, confusion, headache, anxiety, tremors, stimulation, fatigue, depression, insomnia, hallucinations
CV: Orthostatic hypotension, ***ECG changes, tachycardia,*** hypotension
GI: Constipation, nausea, vomiting, anorexia, diarrhea
EENT: Blurred vision, tinnitus, mydriasis
INTEG: Rash, dermatitis, itching

Contraindications: Hypersensitivity to benzodiazepines, narrow-angle glaucoma, psychosis, pregnancy category D, child <18 yr, ritonavir, indinavir
Precautions: Elderly, debilitated, hepatic disease, renal disease
Pharmacokinetics:
PO: Onset 30 min, duration 2-3 hr
IM: Onset 15-30 min, duration 1-1.5 hr
IV: Onset 1-5 min, duration 15 min, half-life 20-50 hr; metabolized by liver; excreted by kidneys; crosses placenta, excreted in breast milk; more effective by mouth

🦷 **Drug interactions of concern to dentistry:**
• Increased effects of diazepam: alcohol, all CNS depressants
• Increased serum levels and prolonged effect of benzodiazepines: erythromycin, clarithromycin, ketoconazole, itraconazole, fluconazole, miconazole (systemic)

DENTAL CONSIDERATIONS
General:
• Assess salivary flow as a factor in caries, periodontal disease, and candidiasis.
• After supine positioning, have patient sit upright for at least 2 min before standing to avoid orthostatic hypotension.
• Psychologic and physical dependence may occur with chronic administration.
• Geriatric patients are more susceptible to drug effects; use lower dose.
• Have someone drive patient to and from dental appointment when used for conscious sedation.
• Provide assistance when escorting patient to and from dental chair when dizziness occurs.
• Avoid the use of this drug in a patient with a history of drug abuse or alcoholism.
Teach patient/family:
• Importance of good oral hygiene to prevent soft tissue inflammation
When chronic dry mouth occurs, advise patient:
• To avoid mouth rinses with high alcohol content due to drying effects
• To use daily home fluoride products for anticaries effect
• To use sugarless gum, frequent sips of water, or saliva substitutes

D

diclofenac

(dye-kloe'fen-ak)

Diclofenac potassium: Cataflam
✿ Difenac, Voltaren Rapide
Diclofenac sodium delayed release: Voltaren
✿ Novo-Difenac Apo-Diclo, Nu-Diclo
Diclofenac sodium extended release: Volaren XR
✿ Novo-Difenac SR

Drug class.: Nonsteroidal antiinflammatory

Action: Inhibits prostaglandin synthesis by interfering with cyclooxygenase needed for biosynthesis; possesses analgesic, antiinflammatory, antipyretic properties

Uses: Acute, chronic rheumatoid arthritis, osteoarthritis, ankylosing spondylitis

Dosage and routes:

Osteoarthritis (immediate or delayed release tablets)
• *Adult:* PO 100-150 mg/day in divided doses; chronic therapy 100 mg/day

Rheumatoid arthritis (immediate or delayed release tablets)
• *Adult:* PO 150-200 mg/day in divided doses; chronic therapy 100 mg/day

Ankylosing spondylitis (delayed release tablets)
• *Adult:* PO 100-125 mg/day; give 25 mg qid and 25 mg hs if needed

Analgesia and dysmenorrhea (immediate release tablets)
• *Adult:* PO 50 mg tid or 100 mg first dose followed by 50 mg with a daily first day limit of 200 mg; do not exceed 150 mg/day thereafter

Available forms include: Enteric-coated tabs 25, 50, 75 mg; ext rel tabs 100 mg

Side effects/adverse reactions:

▼ *ORAL:* Dry mouth, stomatitis, bitter taste, lichenoid reaction

CNS: Dizziness, drowsiness, fatigue, tremors, confusion, insomnia, anxiety, depression, nervousness, paresthesia, muscle weakness

*CV: **CHF, dysrhythmias,** tachycardia, peripheral edema, palpitation, hypotension, hypertension, fluid retention

*GI: **Jaundice, cholestatic hepatitis** constipation, flatulence, cramps, peptic ulcer, GI bleeding, nausea, anorexia, vomiting, diarrhea

*RESP: **Bronchospasm, laryngeal edema,** rhinitis, shortness of breath, dyspnea, hemoptysis, pharyngitis

*HEMA: **Blood dyscrasias,** epistaxis, bruising

*GU: **Nephrotoxicity: dysuria, hematuria, oliguria, azotemia, cystitis, UTI***

EENT: Tinnitus, hearing loss, blurred vision

INTEG: Purpura, rash, pruritus, sweating, erythema, petechiae, photosensitivity, alopecia

Contraindications: Hypersensitivity to aspirin, iodides, other nonsteroidal antiinflammatory agents, asthma

Precautions: Pregnancy category B (first, second trimester), lactation, children, bleeding disorders, GI disorders, cardiac disorders, hypersensitivity to other antiinflammatory agents

Pharmacokinetics:

PO: Peak 2-3 hr, elimination half-life 1-2 hr; 90% bound to plasma proteins; metabolized in liver to metabolite; excreted in urine

⚕ **Drug interactions of concern to dentistry:**
• GI ulceration, bleeding: aspirin, alcohol, corticosteroids

---

bold italic = life-threatening conditions

• Nephrotoxicity: acetaminophen (prolonged use)
• Possible risk of decreased renal function: cyclosporine
When prescribed for dental pain:
• Risk of increased effects: oral anticoagulants, oral antidiabetics, lithium, methotrexate
• Decreased antihypertensive effects of diuretics, β-adrenergic blockers, and ACE inhibitors

DENTAL CONSIDERATIONS
General:
• Patients on chronic drug therapy may rarely have symptoms of blood dyscrasias, which can include infection, bleeding, and poor healing.
• Assess salivary flow as a factor in caries, periodontal disease, and candidiasis.
• Avoid prescribing for dental use in last trimester of pregnancy.
• Avoid prescribing aspirin-containing products.
• Consider semisupine chair position for patients with rheumatic disease.

Consultations:
• In a patient with symptoms of blood dyscrasias, request a medical consult for blood studies and postpone dental treatment until normal values are reestablished.
• Medical consult may be required to assess disease control.

Teach patient/family:
• Importance of good oral hygiene to prevent soft tissue inflammation
• Caution to prevent injury when using oral hygiene aids
When chronic dry mouth occurs, advise patient:
• To avoid mouth rinses with high alcohol content due to drying effects

• To use daily home fluoride products for anticaries effect
• To use sugarless gum, frequent sips of water, or saliva substitutes

---

dicloxacillin sodium
(dye-klox-a-sil′in)
Dycill, Dynapen, Pathocil
Drug class.: Penicillinase-resistant penicillin

Action: Interferes with cell wall replication of susceptible organisms; the cell wall, rendered osmotically unstable, swells and bursts from osmotic pressure
Uses: Infections caused by penicillinase-producing *Staphylococcus*
Dosage and routes:
• *Adult:* PO 500 mg-1 g q4-6h
• *Child:* PO 12.5-25 mg/kg in divided doses q6h (up to 40 kg)
Available forms include: Caps 125, 250, 500 mg; powder for oral susp 250 mg/5 ml
Side effects/adverse reactions:
▼ *ORAL: Candidiasis* (superinfection)
CNS: Coma, convulsions, lethargy, hallucinations, anxiety, depression, twitching
GI: Nausea, vomiting, diarrhea, increased AST/ALT, abdominal pain, colitis
HEMA: Bone marrow depression, granulocytopenia, anemia, increased bleeding time
GU: Oliguria, proteinuria, hematuria, vaginitis, moniliasis, glomerulonephritis
Contraindications: Hypersensitivity to penicillins; neonates
Precautions: Hypersensitivity to cephalosporins, pregnancy category B

Pharmacokinetics:

PO: Peak 1 hr, duration 4-6 hr; metabolized in liver; excreted in urine, bile, breast milk; crosses placenta

💊 Drug interactions of concern to dentistry:

• Decreased antimicrobial effectiveness: tetracyclines, erythromycins

When prescribed for dental infection:

• Decreased effect of oral contraceptives

• Increased dicloxacillin concentration: probenecid

DENTAL CONSIDERATIONS

General:

• Take precautions regarding allergy to medication.

• Determine why the patient is taking the drug.

Consultations:

• Concern for drug of choice if dental infection is also present.

Teach patient/family:

• Importance of good oral hygiene to prevent soft tissue inflammation

• Caution to prevent trauma when using oral hygiene aids

When used for dental infection, advise patient:

• Taking birth control pill to use additional method of contraception for duration of cycle

• To report sore throat, oral burning sensation, fever, fatigue, any of which could indicate superinfection

• To take at prescribed intervals and complete dosage regimen

• To immediately notify the dentist if signs or symptoms of infection increase

---

dicyclomine HCl

(dye-sye′kloe-meen)

Antispas, Bentyl, Di-Spaz, Fyclomine

♣ A-Spas, Bentylol, Formulex, Spasmoban

Drug class.: GI anticholinergic

Action: Inhibits muscarinic actions of acetylcholine at postganglionic parasympathetic parasympathetic neuroeffector sites

Uses: Treatment of peptic ulcer disease in combination with other drugs; infant colic

Dosage and routes:

• *Adult:* PO 10-20 mg tid-qid; limit 160 mg/day; IM 20 mg q4-6h

Available forms include: Caps 10, 20 mg; tabs 20 mg; syr 10 mg/5 ml; inj IM 10 mg/ml

Side effects/adverse reactions:

▼ *ORAL: Dry mouth*

CNS: Confusion, stimulation in elderly, **seizures, coma** (child <3 mo), headache, insomnia, dizziness, drowsiness, anxiety, weakness, hallucination

CV: Palpitation, tachycardia

*GI: Constipation, **paralytic ileus,*** heartburn, nausea, vomiting, dysphagia

GU: Hesitancy, retention, impotence

EENT: Blurred vision, photophobia, mydriasis, cycloplegia, increased ocular tension

SYST: Urticaria, rash, pruritus, anhidrosis, fever, allergic reactions

Contraindications: Hypersensitivity to anticholinergics, narrow-angle glaucoma, GI obstruction, myasthenia gravis, paralytic ileus, GI atony, toxic megacolon

Precautions: Hyperthyroidism, CAD, dysrhythmias, CHF, ulcerative colitis, hypertension, hiatal

---

bold italic = life-threatening conditions

hernia, hepatic disease, renal disease, pregnancy category B, urinary retention, prostatic hypertrophy

Pharmacokinetics:

PO: Onset 1-2 hr, duration 3-4 hr; metabolized by liver; excreted in urine

⚗ Drug interactions of concern to dentistry:
• Increased anticholinergic effect: atropine, scopolamine, other anticholinergics and meperidine
• Decreased effect of ketoconazole

DENTAL CONSIDERATIONS

General:
• Assess salivary flow as a factor in caries, periodontal disease, and candidiasis.
• Avoid dental light in patient's eyes; offer dark glasses for patient comfort.

Consultation:
• Physician should be informed if significant xerostomic side effects occur (increased caries, sore tongue, problems eating or swallowing, difficulty wearing prosthesis) so a medication change can be considered.

Teach patient/family:
• Importance of good oral hygiene to prevent soft tissue inflammation

When chronic dry mouth occurs, advise patient:
• To avoid mouth rinses with high alcohol content due to drying effects
• To use daily home fluoride products for anticaries effect
• To use sugarless gum, frequent sips of water, or saliva substitutes

didanosine (also called ddI, dideoxyinosine)

(dye-dan'o-seen)

Videx, Videx EC

Drug class.: Synthetic antiviral, nucleoside analog

Action: Converted by cellular enzymes to active form, which acts as an antimetabolite to inhibit HIV reverse transcriptase and viral replication

Uses: Advanced HIV infections in adults and children who have been unable to use zidovudine or who have not responded to treatment

Dosage and routes:
• *Adult:* PO >75 kg: 300 mg bid tabs or 375 mg bid buffered powder; tabs must be chewed or crushed in water; 50-74 kg: 200 mg bid tabs or 250 mg bid buffered powder; 35-49 kg: 125 mg bid tabs or 167 mg bid buffered powder; or 400 mg once daily

Enteric-coated capsule
• *Adult:* PO Depending on body weight and renal function one capsule daily (swallowed, do not chew) on an empty stomach
• *Child:* PO 1.1-1.4 m^2, 100 mg bid tabs or 125 mg bid pedi powder; 0.8-1.0 m^2, 75 mg bid tabs or 94 mg bid pedi powder; 0.5-0.7 m^2, 50 mg bid tabs or 62 mg bid pedi powder; <0.4 m^2, 25 mg bid tabs or 31 mg bid pedi powder

Available forms include: Tabs, buffered, chewable/dispersible 25, 50, 100, 150, 200 mg; powder for oral sol, buffered 100, 167, 250, 375 mg; powder for oral sol, pedi 2, 4 g; del rel caps 125, 200, 250, 400 mg

Side effects/adverse reactions:

▼ *ORAL:* Stomatitis, dry mouth, taste perversion, candidiasis

CNS: ***Peripheral neuropathy, seizures, CNS depression,*** confusion, anxiety, hypertonia, abnormal thinking, asthenia, insomnia, pain, dizziness, chills, fever, headache

CV: Hypertension, vasodilation, dysrhythmia, syncope, CHF, palpitation

GI: ***Pancreatitis,*** diarrhea, nausea, vomiting, abdominal pain, constipation, dyspepsia, liver abnormalities, flatulence, melena, increased ALT/AST, alk phosphatase, amylase

RESP: Cough, pneumonia, dyspnea, asthma, epistaxis, hypoventilation, sinusitis

HEMA: ***Leukopenia, granulocytopenia, thrombocytopenia, anemia***

GU: Increased bilirubin, uric acid

EENT: Ear pain, otitis, photophobia, visual impairment

INTEG: Rash, pruritus, alopecia, ecchymosis, hemorrhage, petechiae, sweating

MS: Myalgia, arthritis, myopathy, muscular atrophy

Contraindications: Hypersensitivity

Precautions: Renal disease, hepatic disease, pregnancy category B, lactation, children, sodium-restricted diets; pancreatitis (in combination with stavudine)

Pharmacokinetics:

PO: Elimination half-life 1.62 hr; extensive metabolism is thought to occur; administration within 5 min of food decreases absorption

🦷 **Drug interactions of concern to dentistry:**

• Decreased absorption: ketoconazole, dapsone, itraconazole, tetracyclines, fluoroquinolone antibiotics

• Increased risk of pancreatitis: metronidazole, sulfonamides, sulindac, tetracyclines

• Increased risk of peripheral neuropathy: metronidazole, nitrous oxide

DENTAL CONSIDERATIONS

General:

• Monitor vital signs every appointment due to cardiovascular side effects.

• Avoid dental light in patient's eyes; offer dark glasses for patient comfort.

• Patients on chronic drug therapy may rarely have symptoms of blood dyscrasias, which can include infection, bleeding, and poor healing.

Consultations:

• Medical consult may be required to assess patient's ability to tolerate stress.

• In a patient with symptoms of blood dyscrasias, request a medical consult for blood studies and postpone dental treatment until normal values are reestablished.

Teach patient/family:

• Importance of good oral hygiene to prevent soft tissue inflammation

• Caution to prevent injury when using oral hygiene aids

When chronic dry mouth occurs, advise patient:

• To avoid mouth rinses with high alcohol content due to drying effects

• To use daily home fluoride products for anticaries effect

• To use sugarless gum, frequent sips of water, or saliva substitutes

diethylpropion HCl

(dye-eth-il-proe'pee-on)

Tenuate, Tenuate Dospan

Drug class.: Anorexiant, amphetamine-like

Controlled Substance Schedule IV

Action: Stimulates satiety center by acting on adrenergic pathways

Uses: Exogenous obesity

Dosage and routes:

• *Adult:* PO 25 mg/1 hr ac; con rel 75 mg qd midmorning

Available forms include: Tabs 25 mg; susp rel tabs 75 mg

Side effects/adverse reactions:

▼ *ORAL:* Dry mouth, unpleasant taste

CNS: Hyperactivity, restlessness, anxiety, insomnia, dizziness, dysphonia, depression, tremors, headache, blurred vision, incoordination, fatigue, malaise, euphoria, depression, tremor, confusion

CV: Palpitation, tachycardia, hypertension, dysrhythmias, pulmonary hypertension, ECG changes

GI: Nausea, vomiting, anorexia, diarrhea, constipation

HEMA: **Bone marrow depression,** leukopenia, agranulocytosis

GU: Impotence, change in libido, menstrual irregularities, dysuria, polyuria

INTEG: Urticaria

Contraindications: Hypersensitivity, hyperthyroidism, hypertension, glaucoma, angina pectoris, drug abuse, cardiovascular disease, children <12 yr, severe arteriosclerosis, agitated states

Precautions: Convulsive disorders, pregnancy category B, lactation

Pharmacokinetics:

PO: Duration 4 hr

CON REL: Duration 10-14 hr, half-life 1-3.5 hr; metabolized by liver; excreted by kidneys; crosses placenta, excreted in breast milk

Drug interactions of concern to dentistry:

• Dysrhythmia: hydrocarbon inhalation anesthetics

• Decreased effects: barbiturates, tricyclic antidepressants, phenothiazines

DENTAL CONSIDERATIONS

General:

• Monitor vital signs every appointment due to cardiovascular and respiratory side effects.

• Examine for evidence of oral manifestations of blood dyscrasias (infection, bleeding, poor healing).

• Assess salivary flow as a factor in caries, periodontal disease, and candidiasis.

• Psychologic and physical dependence may occur with chronic administration.

• Consider semisupine chair position for patient comfort due to GI effects of disease.

Consultations:

• Medical consult for blood studies (CBC); leukopenic or thrombocytopenic side effects may result in infection, delayed healing, and excessive bleeding. Postpone dental treatment until normal values are maintained.

Teach patient/family:

• Importance of good oral hygiene to prevent soft tissue inflammation

• Caution in use of oral hygiene aids to prevent injury

When chronic dry mouth occurs, advise patient:

• To avoid mouth rinses with high

alcohol content due to drying effects

• To use daily home fluoride products for anticaries effect

• To use sugarless gum, frequent sips of water, or saliva substitutes

---

difenoxin HCl with atropine sulfate

(dye-fen-ox′in)

Motofen

Drug class.: Antidiarrheal

Controlled Substance Schedule IV

Action: Inhibits gastric motility by acting on mucosal receptors responsible for peristalsis

Uses: Acute nonspecific and acute exacerbations of chronic functional diarrhea

Dosage and routes:

• *Adult:* PO 2 mg, then 1 mg after each loose stool; or 1 mg q3-4h as needed, not to exceed 8 mg/24 hr

Available forms include: Tabs 1 mg difenoxin HCl with 0.025 mg atropine sulfate

Side effects/adverse reactions:

▼ *ORAL:* Dry mouth

CNS: Dizziness, drowsiness, headache, fatigue, nervousness, insomnia, confusion

GI: Nausea, vomiting, epigastric distress, constipation

EENT: Burning eyes, blurred vision

Contraindications: Hypersensitivity, pseudomembranous enterocolitis, jaundice, glaucoma, child <2 yr, severe electrolyte imbalances, diarrhea associated with organisms that penetrate intestinal mucosa, MAO inhibitor

Precautions: Hepatic disease, renal disease, ulcerative colitis, pregnancy category C, lactation, severe liver disease

Pharmacokinetics:

PO: Peak 40-60 min, duration 3-4 hr, terminal half-life 12-14 hr; metabolized in liver to inactive metabolite; excreted in urine, feces

Drug interactions of concern to dentistry:

• Increased effects of alcohol: all CNS depressants, opioid analgesics, and anticholinergics

DENTAL CONSIDERATIONS

General:

• This drug product is normally used only for a few doses for acute problems; however, some patients may have to take it for longer time periods as dictated by a contributing disease.

• Assess salivary flow as a factor in caries, periodontal disease, and candidiasis.

Teach patient/family: *When chronic dry mouth occurs, advise patient:*

• To avoid mouth rinses with high alcohol content due to drying effects

• To use daily home fluoride products for anticaries effect

• To use sugarless gum, frequent sips of water, or saliva substitutes

---

diflorasone diacetate

(die-floor′a-sone)

Florone, Florone E, Maxiflor, Psorcon, Psorcon E

Drug class.: Topical corticosteroid, group II high potency

Action: Glucocorticoids have multiple actions that include antiinflammatory and immunosuppressant effects. They inhibit phospholipase A_2, interfering with or

---

reducing the synthesis of prostaglandins and leukotrienes. They also bind to cytoplasmic glucocorticoid receptors (GRs) and enter the cell nucleus to bind with DNA. This results in the synthesis of various enzymes such as collagenase, elastase, and cytokines that play important roles in inflammation and immunosuppression. They also suppress the production of lymphocytes, monocytes, and eosinophils.

Uses: Psoriasis, eczema, contact dermatitis, pruritus

Dosage and routes:

• *Adult and child:* Apply to affected area qd-tid

Available forms include: Cream 0.05%; oint 0.05%

Side effects/adverse reactions:

▼ *ORAL:* Perioral dermatitis (not intraoral)

INTEG: Burning, dryness, itching, irritation, acne, folliculitis, hypertrichosis, hypopigmentation, atrophy, striae, miliaria, allergic contact dermatitis, secondary infection

Contraindications: Hypersensitivity to corticosteroids, fungal infections

Precautions: Pregnancy category C, lactation, viral infections, bacterial infections

DENTAL CONSIDERATIONS

General:

• Determine why the patient is taking the drug.

• Apply lubricant to dry lips for patient comfort before dental procedures.

• Place on frequent recall to evaluate healing response if used on chronic basis.

diflunisal

(dye-floo′ni-sal)

Dolobid

❦ Apo-Diflunisal, Novo-Diflunisal

Drug class.: Salicylate derivative, nonsteroidal antiinflammatory

Action: Inhibits prostaglandin synthesis by interfering with cyclooxygenase needed for biosynthesis; possesses analgesic, antiinflammatory, antipyretic properties

Uses: Mild-to-moderate pain, symptoms of rheumatoid arthritis and osteoarthritis

Dosage and routes:

Pain/fever

• *Adult:* PO loading dose 1 g, then 500-1000 mg/day in 2 divided doses q12h, not to exceed 1500 mg/day

Available forms include: Tabs 250, 500 mg

Side effects/adverse reactions:

▼ *ORAL:* Dry mouth, lichenoid reaction

CNS: **Convulsions,** stimulation, drowsiness, dizziness, confusion, headache, flushing, hallucinations, coma

CV: **Pulmonary edema,** rapid pulse

GI: Nausea, vomiting, GI bleeding, diarrhea, heartburn, **hepatitis,** anorexia

RESP: Wheezing, hyperpnea

HEMA: **Thrombocytopenia, agranulocytosis, leukopenia, neutropenia, hemolytic anemia,** increased pro-time

EENT: Blurred vision, decreased acuity, corneal deposits

INTEG: Rash, urticaria, bruising

ENDO: Hypoglycemia, hyponatremia, hypokalemia

Contraindications: Hypersensitivity to salicylates, GI bleeding,

italic = common side effects

bleeding disorders, children <3 yr, vitamin K deficiency

Precautions: Anemia, hepatic disease, renal disease, Hodgkin's disease, pregnancy category C, lactation

Pharmacokinetics:

PO: Onset 15-30 min, peak 2-3 hr, half-life up to 6 hr; 99% protein bound; metabolized by liver; excreted by kidneys; crosses placenta; excreted in breast milk

🦷 Drug interactions of concern to dentistry:

• Increased risk of GI ulceration and bleeding: aspirin, steroids, alcohol, indomethacin, and other NSAIDs

• Hepatotoxicity, nephrotoxicity: acetaminophen (prolonged use)

DENTAL CONSIDERATIONS

General:

• Patients on chronic drug therapy may rarely have symptoms of blood dyscrasias, which can include infection, bleeding, and poor healing.

• Assess salivary flow as a factor in caries, periodontal disease, and candidiasis.

• Avoid prescribing for dental use in first and last trimester of pregnancy.

Consultations:

• Medical consult may be required to assess disease control.

• In a patient with symptoms of blood dyscrasias, request a medical consult for blood studies and postpone dental treatment until normal values are reestablished.

Teach patient/family:

• Importance of good oral hygiene to prevent soft tissue inflammation

• Caution to prevent injury when using oral hygiene aids

When chronic dry mouth occurs, advise patient:

• To avoid mouth rinses with high alcohol content due to drying effects

• To use daily home fluoride products for anticaries effect

• To use sugarless gum, frequent sips of water, or saliva substitutes

---

digoxin

(di-jox'in)

Digitek, Lanoxicaps, Lanoxin

🍁 Novo-digoxin

Drug class.: Cardiac glycoside

Action: Acts by inhibiting the sodium-potassium ATPase, which makes more calcium available for contractile proteins, resulting in increased cardiac contractility and cardiac output

Uses: CHF, atrial fibrillation, atrial flutter, paroxysmal atrial tachycardia, rapid digitalization in these disorders

Dosage and routes:

• *Adult:* IV 0.5 mg given over >5 min, then PO 0.125-0.5 mg qd in divided doses q4-6h as needed

• *Elderly:* PO 0.125 qd maintenance

• *Child >2 yr:* PO 0.02-0.04 mg/kg divided q8h over 24 hr; maintenance 0.006-0.012 mg/kg qd in divided doses q12h; IV loading dose 0.015-0.035 mg/kg over >5 min

• *Child 1 mo-2 yr:* IV 0.03-0.05 mg/kg in divided doses over >5 min q4-8h; change to PO as soon as possible; PO 0.035-0.060 mg/kg divided in 3 doses over 24 hr; maintenance 0.01-0.02 mg/kg in divided doses q12h

• *Neonates:* IV loading dose 0.02-

0.03 mg/kg over >5 min in divided doses q4-8h; change to PO as soon as possible; PO loading dose 0.035 mg/kg divided q8h over 24 hr; maintenance 0.01 mg/kg in divided doses q12h

• *Premature infants:* IV 0.015-0.025 mg/kg divided in 3 doses over 24 hr, given over >5 min; maintenance 0.003-0.009 mg/kg in divided doses q12h

Available forms include: Caps 0.05, 0.1, 0.2 mg; elix 0.05 mg/ml; tabs 0.125, 0.25, 0.50 mg; inj 0.1, 0.25 mg/ml

Side effects/adverse reactions:

▼ *ORAL:* Sensitive gag reflex

CNS: Headache, drowsiness, apathy, confusion, disorientation, fatigue, depression, hallucinations

CV: Dysrhythmias, hypotension, bradycardia, *AV block*

GI: Nausea, vomiting, anorexia, abdominal pain, diarrhea

EENT: Blurred vision, yellowish-green halos, photophobia, diplopia

MS: Muscular weakness

Contraindications: Hypersensitivity to digitalis, ventricular fibrillation, ventricular tachycardia, carotid sinus syndrome, second- or third-degree heart block

Precautions: Renal disease, acute MI, AV block, severe respiratory disease, hypothyroidism, elderly, pregnancy category C, sinus nodal disease, lactation, hypokalemia

Pharmacokinetics:

IV: Onset 5-30 min, peak 1-5 hr, duration variable, half-life 1.5 days; excreted in urine

🦷 **Drug interactions of concern to dentistry:**

• Hypokalemia: corticosteroids
• Increased digoxin blood levels: erythromycin, clarithromycin, tetracyclines

• Cardiac dysrhythmias: adrenergic agonists, succinylcholine

DENTAL CONSIDERATIONS

General:

• Monitor vital signs every appointment due to cardiovascular side effects.

• After supine positioning, have patient sit upright for at least 2 min to avoid orthostatic hypotension.

• Avoid dental light in patient's eyes; offer dark glasses for patient comfort.

• An increased gag reflex may make dental procedures such as taking radiographs or impressions difficult.

• Use vasoconstrictors with caution, in low doses, and with careful aspiration. Avoid use of gingival retraction cord with epinephrine.

Consultations:

• Stress from dental procedures may compromise cardiovascular function; determine patient risk.

• Medical consult may be required to assess disease control and stress tolerance of patient.

---

dihydrotachysterol (DHT)

(dye-hye-droe-tak-iss′ter-ole)

DHT Intensol, Hytakerol

Drug class.: Vitamin D analog

Action: Increases intestinal absorption of calcium for bones, increases renal tubular absorption of phosphate

Uses: Nutritional supplement, rickets, hypoparathyroidism, pseudohypoparathyroidism, postoperative tetany

Dosage and routes:

Hypoparathyroidism/Tetany

• *Adult:* PO initial dose 0.75-2.5

mg day, given for several days; maintenance dose 0.2-1.75 mg qd as required

Available forms include: Tabs 0.125, 0.2, 0.4 mg; caps 0.125 mg; intensol sol 0.2 mg/ml

Side effects/adverse reactions:

▼ *ORAL:* Dry mouth, metallic taste

CNS: Drowsiness, headache, vertigo, fever, lethargy

GI: Nausea, diarrhea, vomiting, jaundice, anorexia, constipation, cramps

GU: Polyuria, hematuria, hypercalciuria, hyperphosphatemia

EENT: Tinnitus

MS: Myalgia, arthralgia, decreased bone development

Contraindications: Hypersensitivity, renal disease, hyperphosphatemia, hypercalcemia

Precautions: Pregnancy category C, renal calculi, lactation, cardiovascular disease

Pharmacokinetics:

PO: Onset 2 wk; metabolized by liver; excreted in feces (active/inactive)

🐾 **Drug interactions of concern to dentistry:**

• Decreased effect of dihydrotachysterol: prolonged use of corticosteroids, barbiturates

DENTAL CONSIDERATIONS
General:

• Consider semisupine chair position for patient comfort due to GI effects of drug.

• Assess salivary flow as a factor in caries, periodontal disease, and candidiasis.

Teach patient/family: *When chronic dry mouth occurs, advise patient:*

• To avoid mouth rinses with high alcohol content due to drying effects

• Of need for daily home fluoride to prevent caries

• To use sugarless gum, frequent sips of water, or saliva substitutes

D

diltiazem HCl

(dil-tye'a-zem)
Cardizem, Cardizem CD, Cardizem SR, Tiamate, Tiazac
🍁 Apo-Diltaz, Novo-Diltiazem, Nu-Dilitaz, Syn-Diltiazem
Drug class.: Calcium channel blocker

Action: Inhibits calcium ion influx across cell membrane during cardiac depolarization; produces relaxation of coronary vascular smooth muscle; dilates coronary arteries; slows SA/AV node conduction; dilates peripheral arteries

Uses: Chronic stable angina pectoris, vasospastic angina, coronary artery spasm, hypertension, supraventricular tachydysrhythmias

Dosage and routes:

• *Adult:* PO 30 mg qid, increasing dose gradually to 180-360 mg/day in divided doses or 60-120 mg bid; may increase to 240-360 mg/day

• *Adult:* PO sus rel in hypertension 180-240 mg once daily; angina initial dose 120 mg, range may vary from 180-480 mg/day

Available forms include: Tabs 30, 60, 90, 120 mg; sus rel tab 30, 60, 90, 120, 240 mg; sus rel caps 60, 90, 120, 180, 240, 300, 360 mg; inj 5 mg and 10mg/ml in 5 ml, 10 ml vials

Side effects/adverse reactions:

▼ *ORAL:* Dry mouth, gingival overgrowth, altered taste, ulcers

CNS: Headache, fatigue, drowsi-

---

bold italic = life-threatening conditions

ness, dizziness, depression, weakness, insomnia, tremor, paresthesia
*CV: Dysrhythmia, edema, **CHF,*** bradycardia, hypotension, palpitation, heart block, peripheral edema, angina
GI: Nausea, vomiting, diarrhea, gastric upset, constipation, increased liver function studies
*GU: **Acute renal failure,*** nocturia, polyuria
HEMAT: Postoperative hemorrhage
INTEG: Rash, pruritus, flushing, photosensitivity
Contraindications: Sick sinus syndrome, second- or third-degree heart block, hypotension <90 mm Hg systolic, acute MI, pulmonary congestion
Precautions: CHF, hypotension, hepatic injury, pregnancy category C, lactation, children, renal disease
Pharmacokinetics:
PO: Onset 30-60 min, peak 2-3 hr (immediate rel), 6-11 hr (sus rel), half-life 3.5-9 hr; metabolized by liver; excreted in urine (96% as metabolites)

⚷ Drug interactions of concern to dentistry:
• Decreased effect: indomethacin, possibly other NSAIDs, phenobarbital
• Increased effect: parenteral and inhalational general anesthetics or other drugs with hypotensive actions
• Increased effects of carbamazepine, midazolam, triazolam

DENTAL CONSIDERATIONS
General:
• Monitor cardiac status; take vital signs at each appointment because of CV side effects. Consider a stress reduction protocol to prevent stress-induced angina during the dental appointment.

• After supine positioning, have patient sit upright for at least 2 min to avoid orthostatic hypotension.
• Place on frequent recall to monitor gingival condition.
• Limit use of sodium-containing products such as saline IV fluids for patients with a dietary salt restriction.
• Assess salivary flow as a factor in caries, periodontal disease, and candidiasis.
• Consider drug in diagnosis of taste alterations.
Consultations:
• Medical consult may be required to assess disease control.
Teach patient/family:
• Importance of good oral hygiene to prevent soft tissue inflammation and to minimize gingival overgrowth
• Need for frequent oral prophylaxis if gingival overgrowth occurs
When chronic dry mouth occurs, advise patient:
• To avoid mouth rinses with high alcohol content due to drying effects
• To use daily home fluoride products for anticaries effect
• To use sugarless gum, frequent sips of water, or saliva substitutes

---

dimenhydrinate
(dye-men-hye′dri-nate)
Calm-X, Dinate, Dramamine, Dramanate, Hydrate, PMS-Dimenhydrinate, Triptone Caplets
♣ Apo-Dimenhydrinate, Gravol, Gravol L/A, Novo-Dimenate
Drug class.: H$_1$-receptor antagonist

Action: Acts on blood vessels, GI system, respiratory system by competing with histamine for H$_1$-receptor site; decreases allergic response by blocking histamine

Uses: Motion sickness, nausea, vomiting, vertigo

Dosage and routes:

• *Adult:* PO 50-100 mg q4h; IM/IV 50 mg as needed

• *Child 6-12 yr:* PO 25-50 mg q6-8h, limit 150 mg/day

• *Child 2-6 yr:* IM/PO 1.25-25 mg q6-8h, limit 75 mg/day; IM 1.25 mg/kg qid; limit 300 mg/day

Available forms include: Tabs 50 mg; inj 500 mg/ml; liq 12.5/4 ml, 15.62 mg/5ml; supp 50, 100 mg

Side effects/adverse reactions:

▼ ORAL: Dry mouth

CNS: Drowsiness, **convulsions** (young children), restlessness, headache, dizziness, insomnia, confusion, nervousness, tingling, vertigo, hallucinations

CV: Hypertension, hypotension, palpitation

GI: Nausea, anorexia, diarrhea, vomiting, constipation

EENT: Blurred vision, diplopia, nasal congestion, photosensitivity

SYST: Rash, urticaria, fever, chills, flushing

Contraindications: Hypersensitivity to narcotics, shock

Precautions: Children, cardiac dysrhythmias, elderly, asthma, pregnancy category B, prostatic hypertrophy, bladder neck obstruction, narrow-angle glaucoma, stenosing peptic ulcer, pyloroduodenal obstruction

Pharmacokinetics:

IM/PO: Duration 4-6 hr

🐾 **Drug interactions of concern to dentistry:**

• Increased photosensitization: tetracycline

• Increased effects of alcohol, other CNS depressants, anticholinergics

DENTAL CONSIDERATIONS

General:

• Assess salivary flow as a factor in caries, periodontal disease, and candidiasis.

Teach patient/family: *When chronic dry mouth occurs, advise patient:*

• To avoid mouth rinses with high alcohol content due to drying effects

• To use daily home fluoride products for anticaries effect

• To use sugarless gum, frequent sips of water, or saliva substitutes

---

diphenhydramine HCl

(dye-fen-hye′dra-meen)

AllerMax, Banophen, Benadryl, Calm-X, Diphen, Diphen AF, Diphenhist, Genahist, Hyrexin-50, Siladryl, Tusstat, Uni-Bent Unisom, and others

♣ Allerdryl

Drug class.: Antihistamine, H$_1$-receptor antagonist

Action: Acts on blood vessels, GI system, respiratory system by competing with histamine for H$_1$-receptor site; decreases allergic response by blocking histamine

Uses: Allergy symptoms, rhinitis, motion sickness, antiparkinsonism, nighttime sedation, infant colic, nonproductive cough; unlabeled use for dental local anesthesia

Dosage and routes:

• *Adult:* PO 25-50 mg q4-6h, not to exceed 400 mg/day; IM/IV 10-50 mg, not to exceed 400 mg/day

• *Child >12 kg:* PO/IM/IV 5 mg/kg/day in 4 divided doses, not to exceed 300 mg/day

• *Local anesthetic (unapproved use):* INTRAORAL INJ use *only* the l0 mg/ml solution and never >1.5 ml per injection per patient; risk of tissue irritation if more is used; must use sterile technique at all times; no data to support combined use with vasoconstrictor

Available forms include: Caps 25, 50 mg; tabs 50 mg; elix 12.5 mg/5 ml; syr 12.5 mg/5 ml; inj IM/IV 10, 50 mg/ml

Side effects/adverse reactions:

▼ *ORAL:* Dry mouth

CNS: Dizziness, drowsiness, poor coordination, fatigue, anxiety, euphoria, confusion, paresthesia, neuritis

GI: Nausea, anorexia, diarrhea

RESP: Increased thick secretions, wheezing, chest tightness

HEMA: **Thrombocytopenia, agranulocytosis, hemolytic anemia**

GU: Retention, dysuria, frequency

EENT: Blurred vision, dilated pupils, tinnitus, nasal stuffiness, dry nose/throat

INTEG: Photosensitivity

Contraindications: Hypersensitivity to H_1-receptor antagonist, acute asthma attack, lower respiratory tract disease

Precautions: Increased intraocular pressure, renal disease, cardiac disease, hypertension, bronchial asthma, seizure disorder, stenosed peptic ulcers, hyperthyroidism, prostatic hypertrophy, bladder neck obstruction, pregnancy category C

Pharmacokinetics:

PO: Peak 1-3 hr, duration 4-7 hr

IM: Onset 0.5 hr, peak 1-4 hr, duration 4-7 hr

IV: Onset immediate, duration 4-7 hr, half-life 2-7 hr

Metabolized in liver; excreted by kidneys; crosses placenta; excreted in breast milk

🦷 **Drug interactions of concern to dentistry:**

• Increased CNS depression: all CNS depressants, alcohol

• Increased anticholinergic effect: anticholinergics

• Increased plasma levels of labetalol

DENTAL CONSIDERATIONS

General:

• Patients on chronic drug therapy may rarely have symptoms of blood dyscrasias, which can include infection, bleeding, and poor healing.

• Assess salivary flow as a factor in caries, periodontal disease, and candidiasis.

• Consider semisupine chair position for patients with respiratory disease.

Consultations:

• In a patient with symptoms of blood dyscrasias, request a medical consult for blood studies and postpone dental treatment until normal values are reestablished.

Teach patient/family:

• Importance of good oral hygiene to prevent soft tissue inflammation

• Caution to prevent injury when using oral hygiene aids

When chronic dry mouth occurs, advise patient:

• To avoid mouth rinses with high alcohol content due to drying effects

• To use daily home fluoride products for anticaries effect

• To use sugarless gum, frequent sips of water, or saliva substitutes

---

diphenoxylate HCl with atropine sulfate

(dye-fen-ox'i-late)

Logen, Lomanate, Lomotil, Lonox

Drug class.: Antidiarrheal (opioid with atropine)

**Controlled Substance
Schedule V**

Action: Inhibits gastric motility by acting on mucosal receptors responsible for peristalsis

Uses: Simple diarrhea

Dosage and routes:
• *Adult:* PO 2.5-5 mg qid, titrated to patient response
• *Child 2-12 yr:* PO 0.3-0.4 mg/kg/day in divided doses

Available forms include: Tabs 2.5 mg with atropine 0.025 mg; liquid 2.5 mg with atropine 0.025 mg/5 ml in 60 ml

Side effects/adverse reactions:

▼ *ORAL:* Dry mouth

CNS: Drowsiness, headache, sedation, depression, weakness, lethargy, flushing, hyperthermia

CV: Tachycardia

*GI: Nausea, vomiting, **paralytic ileus, toxic megacolon,** abdominal pain, colitis

GU: Urinary retention

EENT: Blurred vision, nystagmus, mydriasis

*SYST: **Angioneurotic edema,** rash, urticaria, pruritus

Contraindications: Hypersensitivity, severe liver disease, pseudomembranous enterocolitis, glaucoma, child <2 yr, electrolyte imbalances

Precautions: Hepatic disease, renal disease, ulcerative colitis, pregnancy category C, lactation, elderly

Pharmacokinetics:

PO: Onset 45-60 min, peak 2 hr, duration 3-4 hr, half-life 2.5 hr, terminal half-life 12-14 hr; metabolized in liver to active form; excreted in urine, feces, breast milk

☙ **Drug interactions of concern to dentistry:**
• Contraindication: MAO inhibitors
• Increased effects of alcohol, all CNS depressants, opioid analgesics, anticholinergics

DENTAL CONSIDERATIONS
General:
• Assess salivary flow as a factor in caries, periodontal disease, and candidiasis.
• Psychologic and physical dependence may occur with chronic administration.
• Consider semisupine chair position for patient comfort due to GI effects of disease.
• This drug product is normally used only for a few doses for acute problems; however, some patients may have to take it for longer time periods as dictated by a contributing disease.

Teach patient/family:
• To avoid mouth rinses with high alcohol content due to drying effects

dipivefrin HCl

(dye-pi've-frin)

AKPro, Propine

Drug class.: Adrenergic agonist

Action: Converted to epinephrine, which decreases aqueous production and increases outflow

Uses: Open-angle glaucoma

Dosage and routes:
• *Adult:* Instill 1 gtt q12h

Available forms include: Sol 0.1%

Side effects/adverse reactions:

CV: Hypertension, tachycardia, dysrhythmias

EENT: Burning, stinging, mydriasis, photophobia

Contraindications: Hypersensitivity, narrow-angle glaucoma

Precautions: Pregnancy category B, lactation, children, aphakia

Pharmacokinetics:

INSTILL: Onset 30 min, peak 1 hr, duration 12 hr

🦷 **Drug interactions of concern to dentistry:**

• Avoid use of anticholinergics such as atropine, scopolamine, and propantheline; use benzodiazepines with caution

DENTAL CONSIDERATIONS

General:

• Avoid dental light in patient's eyes; offer dark glasses for patient comfort.

---

dipyridamole

(dye-peer-id'a-mole)

Persantine

♣ Apo-Dipyridamole, Novodipiradol

Drug class.: Platelet aggregation inhibitor

Action: Specific action unclear; inhibits ability of platelets to aggregate, possibly through effects on adenosine, cAMP, or thromboxane A_2

Uses: Prevention of transient ischemic attack (TIA), inhibition of platelet aggregation to prevent MI, thromboembolism, with warfarin in prosthetic heart valves, prevention of coronary bypass graft occlusion with aspirin

Dosage and routes:

TIA

• *Adult:* PO 75-100 mg qid, 1 hr ac, not to exceed 400 mg qd

Inhibition of platelet aggregation

• *Adult:* PO 50-75 mg qid in combination with aspirin *or* Coumadin, but not both

Available forms include: Tabs 25, 50, 75 mg

Side effects/adverse reactions:

▼ *ORAL:* Gingival bleeding

CNS: Headache, dizziness, weakness, fainting, syncope

CV: Postural hypotension

GI: Nausea, vomiting, anorexia, diarrhea

INTEG: Rash, flushing

Contraindications: Hypersensitivity, hypotension

Precautions: Pregnancy category B, children <12 yr

Pharmacokinetics:

PO: Peak 2-2.5 hr, duration 6 hr; therapeutic response may take several months; metabolized in liver; excreted in bile; undergoes enterohepatic recirculation

🦷 **Drug interactions of concern to dentistry:**

• Additive antiplatelet effects: aspirin and other NSAIDs

DENTAL CONSIDERATIONS

General:

• Monitor vital signs every appointment due to cardiovascular side effects.

• After supine positioning, have patient sit upright for at least 2 min to avoid orthostatic hypotension.

• Avoid prescribing aspirin-containing products, even though ASA/dipyridamole combination drugs are used in some patients.

• Evaluate for clotting ability during gingival instrumentation, because inhibition of platelet aggregation may occur.

• Consider local hemostatic measures to prevent excessive bleeding during instrumentation.

Consultations:

• Medical consult should include partial prothrombin or prothrombin times.

• Medical consult may be required to assess disease control.

Teach patient/family:

• Importance of good oral hygiene to prevent gingival inflammation

---

dirithromycin

(dye-rith'roe-mye-sin)

Dynabac

Drug class.: Macrolide antibiotic

Action: Active product (erythromycylamine) binds to 50S ribosomal subunits of susceptible bacteria to inhibit bacterial growth

Uses: Treatment of acute and secondary bacterial infection of acute bronchitis, community-acquired pneumonia, streptococcal pharyngitis, and uncomplicated skin and skin structure infections

Dosage and routes:

• *Adult and child >12 yr:* PO 500 mg/day for 7-14 days; give with food or within 1 hr of eating; do not crush or chew tablets

Available forms include: Tabs 250 mg

Side effects/adverse reactions:

▼ *ORAL:* Dry mouth, taste alteration, mouth ulcers (all <1%); although not documented, it is reasonable to assume opportunistic oral candidiasis

CNS: Headache, somnolence, dizziness, insomnia

GI: Diarrhea, abdominal pain, nausea, dyspepsia, pseudomembranous colitis

RESP: Dyspnea, cough

GU: Vaginal candidiasis

INTEG: Rash, pruritus, urticaria

MS: Asthenia

Contraindications: Hypersensitivity to macrolide antibiotics

Precautions: Not for *H. influenzae* or *S. pyogenes* infections, pregnancy category C, lactation, child <12 yr

Pharmacokinetics:

PO: Half-life 30-44 hr; after absorption, parent drug is converted to erythromycylamine; plasma protein binding low (15%-30%); excreted in bile

🔔 Drug interactions of concern to dentistry:

• Other drug interactions: data are limited; antacids and histamine H_2 antagonists tend to enhance absorption; refer to erythromycin for potential interacting drugs

DENTAL CONSIDERATIONS

General:

• Do not use in patients at risk for bacteremias due to inadequate serum levels.

• Potential value in dental infections is unknown.

• Determine why the patient is taking the drug.

• Examine for oral manifestations of opportunistic infections.

Consultations:

• Medical consult may be required to assess disease control.

Teach patient/family:

• Alert the patient to the possibility of secondary oral infection and the need to see dentist immediately if infection occurs

---

disopyramide/ disopyramide phosphate

(dye-soe-peer'a-mide)

Norpace, Norpace CR

♣ Rythmodan, Rythmodan-LA

Drug class.: Antidysrhythmic (class Ia)

Action: Prolongs action potential duration and effective refractory period; reduces disparity in refractoriness between normal and infarcted myocardium

Uses: PVCs, ventricular tachycardia, atrial flutter, fibrillation

Dosage and routes:

• *Adult:* PO 100-200 mg q6h, in renal dysfunction 100 mg q6h; sus rel caps 200 mg q12h

• *Child 12-18 yr:* PO 6-15 mg/kg/day, in divided doses q6h

• *Child 4-12 yr:* PO 10-15 mg/kg/day, in divided doses q6h

• *Child 1-4 yr:* PO 10-20 mg/kg/day, in divided doses q6h

• *Child <1 yr:* PO 10-30 mg/kg/day, in divided doses q6h

Available forms include: Caps 100, 150 mg (as phosphate); sus rel caps 100, 150 mg

Side effects/adverse reactions:

▼ *ORAL:* Dry mouth

CNS: Headache, dizziness, psychosis, fatigue, depression, paresthesia, anxiety, insomnia

CV: Hypotension, bradycardia, **CHF, cardiac arrest,** angina, PVCs, tachycardia, increase in QRS and QT segments, edema, weight gain, AV block, syncope, chest pain

GI: Constipation, nausea, anorexia, flatulence, diarrhea, vomiting

HEMA: ***Thrombocytopenia,***

agranulocytosis, anemia (rare), decreased hemoglobin, hematocrit

GU: Retention, hesitancy, impotence, urinary frequency, urgency

EENT: Blurred vision, dry nose/throat/eyes, narrow-angle glaucoma

INTEG: Rash, pruritus, urticaria

MS: Weakness, pain in extremities

META: Hypoglycemia

Contraindications: Hypersensitivity, second- or third-degree heart block, cardiogenic shock, CHF (uncompensated), sick sinus syndrome, QT prolongation

Precautions: Pregnancy category C, lactation, diabetes mellitus, renal disease, children, hepatic disease, myasthenia gravis, narrow-angle glaucoma, cardiomyopathy, conduction abnormalities

Pharmacokinetics:

PO: Peak 30 min-3 hr, duration 6-12 hr, half-life 4-10 hr; metabolized in liver; excreted in feces, urine, breast milk; crosses placenta

🐾 Drug interactions of concern to dentistry:

• Possible increased risk of prolonged QT interval: clarithromycin, erythromycin

• Increased side effects: anticholinergics, alcohol

• Decreased effects: barbiturates, corticosteroids

DENTAL CONSIDERATIONS

General:

• Monitor vital signs every appointment due to cardiovascular side effects.

• After supine positioning, have patient sit upright for at least 2 min before standing to avoid orthostatic hypotension.

• Patients on chronic drug therapy may rarely have symptoms of blood dyscrasias, which can in-

clude infection, bleeding, and poor healing.
• Assess salivary flow as a factor in caries, periodontal disease, and candidiasis.

Consultations:
• In a patient with symptoms of blood dyscrasias, request a medical consult for blood studies and postpone dental treatment until normal values are reestablished.
• Medical consult may be required to assess disease control and patient's ability to tolerate stress.

Teach patient/family:
• Importance of good oral hygiene to prevent soft tissue inflammation
When chronic dry mouth occurs, advise patient:
• To avoid mouth rinses with high alcohol content due to drying effects
• To use daily home fluoride products for anticaries effect
• To use sugarless gum, frequent sips of water, or saliva substitutes

---

disulfiram

(dye-sul'fi-ram)

generic

Drug class.: Aldehyde dehydrogenase inhibitor

Action: Blocks oxidation of alcohol at acetaldehyde stage; accumulation of acetaldehyde produces the disulfiram-alcohol reaction
Uses: Chronic alcoholism (as adjunct)
Dosage and routes:
• *Adult:* PO 250-500 mg qd × 1-2 wk, then 125-500 mg qd
Available forms include: Tabs 250, 500 mg
Side effects/adverse reactions:
▼ *ORAL:* Metallic taste

CNS: Headache, drowsiness, restlessness, dizziness
CV: Dysrhythmias, tachycardia, chest pain, hypotension
GI: Hepatotoxicity, nausea, vomiting
RESP: Respiratory depression, hyperventilation, dyspnea
INTEG: Rash, dermatitis, urticaria
Disulfiram-alcohol reaction: Flushing, throbbing, headache, respiratory difficulty, nausea, vomiting, sweating, thirst, chest pain, palpitation, dyspnea, hyperventilation, tachycardia, confusion, CV collapse, MI, CHF, convulsions, death
Contraindications: Hypersensitivity, alcohol intoxication, psychoses, CV disease, pregnancy category not listed
Precautions: Hypothyroidism, hepatic disease, diabetes mellitus, seizure disorders, nephritis, cerebral damage
Pharmacokinetics:
PO: Onset 1-2 hr; oxidized by liver; excreted unchanged in feces; can affect alcohol metabolism for 1-2 wk after last dose
⚑ Drug interactions of concern to dentistry:
• Increased CNS depression: long-acting benzodiazepines
• Increased disulfiram reaction: alcohol
• Risk of psychosis: metronidazole (do not use), tricyclic antidepressants

DENTAL CONSIDERATIONS
General:
• Be aware of the needs of patients who are in recovery from substance abuse.
• Avoid other addictive drugs, including opioids and benzodiazepines.

Consultations:
• Medical consult may be required to assess disease control.
Teach patient/family:
• To avoid mouth rinses with high alcohol content due to drying effects and drug-drug interaction

---

docosanol
(do-cos′a-nole)
Abreva
Drug class.: Synthetic lipophilic alcohol

Action: A highly lipophilic, fatty alcohol that prevents fusion of lipid-enveloped viruses with cell membranes, thereby blocking viral replication
Uses: Treatment of recurrent herpes labialis (cold sores, fever blisters) on the face or lips; appears to shorten healing time by at least 1 day
Dosage and routes:
• *Adult and child >12 yr:* TOP apply small amount to affected area on face or lips or at the first sign of lesion for 6 × daily until healed
Available forms include: Cream 10%, 2 g tube (OTC product)
Side effects/adverse reactions:
CNS: Headache
INTEG: Site reaction, rash, pruritus, dry skin, acne
Contraindications: Hypersensitivity
Precautions: External use only (not for intraoral use), children <12 yr, avoid application to eyes, pregnancy category B
Pharmacokinetics:
TOP: Negligible absorption
👉 **Drug interactions of concern to dentistry:**
• None reported

DENTAL CONSIDERATIONS
Teach patient/family:
• Apply with finger cot; wash hands before and after use.
• Do not share this medication to prevent potential cross contamination of virus.
• Replace toothbrush after resolution of lesion to prevent reinfection of virus.

---

dofetilide
(doe-fet′il-ide)
Tikosyn
Drug class.: Antidysrhythmic (class III)

Action: Blockade of the cardiac ion channel carrying the rapid components of the delayed rectifier potassium current (I_{kr}); increases the monophasic action potential duration; increases effective refractory period; increases QT interval on ECG; and terminates induced reentrant tachyarrhythmias
Uses: Maintenance of normal sinus rhythm in patients with atrial fibrillation/atrial flutter >1 wk duration, who have been converted to normal sinus rhythm; conversion of atrial fibrillation/atrial flutter to normal sinus rhythm
Dosage and routes:
• *Adult:* PO initial doses are started only in patients placed in an appropriate facility for 3 days for ECG monitoring; must be individualized according to creatinine clearance and QT interval. Usual dose is 0.5 mg bid. Available only to hospitals or other limited institutions and to physicians who have completed proper training program.
Available forms include: Caps 0.125, 0.25, 0.50 mg

---

italic = common side effects

Side effects/adverse reactions:

▼ *ORAL:* Angioedema, facial paralysis

CNS: Headache, dizziness, insomnia, anxiety, syncope

*CV: Chest pain, **ventricular tachycardia, torsade de pointes,*** AV block, angina pectoris, hypertension, palpitation

GI: Diarrhea, flatulence, abdominal pain

RESP: RTI, dyspnea, cough

GU: UTI

INTEG: Rash, sweating

MS: Back pain, arthralgia, asthenia

MISC: Flu syndrome

Contraindications: Hypersensitivity, congenital or acquired QT syndromes (QT interval greater than 440 ms), severe renal impairment, contraindicated with cimetidine, trimethoprim, ketoconazole, prochlorperazine, megestrol, or verapamil

Precautions: Requires dose adjustment in renal impairment, can cause life-threatening ventricular arrhythmias, caution use with CYP450 3A4 enzyme inhibitors, hepatic impairment, abnormal serum potassium or magnesium levels, pregnancy category C, lactation, children <18 yr

Pharmacokinetics:

PO: Bioavailability >90%, peak plasma levels 2-3 hr, steady-state levels 2-3 days, plasma protein binding 60%-70%, excreted (80%) in urine unchanged, excretion involves both glomerular filtration and active tubular secretion, limited metabolism by CYP450 3A4 enzymes

☙ Drug interactions of concern to dentistry:

• Decreased renal excretion: ketoconazole (contraindicated use)

• Not recommended with concurrent use of: phenothiazines, tricyclic antidepressants, SSRIs, or macrolide antiinfectives (erythromycin, clarithromycin), and azole antifungals

• Contraindicated with cimetidine, trimethoprim, ketoconazole, prochlorperazine, megestrol or verapamil

DENTAL CONSIDERATIONS

General:

• Monitor vital signs every appointment due to cardiovascular side effects.

• Delay or avoid dental treatment if patient shows signs of cardiac symptoms or respiratory distress.

• Ensure patient is compliant with drug therapy.

Consultations:

• Patient's physician should be informed about any use of dental drugs.

• Medical consult may be required to assess disease control and patient's ability to tolerate stress.

Teach patient/family:

• Importance of updating health and drug history if physician makes any changes in evaluation or drug regimens

---

dolasetron mesylate

(dol-a′se-tron)

Anzemet

Drug class.: Antinauseant and antiemetic

Action: Acts as an antagonist for serotonin (5HT$_3$) receptors in the CNS; may also reduce afferent stimulus from GI tract

Uses: Control of nausea and vomiting associated with cancer chemotherapy and prevention of post-operative nausea and vomiting

Dosage and routes:

Cancer chemotherapy

• *Adult:* PO 100 mg given within 1 hr of chemotherapy

• *Child 2-16 yr:* PO 1.8 mg/kg given within 1 hr of chemotherapy not to exceed 100 mg

Parenteral chemotherapy

• *Adult:* IV 1.8 mg/kg as a single dose about 30 min before chemo-therapy, alternatively for most pa-tients, a fixed dose of 100 mg can be given over 30 seconds

• *Child 2-16 yr:* IV 1.8 mg/kg as a single dose approximately 30 min before chemotherapy up to a max-imum of 100 mg

Prevention or treatment of postop-erative nausea and vomiting

• *Adult:* PO 100 mg given 2 hr before surgery

• *Child 2-16 yr:* PO 1.2 mg/kg given 2 hr before surgery, not to exceed 100 mg

• *Adult:* IV 12.5 mg as a single dose 15 min before the end of anesthesia or as soon as nausea and vomiting are evident

• *Child 2-16 yr:* IV 0.35 mg/kg with a maximum dose of 12.5 mg (single dose) approximately 15 min before cessation of anesthesia or as soon as nausea and vomiting are present

Available forms include: Tabs 50, 100 mg; inj 20 mg/ml in 0.625 ml, 5 ml vials

Side effects/adverse reactions:

▼ *ORAL: Taste alteration*

CNS: Headache, fatigue, sedation, dizziness, light-headedness, ner-vousness, paresthesia

CV: Bradycardia, tachycardia, al-teration of ECG, orthostatic hypo-tension, hypertension

GI: Increased appetite, nausea, constipation, diarrhea, dyspepsia, flatulence

EENT: Blurred vision

INTEG: Pruritus

META: Elevation of aminotrans-ferases

MISC: Fever, chills

Contraindications: Hypersensi-tivity

Precautions: Previous hypersensi-tivity to other 5-HT$_3$ antagonists, cardiovascular disease, seizure dis-orders, ECG changes, hypokale-mia, hypomagnesemia, diuretics, antiarrhythmics, pregnancy cate-gory B, lactation

Pharmacokinetics:

IV: Metabolized to active metabo-lite, peak plasma concentrations 1 hr, urinary excretion mostly, some fecal excretion

PO: Well absorbed, rapidly metab-olized to active metabolite

🦷 **Drug interactions of concern to dentistry:**

• Does not influence anesthesia re-covery time

DENTAL CONSIDERATIONS

General:

• Monitor patients in recovery to avoid untoward events.

• Patients taking opioids for acute or chronic pain should be given al-ternative analgesics for dental pain.

• Chlorhexidine mouth rinse before and during chemotherapy may re-duce severity of mucositis.

• Palliative medication may be re-quired for management of oral side effects.

Teach patient/family:

• To be aware of oral side effects

• To report excessive nausea and vomiting to dentist for patients recovering from anesthesia after dental treatment

donepezil HCl

(doe-nep'e-zeel)

Aricept

Drug class.: Cholinesterase inhibitor

Action: A centrally acting reversible inhibitor of choline esterase enzyme

Uses: Mild to moderate dementia associated with Alzheimer's disease

Dosage and routes:

• *Adult:* PO initial 5 mg/day; can increase to 10 mg/day after 4-6 wk evaluation at 5 mg dose; take dose in evening just before retiring

Available forms include: Tabs 5, 10 mg

Side effects/adverse reactions:

▼ *ORAL:* Toothache (1%), dry mouth, bad taste, gingivitis, tongue edema, coated tongue

CNS: Insomnia, anorexia, headache, dizziness, depression, abnormal dreams

CV: Syncope, hot flashes, hypotension, hypertension

GI: Nausea, diarrhea, vomiting, anorexia

RESP: Dyspnea

HEMA: Thrombocytopenia, ecchymosis, anemia

GU: Frequency of urination

EENT: Sore throat, dry eyes, blurred vision, earache, tinnitus

INTEG: Pruritus, urticaria

META: Weight decrease, dehydration

MS: Muscle cramps, arthritis

MISC: Fatigue, generalized pain

Contraindications: Hypersensitivity

Precautions: Bradycardia, sick sinus syndrome, GI ulcer disease, bladder obstruction, seizures, asthma, obstructive pulmonary disease, pregnancy category C, lactation, children, hepatic impairment

Pharmacokinetics:

PO: Bioavailability 100%, peak plasma levels 3-4 hr, 96% bound to plasma proteins, hepatic metabolism, active metabolites, urinary excretion

🦷 **Drug interactions of concern to dentistry:**

• Enhanced succinylcholine muscle relaxation during anesthesia

• Risk of GI side effects: NSAIDs

• Action may be inhibited by anticholinergic drugs or enhanced by cholinergic agonists

• Increased blood levels: Ketoconazole, paroxetine

DENTAL CONSIDERATIONS

General:

• Determine why patient is taking the drug.

• Monitor vital signs every appointment due to cardiovascular side effects.

• After supine positioning, have patient sit upright for at least 2 min before standing to avoid orthostatic hypotension.

• Use precaution if sedation or general anesthesia is required.

• Patient on chronic drug therapy may rarely have symptoms of blood dyscrasias, which can include infection, bleeding, and poor healing.

• Drug is used early in the disease; ensure patient or caregiver understands informed consent.

• Place on frequent recall because early attention to dental health is important for Alzheimer's patients.

D

---

bold italic = life-threatening conditions

- Assess salivary flow as factor in caries, periodontal disease, and candidiasis.
- Consider semisupine chair position for patient comfort if GI side effects occur.
- Consultation with physician may be needed if sedation or general anesthesia is required.

Consultations:
- Medical consult may be required to assess disease control and patient's ability to tolerate stress.
- In a patient with symptoms of blood dyscrasias, request a medical consult for blood studies and postpone treatment until normal values are reestablished.

Teach patient/family:
- Importance of good oral hygiene to prevent soft tissue inflammation
- To prevent trauma when using oral hygiene aids
- Use of electric toothbrush if patient has difficulty holding conventional devices

When chronic dry mouth occurs, advise patient:
- To avoid mouth rinses with high alcohol content due to drying effects
- To use daily home fluoride products for anticaries effect
- To use sugarless gum, frequent sips of water, or saliva substitutes

---

dornase alfa
(dor′nase)
Pulmozyme
Drug class.: Recombinant human deoxyribonuclease (DNase)

Action: Reduces sputum viscosity by hydrolyzing extracellular DNA in sputum

Uses: Cystic fibrosis; reduces incidence of pulmonary infections; improves pulmonary function

Dosage and routes:
- *Adult and child >5 yr:* INH inhale 2.5 mg once daily with recommended nebulizer

Available forms include: INH 1.0 mg/ml in 2.5 ml ampules

Side effects/adverse reactions:
CV: Chest pain, **cardiac failure**
GI: Intestinal obstruction, abdominal pain
RESP: Apnea, bronchitis, dyspnea, coughing
EENT: Pharyngitis, laryngitis, conjunctivitis, voice alteration, sinusitis
INTEG: Rash, urticaria
MISC: Flulike symptoms, malaise, weight loss

Contraindications: Hypersensitivity, allergy to Chinese Hamster Ovary cell products

Precautions: Pregnancy category B, lactation, child <5 yr

Pharmacokinetics:
INH: Peak sputum levels 15 min

🦷 **Drug interactions of concern to dentistry:**
- None documented

DENTAL CONSIDERATIONS
General:
- Consider semisupine chair position for patients with respiratory disease.
- Monitor vital signs every appointment due to respiratory and cardiovascular side effects.
- A stress reduction protocol may be required.

Consultations:
- A medical consult may be required to assess disease control.

Teach patient/family:
- Importance of good oral hygiene to prevent soft tissue inflammation

italic = common side effects

dorzolamide HCl

(dor-zole′a-mide)

Trusopt

Drug class.: **Carbonic anhydrase inhibitor**

Action: Reduces intraocular pressure through inhibition of carbonic anhydrase enzyme

Uses: Ocular hypertension, open-angle glaucoma

Dosage and routes:

• *Adult:* Instill 1 gtt in affected eye(s) tid; if other ophthalmic drug products are also used, give the drugs at least 10 min apart

Available forms include: Sol 2% in 5, 10 ml

Side effects/adverse reactions:

▼ *ORAL: Bitter taste*

CNS: Headache

GI: Nausea

EENT: Ocular burning, stinging, conjunctivitis, lid reactions, keratitis, blurred vision, photophobia

INTEG: Skin rashes

Contraindications: Hypersensitivity

Precautions: Allergy to sulfonamides, renal or hepatic impairment, pregnancy category C, lactation, children, oral carbonic anhydrase inhibitors, contact lenses

Pharmacokinetics: Systemically absorbed from the eye

🦷 **Drug interactions of concern to dentistry:**

• Avoid drugs that may exacerbate glaucoma (anticholinergic drugs)

• High-dose salicylates to avoid systemic toxicity

DENTAL CONSIDERATIONS

General:

• Avoid dental light in patient's eyes; offer dark glasses for patient comfort.

• Protect patient's eyes from accidental spatter during dental treatment.

• Check patient's compliance with prescribed drug regimen for glaucoma.

Consultations:

• Medical consult may be required to assess disease control.

doxazosin mesylate

(dox-ay′zoe-sin)

Cardura

♣ Cardura-1, Cardura-2, Cardura-3

Drug class.: **Peripheral α-adrenergic blocker**

Action: Selectively blocks α_1-adrenergic receptors, which results in peripheral vasodilation and lowering of blood pressure; also causes relaxation of smooth muscles of the bladder, prostate, and prostate capsule in benign prostatic hyperplasia; also lowers total cholesterol, LDL, and triglycerides

Uses: Hypertension, benign prostatic hypertrophy

Dosage and routes:

Hypertension

• *Adult:* PO 1 mg qd, increasing up to 16 mg qd if required; usual range 4-16 mg/day

Benign prostatic hypertrophy

• *Adult:* PO initial dose 1 mg/day, depending on symptoms dose can be increased to 2 mg/day; then to 4 mg/day up to a maximum of 8 mg/day

Available forms include: Tabs 1, 2, 4, 8 mg

Side effects/adverse reactions:

▼ *ORAL: Dry mouth*

CNS: Dizziness, headache, weak-

---

ness, fatigue, asthenia, drowsiness, anxiety, depression, vertigo
CV: Palpitation, orthostatic hypotension, tachycardia, edema, dysrhythmias, chest pain
GI: Nausea, vomiting, diarrhea, constipation, abdominal pain
GU: Incontinence, polyuria
EENT: Epistaxis, tinnitus, red sclera, pharyngitis, rhinitis
INTEG: Lichen planus
Contraindications: Hypersensitivity to quinazolines
Precautions: Pregnancy category B, children, lactation, hepatic disease
Pharmacokinetics:
PO: Onset 2 hr, peak 2-6 hr, duration 24 hr, half-life 22 hr; extensively protein bound (98%); metabolized in liver; excreted via bile, feces (<63%) and in urine (9%)
Drug interactions of concern to dentistry:
• Increased hypotensive effects: all CNS depressants
• Reduced effects with indomethacin, NSAIDs, sympathomimetics
• Caution in use of drugs which may cause urinary retention: anticholinergics, opioids
DENTAL CONSIDERATIONS
General:
• Monitor vital signs every appointment due to cardiovascular side effects.
• After supine positioning, have patient sit upright for at least 2 min before standing to avoid orthostatic hypotension.
• Assess salivary flow as a factor in caries, periodontal disease, and candidiasis.
Consultations:
• Medical consult may be required

to assess disease control and patient's ability to tolerate stress.
Teach patient/family: *When chronic dry mouth occurs, advise patient:*
• To avoid mouth rinses with high alcohol content due to drying effects
• To use daily home fluoride products for anticaries effect
• To use sugarless gum, frequent sips of water, or saliva substitutes

---

doxepin HCl (topical)
(dox′e-pin)
Zonalon
Drug class.: Topical antipruritic (tricyclic antidepressant)

Action: Antipruritic mechanism unknown; has antihistaminic activity; also produces drowsiness
Uses: Pruritus associated with eczema, atopic dermatitis, lichen *simplex chronicus*
Dosage and routes:
• *Adult:* TOP apply to affected area qid with intervals of 3-4 days between applications for up to 8 days
Available forms include: Cream 5% in 30 g tube
Side effects/adverse reactions:
▼ *ORAL: Dry mouth, taste alteration, dry lips*
CNS: Drowsiness, headache, fatigue, dizziness, anxiety
INTEG: Burning, stinging, dryness of skin, edema, paresthesia
MISC: Fever
Contraindications: Hypersensitivity, untreated glaucoma, tendency for urinary retention
Precautions: Pregnancy category

B, lactation, children, for external use only, caution in driving car, current use with alcohol or MAO inhibitor

Pharmacokinetics:

TOP: Variable absorption, half-life 28-52 hr; hepatic metabolism; widely distributed; renal excretion

🦷 Drug interactions of concern to dentistry:

• Potential for interactions depends on how much drug is absorbed and duration of use (>8 days)

• Increased anticholinergic effects: anticholinergics, antihistamines, phenothiazines, other tricyclic antidepressants

• Potential risk for increased CNS depression: all CNS depressants

• Increased effects of direct-acting sympathomimetics: epinephrine, levonordefrin

DENTAL CONSIDERATIONS

General:

• Doxepin may be absorbed and produce typical systemic side effects of tricyclic drugs.

• Monitor vital signs every appointment due to cardiovascular side effects.

• Use vasoconstrictors with caution, in low doses, and with careful aspiration.

• Place on frequent recall due to oral side effects.

• Apply lubricant to dry lips for patient comfort before dental procedures.

• Assess salivary flow as a factor in caries, periodontal disease, and candidiasis.

Consultations:

• Medical consult may be required to assess disease control.

Teach patient/family:

• To avoid mouth rinses with high alcohol content due to interaction with alcohol (see precautions) and drying effects

When chronic dry mouth occurs, advise patient:

• Of need for daily home fluoride for anticaries effect

• To use sugarless gum, frequent sips of water, or saliva substitutes

---

doxepin HCl

(dox'e-pin)

Sinequan

♣ Novo-Doxepin, Triadapin

Drug class.: Antidepressant, tricyclic

Action: Inhibits both norepinephrine and serotonin (5-HT) reuptake in synapses in the brain, but the precise antidepressant mechanism remains unclear

Uses: Major depression, anxiety; unapproved: panic disorders

Dosage and routes:

• *Adult:* PO 50-75 mg/day in divided doses; may increase to 150 mg/day or may give daily dose hs; severe depression up to 300 mg

Available forms include: Caps 10, 25, 50, 75, 100, 150 mg; oral conc 10 mg/ml

Side effects/adverse reactions:

▼ *ORAL: Dry mouth, unpleasant taste,* bleeding, stomatitis, lichenoid reaction

CNS: Dizziness, drowsiness, confusion, headache, anxiety, tremors, stimulation, weakness, insomnia, nightmares, EPS (elderly), increased psychiatric symptoms, paresthesia

CV: Orthostatic hypotension, ECG changes, tachycardia, **hypertension,** palpitation

---

bold italic = life-threatening conditions

*GI: Diarrhea, **paralytic ileus, hepatitis,** increased appetite, cramps, epigastric distress, jaundice, nausea, vomiting*

*HEMA: **Agranulocytosis, thrombocytopenia, eosinophilia, leukopenia***

*GU: Retention, **acute renal failure***

EENT: Blurred vision, tinnitus, mydriasis, ophthalmoplegia

INTEG: Rash, urticaria, sweating, pruritus, photosensitivity

Contraindications: Hypersensitivity to tricyclic antidepressants, urinary retention, narrow-angle glaucoma, prostatic hypertrophy

Precautions: Suicidal patients, elderly, pregnancy category C, MAO inhibitors

Pharmacokinetics:

PO: Steady-state 2-8 days, half-life 8-24 hr; metabolized by liver; excreted by kidneys; crosses placenta; excreted in breast milk

⚴ Drug interactions of concern to dentistry:

• Increased anticholinergic effects: anticholinergic blockers, antihistamines, phenothiazines

• Increased effects of direct-acting sympathomimetics (epinephrine, levonordefrin)

• Potential risk of increased CNS depression: alcohol, barbiturates, benzodiazepines, and other CNS depressants

• Decreased antihypertensive effects: clonidine, guanadrel, guanethidine

DENTAL CONSIDERATIONS

General:

• Take vital signs every appointment due to cardiovascular side effects.

• Assess salivary flow as a factor in caries, periodontal disease, and candidiasis.

• Patients on chronic drug therapy may rarely have symptoms of blood dyscrasias, which can include infection, bleeding, and poor healing.

• After supine positioning, have patient sit upright for at least 2 min before standing to avoid orthostatic hypotension.

• Use vasoconstrictors with caution, in low doses, and with careful aspiration. Avoid use of gingival retraction cord with epinephrine.

• Place on frequent recall due to oral side effects.

Consultations:

• In a patient with symptoms of blood dyscrasias, request a medical consult for blood studies and postpone dental treatment until normal values are reestablished.

• Medical consult may be required to assess disease control.

• Physician should be informed if significant xerostomic side effects occur (increased caries, sore tongue, problems eating or swallowing, difficulty wearing prosthesis) so a medication change can be considered.

Teach patient/family:

• Importance of good oral hygiene to prevent soft tissue inflammation

When chronic dry mouth occurs, advise patient:

• To avoid mouth rinses with high alcohol content due to drying effects

• To use daily home fluoride products for anticaries effect

• To use sugarless gum, frequent sips of water, or saliva substitutes

doxycycline hyclate (dental–systemic)

(dox-i-sye'kleen)

Periostat

Drug class.: Tetracycline derivative for nonantibacterial use

Action: Reduces elevated collagenase activity in gingival crevicular fluid of patients with adult periodontitis; no antibacterial effect reported at this dose

Uses: Adjunct to scaling and root planing to promote attachment level gain and reduce pocket depth in adult periodontitis

Dosage and routes:

• *Adult:* PO 20 mg bid as an adjunct to scaling and root planing; may be administered for up to 9 mo; exceeding the recommended dosage may increase risk of side effects, including the development of resistant organisms

Available forms include: Caps 20 mg

Side effects/adverse reactions: Note: In a clinical study of 428 patients there was little to no difference in the incidence of side effects reported between this drug and a placebo. See doxycycline hyclate monograph for typical side effects associated with oral administration. Whether these side effects would occur at doses used in this product is unknown.

Contraindications: Hypersensitivity to tetracyclines

Precautions: Children <8 yr, pregnant and nursing mothers, predisposition to oral or vaginal candidiasis, pregnancy category D; not to be used for antimicrobial effect in periodontitis

Pharmacokinetics: No data available

🐾 **Drug interactions of concern to dentistry:**

• No data reported for this dose form; see doxycycline hyclate monograph for drug interactions reported with tetracyclines

DENTAL CONSIDERATIONS

General:

• Examine for oral manifestation of opportunistic infection

• Should be administered at least 1 hr before morning or evening meals

Teach patient/family:

• To avoid using ingestible sodium bicarbonate products, such as the air-polishing system (ProphyJet), within 2 hr of drug use

doxycycline hyclate/ doxycycline calcium

(dox-i-sye'kleen)

Doxycycline calcium: Vibramycin

Doxycycline hyclate: BioTab, Doryx, Doxy-Caps, Doxychel, Monodox, Vibramycin, Vibra-Tabs

♣ Apo-Doxy, Novodoxylin

Drug class.: Tetracycline, broad-spectrum antiinfective

Action: Inhibits protein synthesis and phosphorylation in microorganisms by binding to 30S ribosomal subunits, reversibly binding to 50S ribosomal subunits; bacteriostatic

Uses: Syphilis, *C. trachomatis*, gonorrhea, lymphogranuloma venereum, uncommon gram-negative/gram-positive organisms, necrotizing ulcerative gingivostomatitis; cutaneous or inhalational anthrax exposure

Dosage and routes:
• *Adult:* PO 100 mg q12h on day 1, then 100 mg/day; IV 200 mg in 1-2 inf on day 1, then 100-200 mg/day
• *Child >8 yr:* PO/IV 4.4 mg/kg/day in divided doses q12h on day 1, then 2.2-4.4 mg/kg/day

Gonorrhea (uncomplicated)
• *Adult:* PO 200 mg, then 100 mg hs and 100 mg bid × 3 days or 300 mg, then 300 mg in 1 hr
• *Disseminated:* 100 mg PO bid × at least 7 days

Chlamydia trachomatis
• *Adult:* PO 100 mg bid × 7 days

Syphilis
• *Adult:* PO 300 mg/day in divided doses × 10 days

Anthrax Exposure
• *Adult:* PO 100 mg bid × 60 days
• *Child <100 lbs:* PO 2.2 mg/kg given bid × 60 days
• *Child >100 lbs:* PO give adult dose (tetracyclines are used in this age group for anthrax only)

Available forms include: Tabs 50, 100 mg; caps 50, 100 mg; syr 50 mg/ml; powder for inj IV 100, 200 mg; powder for oral susp 25 mg/5 ml in 60 ml; syrup 50 mg/5 ml in 60 ml

Side effects/adverse reactions:
▼ *ORAL:* Candidiasis, tooth discoloration, tongue discoloration, dry mouth
CNS: Fever
CV: Pericarditis
GI: Nausea, abdominal pain, vomiting, diarrhea, **hepatotoxicity,** anorexia, enterocolitis, flatulence, abdominal cramps, gastric burning, pancreatitis
HEMA: **Depression of plasma prothrombin activity, eosinophilia, neutropenia, thrombocytopenia, hemolytic anemia**
EENT: Dysphagia
INTEG: Rash, urticaria, photosensitivity, increased pigmentation, **exfoliative dermatitis, angioedema,** pruritus

Contraindications: Hypersensitivity to tetracyclines, children <8 yr, pregnancy category D

Precautions: Hepatic disease, lactation

Pharmacokinetics:
PO: Peak 1.5-4 hr, half-life 15-22 hr; 25%-93% protein bound; excreted in bile

🦷 **Drug interactions of concern to dentistry:**
• Decreased absorption: $NaHCO_3$, other antacids
• Increased rate of metabolism: barbiturates, carbamazepine, hydantoins
• Decreased effect of penicillins, cephalosporins
• May increase the effectiveness of anticoagulants, methotrexate
• Oral contraceptives: advise patient of a potential risk for decreased contraceptive action, to maintain compliance with oral contraceptive use while using antibiotics, and to consider the use of additional nonhormonal contraception

DENTAL CONSIDERATIONS
General:
• Determine why the patient is taking tetracycline.
• Broad-spectrum antibiotics may promote oral or vaginal *Candida* infection.

Consultations:
• Medical consult may be required to assess disease control.

Teach patient/family:
• Can take with milk, food; take with a full glass of water
• To take tetracycline doses 1 hr before or 2 hr after air polishing device (ProphyJet), if used
When used for dental infection, advise patient:
• To report sore throat, oral burning sensation, fever, fatigue, any of which could indicate superinfection
• To take at prescribed intervals and complete dosage regimen
• To immediately notify the dentist if signs or symptoms of infection increase

---

doxycycline hyclate gel
(dox-i-sye'kleen)
Atridox
Drug class.: Tetracycline, antiinfective

Action: Inhibits bacterial protein synthesis due to disruption of transfer RNA and messenger RNA
Uses: For adjunctive treatment of chronic adult periodontitis to increase clinical attachment, reduce probing depth, and reduce bleeding on probing
Dosage and routes:
• *Adult:* TOP mix contents of syringes according to detailed instructions, completing 100 cycles; attach blunt cannula to syringe A and fill the pocket; after it becomes firm, the mixture may be packed further into the pocket with a dental instrument
Available forms include: Syringe 50 mg and delivery system syringe (450 mg), blunt cannula; refrigerate

Side effects/adverse reactions:
▼ *ORAL: Gingival discomfort, pain, loss of attachment, toothache, periodontal abscess, exudate, infection, drainage, swelling, thermal tooth sensitivity, extreme mobility, localized allergic reaction*
CNS: Headache
CV: High blood pressure
GI: Diarrhea
GU: PMS
EENT: Skin infection, photosensitivity
MS: Muscle aches, backache
MISC: Common cold
Contraindications: Hypersensitivity
Precautions: Pregnancy category D, children (tooth staining), lactation, photosensitivity, predisposition to candidiasis
Pharmacokinetics: Gingival crevicular fluid levels peak 2 hr, sustained levels up to 18 hr and decline over 7 days; low serum levels not exceeding 0.1 g/ml
👉 **Drug interactions of concern to dentistry:**
• None specifically identified for this product; unknown whether typical tetracycline interactions occur

DENTAL CONSIDERATIONS
General:
• Examine for oral manifestation of opportunistic infection.
Teach patient/family:
• To be alert to the possibility of secondary oral infection and the need to see dentist immediately if signs of infection occur
• Caution against oral hygiene procedures in treated areas of mouth for 7 days to avoid dislodging product

---

dronabinol

(droe-nab'i-nol)

Marinol

Drug class.: Antiemetic, appetite stimulant

Controlled Substance Schedule III, Canada N

Action: Orally active cannabinoid (Δ^9-tetrahydrocannabinol) with varying effects in the CNS; exact mechanism unknown, may be due to inhibition of vomiting control mechanism in medulla oblongata

Uses: Control nausea, vomiting in selected patients receiving emetogenic cancer chemotherapy; stimulate appetite in AIDS-associated anorexia

Dosage and routes:

Chemotherapy prophylaxis for emesis

• *Adult:* PO 5 mg/m^2 1-3 hr before chemotherapy, then q2-4h for total of 6 doses per day; dose may be increased by 2.5 mg/m^2 if response is not adequate; do not exceed 15 mg/m^2 per dose

Appetite stimulant

• *Adult:* PO initially 2.5 mg bid, before lunch and supper, or 2.5 mg single dose in PM or hs; max dose 20 mg/day; 5 mg doses may be given if tolerated

Available forms include: Gelcaps 2.5, 5, 10 mg

Side effects/adverse reactions:

▼ *ORAL:* Dry mouth

CNS: Dizziness, drowsiness, poor concentration, ataxia, confusion, paranoid reactions, unsteadiness, restlessness, sleep disturbances, psychotomimetic effects

CV: Palpitation, tachycardia, flushing, orthostatic hypotension

GI: Nausea, vomiting, abdominal pain, diarrhea

EENT: Blurred vision, changes in vision

MS: Asthenia, myalgia

MISC: Abstinence syndrome (hot flashes, sweating, rhinorrhea, loose stools, hiccups, anorexia)

Contraindications: Hypersensitivity: marijuana, sesame oil

Precautions: Pregnancy category C, lactation, children, elderly; cardiac disorders, drug abuse, alcoholism, hypertension, manic or depressive state, schizophrenia

Pharmacokinetics:

PO: 90%-95% absorbed after single dose, only 10%-20% reaches systemic circulation due to first-pass hepatic metabolism and high lipid solubility; protein binding (97%); half-life alpha 4 hr; effects 4-24 hr; fecal elimination

🦷 Drug interactions of concern to dentistry:

• Increased CNS depression: alcohol, CNS depressants

• Additive hypertension, tachycardia, possible cardiotoxicity: amphetamines, other sympathomimetics

• Additive tachycardia, drowsiness: atropine, scopolamine, antihistamines, anticholinergic drugs

DENTAL CONSIDERATIONS

General:

• Monitor vital signs every appointment due to cardiovascular side effects.

• After supine positioning, have patient sit upright for at least 2 min to avoid orthostatic hypotension.

• Patients taking opioids for acute

or chronic pain should be given alternative analgesics for dental pain.

• Assess salivary flow as a factor in caries, periodontal disease, and candidiasis.

• Consider semisupine chair position for patient comfort if GI side effects occur.

Teach patient/family: *When chronic dry mouth occurs, advise patient:*

• To avoid mouth rinses with high alcohol content due to drying effects

• To use daily home fluoride products for anticaries effect

• To use sugarless gum, frequent sips of water, or saliva substitutes

---

dyclonine hydrochloride

(dye'kloe-neen)

Dyclone

Drug class.: Topically acting local anesthetic (ketone)

Action: Inhibits nerve impulses from sensory nerves, thus producing local anesthesia; nerve impulses are blocked as a result of decreased nerve membrane permeability to sodium influx

Uses: Topical anesthesia of mucous membranes of mouth, pharynx, larynx, trachea, esophagus, and urethra before a variety of procedures; 0.5% solution may be used to block the gag reflex to relieve the pain of oral ulcers or stomatitis secondary to antineoplastic chemotherapy or radiation

Dosage and routes:

• *Adult:* TOP individualized dose depending on disease or patient need; use lowest effective dose; max recommended dose is 30 ml of a 1% solution (300 mg); usual dosage range is 4-20 ml; reduced dosage is recommended for elderly and pediatric patients

Available forms include: Topical solution 0.5%, 1.0% in 30 ml bottles

(Note: Astra no longer makes this product.)

Side effects/adverse reactions:

INTEG: Allergic reactions (urticaria, edema, contact dermatitis)

*MISC: **Anaphylaxis***

More severe systemic reactions can be observed if excessive absorption leads to toxic doses

Contraindications: Hypersensitivity

Precautions: Do not inject or apply to nasal or conjunctival mucous membranes, pregnancy category C, lactation, children <12 yr

Pharmacokinetics:

TOP: Rapid onset and relatively short duration of action

DENTAL CONSIDERATIONS

General:

• Low incidence of side effects following topical application.

• Expectorate excess solution when used topically.

• Limit area of application, especially in inflamed or denuded areas.

• Dry mucous membranes in area of application before applying solution.

• Symptoms of systemic toxicity include nervousness, nausea, excitement followed by drowsiness, convulsions, and cardiac and respiratory depression.

• Symptoms may vary because they depend on the amount of drug actually absorbed.

Teach patient/family
• To prevent injury while numbness is present
• To avoid chewing gum or eating after dental treatment

---

dyphylline
(dye'fi-lin)

Dilor, Dilor-400, Lufyllin, Lufyllin-400

Drug class.: Xanthine derivative

Action: Relaxes smooth muscle of respiratory system by blocking phosphodiesterase, which increases intracellular AMP

Uses: Bronchial asthma, bronchospasm in chronic bronchitis, COPD, emphysema

Dosage and routes:
• *Adult:* PO 200-800 mg q6h; IM 250-500 mg q6h injected slowly
• *Child >6 yr:* PO 4-7 mg/kg/day in 4 divided doses

Available forms include: Tabs 200, 400 mg; elix 100, 160 mg/15 ml; inj IM 250 mg/ml

Side effects/adverse reactions:
▼ *ORAL:* Bitter taste

CNS: Anxiety, restlessness, insomnia, dizziness, **convulsions,** headache, light-headedness, muscle twitching

CV: Palpitation, sinus tachycardia, hypotension, flushing, dysrhythmias

GI: Nausea, vomiting, anorexia, dyspepsia, epigastric pain

RESP: Tachypnea

INTEG: Flushing, urticaria

MISC: **Albuminuria,** fever, dehydration, hyperglycemia

Contraindications: Hypersensitivity to xanthines, tachydysrhythmias

Precautions: Elderly, CHF, cor pulmonale, hepatic disease, active peptic ulcer disease, diabetes mellitus, hyperthyroidism, hypertension, children, renal disease, pregnancy category C, glaucoma

Pharmacokinetics:
PO: Peak 1 hr, half-life 2 hr; excreted in urine unchanged

🦷 **Drug interactions of concern to dentistry:**
• Increased action: erythromycin, ciprofloxacin
• Increased risk of cardiac dysrhythmia: halothane-inhalation anesthesia, CNS stimulants
• Decreased effect: barbiturates, carbamazepine, ketoconazole
• May decrease sedative effects of benzodiazepines

DENTAL CONSIDERATIONS

General:
• Monitor vital signs every appointment due to cardiovascular and respiratory side effects.
• Consider semisupine chair position for patients with respiratory disease.

---

econazole nitrate (topical)
(e-kone'a-zole)

Spectazole

Drug class.: Local antifungal

Action: Interferes with fungal cell membrane, increasing permeability and leading to leaking of cell nutrients

Uses: Tinea pedis, tinea cruris, tinea corporis, tinea versicolor, cutaneous candidiasis

Dosage and routes:
• *Adult and child:* TOP apply to affected area once daily

E

Cutaneous candidiasis
- *Adult and child:* TOP apply to affected area bid (AM and PM)

Available forms include: Cream 1% in 15, 30, 85 g

Side effects/adverse reactions:

INTEG: Rash, urticaria, stinging, burning, pruritus

Contraindications: Hypersensitivity

Precautions: Pregnancy category C, lactation

DENTAL CONSIDERATIONS
- None

---

efavirenz

(ef-a-vir′enz)

Sustiva

Drug class.: Antiviral (nonnucleoside)

Action: Acts as a reverse transcriptase inhibitor in HIV-1

Uses: For use in HIV-1 infection, only in combination with other HIV-1 antiretroviral agents that the patient has not previously taken

Dosage and routes:
- *Adult:* PO 600 mg qd in combination with a protease inhibitor or nucleoside reverse transcriptase inhibitor or both; avoid high-fat meals with dosing
- *Child >3 yr weighing 10-40 kg:* PO:

Weight (kg)	Dose (daily)
10-<15	200 mg
15-<20	250 mg
20-<25	300 mg
25-<32.5	350 mg
32.5-<40	400 mg
>40	600 mg

Available forms include: Caps 50, 100, 200 mg

Side effects/adverse reactions:

▼ *ORAL:* Dry mouth, altered taste

CNS: Dizziness, somnolence, insomnia, abnormal dreams, confusion, abnormal thinking, impaired concentration, amnesia, agitation, depersonalization, hallucinations, euphoria

CV: Flushing, palpitation, tachycardia, thrombophlebitis

GI: Nausea, vomiting, diarrhea

RESP: Cough, asthma

EENT: Tinnitus, blurred vision

INTEG: Rash, eczema, urticaria

META: Elevation of AST and ALT enzymes

MS: Arthralgia, myalgia

MISC: Fever, fatigue, alcohol intolerance

Contraindications: Hypersensitivity: concurrent use with midazolam, triazolam, or ergot derivatives

Precautions: Must not be used as a single agent for HIV, avoid pregnancy with use, pregnancy category C, lactation, mental illness, substance abuse, caution with alcohol or psychotropic drugs, driving or other hazardous tasks, monitor cholesterol, hepatic impairment

Pharmacokinetics:

PO: Peak plasma levels 5 hr, avoid high-fat meals, hepatic metabolism by cytochrome P-450 enzymes, excreted in both urine and feces; high plasma protein binding (99%)

 Drug interactions of concern to dentistry:
- Contraindicated drugs: midazolam, triazolam

---

bold italic = life-threatening conditions

• Decreased plasma levels of clarithromycin
• Potential for increased levels with ketoconazole, itraconazole (no studies)
• Increased risk of CNS side effects with CNS depressants

DENTAL CONSIDERATIONS
General:
• Examine for oral manifestation of opportunistic infection.
• Monitor vital signs every appointment due to cardiovascular and respiratory side effects.
• Consider semisupine chair position for patient comfort due to GI side effects of drug.
• Assess salivary flow as a factor in caries, periodontal disease, and candidiasis.
• Short appointments and a stress reduction protocol may be required for anxious patients.

Consultations:
• Medical consult may be required to assess disease control.

Teach patient/family:
• To prevent trauma when using oral hygiene aids
• Importance of good oral hygiene to prevent soft tissue inflammation
• To be alert for the possibility of secondary oral infection and to see dentist immediately if signs of infection occur

When chronic dry mouth occurs, advise patient:
• To avoid mouth rinses with high alcohol content due to drying effects
• To use daily home fluoride products for anticaries effect
• To use sugarless gum, frequent sips of water, or saliva substitutes

emedastine difumarate (optic)
(em-e-das'teen)
Emadine
Drug class.: Ophthalmic antihistamine

Action: Selective H_1-antagonist
Uses: Temporary relief of signs and symptoms of allergic conjunctivitis

Dosage and routes:
• *Adult:* Ophth 1 gtt in affected eye up to qid
Available forms include: Ophth sol 0.05% in 5 ml

Side effects/adverse reactions:
▼ *ORAL:* Bad taste
CNS: Headache, abnormal dreams
EENT: Blurred vision, burning, stinging, corneal staining, dry eyes, rhinitis, sinusitis, tearing
INTEG: Dermatitis, pruritus
MS: Asthenia

Contraindications: Hypersensitivity
Precautions: Avoid wearing contact lens if eye is red, wait at least 10 min after application to insert contact lens, pregnancy category B, lactation, no data for use in children <3 yr

Pharmacokinetics:
TOP: Systemic absorption below level for assay; any absorbed drug is metabolized and excreted in urine

Drug interactions of concern to dentistry:
• None reported

DENTAL CONSIDERATIONS
General:
• Protect patient's eyes from accidental spatter during dental treatment.

enalapril maleate

(e-nal'a-pril)
Vasotec, Vasotec IV

Drug class.: Angiotensin-converting enzyme (ACE) inhibitor

Action: Selectively suppresses renin-angiotensin-aldosterone system; inhibits ACE; prevents conversion of angiotensin I to angiotensin II, leading to dilation of arterial and venous vessels

Uses: Hypertension, heart failure adjunct

Dosage and routes:
• *Adult:* PO 5 mg/day; may increase or decrease to desired response range 10-40 mg/day; lower initial dose with a diuretic

Hypertension
• *Adult:* IV 1.25 mg q6h over 5 min

Patients on diuretics
• *Adult:* IV 0.625 over 5 min; may give additional doses of 1.25 mg q6h

Renal impairment
• *Adult:* 1.25 mg q6h with CrCl <3 mg/dl or 0.625 mg if CrCl >3 mg/dl

Available forms include: Tabs 2.5, 5, 10, 20 mg; inj 1.25 mg/ml

Side effects/adverse reactions:
▼ *ORAL:* Loss of taste, oral ulceration (Stevens-Johnson syndrome, rare), dry mouth, angioedema (lips, tongue, mucous membranes), lichenoid drug reaction

CNS: Insomnia, dizziness, paresthesia, headache, fatigue, anxiety

CV: Hypotension, chest pain, tachycardia, dysrhythmias

GI: Nausea, vomiting, colitis, cramps, diarrhea, constipation, pancreatitis, flatulence

RESP: Dyspnea, cough, rales, angioedema

HEMA: Agranulocytosis, neutropenia

GU: Proteinuria, renal failure, increased frequency of polyurea or oliguria

INTEG: Rash, purpura, alopecia

META: Hyperkalemia

Contraindications: Pregnancy category D; can cause serious reactions in second and third trimester; lactation

Precautions: Renal disease, hyperkalemia

Pharmacokinetics:
PO: Peak 1 hr, half-life 11 hr; metabolized by liver to active metabolite; excreted in urine

IV: Onset 5-15 min, peak up to 4 hr

⚡ Drug interactions of concern to dentistry:
• Increased hypotension: alcohol, phenothiazines
• Decreased hypotensive effects: indomethacin and possibly other NSAIDs, sympathomimetics

DENTAL CONSIDERATIONS
General:
• Monitor vital signs every appointment due to cardiovascular side effects.
• After supine positioning, have patient sit upright for at least 2 min before standing to avoid orthostatic hypotension.
• Patients on chronic drug therapy may rarely have symptoms of blood dyscrasias, which can include infection, bleeding, and poor healing.
• Assess salivary flow as a factor in caries, periodontal disease, and candidiasis.
• Limit use of sodium-containing products such as saline IV fluids for those patients with a dietary salt restriction.
• Use vasoconstrictors with cau-

---

bold italic = life-threatening conditions

tion, in low doses, and with careful aspiration.

• Stress from dental procedures may compromise cardiovascular function; determine patient risk.

• Short appointments and a stress reduction protocol may be required for anxious patients.

Consultations:

• Medical consult may be required to assess patient's ability to tolerate stress.

• In a patient with symptoms of blood dyscrasias, request a medical consult for blood studies and postpone dental treatment until normal values are reestablished.

• Take precautions if dental surgery is anticipated and sedation or general anesthesia is required; risk of hypotensive episode.

Teach patient/family:

• Importance of good oral hygiene to prevent soft tissue inflammation

• When chronic dry mouth occurs, advise patient:

• To avoid mouth rinses with high alcohol content due to drying effects

• To use daily home fluoride products for anticaries effect

• To use sugarless gum, frequent sips of water, or saliva substitutes

---

enoxacin
(en-ox′a-sin)
Penetrex

Drug class.: Fluoroquinolone anti-infective

Action: A broad-spectrum bactericidal agent that inhibits the enzymes topoisomerase II (DNA gyrase) and topoisomerase IV, which are required for bacterial DNA replication, transcription repair, and recombination

Uses: Uncomplicated urethral or cervical gonorrhea, uncomplicated and complicated UTIs

Dosage and routes:

Gonorrhea

• *Adult:* PO 400 mg as a single dose

Uncomplicated UTI

• *Adult:* PO 200 mg bid × 7 days

Complicated UTI

• *Adult:* PO 400 mg bid × 14 days

Available forms include: Tabs 200, 400 mg

Side effects/adverse reactions:

▼ *ORAL:* Candidiasis, dry mouth, unusual taste

CNS: Dizziness, headache, fatigue, somnolence, depression, insomnia

GI: Diarrhea, *nausea, vomiting,* anorexia, flatulence, heartburn, increased AST/ALT, ***pseudomembranous colitis***

EENT: Visual disturbances, phototoxicity

INTEG: Rash

MS: Tendinitis

Contraindications: Hypersensitivity to quinolones

Precautions: Pregnancy category C, lactation, children, elderly, renal disease, seizure disorders

Pharmacokinetics:

PO: Peak 1-3 hr, steady state 2 days, half-life 3-6 hr; excreted in urine as unchanged drug, metabolites

Drug interactions of concern to dentistry:

• Decreased absorption of enoxacin: sodium bicarbonate

• Increased action of caffeine, cyclosporine

DENTAL CONSIDERATIONS

General:

• Due to drug interaction, do not

---

use ingestible sodium bicarbonate products, such as the air polishing system (Prophy Jet), unless 2 hr have passed since enoxacin was taken.
- Assess salivary flow as a factor in caries, periodontal disease, and candidiasis.
- Use caution in prescribing caffeine-containing analgesics.
- Avoid dental light in patient's eyes; offer dark glasses for patient comfort.
- Determine why the patient is taking the drug.

Consultations:
- Consult with patient's physician if an acute dental infection occurs and another antiinfective is required.

Teach patient/family:
- Importance of good oral hygiene to prevent gingival inflammation
- To discontinue treatment and inform dentist immediately if patient experiences pain or inflammation of a tendon, and to rest and refrain from exercise

When chronic dry mouth occurs, advise patient:
- To avoid mouth rinses with high alcohol content due to drying effects
- To use daily home fluoride products for anticaries effect
- To use sugarless gum, frequent sips of water, or artificial saliva substitutes

---

enoxaparin sodium
(ee-nox-a-pa'rin)
Lovenox

Drug class.: Heparin-type anticoagulant

Action: Low-molecular-weight heparin having antithrombotic actions with higher anti-Factor X_a activity compared with anti-Factor II_a

Uses: Prevention and treatment of deep vein thrombosis following hip or knee replacement surgery; also used in abdominal and gynecologic surgery; with aspirin in the prevention of ischemic complications of unstable angina and non-Q-wave MI; in combination with warfarin for deep vein thrombosis, with or without pulmonary embolism

Dosage and routes:
- *Adult:* SC 30 mg bid with first dose given 12-24 hr after surgery; or SC 40 mg qd with first dose given 2 hr before surgery

Available forms include: Prefilled syringes 30, 40, 60, 80, 90, 100, 120, 150 mg

Side effects/adverse reactions:
CNS: Confusion
GI: Nausea
*HEMA: Bleeding after surgery, **thrombocytopenia,*** hemorrhage, anemia
INTEG: Edema, hematoma, erythema
MISC: Local pain, irritation, fever

Contraindications: Hypersensitivity, active major bleeding, thrombocytopenia, IM administration

Precautions: Hemorrhage, thrombocytopenia, renal impairment, elderly, pregnancy category B, lactation, children, requires monitoring, GI bleeding

Pharmacokinetics:
SC INJ ONLY: Maximum anti-Factor X_a and antithrombin effect 3-5 hr, activity lasts up to 12 hr; renal excretion

🔖 **Drug interactions of concern to dentistry:**
- Avoid concurrent use of aspirin,

NSAIDs, dipyridamole, sulfinpyrazone
• Use with caution in patients taking olanzapine

DENTAL CONSIDERATIONS
General:
• Determine why patient is taking the drug.
• Product may be used in outpatient therapy. Delay elective dental treatment until patient completes enoxaparin therapy.
• Consider local hemostasis measures to prevent excessive bleeding if dental treatment must be performed.
• Avoid products that affect platelet function, such as aspirin and NSAIDs.
• Antibiotic prophylaxis before dental treatment may be required for joint prothesis. See 1997 ADA guidelines.

Consultations:
• Medical consult should include routine blood counts, including platelet counts and bleeding time.

Teach patient/family:
• Importance of good oral hygiene to prevent soft tissue inflammation
• Caution to prevent trauma when using oral hygiene aids
• To report oral lesions, soreness, or bleeding to dentist

---

entacapone
(en-tak'a-pone)
Comtan
Drug class.: Antiparkinsonian

Action: Inhibits catechol-O-methyltransferase (COMT), decreases peripheral conversion of levodopa to 3-O-methyldopa
Uses: Adjunct to levodopa/carbidopa in the treatment of Parkinson's disease, not used alone

Dosage and routes:
• *Adult:* PO 200 mg with each levodopa/carbidopa dose not to exceed 8 times daily; adjust dose down as symptoms improve
Available forms include: Tabs 200 mg

Side effects/adverse reactions:
▼ *ORAL:* Taste alteration, dry mouth (1%)
CNS: Dyskinesia, hyperkinesia, psychiatric reactions, hallucinations, aggravation of Parkinson's symptoms, hypokinesia, dizziness, anxiety
CV: Orthostatic hypotension, syncope
GI: Nausea, diarrhea, abdominal pain
RESP: Dyspnea
HEMA: Purpura
GU: Discolored urine (brown-orange)
INTEG: Sweating
META: May decrease serum iron levels
*MS: **Rhabdomyolysis,** back pain, fatigue*
Contraindications: Hypersensitivity, nonselective MAO inhibitors
Precautions: Enhanced orthostatic hypotension with levodopa/carbidopa, hepatic impairment, caution in driving, pregnancy category C, lactation, children

Pharmacokinetics:
PO: Rapid absorption, bioavailability 35%, highly plasma protein bound (98%), hepatic metabolism, metabolites excreted mostly (90%) in feces

🥄 Drug interactions of concern to dentistry:
• Increased heart rate, arrhythmias, hypertension: with epinephrine,

norepinephrine, levonordefrin, or other sympathomimetics metabolized by COMT

DENTAL CONSIDERATIONS
General:
• Monitor vital signs every appointment due to cardiovascular side effects.
• Short appointments and a stress reduction protocol may be required for anxious patients.
• Consider semisupine chair position for patient comfort if GI side effects occur.
• Use vasoconstrictor with caution, in low doses and with careful aspiration. Avoid using gingival retraction cord containing epinephrine.
• Assess for presence of extrapyramidal motor symptoms, such as tardive dyskinesia and akathisia. Extrapyramidal motor activity may complicate dental treatment.
• After supine positioning, have patient sit upright for at least 2 min to avoid orthostatic hypotension.
• Assess salivary flow as a factor in caries, periodontal disease, and candidiasis.

Consultations:
• Medical consult may be required to assess disease control and patient's ability to tolerate stress.

Teach patient/family:
• Use of electric toothbrush if patient has difficulty holding conventional devices
• Importance of updating health and drug history if physician makes any changes in evaluation or drug regimens
When chronic dry mouth occurs, advise patient:
• To avoid mouth rinses with high alcohol content due to drying effects

• To use daily home fluoride products for anticaries effect
• To use sugarless gum, frequent sips of water, or saliva substitutes

---

ephedrine sulfate
(e-fed′rin)
generic
Drug class.: Adrenergic, mixed direct and indirect effects

Action: Causes increased contractility and heart rate by acting on β-receptors in the heart; also acts on α-receptors, causing vasoconstriction in blood vessels
Uses: Shock, increased perfusion, hypotension, bronchodilation, nasal decongestant
Dosage and routes:
• *Adult:* IM/SC 25-50 mg, not to exceed 150 mg/24 hr; IV 10-25 mg, not to exceed 150 mg/24 hr
• *Child:* SC/IV 3 mg/kg/day in divided doses q4-6h
Bronchodilation
• *Adult:* PO 12.5-50 mg bid-qid, not to exceed 400 mg/day
• *Child:* PO 2-3 mg/kg/day in 4-6 divided doses
Available forms include: Inj IM/SC/IV 25, 50 mg/ml; caps 25, 50 mg; syr 11, 20 mg/5 ml
Side effects/adverse reactions:
▼ *ORAL:* Dry mouth
CNS: Tremors, *anxiety,* **convulsions, CNS depression,** insomnia, headache, dizziness, confusion, hallucinations
CV: **Dysrhythmias,** palpitation, tachycardia, hypertension, chest pain
GI: Anorexia, nausea, vomiting
GU: Dysuria, urinary retention
Contraindications: Hypersensi-

---

bold italic = life-threatening conditions

tivity to sympathomimetics, narrow-angle glaucoma

Precautions: Pregnancy category C, cardiac disorders, hyperthyroidism, diabetes mellitus, prostatic hypertrophy

Pharmacokinetics:

PO: Onset 15-60 min, duration 2-4 hr

IV: Onset 5 min, duration 2 hr Metabolized in liver; excreted in urine (unchanged); crosses blood-brain barrier, placenta, excreted in breast milk

🦷 Drug interactions of concern to dentistry:

• Decreased pressor effect: haloperidol, phenothiazines, thioxanthenes

• Dysrhythmia: halogenated general anesthetics

DENTAL CONSIDERATIONS

General:

• Monitor vital signs every appointment due to cardiovascular side effects.

• Assess salivary flow as a factor in caries, periodontal disease, and candidiasis.

• Consider semisupine chair position for patients with respiratory disease.

• Consider short appointments and a stress reduction protocol for anxious patients.

Consultations:

• Medical consult may be required to assess disease control and patient's tolerance for stress.

Teach patient/family: *When chronic dry mouth occurs, advise patient:*

• To avoid mouth rinses with high alcohol content due to drying effects

• To use daily home fluoride products for anticaries effect

• To use sugarless gum, frequent sips of water, or saliva substitutes

---

epinephrine/ epinephrine bitartrate/ epinephrine HCl

(ep-i-nef′rin)

Epinephrine HCl inj: Adrenalin Chloride, Ana-Guard, EpiPen Auto-Injector, EpiPen Jr., Sus-Phrine Suspension

Epinephrine HCl inh: Adrenalin, Bronkaid Mist, Primatine Mist

♣ Bronkaid Mistometer

Epinephrine bitartrate inh: AsthmaHaler, Primatene Mist Suspension

Racemic epinephrine: Asthma Nefrin, MicroNefrin, Nephron, S-2

Epinephrine HCl ophthalmic: Epiferin, Glaucon

Epinephrine borate ophthalmic: Epinal

Drug class.: Adrenergic agonist, catecholamine

Action: Acts on both α- and β-adrenergic receptors; magnitude of response depends on specific receptors activated, tissue innervated, and the dose and rate of administration; effects on the cardiovascular system include peripheral vasoconstriction, stimulation of cardiac muscle, and, in the pulmonary system, relaxation of bronchial smooth muscles. Epinephrine elevates systemic blood pressure, increases the strength and rate of cardiac contraction; action on β_2-adrenergic receptors reduces bronchial congestion by relaxing bronchial smooth muscle mediated through cyclic AMP; application to the eye results in mydriasis and reduction in intraocular pressure.

Uses: Acute asthmatic attacks, hemostasis, bronchospasm, anaphylaxis, allergic reactions, cardiac arrest, vasopressor

Dosage and routes:

• *Adult:* Bronchial asthma, allergic reactions, angioedema, urticaria, serum sickness, anaphylaxis (give SC: 0.1-0.25 mg; if given IM do not administer in buttocks)

Cardiopulmonary resuscitation: applicable when other CPR measures have failed; IV or intracardially administer 1-10 ml of a 1:10,000 solution (use diluted solutions or dilute more concentrated solutions) and support with CPR measures.

• *Child:* Bronchial asthma and allergic reactions the usual dose is 0.01 mg/kg or 0.3 mg/m^2 to a maximum of 0.5 mg

Asthma

• *Adult and child:* INH 1-2 puffs of 1:100 or 2.25% racemic q15min

Hemostasis

• *Adult:* TOP 1:50,000-1:1000 applied as needed to stop bleeding; OPHTH: 1 gtt in affected eye(s) daily; dose may need to be adjusted for each patient

Available forms include: Aerosol 0.16, 0.2, 0.25 mg/spray; inj IM/ IV/SC 1:1000 (1 mg/ml), inj 1:2000 (5 mg/ml); suspension for injection 1:200 (5 mg/ml), 0.01 mg/ml (1:100,000), 0.01 mg/ml (1:10.000); sol for nebuliz 1:100, 1.25% 2.25% (base)

Side effects/adverse reactions:

CNS: Tremors, anxiety, **cerebral hemorrhage,** insomnia, headache, dizziness, confusion, hallucinations

CV: **Dysrhythmias,** palpitations, tachycardia, hypertension, increased T wave

GI: Anorexia, nausea, vomiting

RESP: Dyspnea

GU: Urinary retention

Contraindications: Hypersensitivity to sympathomimetics, narrow-angle glaucoma

Precautions: Pregnancy category C, cardiac disorders, hyperthyroidism, diabetes mellitus, prostatic hypertrophy

Pharmacokinetics:

SC: Onset 3-5 min, duration 20 min

PO/INH: Onset 1 min

⚖ Drug interactions of concern to dentistry:

• Hypotension, tachycardia: haloperidol, loxapine, phenothiazines, thioxanthenes

• Ventricular dysrhythmia: hydrocarbon-inhalation anesthetics, CNS stimulants, tricyclic antidepressants

• With larger doses of epinephrine risk of hypertension followed by bradycardia with β-adrenergic antagonists

DENTAL CONSIDERATIONS

General:

• Monitor vital signs every appointment due to cardiovascular side effects.

• Assess salivary flow as a factor in caries, periodontal disease, and candidiasis.

• Consider semisupine chair position for patients with respiratory disease.

• Acute asthmatic episodes may be precipitated in the dental office. Sympathomimetic inhalants should be available for emergency use; a stress reduction protocol may be required.

---

bold italic = life-threatening conditions

eprosartan

(ep-roe-sar'tan)
Teveten

Drug class.: Antihypertensive, angiotensin II receptor (AT₁) antagonist

Note: Although approved in 1997, its marketing was delayed until 1999

Action: A selective antagonist for angiotensin II receptor sites (AT_1); antagonizes the vasoconstrictor- and aldosterone-secreting effects of angiotensin

Uses: Hypertension as a single drug or in combination with other antihypertensive drugs; may also be used in congestive heart failure or chronic renal failure

Dosage and route:
• *Adult:* PO initial 600 mg qd, can also be given bid in daily doses ranging from 400-800 mg

Available forms include: Tabs 400, 600 mg

Side effects/adverse reactions: Information was not available. However, side effects reported with other angiotensin receptor antagonists have included taste alterations, insomnia, dizziness, a low incidence of palpitation, peripheral edema, hypotension, cough, and urinary frequency. The relationship of these side effects to this drug is unknown.

Contraindications: Hypersensitivity, pregnancy second and third trimester

Precautions: This group of drugs has a general warning about their use during the second and third trimesters of pregnancy

Pharmacokinetics: Not metabolized by cytochrome P-450 isoenzyme system

🦷 **Drug interactions of concern to dentistry:** Unknown, but ketoconazole may inhibit the metabolism of other similar drugs

DENTAL CONSIDERATIONS:
General:
• Monitor vital signs every appointment due to cardiovascular side effects.
• Stress from dental procedures may compromise cardiovascular function; determine patient risk.
• Limit use of sodium-containing products such as saline IV fluids for those patients with a dietary salt restriction.
• Short appointments and a stress reduction protocol may be required for anxious patients.
• Use precaution if sedation or general anesthesia is required; risk of hypotensive episode.

Consultations:
• Medical consult may be required to assess disease control and patient's ability to tolerate stress.

Teach patient/family:
• Importance of updating health and drug history if physician makes any changes in evaluation or drug regimens

ergoloid mesylate

(er'goe-loid) (mess'i-late)
Gerimal, Hydergine, Hydergine LC

Drug class.: Ergot alkaloids

Action: May increase cerebral metabolism and blood flow

Uses: Senile dementia, Alzheimer's dementia, multiinfarct dementia, primary progressive dementia

Dosage and routes:

• *Adult:* PO/SL 1 mg tid; may increase to 4.5-12 mg/day

Available forms include: Tabs SL 0.5, 1 mg; tabs 0.5, 1 mg; caps 1 mg; liq 1 mg/ml

Side effects/adverse reactions:

▼ *ORAL:* Sublingual irritation (SL tablet)

CNS: Dizziness, syncope, headache, anorexia

CV: Bradycardia, orthostatic hypotension

GI: Nausea, vomiting

EENT: Blurred vision, nasal stuffiness

INTEG: Skin rash, flushing

Contraindications: Hypersensitivity to ergot preparations; psychosis

Precautions: Acute intermittent porphyria, pregnancy category C

Pharmacokinetics:

PO: Peak 1 hr, half-life 3.5 hr; metabolized in liver; excreted as metabolites in feces; crosses blood-brain barrier

DENTAL CONSIDERATIONS

General:

• Monitor vital signs every appointment due to cardiovascular side effects.

• After supine positioning, have patient sit upright for at least 2 min before standing to avoid orthostatic hypotension.

• Consider semisupine chair position for patient comfort due to GI effects of drug.

Teach patient/family:

• Use of electric toothbrush if patient is unable to carry out oral hygiene procedures

ergotamine tartrate

(er-got′a-meen)

Ergomar

♣ Gynergen

Drug class.: α-adrenergic blocker

Action: By a direct action, constricts vascular smooth muscle in peripheral and cranial blood vessels; relaxes uterine muscle

Uses: Vascular headache (migraine or histamine), cluster headache

Dosage and routes:

• *Adult:* SL 2 mg, then 1-2 mg qh or q0.5h, not to exceed 6 mg/day or 10 mg/wk

Available forms include: SL tabs 2 mg

Side effects/adverse reactions:

CNS: Numbness in fingers/toes, headache, weakness, visual changes

CV: Transient tachycardia, chest pain, bradycardia, edema, claudication, increase or decrease in BP

GI: Nausea, vomiting

MS: Muscle pain

Contraindications: Hypersensitivity to ergot preparations, occlusion (peripheral, vascular), CAD, hepatic disease, renal disease, peptic ulcer, hypertension, pregnancy category X

Precautions: Lactation, children, anemia

Pharmacokinetics:

PO: Peak 30 min-3 hr; metabolized in liver; excreted as metabolites in feces; crosses blood-brain barrier; excreted in breast milk

Drug interactions of concern to dentistry:

• Increased vasoconstriction: vasoconstrictor in local anesthetics

---

• Suspected increased risk of ergotism: erythromycin, clarithromycin, troleandomycin
• Use anticholinergic with caution in the elderly

DENTAL CONSIDERATIONS
General:
• Monitor vital signs every appointment due to cardiovascular side effects.

Teach patient/family:
• Use of electric toothbrush if patient has difficulty holding conventional devices

---

erythromycin (ophthalmic)
(er-ith-roe-mye′sin)
Ilotycin Ophthalmic
Drug class.: Antiinfective

Action: Inhibits bacterial protein synthesis
Uses: Infection of external eye, prophylaxis of neonatal conjunctivitis and ophthalmia neonatorum
Dosage and routes:
• *Adult and child:* Oint apply qd-qid as needed
Ophthalmia neonatorum
• *Neonates:* Apply oint to conjunctival sacs immediately after delivery
Available forms include: Oint 0.5% in 3.5 g
Side effects/adverse reactions:
EENT: Poor corneal wound healing, temporary visual haze, irritation, overgrowth of nonsusceptible organisms, irritation
Contraindications: Hypersensitivity
Precautions: Antibiotic hypersensitivity, pregnancy category B, lactation

DENTAL CONSIDERATIONS
General:
• Avoid dental light in patient's eyes; offer dark glasses for patient comfort.
• Protect patient's eyes from accidental spatter during dental treatment.

---

erythromycin (topical)
(er-ith-roe-mye′sin)
Akne-mycin, Emgel, Erygel
Drug class.: Macrolide antibacterial (topical)

Action: Interferes with bacterial protein synthesis to inhibit bacterial growth
Uses: Acne vulgaris
Dosage and routes:
• *Adult and child >12 yr:* Top apply to affected area tid to qid
Available forms include: Top oint 2%; gel 2%
Side effects/adverse reactions:
INTEG: Rash, urticaria, stinging, burning, pruritus, dry/scaly/oily skin
EENT: Eye irritation, tenderness
Contraindications: Hypersensitivity
Precautions: Pregnancy category C, lactation
DENTAL CONSIDERATIONS
• None indicated

---

     italic = common side effects

erythromycin base/
erythromycin estolate/
erythromycin
ethylsuccinate/
erythromycin
gluceptate/
erythromycin
lactobionate/
erythromycin stearate
(er-ith-roe-mye'sin)

Erythromycin base: E-Base, E-Mycin, Eryc, Ery-Tab, Erythromycin Filmtabs, PCE Dispertab
♣ Apo-Erythro, Apo-Erythro-EC, Erybid, Erythromid, Novo-Rythro EnCap
Erythromycin estolate: Ilosone
♣ Novo-Erythro
Erythromycin stearate: Erythrocin Stearate
♣ Apo-Erythro-S
Erythromycin ethylsuccinate: EES 200, EES 400, EES Granules, EryPed
♣ Apo-Erythro-ES, Novo-Rythro
Erythromycin lactobionate inj: Erythrocin
Erythromycin gluceptate inj: Ilotycin

Drug class.: Macrolide antibiotic

Action: Binds to 50S ribosomal subunits of susceptible bacteria and suppresses protein synthesis

Uses: Infections caused by *N. gonorrhoeae;* mild-to-moderate respiratory tract, skin, soft tissue infections caused by *S. pneumoniae, M. pneumoniae, C. diphtheriae, B. pertussis, L. monocytogenes, S. pyogenes;* syphilis; legionnaire's disease; *C. trachomatis; H. influenzae;* endocarditis prophylaxis

Dosage and routes:
Soft tissue infections
• *Adult:* PO 250-500 mg q6h (base, estolate, stearate); PO 400-800 mg q6h (ethylsuccinate); IV inf 15-20 mg/kg/day (lactobionate)
• *Child:* PO 30-50 mg/kg/day in divided doses q6h (salts); IV 15-20 mg/kg/day in divided doses q4-6h (lactobionate)

Available forms include: Base: enteric-coated tabs 250, 333, 500 mg; film-coated tabs 250, 500 mg; estolate: tabs 500 mg; caps 250 mg; susp 125, 250 mg/5 ml; stearate: film-coated tabs 250, 500 mg; ethylsuccinate: chew tabs 200 mg; susp 100 mg/2.5 ml, 200, 400 mg/5 ml; susp 200, 400 mg; powder for susp; 200 and 400 mg/5 ml; powder for inj; 500 mg and 1 g

Side effects/adverse reactions:
▼ *ORAL:* Candidiasis, lichenoid reaction
GI: Nausea, vomiting, diarrhea, **hepatotoxicity,** abdominal pain, heartburn, anorexia, pruritus ani, pseudomembranous colitis
GU: Vaginitis, moniliasis
EENT: Hearing loss, tinnitus
INTEG: Rash, urticaria, pruritus, thrombophlebitis (IV site), hypersensitivity

Contraindications: Hypersensitivity, erythromycin estolate in preexisting hepatic disease, cisipride, sparfloxacin, pimozide
Precautions: Pregnancy category B, hepatic disease, lactation
Pharmacokinetics:
PO: Peak 4 hr, duration 6 hr, half-life 1-3 hr; metabolized in liver; excreted in bile, feces
🦷 **Drug interactions of concern to dentistry:**
• Increased duration of alfentanil, cyclosporine

---

bold italic = life-threatening conditions

• Increased serum levels: indinavir, digoxin
• Decreased action of clindamycin, penicillins, lincomycin
• Increased serum levels of alfentanil, carbamazepine, theophylline (and other methylxanthines) and felodipine (possibly with other calcium blockers in the dihydropyridine class), ergotamine, oral anticoagulants
• Risk of rhabdomyolysis: HMG-CoA reductase inhibitors
• Oral contraceptives: advise patient of a potential risk for decreased contraceptive action, to maintain compliance with oral contraceptive use while using antibiotics, and to consider the use of additional nonhormonal contraception
• May increase the effects of certain benzodiazepines: alprazolam, diazepam, midazolam, and triazolam
• Risk of increased QT interval—use with caution in patients taking gatifloxacin, moxifloxacin, pimozide, disopyramide
• Possible serotonin syndrome with selective serotonin reuptake inhibitors

DENTAL CONSIDERATIONS
General:
• Alternative drug of choice for mild infection due to a susceptible organism in patients who are allergic to penicillin.
• Determine why the patient is taking the drug.
• Estolate salt form not indicated for adults due to risk of cholestatic jaundice.

Teach patient/family:
• To take oral drug with full glass of water; take with food if GI symptoms occur (estolate, ethylsuccinate, and coated tabs only)
When used for dental infection, advise patient:
• To report sore throat, oral burning sensation, fever, fatigue, any of which could indicate superinfection
• To take at prescribed intervals and complete dosage regimen
• To immediately notify the dentist if signs or symptoms of infection increase

---

esomeprazole magnesium
(es-oh-me′pray-sol)
Nexium
Drug class.: Antisecretory, proton pump inhibitor

Action: Suppresses gastric acid secretion by inhibiting hydrogen/potassium ATPase enzyme system in the gastric parietal cell; characterized as a gastric acid pump inhibitor because it blocks the final step of acid production
Uses: Gastroesophageal reflux disease (GERD), healing and maintenance of erosive esophagitis and *H. pylori* eradication in combination with antibiotics
Dosage and routes:
Healing of erosive esophagitis
• *Adult:* PO 20 or 40 mg/day × 4-8 wk; some may require 16 wk
Maintenance of healing of erosive esophagitis
• *Adult:* PO 20 mg/day × 4 wk
Symptomatic GERD
• *Adult:* PO 20 mg/day × 4 wk
H. pylori eradication to reduce risk of duodenal ulcer recurrence
• *Adult:* PO 40 mg/day × 10 days,

---

with amoxicillin 1000 mg bid × 10 days and clarithromycin 500 mg bid × 10 days

Available forms include: Del rel caps 20, 40 mg (do not chew or crush)

Side effects/adverse reactions:

▼ *ORAL: Dry mouth,* ulcerative stomatitis, taste loss

CNS: Headache, anorexia, apathy, nervousness, sleep disorder

CV: Flushing, hypertension, tachycardia

GI: Nausea, diarrhea, flatulence, abdominal pain, constipation, dyspepsia

RESP: Asthma aggravated, cough, dyspnea, laryngeal swelling

HEMA: Anemia, leukocytosis, leukopenia, thrombocytopenia

GU: Dysmenorrhea, vaginitis, dysuria, polyuria

EENT: Earache, tinnitus, conjunctivitis, abnormal vision

INTEG: Acne, dermatitis, pruritus, urticaria, angioedema

ENDO: Goiter

META: Glycosuria, hyperuricemia, hyponatremia, ↑alkaline phosphatase

MS: Back pain, chest pain, arthralgia

MISC: Asthenia, flulike symptoms

Contraindications: Hypersensitivity

Precautions: Presence of gastric malignancy, atrophic gastritis, pregnancy category B, lactation, use in pediatric patients has not been studied, severe hepatic impairment, allergic reactions to related proton pump inhibitors

Pharmacokinetics:

PO: Take 1 hr before meals; peak plasma levels 1.5 hr; bioavailability ~90%, highly plasma protein bound (97%); extensive hepatic metabolism (CYP 2C19 major, CYP 3A4 lesser); 80% of metabolites excreted in urine with 2% in feces

🦷 **Drug interactions of concern to dentistry:**

• May interfere with absorption of drugs where gastric pH is an important factor in bioavailability (e.g., iron products, ketoconazole)

DENTAL CONSIDERATIONS

General:

• Assess salivary flow as a factor in caries, periodontal disease, and candidiasis.

• Question patient about tolerance of NSAIDs or aspirin related to GI disease.

• To be aware of oral side effects and potential sequelae.

• Consider semisupine chair position for patient comfort due to GI side effects of disease.

• Patient on chronic drug therapy may rarely present with symptoms of blood dyscrasias, which can include infection, bleeding, and poor healing.

Consultations:

• In a patient with symptoms of blood dyscrasias, request a medical consult for blood studies and postpone treatment until normal values are reestablished.

Teach patient/family:

• To prevent trauma when using oral hygiene aids

• Importance of good oral hygiene to prevent soft tissue inflammation/infection

• Place on frequent recall due to oral side effects and oral effects of reflux disease

---

bold italic = life-threatening conditions

When chronic dry mouth occurs advise patient:

• To avoid mouth rinses with high alcohol content due to drying effects

• To use daily home fluoride products for anticaries effect

• To use sugarless gum, frequent sips of water, or saliva substitutes

---

estazolam

(es-ta′zoe-lam)
ProSom

Drug class.: Benzodiazepine, sedative-hypnotic

Controlled Substance Schedule IV (US)

Action: Produces CNS depression by interacting with a benzodiazepine receptor to facilitate the action of the inhibitory neurotransmitter γ-aminobutyric acid (GABA)

Uses: Insomnia

Dosage and routes:

• *Adult:* PO 1-2 mg hs

Available forms include: Tabs 1, 2 mg

Side effects/adverse reactions:

▼ *ORAL:* Dry mouth, taste alteration, oral ulceration

CNS: Lethargy, drowsiness, daytime sedation, dizziness, confusion, light-headedness, headache, anxiety, irritability, weakness, tremors, depression, lack of coordination

CV: Chest pain, pulse changes, palpitation, tachycardia

GI: Nausea, vomiting, diarrhea, heartburn, abdominal pain, constipation, anorexia

HEMA: **Leukopenia, granulocytopenia** (rare)

INTEG: Dermatitis, allergy, sweating, flushing, pruritus

MISC: Joint pain, congestion

Contraindications: Hypersensitivity to benzodiazepines, pregnancy category X, sleep apnea, ritonavir

Precautions: Hepatic disease, renal disease, suicidal individuals, drug abuse, elderly, psychosis, child <18 yr, lactation, depression, pulmonary insufficiency, narrow-angle glaucoma

Pharmacokinetics:

PO: Onset 15-45 min, peak 1.5-2 hr, duration 7-8 hr; metabolized by liver; excreted by kidneys (inactive/active metabolites); crosses placenta; excreted in breast milk

⚕ Drug interactions of concern to dentistry:

• Increased CNS depression: alcohol, all CNS depressants

• Increased serum levels and prolonged effect of benzodiazepines: ketoconazole, itraconazole, fluconazole, and miconazole (systemic), indinavir

DENTAL CONSIDERATIONS

General:

• Psychologic and physical dependence may occur with chronic administration.

• Geriatric patients are more susceptible to drug effects; use lower dose.

• Avoid the use of this drug in a patient with a history of drug abuse or alcoholism.

Teach patient/family:

• To avoid mouth rinses with high alcohol content due to drying effects

esterified estrogens

Estratab, Menest
♣ Neo-Estrone
Drug class.: Synthetic estrogen

Action: Required for the development, maintenance, and adequate function of the female reproductive system by increasing synthesis of DNA, RNA, and selected proteins; decreases the release of gonadotropin-releasing hormone; inhibits ovulation and helps maintain bone structure

Uses: Menopause, breast cancer, prostatic cancer, hypogonadism, ovariectomy, primary ovarian failure, osteoporosis prevention

Dosage and routes:

Menopause
• *Adult:* PO 0.30-3.75 mg qd 3 wk on, 1 wk off

Hypogonadism/ovariectomy/ovarian failure
• *Adult:* PO 2.5 mg qd-tid 3 wk on, 1 wk off

Prostatic cancer
• *Adult:* PO 1.25-2.50 mg tid

Breast cancer
• *Adult:* PO 10 mg tid × 3 mo or longer

Available forms include: Tabs 0.3, 0.625, 1.25, 2.5 mg

Side effects/adverse reactions:

▼ *ORAL:* Exacerbates gingivitis, bleeding

CNS: Dizziness, headache, migraines, depression

*CV: **Thromboembolism, stroke, pulmonary embolism, MI,*** hypertension, thrombophlebitis, edema

GI: Nausea, cholestatic jaundice, vomiting, diarrhea, anorexia, pancreatitis, cramps, constipation, increased appetite, increased weight

GU: Gynecomastia, testicular atrophy, impotence, amenorrhea, cervical erosion, breakthrough bleeding, dysmenorrhea, vaginal candidiasis, breast changes

EENT: Contact lens intolerance, increased myopia, astigmatism

INTEG: Rash, urticaria, acne, hirsutism, alopecia, oily skin, seborrhea, purpura, melasma

META: Folic acid deficiency, hypercalcemia, hyperglycemia

Contraindications: Breast cancer, thromboembolic disorders, reproductive cancer, vaginal bleeding (abnormal, undiagnosed), pregnancy category X

Precautions: Hypertension, asthma, blood dyscrasias, gallbladder disease, CHF, diabetes mellitus, bone disease, depression, migraine headache, convulsive disorders, hepatic disease, renal disease, family history of cancer of breast or reproductive tract

Pharmacokinetics:

PO: Degraded in liver, excreted in urine, crosses placenta, excreted in breast milk

👍 **Drug interactions of concern to dentistry:**
• Increased action of corticosteroids

DENTAL CONSIDERATIONS

General:
• Place on frequent recall to evaluate gingival condition.
• Monitor vital signs every appointment due to cardiovascular side effects.

Teach patient/family:
• Importance of good oral hygiene to prevent gingival inflammation

---

bold italic = life-threatening conditions

estradiol/estradiol cypionate/estradiol valerate

(es-tra-dye′ole)

Estradiol: Estrace

Estradiol cypionate: depGynogen, Depo-Estriadol, DepoGen

Estradiol valerate: Delestrogen, Gynogen LA 20, Valergen 40, Valergen 20, Estra-L 40

♣ Femogex

Drug class.: Estrogen

Action: Required for the development, maintenance, and adequate function of the female reproductive system by increasing synthesis of DNA, RNA, and selected proteins; decreases the release of gonadotropin-releasing hormone; inhibits ovulation and helps maintain bone structure

Uses: Menopause, breast cancer, prostatic cancer, atrophic vaginitis, kraurosis vulvae, hypogonadism, ovariectomy, primary ovarian failure, prevention of osteoporosis and menopause-related vasomotor symptoms

Dosage and routes:

Menopause/hypogonadism/ovariectomy/ovarian failure

• *Adult:* PO 1-2 mg qd 3 wk on, 1 wk off or 5 days on, 2 days off; IM 0.2-1 mg qwk

Prostatic cancer

• *Adult:* IM 30 mg q1-2wk (valerate); PO 1-2 mg tid (oral estradiol)

Breast cancer

• *Adult:* PO 10 mg tid × 3 mo or longer

Atropic vaginitis

• *Adult:* Vag cream 2-4 g qd × 1-2 wk, then 1 g 1-3× weekly

Kraurosis valvae

• *Adult:* IM 1-1.5 mg 1-2× weekly

Available forms include: Estradiol—tabs 0.5, 1, 2 mg; cypionate—inj IM 5 mg/ml; valerate—inj IM 10, 20, 40 mg/ml

Side effects/adverse reactions:

▼ *ORAL:* Exacerbates gingivitis, bleeding

CNS: Dizziness, headache, migraines, depression

CV: **Thromboembolism, stroke, pulmonary embolism, MI,** hypertension, thrombophlebitis, edema

GI: Nausea, **cholestatic jaundice,** vomiting, diarrhea, anorexia, pancreatitis, cramps, constipation, increased appetite, increased weight

GU: Gynecomastia, testicular atrophy, impotence, amenorrhea, cervical erosion, breakthrough bleeding, dysmenorrhea, vaginal candidiasis, breast changes

EENT: Contact lens intolerance, increased myopia, astigmatism

INTEG: Rash, urticaria, acne, hirsutism, alopecia, oily skin, seborrhea, purpura, melasma

META: Folic acid deficiency, hypercalcemia, hyperglycemia

Contraindications: Breast cancer, thromboembolic disorders, reproductive cancer, vaginal bleeding (abnormal, undiagnosed), pregnancy category X

Precautions: Hypertension, asthma, blood dyscrasias, gallbladder disease, CHF, diabetes mellitus, bone disease, depression, migraine headache, convulsive disorders, hepatic disease, renal disease, family history of cancer of breast or reproductive tract

Pharmacokinetics:

PO: Well absorbed; moderate-to-high protein binding; hepatic metabolism with primary renal excretion

🦷 **Drug interactions of concern to dentistry:**
• Increased action of corticosteroids

DENTAL CONSIDERATIONS
General:
• Place on frequent recall to evaluate gingival condition.
• Monitor vital signs due to cardiovascular side effects.

Teach patient/family:
• Importance of good oral hygiene to prevent gingival inflammation

---

estradiol transdermal system

(es-tra-dye'ole)

Alora, Climara, Esclim, Estraderm, FemPatch, Vivelle-Dot
♣ Vivelle

Drug class.: Estrogen

Action: Required for the development, maintenance, and adequate function of the female reproductive system by increasing synthesis of DNA, RNA, and selected proteins; decreases the release of gonadotropin-releasing hormone; inhibits ovulation and helps maintain bone structure

Uses: Menopause, breast cancer, prostatic cancer, abnormal uterine bleeding, hypogonadism, ovariectomy, primary ovarian failure, osteoporosis

Dosage and routes:
Menopause
• *Adult:* 0.05 mg twice weekly; apply patch to skin
Postmenopausal bone loss
• *Adult:* 0.05 mg daily (one patch weekly)

Available forms include: Transdermal system patches with release rates of 0.025, 0.0375, 0.05, 0.075, 0.1 mg/24 hr

Side effects/adverse reactions:
▼ *ORAL:* Exacerbates gingivitis, bleeding
CNS: Dizziness, headache, migraines, depression
CV: ***Thromboembolism, stroke, pulmonary embolism, MI,*** hypertension, thrombophlebitis, edema
*GI: Nausea, **cholestatic jaundice,*** vomiting, diarrhea, anorexia, pancreatitis, cramps, constipation, increased appetite, increased weight
GU: Gynecomastia, testicular atrophy, impotence, amenorrhea, cervical erosion, breakthrough bleeding, dysmenorrhea, vaginal candidiasis, breast changes
EENT: Contact lens intolerance, increased myopia, astigmatism
INTEG: Rash, urticaria, acne, hirsutism, alopecia, oily skin, seborrhea, purpura, melasma
META: Folic acid deficiency, hypercalcemia, hyperglycemia

Contraindications: Breast cancer, thromboembolic disorders, reproductive cancer, genital bleeding (abnormal, undiagnosed), pregnancy category X

Precautions: Hypertension, asthma, blood dyscrasias, gallbladder disease, CHF, diabetes mellitus, bone disease, depression, migraine headache, convulsive disorders, hepatic disease, renal disease, family history of cancer of the breast or reproductive tract

Pharmacokinetics:
TOP: Absorbed through the skin at a release rate of 0.05 or 1.0 mg/24 hr; hepatic metabolism and renal excretion; serum levels in 4 hr

---

bold italic = life-threatening conditions

Drug interactions of concern to dentistry:
• Increased action of corticosteroids

DENTAL CONSIDERATIONS

General:
• Place on frequent recall to evaluate gingival condition.
• Monitor vital signs due to cardiovascular side effects.

Teach patient/family:
• Importance of good oral hygiene to prevent gingival inflammation

---

estrogenic substances, conjugated

Premarin
♣ CES, Congest, Conjugated Estrogen CDS

Drug class.: Estrogen

Action: Required for the development, maintenance, and adequate function of the female reproductive system by increasing synthesis of DNA, RNA, and selected proteins; decreases the release of gonadotropin-releasing hormone; inhibits ovulation and helps maintain bone structure

Uses: Menopause, breast cancer, prostatic cancer, abnormal uterine bleeding, hypogonadism, ovariectomy, primary ovarian failure, osteoporosis

Dosage and routes:

Menopause
• *Adult:* PO 0.3-1.25 mg qd 3 wk on, 1 wk off

Prostatic cancer
• *Adult:* PO 1.25-2.5 mg tid

Breast cancer
• *Adult:* PO 10 mg tid × 3 mo or longer

Abnormal uterine bleeding
• *Adult:* IV/IM 25 mg, repeat in 6-12 hr

Ovariectomy/primary ovarian failure/osteoporosis
• *Adult:* PO 1.25 mg qd 3 wk on, 1 wk off

Hypogonadism
• *Adult:* PO 2.5 mg bid-tid × 20 days/mo

Available forms include: Tabs 0.3, 0.625, 0.9, 1.25, 2.5 mg

Side effects/adverse reactions:

▼ *ORAL:* Exacerbates gingivitis, bleeding

CNS: Dizziness, headache, migraine, depression

CV: **Thromboembolism, stroke, pulmonary embolism, MI,** hypertension, thrombophlebitis, edema

*GI: Nausea, **cholestatic jaundice,** vomiting, diarrhea, anorexia, pancreatitis, cramps, constipation, increased appetite, increased weight

GU: Gynecomastia, testicular atrophy, impotence, amenorrhea, cervical erosion, breakthrough bleeding, dysmenorrhea, vaginal candidiasis, breast changes

EENT: Contact lens intolerance, increased myopia, astigmatism

INTEG: Rash, urticaria, acne, hirsutism, alopecia, oily skin, seborrhea, purpura, melasma

META: Folic acid deficiency, hypercalcemia, hyperglycemia

Contraindications: Breast cancer, thromboembolic disorders, reproductive cancer, vaginal bleeding (abnormal, undiagnosed), pregnancy category X, lactation

Precautions: Hypertension, asthma, blood dyscrasias, gallbladder disease, CHF, diabetes mellitus, bone disease, depression, migraine headache, convulsive disorders, hepatic disease, renal disease, family history of cancer of breast or reproductive tract

Pharmacokinetics:

PO: Well absorbed; moderate-to-high protein binding; hepatic metabolism with primary renal excretion

🦷 Drug interactions of concern to dentistry:
• Increased action of corticosteroids

DENTAL CONSIDERATIONS

General:
• Place on frequent recall to evaluate gingival condition.
• Monitor vital signs due to cardiovascular side effects.

Teach patient/family:
• Importance of good oral hygiene to prevent gingival inflammation

---

estrogens A, conjugated synthetic

(es'troe-jenz)

Cenestin

Drug class.: Estrogens (nine synthetic estrogens expressed as alphabetical A for this combination)

Action: Reacts with estrogenic receptors; responsible for development and maintenance of female reproductive system and secondary sex characteristics, acts to reduce elevated levels of LH and FSH in postmenopausal women

Uses: Control of vasomotor symptoms, such as hot flashes and sweating in menopausal women

Dosage and routes:
• *Adult:* PO initial dose 0.625 mg; doses can be titrated to 1.25 mg; reassess use q3-6mo; discontinue asap

Available forms include: Tabs 0.625, 0.9 mg

Side effects/adverse reactions:

CNS: Headache

CV: Depression, insomnia, dizziness, nervousness, paresthesia

GI: Abdominal pain, flatulence, nausea, diarrhea

GU: Metrorrhagia, vagal bleeding changes

MS: Back pain, myalgia

MISC: Breast pain

Contraindications: Undiagnosed genital bleeding, breast cancer, estrogen-dependent neoplasm, active thrombophlebitis or thromboembolic disorders; pregnancy

Precautions: Endometrial cancer risk, venous thromboembolism, gallbladder disease, elevated BP, hyperlipoproteinemia, impaired liver function, lactation, pediatric patients, hypercalcemia

Pharmacokinetics:

PO: Well absorbed, maximum plasma levels in 4-16 hr; metabolized in liver, enterohepatic circulation

🦷 Drug interactions of concern to dentistry:
• None reported for dental drugs

DENTAL CONSIDERATIONS

General:
• Consider semisupine chair position for patient comfort if GI side effects occur.

Teach patient/family:
• Importance of good oral hygiene to prevent soft tissue inflammation

---

estropipate

(es'troe-pih-pate)

Ogen, Ortho-Est

Drug class.: Estrogen (piperazine estrone sulfate)

Action: Required for the development, maintenance, and adequate

---

bold italic = life-threatening conditions

function of the female reproductive system by increasing synthesis of DNA, RNA, and selected proteins; decreases the release of gonadotropin-releasing hormone; inhibits ovulation and helps maintain bone structure

Uses: Vasomotor symptoms of menopause, atrophic vaginitis, primary female hypogonadism, primary ovarian failure, estrogen imbalance, advanced prostatic carcinoma, ovariectomy

Dosage and routes:

Menopause

• *Adult:* 0.625-5 mg daily

Hypogonadism

• *Adult:* 1.25-7.5 mg/day × 3 wk; rest 8-10 days

Available forms include: Tabs 0.625, 1.25, 2.5, 5 mg

Side effects/adverse reactions:

▼ *ORAL:* Exacerbates gingivitis, bleeding

CNS: Dizziness, headache, migraine, depression

CV: **Thromboembolism, stroke, pulmonary embolism, MI,** hypertension, thrombophlebitis, edema

*GI: Nausea, **cholestatic jaundice,** vomiting, diarrhea, anorexia, pancreatitis, cramps, constipation, increased appetite, increased weight

GU: Gynecomastia, testicular atrophy, impotence, amenorrhea, cervical erosion, breakthrough bleeding, dysmenorrhea, vaginal candidiasis, breast changes

EENT: Contact lens intolerance, increased myopia, astigmatism

INTEG: Rash, urticaria, acne, hirsutism, alopecia, oily skin, seborrhea, purpura, melasma

META: Folic acid deficiency, hypercalcemia, hyperglycemia

Contraindications: Breast cancer, thromboembolic disorders, reproductive cancer, vaginal bleeding (abnormal, undiagnosed), pregnancy category X, lactation

Precautions: Hypertension, asthma, blood dyscrasias, gallbladder disease, CHF, diabetes mellitus, bone disease, depression, migraine headache, convulsive disorders, hepatic disease, renal disease, family history of cancer of breast or reproductive tract

Pharmacokinetics:

PO: Well absorbed; moderate-to-high protein binding; hepatic metabolism with primary renal excretion

⚖ Drug interactions of concern to dentistry:

• Increased action of corticosteroids

DENTAL CONSIDERATIONS

General:

• Place on frequent recall to evaluate gingival condition.

• Monitor vital signs due to cardiovascular side effects.

Teach patient/family:

• Importance of good oral hygiene to prevent gingival inflammation

---

etanercept

(e-tan'er-cept)

Enbrel

Drug class.: Antiinflammatory and immunomodulator; biologic response modifier

Action: This drug consists of the extracellular ligand-binding protein of tumor necrosis factor (TNF) receptor linked to the Fc portion of human IgG1 that specifically binds to TNF and blocks its interaction with cell surfaces.

Uses: Reduction in signs and symptoms of moderately to severely active rheumatoid arthritis in patients with an inadequate response to one or more disease-modifying antirheumatic drugs; also approved for initial therapy

Dosage and routes:
• *Adult:* SC 25 mg twice weekly; can be given with other drugs used in rheumatoid arthritis treatment
• *Child:* Limited use in children at doses of 0.4 mg/kg (limit 25 mg) 2 × weekly × 3 mo

Available forms include: 25 mg single-use vial kit

Side effects/adverse reactions:

CNS: Headache, dizziness, asthenia

*CV: **MI, myocardial ischemia, cerebral ischemia** (all rare but life-threatening reactions)*

GI: Abdominal pain, vomiting in children

RESP: Sinusitis, URI, cough, pharyngitis, rhinitis

INTEG: Injection site reactions, rash

*MISC: Infections, positive ANA readings, **pancytopenia,** allergic reactions*

Contraindications: Hypersensitivity, use of live vaccines

Precautions: Risk of new malignancies and infrequent severe cardiovascular events, discontinue if serious infection occurs, immunosuppression risk, caution with pre-existing demyelinating disorders, pregnancy category B, lactation, viral infections, children <4 yr

Pharmacokinetics:

SC: Half-life 115 hr, maximum plasma levels 72 hr, no information on metabolism or excretion

🦷 **Drug interactions of concern to dentistry:**
• No studies have been conducted.

DENTAL CONSIDERATIONS

General:
• Monitor vital signs every appointment due to potential cardiovascular side effects
• Consider semisupine chair position for patient comfort due to GI side effects of drug
• If acute oral infection occurs, inform physician.
• Note elevated ANA levels if diagnosing Sjögren's syndrome.

Consultations:
• Consult if needed.

Teach patient/family:
• Importance of good oral hygiene to prevent soft tissue inflammation
• Use of electric toothbrush if patient has difficulty holding conventional devices

---

ethacrynate sodium/ ethacrynic acid
(eth-a-kri′nate)
Edecrin, Edecrin Sodium
Drug class.: Loop diuretic

Action: Acts on loop of Henle by increasing excretion of chloride, sodium

Uses: Pulmonary edema, edema in CHF, liver disease, nephrotic syndrome, ascites, hypertension

Dosage and routes:
• *Adult:* PO 50-200 mg/day; may give up to 200 mg bid
• *Child:* PO 25 mg, increased by 25 mg/day until desired effect occurs

Pulmonary edema
• *Adult:* IV 50 mg given over several minutes or 0.5-1.0 mg/kg

Available forms include: Tabs 25, 50 mg; powder for inj 50 mg

---

bold italic = life-threatening conditions

Side effects/adverse reactions:

▼ *ORAL:* Dry mouth, increased thirst

CNS: Headache, fatigue, weakness, vertigo

*CV: **Circulatory collapse,*** chest pain, hypotension, ECG changes

*GI: **GI bleeding, severe diarrhea, acute pancreatitis,*** nausea, vomiting, anorexia, cramps, upset stomach, abdominal pain, jaundice

HEMA: ***Thrombocytopenia, agranulocytosis, leukopenia, neutropenia***

GU: Polyuria, renal failure, glycosuria

*EENT: **Loss of hearing,*** ear pain, tinnitus, blurred vision

*INTEG: Rash, pruritus, **Stevens-Johnson syndrome,*** sweating, purpura, photosensitivity

ENDO: Hyperglycemia

MS: Cramps, arthritis, stiffness

ELECT: Hypokalemia, hypochloremic alkalosis, hypomagnesemia, hyperuricemia, hypocalcemia, hyponatremia

Contraindications: Hypersensitivity to sulfonamides, anuria, hypovolemia, lactation, electrolyte depletion, infants

Precautions: Dehydration, ascites, severe renal disease, pregnancy category D, hypoproteinemia

Pharmacokinetics:

PO: Onset 0.5 hr, peak 2 hr, duration 6-8 hr

IV: Onset 5 min, peak 15-30 min, duration 2 hr

Half-life 30-70 min, excreted by kidneys, crosses placenta

👆 **Drug interactions of concern to dentistry:**

• Masked ototoxicity: phenothiazines

• Decreased antihypertensive effect: NSAIDs, especially indomethacin

DENTAL CONSIDERATIONS

General:

• Monitor vital signs every appointment due to cardiovascular side effects.

• Patients on chronic drug therapy may rarely have symptoms of blood dyscrasias, which can include infection, bleeding, and poor healing.

• Assess salivary flow as a factor in caries, periodontal disease, and candidiasis.

• After supine positioning, have patient sit upright for at least 2 min before standing to avoid orthostatic hypotension.

• Patients on high-potency diuretics should be monitored for serum K^+ levels.

Consultations:

• In a patient with symptoms of blood dyscrasias, request a medical consult for blood studies and postpone dental treatment until normal values are reestablished.

• Medical consult may be required to assess disease control.

Teach patient/family:

• Importance of good oral hygiene to prevent gingival inflammation

When chronic dry mouth occurs, advise patient:

• To avoid mouth rinses with high alcohol content due to drying effects

• To use daily home fluoride products for anticaries effect

• To use sugarless gum, frequent sips of water, or saliva substitutes

---

ethambutol HCl

(e-tham'byoo-tole)

Myambutol

✦ Etibi

Drug class.: Antitubercular

Action: Inhibits RNA synthesis, decreases tubercle bacilli replication

Uses: Pulmonary TB, as an adjunct

Dosage and routes:

• *Adult and child >13 yr:* PO 15 mg/kg/day as a single dose

Re-treatment

• *Adult and child >13 yr:* PO 25 mg/kg/day as single dose × 2 mo with at least one other drug, then decrease to 15 mg/kg/day as single dose

Available forms include: Tabs 100, 400 mg

Side effects/adverse reactions:

▼ *ORAL:* Lichenoid reaction

CNS: Headache, confusion, fever, malaise, dizziness, disorientation, hallucinations, peripheral neuritis

GI: Abdominal distress, anorexia, nausea, vomiting

EENT: Blurred vision, optic neuritis, photophobia, decreased visual acuity

INTEG: Dermatitis, pruritus

META: Elevated uric acid, acute gout, liver function impairment

MISC: **Thrombocytopenia,** joint pain

Contraindications: Hypersensitivity, optic neuritis, child <13 yr

Precautions: Pregnancy category D, renal disease, diabetic retinopathy, cataracts, ocular defects, hepatic disorders, hematopoietic disorders

Pharmacokinetics:

PO: Peak 2-4 hr, half-life 3 hr; metabolized in liver; excreted in urine (unchanged drug/inactive metabolites); excreted unchanged in feces

DENTAL CONSIDERATIONS

General:

• Examine for evidence of oral signs of disease.

• Avoid dental light in patient's eyes; offer dark glasses for patient comfort.

• Determine why the patient is taking the drug.

Consultations:

• Medical consult is required to assess patient's current status; avoid elective dental procedures in active infections.

Determine that noninfectious status exists by ensuring the following:

• Anti-TB drugs have been taken for longer than 3 wk.

• Culture confirms antibiotic susceptibility to TB microorganisms.

• Patient has had 3 consecutive negative sputum smears.

• Patient is not in the coughing stage.

Teach patient/family:

• Importance of taking medication for full length of prescribed therapy to ensure effectiveness of treatment and to prevent the emergence of resistant forms of microbes

ethinyl estradiol

(eth'in-il) (ess-tra-dye'ole)

Estinyl

Drug class.: Nonsteroidal synthetic estrogen

Action: Needed for adequate functioning of female reproductive system; affects release of pituitary gonadotropins; inhibits ovulation; promotes adequate calcium use in bone structures

Uses: Menopause, prostatic cancer, breast cancer, hypogonadism, estrogen deficiency, postmenopausal osteoporosis; unapproved: postcoital contraceptive

Dosage and routes:

Menopause
• *Adult:* PO 0.02-0.5 mg qd 3wk on, 1 wk off

Prostatic cancer
• *Adult:* PO 0.15-2 mg qd

Hypogonadism
• *Adult:* PO 0.05 mg qd-tid × 2 wk/mo, then 2 wk progesterone, then 3-6 mo cycles, then 2 mo off

Breast cancer
• *Adult:* PO 1 mg tid

Available forms include: Tabs 0.02, 0.05, 0.5 mg

Side effects/adverse reactions:

▼ *ORAL:* Exacerbates gingivitis, bleeding

CNS: Dizziness, headache, migraine, depression

CV: **Thromboembolism, stroke, pulmonary embolism, MI,** hypertension, thrombophlebitis, edema

GI: Nausea, **cholestatic jaundice,** vomiting, diarrhea, anorexia, pancreatitis, cramps, constipation, increased appetite, increased weight

GU: Gynecomastia, testicular atrophy, impotence, amenorrhea, cervical erosion, breakthrough bleeding, dysmenorrhea, vaginal candidiasis, breast changes

EENT: Contact lens intolerance, increased myopia, astigmatism

INTEG: Rash, urticaria, acne, hirsutism, alopecia, oily skin, seborrhea, purpura, melasma

META: Folic acid deficiency, hypercalcemia, hyperglycemia

Contraindications: Breast cancer, thromboembolic disorders, reproductive cancer, vaginal bleeding (abnormal, undiagnosed), pregnancy category X

Precautions: Hypertension, asthma, blood dyscrasias, gallbladder disease, CHF, diabetes mellitus, bone disease, depression, migraine headache, convulsive disorders, hepatic disease, renal disease, family history of cancer of the breast or reproductive tract

Pharmacokinetics:

PO: Degraded in liver; excreted in urine; crosses placenta; excreted in breast milk

Drug interactions of concern to dentistry:

• Increased action of corticosteroids

DENTAL CONSIDERATIONS

General:

• Place on frequent recall to evaluate gingival condition.

• Monitor vital signs due to cardiovascular side effects.

Teach patient/family:

• Importance of good oral hygiene to prevent gingival inflammation

---

ethionamide

(e-thye-on-am'ide)

Trecator-SC

Drug class.: Antitubercular

Action: Bacteriostatic against *M. tuberculosis;* may inhibit protein synthesis

Uses: Pulmonary, extrapulmonary tuberculosis when other antitubercular drugs have failed

Dosage and routes:
• *Adult:* PO 500 mg-1 g qd in divided doses, with another antitubercular drug and pyridoxine
• *Child:* PO 15-20 mg/kg/day in 3-4 doses, not to exceed 1 g
Available forms include: Tabs 250 mg

Side effects/adverse reactions:
▼ *ORAL:* Metallic taste, stomatitis, salivation
CNS: Anorexia, **convulsions,** headache, drowsiness, tremors, depression, psychosis, dizziness, peripheral neuritis
CV: Severe postural hypotension
GI: Anorexia, nausea, vomiting, diarrhea, hepatitis, jaundice, hypoglycemia
HEMA: **Thrombocytopenia,** purpura
EENT: Blurred vision, optic neuritis
INTEG: Dermatitis, alopecia, acne
MS: Asthenia
MISC: Gynecomastia, impotence, menorrhagia, difficulty managing diabetes mellitus, hypothyroidism

Contraindications: Hypersensitivity, severe hepatic disease

Precautions: Pregnancy category D, renal disease, diabetic retinopathy, cataracts, ocular defects, child <13 yr

Pharmacokinetics:
PO: Peak 3 hr, duration 9 hr, half-life 3 hr; metabolized in liver; excreted in urine (unchanged drug/inactive); crosses placenta

🖐 Drug interactions of concern to dentistry:
• None reported

DENTAL CONSIDERATIONS
General:
• Monitor vital signs every appointment due to cardiovascular side effects.

• After supine positioning, have patient sit upright for at least 2 min before standing to avoid orthostatic hypotension.
• Consider semisupine chair position for patient comfort due to GI effects of disease.
• Evaluate for clotting ability during gingival instrumentation.
• Examine for evidence of oral manifestations of blood dyscrasias (infection, bleeding, poor healing).
• Palliative treatment may be required for oral side effects.
• Examine for evidence of oral signs of disease.

Consultations:
• Medical consult for blood studies (CBC); leukopenic or thrombocytopenic side effects may result in infection, delayed healing, and excessive bleeding. Postpone elective dental treatment until normal values are maintained. Instruct patient to take with meals to decrease GI symptoms.
• Medical consult may be required to assess disease control and determine infectious nature of disease.

Teach patient/family:
• Importance of good oral hygiene to prevent soft tissue inflammation
• Caution in use of oral hygiene aids to prevent injury

---

ethosuximide

(eth-oh-sux′i-mide)
Zarontin
Drug class.: Anticonvulsant

Action: Suppresses spike and wave formation in absence seizures (petit mal); decreases amplitude, frequency, duration, spread of discharge in minor motor seizures
Uses: Absence seizures (petit mal);

---

bold italic = life-threatening conditions

unapproved: complex partial seizures

Dosage and routes:
• *Adult and child >6 yr:* PO 250 mg bid initially; may increase by 250 mg q4-7d, not to exceed 1.5 g/day
• *Child 3-6 yr:* PO 250 mg/day or 125 mg bid; may increase by 250 mg q4-7d, not to exceed 1.5 g/day
Available forms include: Caps 250 mg; syr 250 mg/5 ml

Side effects/adverse reactions:
▼ *ORAL:* Gingival bleeding, ulcerations (Stevens-Johnson syndrome); swelling of tongue and gingival enlargement (rare)
CNS: Drowsiness, dizziness, fatigue, euphoria, lethargy, anxiety, aggressiveness, irritability, depression, insomnia, headache
GI: Nausea, vomiting, heartburn, anorexia, diarrhea, abdominal pain, cramps, constipation, hiccups, weight loss
HEMA: Agranulocytosis, aplastic anemia, thrombocytopenia, leukocytosis, eosinophilia, pancytopenia
GU: Hematuria, renal damage, vaginal bleeding
EENT: Myopia
INTEG: Stevens-Johnson syndrome, urticaria, pruritic erythema, hirsutism

Contraindications: Hypersensitivity to succinimide derivatives, blood dyscrasias

Precautions: Lactation, pregnancy category not established, hepatic disease, renal disease

Pharmacokinetics:
PO: Peak 1-7 hr, steady state 4-7 days, half-life 24-60 hr; metabolized by liver; excreted in urine, bile, feces

🦷 **Drug interactions of concern to dentistry:**
• Enhanced CNS depression: CNS depressants, alcohol
• Decreased effects: phenothiazines, thioxanthenes, barbiturates

DENTAL CONSIDERATIONS
General:
• Patients on chronic drug therapy may rarely have symptoms of blood dyscrasias, which can include infection, bleeding, and poor healing.
• Talk with patient to ascertain seizure frequency and how well seizures are controlled. A stress reduction protocol may be required.

Consultations:
• In a patient with symptoms of blood dyscrasias, request a medical consult for blood studies and postpone dental treatment until normal values are reestablished.
• Medical consult may be required to assess disease control and patient's ability to tolerate stress.

Teach patient/family:
• Importance of good oral hygiene to prevent gingival inflammation
• To avoid mouth rinses with high alcohol content due to drying effects

---

ethotoin
(eth'oh-toyin)
Peganone
Drug class.: Hydantoin derivative anticonvulsant

Action: Inhibits spread of seizure activity in motor cortex
Uses: Generalized tonic-clonic or complex-partial seizures
Dosage and routes:
• *Adult:* PO 250 mg qid initially;

italic = common side effects

may increase over several days to 3 g/day in divided doses

• *Child:* PO 250 mg bid; may increase to 250 mg qid, not to exceed 3 g/day

Available forms include: Tabs 250, 500 mg

Side effects/adverse reactions:

▼ *ORAL:* Gingival overgrowth (rare), gingival bleeding

CNS: Fatigue, insomnia, numbness, fever, headache, dizziness

CV: Chest pain

GI: Nausea, vomiting, diarrhea

*HEMA: **Agranulocytosis, thrombocytopenia, leukopenia, pancytopenia, megaloblastic anemia,** lymphadenopathy*

EENT: Nystagmus, diplopia

INTEG: Rash

Contraindications: Hypersensitivity to hydantoins, blood dyscrasias, hematologic disease, hepatic disease

Precautions: Pregnancy category C, lactation, geriatric patients

Pharmacokinetics:

PO: Half-life 3-9 hr, rapid oral absorption; metabolized by liver; excreted in urine

Drug interactions of concern to dentistry:

• Decreased effects: barbiturates, carbamazepine

• Increased effects: ketoconazole, fluconazole, metronidazole

• Hepatotoxicity: acetaminophen (chronic, high doses only)

• Decreased effects of corticosteroids, doxycycline

DENTAL CONSIDERATIONS

General:

• Patients on chronic drug therapy may rarely have symptoms of blood dyscrasias, which can include infection, bleeding, and poor healing.

• Place on frequent recall to evaluate gingival condition and self-care.

• Short appointments and a stress reduction protocol may be required for anxious patients.

• Determine type of epilepsy, seizure frequency, and quality of seizure control. A stress reduction protocol may be required.

• Consider semisupine chair position for patient comfort if GI side effects occur.

Consultations:

• In a patient with symptoms of blood dyscrasias, request a medical consult for blood studies and postpone dental treatment until normal values are reestablished.

• Medical consult may be required to assess disease control and patient's ability to tolerate stress.

Teach patient/family:

• Importance of good oral hygiene to prevent soft tissue inflammation and minimize gingival overgrowth

• Caution patient to prevent trauma when using oral hygiene aids

---

etidocaine HCl (local)

(et-ee'doe-kane)

Duranest, Duranest MPF

With vasoconstrictor: Duranest with Epinephrine, Duranest MPF

Drug class.: Amide, local anesthetic

Action: Inhibits ion fluxes across membranes, particularly sodium transport across cell membrane; decreases rise of depolarization phase of action potential; blocks nerve action potential

Uses: Local dental anesthetic, peripheral nerve block, caudal anes-

---

bold italic = life-threatening conditions

thetic, central neural block, vaginal block

Dosage and routes:
Dental injection: infiltration or conduction block
• *Etidocaine 1.5% with epinephrine 1:200,000:* Max dose limit recommended is 5.5 mg/kg, not to exceed 400 mg max dose for healthy patients; doses must be adjusted downward for medically compromised, debilitated, or elderly patients and for each individual patient. The package insert indicates that 0.5-2.5 dental cartridges are usually adequate. **Always use the lowest effective dose, a slow injection technique, and a careful aspiration technique.**

Example calculations illustrating amount of drug administered per dental cartridge

# of cartridges (1.8 ml)	mg of etidocaine (0.5%)	mg (µg) of vasoconstrictor (1:200,000)
1	27	0.009 (9)
2	54	0.018 (18)
4	108	0.036 (36)
6	162	0.054 (54)

Maximum dose is cited from the *USP-DI,* ed 16, 1996, US Pharmacopeial Convention, Inc. Doses may differ in other published reference resources.

• Package insert does not list approved doses for pediatric patients
Available forms include: Inj 1.5%; inj with epinephrine 1:200,000 1% dental cartridge

Side effects/adverse reactions:
▼ *ORAL:* Numbness, tingling, trismus
CNS: ***Convulsions, loss of consciousness,*** drowsiness, disorientation, tremors, shivering, anxiety, restlessness
CV: ***Myocardial depression, cardiac arrest, dysrhythmias,*** bradycardia, hypotension, hypertension, fetal bradycardia
GI: Nausea, vomiting
RESP: ***Status asthmaticus, respiratory arrest, anaphylaxis***
EENT: Blurred vision, tinnitus, pupil constriction
INTEG: Rash, urticaria, allergic reactions, edema, burning, skin discoloration at injection site, tissue necrosis

Contraindications: Hypersensitivity, cross-sensitivity with other amides rare, child <12 yr, elderly, severe liver disease

Precautions: Elderly, severe drug allergies, pregnancy category B, children (risk of injury due to long duration)

Pharmacokinetics:
INJ: Onset 2-8 min, duration 1.5-9 hr; metabolized by liver; excreted in urine (metabolites)

Drug interactions of concern to dentistry:
• CNS depressants: may see increased risk of CNS depression with all CNS depressants, especially in children and when larger doses are used; avoid placing dental cartridges in disinfectant solutions with heavy metals or surface-active agents; after injection, may see release of metal ions into local anesthetic solutions with tissue irritation

• Avoid excessive exposure of dental cartridges to light or heat; hastens deterioration of vasoconstrictor; color change in local anesthetic solution indicates breakdown of vasoconstrictor

• Risk of cardiovascular side effects: rapid intravascular administration of local anesthetic containing vasoconstrictor, either alone or in patients taking tricyclic antidepressants, MAO inhibitors, digitalis drugs, cocaine, phenothiazines, β-blockers, and in the presence of halogenated-hydrocarbon general anesthetics; use smallest effective vasoconstrictor dose and careful aspiration techniques

• Avoid use of vasoconstrictors in patients with uncontrolled hyperthyroidism, diabetes, angina, or hypertension; refer these patients for medical treatment before elective dental procedures

DENTAL CONSIDERATIONS

General:

• Monitor vital signs every appointment due to cardiovascular side effects.

• Lubricate dry lips before injection or dental treatment as required.

Teach patient/family:

• To use care to prevent injury while numbness exists by not chewing gum or eating after dental anesthesia

• That numbness with this drug is expected to last for a considerable period

• To report any signs of infection, muscle pain, or fever to dentist when feeling returns

• To report any unusual soft tissue reactions

---

etidronate disodium

(e-ti-droe′nate)

Didronel, Didronel IV

Drug class.: Antihypercalcemic

Action: Decreases bone resorption and new bone development (accretion)

Uses: Paget's disease, heterotopic ossification, hypercalcemia of malignancy

Dosage and routes:

Paget's disease

• *Adult:* PO 5-10 mg/kg/day 2 hr ac with water, not to exceed 20 mg/kg/day, max 6 mo

Heterotropic ossification

• *Adult:* PO 20 mg/kg qd × 2 wk, then 10 mg/kg/day for 10 wk, total 12 wk

Available forms include: Tabs 200, 400 mg; inj 50 mg/ml in 6 ml

Side effects/adverse reactions:

▼ *ORAL:* Altered taste (parenteral administration)

GI: Nausea, diarrhea

MS: Bone pain, hypocalcemia, decreased mineralization of nonaffected bones

Contraindications: Pathologic fractures, children, colitis, severe renal disease with creatinine >5 mg/dl, cardiac failure

Precautions: Pregnancy category C, renal disease, lactation, restricted vitamin D/calcium

Pharmacokinetics: Therapeutic response: 1-3 mo; not metabolized; excreted in urine, feces

DENTAL CONSIDERATIONS

General:

• Be aware of the oral manifestations of Paget's disease (macrognathia, alveolar pain).

---

bold italic = life-threatening conditions

Consultations:
• Medical consult may be required to assess disease control.

---

etodolac

(e-toe-doe'lack)

Lodine, Lodine XL

Drug class.: Nonsteroidal antiinflammatory

Action: Inhibits prostaglandin synthesis by interfering with cyclooxygenase needed for biosynthesis; possesses analgesic, antiinflammatory, antipyretic properties

Uses: Mild-to-moderate pain, osteoarthritis, rheumatoid arthritis

Dosage and routes:

Osteoarthritis
• *Adult:* PO initial dose 300 mg bid or 400-500 mg bid, then adjust dose to 600-1200 mg/day in divided doses; do not exceed 1200 mg/day; patients <60 kg, not to exceed 20 mg/kg; ext rel 400-1200 mg qd

Analgesia
• *Adult:* PO 200-400 q6-8h prn for acute pain; do not exceed 1200 mg/day; patients <60 kg, not to exceed 20 mg/kg

Available forms include: Caps 200, 300, 400 mg; ext rel tabs 400, 500, 600 mg; tabs 400, 500 mg

Side effects/adverse reactions:

▼ *ORAL:* Stomatitis, lichenoid reaction, dry mouth, bitter taste
CNS: Dizziness, headache, drowsiness, fatigue, tremors, confusion, insomnia, anxiety, depression, light-headedness, vertigo
CV: Tachycardia, peripheral edema, fluid retention, palpitation, dysrhythmias, CHF

*GI: Nausea, anorexia, **cholestatic hepatitis, GI bleeding,** vomiting,* diarrhea, jaundice, constipation, flatulence, cramps, peptic ulcer, dyspepsia
RESP: Bronchospasm
*HEMA: **Blood dyscrasias***
*GU: **Nephrotoxicity: dysuria, hematuria, oliguria, azotemia,** cysti*tis, UTI
EENT: Tinnitus, hearing loss, blurred vision
INTEG: Erythema, urticaria, purpura, rash, pruritus, sweating, angioedema

Contraindications: Hypersensitivity; patients in whom aspirin, iodides, or other nonsteroidal antiinflammatories have produced asthma, rhinitis, urticaria, nasal polyps, angioedema, bronchospasm

Precautions: Pregnancy category C, lactation, children, bleeding disorders, GI disorders, cardiac disorders, elderly, renal, hepatic disorders

Pharmacokinetics:

PO: Onset 30 min, peak 1-2 hr, half-life 7 hr; serum protein binding >90%; metabolized by liver (metabolites excreted in urine)

⚘ Drug interactions of concern to dentistry:
• GI ulceration, bleeding: aspirin, alcohol, corticosteroids
• Decreased action: salicylates
• Nephrotoxicity: acetaminophen (prolonged use)
• Possible risk of decreased renal function: cyclosporine
When prescribed for dental pain:
• Risk of increased effects: oral anticoagulants, oral antidiabetics, lithium, methotrexate
• Decreased effects of diuretics

DENTAL CONSIDERATIONS
General:
• Patients on chronic drug therapy may rarely have symptoms of blood dyscrasias, which can include infection, bleeding, and poor healing.
• Assess salivary flow as a factor in caries, periodontal disease, and candidiasis.
• Avoid prescribing for dental use in last trimester of pregnancy.
• Avoid prescribing aspirin-containing products.
• Consider semisupine chair position for patients with arthritic disease.

Consultations:
• In a patient with symptoms of blood dyscrasias, request a medical consult for blood studies and postpone dental treatment until normal values are reestablished.
• Medical consult may be required to assess disease control.

Teach patient/family:
• To avoid mouth rinses with high alcohol content due to drying effects

---

famciclovir
(fam-sye′kloe-veer)
Famvir

Drug class.: Antiviral

Action: Converted to active metabolite, penciclovir triphosphate, which inhibits DNA viral synthesis and replication

Uses: Acute herpes zoster (shingles) infection; recurrent genital herpes; recurrent herpes simplex virus infections in HIV-infected patients

Dosage and routes:
Shingles
• *Adult:* PO 500 mg tid × 7 days, start soon after symptoms appear; reduce doses in renal impairment
Recurrent genital herpes
• *Adult:* PO 125 mg bid/5 days; initiate therapy at first sign or symptom
Available forms include: Tabs 125, 250, 500 mg

Side effects/adverse reactions:
CNS: Headache, fatigue, dizziness, paresthesia
GI: Nausea, diarrhea, vomiting
EENT: Sinusitis, pharyngitis
INTEG: Pruritus
MS: Arthralgia, back pain
MISC: Fever

Contraindications: Hypersensitivity

Precautions: Pregnancy category B, children <18 yr, lactation, elderly, hepatic and renal function impairment

Pharmacokinetics:
PO: Peak plasma levels less than 1 hr; after PO absorption, converted to penciclovir; low plasma protein binding (20%-25%); renal excretion

🐾 Drug interactions of concern to dentistry:
• None reported in otherwise uncompromised patients

DENTAL CONSIDERATIONS
General:
• Determine why the patient is taking the drug.
• Consider semisupine chair position for patient comfort due to GI effects of drug.
• Awareness of general discomfort associated with shingles; acute symptoms may preclude patient's routine dental visit or mandate short appointments.

---

bold italic = life-threatening conditions

Consultations:

• Medical consult may be required to assess patient's ability to tolerate stress.

• Medical consult may be required to assess disease control.

---

famotidine

(fa-moe'te-deen)

Pepcid, Pepcid IV, Pepcid RPD
♣ Acid Control, Apo-Famotidine, Dysep HB, Gen-Famotidine, Nu-Famotidine, Ulcidine-HB
OTC: Mylanta-AR, Pepcid AC Acid Controller

Drug class.: H_2 histamine receptor antagonist

Action: Inhibits histamine at H_2-receptor site in parietal cells, which inhibits gastric acid secretion

Uses: Short-term treatment of active duodenal ulcer, maintenance therapy for duodenal ulcer, Zollinger-Ellison syndrome, multiple endocrine adenomas, gastric ulcers

Dosage and routes:
Duodenal ulcer
• *Adult:* PO 40 mg qd hs × 4-8 wk, then 20 mg qd hs if needed (maintenance); IV 20 mg q12h if unable to take PO

Hypersecretory conditions
• *Adult:* PO 20 mg q6h, may give 160 mg q6h if needed; IV 20 mg q12h if unable to take PO

GERD
• *Adult:* PO 20 mg bid up to 6 wk, if ulcerations/erosions present 20-40 mg bid up to 12 wk

Gastric distress (OTC):
• *Adult and child >12 yr:* PO prophylaxis 10 mg 15 min ac; treatment 10 mg once or twice daily (limit 20 mg/day)

Available forms include: Tabs 10 mg (OTC) and 20, 40 mg; powder for oral susp 40 mg/5 ml; oral disintegrating tab 20, 40 mg, inj IV 10 mg/ml; tabs chewable 10 mg

Side effects/adverse reactions:

▼ *ORAL: Dry mouth,* taste changes

CNS: Headache, dizziness, paresthesia, seizure, depression, anxiety, somnolence, insomnia, fever

GI: Constipation, nausea, vomiting, anorexia, cramps, abnormal liver enzymes

RESP: Bronchospasm

HEMA: Thrombocytopenia

EENT: Tinnitus, orbital edema

INTEG: Rash

MS: Myalgia, arthralgia

Contraindications: Hypersensitivity

Precautions: Pregnancy category B, lactation, children, severe renal disease, severe hepatic function, elderly

Pharmacokinetics:

PO: Peak 1-3 hr, half-life 2.5-3.5 hr; plasma protein binding 15%-20%; metabolized in liver (active metabolites); excreted by kidneys

🦷 **Drug interactions of concern to dentistry:**

• Decreased absorption of ketoconazole or itraconazole (take doses 2 hr apart)

DENTAL CONSIDERATIONS
General:

• Avoid prescribing aspirin-containing products in patients with active GI disease.

• Consider semisupine chair position for patient comfort due to GI effects of disease.

- Assess salivary flow as a factor in caries, periodontal disease, and candidiasis.
Teach patient/family:
- Importance of good oral hygiene to prevent gingival inflammation
When chronic dry mouth occurs, advise patient:
- To avoid mouth rinses with high alcohol content due to drying effects
- To use daily home fluoride products for anticaries effect
- To use sugarless gum, frequent sips of water, or saliva substitutes

---

felbamate

(fel'ba-mate)
Felbatol

Drug class.: Anticonvulsant (carbamate derivative)

Action: Anticonvulsant action is unclear
Uses: Used alone or as adjunct therapy in partial seizures; also for partial seizures associated with Lennox-Gastaut syndrome in children
Dosage and routes:
- *Adult and child >14 yr:* PO (used alone) 1200 mg/day in 3 or 4 divided doses; increase dose by 600 mg increments q2wk; 3600 mg/day usual dose
- *Child 2-14 yr:* PO with Lennox-Gastaut syndrome (adjunctive) 15 mg/kg/day in 3-4 divided doses; reduce dose of other anticonvulsant drugs by 20%; increase dose by 15 mg/kg/day up to 45 mg/kg/day while further reducing the dose of other anticonvulsant drugs
Adjunctive therapy: PO reduce doses of other anticonvulsants by one third; then 1200 mg/day in 3 or

4 divided doses with 1200 mg increments to 3600 mg; doses of other anticonvulsants must be further reduced
Available forms include: Tabs 400, 600 mg; susp 600 mg/5 ml in 240, 960 ml sizes
Side effects/adverse reactions:
▼ *ORAL: Facial edema,* buccal mucous membrane swelling (rare), dry mouth
CNS: Insomnia, headache, somnolence, dizziness, ataxia, fatigue, anorexia, abnormal gait
CV: Palpitation, tachycardia
GI: Vomiting, diarrhea, nausea, constipation, dyspepsia
RESP: Dyspnea, upper respiratory infection, rhinitis
*HEMA: **Aplastic anemia,*** agranulocytosis, granulocytopenia, lymphadenopathy, leukopenia, thrombocytopenia
GU: UTI, incontinence (children)
EENT: Blurred vision
INTEG: Acne, rash, pruritus, photosensitivity reaction
MS: Tremor, abnormal gait
Contraindications: Hypersensitivity
Precautions: Pregnancy category C, lactation
Pharmacokinetics:
PO: Peak plasma levels 1-3 hr; 20%-25% protein bound; up to 40% excreted in urine unchanged
🦷 Drug interactions of concern to dentistry:
- Decreased effects of carbamazepine
- Increased photosensitization: drugs causing photosensitivity (e.g., tetracyclines)

DENTAL CONSIDERATIONS
General:
- Examine for evidence of oral

manifestations of blood dyscrasia (infection, bleeding, poor healing).

• Short appointments and a stress reduction protocol may be required for anxious patients.

• Determine type of epilepsy, seizure frequency, and quality of seizure control. A stress reduction protocol may be required.

• Assess salivary flow as a factor in caries, periodontal disease, and candidiasis.

• Monitor vital signs every appointment due to cardiovascular side effects.

• Advise patient if dental drugs prescribed have a potential for photosensitivity.

Consultations:

• Medical consult may be required to assess disease control.

• Medical consult may be required to assess patient's ability to tolerate stress.

Teach patient/family:

• Importance of good oral hygiene to prevent soft tissue inflammation

• Caution to prevent injury when using oral hygiene aids

• Use of electric toothbrush if patient has difficulty holding conventional devices

When chronic dry mouth occurs, advise patient:

• To avoid mouth rinses with high alcohol content due to drying effects

• To use daily home fluoride products for anticaries effect

• To use sugarless gum, frequent sips of water, or saliva substitutes

felodipine

(fel-loe′di-peen)
Plendil
♣ Renedil

Drug class.: Calcium channel blocker

Action: Inhibits calcium ion influx across cell membrane during cardiac depolarization; produces relaxation of coronary vascular smooth muscle, dilates coronary arteries, decreases SA/AV node conduction, dilates peripheral arteries

Uses: Essential hypertension, alone or with other antihypertensives, chronic angina pectoris

Dosage and routes:

• *Adult:* PO 5 mg qd initially, usual range 5-10 mg qd; do not exceed 20 mg qd; do not adjust dosage at intervals of <2 wk

Available forms include: Ext rel tabs 2.5, 5, 10 mg

Side effects/adverse reactions:

▼ *ORAL:* Gingival enlargement, dry mouth

CNS: Headache, fatigue, drowsiness, dizziness, anxiety, depression, nervousness, insomnia, lightheadedness, paresthesia, tinnitus, psychosis, somnolence

*CV: **MI, pulmonary edema,** dysrhythmia, edema, CHF, hypotension, palpitation, tachycardia, syncope, AV block, angina

GI: Nausea, vomiting, diarrhea, gastric upset, constipation, increased liver function studies

HEMA: Anemia

GU: Nocturia, polyuria

INTEG: Rash, pruritus

MISC: Flushing, sexual difficulties,

cough, nasal congestion, shortness of breath, wheezing, epistaxis, respiratory infection, chest pain

Contraindications: Hypersensitivity, sick sinus syndrome, second- or third-degree heart block

Precautions: CHF, hypotension <90 mm Hg systolic, hepatic injury, pregnancy category C, lactation, children, renal disease, elderly

Pharmacokinetics:
PO: Peak plasma levels 2.5-5 hr, elimination half-life 11-16 hr; highly protein bound; >99% metabolized in liver; 0.5% excreted unchanged in urine

Drug interactions of concern to dentistry:
• Decreased effect: indomethacin, possibly other NSAIDs, phenobarbital
• Increased effect: parenteral and inhalational general anesthetics or other drugs with hypotensive actions
• Increased effects of nondepolarizing muscle relaxants
• Increased effects of carbamazepine
• Increased plasma levels of itraconazole

DENTAL CONSIDERATIONS
General:
• Monitor cardiac status; take vital signs at each appointment because of CV side effects. Consider a stress reduction protocol to prevent stress-induced angina during the dental appointment.
• After supine positioning, have patient sit upright for at least 2 min before standing to avoid orthostatic hypotension at dismissal.
• Place on frequent recall to monitor gingival condition.
• Limit use of sodium-containing

products such as saline IV fluids for patients with a dietary salt restriction.
• Assess salivary flow as a factor in caries, periodontal disease, and candidiasis.
• Use vasoconstrictors with caution, in low doses, and with careful aspiration. Avoid use of gingival retraction cord with epinephrine.

Consultations:
• Medical consult may be required to assess disease control.

Teach patient/family:
• Importance of good oral hygiene to prevent gingival inflammation and minimize hyperplasia
• Need for frequent oral prophylaxis if hyperplasia occurs
When chronic dry mouth occurs, advise patient:
• To avoid mouth rinses with high alcohol content due to drying effects
• To use daily home fluoride products for anticaries effect
• To use sugarless gum, frequent sips of water, or saliva substitutes

---

fenofibrate (micronized)
(fen-o-fye'brate)
Tricor
Drug class.: Antihyperlipidemic

Action: Inhibits biosynthesis of triglyceride synthesis, reducing VLDL, and stimulates the catabolism of triglyceride-rich lipoprotein (ULDL); reduces serum uric acid levels

Uses: Hyperlipidemia, types IV and V, as an adjunct to diet therapy

Dosage and routes:
• *Adult:* PO initial dose 67-200 mg

daily in conjunction with tri-glyceride-lowering diet; max dose 200 mg/d

• *Elderly:* Limit initial dose to 67 mg daily

Available forms include: Caps 67, 134, 200 mg

Side effects/adverse reactions:

CNS: Headache, dizziness, paresthesia, insomnia, increased appetite

CV: Arrhythmia

GI: Dyspepsia, flatulence, nausea, vomiting, abdominal pain, constipation, diarrhea, pancreatitis

RESP: Flulike syndrome, cough

HEMA: **Thrombocytopenia, agranulocytosis** (very rare)

GU: Decreased libido, polyuria, vaginitis

EENT: Rhinitis, sinusitis, earache, blurred vision, photosensitivity

INTEG: Pruritus, rash

METAB: Elevated BUN and creatinine

MS: Asthenia, myositis, rhabdomyolysis (rare)

MISC: Fatigue, localized pain, hypersensitivity

Contraindications: Hypersensitivity, hepatic or severe renal dysfunction, primary biliary cirrhosis, preexisting gallbladder disease

Precautions: Monitor liver function; may lead to cholelithiasis; can be associated with myositis, myopathy, or rhabdomyolysis; pregnancy category C, avoid if lactating; safe use in children unknown; discontinue use if no response in 2 mo; increased anticoagulant effect with oral anticoagulants

Pharmacokinetics:

PO: Well absorbed, increased absorption with food, peak plasma levels 6-8 hr, highly plasma protein bound (99%); hepatic metabolism, active metabolite; excreted largely in urine (60%)

🦷 **Drug interactions of concern to dentistry:**

• No dental drug interactions reported

DENTAL CONSIDERATIONS

General:

• Monitor vital signs every appointment due to cardiovascular and respiratory side effects.

• Consider semisupine chair position for patient comfort due to GI side effects of drug.

• Patients on chronic drug therapy may rarely have symptoms of blood dyscrasias, which can include infection, bleeding, and poor healing.

• Avoid dental light in patient's eyes; offer dark glasses for patient comfort.

Consultations:

• In a patient with symptoms of blood dyscrasias, request a medical consult for blood studies and postpone treatment until normal values are reestablished.

Teach patient/family:

• Use of electric toothbrush if patient has difficulty holding conventional devices

• To prevent trauma when using oral hygiene aids

---

fenoprofen calcium

(fen-oh-proe'fen)

Nalfon

Drug class.: Nonsteroidal antiinflammatory, propionic acid derivative

---

Action: Inhibits prostaglandin synthesis by interfering with cyclooxygenase needed for biosynthesis; possesses analgesic, antiinflammatory, antipyretic properties

Uses: Mild-to-moderate pain, osteoarthritis, rheumatoid arthritis, acute gout, arthritis, ankylosing spondylitis, nonrheumatic inflammation, dysmenorrhea

Dosage and routes:
Pain (mild to moderate)
• *Adult:* PO 200 mg q4-6h as needed
Arthritis
• *Adult:* PO 300-600 mg qid, not to exceed 3.2 g/day
Available forms include: Caps 200, 300 mg; tabs 600 mg

Side effects/adverse reactions:
▼ *ORAL:* Dry mouth, bleeding, stomatitis, lichenoid reaction
CNS: Dizziness, headache, drowsiness, fatigue, tremors, confusion, insomnia, anxiety, depression
CV: Tachycardia, peripheral edema, palpitation, dysrhythmias
GI: ***Cholestatic hepatitis,*** nausea, anorexia, vomiting, diarrhea, jaundice, constipation, flatulence, cramps, peptic ulcer
HEMA: ***Blood dyscrasias,*** increased bleeding time
GU: ***Nephrotoxicity: dysuria, hematuria, oliguria, azotemia***
EENT: Tinnitus, hearing loss, blurred vision
INTEG: Purpura, rash, pruritus, sweating

Contraindications: Hypersensitivity, asthma, severe renal disease, severe hepatic disease

Precautions: Pregnancy category not established (use not recommended); lactation, children, bleeding disorders, GI disorders, cardiac disorders, hypersensitivity to other antiinflammatory agents

Pharmacokinetics:
PO: Peak 2 hr, half-life 3-3.5 hr; 99% plasma protein binding; metabolized in liver; excreted in urine (metabolites), breast milk

🦷 **Drug interactions of concern to dentistry:**
• GI bleeding, ulceration: salicylates, alcohol, corticosteroids, other NSAIDs
• May decrease effects of fenoprofen: phenobarbital
• Nephrotoxicity: acetaminophen (prolonged use)
• Possible risk of decreased renal function: cyclosporine

DENTAL CONSIDERATIONS
General:
• Assess salivary flow as a factor in caries, periodontal disease, and candidiasis.
• Avoid prescribing for dental use in pregnancy.
• Possibility of cross-allergenicity when patient is allergic to aspirin.

Consultations:
• Medical consult may be required to assess disease control.

Teach patient/family:
• Importance of good oral hygiene to prevent gingival inflammation
• Caution to prevent injury when using oral hygiene aids
When chronic dry mouth occurs, advise patient:
• To avoid mouth rinses with high alcohol content due to drying effects
• To use daily home fluoride products for anticaries effect
• To use sugarless gum, frequent sips of water, or saliva substitutes

---

bold italic = life-threatening conditions   *For periodic updates, visit* **www.mosby.com**

fentanyl transdermal system

(fen'ta-nil)

Duragesic 25, 50, 75, 100 Transdermal Patches

Oral transmucosal fentanyl citrate: Actiq (lozenges)

Drug class.: Narcotic analgesics

Controlled Substance Schedule II, Canada N

Action: Interacts with opioid receptors in the CNS to alter pain perception

Uses: Management of chronic pain when opioids are necessary; transmucosal form: only for management of breakthrough cancer pain in patients with malignancies who are using or tolerant to opioids

Dosage and routes:

Chronic pain

• *Adult only:* One patch every 72 hr; dose depends on need for pain control; titrate as required

Transmucosal form:

• *Adult only:* Dose must be titrated starting with lowest dose size (must be kept secure from children)

Available forms include: Number on patch 25, 50, 75 and 100 refers to µg/hr/fentanyl-release rate; lozenges, transmucosal matrix attached to a radiopaque holder to be dissolved in mouth 200, 400, 600, 800, 1200, 1600 µg; lozenges on a stick 200, 400, 600, 800, 1200, 1600 µg

Side effects/adverse reactions:

▼ *ORAL:* Dry mouth

CNS: Dizziness, delirium, euphoria

CV: **Bradycardia, arrest,** hypotension or hypertension

GI: Nausea, vomiting

RESP: **Respiratory depression, arrest, laryngospasm**

EENT: Blurred vision, miosis

MS: Muscle rigidity

Contraindications: Hypersensitivity to opiates, myasthenia gravis

Precautions: Elderly, respiratory depression, increased intracranial pressure, seizure disorders, severe respiratory disorders, cardiac dysrhythmias, pregnancy category C

Pharmacokinetics:

TD: Dosage adjusted according to opioid tolerance if patient has been taking opioids (2.5 mg of transdermal fentanyl is equivalent to approximately 90 mg oral morphine in 24 hr); peak serum levels take up to 24 hr after applied; liver metabolism; renal excretion of metabolites

⚕ Drug interactions of concern to dentistry:

• Effects may be increased with other CNS depressants: alcohol, narcotics, sedative/hypnotics, skeletal muscle relaxants, chlorpromazine

• Additive hypotension: nitrous oxide, benzodiazepines, phenothiazines

• Increased anticholinergic effect: anticholinergics

• Contraindication: MAO inhibitors

DENTAL CONSIDERATIONS

General:

• Monitor vital signs every appointment due to cardiovascular and respiratory side effects.

• After supine positioning, have patient sit upright for at least 2 min

before standing to avoid orthostatic hypotension.
• Assess salivary flow as a factor in caries, periodontal disease, and candidiasis.
• Psychologic and physical dependence may occur with chronic administration.
• Determine why the patient is taking the drug.
• Consider alternative drugs to opioids and NSAIDs for management of dental pain.

Consultations:
• Medical consult may be required to assess disease control.

Teach patient/family:
• Importance of good oral hygiene to prevent gingival inflammation
• To avoid mouth rinses with high alcohol content due to drying effects

---

ferrous fumarate/ ferrous gluconate/ ferrous sulfate

(fer'us fyoo'ma-rate; gloo'koe-nate)

Ed-in-sol, Femiron, Feosol, Feostat, Feratab, Fer-gen-sol, Fergon, Fer-in-Sol, Fer-Iron, Fumerin, Hemocyte, Ircon, Slow-Fe, Vitron-C

♣ Fero-Grad, Fertinic, Nephro-Fer, Novoferrogluc, Novoferro-sulfa, Novofumar, Palafer

Drug class.: Hematinic, iron preparation

Action: Replaces iron stores needed for red blood cell development, energy and O_2 transport, utilization

Uses: Iron deficiency anemia, prophylaxis for iron deficiency in pregnancy

Dosage and routes:
Fumarate
• *Adult:* PO 200 mg tid-qid
• *Child 2-12 yr:* PO 3 mg/kg/day (elemental iron) tid-qid
• *Child 6 mo-2 yr:* PO up to 6 mg/kg/day (elemental iron) tid-qid
• *Infants:* PO 10-25 mg/day (elemental iron) tid-qid
Gluconate
• *Adult:* PO 200-600 mg tid
• *Child 6-12 yr:* 300-900 mg qd
• *Child <6 yr:* 100-300 mg qd
Sulfate
• *Adult:* PO 0.750-1.5 g/day in divided doses tid
• *Child 6-12 yr:* 600 mg/day in divided doses
Pregnancy
• *Adult:* PO 300-600 mg/day in divided doses

Available forms include:
• *Fumarate:* Tabs 63, 200, 324, 325, 350 mg; chew tabs 100 mg; con rel tabs 300 mg; oral susp 100 mg/5 ml, drops 45 mg/0.6 ml
• *Gluconate:* Tabs 240, 325 mg
• *Sulfate:* Tabs 187, 200, 324, 325 mg; slow rel tabs 160 mg; ext rel caps 160 mg; syr 90 mg/5 ml; elixir 220 mg/5 ml; drops 75 mg/0.6 ml

Side effects/adverse reactions:
▼ *ORAL:* Extrinsic stain on teeth (liquid form)
GI: Nausea, constipation, epigastric pain, black and red tarry stools, vomiting, diarrhea

Contraindications: Hypersensitivity, ulcerative colitis/regional enteritis, hemosiderosis/hemochromatosis, peptic ulcer disease, hemolytic anemia, cirrhosis

---

bold italic = life-threatening conditions

Precautions: Long-term anemia, pregnancy category A

Pharmacokinetics:

PO: Excreted in feces, urine, skin, breast milk; enters bloodstream; bound to transferrin; crosses placenta

🐾 **Drug interactions of concern to dentistry:**

• Decreased absorption of tetracycline, zinc, ciprofloxacin

DENTAL CONSIDERATIONS

Teach patient/family:

• If patient is using hydrogen peroxide as a dentifrice to remove extrinsic stain, caution against frequent use to avoid peroxide-related soft tissue injury

• That liquid iron preparation taken through straw followed by rinsing mouth can reduce staining

---

fexofenadine HCl

(fex-oh-fen'a-deen)
Allegra

Drug class.: Antihistamine, nonsedating

Action: Antagonist for histamine (H_1) receptors; active metabolite of terfenadine

Uses: Seasonal allergic rhinitis

Dosage and routes:

• *Adult and child >12 yr:* PO 60 mg bid or 180 mg qd

• *Child 6-11 yr:* PO 30 mg bid

• *Adult >65 yr:* PO 60 mg qd

Renal dysfunction

• *Adult and child >12 yr:* PO 60 mg/d

• *Child 6-11 yr:* PO 30 mg/d

Available forms include: Caps 60 mg; tabs 30, 60, 180 mg

Side effects/adverse reactions:

CNS: Drowsiness, headache

GI: Nausea, dyspepsia

GU: Dysmenorrhea

EENT: Throat irritation

MISC: Fatigue

Contraindications: Hypersensitivity; troglitazone

Precautions: Reduce dose in elderly, renally impaired, pregnancy category C, lactation, child <12 yr

Pharmacokinetics:

PO: Well absorbed, peak plasma levels 2.6 hr; 60%-70% plasma protein bound; excreted mainly in feces; only 5% of dose is metabolized

🐾 **Drug interactions of concern to dentistry:**

• Elevated plasma levels with erythromycin, ketoconazole

DENTAL CONSIDERATIONS

General:

• Consider semisupine chair position for patient comfort due to GI effects of drug.

---

finasteride

(fi-nas'ter-ide)
Propecia (hair growth product),
Proscar

Drug class.: Synthetic steroid

Action: Competitive inhibitor of type II 5-α-reductase, an enzyme that converts testosterone to 5-α-dihydrotestosterone; this enzyme is found in the liver, skin, and scalp

Uses:

Proscar: Symptomatic benign prostatic hyperplasia, reduce risk for acute urinary retention and surgery

Propecia: Treatment of male pattern baldness in men 18-41 yr

Dosage and routes:

Prostatic hypertrophy

• *Adult:* PO 5 mg day, reassess in 6-12 mo

Male pattern baldness
• *Adult:* PO 1 mg daily; several months of therapy may be required, minimum 3 mo

Available forms include: Tabs 1 mg (Propecia), 5 mg (Proscar)

Side effects/adverse reactions:
GU: Impotence, decreased libido, decreased ejaculate volume
INTEG: Skin rash
MISC: Gynecomastia, allergic reactions

Contraindications: Hypersensitivity, pregnancy, lactation, children, prostate cancer, obstructive urinary disease

Precautions: Pregnancy category X, lactation, lower PSA levels do not suggest absence of prostate cancer; women should avoid drug/semen contact

Pharmacokinetics:
PO: Peak levels 1-2 hr, half-life 6 hr; highly protein bound; liver metabolism; metabolites excreted in feces, urine

⚕ Drug interactions of concern to dentistry:
• Opioids and anticholinergic drugs may enhance urinary retention; use alternative analgesics (NSAIDs)

DENTAL CONSIDERATIONS
Consultations:
• Determine why patient is taking the drug; for prostatic hyperplasia or male pattern baldness.
• Medical consult may be required to assess disease control.

---

flavoxate HCl
(fla-vox′ate)
Urispas
Drug class.: Antispasmatic

Action: Relaxes smooth muscles in urinary tract

Uses: Relief of nocturia, incontinence, suprapubic pain, dysuria, frequency associated with urologic conditions (symptomatic only)

Dosage and routes:
• *Adult and child >12 yr:* PO 100-200 mg tid-qid

Available forms include: Tabs 100, 200 mg

Side effects/adverse reactions:
▼ *ORAL:* Dry mouth
CNS: Anxiety, restlessness, dizziness, convulsions, headache, drowsiness, confusion, decreased concentration
CV: Palpitation, sinus tachycardia, hypotension
GI: Nausea, vomiting, anorexia, abdominal pain, constipation
HEMA: **Leukopenia, eosinophilia**
GU: Dysuria
EENT: Blurred vision, increased intraocular tension, dry throat
INTEG: Urticaria, dermatitis

Contraindications: Hypersensitivity, GI obstruction, GI hemorrhage, GU obstruction

Precautions: Pregnancy category B, lactation, suspected glaucoma, children <12 yr

Pharmacokinetics: Excreted in urine

⚕ Drug interactions of concern to dentistry:
• Increased anticholinergic effect: anticholinergic drugs

DENTAL CONSIDERATIONS
General:
• Assess salivary flow as a factor in caries, periodontal disease, and candidiasis.

Teach patient/family:
• Importance of good oral hygiene to prevent gingival inflammation
• To avoid mouth rinses with high alcohol content due to drying effects

---

bold italic = life-threatening conditions

flecainide acetate

(fle-kay'nide)
Tambocor

Drug class.: Antidysrhythmic (Class IC)

Action: Decreases conduction in all parts of the heart, with greatest effect on His-Purkinje system, which stabilizes cardiac membrane

Uses: Life-threatening ventricular dysrhythmias, sustained supraventricular tachycardia

Dosage and routes:

• *Adult:* PO 100 mg q12h, may increase q4d by 50 mg q12h to desired response, not to exceed 400 mg/day

Available forms include: Tabs 50, 100, 150 mg

Side effects/adverse reactions:

▼ *ORAL:* Changes in taste, dry mouth

CNS: Headache, dizziness, involuntary movement, confusion, psychosis, restlessness, irritability, paresthesia, ataxia, flushing, somnolence, depression, anxiety, malaise

CV: Hypotension, bradycardia, heart block, cardiovascular collapse, cardiac arrest, dysrhythmias, CHF, fatal ventricular tachycardia, angina, PVC

GI: Nausea, vomiting, anorexia, constipation, abdominal pain, flatulence

RESP: Respiratory depression, dyspnea

HEMA: Leukopenia, thrombocytopenia

GU: Impotence, decreased libido, polyuria, urinary retention

EENT: Blurred vision, hearing loss, tinnitus

INTEG: Rash, urticaria, edema, swelling

Contraindications: Hypersensitivity, severe heart block, cardiogenic shock, nonsustained ventricular dysrhythmias, frequent PVCs, non–life-threatening dysrhythmias

Precautions: Pregnancy category C, lactation, children, renal disease, liver disease, CHF, respiratory depression, myasthenia gravis

Pharmacokinetics:

PO: Peak 3 hr, half-life 12-27 hr; metabolized by liver; excreted unchanged by kidneys (10%); excreted in breast milk

⚡ Drug interactions of concern to dentistry:

• No specific interactions are reported with dental drugs; however, any drug that could affect the cardiac action of flecainide (e.g., other local anesthetics, vasoconstrictors, and anticholinergics) should be used in the least effective dose.

DENTAL CONSIDERATIONS
General:

• Monitor vital signs every appointment due to cardiovascular and respiratory side effects.

• Assess salivary flow as a factor in caries, periodontal disease, and candidiasis.

• Stress from dental procedures may compromise cardiovascular function; determine patient risk.

• Use vasoconstrictors with caution, in low doses, and with careful aspiration. Avoid use of gingival retraction cord with epinephrine.

Consultations:

• Medical consult may be required to assess disease control and patient's ability to tolerate stress.

Teach patient/family:
• Importance of good oral hygiene to prevent gingival inflammation
• To avoid mouth rinses with high alcohol content due to drying effects

---

fluconazole

(floo-koe′na-zole)
Diflucan
Drug class.: Antifungal

Action: Inhibits ergosterol biosynthesis, causes direct damage to membrane phospholipids
Uses: Oropharyngeal candidiasis, chronic mucocutaneous candidiasis, urinary candidiasis, cryptococcal meningitis
Dosage and routes:
• *Pediatric doses:* PO 3 mg/kg (equivalent to 100 mg adult dose), 6 mg/kg (equivalent to 200 mg adult dose), 12 mg/kg (equivalent to 400 mg adult dose)
Esophageal candidiasis
• *Child:* PO 6 mg/kg on day 1, then 3 mg/kg qd up to 3-wk minimum, then for 2 wk following resolution
Oropharyngeal candidiasis
• *Adult:* PO 200 mg first day, then 100 mg daily
• *Child:* PO 6 mg/kg on day 1, then 3 mg/kg qd up to 2 wk
Serious fungal infections
• *Adult:* IV 400 mg initially, then 200 mg/day; adjust dose downward for renal impairment
• *Adult:* PO 400 mg daily; or 400 mg first day, then 200 mg daily × 4 wk
Vaginal candidiasis
• *Adult:* PO 150 mg as a single dose
Available forms include: Tabs 50, 100, 150, 200 mg; IV inj 200, 400 mg; powder oral susp 10 mg/ml, 40 mg/ml
Side effects/adverse reactions:
CNS: **Headache,** seizures
GI: Nausea, vomiting, diarrhea, cramping, flatus, increased AST/ALT
HEMA: **Agranulocytosis, hepatic failure,** leukopenia, thrombocytopenia, hepatitis
INTEG: **Toxic epidermal necrolysis** (Stevens-Johnson syndrome, rare*), skin rash,* exfoliative skin disorders
META: Rare abnormal liver function, elevated cholesterol, triglycerides
MS: **Anaphylaxis**
Contraindications: Hypersensitivity
Precautions: Renal disease, pregnancy category C
Pharmacokinetics:
PO/IV: Bioavailability more than 90%, peak plasma levels 1-2 hr, with loading doses see quicker steady-state levels; low plasma protein binding (12%); minimal metabolism; 80% excreted unchanged in urine
Drug interactions of concern to dentistry:
• Increased plasma levels of oral hypoglycemics: theophylline, cyclosporine, tacrolimus
• Inhibits metabolism of certain benzodiazepines: alprazolam, chlordiazepoxide, clonazepam, clorazepate, diazepam, estazolam, flurazepam, halazepam, midazolam, triazolam, quazepam, zolpidem
• Increased anticoagulant effect: may inhibit metabolism of warfarin
• Suspected risk of increased neurological side effects: haloperidol, tricyclic antidepressants

---

bold italic = life-threatening conditions

DENTAL CONSIDERATIONS
General:
• Culture may be required to confirm fungal organism.
• Patient on chronic drug therapy may rarely present with symptoms of blood dyscrasias, which can include infection, bleeding, and poor healing.

Consultations:
• In a patient with symptoms of blood dyscrasias, request a medical consult for blood studies and postpone treatment until normal values are reestablished.

Teach patient/family:
• That long-term therapy may be needed to clear infection
• To prevent reinoculation of *Candida* infection, dispose of toothbrush or other contaminated oral hygiene devices used during period of infection

---

flucytosine
(floo-sye'toe-seen)
Ancobon
✦ Ancotil
Drug class.: Antifungal

Action: Converted to fluorouracil after entering fungi, thus inhibiting DNA and RNA synthesis
Uses: *Candida* infections (septicemia, endocarditis, pulmonary and urinary tract infections), *Cryptococcus* (meningitis, pulmonary and urinary tract infections)
Dosage and routes:
• *Adult and child >50 kg:* PO 50-150 mg/kg/day q6h
Available forms include: Caps 250, 500 mg
Side effects/adverse reactions:
▼ *ORAL:* Bleeding (if bone marrow depression occurs), stomatitis

CNS: Headache, confusion, dizziness, sedation
GI: Nausea, vomiting, anorexia, **bowel perforation** (rare), diarrhea, cramps, enterocolitis, increased AST/ALT, alk phosphatase
RESP: **Respiratory arrest,** chest pain, dyspnea
HEMA: **Thrombocytopenia, agranulocytosis, anemia, leukopenia, pancytopenia**
GU: Increased BUN, creatinine
INTEG: Rash, photosensitivity, urticaria
Contraindications: Hypersensitivity
Precautions: Renal disease, bone marrow depression, blood dyscrasias, radiation/chemotherapy, pregnancy category C
Pharmacokinetics:
PO: Peak 2.5-6 hr, half-life 3-6 hr; excreted in urine (unchanged); well distributed to CSF, aqueous humor, joints

⚕ Drug interactions of concern to dentistry:
• None

DENTAL CONSIDERATIONS
General:
• Patients on chronic drug therapy may rarely have symptoms of blood dyscrasias, which can include infection, bleeding, and poor healing.
• Examine for evidence of oral *Candida* infection.

Consultations:
• Medical consult may be required to assess disease control.
• In a patient with symptoms of blood dyscrasias, request a medical consult for blood studies and postpone dental treatment until normal values are reestablished.

italic = common side effects

Teach patient/family:
• Importance of good oral hygiene to prevent gingival inflammation

---

fludrocortisone acetate

(floo-droe-kor´ti-sone)
Florinef Acetate

Drug class.: Glucocorticoid and mineralocorticoid

Action: Glucocorticoids have multiple actions that include antiinflammatory and immunosuppressant effects. They inhibit phospholipase A_2, interfering with or reducing the synthesis of prostaglandins and leukotrienes. They also bind to cytoplasmic glucocorticoid receptors (GRs) and enter the cell nucleus to bind with DNA. This results in the synthesis of various enzymes such as collagenase, elastase, and cytokines that play important roles in inflammation and immunosuppression. They also suppress the production of lymphocytes, monocytes, and eosinophils.

Uses: Adrenal insufficiency (Addison's disease), salt-losing adrenogenital syndrome

Dosage and routes:
• *Adult:* PO 0.1-0.2 mg/day
• *Pediatric:* PO 0.05-0.10 mg/day
Available forms include: Tabs 0.1 mg

Side effects/adverse reactions:
*CNS: **Flushing, sweating,*** headache
*CV: Hypertension, **circulatory collapse, thrombophlebitis, embolism,*** tachycardia, edema, enlargement of heart
MS: Fractures, osteoporosis, weakness

Contraindications: Hypersensitivity, acute glomerulonephritis, amebiasis

Precautions: Pregnancy category C, osteoporosis, CHF

Pharmacokinetics:
PO: Half-life 3.5 hr, duration 1-2 days; highly protein bound; metabolized by liver; excreted in urine

⚡ Drug interactions of concern to dentistry:
• Decreased action: barbiturates
• Increased side effects: sodium-containing food or sodium-containing polishing devices
• Decreased effects of salicylates

DENTAL CONSIDERATIONS
General:
• Patients with Addison's disease are more susceptible to stress and may require supplemental systemic glucocorticoids before dental treatment.
• Patients who have been or are currently on chronic steroid therapy (>2 wk) may require supplemental steroids for dental treatment.
• Evaluate vital signs at each appointment due to nature of disease.
• Short appointments and a stress reduction protocol may be required for anxious patients.
• Patients with Addison's disease must be evaluated closely for presence of oral infection.
• Do not use ingestible sodium bicarbonate products, such as the air polishing system (Prophy Jet), or IV saline fluids for patients on a salt-restriction regimen.
• Place on frequent recall to evaluate healing response.
• Use precautions if dental surgery is anticipated and conscious sedation or general anesthesia is required.

---

bold italic = life-threatening conditions

• Monitor patient for any signs of inadequate management of disease such as potassium depletion, muscle weakness, paresthesia, fatigue, nausea, depression, polyuria, and edema.

Consultations:

• Medical consult is required to assess disease control and stress tolerance of the patient.

• Consult may be required to confirm steroid dose and duration of use.

Teach patient/family:

• That identification as a steroid user should be carried

• To report to the dental office any signs that might indicate an oral infection

---

flumazenil

(floo-may′ze-nil)

Anexate, Romazicon

Drug class.: Benzodiazepine receptor antagonist

Action: Antagonizes the actions of benzodiazepines on the CNS; competitively inhibits the activity at the benzodiazepine recognition site on the GABA/benzodiazepine receptor complex

Uses: Reversal of the sedative effects of benzodiazepines

Dosage and routes:

Reversal of conscious sedation or in general anesthesia

• *Adult:* IV 0.2 mg (2 ml) given over 15-30 sec; wait 45-60 sec for desired response, then give 0.2 mg (2 ml) if consciousness does not occur; may be repeated at 60 sec intervals as needed, up to 4 additional times (max total dose 1 mg); dose is to be individualized

Management of suspected benzodiazepine overdose

• *Adult:* IV 0.2 mg (2 ml) given over 15-30 sec; wait 45-60 sec for desired response, then give 0.2 mg (2 ml) over 30 sec if consciousness does not occur; further doses of 0.5 mg (5 ml) can be given over 30 sec at intervals of 1 min up to cumulative dose of 3 mg in 1 hr

Available forms include: Inj 0.1 mg/ml in 5 ml and 10 ml vials

Side effects/adverse reactions:

CNS: **Convulsions,** dizziness, agitation, emotional lability, confusion, somnolence

CV: Hypertension, palpitation, cutaneous vasodilation, dysrhythmias, bradycardia, tachycardia, chest pain

GI: Nausea, vomiting, hiccups

EENT: Abnormal vision, blurred vision, tinnitus

SYST: Headache, injection site pain, increased sweating, fatigue, rigors

Contraindications: Hypersensitivity to this drug or benzodiazepines, serious cyclic antidepressant overdose, patients given benzodiazepine for control of life-threatening condition

Precautions: Pregnancy category C, lactation, children, elderly, renal disease, seizure disorders, head injury, labor and delivery, hepatic disease, hypoventilation, panic disorder, drug and alcohol dependency, ambulatory patients

Pharmacokinetics:

IV: Terminal half-life 41-79 min; metabolized in liver

🦷 **Drug interactions of concern to dentistry:**

• May not be effective: mixed drug overdosage

DENTAL CONSIDERATIONS
General:
• Monitor vital signs every appointment due to cardiovascular side effects.
• Monitor for resedation; duration of antagonism is short compared with benzodiazepines.
Teach patient/family:
• To be alert for possible resedation when discharged from office

---

flunisolide
(floo-niss'oh-lide)

Oral inh aerosol: Aerobid, Aerobid-M
♣ Bronalide
Nasal sol: Nasalide, Nasarel
♣ Rhinalar

Drug class.: Synthetic glucocorticoid

Action: Glucocorticoids have multiple actions that include antiinflammatory and immunosuppressant effects. They inhibit phospholipase A_2, interfering with or reducing the synthesis of prostaglandins and leukotrienes. They also bind to cytoplasmic glucocorticoid receptors (GRs) and enter the cell nucleus to bind with DNA. This results in the synthesis of various enzymes such as collagenase, elastase, and cytokines that play important roles in inflammation and immunosuppression. They also suppress the production of lymphocytes, monocytes, and eosinophils.
Uses: Rhinitis (seasonal or perennial)
Dosage and routes:
• *Adult:* INSTILL 2 sprays in each nostril bid, then increase to tid if needed; not to exceed 8 sprays in each nostril per day INH 2 inhalations bid (AM and PM), limit to 4 inh/day
• *Child 6-15 yr:* INSTILL 1 spray in each nostril tid or 2 sprays bid; not to exceed 4 sprays in each nostril per day INH 2 inhalations bid

Available forms include: Aerosol 250 µg/spray; nasal sol 0.025% in 25 ml
Side effects/adverse reactions:
▼ *ORAL:* Dry mouth, candidiasis, loss of taste sensation
CNS: Headache, dizziness
EENT: Nasal irritation, dryness, rebound congestion, epistaxis, sneezing
INTEG: Urticaria
SYST: **CHF, convulsions,** increased sodium, hypertension
Contraindications: Hypersensitivity, child <12 yr, fungal, bacterial infection of nose
Precautions: Lactation, pregnancy category C
Pharmacokinetics:
AERO: Effective response time 1-4 wk; metabolized in liver; excreted in urine and feces
DENTAL CONSIDERATIONS
General:
• Examine oral cavity for evidence of drug side effects.
• Assess salivary flow as a factor in caries, periodontal disease, and candidiasis.
• Evaluate respiration characteristics and rate.
• Consider semisupine chair position for patients with respiratory disease.
• Determine dose and duration of

---

bold italic = life-threatening conditions

steroid therapy for each patient to assess risk for stress tolerance and immunosuppression.

• Acute asthmatic episodes may be precipitated in the dental office. Sympathomimetic inhalants should be available for emergency use. A stress reduction protocol may be required.

• Consider the drug in the diagnosis of taste alterations.

Consultations:

• Medical consult may be required to assess disease control.

Teach patient/family:

• Importance of good oral hygiene to prevent soft tissue inflammation
• Caution to prevent injury when using oral hygiene aids
• Importance of gargling, rinsing mouth with water, and expectorating after each aerosol dose

When chronic dry mouth occurs, advise patient:

• To use daily home fluoride products for anticaries effect
• To avoid mouth rinses with high alcohol content due to drying effects
• To use sugarless gum, frequent sips of water, or saliva substitutes

---

fluocinonide
(floo-oh-sin′oh-nide)

Cream: Fluocin, Fluonex, Licon, Lidex, Lidex-E
✤ Lidemol, Lyderm
Ointment: Lidex
Solution: Lidex
Gel: Lidex
✤ Topsyn

Drug class.: Topical corticosteroid, synthetic fluorinated agent, group II potency

Action: Glucocorticoids have mul-tiple actions that include antiin-flammatory and immunosuppressant effects. They inhibit phospholipase A_2, interfering with or reducing the synthesis of prostaglandins and leukotrienes. They also bind to cytoplasmic glucocorticoid receptors (GRs) and enter the cell nucleus to bind with DNA. This results in the synthesis of various enzymes such as collagenase, elastase, and cytokines that play important roles in inflammation and immunosuppression. They also suppress the production of lymphocytes, monocytes, and eosinophils.

Uses: Psoriasis, eczema, contact dermatitis, pruritus, oral lichen planus lesions

Dosage and routes:

• *Adult and child:* Apply to affected area tid-qid

Available forms include: Oint 0.5%; cream 0.05%; sol 0.05% in 20, 60 ml; gel 0.05% in 15, 30, 60, and 120 g tubes

Side effects/adverse reactions:

▼ *ORAL:* Thinning of mucosa, stinging sensation (oral application)

INTEG: Burning, dryness, itching, irritation, acne, folliculitis, hypertrichosis, perioral dermatitis, hypopigmentation, atrophy, striae, miliaria, allergic contact dermatitis, secondary infection

Contraindications: Hypersensitivity to corticosteroids, fungal infections

Precautions: Pregnancy category C, lactation, viral infections, bacterial infections

DENTAL CONSIDERATIONS
General:

• Place on frequent recall to evaluate healing response.

Teach patient/family:
• When used for oral lesions, to return for oral evaluation if response of oral tissues has not occurred in 7-14 days
• That use on oral herpetic ulcerations is contraindicated
• Importance of good oral hygiene to prevent soft tissue inflammation
• To apply at bedtime or after meals for maximum effect
• To apply with cotton-tipped applicator by pressing, not rubbing, paste on lesion

---

fluorouracil (topical)
(flure-oh-yoor'a-sil)
Efudex, Fluoroplex, 5-FU
Drug class.: Topical antineoplastic

Action: Inhibits synthesis of DNA and RNA in susceptible cells
Uses: Keratosis (multiple/actinic), basal cell carcinoma; unapproved: condyloma acuminatum
Dosage and routes:
• *Adult and child:* TOP apply to affected area bid
Available forms include: Sol 1%, 2%, 5%; cream 1%, 5%
Side effects/adverse reactions:
▼ *ORAL:* Stomatitis, medicinal taste, lichenoid reaction
CNS: Insomnia, irritability
EENT: Lacrimation, soreness
INTEG: Pain, burning, pruritus, contact dermatitis, scaling, swelling, soreness, hyperpigmentation
Contraindications: Hypersensitivity, pregnancy
Precautions: Pregnancy category X, occlusive dressings, lactation, children, excessive exposure to sunlight

Pharmacokinetics:
TOP: No significant absorption, onset 2-3 days; treatment may last up to 12 wk; healing may be delayed for 1-2 mo
🦷 **Drug interactions of concern to dentistry:**
• None reported, but limit drugs that may also produce photosensitivity reaction
DENTAL CONSIDERATIONS
General:
• Be aware of patient's disease and avoid treated areas to prevent further irritation.

---

fluoxetine
(floo-ox'e-teen)
Prozac, Prozac Weekly, Sarafem
Drug class.: Antidepressant

Action: Inhibits CNS neuron uptake of serotonin, but not norepinephrine
Uses: Major depressive disorder, bulimia, obsessive-compulsive disorder, premenstrual tension, geriatric depression in patients >65 yr, premenstrual dysphoric disorder (Sarafem)
Dosage and routes:
Depression
• *Adult:* PO 20 mg qd in AM; after several weeks if no clinical improvement is noted, dose may be increased to 20 mg bid, not to exceed 80 mg/day; Prozac Weekly 90 mg del rel capsule only for stabilized patients requiring maintenance therapy
Obsessive-compulsive disorder
• *Adult:* PO initial 20 mg qd in AM; if no improvement after several weeks dose may be increased to 20 mg bid, not to exceed 80 mg/day

---

bold italic = life-threatening conditions

Bulimia

• *Adult:* PO 60 mg qd in AM; can start with lower dose and gradually increase to 60 mg/day

Available forms include: Tabs 10 mg; caps 10, 20, 40 mg; del rel caps 90 mg

Side effects/adverse reactions:

▼ *ORAL: Dry mouth, taste changes*

CNS: Headache, nervousness, insomnia, drowsiness, anxiety, tremor, dizziness, fatigue, sedation, poor concentration, abnormal dreams, agitation, convulsions, apathy, euphoria, hallucinations, delusions, psychosis

CV: Hot flashes, palpitation, MI, angina pectoris, hemorrhage, tachycardia, first-degree AV block, bradycardia, thrombophlebitis

GI: Nausea, diarrhea, anorexia, dyspepsia, constipation, cramps, vomiting, flatulence, decreased appetite

RESP: Infection, pharyngitis, nasal congestion, sinus headache, sinusitis, cough, dyspnea, bronchitis, asthma, hyperventilation, pneumonia

GU: Dysmenorrhea, decreased libido, abnormal ejaculation, urinary frequency, UTI, amenorrhea, cystitis, impotence

EENT: Visual changes, ear/eye pain, photophobia, tinnitus

INTEG: Sweating, rash, pruritus, acne, alopecia, urticaria

MS: Pain, arthritis, twitching

SYST: Asthenia, viral infection, fever, allergy, chills

Contraindications: Hypersensitivity, MAO inhibitors

Precautions: Pregnancy category B, lactation, children, elderly

Pharmacokinetics:

PO: Peak 6-8 hr, half-life 2-7 days; metabolized in liver; excreted in urine

⚕ Drug interactions of concern to dentistry:

• Increased CNS depression: alcohol, all CNS depressants

• Increased side effects: highly protein-bound drugs (aspirin)

• Increased half-life of diazepam

• Possible "serotonin syndrome" with macrolide antibiotics

DENTAL CONSIDERATIONS

General:

• Monitor vital signs every appointment due to cardiovascular side effects.

• Assess salivary flow as a factor in caries, periodontal disease, and candidiasis.

Consultations:

• Medical consult may be required to assess disease control and patient's ability to tolerate stress.

• Physician should be informed if significant xerostomic side effects occur (increased caries, sore tongue, problems eating or swallowing, difficulty wearing prosthesis) so a medication change can be considered.

Teach patient/family:

• To use electric toothbrush if patient has difficulty holding conventional devices

When chronic dry mouth occurs, advise patient:

• To avoid mouth rinses with high alcohol content due to drying effects

• To use daily home fluoride products for anticaries effect

• To use sugarless gum, frequent sips of water, or saliva substitutes

fluoxymesterone

(floo-ox-i-mes'te-rone)

Halotestin

Drug class.: Androgenic anabolic steroid

Controlled Substance Schedule III

Action: Increases weight by building body tissue; increases potassium, phosphorus, chloride, nitrogen levels; increases bone development

Uses: Impotence from testicular deficiency, hypogonadism, breast engorgement, palliative treatment of female breast cancer

Dosage and routes:

Hypogonadism/impotence

• *Adult:* PO 2-20 mg qd

Breast engorgement

• *Adult:* PO 2.5 mg qd, then 5-10 mg qd × 5 days

Breast cancer

• *Adult:* PO 10-40 mg qd in divided doses until therapeutic effect occurs; dosage should then be reduced

Available forms include: Tabs 2, 5, 10 mg

Side effects/adverse reactions:

▼ *ORAL:* Reddish spots on mucosa (high dose)

CNS: Dizziness, headache, fatigue, tremors, paresthesia, flushing, sweating, anxiety, lability, insomnia

CV: Increased BP

GI: **Cholestatic jaundice,** nausea, vomiting, constipation, weight gain

GU: **Hematuria,** amenorrhea, vaginitis, decreased libido, decreased breast size, clitoral hypertrophy, testicular atrophy

EENT: Carpal tunnel syndrome, conjunctival edema, nasal congestion

INTEG: Rash, acneiform lesions, oily hair/skin, flushing, sweating, acne vulgaris, alopecia, hirsutism

ENDO: Abnormal GTT

MS: Cramps, spasms

Contraindications: Severe renal disease, severe cardiac disease, severe hepatic disease, hypersensitivity, pregnancy category X, lactation, genital bleeding (abnormal)

Precautions: Diabetes mellitus, CV disease, MI

Pharmacokinetics:

PO: Metabolized in liver; excreted in urine; crosses placenta; excreted in breast milk

🖘 Drug interactions of concern to dentistry:

• Edema: corticosteroids

DENTAL CONSIDERATIONS

General:

• Monitor vital signs every appointment due to cardiovascular side effects.

• Patients receiving chemotherapy may require palliative treatment for stomatitis.

Teach patient/family:

• Importance of good oral hygiene to prevent soft tissue inflammation

• Caution the patient in use of dental hygiene aids to prevent trauma

---

fluphenazine decanoate/ fluphenazine enanthate/ fluphenazine HCl

(floo-fen'a-zeen)

Permitil, Permitil Concentrate HCl, Prolixin Concentrate, Prolixin Decanoate, Prolixin Enanthate ♣ Apo-Fluphenazine, Modecate, Modecate Concentrate, Moditen HCl

Drug class.: Phenothiazine antipsychotic

Action: Blocks neurotransmission at dopaminergic synapses in the cerebral cortex, hypothalamus, and limbic system; exhibits strong peripheral α-adrenergic, anticholinergic blocking action; mechanism for antipsychotic effects is unclear

Uses: Psychotic disorders, schizophrenia; unapproved: adjunct to tricyclic antidepressants in neurogenic pain

Dosage and routes:

Enanthate, decanoate

• *Adult and child >12 yr:* SC 12.5-25 mg q1-3wk

HCl

• *Adult:* PO 2.5-10 mg in divided doses q6-8h, not to exceed 20 mg qd; IM initially 1.25 mg, then 2.5-10 mg in divided doses q6-8h

Available forms include: HCl–tabs 1, 2.5, 5, 10 mg; elix 2.5 mg/5 ml; conc 5 mg/ml; inj IM 2.5 mg/ml; enanthate, decanoate–inj SC/IM 25 mg/ml

Side effects/adverse reactions:

▼ *ORAL: Dry mouth,* lichenoid reaction

CNS: Extrapyramidal symptoms: pseudoparkinsonism, akathisia, dystonia, *tardive dyskinesia,* drowsiness, headache, **neuroleptic malignant syndrome,** seizures

CV: Orthostatic hypotension, **cardiac arrest, tachycardia,** hypertension, ECG changes

GI: **Paralytic ileus, hepatitis,** nausea, vomiting, anorexia, constipation, diarrhea, jaundice, weight gain

RESP: **Respiratory depression,** laryngospasm, dyspnea

HEMA: **Leukopenia, leukocytosis, agranulocytosis,** anemia

GU: Urinary retention, urinary frequency, enuresis, impotence, amenorrhea, gynecomastia

EENT: Blurred vision, glaucoma, dry eyes

INTEG: Rash, photosensitivity, dermatitis

Contraindications: Hypersensitivity, circulatory collapse, liver damage, cerebral arteriosclerosis, coronary disease, severe hypertension/hypotension, blood dyscrasias, coma, child <12 yr, brain damage, bone marrow depression, alcohol and barbiturate withdrawal states

Precautions: Pregnancy category not established, lactation, seizure disorders, hypertension, hepatic disease, cardiac disease

Pharmacokinetics:

PO/IM: HCl–onset 1 hr, peak 2-4 hr, duration 6-8 hr

SC: Enanthate–onset 1-2 days, peak 2-3 days, duration 1-3 wk, half-life 3.5-4 days; decanoate–onset 1-3 days, peak 1-2 days, duration >4 wk, half-life (single dose) 6.8-9.6 days, (multiple dose) 14.3 days; metabolized by liver; excreted in urine (metabolites); crosses placenta; excreted in breast milk

italic = common side effects

🦷 **Drug interactions of concern to dentistry:**

• Increased sedation: other CNS depressants, alcohol, barbiturate anesthetics, opioid analgesics

• Hypotension, tachycardia: epinephrine

• Increased extrapyramidal effects: phenothiazines and related drugs (haloperidol, droperidol), metoclopramide

• Additive photosensitization: tetracyclines

• Increased anticholinergic effects: anticholinergics

DENTAL CONSIDERATIONS

General:

• Monitor vital signs every appointment due to cardiovascular side effects.

• Patients on chronic drug therapy may rarely have symptoms of blood dyscrasias, which can include infection, bleeding, and poor healing.

• After supine positioning, have patient sit upright for at least 2 min before standing to avoid orthostatic hypotension.

• Assess salivary flow as a factor in caries, periodontal disease, and candidiasis.

• Avoid dental light in patient's eyes; offer dark glasses for patient comfort.

• Assess for presence of extrapyramidal motor symptoms, such as tardive dyskinesia and akathisia. Extrapyramidal motor activity may complicate dental treatment.

• Geriatric patients are more susceptible to drug effects; use a lower dose.

• Use vasoconstrictors with caution, in low doses, and with careful aspiration.

Consultations:

• In a patient with symptoms of blood dyscrasias, request a medical consult for blood studies and postpone dental treatment until normal values are reestablished.

• Take precautions if dental surgery is anticipated and anesthesia is required.

• If signs of tardive dyskinesia or akathisia are present, refer to physician.

• Physician should be informed if significant xerostomic side effects occur (increased caries, sore tongue, problems eating or swallowing, difficulty wearing prosthesis) so a medication change can be considered.

Teach patient/family:

• Importance of good oral hygiene to prevent soft tissue inflammation

• Caution to prevent injury when using oral hygiene aids

• To use electric toothbrush if patient has difficulty holding conventional devices

When chronic dry mouth occurs, advise patient:

• To avoid mouth rinses with high alcohol content due to drying effects

• To use daily home fluoride products for anticaries effect

• To use sugarless gum, frequent sips of water, or saliva substitutes

---

flurandrenolide
(flure-an-dren′oh-lide)
Cordran, Cordran SP
♣ Dreison-1/4, Drenison
Drug class.: Topical corticosteroid, group III medium potency

Action: Glucocorticoids have multiple actions that include antiin-

---

flammatory and immunosuppressant effects. They inhibit phospholipase A_2, interfering with or reducing the synthesis of prostaglandins and leukotrienes. They also bind to cytoplasmic glucocorticoid receptors (GRs) and enter the cell nucleus to bind with DNA. This results in the synthesis of various enzymes, such as collagenase, elastase, and cytokines, that play important roles in inflammation and immunosuppression. They also suppress the production of lymphocytes, monocytes, and eosinophils.

Uses: Corticosteroid-responsive dermatoses, pruritus

Dosage and routes:
• *Adult and child:* TOP apply to affected area tid-qid; apply tape q12-24h

Available forms include: Oint 0.025%, 0.05%; cream 0.025%, 0.05%; lotion 0.05%; tape 4 $\mu g/cm^2$

Side effects/adverse reactions:
▼ *ORAL:* Perioral dermatitis
INTEG: Burning, dryness, itching, irritation, acne, folliculitis, hypertrichosis, hypopigmentation, atrophy, striae, miliaria, allergic contact dermatitis, secondary infection

Contraindications: Hypersensitivity to corticosteroids, fungal infections, viral infections

Precautions: Pregnancy category C, lactation, viral infections, bacterial infections

DENTAL CONSIDERATIONS
General:
• Determine why the patient is taking the drug.

• Apply lubricant to dry lips for patient comfort before dental procedures.
• Place on frequent recall to evaluate healing response when used on chronic basis.

---

flurazepam HCl
(flur-az′e-pam)
Dalmane
♣ Apo-Flurazepam, Novoflupam, Somnol
Drug class.: Benzodiazepine, sedative-hypnotic

Controlled Substance Schedule IV
Action: Produces CNS depression by interacting with a benzodiazepine receptor to facilitate the action of the inhibitory neurotransmitter γ-aminobutyric acid (GABA)
Uses: Insomnia

Dosage and routes:
• *Adult:* PO 15-30 mg hs, may repeat dose once if needed
• *Geriatric:* PO 15 mg hs, may increase if needed

Available forms include: Caps 15, 30 mg

Side effects/adverse reactions:
▼ *ORAL:* Dry mouth (infrequent)
CNS: Lethargy, drowsiness, daytime sedation, dizziness, confusion, light-headedness, headache, anxiety, irritability
CV: Chest pain, pulse changes
GI: Nausea, vomiting, diarrhea, heartburn, abdominal pain, constipation
HEMA: Leukopenia, granulocytopenia (rare)

Contraindications: Hypersensitivity to benzodiazepines, pregnancy category X, lactation, inter-

italic = common side effects

mittent porphyria, uncontrolled pain, ritonavir

Precautions: Anemia, hepatic disease, renal disease, suicidal individuals, drug abuse, elderly, psychosis, child <15 yr

Pharmacokinetics:

PO: Onset 15-45 min, duration 7-8 hr, half-life 47-100 hr, additional 100 hr for active metabolites; metabolized by liver; excreted by kidneys (inactive/active metabolites); crosses placenta; excreted in breast milk

⚜ Drug interactions of concern to dentistry:

• Increased sedation: alcohol, CNS depressants

• Increased serum levels and prolonged effect of benzodiazepines: ketoconazole, itraconazole, fluconazole, and miconazole (systemic), indinavir

DENTAL CONSIDERATIONS

General:

• Assess salivary flow as a factor in caries, periodontal disease, and candidiasis.

• Psychologic and physical dependence may occur with chronic administration.

• Geriatric patients are more susceptible to drug effects; use lower dose.

Consultations:

• Medical consult may be required to assess disease control.

Teach patient/family:

• To avoid mouth rinses with high alcohol content due to drying effects

flurbiprofen

(flure-bi′proe-fen)

Ansaid

♣ Apo-Flurbiprofen, Froben, Froben SR, Novo-Flurbiprofen, Nu-Flurbiprofen

Drug class.: Nonsteroidal antiinflammatory

Action: Inhibits prostaglandin synthesis by interfering with cyclooxygenase needed for biosynthesis; possesses analgesic, antiinflammatory, antipyretic properties

Uses: Acute, long-term treatment of rheumatoid arthritis, osteoarthritis; unapproved: mild-to-moderate pain

Dosage and routes:

• *Adult:* PO 200-300 mg daily in divided doses bid, tid, or qid

Available forms include: Tabs 50, 100 mg

Side effects/adverse reactions:

▼ *ORAL:* Dry mouth, stomatitis, lichenoid reaction

CNS: Dizziness, drowsiness, fatigue, tremors, confusion, anxiety, myalgia, insomnia, depression, convulsions, malaise, nervousness, paresthesias

CV: Tachycardia, peripheral edema, palpitation, chest pain

GI: ***Jaundice, cholestatic hepatitis,*** nausea, anorexia, vomiting, diarrhea, constipation, flatulence, cramps, peptic ulcer, dyspepsia, indigestion

RESP: ***Bronchospasm,*** dyspnea, hemoptysis, rhinitis, shortness of breath

HEMA: ***Blood dyscrasias, bone marrow depression***

---

bold italic = life-threatening conditions   *For periodic updates, visit* **www.mosby.com**

*GU: **Nephrotoxicity: dysuria, hematuria, oliguria, azotemia, cystitis, UTI, nocturia, renal insufficiency***
EENT: Tinnitus, hearing loss, blurred vision
INTEG: Purpura, rash, pruritus, erythema, urticaria, petechiae, ecchymosis, photosensitivity, exfoliative dermatitis, alopecia, eczema
Contraindications: Hypersensitivity, hypersensitivity to other antiinflammatory agents
Precautions: Pregnancy category B, first or second trimester, lactation, children, bleeding disorders, GI disorders, cardiac disorders, severe renal disease, severe hepatic disease
Pharmacokinetics:
PO: Peak 1.5 hr, half-life 6 hr; metabolized in liver; excreted in urine (metabolites), breast milk
🦷 **Drug interactions of concern to dentistry:**
• GI ulceration, bleeding: aspirin, alcohol, corticosteroids
• Decreased action: salicylates
• Nephrotoxicity: acetaminophen (prolonged use)
When prescribed for dental pain:
• Risk of increased effects: oral anticoagulants, oral antidiabetics, lithium, methotrexate
• Decreased effects of diuretics
DENTAL CONSIDERATIONS
General:
• Patients on chronic drug therapy may rarely have symptoms of blood dyscrasias, which can include infection, bleeding, and poor healing.
• Assess salivary flow as a factor in caries, periodontal disease, and candidiasis.
• Avoid prescribing for dental use in last trimester of pregnancy.

• Avoid prescribing aspirin-containing products.
• Consider semisupine chair position for patients with arthritic disease.
Consultations:
• Medical consult may be required to assess disease control.
• In a patient with symptoms of blood dyscrasias, request a medical consult for blood studies and postpone dental treatment until normal values are reestablished.
Teach patient/family:
• Importance of good oral hygiene to prevent soft tissue inflammation
• Caution to prevent injury when using oral hygiene aids
When chronic dry mouth occurs, advise patient:
• To avoid mouth rinses with high alcohol content due to drying effects
• To use daily home fluoride products for anticaries effect
• To use sugarless gum, frequent sips of water, or saliva substitutes

---

flurbiprofen sodium
(flure-bi′proe-fen)
Ocufen

Drug class.: Nonsteroidal antiinflammatory ophthalmic

Action: Inhibits enzyme system necessary for biosynthesis of prostaglandins; inhibits miosis
Uses: Inhibition of intraoperative miosis, corneal edema
Dosage and routes:
• *Adult:* 1 gtt q0.5h 2 hr before surgery (4 gtt total)
Available forms include: Sol 0.03%

Side effects/adverse reactions:
EENT: Burning, stinging in the eye, eye irritation/bleeding/redness

Contraindications: Hypersensitivity, epithelial herpes simplex keratitis

Precautions: Pregnancy category C, lactation, child, aspirin or nonsteroidal antiinflammatory drug hypersensitivity, allergy, bleeding disorder

DENTAL CONSIDERATIONS
General:
• Avoid dental light in patient's eyes; offer dark glasses for patient comfort.

---

flutamide
(floo'ta-mide)
Eulexin
✤ Euflex
Drug class.: Antineoplastic

Action: Interferes with testosterone at the cellular level; inhibits androgen uptake by inhibiting nuclear binding or by interfering with androgen in target tissues

Uses: Metastatic prostatic carcinoma, stage D2; early-stage prostate cancer, stages B2 and C, in combination with LHRH agonistic analogs (leuprolide) and radiation

Dosage and routes:
• *Adult:* PO 250 mg q8h, for a daily dose of 750 mg

Available forms include: Caps 125 mg

Side effects/adverse reactions:
CNS: Hot flashes, drowsiness, confusion, depression, anxiety
*GI: Diarrhea, nausea, vomiting, **hepatitis, liver failure,*** increased liver function studies, anorexia

GU: Decreased libido, impotence, gynecomastia
INTEG: Irritation at site, rash, photosensitivity
MISC: Edema, hematopoietic symptoms, neuromuscular and pulmonary symptoms, hypertension

Contraindications: Hypersensitivity, severe hepatic impairment, pregnancy category D

Precautions: Liver toxicity, monitoring requirements for hepatic injury, women

Pharmacokinetics: Rapidly and completely absorbed, half-life 6 hr, geriatric half-life 8 hr; 94% bound to plasma proteins; excreted in urine and feces as metabolites

DENTAL CONSIDERATIONS
General:
• Talk with patient about any pain medication being taken.
• Avoid drugs (anticholinergics) that could exacerbate urinary retention (if present).

---

fluticasone propionate
(floo-tik'a-sone)
Cutivate (topical), Flonase (nasal spray), Flovent (inhaler), Flovent Rotadisk (inh powder)
Drug class.: Synthetic corticosteroid, medium potency

Action: Glucocorticoids have multiple actions that include antiinflammatory and immunosuppressant effects. They inhibit phospholipase A_2, interfering with or reducing the synthesis of prostaglandins and leukotrienes. They also bind to cytoplasmic glucocorticoid receptors (GRs) and enter the cell nucleus to bind with DNA. This results in the synthesis of various

---

bold italic = life-threatening conditions

enzymes such as collagenase, elastase, and cytokines that play important roles in inflammation and immunosuppression. They also suppress the production of lymphocytes, monocytes, and eosinophils.

Uses: Topical for inflammation of corticosteroid-responsive skin disorders, eczema; spray for seasonal and perennial allergic rhinitis; inhaler for asthma

Dosage and routes:

• *Adult:* TOP apply to affected areas bid, 0.05% cream once daily dosing; instill nasal spray, 2 sprays in each nostril once daily; initial dose can also be given in 2 equal doses bid; reduce to 1 spray for maintenance; inh 1 puff bid

• *Child >12 yr:* Instill nasal spray, 1 spray in each nostril

• *Child >4 yr:* INH breath-activated powder

Available forms include: Oint 0.005%; cream 0.05%; nasal spray 50 μg per actuation; inhaler 44, 110, 220 μg per puff; inh powder 50, 100, 250 μg

Side effects/adverse reactions:

INTEG: Burning, dryness, itching, irritation, acne, folliculitis, hypertrichosis, perioral dermatitis, hypopigmentation, atrophy, striae, miliaria, allergic contact dermatitis, secondary infections

Contraindications: Hypersensitivity, viral and fungal infections

Precautions: Pregnancy category C, lactation, bacterial infections; avoid spray in child <12 yr

DENTAL CONSIDERATIONS

General:

• Examine oral cavity for evidence of opportunistic candidiasis in patients using the spray.

• Allergic rhinitis may be a factor in mouth breathing and drying of oral tissues.

Teach patient/family:

• That use of topical preparations on herpetic ulcerations is contraindicated

• Importance of gargling, rinsing mouth with water, and expectorating after each aerosol use

---

fluvastatin sodium

(floo′va-sta-tin)

Lescol, Lescol XL

Drug class.: Cholesterol-lowering agent, antihyperlipidemic

Action: Inhibits HMG-CoA reductase enzyme, which reduces cholesterol synthesis; reduced synthesis of VLDL; plasma triglyceride levels may also be decreased

Uses: As an adjunct in homozygous familial hypercholesterolemia, mixed hyperlipidemia, elevated serum triglyceride levels and type IV hyperproteinemia, also reduces total cholesterol LDL-C, apo B and triglyceride levels; patient should first be placed on cholesterol-lowering diet

Dosage and routes:

• *Adult:* PO initial 20-40 mg/day hs; dosage range 20-80 mg/d; ext rel tabs 80 mg as starting dose. With larger goal for LDL reduction 80 mg/day hs can be used.

Available forms include: Caps 20, 40 mg; ext rel tabs 80 mg

Side effects/adverse reactions:

▼ *ORAL:* Taste alteration (rare)

CNS: Fatigue, headache, dizziness, insomnia

GI: **Nausea, diarrhea, dyspepsia, abdominal pain, constipation, flatulence,** elevated transaminase levels

RESP: Upper respiratory infection, bronchitis, coughing

GU: Decreased libido

EENT: Rhinitis, sinusitis, pharyngitis

INTEG: Rash, pruritus

MS: Muscle pain, back pain, arthropathy, **rhabdomyolysis,** *myopathy*

MISC: Photosensitivity, **anaphylaxis**

Contraindications: Hypersensitivity, active liver disease, pregnancy, lactation, child <18 yr

Precautions: Pregnancy category X; liver dysfunction; alcoholism; severe acute infection; metabolic, endocrine, or electrolyte disorders; uncontrolled seizures; alterations in liver function tests may be observed with use

Pharmacokinetics:

PO: Good absorption; first-pass metabolism; highly protein bound, hepatic metabolism; excreted in feces

Drug interactions of concern to dentistry:

• No specific interactions reported but (as with other drugs in this class) should not be used with erythromycin, itraconazole, or cyclosporine

DENTAL CONSIDERATIONS

General:

• Consider semisupine chair position for patient comfort due to GI, musculoskeletal, and respiratory side effects.

fluvoxamine maleate

(floo-vox′a-meen)

Luvox

Drug class.: Selective serotonin reuptake inhibitor, antidepressant

Action: Selectively inhibits the reuptake of serotonin in CNS neurons

Uses: Obsessive-compulsive disorder and panic disorder

Dosage and routes:

• *Adult:* PO initial dose 50 mg hs, increase by 50 mg increments slowly q4-7d as required in 2 divided doses; limit 300 mg/day

• *Child 8-17 yr:* PO 25 mg hs; can increase dose in 25 mg increments q 4-7 days in two divided doses, limit 200 mg/day

Available forms include: Tabs 25, 50, 100 mg

Side effects/adverse reactions:

▼ *ORAL: Dry mouth,* dysphagia, increased salivation (rare)

CNS: Somnolence, asthenia, nervousness, dizziness, headache, agitation, anxiety, suicidal ideation, anorexia

CV: Postural hypotension, palpitation, hypertension, syncope, tachycardia

GI: Nausea, dyspepsia, diarrhea

GU: Sexual dysfunction

RESP: Dyspnea

MS: Dystonic symptoms

Contraindications: Hypersensitivity, MAO inhibitors, alcohol

Precautions: Pregnancy category C, lactation, renal and hepatic impairment, epilepsy

Pharmacokinetics:

PO: Rapid absorption, peak plasma

---

bold italic = life-threatening conditions

levels 5 hr; plasma protein binding 77%; hepatic metabolism; urinary excretion

🦷 Drug interactions of concern to dentistry:

• Increased plasma levels of tricyclic antidepressants, carbamazepine, benzodiazepine; reduce doses of alprazolam, diazepam, midazolam, and triazolam by one half

DENTAL CONSIDERATIONS
General:

• After supine positioning, have patient sit upright for at least 2 min to avoid orthostatic hypotension.

• Assess salivary flow as a factor in caries, periodontal disease, and candidiasis.

• Consider semisupine chair position for patient comfort due to GI effects of drug.

Consultations:

• Medical consult may be required to assess patient's ability to tolerate stress.

• Physician should be informed if significant xerostomic side effects occur (increased caries, sore tongue, problems eating or swallowing, difficulty wearing prosthesis) so a medication change can be considered.

Teach patient/family:

When chronic dry mouth occurs, advise patient:

• To avoid mouth rinses with high alcohol content due to drying effects

• To use daily home fluoride products for anticaries effect

• To use sugarless gum, frequent sips of water, or saliva substitutes

folic acid (vitamin B₉)
(foe′lic)
Folvite
♣ Apo-Folic, Novo-Folacid

Drug class.: Water-soluble B vitamin

Action: Needed for erythropoiesis; increases RBC, WBC, and platelet formation in megaloblastic anemias

Uses: Megaloblastic or macrocytic anemia caused by folic acid deficiency; liver disease; alcoholism; hemolysis; intestinal obstruction; pregnancy

Dosage and routes:

Chemical supplement
• *Adult:* PO/IM/SC 0.1 mg qd
• *Child:* PO 0.05 mg qd

Megaloblastic/macrocytic anemia
• *Adult and child >4 yr:* PO/SC/IM 1 mg qd × 4-5 days
• *Child <4 yr:* PO/SC/IM 0.3 mg or less qd
• *Infant* PO/SC/IM 0.1 mg qd
• *Pregnancy/lactation:* PO/SC/IM 0.8 mg qd

Prevention of megaloblastic/macrocytic anemia
• *Pregnancy:* PO/SC/IM 1 mg qd

Available forms include: Tabs 0.4, 0.8, 1 mg; inj SC/IM 5 mg/ml

Side effects/adverse reactions:

RESP: Bronchospasm (rare allergic reaction)

Contraindications: Hypersensitivity, anemias other than megaloblastic/macrocytic anemia, vitamin B₁₂ deficiency anemia

Precautions: Pregnancy category A

---

italic = common side effects

Pharmacokinetics:

PO: Peak 0.5-1 hr; bound to plasma proteins; excreted in breast milk; methylated in liver; excreted in urine (small amounts)

🦷 Drug interactions of concern to dentistry:

• Increased metabolism of phenobarbital

DENTAL CONSIDERATIONS

General:

• Deficiency in folic acid; glossitis may be a symptom of folic acid deficiency.

---

formoterol fumarate inhalation powder

(for-moh'te-rol)

Foradil Aerolizer

Drug class.: Selective B$_2$-adrenergic bronchodilator

Action: A long-acting, selective B$_2$-adrenergic agonist that acts locally in the lung as a bronchodilator, resulting in bronchial smooth muscle relaxation and inhibition of release of inflammatory mediators

Uses: Long-term treatment of asthma and prevention of bronchospasm in adults and children >5 yr; prevention of exercise-induced bronchospasm in adults and children >12 yr

Dosage and routes:

Maintenance treatment of asthma

• *Adult and child >5 yr:* INH: Inhale the contents of one capsule (12 µg) q12h using the Aerolizer Inhaler System, do not exceed this dose; not for oral use

Prevention of exercise-induced bronchospasm (EIB)

• *Adult and child >12 yr:* INH: Inhale the contents of one capsule (12 µg) 15 min before exercise, administered on prn basis

Available forms include: Caps 12 µg for use only by inhalation in the Aerolizer Inhaler System

Side effects/adverse reactions:

▼ *ORAL:* Dry mouth, irritation of mouth and throat, taste alteration

CNS: Tremor, *dizziness, insomnia,* nervousness, headache

CV: Angina, hypertension, tachycardia, arrhythmias, palpitation

GI: Nausea, dyspepsia, abdominal pain, vomiting

RESP: Bronchitis, URI, dyspnea, exacerbation of asthma, coughing

EENT: Tonsillitis

INTEG: Rash, urticaria

META: Hypokalemia, hyperglycemia, metabolic acidosis

MISC: Viral infection, ***immediate hypersensitivity reaction (anaphylaxis), angioedema***

Contraindications: Hypersensitivity

Precautions: Not for acute asthma symptoms, not for use in life-threatening situations; paradoxical bronchospasm may occur with use; not a substitute for corticosteroids; cardiovascular disease (coronary insufficiency, cardiac arrhythmias, hypertension), hyperthyroidism, seizures, hypokalemia, pregnancy category C, lactation

Pharmacokinetics:

INH: Rapid absorption, peak plasma levels 5 min; plasma protein binding 61%-64%; extensive hepatic metabolism, excreted mostly in urine (62%) and in feces (34%), onset 1-3 min, peak effects 2 hr with duration 8-12 hr

🦷 Drug interactions of concern to dentistry:

• Avoid MAO inhibitors, tricyclic

---

bold italic = life-threatening conditions

antidepressants, or drugs that prolong the QT interval

DENTAL CONSIDERATIONS

General:

• Monitor vital signs every appointment due to cardiovascular side effects.

• Assess salivary flow as a factor in caries, periodontal disease, and candidiasis.

• Consider semisupine chair position for patient comfort due to respiratory side effects of disease.

• Short midday appointments and a stress reduction protocol may be required for anxious patients.

• Have patient bring personal short-acting bronchodilator to appointment for use in emergency.

• Acute asthmatic episodes may be precipitated in the dental office. Rapid-acting sympathomimetic inhalants should be available for emergency use.

• Avoid prescribing aspirin-containing products.

Consultations:

• Medical consult may be required to assess disease control.

• Medical consult may be required to assess disease control and patient's ability to tolerate stress.

Teach patient/family:

• Importance of gargling, rinsing mouth with water, and expectorating after each aerosol dose

When chronic dry mouth occurs, advise patient:

• To avoid mouth rinses with high alcohol content due to drying effects

• To use daily home fluoride products for anticaries effect

• To use sugarless gum, frequent sips of water, or saliva substitutes

foscarnet sodium/ phosphonoformic acid

(foss-car'net)

Foscavir

Drug class.: Antiviral

Action: Antiviral activity is produced by selective inhibition at the pyrophosphate binding site of viral DNA polymerase, preventing replication of herpes simplex virus (HSV)

Uses: Treatment of cytomegalovirus (CMV) retinitis in AIDS; unapproved: life-threatening CMV disease, acyclovir-resistant herpes simplex I mucocutaneous diseases, and acyclovir-resistant HSV in immunocompromised patients

Dosage and routes:

• *Adult:* IV inf 60 mg/kg given over at least 1 hr q8h × 2-3 wk initially, then 90-120 mg/kg/day over 2 hr

HSV

• *Adult:* IV inf 40 mg/kg bid × 3 wk

Available forms include: Inj 24 mg/ml in 250, 500 ml bottles

Side effects/adverse reactions:

▼ *ORAL:* Glossitis, stomatitis, facial edema, dry mouth, ulcerative stomatitis, taste perversion

CNS: **Seizures, coma, paralysis, tetany,** fever, dizziness, headache, fatigue, neuropathy, tremor, ataxia, dementia, stupor, EEG abnormalities, vertigo, abnormal gait, hypertonia, extrapyramidal disorders, hemiparesis, hyperreflexia paraplegia, hyporeflexia, neuralgia, neuritis, cerebral edema, paresthesia, depression, confusion, anxiety, insomnia, somnolence, amnesia, hallucinations, agitation

*CV: **Cardiac arrest,*** hypertension, palpitations, ECG abnormalities, first-degree AV block, nonspecific ST-T segment changes, hypotension, cerebrovascular disorder, cardiomyopathy, bradycardia, dysrhythmias

*GI: **Pseudomembranous colitis, paralytic ileus, esophageal ulceration, hepatitis,*** nausea, vomiting, anorexia, abdominal pain, constipation, dysphagia, rectal hemorrhage, melena, flatulence, pancreatitis, enteritis, enterocolitis, proctitis, increased amylases, gastroenteritis, duodenal ulcer, abnormal A-G ratio, increased AST/ALT, cholecystitis, dyspepsia, tenesmus, hepatosplenomegaly, jaundice

*RESP: **Pulmonary infiltration, pneumothorax, hemoptysis, bronchospasm, respiratory depression, pleural effusion, pulmonary hemorrhage,*** rhinitis, coughing, dyspnea, pneumonia, sinusitis, pharyngitis, bronchitis, stridor

*HEMA: **Granulocytopenia, leukopenia, thrombocytopenia, thrombosis, pulmonary embolism, coagulation disorders, decreased prothrombin, hypochromic anemia, pancytopenia, hemolysis, leukocytosis,*** lymphadenopathy, epistaxis, lymphopenia, anemia, platelet abnormalities

*GU: **Acute renal failure, glomerulonephritis, toxic nephropathy, nephrosis, renal tubular disorders, pyelonephritis, uremia, hematuria, albuminuria,*** dysuria, polyuria, decreased CCr, increased serum creatinine

EENT: Visual field defects, vocal cord paralysis, speech disorders, eye pain, conjunctivitis, tinnitus, otitis

INTEG: Rash, sweating, pruritus, skin ulceration, seborrhea, skin discoloration, alopecia, acne, dermatitis, pain/inflammation at injection site, facial edema, dry skin, urticaria

MS: Arthralgia, myalgia

*SYST: **Sepsis, death, ascites,*** hypokalemia, hypocalcemia, hypomagnesemia, increased alk phosphatase, LDH, BUN, acidosis, hypophosphatemia, hyperphosphatemia, dehydration, glycosuria, increased creatine phosphokinase, hypervolemia, infection, hyponatremia, hypochloremia, hypercalcemia

Contraindications: Hypersensitivity

Precautions: Pregnancy category C, lactation, children, elderly, renal disease, seizure disorders, electrolyte/mineral imbalances, severe anemia

Pharmacokinetics:
IV: Half-life 2-8 hr in normal renal function; 14%-17% plasma protein bound

🥄 Drug interactions of concern to dentistry:
• No specific interactions, but nephrotoxic drugs (acyclovir) should be avoided

DENTAL CONSIDERATIONS
General:
• Examine for oral manifestations of opportunistic infections.
• Examine for evidence of oral manifestations of blood dyscrasias (infection, bleeding, poor healing).
• Consider local hemostasis measures to prevent excessive bleeding.
• Assess salivary flow as a factor in caries, periodontal disease, and candidiasis.
• Monitor vital signs every appointment due to cardiovascular and respiratory side effects.

---

bold italic = life-threatening conditions

• Place on frequent recall to evaluate healing response.

Consultations:

• Medical consult for blood studies (CBC); leukopenic or thrombocytopenic side effects may result in infection, delayed healing, and excessive bleeding. Postpone elective dental treatment until normal values are maintained.

• Medical consult may be required to assess disease control.

Teach patient/family:

• Caution in use of oral hygiene aids to prevent injury

• That secondary oral infection may occur; must see dentist immediately if infection occurs

• Importance of good oral hygiene to prevent soft tissue inflammation

• Use of electric toothbrush if patient has difficulty holding conventional devices due to extrapyramidal side effects

When chronic dry mouth occurs, advise patient:

• To avoid mouth rinses with high alcohol content due to drying effects

• To use daily home fluoride products for anticaries effect

• To use sugarless gum, frequent sips of water, or saliva substitutes

---

fosfomycin tromethamine

(fos-foe-mye′sin)
Monurol

Drug class.: Antiinfective (phosphonic acid derivative)

Action: Broad-spectrum and bactericidal against a wide range of gram-positive aerobic microorganisms associated with GU infections; inactivates the enzyme diphosphate acetylglucosamine to interfere with cell wall synthesis

Uses: Uncomplicated UTIs in women due to susceptible strains of *E. coli* and *Enterococcus faecalis*

Dosage and routes:

• *Women >18 yr:* PO one sachet with or without food; mix contents of one sachet with water to take

Available forms include: Sachet 3 g

Side effects/adverse reactions:

▼ *ORAL:* Dry mouth (<1%)

CNS: Headache, dizziness, migraine, somnolence

GI: Diarrhea, nausea, dyspepsia

RESP: Asthma (rare)

HEMA: **Angioedema (rare), aplastic anemia**

GU: Vaginitis

EENT: Rhinitis, pharyngitis

INTEG: Rash

ENDO: Menstrual disorder

MS: Asthenia, myalgia

MISC: Fever

Contraindications: Hypersensitivity

Precautions: Renal impairment, one dose per single episode of cystitis, pregnancy category B, lactation, children <12 yr

Pharmacokinetics:

PO: Peak plasma levels >2 hr; not plasma protein bound; widely distributed to GU tissues; excreted unchanged in urine and feces

 Drug interactions of concern to dentistry:

• Lowered serum concentrations: metoclopramide

DENTAL CONSIDERATIONS

General:

• Determine why patient is taking the drug.

• Consider semisupine chair position for patient comfort if GI side effects occur.

Teach patient/family:

When chronic dry mouth occurs, advise patient:

• To avoid mouth rinses with high alcohol content due to drying effects

• To use daily home fluoride products for anticaries effect

• To use sugarless gum, frequent sips of water, or saliva substitutes

---

fosinopril

(foe-sin′oh-pril)

Monopril

Drug class.: Angiotension-converting enzyme (ACE) inhibitor

Action: Selectively suppresses renin-angiotensin-aldosterone system; inhibits ACE; prevents conversion of angiotensin I to angiotensin II; results in dilation of arterial, venous vessels

Uses: Hypertension, alone or in combination with thiazide diuretics

Dosage and routes:

• *Adult:* PO 10 mg qd initially, then 20-40 mg/day divided bid or qd

Available forms include: Tabs 10, 20 mg

Side effects/adverse reactions:

▼ *ORAL:* Taste disturbances, angioedema (lips, tongue), dry mouth

CNS: Insomnia, paresthesia, headache, dizziness, fatigue, memory disturbance, tremor, mood change

CV: Hypotension, chest pain, palpitation, angina, orthostatic hypotension

GI: Nausea, constipation, vomiting, diarrhea

RESP: Bronchospasm, cough, sinusitis, dyspnea

HEMA: Eosinophilia, leukopenia, neutropenia, decreased Hct/Hgb

GU: Proteinuria, increased BUN/creatinine, decreased libido

INTEG: Angioedema, rash, flushing, sweating, photosensitivity, pruritus

MS: Arthralgia, myalgia

META: Hyperkalemia

Contraindications: Hypersensitivity to ACE inhibitors, pregnancy category D, lactation, children

Precautions: Impaired liver function, hypovolemia, blood dyscrasias, CHF, COPD, asthma, elderly

Pharmacokinetics:

PO: Onset 1 hr, peak 3 hr, half-life 12 hr; serum protein binding 97%; metabolized by liver; metabolites excreted in urine, feces

🦷 **Drug interactions of concern to dentistry:**

• Increased hypotension: alcohol, phenothiazines

• Decreased hypotensive effects: indomethacin and possibly other NSAIDs, sympathomimetics

DENTAL CONSIDERATIONS

General:

• Monitor vital signs every appointment due to cardiovascular and respiratory side effects.

• After supine positioning, have patient sit upright for at least 2 min before standing to avoid orthostatic hypotension.

• Patients on chronic drug therapy may rarely have symptoms of blood dyscrasias, which can include infection, bleeding, and poor healing.

• Assess salivary flow as a factor in caries, periodontal disease, and candidiasis.

• Limit use of sodium-containing products such as saline IV fluids for patients with a dietary salt restriction.

• Stress from dental procedures may compromise cardiovascular function; determine patient risk.

• Short appointments and a stress reduction protocol may be required for anxious patients.

Consultations:

• Medical consult may be required to assess disease control and patient's ability to tolerate stress.

• In a patient with symptoms of blood dyscrasias, request a medical consult for blood studies and postpone dental treatment until normal values are reestablished.

• Take precautions if dental surgery is anticipated and sedation or general anesthesia is required (risk of hypotensive episode).

Teach patient/family:

• Importance of good oral hygiene to prevent soft tissue inflammation

• Caution to prevent injury when using oral hygiene aids

When chronic dry mouth occurs, advise patient:

• To avoid mouth rinses with high alcohol content due to drying effects

• To use daily home fluoride products for anticaries effect

• To use sugarless gum, frequent sips of water, or saliva substitutes

---

fosphenytoin sodium
(fos'fen-i-toyn)
Cerebyx

Drug class.: Hydantoin-anticonvulsant

Action: Prodrug converted to phenytoin after injection; phenytoin inhibits spread of seizure activity in motor cortex

Uses: Control of generalized convulsive status epilepticus; prevention and treatment of seizures during neurosurgery; short-term substitute for oral phenytoin

Dosage and routes:

• *Adult:* IV loading dose, 15-20 mg phenytoin sodium equivalents (PE/kg) at 100-150 mg PE/min; effect is not immediate, may require use of IV benzodiazepine

• *Adult:* IV maintenance dose, IM 4-6 mg/PE/kg per day

Substitution for oral phenytoin

• *Adult:* IV, IM at the same total daily dose for phenytoin

Available forms include: Inj 10 ml (750 mg of fosphenytoin sodium equivalent to 500 mg phenytoin); 2 ml (150 mg of fosphenytoin equivalent to 100 mg of phenytoin)

Side effects/adverse reactions:

▼ *ORAL:* Dry mouth, taste perversion, gingival overgrowth

CNS: Nystagmus, dizziness, paresthesia, headache, somnolence, ataxia, tremor, extrapyramidal syndrome

CV: Hypotension, bradycardia, vasodilation, tachycardia

GI: Nausea, vomiting, constipation

HEMA: **Thrombocytopenia, anemia, leukopenia,** petechia

EENT: Tinnitus, diplopia

INTEG: Pruritus, rash

MS: Asthenia, back pain

META: Hypokalemia

Contraindications: Hypersensitivity to hydantoin drugs; sinus bradycardia, S-A block, second- and third-degree AV block; Adams-Stokes syndrome, abrupt discontinuation

Precautions: IV–do not exceed injection rate of 150 mg PE/min, risk of seizures with abrupt withdrawal; hypotension, severe myocardial insufficiency, phosphate restriction; thyroid, renal, or hepatic disease; elderly, pregnancy category D, lactation, pediatric use

Pharmacokinetics:
IV: Highly protein bound (95%-99%); converted to phenytoin; metabolized in liver; renal excretion
IM: Completely bioavailable, peak levels 30 min

🐝 Drug interactions of concern to dentistry:
• Increased phenytoin levels: benzodiazepines (chlordiazepoxide, diazepam), halothane, salicylates
• Increased CNS depression: benzodiazepines, H_1-blocker antihistamines, opiate agonists
• Decreased phenytoin levels: carbamazepine
• Decreased effectiveness of corticosteroids

DENTAL CONSIDERATIONS
General:
• This drug is intended for short-term use in an emergency department or hospital setting. Patient will probably return to oral phenytoin or other anticonvulsant after hospital care.
• Use precaution if sedation or general anesthesia is required; risk of hypotensive episode.

Consultations:
• Determine type of epilepsy, seizure frequency, and quality of seizure control. A stress reduction protocol may be required.
• Medical consult may be required to assess disease control and patient's ability to tolerate stress.

Teach patient/family:
• Importance of updating health and drug history if physician makes any changes in evaluation or drug regimens

frovatriptan succinate
(froe-va-trip′tan)
Frova
Drug class.: Serotonin agonist

Action: A selective serotonin agonist for $5\text{-}HT_{1D}$ and $5\text{-}HT_{1B}$ serotonin receptors on intracranial blood vessels
Uses: Acute treatment of migraine with or without aura

Dosage and routes:
• *Adult:* PO 2.5 mg
Available forms include: Tabs 2.5 mg

Side effects/adverse reactions: Limited information, side effect profile unavailable at publication time

Contraindications: Hypersensitivity, ischemic heart disease (angina, MI), Prinzmetal's variant angina, uncontrolled hypertension within 24 hr of use of ergotamine or other $5HT_1$ agonist, hemiplegic or basilar migraine, prophylactic therapy of migraine, Wolff-Parkinson-White syndrome, accessory conduction arrhythmias, MAOIs

Precautions: Renal impairment, hypertension, coronary artery disease, hypercholesterolemia, smokers, diabetes mellitus, men >40 yr, asthma, allergies, pregnancy category C, lactation, children, serotonin syndrome

Pharmacokinetics:
PO: Peak blood levels 2-4 hr; bioavailability 24%-30%; hepatic metabolism; urinary excretion

🐝 Drug interactions of concern to dentistry:
• Potential serotonin crisis: SSRIs, ergot-containing drugs (avoid use within 24 hr of taking this drug)

---

bold italic = life-threatening conditions

• Decreased plasma levels: cimetidine

DENTAL CONSIDERATIONS
General:
• This is an acute-use drug; it is doubtful that patients will present for dental treatment during acute migraine attacks.
• Be aware of patient's disease, its severity, and frequency, when known.
• Advise patient if dental drugs prescribed have a potential for photosensitivity.

Consultations:
• If treating chronic orofacial pain, consult with physician of record.
• Medical consult may be required to assess disease control and patient's ability to tolerate stress.

Teach patient/family:
• That dryness of the mouth may occur when taking this drug; avoid mouth rinses with high alcohol content due to additional drying effects
• Importance of updating health and drug history if physician makes any changes in evaluation or drug regimens

---

furosemide

(fur-oh'se-mide)
Furoside, Lasix, Lasix Special, Myrosemide
♣ Apo-Furosemide, Novosemide, Uritol
Drug class.: Loop diuretic

Action: Acts on loop of Henle to decrease the reabsorption of chloride and sodium with resultant diuresis
Uses: Pulmonary edema, edema in CHF, liver disease, nephrotic syndrome, ascites, hypertension

Dosage and routes:
• *Adult:* PO 20-80 mg/day in AM, may give another dose in 6 hr, up to 600 mg/day; IM/IV 20-40 mg, increased by 20 mg q2h until desired response
• *Child:* PO/IM/IV 2 mg/kg, may increase by 1-2 mg/kg q6-8h up to 6 mg/kg
Pulmonary edema
• *Adult:* IV 40 mg given over several minutes, repeated in 1 hr; increase to 80 mg if needed
Available forms include: Tabs 20, 40, 80 mg; oral sol 10 mg/ml, 40 mg/5 ml; inj IM/IV 10 mg/ml
Side effects/adverse reactions:
▼ *ORAL:* Dry mouth, increased thirst, lichenoid drug reaction
CNS: Headache, fatigue, weakness, vertigo, paresthesia
CV: **Circulatory collapse,** orthostatic hypotension, chest pain, ECG changes
GI: Nausea, diarrhea, vomiting, anorexia, cramps, gastric irritations, pancreatitis
HEMA: **Thrombocytopenia, agranulocytosis, leukopenia, neutropenia, anemia**
GU: Polyuria, **renal failure,** glycosuria
EENT: Loss of hearing, ear pain, tinnitus, blurred vision
INTEG: **Rash, pruritus, Stevens-Johnson syndrome,** purpura, sweating, photosensitivity, urticaria
ENDO: **Hyperglycemia**
MS: Cramps, arthritis, stiffness
ELECT: Hypokalemia, hypochloremic alkalosis, hypomagnesemia, hyperuricemia, hypocalcemia, hyponatremia
Contraindications: Hypersensitivity to sulfonamides, anuria, hy-

povolemia, infants, lactation, electrolyte depletion

Precautions: Diabetes mellitus, dehydration, ascites, severe renal disease, pregnancy category C

Pharmacokinetics:

PO: Onset 1 hr, peak 1-2 hr, duration 6-8 hr

IV: Onset 5 min, peak 0.5 hr, duration 2 hr

Excreted in urine, feces, breast milk; crosses placenta

⚷ Drug interactions of concern to dentistry:

• Increased electrolyte imbalance: corticosteroids

• Masked ototoxicity: phenothiazines

• Decreased antihypertensive effect: NSAIDs, especially indomethacin

DENTAL CONSIDERATIONS
General:

• Monitor vital signs every appointment due to cardiovascular side effects.

• Patients on chronic drug therapy may rarely have symptoms of blood dyscrasias, which can include infection, bleeding, and poor healing.

• Assess salivary flow as a factor in caries, periodontal disease, and candidiasis.

• After supine positioning, have patient sit upright for at least 2 min before standing to avoid orthostatic hypotension.

• Patients on high-potency diuretics should be monitored for serum K⁺ levels.

Consultations:

• In a patient with symptoms of blood dyscrasias, request a medical consult for blood studies and postpone dental treatment until normal values are reestablished.

• Medical consult may be required to assess disease control.

Teach patient/family:

• Importance of good oral hygiene to prevent soft tissue inflammation

• Caution to prevent injury when using oral hygiene aids

When chronic dry mouth occurs, advise patient:

• To use daily home fluoride products for anticaries effect

• To avoid mouth rinses with high alcohol content due to drying effects

• To use sugarless gum, frequent sips of water, or saliva substitutes

---

gabapentin

(ga′ba-pen-tin)

Neurontin

Drug class.: Anticonvulsant

Action: Anticonvulsant action is unclear

Uses: Adjunctive therapy in patients 12 yr or older with partial seizures with or without secondary generalization and as adjunctive therapy for partial seizures in children 3-12 yr; unlabeled use neuropathic pain, bipolar disorder, migraine prophylaxis, tremors of multiple sclerosis

Dosage and routes:

• *Adult and child >12 yr:* PO titration to 900-1800 mg/day in 3 equal doses; start 300 mg on day 1, 300 mg bid on day 2, 300 mg tid on day 3, can be increased to 1800 mg/day with titration of doses; doses up to 3600 mg/day have been used

• *Child 3-12 yr:* PO initial dose 10 mg to 15 mg/dg/day in 3 equal doses; titrated dose upward over 3-day period

Available forms include: Caps 100, 300, 400 mg; tabs 600 mg; oral sol 250 mg/5 ml

Side effects/adverse reactions:

▼ *ORAL:* Dry mouth, glossitis, gingivitis, stomatitis (infrequent)

CNS: Somnolence, dizziness, ataxia, fatigue, nystagmus

CV: Hypertension, palpitation, tachycardia

GI: Dyspepsia, constipation

RESP: Pharyngitis, coughing

HEMA: Leukopenia, purpura

GU: Impotence

EENT: Rhinitis, blurred vision

INTEG: Pruritus

MS: Myalgia

MISC: Edema

Contraindications: Hypersensitivity

Precautions: Pregnancy category C, lactation, renal function impairment, children <12 yr, elderly

Pharmacokinetics: Bioavailability decreases as dose increases; low protein binding 3%; renal excretion primary

🦷 Drug interactions of concern to dentistry:

• None reported at this time, but, because CNS side effects are common, the use of anxiolytic sedative drugs may potentially increase the CNS side effects.

DENTAL CONSIDERATIONS

General:

• Early-morning appointments and a stress reduction protocol may be required for anxious patients.

• Place on frequent recall due to oral side effects.

• Monitor vital signs every appointment due to cardiovascular side effects.

• Assess salivary flow as a factor in caries, periodontal disease, and candidiasis.

• Determine type of epilepsy and quality of seizure control.

Consultations:

• Medical consult may be required to assess disease control.

• Medical consult may be required to assess patient's ability to tolerate stress.

Teach patient/family:

• Importance of good oral hygiene to prevent soft tissue inflammation

• Caution in use of oral hygiene aids to prevent injury

When chronic dry mouth occurs, advise patient:

• To avoid mouth rinses with high alcohol content due to drying effects

• To use daily home fluoride products for anticaries effect

• To use sugarless gum, frequent sips of water, or saliva substitutes

---

galantamine (HBr)

(ga-lan'ta-meen)

Reminyl

Drug class.: Cholinesterase inhibitor

Action: Exact mechanism unclear, but it is thought to be a competitive, long-acting, and reversible inhibitor of acetylcholinesterase enzyme; inhibits acetylcholinesterase activity at peripheral and central cholinergic synapses and in PNS; potentiates nicotinic receptor response to acetylcholine

Uses: Mild to moderate dementia of Alzheimer's disease

Dosage and routes:

• *Adult:* PO starting dose is 4 mg bid; increase dose to 8 mg bid after a 4-wk minimum treatment period; increases to 12 mg bid should be attempted only after a minimum of

4 wk; increase dose only if the lower dose is tolerated; dose range 16-24 mg/day in two equal doses preferably with AM and PM meals; with moderate renal or hepatic impairment dose should not exceed 16 mg/day (severe impairment do not use)

Available forms include: Tabs 4, 8, 12 mg

Side effects/adverse reactions:

CNS: Anorexia, dizziness, headache, tremor, depression, insomnia, somnolence, agitation, confusion, fatigue

CV: Syncope, bradycardia, peripheral edema, chest pain

GI: Nausea, vomiting, diarrhea, abdominal pain, dyspepsia, constipation, flatulence

RESP: URI, bronchitis

HEMA: Anemia

GU: UTI, hematuria, incontinence

EENT: Rhinitis

ENDO: Weight loss, sweating

Contraindications: Hypersensitivity, severe hepatic or renal impairment

Precautions: Potentiation of succinylcholine-like neuromuscular blocking drugs, obstructive GI disease, Parkinson's disease, epilepsy, cardiac conduction disorders, AV block, bradycardia, history of GI ulcer, hypersecretory disorders (gastric), bladder outflow obstruction, COPD, asthma, moderate hepatic impairment, moderate renal impairment, pregnancy category B, lactation, pediatric use

Pharmacokinetics:

PO Absolute bioavailability ~90%, peak plasma levels 1 hr, plasma protein binding 18%; hepatic metabolism (CYP450 2D6 and CYP450 3A4); unchanged drug and glucuronate metabolites, excreted in urine

⚖ Drug interactions of concern to dentistry:

• Increased plasma levels: ketoconazole

• Increased bioavailability: cimetidine, paroxetine

• Enhanced succinylcholine muscle relaxation during anesthesia

• Action may be inhibited by anticholinergic drugs or enhanced by cholinergic agonists

DENTAL CONSIDERATIONS

General:

• Monitor vital signs every appointment due to cardiovascular side effects.

• After supine positioning, have patient sit upright for 2 or more minutes to avoid orthostatic hypotension.

• Drug is used early in the disease; ensure that patient or caregiver understands informed consent.

• Place on frequent recall because early attention to dental health is important for Alzheimer's patients.

• Consider semisupine chair position for patient comfort if GI side effects occur.

Consultations:

• Consultation with physician may be needed if sedation or general anesthesia is required.

• Medical consult may be required to assess disease control and patient's ability to tolerate stress.

Teach patient/family:

• Importance of good oral hygiene to prevent soft tissue inflammation

• To assist patient or caregiver with oral home-care regimen as cognitive ability declines

---

bold italic = life-threatening conditions

• Use of electric toothbrush if patient has difficulty holding conventional devices
• Importance of updating health and drug history if physician makes any changes in evaluation or drug regimens

ganciclovir

(gan-sye'kloe-veer)
Cytovene, Cytovene IV, DHPG, Vitrasert implant

Drug class.: Antiviral, nucleoside analog

Action: Inhibits replication of most herpes viruses in vitro; phosphorylated by CMV protein kinase to triphosphate forms; inhibits viral DNA polymerase and is incorporated into viral DNA, resulting in termination of elongation of viral DNA

Uses: Prevention and treatment of CMV retinitis in patients with AIDS or organ transplants; life-threatening CMV disease and CMV polyradiculopathy in patients with AIDS

Dosage and routes:
Induction treatment
• *Adult:* IV 5 mg/kg given over 1 hr, q12h × 2-3 wk
Maintenance treatment
• *Adult:* IV inf 5 mg/kg given over 1 hr, qd × 7 days/wk; or 6 mg/kg qd × 5 days/wk; dosage must be reduced in renal impairment
• *Adult:* PO 1000 mg tid with food or 500 mg q3h (for 6 doses) during waking hours and with food
Available forms include: Caps 250, 500 mg; vials 500 mg; intraocular implant 4.5 mg

Side effects/adverse reactions:
*CNS: Fever, **coma,** chills,* confusion, abnormal thoughts, dizziness, bizarre dreams, headache, psychosis, tremors, somnolence, paresthesia
CV: Dysrhythmia, hypertension/hypotension
*GI: Abnormal LFTs, **hemorrhage,*** nausea, vomiting, anorexia, diarrhea, abdominal pain
RESP: Dyspnea
*HEMA: **Granulocytopenia, thrombocytopenia, irreversible neutropenia, anemia, eosinophilia***
*GU: **Hematuria,*** increased creatinine/BUN
EENT: Retinal detachment in CMV retinitis
INTEG: Rash, alopecia, pruritus, urticaria, pain at site, phlebitis

Contraindications: Hypersensitivity to acyclovir or ganciclovir
Precautions: Preexisting cytopenia, renal function impairment, pregnancy category C, lactation, children <6 mo, elderly, platelet count <25,000/mm^3

Pharmacokinetics:
PO/IV: Half-life 3-4.5 hr; excreted by the kidneys (unchanged drug); crosses blood-brain barrier

⚕ Drug interactions of concern to dentistry:
• Increased risk of blood dyscrasias: dapsone, carbamazepine, phenothiazines
• Increased risk of seizures: imipenem/cilastatin (Primaxin)
• Low platelet counts may prevent the use of aspirin, NSAIDs

DENTAL CONSIDERATIONS
General:
• Examine for oral manifestations of opportunistic infection.
• Examine for evidence of oral

manifestations of blood dyscrasias (infection, bleeding, poor healing).
• Place on frequent recall to evaluate healing response.
• Consider local hemostasis measures to prevent excessive bleeding.
• Monitor vital signs every appointment due to cardiovascular and respiratory side effects.

Consultations:
• Medical consult for blood studies (CBC); leukopenic or thrombocytopenic side effects may result in infection, delayed healing, and excessive bleeding. Postpone elective dental treatment until normal values are maintained.
• Medical consult may be required to assess disease control.

Teach patient/family:
• Caution in use of oral hygiene aids to prevent injury
• That secondary oral infection may occur; must see dentist immediately if infection occurs
• Importance of good oral hygiene to prevent soft tissue inflammation

---

gatifloxacin
(gat-i-flox′a-sin)
Tequin
Drug class.: Fluoroquinolone anti-infective

Action: A broad-spectrum bactericidal agent that inhibits the enzymes topoisomerase II (DNA gyrase) and topoisomerase IV required for bacterial DNA replication, transcription repair, and recombination
Uses: Acute bacterial exacerbation of chronic bronchitis caused by *S. pneumoniae, H. influenzae, H. parainfluenzae, M. catarrhalis,* or *S. aureus;* acute sinusitis (*S. pneu-moniae, H. influenzae*); community-acquired pneumonia (*S. pneumoniae, H. influenzae, H. parainfluenza, M. catarrhalis, M. pneumoniae, C. pneumoniae, L. pneumoniae,* or *S. aureus;* complicated or uncomplicated UTI (*E. coli, K. pneumoniae,* or *P. mirabilis*); pyelonephritis (*E. coli*), acute uncomplicated rectal infections in women or uncomplicated urethral or cervical gonorrhea (*N. gonorrhoeae*)

Dosage and routes:
Uncomplicated uretheral gonorrhae in men or rectal gonorrhae in women
• *Adult and child >18 yr:* PO or IV inf 200-400 mg qd as a single dose; for PO doses take at least 4 hr before or 8 hr after antacids (Mg^{2+}, Al^{3+}), sucralfate, metal cations (Fe^{2+}, Zn^{2+}), or didanosine

Other infections
• *Adult and child >18 yr:* PO or IV inf 200-400 mg qd for 3-14 days depending on type of infection; for PO doses take at least 4 hr before or 8 hr after antacids (Mg^{2+}, Al^{3+}), sucralfate, metal cations (Fe^{2+}, Zn^{2+}), or didanosine

Available forms include: Tabs 200, 400 mg; single-use vials 200, 400 mg; premix parenteral sol 200, 400 mg

Side effects/adverse reactions:
▼ *ORAL:* Candidiasis, glossitis, stomatitis, mouth ulcers, taste perversion
CNS: **Headache, dizziness,** insomnia, tremor, nervousness
CV: **Prolonged QT interval,** palpitation, peripheral edema, vasodilation
GI: Nausea, diarrhea, abdominal pain, antibiotic associated pseudomembranous colitis
RESP: Dyspnea, bronchospasm

HEMA: Neutropenia

GU: Vaginitis, dysuria, hematuria

EENT: Vertigo, pharyngitis, abnormal vision, tinnitus

INTEG: Rash, sweating, photosensitivity

META: Increased ALT, AST, alk phosphatase levels

MS: Back pain, chest pain, risk of tendon rupture

MISC: Injection site reactions, chills fever, allergic reaction

Contraindications: Hypersensitivity to fluoroquinolones

Precautions: Reduce dose with creatinine clearance <40 ml/min; probenecid increases half life; children <18 yr, pregnancy category C, lactation, seizure history, avoid use with class IA and III antiarrhythmics; many prolong QT interval; cross resistance with other fluoroquinolones, diabetes

Pharmacokinetics:

PO: Well absorbed, bioavailability 96%, peak plasma levels 1-2 hr, kinetics of IV dose after 1 hr inf are similar to oral doses; steady-state levels in 3 days PO or third dose IV; plasma protein binding 20%, widely distributed, limited metabolism; excreted unchanged mainly in urine

⚕ Drug interactions of concern to dentistry:

• Caution use: erythromycin and tricyclic antidepressants (no data, risk of ↑ QT interval)

• Decreased absorption: divalent and trivalent cations, iron and zinc salts

• Increased risk of CNS stimulation and seizures: NSAIDs

DENTAL CONSIDERATIONS

General:

• Determine why patient is taking the drug.

• Monitor vital signs every appointment due to cardiovascular side effects.

• Examine for oral manifestation of opportunistic infection.

• Advise patient if dental drugs prescribed have a potential for photosensitivity.

• Ruptures of the shoulder, hand, and Achilles tendons that required surgical repair or resulted in prolonged disability have been reported with the use of fluoroquinolones. Question patient about history of side effects associated with fluoroquinolone use.

Consultations:

• Physician consult is advised in the presence of an acute dental infection requiring another antibiotic.

Teach patient/family:

If used for dental infection:

• To minimize exposure to sunlight and wear sunscreen if sun exposure is planned

• To discontinue treatment and inform dentist immediately if patient experiences pain or inflammation of a tendon, and to rest and refrain from exercise

---

gemfibrozil

(jem-fi'broe-zil)

Lopid

♣ Apo-Gemfibrozil, Gen-Fibro, Novo-Gemfibrozil, Nu-Gemfibrozil

Drug class.: Antihyperlipidemic

Action: Reduces plasma triglyceride and very-low-density lipoprotein (VLDL) levels, possibly through inhibition of peripheral lipolysis and decreased hepatic extraction of free fatty acids; HDL levels increase

Uses: Types IIb, IV, V hyperlipidemia

Dosage and routes:
• *Adult:* PO 1200 mg in divided doses bid 30 min before AM and PM meals

Available forms include: Tabs 600 mg

Side effects/adverse reactions:
CNS: Dizziness, blurred vision
GI: Nausea, vomiting, dyspepsia, diarrhea, abdominal pain
HEMA: **Leukopenia, anemia, eosinophilia**
INTEG: Rash, urticaria, pruritus

Contraindications: Severe hepatic disease, preexisting gallbladder disease, severe renal disease, primary biliary cirrhosis, hypersensitivity

Precautions: Monitor hematologic and hepatic function, pregnancy category B, lactation

Pharmacokinetics:
PO: Peak 1-2 hr, half-life 1.5 hr; plasma protein binding >90%; excreted in urine; metabolized in liver

DENTAL CONSIDERATIONS
General:
• Patients on chronic drug therapy may rarely have symptoms of blood dyscrasias, which can include infection, bleeding, and poor healing.

Consultations:
• In a patient with symptoms of blood dyscrasias, request a medical consult for blood studies and postpone dental treatment until normal values are reestablished.

gentamicin sulfate (ophthalmic)
(jen-ta-mye'sin)
Garamycin Ophthalmic, Genoptic, Genoptic SOP, Gentacidin, Gentak

Drug class.: Aminoglycoside antiinfective ophthalmic

Action: Inhibits bacterial protein synthesis

Uses: Infection of external eye

Dosage and routes:
• *Adult and child:* Instill 1 gtt q4h; top apply oint to conjunctival sac bid (can use 1 gtt qh for severe infections)

Available forms include: Oint, sol 3%

Side effects/adverse reactions:
EENT: Poor corneal wound healing, temporary visual haze, overgrowth of nonsusceptible organisms

Contraindications: Hypersensitivity

Precautions: Antibiotic hypersensitivity, pregnancy category C

DENTAL CONSIDERATIONS
General:
• Avoid dental light in patient's eyes; offer dark glasses for patient comfort.
• Protect patient's eyes from accidental spatter during dental treatment.

glimepiride
(glye'me-pye-ride)
Amaryl

Drug class.: Oral antidiabetic (second generation)

Action: Causes functioning β-cells in pancreas to release insulin, lead-

---

ing to drop in blood glucose levels; may also play a role in increased sensitivity of peripheral tissues to insulin

Uses: Stable adult-onset diabetes mellitus (type II); may also be used with insulin or metformin where diet and exercise are not effective in controlling hyperglycemia

Dosage and routes:
• *Adult:* PO usual initial dose 1-2 mg once daily with breakfast or first meal of the day; maintenance dose range 1-4 mg daily; max daily dose 8 mg; adjust dose increments at no more than 2 mg every 1-2 wk

Insulin supplementation
• *Adult:* PO 8 mg daily with first main meal; start low-dose insulin and adjust dose according to patient response

Available forms include: Tabs 1, 2, 4 mg

Side effects/adverse reactions:
CNS: Dizziness, headache
GI: Nausea, abdominal pain, cholestatic jaundice, vomiting, diarrhea
*HEMA: **Leukopenia, agranulocytosis, thrombocytopenia, hemolytic anemia, pancytopenia***
EENT: Blurred vision, changes in accommodation
INTEG: Pruritus, erythema, urticaria, rash, photosensitivity
META: Hyponatremia, hypoglycemia
MISC: Asthenia

Contraindications: Hypersensitivity, diabetic ketoacidosis

Precautions: Malnourished; adrenal, pituitary, or hepatic insufficiency; hypoglycemia recognition in elderly or in those taking β-blockers; increased risk of cardiovascular mortality has been reported in patients using oral hypoglycemics; alcohol use; pregnancy category C, lactation; children

Pharmacokinetics:
PO: Good oral absorption, peak plasma levels 2-3 hr; plasma protein binding 99.5%; extensive hepatic metabolism; excreted in urine (60%) and feces (40%)

Drug interactions of concern to dentistry:
• Risk of potentiation of hypoglycemic effects: NSAIDs, salicylates, sulfonamides, β-adrenergic blockers, ketoconazole

DENTAL CONSIDERATIONS
General:
• Short appointments and a stress reduction protocol may be required for anxious patients.
• Question patient about self-monitoring of drug's antidiabetic effect, including blood glucose values or finger-stick records.
• Ensure that patient is following prescribed diet and regularly takes medication.
• Patients on chronic drug therapy may rarely have symptoms of blood dyscrasias, which can include infection, bleeding, and poor healing.
• Diabetics may be more susceptible to infection and have delayed wound healing.
• Place on frequent recall to evaluate healing response.
• Advise patient if dental drugs prescribed have a potential for photosensitivity.

Consultations:
• Medical consult may be required to assess disease control.
• In a patient with symptoms of blood dyscrasias, request a medical

consult for blood studies and post-pone treatment until normal values are reestablished.

• Medical consult may include data from patient's blood glucose monitoring, including glycosylated hemoglobin or HbA_{1c} testing.

Teach patient/family:

• Importance of good oral hygiene to prevent soft tissue inflammation

• Caution to prevent trauma when using oral hygiene aids

• Importance of updating health and drug history if physician makes any changes in evaluation or drug regimens

---

glipizide

(glip'i-zide)

Glucotrol, Glucotrol XL

Drug class.: Oral antidiabetic (second generation)

Action: Causes functioning β-cells in pancreas to release insulin, leading to drop in blood glucose levels; may improve insulin binding to insulin receptors or increase the number of insulin receptors; not effective if patient lacks functioning β-cells

Uses: Stable adult-onset diabetes mellitus (type II)

Dosage and routes:

• *Adult:* PO 5 mg/day initially, then increased to desired response; max 15 mg once-a-day dose, 40 mg/day in divided doses

• *Elderly:* PO 2.5 mg initially, then increased to desired response; max 40 mg/day in divided doses or 15 mg once-a-day dose

Available forms include: Tabs 5, 10 mg; ext rel 5, 10 mg

Side effects/adverse reactions:

CNS: Headache, weakness, dizziness, drowsiness, tinnitus, fatigue, vertigo

*GI: **Hepatotoxicity, cholestatic jaundice,*** nausea, vomiting, diarrhea, heartburn

*HEMA: **Leukopenia, thrombocytopenia, agranulocytosis, aplastic anemia,*** pancytopenia, hemolytic anemia, increased AST/ALT, alk phosphatase

INTEG: Rash, allergic reactions, pruritus, urticaria, eczema, photosensitivity, erythema

*ENDO: **Hypoglycemia***

Contraindications: Hypersensitivity to sulfonylureas, juvenile or brittle diabetes

Precautions: Pregnancy category C, elderly, cardiac disease, severe renal disease, severe hepatic disease, thyroid disease

Pharmacokinetics:

PO: Completely absorbed by GI route, onset 1-1.5 hr, duration 10-24 hr, half-life 2-4 hr; 90%-95% is plasma protein bound; metabolized in liver; excreted in urine

Drug interactions of concern to dentistry:

• Increased hypoglycemic effects: salicylates, ketoconazole

• Decreased action of glipizide: corticosteroids

• Disulfiram-like reaction: alcohol

DENTAL CONSIDERATIONS

General:

• Monitor vital signs every appointment due to cardiovascular side effects.

• Patients on chronic drug therapy may rarely have symptoms of blood dyscrasias, which can include infection, bleeding, and poor healing.

• Short appointments and a stress reduction protocol may be required for anxious patients.

• Place on frequent recall to evaluate healing response.

• Diabetics may be more susceptible to infection and have delayed wound healing.

• Question patient about self-monitoring of drug's antidiabetic effect, including blood glucose values or finger-stick records.

• Ensure that patient is following prescribed diet and regularly takes medication.

• Avoid prescribing aspirin-containing products.

Consultations:

• In a patient with symptoms of blood dyscrasias, request a medical consult for blood studies and postpone dental treatment until normal values are reestablished.

• Medical consult may be required to assess disease control.

• Medical consult may include data from patient's blood glucose monitoring, including glycosylated hemoglobin or HbA_{1c} testing.

Teach patient/family:

• Importance of good oral hygiene to prevent soft tissue inflammation

• Caution to prevent injury when using oral hygiene aids

• To avoid mouth rinses with high alcohol content due to drying effects

---

glucagon

(gloo'ka-gon)
Glucagon Emergency Kit

Drug class.: Antihypoglycemic, hormone

Action: A (rDNA) polypeptide hormone, identical to human pancreatic glucagon, that increases blood glucose and relaxes the smooth muscle of the GI tract

Uses: Severe hypoglycemia; as a diagnostic aid to facilitate in the radiologic examination of the GI tract by relaxing smooth muscle

Dosage and routes:

Severe hypoglycemia

• *Adult and child >20 kg (44 lb):* IV, SC, or IM 1 mg

• *Child <20 kg (44 lb):* IV, SC, or IM 0.5 mg; use only freshly reconstituted, water-clear solution; discard any unused quantity; do not exceed concentration of 1 mg/ml

Available forms include: Emergency and diagnostic kits: each contain 1 mg powder with 1 ml dilutent

Side effects/adverse reactions:

CV: Transient increase in blood pressure, pulse rate

GI: Nausea, vomiting

MISC: Generalized allergic reactions

Contraindications: Hypersensitivity; patients with known pheochromocytoma

Precautions: For type I diabetes give supplemental carbohydrates as soon as possible; insulinoma, starvation, glycogen depletion, adrenal insufficiency, chronic hypoglycemia, pregnancy category B, lactation

Pharmacokinetics:

PARENTERAL: Peak levels in 20 min (SC) or 13 min (IM); extensively metabolized in liver, kidney, and plasma

🥄 **Drug interactions of concern to dentistry:**

• Patients taking β-adrenergic blockers: may be expected to have a transient but greater increase in blood pressure and pulse

---

italic = common side effects

DENTAL CONSIDERATIONS
General:
• Glucagon may be used as an emergency drug for severe hypoglycemia. Patients should be closely monitored and referred immediately for evaluation.
• IV glucose may be required for patients nonresponsive to glucagon.
• Unconscious patients should awaken within 15 min or less.

---

glyburide
(glye'byoor-ide)
DiaBeta, Glynase PresTab, Micronase
✦ Albert Glyburide, Apo-Glyburide, Euglucon, Gen-Glybe, Novo-Glyburide, Nu-Glyburide

Drug class.: Oral antidiabetic (second generation)

Action: Causes functioning β-cells in pancreas to release insulin, leading to drop in blood glucose levels; may improve insulin binding to insulin receptors and increase number of insulin receptors; not effective if patient lacks functioning β-cells

Uses: Stable adult-onset diabetes mellitus (type II)

Dosage and routes:
• *Adult:* PO 2.5-5 mg/day initially, then increased to desired response; limit 20 mg/day
• *Elderly:* PO 1.25 mg initially, then increased to desired response; max 20 mg/day; maintenance 1.25-20 mg qd
Available forms include: Tabs 1.25, 1.5, 2.5, 3, 4.5, 5, 6 mg

Side effects/adverse reactions:
*CNS: **Headache, weakness,*** paresthesia, tinnitus, fatigue, vertigo

*GI: **Hepatotoxicity, cholestatic jaundice,*** nausea, fullness, heartburn, vomiting, diarrhea
*HEMA: **Leukopenia, thrombocytopenia, agranulocytosis, aplastic anemia,*** increased AST/ALT, alk phosphatase
INTEG: Rash, allergic reactions, pruritus, urticaria, eczema, photosensitivity, erythema
*ENDO: **Hypoglycemia***
MS: Joint pains

Contraindications: Hypersensitivity to sulfonylureas, juvenile or brittle diabetes

Precautions: Pregnancy category B, elderly, cardiac disease, severe renal disease, severe hepatic disease, thyroid disease, severe hypoglycemia reactions

Pharmacokinetics:
PO: Completely absorbed by GI route, onset 2-4 hr, peak 2-8 hr, duration 24 hr, half-life 10 hr; 90%-95% is plasma protein bound; metabolized in liver; excreted in urine, feces (metabolites); crosses placenta

🥄 **Drug interactions of concern to dentistry:**
• Increased hypoglycemic effects: NSAIDs, salicylates, ketoconazole
• Decreased action of glyburide: corticosteroids
• Disulfiram-like reaction: alcohol

DENTAL CONSIDERATIONS
General:
• Monitor vital signs every appointment due to cardiovascular side effects.
• Patients on chronic drug therapy may rarely have symptoms of blood dyscrasias, which can include infection, bleeding, and poor healing.
• Place on frequent recall to evaluate healing response.

---

bold italic = life-threatening conditions

• Ensure that patient is following prescribed diet and regularly takes medication.

• Short appointments and stress reduction protocol may be required for anxious patients.

• Patients with diabetes may be more susceptible to infection and have delayed wound healing.

• Question patient about self-monitoring of drug's antidiabetic effect, including blood glucose values or finger-stick records.

• Avoid prescribing aspirin-containing products.

Consultations:

• In a patient with symptoms of blood dyscrasias, request a medical consult for blood studies and postpone dental treatment until normal values are reestablished.

• Medical consult may be required to assess disease control.

• Medical consult may include data from patient's blood glucose monitoring, including glycosylated hemoglobin or HbA_{1c} testing.

Teach patient/family:

• Importance of good oral hygiene to prevent soft tissue inflammation

• Caution to prevent injury when using oral hygiene aids

• To avoid mouth rinses with high alcohol content due to drying effects

---

glycopyrrolate
(glye-koe-pye'roe-late)
Robinul, Robinul Forte
Drug class.: Anticholinergic

Action: Inhibits acetylcholine at receptor sites in autonomic nervous system, which controls secretions, free acids in stomach

Uses: Decreased secretions before surgery, reversal of neuromuscular blockade, peptic ulcer disease, irritable bowel syndrome

Dosage and routes:

Preoperatively

• *Adult:* IM 0.002 mg/lb 0.5-1 hr before surgery

• *Child 2-12 yr:* IM 0.002-0.004 mg/lb

• *Child <2 yr:* IM 0.004 mg/lb

Reversal of neuromuscular blockage

• *Adult:* IV 0.2 mg for each 1 mg of neostigmine or 5 mg IV of pyridostigmine simultaneously

GI disorders

• *Adult:* PO 1-2 mg bid-tid; IM/IV 0.1-0.2 mg tid-qid, titrated to patient response

Available forms include: Tabs 1, 2 mg; inj 0.2 mg/ml

Side effects/adverse reactions:

▼ *ORAL: Dry mouth*

CNS: Confusion, anxiety, restlessness, irritability, delusions, hallucinations, headache, sedation, depression, incoherence, dizziness, lethargy, flushing, weakness

CV: Palpitation, tachycardia, postural hypotension, paradoxic bradycardia

GI: Constipation, nausea, vomiting, abdominal distress, paralytic ileus

GU: Hesitancy, retention, impotence

EENT: Blurred vision, photophobia, dilated pupils, difficulty swallowing, increased intraocular pressure, mydriasis, cycloplegia

INTEG: Urticaria, allergic reactions

MISC: Suppression of lactation, nasal congestion, decreased sweating

Contraindications: Hypersensitivity, narrow-angle glaucoma, myasthenia gravis, GI/GU obstruction, child <3 yr, tachycardia, myocardial ischemia, hepatic disease, ulcerative colitis, toxic megacolon

Precautions: Pregnancy category C, elderly, lactation, prostatic hypertrophy, renal disease, CHF, pulmonary disease, hyperthyroidism

Pharmacokinetics:

PO: Peak 1 hr, duration 6 hr

IM: Peak 30-45 min, duration 7 hr

IV: Peak 10-15 min, duration 4 hr, excreted in urine, bile, feces (unchanged)

⚘ Drug interactions of concern to dentistry:

• Increased anticholinergic effect: antihistamines, phenothiazines, meperidine, haloperidol, scopolamine, atropine

• Do not mix with diazepam, pentobarbital, in syringe or solution

• Constipation, urinary retention: opioid analgesics

• Reduced absorption of ketoconazole

DENTAL CONSIDERATIONS

General:

• Avoid dental light in patient's eyes; offer dark glasses for patient comfort.

• Assess salivary flow as a factor in caries, periodontal disease, and candidiasis.

Consultation:

• Physician should be informed if significant xerostomic side effects occur (increased caries, sore tongue, problems eating or swallowing, difficulty wearing prosthesis) so a medication change can be considered.

Teach patient/family:

When chronic dry mouth occurs, advise patient:

• To avoid mouth rinses with high alcohol content due to drying effects

• To use daily home fluoride products for anticaries effect

• To use sugarless gum, frequent sips of water, or saliva substitutes

---

griseofulvin microsize/ griseofulvin ultramicrosize

(gri-see-oh-ful'vin)

Fulvicin P/G, Fulvicin U/F, Grifulvin V, Grisactin, Grisactin Ultra, Gris-PEG

♣ Grisovin-FP

Drug class.: Antifungal

Action: Arrests fungal cell division at metaphase; binds to human keratin, making it resistant to disease

Uses: Mycotic infections: tinea corporis, tinea pedis, tinea cruris, tinea barbae, tinea capitis, tinea unguium if caused by *Epidermophyton, Microsporum, Trichophyton*

Dosage and routes:

• *Adult:* PO 250-500 mg qd in single or divided doses (microsize), 125-375 mg bid (ultramicrosize)

• *Child:* PO 11 mg/kg/day or 300 mg/m^2/day (microsize) or 7.3 mg/kg/day (ultramicrosize)

Available forms include: Microcaps 250 mg; tabs 250, 500 mg; oral susp 125 mg/ml; ultratabs 125, 165, 250, 330 mg

Side effects/adverse reactions:

▼ *ORAL:* Dry mouth, candidiasis, furry tongue, lichenoid lesions, taste alteration

---

bold italic = life-threatening conditions   *For periodic updates, visit* **www.mosby.com**

CNS: Headache, peripheral neuritis, paresthesia, confusion, dizziness, fatigue, insomnia, psychosis
GI: Nausea, vomiting, anorexia, diarrhea, cramps, flatulence
*HEMA: **Leukopenia, granulocytopenia, neutropenia, monocytosis***
GU: Proteinuria, cylindruria, precipitate porphyria
EENT: Blurred vision, transient hearing loss
INTEG: Rash, urticaria, photosensitivity, lichen planus, angioedema
Contraindications: Hypersensitivity, porphyria, hepatic disease, lupus erythematosus
Precautions: Penicillin sensitivity, pregnancy category C
Pharmacokinetics:
PO: Peak 4 hr, half-life 9-24 hr; metabolized in liver; excreted in urine (inactive metabolites), feces, perspiration
⚕ Drug interactions of concern to dentistry:
• Decreased absorption: barbiturates
• Additive photosensitization: tetracycline
• Potentiation of alcohol
DENTAL CONSIDERATIONS
General:
• Assess salivary flow as a factor in caries, periodontal disease, and candidiasis.
Teach patient/family:
When chronic dry mouth occurs, advise patient:
• To use daily home fluoride products for anticaries effect
• To avoid mouth rinses with high alcohol content due to drying effects
• To use sugarless gum, frequent sips of water, or saliva substitutes

guaifenesin

(gwye-fen'e-sin)
Anti-Tuss, Benylin-E, Breonesin, Duratuss-G, Fenesin, GeeGee, Genatuss, GG-Cen, Glycotuss, Glytuss, Guaifenex LA, Guaituss, Gylate, Humibid LA, Humibid Sprinkle, Hytuss, Hytuss 2X, Mytussin, Organidin NR, Robitussin, Scot-Tussin, Siltussin, Tusibron, Tussin, Uni-Tussin, *and many others*
♣ Balminil, Resyl
Drug class.: Expectorant

Action: Acts as an expectorant by stimulating a mucosal reflex to increase the production of less-viscous lung mucus
Uses: Dry, nonproductive cough
Dosage and routes:
• *Adult:* PO 200-400 mg q4-6h, not to exceed 1-2 g/day
• *Child 6-12 yr:* PO 100-200 mg q4h; max dose 1200 mg day
Available forms include: Tabs 100, 200, 1200 mg; caps 200 mg; syr 100 mg/5 ml; ext rel caps 300, 600 mg; ext rel tabs 600 mg; liquid 100, 200 mg/5 ml
Side effects/adverse reactions:
CNS: Drowsiness
GI: Nausea, anorexia, vomiting
Contraindications: Hypersensitivity, persistent cough
Precautions: Pregnancy category C
DENTAL CONSIDERATIONS
General:
• Consider semisupine chair position for patients with respiratory disease.
• Elective dental treatment may be precluded by significant coughing episodes.

guanabenz acetate
(gwahn'a-benz)
Wytensin
Drug class.: Centrally acting antihypertensive

Action: Stimulates central α_2-adrenergic receptors, resulting in decreased sympathetic outflow from brain
Uses: Hypertension
Dosage and routes:
• *Adult:* PO 4 mg bid, increasing in increments of 4-8 mg/day q1-2wk, not to exceed 32 mg bid
Available forms include: Tabs 4, 8 mg
Side effects/adverse reactions:
▼ *ORAL: Dry mouth*
CNS: Drowsiness, dizziness, sedation, headache, depression, weakness
CV: Severe rebound hypertension, chest pain, dysrhythmias, palpitation
GI: Nausea, diarrhea, constipation
GU: Impotence
EENT: Nasal congestion, blurred vision
Contraindications: Hypersensitivity to guanabenz
Precautions: Pregnancy category C, lactation, children <12 yr, severe coronary insufficiency, recent MI, cerebrovascular disease, severe hepatic or renal failure
Pharmacokinetics:
PO: Peak 2-4 hr, half-life 6 hr; excreted in urine
Drug interactions of concern to dentistry:
• Increased CNS depression: alcohol, all CNS depressants
• Decreased hypotensive effects: NSAIDs, especially indomethacin, sympathomimetics

DENTAL CONSIDERATIONS
General:
• Monitor vital signs every appointment due to cardiovascular side effects.
• Limit use of sodium-containing products such as saline IV fluids for patients with a dietary salt restriction.
• Assess salivary flow as a factor in caries, periodontal disease, and candidiasis.
• Stress from dental procedures may compromise cardiovascular function; determine patient risk.
• Short appointments and a stress reduction protocol may be required for anxious patients.
Consultations:
• Medical consult may be required to assess disease control and patient's ability to tolerate stress.
Teach patient/family:
When chronic dry mouth occurs, advise patient:
• To avoid mouth rinses with high alcohol content due to drying effects
• To use daily home fluoride products for anticaries effect
• To use sugarless gum, frequent sips of water, or saliva substitutes

guanadrel sulfate
(gwahn'a-drel)
Hylorel
Drug class.: Antihypertensive

Action: Inhibits sympathetic vasoconstriction by inhibiting release of norepinephrine; depletes norepinephrine stores in adrenergic nerve endings
Uses: Hypertension
Dosage and routes:
• *Adult:* PO 5 mg bid, adjusted to

---

bold italic = life-threatening conditions

desired response, may need 20-75 mg/day in divided doses

Available forms include: Tabs 10, 25 mg

Side effects/adverse reactions:

▼ *ORAL:* Dry mouth

CNS: Drowsiness, fatigue, weakness, feeling of faintness, insomnia, dizziness, mental changes, memory loss, hallucinations, *depression,* anxiety, *confusion, paresthesias, headache*

CV: Orthostatic hypotension, bradycardia, CHF, palpitation, chest pain, tachycardia, dysrhythmias

GI: Nausea, cramps, diarrhea, constipation, anorexia, indigestion

RESP: Bronchospasm, dyspnea, cough, rales, shortness of breath

GU: Ejaculation failure, impotence, dysuria, nocturia, frequency

EENT: Nasal stuffiness, tinnitus, visual changes, sore throat, double vision, dry/burning eyes

INTEG: Rash, purpura, alopecia

MS: Leg cramps, aching, pain, inflammation

Contraindications: Hypersensitivity, pregnancy category B, pheochromocytoma, lactation, CHF, child <18 yr

Precautions: Elderly, bronchial asthma, peptic ulcer, electrolyte imbalances, vascular disease

Pharmacokinetics:

PO: Onset 0.5-2 hr, peak 1.5-2 hr, duration 4-14 hr, half-life 10-12 hr; excreted in urine (50% unchanged)

🦷 **Drug interactions of concern to dentistry:**

• Increased orthostatic hypotension: alcohol, opioid analgesics, barbiturates, phenothiazines, haloperidol

• Decreased hypotensive effect: ephedrine, sympathomimetics, NSAIDs, indomethacin, tricyclic antidepressants

DENTAL CONSIDERATIONS

General:

• Monitor vital signs every appointment due to cardiovascular side effects.

• After supine positioning, have patient sit upright for at least 2 min before standing to avoid orthostatic hypotension.

• Limit use of sodium-containing products such as saline IV fluids for patients with a dietary salt restriction.

• Stress from dental procedures may compromise cardiovascular function; determine patient risk.

• Short appointments and a stress reduction protocol may be required for anxious patients.

• Assess salivary flow as a factor in caries, periodontal disease, and candidiasis.

Consultations:

• Medical consult may be required to assess disease control and patient's ability to tolerate stress.

Teach patient/family:

When chronic dry mouth occurs, advise patient:

• To avoid mouth rinses with high alcohol content due to drying effects

• To use daily home fluoride products for anticaries effect

• To use sugarless gum, frequent sips of water, or saliva substitutes

---

guanethidine sulfate

(gwahn-eth′i-deen)

Ismelin

♣ Apo-Guanethidine

Drug class.: Antihypertensive

Action: Inhibits norepinephrine

release, depleting norepinephrine stores in adrenergic nerve endings

Uses: Moderate-to-severe hypertension

Dosage and routes:
• *Adult:* PO 10 mg qd, increase by 10 mg qwk at monthly intervals; may require 25-50 mg qd
• *Adult (hospitalized):* 25-50 mg; may increase by 25-50 mg/day or qod
• *Child:* PO 200 μg/kg/day; increase q7-10d; not to exceed 3000 μg/kg/24 hr

Available forms include: Tabs 10, 25 mg

Side effects/adverse reactions:
▼ *ORAL:* Dry mouth, salivary gland pain or swelling
CNS: Depression
CV: Orthostatic hypotension, dizziness, weakness, lassitude, bradycardia, **CHF,** fatigue, angina, heart block, chest paresthesia
GI: Nausea, vomiting, *diarrhea,* constipation, weight gain, anorexia
RESP: Dyspnea
*HEMA: **Thrombocytopenia, leukopenia***
GU: Ejaculation failure, impotence, nocturia, edema, retention, increased BUN
EENT: Nasal congestion, ptosis, blurred vision
INTEG: Dermatitis, loss of scalp hair

Contraindications: Hypersensitivity, pheochromocytoma, recent MI, CHF, cardiac failure, sinus bradycardia

Precautions: Pregnancy category B, lactation, peptic ulcer, asthma

Pharmacokinetics:
PO: Therapeutic level 1-3 wk, half-life 5 days; metabolized by liver; excreted in urine (metabolites), breast milk

🦷 **Drug interactions of concern to dentistry:**
• Increased orthostatic hypotension: alcohol, opioid analgesics, barbiturates, phenothiazines, haloperidol
• Decreased hypotensive effect: ephedrine, NSAIDs, indomethacin, sympathomimetics, tricyclic antidepressants

DENTAL CONSIDERATIONS

General:
• Monitor vital signs every appointment due to cardiovascular and respiratory side effects.
• Patients on chronic drug therapy may rarely have symptoms of blood dyscrasias, which can include infection, bleeding, and poor healing.
• Assess salivary flow as a factor in caries, periodontal disease, and candidiasis.
• After supine positioning, have patient sit upright for at least 2 min before standing to avoid orthostatic hypotension.
• Limit use of sodium-containing products such as saline IV fluids for patients with a dietary salt restriction.
• Stress from dental procedures may compromise cardiovascular function; determine patient risk.
• Short appointments and a stress reduction protocol may be required for anxious patients.
• Use vasoconstrictors with caution, in low doses, and with careful aspiration. Avoid using gingival retraction cord with epinephrine.
• Consider semisupine chair position for patients with respiratory distress.

Consultations:
• Medical consult may be required

G

---

bold italic = life-threatening conditions

to assess disease control and patient's ability to tolerate stress.
• In a patient with symptoms of blood dyscrasias, request a medical consult for blood studies and postpone dental treatment until normal values are reestablished.

Teach patient/family:
• Importance of good oral hygiene to prevent soft tissue inflammation
• Caution to prevent injury when using oral hygiene aids

When chronic dry mouth occurs, advise patient:
• To avoid mouth rinses with high alcohol content due to drying effects
• To use daily home fluoride products for anticaries effect
• To use sugarless gum, frequent sips of water, or saliva substitutes

---

halcinonide

(hal-sin'oh-nide)
Halog, Halog-E
Drug class.: Corticosteroid, synthetic topical

Action: Glucocorticoids have multiple actions that include antiinflammatory and immunosuppressant effects. They inhibit phospholipase A_2, interfering with or reducing the synthesis of prostaglandins and leukotrienes. They also bind to cytoplasmic glucocorticoid receptors (GRs) and enter the cell nucleus to bind with DNA. This results in the synthesis of various enzymes such as collagenase, elastase, and cytokines that play important roles in inflammation and immunosuppression. They also suppress the production of lymphocytes, monocytes, and eosinophils.

Uses: Inflammation of corticosteroid-responsive dermatoses

Dosage and routes:
• *Adult:* TOP apply to affected area bid-tid

Available forms include: Cream 0.025%, 0.1%; oint 0.1%; sol 0.1%

Side effects/adverse reactions:
▼ *ORAL:* Thinning of mucosa, stinging sensation (local application)
INTEG: Acne, atrophy, epidermal thinning, purpura, striae

Contraindications: Hypersensitivity, viral infections, fungal infections

Precautions: Pregnancy category C

DENTAL CONSIDERATIONS
General:
• Place on frequent recall to evaluate healing response when used on chronic basis.

Teach patient/family:
• Importance of good oral hygiene to prevent soft tissue inflammation
• When used for oral lesions, to return for oral evaluation if response of oral tissues has not occurred in 7-14 days
• To apply at bedtime or after meals for maximum effect
• To apply with cotton-tipped applicator by pressing, not rubbing, paste on lesion
• That use on oral herpetic ulcerations is contraindicated

---

halobetasol propionate

(hal-oh-bay'ta-sol)
Ultravate
Drug class.: Topical corticosteroid, group VI potency

Action: Glucocorticoids have multiple actions that include antiin-flammatory and immunosuppres-sant effects. They inhibit phos-pholipase A_2, interfering with or reducing the synthesis of prosta-glandins and leukotrienes. They also bind to cytoplasmic glucocor-ticoid receptors (GRs) and enter the cell nucleus to bind with DNA. This results in the synthesis of various enzymes such as collage-nase, elastase, and cytokines that play important roles in inflamma-tion and immunosuppression. They also suppress the production of lymphocytes, monocytes, and eo-sinophils.

Uses: Psoriasis, eczema, contact dermatitis, pruritus

Dosage and routes:
• *Adult and child:* Apply to af-fected area tid-qid

Available forms include: Cream 0.05%; oint 0.005%

Side effects/adverse reactions:
INTEG: Burning, dryness, itching, irritation, acne, folliculitis, hyper-trichosis, perioral dermatitis, hy-popigmentation, atrophy, striae, miliaria, allergic contact dermati-tis, secondary infection

Contraindications: Hypersensi-tivity to corticosteroids, fungal in-fections

Precautions: Pregnancy category C, lactation, viral infections, bacte-rial infections

DENTAL CONSIDERATIONS
Teach patient/family:
• That use on oral herpetic ulcer-ations is contraindicated

haloperidol/haloperidol decanoate
(ha-loe-per′i-dole)
Haldol
♣ Apo-Haloperidol, Novoperi-dol, Peridol, PMS Haloperidol
Drug class.: Antipsychotic/butyro-phenone

Action: Blocks neurotransmission at dopaminergic synapses in the cerebral cortex, hypothalamus, and limbic system; exhibits strong pe-ripheral α-adrenergic and anticho-linergic blocking action; mecha-nism for antipsychotic effects is unclear

Uses: Psychotic disorders, con-trol of tics and vocal utterances in Tourette's syndrome, short-term treatment of hyperactive chil-dren showing excessive motor ac-tivity; unapproved: autism and chemotherapy-induced nausea and vomiting

Dosage and routes:
Psychosis
• *Adult:* PO 0.5-5 mg bid or tid initially, depending on severity of condition, dose is increased to de-sired dose, max 100 mg/day; IM 2-5 mg q1-8h
• *Child 3-12 yr:* PO/IM 0.05-0.15 mg/kg/day
• *Decanoate:* Initial dose IM is 10-15× daily PO dose q4wk; do not administer IV; not to exceed 100 mg

Chronic schizophrenia
• *Adult:* IM 10-15× PO dose q4wk (decanoate)
• *Child 3-12 yr:* PO/IM 0.05-0.15 mg/kg/day

Tics/vocal utterances
• *Adult:* PO 0.5-5 mg bid or tid,

---

bold italic = life-threatening conditions

increased until desired response occurs

• *Child 3-12 yr:* PO 0.05-0.075 mg/kg/day

Hyperactive children

• *Child 3-12 yr:* PO 0.05-0.075 mg/kg/day

Available forms include: Tabs 0.5, 1, 2, 5, 10, 20 mg; conc 2 mg/ml; inj IM 5 mg/ml, 50, 100 mg in 1 ml amps; 5 ml vials

Side effects/adverse reactions:

▼ *ORAL: Dry mouth, tardive dyskinesia (tongue, lip movements),* sore throat, mouth

*CNS: Extrapyramidal symptoms: pseudoparkinsonism, akathisia, dystonia, tardive dyskinesia, drowsiness, headache, **seizures, neuroleptic malignant syndrome,*** confusion

*CV: Orthostatic hypotension, **cardiac arrest, tachycardia,*** hypertension, ECG changes

*GI: Nausea, vomiting, anorexia, constipation, **ileus, hepatitis,*** diarrhea, jaundice, weight gain

*RESP: **Laryngospasm, respiratory depression,*** dyspnea

GU: Urinary retention, urinary frequency, enuresis, impotence, amenorrhea, gynecomastia

EENT: Blurred vision, glaucoma, dry eyes

INTEG: Rash, photosensitivity, dermatitis

Contraindications: Hypersensitivity, blood dyscrasias, coma, child <3 yr, brain damage, bone marrow depression, alcohol and barbiturate withdrawal states, Parkinson's disease, angina, epilepsy, urinary retention, narrow-angle glaucoma

Precautions: Pregnancy category C, lactation, seizure disorders, hypertension, hepatic disease, cardiac disease

Pharmacokinetics:

PO: Onset erratic, peak 2-6 hr, half-life 24 hr

IM: Onset 15-30 min, peak 15-20 min, half-life 21 hr; decanoate—peak 4-11 days, half-life 3 wk Metabolized by liver; excreted in urine, bile; crosses placenta; excreted in breast milk

🦷 **Drug interactions of concern to dentistry:**

• Increased sedation: other CNS depressants, alcohol, barbiturate anesthetics, opioid analgesics

• Hypotension, tachycardia: epinephrine

• Increased extrapyramidal effects: phenothiazines and related drugs (haloperidol, droperidol), metoclopramide

• Additive photosensitization: tetracyclines

• Increased anticholinergic effects: anticholinergics

• Suspected increase in neurological side effects: fluconazole, itraconazole, ketoconazole

DENTAL CONSIDERATIONS
General:

• Monitor vital signs every appointment due to cardiovascular side effects.

• After supine positioning, have patient sit upright for at least 2 min before standing to avoid orthostatic hypotension.

• Assess salivary flow as a factor in caries, periodontal disease, and candidiasis.

• Avoid dental light in patient's eyes; offer dark glasses for patient comfort.

• Assess for presence of extrapyramidal motor symptoms, such as tardive dyskinesia and akathisia. Extrapyramidal motor activity may complicate dental treatment.
• Geriatric patients are more susceptible to drug effects; use lower dose.
• Use vasoconstrictors with caution, in low doses, and with careful aspiration. Avoid use of gingival retraction cord with epinephrine.
Consultations:
• Take precautions if dental surgery is anticipated and anesthesia is required.
• If signs of tardive dyskinesia or akathisia are present, refer to physician.
• Physician should be informed if significant xerostomic side effects occur (increased caries, sore tongue, problems eating or swallowing, difficulty wearing prosthesis) so a medication change can be considered.
Teach patient/family:
• Importance of good oral hygiene to prevent soft tissue inflammation
• Caution to prevent injury when using oral hygiene aids
• To use electric toothbrush if patient has difficulty holding conventional devices
When chronic dry mouth occurs, advise patient:
• To avoid mouth rinses with high alcohol content due to drying effects
• To use daily home fluoride products for anticaries effect
• To use sugarless gum, frequent sips of water, or saliva substitutes

heparin calcium/ heparin sodium
(hep'a-rin)
Heparin sodium: generic, Hep Lock, Hep-Lock Flush, Hep-Lock U/P
✦ *Heparin calcium:* Calcilean, Calciparine
Drug class.: Anticoagulant

Action: Acts in combination with antithrombin III (heparin cofactor) to inhibit thrombosis; inactivates Factor Xa and inhibits conversion of prothrombin to thrombin; affects both intrinsic and extrinsic clotting pathways
Uses: Anticoagulant in thrombosis, embolism (both prevention and treatment), coagulopathies, deep vein thrombosis, prevention of clotting when extracorporeal circulation is required (cardiac surgery), dialysis, maintenance of patency of indwelling IV lines
Dosage and routes: General doses listed, all doses must be individualized to patient and circumstance
• *Adult:* SC 10,000-20,000 U (USP) initially, then 8000-10,000 U q8h or 15,000 U q12h; IV 10,000 U initially, then 5000-10,000 U q4-6h; IV inf 20,000-40,000 U in 1 L of normal saline over 24 hr
• *Child:* IV 50 U/kg initially, then 100 U/kg by IV drip q4h or 20,000 U/m² over 24 hr by continuous infusion
Available forms include: Amps 1000, 5000, 10,000 U/ml; vials 1000, 2000, 2500, 5000, 10,000, 20,000, 40,000 U/ml; unit dose 1000, 2500, 5000, 7500, 10,000,

20,000 U/dose; heparin lock flush 10, 100 U/ml; heparin calcium 5000 U/dose

Side effects/adverse reactions:

▼ *ORAL:* Bleeding, stomatitis

CNS: Fever, chills

GI: Diarrhea, **hepatitis,** nausea, vomiting, anorexia, abdominal cramps

GU: **Hematuria**

HEMA: **Hemorrhage, thrombocytopenia**

INTEG: Rash, hives, itching, allergies

Contraindications: Hypersensitivity, hemophilia, leukemia with bleeding, peptic ulcer disease, thrombocytopenic purpura, hepatic disease (severe), renal disease (severe), blood dyscrasias, pregnancy, severe hypertension, subacute bacterial endocarditis, acute nephritis

Precautions: Hematoma (IM); elderly; pregnancy category C; lactation; hyperkalemia; monitor APTT, PTT, WBC, ACT; endocarditis; trauma; alcoholism; prolongs intrinsic clotting pathway approximately 4-6 hr after each dose

Pharmacokinetics:

IV: Peak 5 min, duration 2-6 hr

SC: Onset 20-60 min, duration 8-12 hr, half-life 1.5 hr (variable depending on dose); 95% bound to plasma proteins; excreted in urine

🐝 **Drug interactions of concern to dentistry:**

• Increased risk of bleeding: salicylates, NSAIDs, parenteral penicillins, glucocorticoids, certain cephalosporins (cefamandole, cefoperazone, cefotetan)

DENTAL CONSIDERATIONS

General:

• Heparin is used only in hospitalized patients or during dialysis. A medical consult is necessary if oral and maxillofacial surgery or trauma treatment is required. May need to defer treatment.

• Avoid products that affect platelet function, such as aspirin and NSAIDs.

• Consider local hemostasis measures to prevent excessive bleeding.

• Take precautions if dental surgery or intubation for general anesthesia is anticipated.

Consultations:

• Medical consult may be required to assess disease control and patient's ability to tolerate stress.

• Medical consult should include ACT, partial prothrombin, and prothrombin times.

Teach patient/family:

• Caution to prevent trauma when using oral hygiene aids

• Importance of good oral hygiene to prevent soft tissue inflammation

• To report oral lesions, soreness, or bleeding

---

homatropine hydrobromide (optic)

(hoe-ma′troe-peen)

AK-Homatropine, Isopto Homatropine

♣ Minims Homatropine

Drug class.: Mydriatic (topical)

Action: Blocks response of iris sphincter muscle and muscle of accommodation of ciliary body to cholinergic stimulation, resulting in dilation and paralysis of accommodation

Uses: Cycloplegic refraction, uveitis, mydriatic lens opacities

Dosage and routes:

• *Adult and child:* Instill 1 gtt, repeat in 5-10 min for refraction or 1 gtt bid or tid for uveitis

Available forms include: Sol 2%, 5%

Side effects/adverse reactions:

CNS: Confusion, somnolence, flushing, fever

CV: Tachycardia

EENT: Blurred vision, photophobia, increased intraocular pressure, irritation, edema

Contraindications: Hypersensitivity, children <6 yr, narrow-angle glaucoma, increased intraocular pressure, infants

Precautions: Children, elderly, hypertension, hyperthyroidism, diabetes, pregnancy category C

Pharmacokinetics:

INSTILL: Peak 0.5-1 hr, duration 1-3 days

🦷 Drug interactions of concern to dentistry:

• Avoid concurrent use with pilocarpine

• Increased anticholinergic effects with other anticholinergic drugs (when significant absorption from the eye occurs)

DENTAL CONSIDERATIONS

General:

• Avoid dental light in patient's eyes; offer dark glasses for patient comfort.

• Protect patient's eyes from accidental spatter during dental treatment.

hydralazine HCl

(hye-dral'a-zeen)

Apresoline

♣ Novo-Hylazin

Drug class.: Antihypertensive, direct-acting peripheral vasodilator

Action: Dilates arteriolar smooth muscle by direct relaxation; reduction in blood pressure with reflex increases cardiac function

Uses: Essential hypertension; parenteral: severe essential hypertension

Dosage and routes:

• *Adult:* PO 10 mg qid 2-4 days, then 25 mg for rest of first wk, then 50 mg qid individualized to desired response, not to exceed 300 mg; IV/IM bol 20-40 mg q4-6h, administer PO asap; IM 20-40 mg q4-6h

• *Child:* PO 0.75 mg/kg qd 0.75-3 mg/kg/day in 4 divided doses; max 7.5 mg/kg/24 hr; IV bol 0.1-0.2 mg/kg q4-6h; IM 0.1-0.2 mg/kg q4-6h

Available forms include: Inj IV/IM 20 mg/ml; tabs 10, 25, 50, 100 mg

Side effects/adverse reactions:

CNS: Headache, tremors, dizziness, anxiety, peripheral neuritis, depression

*CV: Palpitation, reflex tachycardia, angina, **shock,** edema, rebound hypertension

GI: Nausea, vomiting, anorexia, diarrhea, constipation

*HEMA: **Leukopenia, agranulocytosis,*** anemia

GU: Impotence, urinary retention, sodium, water retention

INTEG: Rash, pruritus

---

bold italic = life-threatening conditions   *For periodic updates, visit* **www.mosby.com**

MISC: Lupuslike symptoms, nasal congestion, muscle cramps

Contraindications: Hypersensitivity to hydralazines, CAD, mitral valvular rheumatic heart disease, rheumatic heart disease

Precautions: Pregnancy category C, CVA, advanced renal disease

Pharmacokinetics:
PO: Onset 20-45 min, peak 1-2 hr, duration 2-4 hr
IV: Onset 5-20 min, peak 10-80 min, duration 2-6 hr, half-life 2-8 hr
Metabolized by liver; <10% present in urine

🦷 **Drug interactions of concern to dentistry:**
• Increased tachycardia, angina: IV sympathomimetics (epinephrine, norepinephrine)
• Reduced effects: NSAIDs, indomethacin

DENTAL CONSIDERATIONS
General:
• Monitor vital signs every appointment due to cardiovascular side effects.
• Patients on chronic drug therapy may rarely have symptoms of blood dyscrasias, which can include infection, bleeding, and poor healing.
• Limit use of sodium-containing products such as saline IV fluids for patients with a dietary salt restriction.
• After supine positioning, have patient sit upright for at least 2 min to avoid orthostatic hypotension.

Consultations:
• In a patient with symptoms of blood dyscrasias, request a medical consult for blood studies and postpone dental treatment until normal values are reestablished.

• Medical consult may be required to assess disease control and patient's ability to tolerate stress.

Teach patient/family:
• Importance of good oral hygiene to prevent soft tissue inflammation
• Caution to prevent injury when using oral hygiene aids

---

hydrochlorothiazide (HTCZ)
(hye-droe-klor-oh-thye'a-zide)
Esidrix, Ezide, HydroDIURIL, Hydro-Par, Microzide, Oretic
🍁 Apo-Hydro, Diuchlor H, Neo-Codema, Novo-Hydrazide, Urozide

Drug class.: Thiazide diuretic

Action: Acts on distal tubule by increasing excretion of water, sodium, chloride, potassium

Uses: Edema, hypertension, diuresis, CHF

Dosage and routes:
• *Adult:* PO 12.5-100 mg/day; up to 200 mg/d
• *Child >6 mo:* PO 2.2 mg/kg/day in divided doses
• *Child <6 mo:* PO up to 3.3 mg/kg/day in divided doses

Available forms include: Tabs 12.5, 25, 50, 100 mg; sol 50 mg/5 ml, 100 mg/ml

Side effects/adverse reactions:
▼ *ORAL: Dry mouth, increased thirst,* lichenoid reaction
CNS: Dizziness, fatigue, weakness, drowsiness, paresthesia, anxiety, depression, headache
CV: Irregular pulse, orthostatic hypotension, palpitation, volume depletion
GI: Nausea, vomiting, anorexia,

hepatitis, constipation, diarrhea, cramps, pancreatitis, GI irritation

HEMA: **Aplastic anemia, hemolytic anemia, leukopenia, agranulocytosis, thrombocytopenia, neutropenia**

GU: Frequency, uremia, glucosuria, polyuria

EENT: Blurred vision

INTEG: Rash, urticaria, purpura, photosensitivity, fever

META: Hyperglycemia, hyperuricemia, increased creatinine, BUN

ELECT: Hypokalemia, hypercalcemia, hyponatremia, hypochloremia, hypomagnesemia

Contraindications: Hypersensitivity to thiazides or sulfonamides, anuria, renal decompensation, hypomagnesemia

Precautions: Hypokalemia, renal disease, pregnancy category D, hepatic disease, gout, COPD, lupus erythematosus, diabetes mellitus

Pharmacokinetics:

PO: Onset 2 hr, peak 4 hr, duration 6-12 hr; excreted unchanged by kidneys; crosses placenta; enters breast milk

⚕ Drug interactions of concern to dentistry:

• Increased photosensitization: tetracycline

• Decreased hypotensive response: NSAIDs, especially indomethacin

DENTAL CONSIDERATIONS

General:

• Monitor vital signs every appointment due to cardiovascular side effects.

• Patients on chronic drug therapy may rarely have symptoms of blood dyscrasias, which can include infection, bleeding, and poor healing.

• After supine positioning, have patient sit upright for at least 2 min before standing to avoid orthostatic hypotension.

• Assess salivary flow as a factor in caries, periodontal disease, and candidiasis.

• Limit use of sodium-containing products such as saline IV fluids for patients with a dietary salt restriction.

• Stress from dental procedures may compromise cardiovascular function; determine patient risk.

• Short appointments and a stress reduction protocol may be required for anxious patients.

• Patients taking diuretics should be monitored for serum K^+ levels.

Consultations:

• In a patient with symptoms of blood dyscrasias, request a medical consult for blood studies and postpone dental treatment until normal values are reestablished.

• Medical consult may be required to assess disease control and patient's ability to tolerate stress.

• Physician should be informed if significant xerostomic side effects occur (increased caries, sore tongue, problems eating or swallowing, difficulty wearing prosthesis) so a medication change can be considered.

Teach patient/family:

• Importance of good oral hygiene to prevent soft tissue inflammation

• Caution to prevent injury when using oral hygiene aids

When chronic dry mouth occurs, advise patient:

• To avoid mouth rinses with high alcohol content due to drying effects

• To use daily home fluoride products for anticaries effect

---

bold italic = life-threatening conditions

• To use sugarless gum, frequent sips of water, or saliva substitutes

---

hydrocodone bitartrate

(hye-droe-koe'done)
Hycodan
♣ Robidone
Drug class.: Narcotic analgesic

Controlled Substance Schedule III, Canada N

Action: Interacts with opioid receptors in the CNS to alter pain perception; acts directly on cough center in medulla to suppress cough

Uses: Hyperactive and nonproductive cough; mild-to-moderate pain; normally used in combination with aspirin or acetaminophen for posttreatment pain control

Dosage and routes:

• *Adult:* PO 5 mg q4h prn or 10 mg q12h (long-acting)
• *Child:* PO 0.15 mg/kg q6h

Available forms include: Caps 5 mg; susp 5 mg/ml; tabs 5, 10 mg (long-acting); some dose forms not available in United States

Side effects/adverse reactions:

▼ *ORAL:* Dry mouth

CNS: **Convulsions,** drowsiness, dizziness, light-headedness, confusion, headache, sedation, euphoria, dysphoria, weakness, hallucinations, disorientation

CV: **Circulatory depression,** palpitation, tachycardia, bradycardia, change in BP, syncope

GI: Nausea, vomiting, anorexia, constipation, cramps

RESP: **Respiratory depression**

GU: Increased urinary output, dysuria, urinary retention

EENT: Tinnitus, blurred vision, miosis, diplopia

INTEG: Rash, urticaria, flushing, pruritus

Contraindications: Hypersensitivity, addiction (narcotic)

Precautions: Addictive personality, pregnancy category C, lactation, increased intracranial pressure, MI (acute), severe heart disease, respiratory depression, hepatic disease, renal disease, child <18 yr

Pharmacokinetics: Onset 10-20 min, duration 3-6 hr, half-life 3-4 hr; metabolized in liver; excreted in urine; crosses placenta

🦷 Drug interactions of concern to dentistry:

• Increased CNS depression: alcohol, other opioids, phenothiazines, sedative/hypnotics, skeletal muscle relaxants, general anesthetics
• Contraindication: MAO inhibitors
• Increased effects of anticholinergics

DENTAL CONSIDERATIONS

General:

• Monitor vital signs every appointment due to cardiovascular and respiratory side effects.
• After supine positioning, have patient sit upright for at least 2 min to avoid orthostatic hypotension.
• Psychologic and physical dependence may occur with chronic administration.
• Determine why the patient is taking the drug.

Teach patient/family:

• To avoid mouth rinses with high alcohol content due to drying effects

hydrocortisone/ hydrocortisone acetate/hydrocortisone buteprate/ hydrocortisone butyrate/ hydrocortisone valerate

(hye-droe-kor′ti-sone)

Hydrocortisone: Ala-Cort, Cortaid, Cort-Dome, Cortifair, Cortizone-5, Cortizone-10, Delcort, Dermacort, Dermolate, Dermtex HC, Hycort, Hydro-Tex, Hytone, Nutracort, Penecort, Procort, Synacort, Tegrin-HC
♣ Cortef, Emo-Cort, Lemoderm Cortate, Prevex-HC, Unicort
Hydrocortisone acetate: Anusol HC, Cortaid, Corticaine, Gynecort, Lanacort-5
♣ Cortacet, Corticreme, Hyderm, Novohydrocort
Hydrocortisone buteprate: Pandel
Hydrocortisone butyrate: Locoid Cream, Locoid Ointment
Hydrocortisone valerate: Wescort Cream, Westcort Ointment
Drug class.: Topical corticosteroid

Action: Interacts with steroid cytoplasmic receptors to induce antiinflammatory effects; possesses antipruritic, antiinflammatory actions
Uses: Psoriasis, eczema, contact dermatitis, pruritus
Dosage and routes:
• *Adult and child >2 yr:* Apply to affected area qd-qid
Available forms include: Hydrocortisone: oint 0.5%, 1%, 2.5%;

cream 0.5%, 1%, 2.5%; lotion 0.25%, 0.5%, 1%, 2%, 2.5%; gel 1%; sol 1%; aerosol/pump spray 1.0%; acetate: oint 0.5%, 1%, 2.5%; cream 0.5%; lotion 0.05%; valerate: oint 0.2%; cream 0.2%; buteprate: cream 0.1% in 15 and 45 g; butyrate: oint 0.1%, cream 0.1% (many others)
Side effects/adverse reactions:
▼ *ORAL:* Thinning of mucosa, stinging sensation (oral application site)
INTEG: Burning, dryness, itching, irritation, acne, folliculitis, hypertrichosis, perioral dermatitis, hypopigmentation, atrophy, striae, miliaria, allergic contact dermatitis, secondary infection
Contraindications: Hypersensitivity to corticosteroids, fungal infections, herpetic infections
Precautions: Pregnancy category C, lactation, viral infections, bacterial infections
DENTAL CONSIDERATIONS
General:
• Place on frequent recall to evaluate healing response if used on a chronic basis.
Teach patient/family:
• Importance of good oral hygiene to prevent soft tissue inflammation
• To apply at bedtime or after meals for maximum effect
• That use on oral herpetic ulcerations is contraindicated
• To apply with cotton-tipped applicator by pressing, not rubbing, paste on lesion
• That when used for oral lesions, to return for oral evaluation if response of oral tissues has not occurred in 7-14 days

bold italic = life-threatening conditions   *For periodic updates, visit* www.mosby.com

hydrocortisone/ hydrocortisone acetate/ hydrocortisone cypionate/ hydrocortisone sodium phosphate/ hydrocortisone sodium succinate

(hye-dro-kor′ti-sone)

Hydrocortisone (tab): Cortef, Hydrocortone

Hydrocortisone cypionate (oral susp): Cortef

Hydrocortisone sodium phosphate (IV/IM/SC): Hydrocortone Phosphate

Hydrocortisone sodium succinate (IV/IM): A-Hydrocort, Solu-Cortef

Hydrocortisone acetate (intraarticular, soft tissue only): Hydrocortone Acetate

Hydrocortisone acetate (rectal): Cortiform

Hydrocortisone (rectal): Cortenema

Drug class.: Corticosteroid

Action: Glucocorticoids have multiple actions that include antiinflammatory and immunosuppressant effects. They inhibit phospholipase A_2, interfering with or reducing the synthesis of prostaglandins and leukotrienes. They also bind to cytoplasmic glucocorticoid receptors (GRs) and enter the cell nucleus to bind with DNA. This results in the synthesis of various enzymes such as collagenase, elastase, and cytokines that play important roles in inflammation and immunosuppression. They also suppress the production of lymphocytes, monocytes, and eosinophils.

Uses: Severe inflammation, shock, adrenal insufficiency, ulcerative colitis, collagen disorders

Dosage and routes:

Adrenal insufficiency/inflammation

• *Adult:* PO 5-30 mg bid-qid; IM/IV 100-250 mg (succinate), then 50-100 mg IM as needed; IM/IV 15-240 mg q12h (phosphate)

Shock

• *Adult:* 500 mg-2 g q2-6h (succinate)

• *Child:* IM/IV 0.16-1 mg/kg bid-tid (succinate)

Colitis

• *Adult:* Enema 100 mg nightly for 21 days

Available forms include: Retention enema 100 mg/60 ml; tabs 5, 10, 20 mg; inj 50 mg/ml; succinate inj 100, 250, 500, 1000 mg/vial; phosphate inj 50 mg/ml; acetate inj 25, 50 mg/ml; oral susp 10 mg/5 ml in 120 ml

Side effects/adverse reactions:

▼ *ORAL:* Dry mouth, poor wound healing, petechiae, candidiasis

CNS: Depression, flushing, sweating, headache, mood changes

*CV: Hypertension, **circulatory collapse, thrombophlebitis, embolism,** tachycardia, edema*

*GI: Diarrhea, nausea, **pancreatitis, GI hemorrhage,*** increased appetite, abdominal distention

*HEMA: **Thrombocytopenia***

EENT: Fungal infections, increased intraocular pressure, blurred vision

INTEG: Acne, poor wound healing, ecchymosis, petechiae

MS: Fractures, osteoporosis, weakness

Contraindications: Psychosis, hypersensitivity, idiopathic thrombocytopenia, acute glomerulonephritis, amebiasis, fungal infections, nonasthmatic bronchial disease, child <2 yr, AIDS, TB

Precautions: Pregnancy category C, diabetes mellitus, glaucoma, osteoporosis, seizure disorders, ulcerative colitis, CHF, myasthenia gravis, renal disease, esophagitis, peptic ulcer, rifampin

Pharmacokinetics:

PO: Onset 1-2 hr, peak 1 hr, duration 1-1.5 days

IM/IV: Onset 20 min, peak 4-8 hr, duration 1-1.5 days

REC: Onset 3-5 days

Metabolized by liver, excreted in urine (17-OHCH, 17-KS), crosses placenta

Drug interactions of concern to dentistry:

• Decreased action: barbiturates, rifabutin, rifampin

• Increased GI side effects: alcohol, salicylates, NSAIDs

• Increased action: ketoconazole, macrolide antibiotics

DENTAL CONSIDERATIONS

General:

• Monitor vital signs every appointment due to cardiovascular side effects.

• Patients on chronic drug therapy may rarely have symptoms of blood dyscrasias, which can include infection, bleeding, and poor healing.

• Assess salivary flow as a factor in caries, periodontal disease, and candidiasis.

• Place on frequent recall to evaluate healing response.

• Prophylactic antibiotics may be indicated to prevent infection if surgery or deep scaling is planned.

• Avoid prescribing aspirin-containing products.

• Symptoms of oral infections may be masked.

• Determine dose and duration of steroid therapy for each patient to assess the risk for stress tolerance and immunosuppression.

• Patients who have been or are currently on chronic steroid therapy >2 wk may require supplemental steroids for dental treatment.

• Determine why the patient is taking the drug.

Consultations:

• In a patient with symptoms of blood dyscrasias, request a medical consult for blood studies and postpone dental treatment until normal values are reestablished.

• Medical consult may be required to assess disease control and patient's ability to tolerate stress.

• Consult may be required to confirm steroid dose and duration of use.

Teach patient/family:

• Importance of good oral hygiene to prevent soft tissue inflammation

• Caution to prevent injury when using oral hygiene aids

When chronic dry mouth occurs, advise patient:

• To avoid mouth rinses with high alcohol content due to drying effects

• To use sugarless gum, frequent sips of water, or saliva substitutes

• To use daily home fluoride products for anticaries effect

H

hydromorphone HCl

(hye-droe-mor'fone)

Dilaudid, Dilaudid-5, Dilaudid HP
♣ PMS-Hydromorphone

Drug class.: Synthetic narcotic analgesic

Controlled Substance Schedule II, Canada N

Action: Inhibits ascending pain pathways in CNS, increases pain threshold, alters pain perception

Uses: Moderate-to-severe pain

Dosage and routes:

• *Adult:* PO 1-10 mg q3-6h depending on pain severity and dose form; IM/SC/IV 2-4 mg q4-6h; rec 3 mg hs prn

Available forms include: Inj IM/IV 1, 2, 3, 4, 10 mg/ml; tabs 1, 2, 3, 4, 8 mg; rec supp 3 mg; liquid 5 mg/5 ml

Side effects/adverse reactions:

▼ *ORAL:* Dry mouth

CNS: Drowsiness, dizziness, confusion, headache, sedation, euphoria

CV: Palpitation, bradycardia, change in BP

GI: Nausea, vomiting, anorexia, constipation, cramps

*RESP: **Respiratory depression***

GU: Increased urinary output, dysuria, urinary retention

EENT: Tinnitus, blurred vision, miosis, diplopia

INTEG: Rash, urticaria, bruising, flushing, diaphoresis, pruritus

Contraindications: Hypersensitivity, addiction (narcotic), MAO inhibitors

Precautions: Addictive personality, pregnancy category C, lactation, increased intracranial pressure, MI (acute), severe heart disease, respiratory depression, hepatic disease, renal disease, child <18 yr

Pharmacokinetics:

PO: Onset 15-30 min, peak 0.5-1.5 hr, duration 4-5 hr; metabolized by liver; excreted by kidneys; crosses placenta; excreted in breast milk

🏥 **Drug interactions of concern to dentistry:**

• Effects may be increased with other CNS depressants: alcohol, narcotics, sedative/hypnotics, skeletal muscle relaxants

• Increased effects of anticholinergic drugs

DENTAL CONSIDERATIONS

General:

• Monitor vital signs every appointment due to cardiovascular and respiratory side effects.

• After supine positioning, have patient sit upright for at least 2 min to avoid orthostatic hypotension.

• Assess salivary flow as a factor in caries, periodontal disease, and candidiasis.

• Psychologic and physical dependence may occur with chronic administration.

• Determine why the patient is taking the drug.

• Avoid in patients with chronic obstructive pulmonary disease.

Teach patient/family:

• To avoid mouth rinses with high alcohol content due to drying effects

hydroxychloroquine sulfate

(hye-drox-ee-klor'oh-kwin)

Plaquenil Sulfate

Drug class.: Antimalarial

Action: Inhibits parasite replications and transcription of DNA to

RNA by forming complexes with DNA of parasite

Uses: Malaria caused by *P. vivax, P. malariae, P. ovale, P. falciparum* (some strains); lupus erythematosus; rheumatoid arthritis

Dosage and routes:

Malaria

• *Adult and child:* PO 5 mg/kg/wk on same day of week, not to exceed 400 mg; treatment should begin 2 wk before entering endemic area, continue 8 wk after leaving; if treatment begins after exposure, 800 mg for adult, 10 mg/kg for children in 2 divided doses 6 hr apart

Lupus erythematosus

• *Adult:* PO 400 mg qd-bid, length depends on patient response; maintenance 200-400 mg qd

Rheumatoid arthritis

• *Adult:* PO 400-600 mg qd, then 200-300 mg qd after good response

Available forms include: Tabs 200 mg

Side effects/adverse reactions:

▼ *ORAL:* Discoloration of mucosa, lichenoid lesions

CNS: Convulsions, headache, stimulation, fatigue, irritability, bad dreams, dizziness, confusion, psychosis, decreased reflexes

CV: Asystole with syncope, hypotension, heart block

GI: Nausea, vomiting, anorexia, diarrhea, cramps

HEMA: Thrombocytopenia, agranulocytosis, hemolytic anemia, leukopenia

EENT: Blurred vision, corneal changes, retinal changes, difficulty focusing, tinnitus, vertigo, deafness, photophobia, corneal edema

INTEG: Exfoliative dermatitis, alopecia, pruritus, pigmentation changes, skin eruptions, lichen planus-like eruptions, eczema

Contraindications: Hypersensitivity, retinal field changes, porphyria, children (long-term)

Precautions: Blood dyscrasias, severe GI disease, neurologic disease, alcoholism, hepatic disease, G6PD deficiency, psoriasis, eczema, pregnancy category C

Pharmacokinetics:

PO: Peak 1-2 hr, half-life 3-5 days; metabolized in liver; excreted in urine, feces, breast milk; crosses placenta

🦷 **Drug interactions of concern to dentistry:**

• Hepatotoxicity: alcohol, hepatotoxic drugs

DENTAL CONSIDERATIONS

General:

• Patients on chronic drug therapy may rarely have symptoms of blood dyscrasias, which can include infection, bleeding, and poor healing.

• Avoid dental light in patient's eyes; offer dark glasses for patient comfort.

• Determine why the patient is taking the drug.

Consultations:

• In a patient with symptoms of blood dyscrasias, request a medical consult for blood studies and postpone dental treatment until normal values are reestablished.

Teach patient/family:

• Importance of good oral hygiene to prevent soft tissue inflammation

• To avoid mouth rinses with high alcohol content due to drying effects

---

bold italic = life-threatening conditions   *For periodic updates, visit* **www.mosby.com**

hydroxyurea

(hye-drox-ee-your-ee′a)

Droxia, Hydrea

Drug class.: Antineoplastic

Action: Acts by inhibiting DNA synthesis without interfering with the synthesis of RNA or protein

Uses: Melanoma, chronic myelocytic leukemia, recurrent or metastatic ovarian cancer, in combination with irradiation therapy for carcinomas of the head and neck (except the lip); sickle cell anemia

Dosage and routes:

Sickle cell anemia

• *Child:* PO 15 mg/kg/day single dose, titrated at 12 wk up to 35 mg/kg/day; monitor CBC q2wk

Solid tumors

• *Adult:* PO 80 mg/kg as a single dose q3d or 20-30 mg/kg as a single dose daily for continuous therapy

With radiation

• *Adult:* PO 80 mg/kg as a single dose q3d

Available forms include: Caps 500 mg

Side effects/adverse reactions:

▼ *ORAL:* Stomatitis, mucositis (with irradiation), lichenoid reaction

CNS: **Convulsions,** anorexia, headache, confusion, hallucinations, dizziness

CV: Angina, ischemia

GI: Nausea, vomiting, anorexia, diarrhea, constipation

HEMA: **Leukopenia, anemia, thrombocytopenia**

GU: Increased BUN, uric acid, creatinine, temporary renal function impairment

INTEG: *Rash,* urticaria, pruritus, dry skin, facial erythema

Contraindications: Hypersensitivity, leukopenia ($<2500/mm^3$), thrombocytopenia ($<100,000/mm^3$), anemia (severe), marked bone marrow depression

Precautions: Pregnancy category D, monitor blood counts and hemoglobin, renal impairment, elderly

Pharmacokinetics:

PO: Readily absorbed with PO use, peak level in 2 hr; 80% excreted in urine

⚕ Drug interactions of concern to dentistry:

• None reported

DENTAL CONSIDERATIONS

General:

• Patients receiving chemotherapy may be taking chronic opioids for pain. Consider NSAIDs for dental pain management.

• Patients receiving chemotherapy may require palliative therapy for stomatitis.

• Patients on chronic drug therapy may rarely have symptoms of blood dyscrasias, which can include infection, bleeding, and poor healing.

Consultations:

• Medical consult may be required to assess disease control.

• In a patient with symptoms of blood dyscrasias, request a medical consult for blood studies and postpone dental treatment until normal values are reestablished.

Teach patient/family:

• That secondary oral infection may occur; must see dentist immediately if infection occurs

When chronic dry mouth occurs, advise patient:

• To avoid mouth rinses with high alcohol content due to drying effects

italic = common side effects

• To use sugarless gum, frequent sips of water, or saliva substitutes
• To use daily home fluoride products for anticaries effect

---

hydroxyzine HCl/ hydroxyzine pamoate

(hye-drox′i-zeen)

Atarax, Vistaril, Vistaril IM
♣ Apo-Hydroxyzine, Multipax, Novo-Hydroxyzin

Drug class.: Antianxiety antihistamine

Action: Depresses subcortical levels of CNS, antagonist for histamine H_1-receptors
Uses: Anxiety, preoperatively/postoperatively to prevent nausea and vomiting, to potentiate narcotic analgesics, sedation, pruritus
Dosage and routes:
• *Adult:* PO 25 mg tid-qid
• *Child >6 yr:* 50-100 mg/day in divided doses
• *Child <6 yr:* Up to 50 mg/day in divided doses
Preoperatively/postoperatively
• *Adult:* IM 25-100 mg q4-6h
• *Child:* IM 1.1 mg/kg q4-6h
Available forms include: Tabs 10, 25, 50, 100 mg; caps 25, 50, 100 mg; syr 10 mg/5 ml; oral susp 25 mg/5 ml; inj IM 25 mg/ml, 50 mg/5 ml
Side effects/adverse reactions:
▼ *ORAL:* Dry mouth
CNS: Dizziness, drowsiness, confusion, headache, tremors, fatigue, depression, convulsions
Contraindications: Hypersensitivity, pregnancy category not established, avoid in pregnancy
Precautions: Elderly, debilitated, hepatic disease, renal disease

Pharmacokinetics:
PO: Onset 15-30 min, duration 4-6 hr, half-life 3 hr
🦷 **Drug interactions of concern to dentistry:**
• Increased CNS depressant effect: alcohol, all CNS depressants
• Increased anticholinergic effects: other antihistamines, anticholinergics, opioid analgesics
DENTAL CONSIDERATIONS
General:
• Potentiates other CNS depressant drugs. When used in combination, the dose of other CNS depressants should be reduced by one half.
• Assess salivary flow as a factor in caries, periodontal disease, and candidiasis.
• Geriatric patients are more susceptible to drug effects; use lower dose.
• Have someone drive patient to and from dental appointment if the drug is prescribed for dental therapy.
Teach patient/family: *When chronic dry mouth occurs, advise patient:*
• To avoid mouth rinses with high alcohol content due to drying effects
• To use sugarless gum, frequent sips of water, or saliva substitutes
• To use daily home fluoride products for anticaries effect

---

hyoscyamine sulfate

(hye-oh-sye′a-meen)

Anaspaz, Cystospaz-M, Gastrosed, Levbid, Levsin, Levsinex, Neoquess

Drug class.: Anticholinergic

Action: Inhibits muscarinic actions of acetylcholine at postgan-

---

glionic parasympathetic neuroeffector sites

Uses: Treatment of peptic ulcer disease in combination with other drugs, other GI disorders, other spastic disorders such as parkinsonism, preoperatively to reduce secretions, GU disorders (cystitis, renal colic), partial heart block

Dosage and routes:
• *Adult:* PO/SL 0.125-0.25 mg tid-qid ac, hs; time rel 0.375 q12h; IM/SC/IV 0.25-0.5 mg q6h
• *Child 2-10 yr:* One-half adult dose
• *Child <2 yr:* One-fourth adult dose

Available forms include: Tabs 0.125, 0.13, 0.15 mg; time rel caps 0.375 mg; ext rel tabs 0.375; sol 0.125 mg/ml; elix 0.125 mg/5 ml; inj IM/IV/SC 0.5 mg/ml

Side effects/adverse reactions:
▼ *ORAL: Dry mouth*
CNS: Confusion, stimulation in elderly, headache, insomnia, dizziness, drowsiness, anxiety, weakness, hallucination
CV: Palpitation, tachycardia
GI: Constipation, paralytic ileus, heartburn, nausea, vomiting, dysphagia
GU: Hesitancy, retention, impotence
EENT: Blurred vision, photophobia, mydriasis, cycloplegia, increased ocular tension
INTEG: Urticaria, rash, pruritus, anhidrosis, fever, allergic reactions

Contraindications: Hypersensitivity to anticholinergics, narrow-angle glaucoma, GI obstruction, myasthenia gravis, paralytic ileus, GI atony, toxic megacolon, prostatic hypertrophy

Precautions: Hyperthyroidism, CAD, dysrhythmias, CHF, ulcerative colitis, hypertension, hiatal hernia, hepatic disease, renal disease, pregnancy category C, urinary retention

Pharmacokinetics:
PO: Duration 4-6 hr; metabolized by liver, excreted in urine, half-life 3.5 hr

Drug interactions of concern to dentistry:
• Increased anticholinergic effect: other anticholinergics, opioid analgesics
• Decreased effect of phenothiazines, ketoconazole

DENTAL CONSIDERATIONS
General:
• After supine positioning, have patient sit upright for at least 2 min to avoid orthostatic hypotension.
• Assess salivary flow as a factor in caries, periodontal disease, and candidiasis.
• Avoid dental light in patient's eyes; offer dark glasses for patient comfort.

Consultation:
• Physician should be informed if significant xerostomic side effects occur (increased caries, sore tongue, problems eating or swallowing, difficulty wearing prosthesis) so a medication change can be considered.

Teach patient/family:
• Importance of good oral hygiene to prevent soft tissue inflammation
When chronic dry mouth occurs, advise patient:
• To avoid mouth rinses with high alcohol content due to drying effects
• To use sugarless gum, frequent sips of water, or artificial saliva substitutes
• To use daily home fluoride products for anticaries effect

ibuprofen

(eye-byoo-proe'fen)

Ibifon, IBU, Ibuprohm, Motrin, Rufen

✤ Amersol

OTC: Advil, Advil Migraine, Children's Advil, Children's Motrin, Genpril, Haltran, Junior Strength Motrin, Menadol, Midol Maximum, Motrin Migraine Pain, Nuprin

✤ Actiprofen,   Apo-Ibuprofen, Novo-Profen, Nu-Ibuprofen

Susp: Children's Advil, Children's Motrin Oral Drops, Infant's Motrin, PediaCare, PediaCare Fever

✤ Children's Apo-Ibuprofen

Drug class.: Nonsteroidal antiinflammatory

Action: Inhibits prostaglandin synthesis by interfering with cyclooxygenase needed for biosynthesis; possesses analgesic, antiinflammatory, antipyretic properties

Uses: Rheumatoid arthritis, osteoarthritis, primary dysmenorrhea, gout, mild-to-moderate pain, fever

Dosage and routes:

Arthritis

• *Adult:* PO 200-800 mg qid, not to exceed 3.2 g/day

• *Child 2-11 yr:* PO oral suspension (OTC) for fever and minor aches and pain, toothache; 7.5 mg/kg up to qid; max daily dose 30 mg/kg

Mild to moderate pain

• *Adult:* PO 400 mg q4-6h

Dysmenorrhea

• *Adult:* PO 400 mg q4h

Antipyretic use only

• *Child 6 mo-12 yr:* 5 mg/kg for temperature <102.5° F;

10 mg/kg for higher temperature q4-6h

Available forms include: Tabs 100, 200 (OTC), 300, 400, 600, 800 mg; chew tabs 50, 100 mg; OTC susp 100 mg/5 ml in 60, 120, and 480 ml volumes; caps 100 mg; oral drops 40 mg/ml in 15 ml

Side effects/adverse reactions:

▼ *ORAL:* Dry mouth, bleeding, stomatitis, lichenoid reaction

CNS: Dizziness, drowsiness, fatigue, tremors, confusion, insomnia, anxiety, depression

CV: Tachycardia, peripheral edema, palpitation, dysrhythmias

GI: **Cholestatic hepatitis,** nausea, anorexia, vomiting, diarrhea, jaundice, constipation, flatulence, cramps, peptic ulcer

HEMA: **Blood dyscrasias**

GU: **Nephrotoxicity: dysuria, hematuria, oliguria, azotemia**

EENT: Tinnitus, hearing loss, blurred vision

INTEG: Purpura, rash, pruritus, sweating

Contraindications: Hypersensitivity, asthma, severe renal disease, severe hepatic disease, alcohol

Precautions: Pregnancy category not established (use not recommended), lactation, children, bleeding disorders, GI disorders, cardiac disorders, hypersensitivity to other antiinflammatory agents

Pharmacokinetics:

PO: Peak 1-2 hr, half-life 2-4 hr; 90%-99% plasma-protein binding; metabolized in liver (inactive metabolites); excreted in urine (inactive metabolites)

🦷 **Drug interactions of concern to dentistry:**

• GI ulceration, bleeding: aspirin, alcohol (3 or more drinks/day), corticosteroids

---

bold italic = life-threatening conditions

• Decreased action: salicylates
• Nephrotoxicity: acetaminophen (prolonged use)
• Possible risk of decreased renal function: cyclosporine
When prescribed for dental pain:
• Risk of increased effects: oral anticoagulants, oral antidiabetics, lithium, methotrexate
• Decreased antihypertensive effects of diuretics, β-adrenergic blockers, and ACE inhibitors

DENTAL CONSIDERATIONS

General:
• Patients on chronic drug therapy may rarely have symptoms of blood dyscrasias, which can include infection, bleeding, and poor healing.
• Assess salivary flow as a factor in caries, periodontal disease, and candidiasis.
• Avoid prescribing aspirin-containing products.
• Consider semisupine chair position for patients with arthritic disease.

Consultations:
• In a patient with symptoms of blood dyscrasias, request a medical consult for blood studies and postpone dental treatment until normal values are reestablished.
• Medical consult may be required to assess disease control.

Teach patient/family:
• To follow labeled directions for OTC products
• Importance of good oral hygiene to prevent soft tissue inflammation
• Caution to prevent injury when using oral hygiene aids
When chronic dry mouth occurs, advise patient:
• To avoid mouth rinses with high

alcohol content due to drying effects
• To use sugarless gum, frequent sips of water, or saliva substitutes
• To use daily home fluoride products for anticaries effect

---

imatinib mesylate

(im-at′i-nib)
Gleevec
Drug class.: Antineoplastic

Action: Inhibits protein-tyrosine kinase, notably Bcr-Abl tyrosine kinase (the abnormal tyrosine kinase) in chronic myeloid leukemia; inhibits proliferation and induces apoptosis (programmed cell death) in Bcr-Abl positive cell lines

Uses: Chronic myeloid leukemia (CML) in blast crisis, accelerated phase or chronic phase after failure of interferon-alpha therapy

Dosage and routes:
• *Adult:* PO 400 mg/day for patients in chronic phase; 600 mg/day for patients in blast crisis or accelerated phases; dose is administered once daily with a meal and large glass of water

Available forms include: Caps 100 mg

Side effects/adverse reactions:

CNS: Headache, fatigue, anorexia, weakness

CV: Neutropenia, thrombocytopenia, anemia, potentially serious edema

GI: Nausea, vomiting, diarrhea, dyspepsia, abdominal pain

*RESP: **Pleural effusion,*** pulmonary edema, cough, dyspnea, pneumonia

---

HEMA: Hemorrhage (CNS, GI), epistaxis
EENT: Nasopharyngitis
INTEG: Rash, pruritus, petechiae
ENDO: Hypokalemia, elevation of transaminase, bilirubin, AST, ALT, creatinine, alk phosphatase
META: Weight gain
MS: Muscle cramps, pain, arthralgia
MISC: Edema (lower limbs, periorbital tissues), ascites, fever
Contraindications: Hypersensitivity, pregnancy not advised while taking this drug
Precautions: Fluid retention, edema risk; neutropenia, thrombocytopenia, GI irritation, liver function abnormalities; pregnancy category D, safety in lactation or pediatric patients has not been studied
Pharmacokinetics:
PO: Mean absolute bioavailability 95%; plasma protein binding 95%; metabolized by cytochrome P450 3A4 enzymes; active metabolite, excreted mainly in feces 68%, urine 13%
⚖ Drug interactions of concern to dentistry:
• Increased plasma levels with CYP 3A4 inhibitors: ketoconazole; possibly macrolide antibiotics, itraconazole
• Increased concentration of drugs metabolized by CYP 3A4, such as benzodiazepines
• Use acetaminophen with caution or avoid if hepatotoxicity is present
• Possible decrease in plasma concentrations: dexamethasone, carbamazepine, St. John's Wort

DENTAL CONSIDERATIONS
General:
• Prophylactic or therapeutic antibiotics may be indicated to prevent or treat infection if surgery or periodontal débridement is required.
• Patients taking opioids for acute or chronic pain should be given alternative analgesics for dental pain.
• Short appointments and a stress reduction protocol may be required for anxious patients.
• Consider local hemostasis measures to control excessive bleeding.
• Patient on chronic drug therapy may rarely present with symptoms of blood dyscrasias, which can include infection, bleeding, and poor healing.
• Consider semisupine chair position for patient comfort if GI side effects occur.
Consultations:
• In a patient with symptoms of blood dyscrasias, request a medical consult for blood studies and postpone treatment until normal values are reestablished.
• Consultation with physician may be needed if sedation or general anesthesia is required.
• Medical consult should include routine blood counts including platelet counts and bleeding time.
Teach patient/family:
• Importance of good oral hygiene to prevent soft tissue inflammation/infection
• To inform dentist of unusual bleeding episodes following dental treatment

imipramine HCl/imipramine pamoate

(im-ip'ra-meen)

Imipramine HCl: Tofranil
♣ Apo-Imipramine, Impril, Novopramine
Imipramine pamoate: Tofranil-PM Capsules

Drug class.: Antidepressant (tricyclic)

Action: Inhibits both norepinephrine and serotonin (5-HT) uptake in the brain, although the precise antidepressant mechanism remains unclear

Uses: Depression, enuresis in children; unapproved: neurogenic pain, panic disorder, migraine headache

Dosage and routes:
• *Adult:* PO/IM 75-100 mg/day in divided doses; may increase by 25-50 mg to 200 mg, not to exceed 300 mg/day; may give daily dose hs
• *Child:* PO 25-75 mg/day

Available forms include: Tabs 10, 25, 50 mg; caps 75, 100, 125 mg

Side effects/adverse reactions:

▼ *ORAL: Dry mouth, unpleasant taste,* stomatitis

CNS: Dizziness, drowsiness, confusion, headache, anxiety, tremors, stimulation, weakness, insomnia, nightmares, EPS (elderly), increased psychiatric symptoms, paresthesia

CV: Orthostatic hypotension, ECG changes, tachycardia, **hypertension,** palpitation

GI: Diarrhea, **paralytic ileus, hepatitis,** nausea, vomiting, increased appetite, cramps, epigastric distress, jaundice

HEMA: **Agranulocytosis, thrombocytopenia, eosinophilia, leukopenia**

GU: Retention, **acute renal failure**

EENT: Blurred vision, tinnitus, mydriasis

INTEG: Rash, urticaria, sweating, pruritus, photosensitivity

Contraindications: Hypersensitivity to tricyclic antidepressants, recovery phase of MI, convulsive disorders, prostatic hypertrophy

Precautions: Suicidal patients, severe depression, increased intraocular pressure, narrow-angle glaucoma, urinary retention, cardiac disease, hepatic disease, hyperthyroidism, electroshock therapy, elective surgery, elderly, pregnancy category B, MAO inhibitors

Pharmacokinetics:

PO: Steady state 2-5 days, half-life 6-20 hr; metabolized by liver; excreted by kidneys, feces; crosses placenta; excreted in breast milk

🦷 **Drug interactions of concern to dentistry:**
• Increased anticholinergic effects: muscarinic blockers, antihistamines, phenothiazines
• Increased effects of direct-acting sympathomimetics (epinephrine, levonordefrin)
• Potential risk of increased CNS depression: alcohol, barbiturates, benzodiazepines, and other CNS depressants
• Decreased antihypertensive effects: clonidine, guanadrel, guanethidine

DENTAL CONSIDERATIONS

General:
• Monitor vital signs every appointment due to cardiovascular side effects.

• Assess salivary flow as a factor in caries, periodontal disease, and candidiasis.

• Patients on chronic drug therapy may rarely have symptoms of blood dyscrasias, which can include infection, bleeding, and poor healing.

• After supine positioning, have patient sit upright for at least 2 min to avoid orthostatic hypotension.

• Use vasoconstrictors with caution, in low doses, and with careful aspiration. Avoid use of gingival retraction cord with epinephrine.

• Place on frequent recall due to oral side effects.

Consultations:

• In a patient with symptoms of blood dyscrasias, request a medical consult for blood studies and postpone dental treatment until normal values are reestablished.

• Medical consult may be required to assess disease control.

• Physician should be informed if significant xerostomic side effects occur (increased caries, sore tongue, problems eating or swallowing, difficulty wearing prosthesis) so a medication change can be considered.

Teach patient/family:

• Importance of good oral hygiene to prevent soft tissue inflammation

• Caution to prevent injury when using oral hygiene aids

When chronic dry mouth occurs, advise patient:

• To avoid mouth rinses with high alcohol content due to drying effects

• To use sugarless gum, frequent sips of water, or saliva substitutes

• To use daily home fluoride products for anticaries effect

imiquimod
(i-mi-kwi′mod)
Aldara

Drug class.: Immune response modifier

Action: Mechanism is unknown; imiquimod induces cytokines including interferon-α in animal studies

Uses: External genital and perianal warts, condylomata acuminata; unapproved: refractory common and plantar warts

Dosage and routes:

• *Adult:* TOP apply cream 3 days per week at bedtime, leave on the skin for 6-10 hr; remove cream with mild soap and water after treatment; max duration of treatment 16 wk; cream is applied in a thin layer to the wart and rubbed in until no longer visible

Available forms include: Cream 5% in packets containing 250 mg of cream, 12 packets/box

Side effects/adverse reactions:

CNS: Headache, fatigue, fever

GI: Diarrhea

INTEG: Erythema, erosion, flaking, edema, induration, ulceration, scabbing, vesicles

MS: Myalgia

MISC: Fungal infection, flulike symptoms

Contraindications: None listed

Precautions: Has not been evaluated in papilloma viral diseases, cream may weaken condoms and diaphragms, external use only, pregnancy category B, lactation, children <18 yr

---

Pharmacokinetics:

TOP: Minimal cutaneous absorption

🦷 **Drug interactions of concern to dentistry:**
• None reported

DENTAL CONSIDERATIONS

General:
• Oral manifestations of the disease may occur in the oral mucosa.
• Patient may have history of other STDs.

Consultations:
• Medical consult may be required to assess disease control.

Teach patient/family:
• To report oral lesions to the dentist
• Importance of updating health and drug history if physician makes any changes in evaluation or drug regimens

---

indapamide

(in-dap'a-mide)

Lozol

♣ Lozide

Drug class.: Diuretic, thiazide-like

Action: Acts on distal tubule by increasing excretion of water, sodium, chloride, potassium

Uses: Edema, hypertension

Dosage and routes:
• *Adult:* PO 2.5 mg qd in AM, may be increased to 5 mg qd if needed

Available forms include: Tabs 1.25, 2.5 mg

Side effects/adverse reactions:

▼ *ORAL:* Dry mouth

CNS: Headache, dizziness, fatigue, weakness, paresthesia, depression

CV: Orthostatic hypotension, volume depletion, palpitation

GI: Nausea, diarrhea, vomiting, anorexia, cramps, constipation, pancreatitis, abdominal pain, jaundice, hepatitis

HEMA: **Thrombocytopenia, agranulocytosis, leukopenia, neutropenia, anemia**

GU: Polyuria, dysuria, frequency

EENT: Loss of hearing, tinnitus, blurred vision, nasal congestion, increased intraocular pressure

INTEG: Rash, pruritus, photosensitivity, alopecia, urticaria

MS: Cramps

ELECT: Hypochloremic alkalosis, hypomagnesemia, hyperuricemia, hypercalcemia, hyponatremia, hypokalemia, hyperglycemia

Contraindications: Hypersensitivity, anuria

Precautions: Hypokalemia, dehydration, ascites, hepatic disease, severe renal disease, pregnancy category B

Pharmacokinetics:

PO: Onset 1-2 hr, peak 2 hr, duration up to 36 hr, half-life 14-18 hr; excreted in urine, feces

🦷 **Drug interactions of concern to dentistry:**
• Increased photosensitization: tetracycline
• Decreased hypotensive response: NSAIDs, especially indomethacin

DENTAL CONSIDERATIONS

General:
• Monitor vital signs every appointment due to cardiovascular side effects.
• Patients on chronic drug therapy may rarely have symptoms of blood dyscrasias, which can include infection, bleeding, and poor healing.
• After supine positioning, have patient sit upright for at least 2 min before standing to avoid orthostatic hypotension.

• Assess salivary flow as a factor in caries, periodontal disease, and candidiasis.
• Limit use of sodium-containing products such as saline IV fluids for patients with a dietary salt restriction.
• Stress from dental procedures may compromise cardiovascular function; determine patient risk.
• Short appointments and a stress reduction protocol may be required for anxious patients.
• Patients on diuretic therapy should be monitored for serum K^+ levels.

Consultations:
• In a patient with symptoms of blood dyscrasias, request a medical consult for blood studies and postpone dental treatment until normal values are reestablished.
• Medical consult may be required to assess disease control and patient's ability to tolerate stress.

Teach patient/family:
• Importance of good oral hygiene to prevent soft tissue inflammation
• Caution to prevent injury when using oral hygiene aids
When chronic dry mouth occurs, advise patient:
• To avoid mouth rinses with high alcohol content due to drying effects
• To use sugarless gum, frequent sips of water, or saliva substitutes
• To use daily home fluoride products for anticaries effect

---

indinavir sulfate
(in-din′a-veer)
Crixivan
Drug class.: Antiviral

Action: Inhibits HIV protease enzyme, preventing cleavage of viral polyproteins and formation of immature noninfectious viral particles
Uses: HIV infection; prophylaxis after needle stick with AZT and lamivudine within 2 hr of needle stick

Dosage and routes:
• *Adult:* PO 800 mg q8h without food, 1 hr before or 2 hr after meal, force fluids; reduce dose to 600 mg q8h with concurrent use of ketoconazole
Available forms include: Caps 200, 400 mg

Side effects/adverse reactions:
▼ *ORAL: Dry mouth, taste alteration,* aphthous stomatitis, gingivitis
CNS: Headache, insomnia, dizziness, somnolence
CV: Palpitation
GI: Abdominal pain, nausea, diarrhea, vomiting, acid regurgitation
RESP: Upper respiratory infection, cough
HEMA: **Hyperbilirubinemia,** anemia, lymphadenopathy
GU: Nephrolithiasis, flank pain, hematuria
EENT: Pharyngitis, blurred vision
INTEG: Rash, dry skin, dermatitis
MS: Asthenia, fatigue, back pain
Contraindications: Hypersensitivity; concurrent use with triazolam, midazolam, alprazolam, chlordiazepoxide, clonazepam, chlorazepate, diazepam, estazolam, flurazepam, halazepam, quazepam
Precautions: Nephrolithiasis (requires adequate hydration), hyperbilirubinemia, serum transaminase elevation, hepatic impairment, dose reduction of rifabutin required, pregnancy category C, lactation, children

---

bold italic = life-threatening conditions

Pharmacokinetics:
PO: Rapid absorption, food reduces absorption, 60% plasma protein bound, peak plasma levels 1 hr, hepatic metabolism, urinary and GI excretion

🦷 **Drug interactions of concern to dentistry:**
• Contraindicated with triazolam, midazolam
• Reduce dose when given with ketoconazole
• Increased blood levels of: clarithromycin

DENTAL CONSIDERATIONS
General:
• Consider semisupine chair position when GI side effects occur.
• Assess salivary flow as a factor in caries, periodontal disease, candidiasis.
• Monitor vital signs every appointment due to cardiovascular side effects.
• Examine for oral manifestation of opportunistic infection.
• Patients with gastroesophageal reflux may have oral symptoms, including burning mouth, secondary candidiasis, and signs of tooth erosion.
Consultations:
• Medical consult may be required to assess disease control.
Teach patient/family:
• Importance of good oral hygiene to prevent soft tissue inflammation
• To report oral lesions, soreness, or bleeding to dentist
• Importance of updating health history/drug record if physician makes any changes in evaluation or drug regimens
When chronic dry mouth occurs, advise patient:
• To avoid mouth rinses with high alcohol content due to drying effects
• To use daily home fluoride products for anticaries effect
• To use sugarless gum, frequent sips of water, or saliva substitutes

---

indomethacin/ indomethacin sodium trihydrate
(in-doe-meth′a-sin)
Indameth, Indocin, Indocin SR
♣ Apo-Indomethacin, Indocid, Indocid SR, Novo-Methacin, Nu-Indo
Drug class.: Nonsteroidal antiinflammatory

Action: Inhibits prostaglandin synthesis by interfering with cyclooxygenase needed for biosynthesis; possesses analgesic, antiinflammatory, antipyretic properties
Uses: Rheumatoid arthritis, osteoarthritis, ankylosing rheumatoid spondylitis, acute gouty arthritis; unapproved: closure of patent ductus arteriosus in premature infants
Dosage and routes:
Arthritis
• *Adult:* PO/REC 25 mg bid-tid, may increase by 25 mg/day q1wk, not to exceed 200 mg/day; sus rel 75 mg qd, may increase to 75 mg bid
Acute arthritis
• *Adult:* PO/REC 50 mg tid; use only for acute attack, then reduce dose
Available forms include: Caps 25, 50 mg; ext rel caps 75 mg; susp 25

---

mg/5 ml; rec supp 50 mg; powder for inj 1 mg vial

Side effects/adverse reactions:

▼ *ORAL:* Dry mouth, bleeding, stomatitis, lichenoid reaction

CNS: Dizziness, drowsiness, fatigue, tremors, confusion, insomnia, anxiety, depression

CV: Tachycardia, peripheral edema, palpitation, dysrhythmias

GI: **Cholestatic hepatitis,** nausea, anorexia, vomiting, diarrhea, jaundice, constipation, flatulence, cramps, peptic ulcer

HEMA: **Blood dyscrasias**

GU: **Nephrotoxicity: dysuria, hematuria, oliguria, azotemia**

EENT: Tinnitus, hearing loss, blurred vision

INTEG: Purpura, rash, pruritus, sweating

Contraindications: Hypersensitivity, asthma, severe renal disease, severe hepatic disease

Precautions: Pregnancy category not listed (use not recommended), lactation, children, bleeding disorders, GI disorders, cardiac disorders, hypersensitivity to other anti-inflammatory agents, depression

Pharmacokinetics:

PO: Onset 1-2 hr, peak 3 hr, duration 4-6 hr; 99% plasma-protein binding; metabolized in liver, kidneys; excreted in urine, bile, feces, breast milk; crosses placenta

🥄 **Drug interactions of concern to dentistry:**

• Increased GI bleeding, ulceration: corticosteroids, alcohol, aspirin, other NSAIDs

• Renal toxicity: acetaminophen (high doses, prolonged use)

• Possible risk of decreased renal function: cyclosporine

When prescribed for dental pain:

• Risk of increased effects: oral anticoagulants, oral antidiabetics, lithium, methotrexate

• Decreased antihypertensive effects of diuretics, β-adrenergic blockers, and ACE inhibitors

DENTAL CONSIDERATIONS

General:

• Avoid prescribing aspirin-containing products.

• Patients on chronic drug therapy may rarely have symptoms of blood dyscrasias, which can include infection, bleeding, and poor healing.

• Assess salivary flow as a factor in caries, periodontal disease, and candidiasis.

• Consider semisupine chair position for patients with arthritic disease.

Consultations:

• In a patient with symptoms of blood dyscrasias, request a medical consult for blood studies and postpone dental treatment until normal values are reestablished.

• Medical consult may be required to assess disease control.

Teach patient/family:

• Importance of good oral hygiene to prevent soft tissue inflammation

• Caution to prevent injury when using oral hygiene aids

When chronic dry mouth occurs, advise patient:

• To avoid mouth rinses with high alcohol content due to drying effects

• To use sugarless gum, frequent sips of water, or saliva substitutes

• To use daily home fluoride products for anticaries effect

---

bold italic = life-threatening conditions   *For periodic updates, visit* **www.mosby.com**

infliximab

(in-flix'i-mab)

Remicade

Drug class.: Antiinflammatory

Action: A monoclonal antibody to tumor necrosis factor alpha (TNF_α) and is believed to prevent TNF_α receptor binding resulting in reduced infiltration of inflammatory cells and reduced cytokine levels

Uses: Reduces signs and symptoms, progression of structural damage in rheumatoid arthritis in combination with methotrexate; reduction in signs and symptoms in patients with Crohn's disease with inadequate response to conventional therapy

Dosage and routes:

Rheumatoid arthritis

• *Adult:* IV 3 mg/kg infusion followed by additional doses at 2 and 6 wk, then q8wk; used with methotrexate; doses up to 10 mg/kg have been used

Crohn's disease

• *Adult:* IV 5 mg/kg infusion; with fistulizing disease follow with doses at 2 and 6 wk

Available forms include: Vial 100 mg in 20 ml

Side effects/adverse reactions:

▼ *ORAL: Facial lip edema*

CNS: Headache, dizziness, fatigue

CV: Syncope (rare), hypotension or hypertension, chest pain, arrhythmia

GI: Nausea, diarrhea, abdominal pain, vomiting, dyspepsia

RESP: UTI, sinusitis, bronchitis, latent TB, coughing, pneumonia

HEMA: Development of antinuclear antibodies (ANA), **lymphoma**

GU: UTI

EENT: Sore throat, pharyngitis, rhinitis

INTEG: Rash, pruritus, LE

META: Transient elevation of AST, ALT

MS: Myalgia, arthralgia

MISC: Infusion reaction, fever

Contraindications: Hypersensitivity to murine proteins, active infection

Precautions: Risk of serious infections, risk of autoimmunity, chronic use increases risk of lymphoma, do not give live vaccines to patients taking this drug, patients should be tested for TB before starting therapy, pregnancy category B, no data on lactation or pediatric use

Pharmacokinetics:

IV: Peak levels at end of infusion; detectable levels up to 12 wk, no data on metabolism or excretion

🦷 Drug interactions of concern to dentistry:

• No drug interaction studies conducted

DENTAL CONSIDERATIONS

General:

• Determine why patient is taking the drug.

• Question patient about other drugs being taken.

• Examine for oral manifestation of opportunistic infection.

• Report oral infections to patient's physician, treat infections aggressively.

Consultations:

• Medical consult may be required to assess disease control and patient's ability to tolerate stress.

Teach patient/family:
• Importance of good oral hygiene to prevent soft tissue inflammation/infection
• To immediately report any signs/symptoms of oral infection

---

insulin
(in'su-lin)
rapid acting insulin
Insulin injection USP (pork): Iletin II Regular
♣ Iletin, Iletin II
Insulin human injection USP: Humulin-R, Novolin R, Novolin R Pen Fill, Novolin R Prefilled, Velosulin BR
♣ Novolin ge Toronto
Insulin analog solution: insulin lispro (Humalog) and insulin aspart (Novolog)
intermediate acting insulin
Isophane insulin suspension (pork): NPH Iletin II
♣ Iletin NPH, Iletin II NPH, Novolin ge NPH
Isophane insulin suspension, human: Humulin N, Novolin N, Novolin N Pen Fill, Novolin N Prefilled
♣ Novolin ge NPH
Insulin zinc suspension (pork): Lente Iletin II
♣ Iletin, Iletin II, Novolin ge Lente
Insulin zinc suspension, human: Humulin L, Novolin L
long acting insulin
Insulin zinc suspension, human extended: Humulin U Ultralente
♣ Novolin ge Ultralente
Insulin analog solution: insulin glargine solution (Lantus)

combination insulin products
Isophane insulin suspension and insulin, human: Humulin 50/50, Humulin 70/30, Novolin 70/30, Novolin 70/30 Pen Fill, Novolin 70/30 Prefilled
♣ Humulin 30/70, Novolin ge 50/50, Novolin ge 30/70
Insulin analog with protamine: Humalog Mix 50/50, Humalog Mix 75/25
insulin injection concentrated, human
Insulin (human): Humulin R Regular U-500

Drug class.: Hormone, antidiabetic

Action: Decreases blood glucose; stimulates glucose uptake in skeletal muscle, fat and other tissues, decreases hepatic glucose production, inhibits lipolysis and proteolysis
Uses: Severe ketoacidosis, type 1 (IDDM) and type 2 (NIDDM—when diet, weight control, exercise or oral hypoglycemics are not sufficient); hyperkalemia, hyperalimentation
Dosage and routes:
• *Adult:* SC/IV/IM dosage individualized by blood, urine glucose qd-tid; dose range for adults or child 0.5-1.0 units/kg/day. Type of insulin selected varies with patient need.
Available forms include: 100 U/ml in multiple dose vials (10 ml) or prefilled pens and cartridges for NovoPen units
Side effects/adverse reactions: These reactions may reflect either the disease or inappropriate insulin doses.

---

bold italic = life-threatening conditions

▼ *ORAL:* Dry mouth (rarely a problem)

CNS: Headache, lethargy, tremors, weakness, fatigue, delirium, sweating

CV: Tachycardia, palpitation

GI: Hunger, nausea

EENT: Blurred vision

INTEG: Flushing, rash, urticaria, warmth, lipodystrophy, lipohypertrophy

META: Hypoglycemia

SYST: **Anaphylaxis,** local allergic reactions

Contraindications: Hypersensitivity to protamine and/or animal source insulin; hypoglycemia

Precautions: Change in type of insulin requires monitoring, dose adjustment for human insulin in renal failure, pregnancy category B, glargine and aspart pregnancy category C, dose intervals in elderly, insulin resistance, lipodystrophy, lipohypertrophy, changes in thyroid function

Pharmacokinetics: Depends on type of insulin used; regular insulin, insulin lispro, insulin aspart, and prompt insulin zinc suspension have rapid onset and short duration; NPH insulin and zinc insulin suspensions are intermediate acting, and protamine zinc insulin and extended zinc insulin are long acting

🦷 **Drug interactions of concern to dentistry:**

• Increased hypoglycemia: salicylates and NSAIDs (large doses and chronic use), alcohol

• Hyperglycemia: corticosteroids, epinephrine

DENTAL CONSIDERATIONS

General:

• Monitor vital signs every appointment due to cardiovascular effects of hypoglycemia.

• Place on frequent recall to evaluate healing response.

• Diabetics may be more susceptible to infection and have delayed wound healing.

• Assess salivary flow as a factor in caries, periodontal disease, and candidiasis.

• Prophylactic antibiotics may be indicated in uncontrolled diabetics to prevent infection if surgery or deep scaling is planned.

• Ensure that patient is following prescribed diet and regularly takes medication.

• Question patient about self-monitoring of drug's antidiabetic effect, including blood glucose values or finger-stick records.

• Keep a readily available source of sugar or fruit juice in case of insulin overdose.

Consultations:

• Medical consult may be required to assess disease control and patient's tolerance for stress.

• Medical consult may include data from patient's blood glucose monitoring, including glycosylated hemoglobin or HbA_{1c} testing.

Teach patient/family:

• Importance of good oral hygiene to prevent soft tissue inflammation

• Caution to prevent injury when using oral hygiene aids

• To avoid mouth rinses with high alcohol content due to drying effects

interferon alfa-2a/ interferon alfa-2b/ interferon alfa-n1/ interferon alfa-n3/ interferon beta-1a

(in-ter-feer′on)

Interferon alfa-2a: Roferon A
Interferon alfa-2b: Intron A
♣ *Interferon alfa-n1:* Wellferon
Interferon alfa-n3: Alferon N
Interferon beta-1a: Avonex
Peginterferon alfa-2b: Peg-In-tron

Drug class.: Biologic response modifier

Action: Antiviral action inhibits viral replication by reprogramming virus; antitumor action suppresses cell proliferation; immunomodulating action phagocytizes target cells

Uses: Hairy cell leukemia in persons >18 yr, condyloma acuminatum, metastatic melanoma, AIDS, Kaposi's sarcoma, bladder carcinoma, lymphomas, malignant myeloma, mycosis fungoides, laryngeal papillomatosis, chronic hepatitis C, chronic hepatitis B in pediatric patients <1 yr

Dosage and routes:
• *Adult:* SC/IM (interferon alfa-2a) 3 million IU × 16-24 wk, then 3 million IU 3 × weekly maintenance; SC/IM (interferon alfa-2b) 2 million IU/m² 3 × weekly; if severe adverse reactions occur, dose should be reduced by one half; doses will vary to some extent with disease being treated

Condyloma acuminatum (veneral/ genital warts)
• *Adult:* SC/IM (interferon alfa-n3) 0.05 ml (250,000 IU) intralesional,

given 2 × weekly × 8 wk; not to exceed 0.5 ml (2.5 million IU); inject into base of wart

Multiple sclerosis
• *Adult:* IM interferon beta-1a 30 μg weekly

Chronic hepatitis C (Peginterferon)
• *Adult:* SC qwk × 1 yr according to the following schedule: Dose modifications required if serious adverse reactions occur.

Wt (Kg)	μg of peginterferon
37-45	40
46-56	50
57-72	64
73-88	80
89-106	96
107-136	120
137-160	150

Available forms include: Interferon alfa-2a inj 3, 6, 9, 36 million IU/vial; alfa-2b inj 3, 5, 10, 18, 25, 50 million IU/vial; alfa-n3 inj 5 million IU/1 ml vial with 3.3 mg/ml phenol and 1 mg/ml human albumin

Side effects/adverse reactions:
▼ *ORAL: Taste changes,* dry mouth, stomatitis
CNS: Dizziness, confusion, numbness, paresthesia, **convulsions, coma,** *hallucinations, amnesia, anxiety, mood changes*
CV: Edema, hypotension, **CHF, MI, CVA,** *hypertension, chest pain, palpitation, dysrhythmias*
GI: Weight loss
GU: Impotence
INTEG: Rash, dry skin, itching, alopecia, flushing

MISC: Flulike syndrome: fever, fatigue, myalgias, headache, chills
Contraindications: Hypersensitivity

Precautions: Severe hypotension, dysrhythmia, tachycardia, pregnancy category C, lactation, children, severe renal or hepatic disease, convulsion disorder, thrombophlebitis, coagulation disorders, hemophilia

Pharmacokinetics:
SC/IM: Half-life (interferon alfa-2a) 3.7-8.5 hr, peak 3-4 hr; half-life (interferon alfa-2b) 2-7 hr, peak 6-8 hr; alfa-n3: no detectable plasma levels

🦷 **Drug interactions of concern to dentistry:**
• None reported

DENTAL CONSIDERATIONS
General:
• Determine why the patient is taking the drug.
• Monitor vital signs every appointment due to cardiovascular side effects.
• After supine positioning, have patient sit upright for at least 2 min to avoid orthostatic hypotension.
• Palliative medication may be required for oral side effects.
• Assess salivary flow as a factor in caries, periodontal disease, and candidiasis.

Consultations:
• Medical consult may be required to assess disease control.

Teach patient/family:
• Importance of good oral hygiene to prevent soft tissue inflammation
• To report oral lesions, soreness, or bleeding to dentist
When chronic dry mouth occurs, advise patient:

• To avoid mouth rinses with high alcohol content due to drying effects
• To use sugarless gum, frequent sips of water, or saliva substitutes
• To use daily home fluoride products for anticaries effect
• Importance of updating medical/drug record if physician makes any changes in evaluation or drug regimen

---

interferon gamma-1b
(in-ter-fer′on)
Actimmune
Drug class.: Biologic response modifier

Action: Species-specific protein synthesized in response to viruses, potent phagocyte-activating effects, stimulates superoxide anion production, enhances oxidative metabolism of macrophages, enhances antibody-dependent cellular cytotoxicity, enhances natural killer cell activity

Uses: Serious infections associated with chronic granulomatous disease

Dosage and routes:
• *Adult:* SC 50 µg/m^2 (1.5 million U/m^2) for patients with a surface area >0.5 m^2; 1.5 µg/kg/dose for patients with a surface area <0.5/ m^2; give on Monday, Wednesday, Friday for dosing 3 × weekly

Available forms include: Inj 100 µg (2 million U) single-dose vial

Side effects/adverse reactions:
CNS: Headache, fatigue, fever, chills, depression, confusion, seizures

CV: Hypotension, syncope, tachycardia, heart block

GI: Nausea, anorexia, diarrhea,

vomiting, abdominal pain, weight loss, GI bleeding
RESP: Bronchospasm, tachypnea
HEMA: **Leukopenia, thrombocytopenia,** deep vein thrombosis
INTEG: Rash, pain at injection site
MS: Myalgia, arthralgia
META: Hyponatremia, hyperglycemia

Contraindications: Hypersensitivity to interferon gamma, *E. coli*–derived products

Precautions: Pregnancy category C, cardiac disease, seizure disorders, CNS disorders, myelosuppression, lactation, children <1 yr; monitor hematologic values q3mo

Pharmacokinetics:
SC: Slow absorption, peak 7 hr, elimination half-life 5.9 hr; dose absorbed 89%

🦷 **Drug interactions of concern to dentistry:**
• None reported

DENTAL CONSIDERATIONS
General:
• Determine why the patient is taking the drug.
• Patients on chronic drug therapy may rarely have symptoms of blood dyscrasias, which can include infection, bleeding, and poor healing.
• Ask patient about side effects associated with drug use (abnormal hematologic values).
• Consider semisupine chair position for patient comfort if GI side effects occur.
• Place on frequent recall to evaluate healing response.

Consultations:
• In a patient with symptoms of blood dyscrasias, request a medical consult for blood studies and postpone dental treatment until normal values are reestablished.

• Medical consult may be required to assess disease control and patient's ability to tolerate stress.

Teach patient/family:
• Importance of good oral hygiene to prevent soft tissue inflammation
• Caution to prevent trauma when using oral hygiene aids
• Importance of updating medical history/drug record if physician makes any changes in evaluation or drug regimens

---

ipratropium bromide
(i-pra-troe′pee-um)
Atrovent
🍁 Apo-Ipravent, Kendral-Ipratropium
Drug class.: Anticholinergic bronchodilator

Action: Inhibits interaction of acetylcholine at receptor sites on the bronchial smooth muscle, resulting in bronchodilation

Uses: Bronchodilation during bronchospasm in those with COPD, bronchitis, emphysema, asthma; not for rapid bronchodilation, maintenance treatment only; rhinorrhea, rhinorrhea associated with allergic and nonallergic perennial rhinitis in children age 6-11 yr

Dosage and routes:
• *Adult and child >5 yr:* INH 2 inh 4 × daily, not to exceed 12 inh/24 hr; SOLN 500 µg nebulized at 6-8 hr intervals

Available forms include: Nasal spray 0.06% (42 µg/spray); aerosol 18 µg/actuation; Canada 20 µg/actuation, 200 inh/container; sol for INH 0.02% (500 µg/vial)

Side effects/adverse reactions:
▼ *ORAL: Dry mouth,* stomatitis, metallic taste

CNS: Anxiety, dizziness, headache
CV: Palpitation
GI: Nausea, vomiting, cramps
RESP: Cough, worsening of symptoms
EENT: Blurred vision, nasal dryness, nasal bleeding
INTEG: Rash
Contraindications: Hypersensitivity to this drug or atropine
Precautions: Pregnancy category B, lactation, children <12 yr, narrow-angle glaucoma, prostatic hypertrophy, bladder neck obstruction
Pharmacokinetics: Onset 5-15 min, duration 3-4 hr, half-life 2 hr; does not cross blood-brain barrier

⚕ Drug interactions of concern to dentistry:
• Increased effects of anticholinergic drugs

DENTAL CONSIDERATIONS
General:
• Monitor vital signs every appointment due to cardiovascular and respiratory side effects.
• Assess salivary flow as a factor in caries, periodontal disease, and candidiasis.
• Acute asthmatic episodes may be precipitated in the dental office. Sympathomimetic inhalants should be available for emergency use.
• Consider semisupine chair position for patients with respiratory disease.
• Place on frequent recall due to oral side effects.
Consultations:
• Medical consult may be required to assess disease control and patient's ability to tolerate stress.
Teach patient/family:
• For inhalation dosage forms, rinse mouth with water after each dose to prevent dryness

When chronic dry mouth occurs, advise patient:
• To avoid mouth rinses with high alcohol content due to drying effects
• To use sugarless gum, frequent sips of water, or saliva substitutes
• To use daily home fluoride products for anticaries effect

---

irbesartan
(ir-be-sar′tan)
Avapro
Drug class.: Angiotensin II receptor antagonist, antihypertensive

Action: Acts as a competitive antagonist for angiotensin II (AT_1) receptors, inhibiting both vasoconstrictor and aldosterone secreting effects
Uses: Hypertension alone or in combination with other antihypertensive drugs
Dosage and routes:
• *Adult:* PO initial 150 mg qd; some patients may require 300 mg/day; initial dose for volume- or salt-depleted patients is 75 mg/day
Available forms include: Tabs 75, 150, 300 mg
Side effects/adverse reactions:
CNS: Fatigue, headache, dizziness, anxiety
CV: Orthostatic hypotension, increased heart rate
GI: Diarrhea, dyspepsia, heartburn, nausea, vomiting
RESP: URI, pharyngitis
EENT: Rhinitis
INTEG: Rash, urticaria, pruritus
MS: Musculoskeletal trauma, muscle ache
Contraindications: Hypersensitivity, pregnancy (second, third trimester)

italic = common side effects

Precautions: Hypersensitivity to other angiotensin II receptor antagonists, pregnancy category C, volume- or salt-depleted patients, renal impairment, lactation, children

Pharmacokinetics:

PO: Bioavilaility 60%-80%, rapid absorption, peak serum levels 1.5-2 hr, 90% protein bound, hepatic metabolism, both biliary and renal excretion

Drug interactions of concern to dentistry:

• None reported

DENTAL CONSIDERATIONS

General:

• Monitor vital signs every appointment due to cardiovascular side effects.

• Limit use of sodium-containing products such as saline IV fluids for those patients with a dietary salt restriction.

• Stress from dental procedures may compromise cardiovascular function; determine patient risk.

• Short appointments and a stress reduction protocol may be required for anxious patients.

• Use precaution if sedation or general anesthesia is required; risk of hypotensive episode.

• After supine positioning, have patient sit upright for at least 2 min before standing to avoid orthostatic hypotension.

• Consider semisupine chair position for patient comfort if GI side effects occur.

Consultations:

• Consultation with physician may be needed if sedation or general anesthesia is required.

• Medical consult may be required to assess disease control and pa-tient's ability to tolerate stress; there is risk for a hypotensive episode.

Teach patient/family: Importance of updating health and drug history if physician makes any changes in evaluation or drug regimens

---

isocarboxazid

(eye-soe-kar-box′a-zid)

Marplan

Drug class.: Antidepressant—monoamine oxidase inhibitor

Action: Increases concentrations of endogenous norepinephrine, se-rotonin, and dopamine in CNS storage sites by nonselective inhi-bition of MAO enzymes; the pre-cise antidepressant mechanism is unknown

Uses: Depression

Dosage and routes:

• *Adult:* PO 10 mg/bid, if tolerated can increase dose 10 mg every 2-4 days to 40 mg by end of first wk; max daily dose 60 mg in divided doses

Available forms include: Tabs 10 mg

Side effects/adverse reactions:

▼ *ORAL: Dry mouth*

CNS: Dizziness, sedation, hypo-mania, headache, mania, insom-nia, anxiety, tremors, stimulation, weakness, agitation, convulsions, increased neuromuscular activity

CV: Orthostatic hypotension, syn-cope, palpitation, tachycardia

GI: Constipation, nausea, diar-rhea, abdominal pain

*HEMA: **Agranulocytosis, thrombo-cytopenia,*** spider telangiectases, anemia (rare)

GU: Sexual dysfunction, urinary retention

EENT: Blurred vision, ocular toxicity

INTEG: Rash

ENDO: **SIADH-like syndrome,** hyperprolactinemia

META: Hepatic function abnormalities

MISC: Weight gain

Contraindications: Hypersensitivity to MAO inhibitors, elderly, hypertension, CHF, severe hepatic disease, pheochromocytoma, severe renal disease, severe cardiac disease, foods with high tryptophan or tyramine content, excessive caffeine, sympathomimetics, meperidine

Precautions: Suicidal patients, concurrent use with other antidepressants (patients must stop taking MAO inhibitor 14 days before initiating therapy with other antidepressants), general anesthesia, severe depression, schizophrenia, diabetes mellitus, pregnancy category C, lactation, children <16 yr

Pharmacokinetics:

PO: Good absorption; maximum MAO inhibition 5-10 days, duration up to 2 wk; metabolized by liver; excreted by kidneys

♣ Drug interactions of concern to dentistry:

• Increased pressor effects: indirect-acting sympathomimetics (ephedrine)

• Hyperpyretic crisis, convulsions, hypertensive episode: meperidine, possibly other opioids, carbamazepine

• Increased anticholinergic effects: anticholinergics, antihistamines

• Increased effects of alcohol, barbiturates, benzodiazepines, CNS depressants, SSRIs, tricyclic antidepressants, cyclobenzaprine, bupropion, buspirone, dextromethorphan, antihypertensives

DENTAL CONSIDERATIONS

General:

• Monitor vital signs every appointment due to cardiovascular side effects.

• After supine positioning, have patient sit upright for at least 2 min to avoid orthostatic hypotension.

• Patients on chronic drug therapy may rarely have symptoms of blood dyscrasias, which can include infection, bleeding, and poor healing.

• Consider semisupine chair position for patient comfort if GI side effects occur.

• Assess salivary flow as a factor in caries, periodontal disease, and candidiasis.

• Hypertensive episodes are possible even though there are no specific contraindications to vasoconstrictor use in local anesthetics.

• Short appointments and a stress reduction protocol may be required for anxious patients.

Consultations:

• Medical consult may be required to assess disease control and patient's ability to tolerate stress.

• In a patient with symptoms of blood dyscrasias, request a medical consult for blood studies and postpone treatment until normal values are reestablished.

Teach patient/family: *When chronic dry mouth occurs, advise patient:*

• To avoid mouth rinses with high alcohol content due to drying effects

• To use daily home fluoride products for anticaries effect
• To use sugarless gum, frequent sips of water, or saliva substitutes

isoetharine HCl

(eye-soe-eth'a-reen)
Isoetharine
Drug class.: Adrenergic β₂-agonist

Action: Causes bronchodilation by β₂ stimulation, resulting in increased levels of cAMP and causing relaxation of bronchial smooth muscle with little effect on heart rate
Uses: Bronchospasm, asthma
Dosage and routes:
• *Adult:* IPPB 0.5 ml diluted 1:3 with NS
Available forms include: Sol for inh 1%
Side effects/adverse reactions:
▼ *ORAL:* Dry mouth
CNS: Tremors, anxiety, insomnia, headache, dizziness, stimulation
*CV: **Cardiac arrest,*** palpitation, tachycardia, hypertension, dysrhythmias
GI: Nausea
META: Hyperglycemia
Contraindications: Hypersensitivity to sympathomimetics, narrow-angle glaucoma
Precautions: Pregnancy category C, cardiac disorders, hyperthyroidism, diabetes mellitus, prostatic hypertrophy
Pharmacokinetics:
INH: Onset immediate, peak 5-15 min, duration 1-4 hr; metabolized in liver, GI tract, lungs; excreted in urine

Drug interactions of concern to dentistry:
• Increased effects of both drugs: other sympathomimetics
• Increased dysrhythmia: halogenated hydrocarbon anesthetics
DENTAL CONSIDERATIONS
General:
• Assess salivary flow as a factor in caries, periodontal disease, and candidiasis.
• Consider semisupine chair position for patients with respiratory disease.
• Acute asthmatic episodes may be precipitated in the dental office. Sympathomimetic inhalants should be available for emergency use.
Consultations:
• Medical consult may be required to assess disease control and patient's ability to tolerate stress.
Teach patient/family:
• For inhalation dosage forms, rinse mouth with water after each dose to prevent dryness
When chronic dry mouth occurs, advise patient:
• To avoid mouth rinses with high alcohol content due to drying effects
• To use sugarless gum, frequent sips of water, or saliva substitutes
• To use daily home fluoride products for anticaries effect

isoniazid (INH)

(eye-soe-nye'a-zid)
Nydrazid
🍁 Isotamine, PMS-Isoniazid
Drug class.: Antitubercular

Action: Bactericidal interference with lipid, nucleic acid biosynthesis

---

bold italic = life-threatening conditions   *For periodic updates, visit* **www.mosby.com**

Uses: Treatment/prevention of TB

Dosage and routes:

Treatment

• *Adult:* PO/IM 5 mg/kg qd as single dose for 9 mo-2 yr, not to exceed 300 mg/day

• *Child and infant:* PO/IM 10-20 mg/kg qd as single dose for 18-24 mo, not to exceed 300 mg/day

Prevention

• *Adult:* PO 300 mg qd as single dose for 12 mo; IM 5 mg/kg (300 mg) qd

• *Child and infant:* PO/IM 10 mg/kg qd as single dose for 12 mo, not to exceed 300 mg/day

Available forms include: Tabs 100, 300 mg; inj 100 mg/ml; powder, syr 50 mg/5 ml

Side effects/adverse reactions:

▼ *ORAL:* Lichenoid reaction

CNS: Peripheral neuropathy, **toxic encephalopathy, convulsions,** memory impairment, psychosis

GI: **Jaundice, fatal hepatitis,** nausea, vomiting, epigastric distress

HEMA: **Agranulocytosis, hemolytic anemia, aplastic anemia, thrombocytopenia, eosinophilia, methemoglobinemia**

EENT: Blurred vision, optic neuritis

INTEG: Hypersensitivity: fever, skin eruptions, lymphadenopathy, vasculitis

MISC: Dyspnea, B_6 deficiency, pellagra, hyperglycemia, metabolic acidosis, gynecomastia, rheumatic syndrome, SLE-like syndrome

Contraindications: Hypersensitivity, optic neuritis

Precautions: Pregnancy category C; renal disease; diabetic retinopathy cataracts; ocular defects; hepatic disease; fatal hepatitis, especially in Black, Hispanic women; child <13 yr

Pharmacokinetics:

PO: Peak 1-2 hr, duration 6-8 hr

IM: Peak 45-60 min Metabolized in liver, excreted in urine (metabolites), crosses placenta, excreted in breast milk

Drug interactions of concern to dentistry:

• Increased hepatotoxicity: alcohol, acetaminophen, carbamazepine

• Decreased effectiveness: glucocorticoids, especially prednisolone

• Increased plasma concentration: benzodiazepines, alfentanil

• Decreased effect of ketoconazole, miconazole

DENTAL CONSIDERATIONS

General:

• Patients on chronic drug therapy may rarely have symptoms of blood dyscrasias, which can include infection, bleeding, and poor healing.

• Medical consult may be required to assess disease control.

• Examine for evidence of oral signs of disease.

Consultations:

• In a patient with symptoms of blood dyscrasias, request a medical consult for blood studies and postpone dental treatment until normal values are reestablished.

Teach patient/family:

• Caution to prevent injury when using oral hygiene aids

---

isoproterenol HCl/isoproterenol sulfate

(eye-soe-proe-ter'e-nole)

Isuprel, Isuprel Mistometer

♣ Medihaler-Iso

Drug class.: Adrenergic β_1- and β_2-agonist

Action: Has β_1 and β_2 actions;

relaxes bronchial smooth muscle and dilates the trachea and main bronchi by increasing levels of cAMP, which relaxes smooth muscles; causes increased contractility and heart rate by acting on β-receptors in heart

Uses: Bronchospasm, asthma, heart block, bradycardia, shock

Dosage and routes:

Asthma, bronchospasm

• *Adult:* SL 10-20 mg q6-8h HCl; inh 1 puff, may repeat in 2-5 min, maintenance 1-2 puffs 4-6 × daily

• *Child:* SL 5-10 mg q6-8h HCl; inh 1 puff, may repeat in 2-5 min, maintenance 1-2 puffs 4-6 × daily

Heart block/bradycardia

• *Adult:* IV 0.02-0.06 mg, then 0.01-0.2 mg or 5 µg/min HCl; IM 0.2 mg, then 0.02-1 mg as needed HCl

• *Child:* IV/IM one-half beginning adult dose

Shock

• *Adult and child:* IV inf 0.5-5 µg/min 1 mg/500 ml D₅W, titrate to BP, CVP, and hourly urine output

Available forms include: Sol for nebuliz 1:200 (0.5%), 1:100 (1%); aerosol 0.25%, 0.2%; inj IV/IM 1:5000 (0.2 mg/ml), 1:50,000 (0.2 mg/ml)

Side effects/adverse reactions:

▼ *ORAL:* Dry mouth, altered taste

CNS: Tremors, anxiety, insomnia, headache, dizziness, stimulation

CV: Cardiac arrest, palpitation, tachycardia, hypertension

GI: Nausea, vomiting

RESP: Bronchial irritation, edema, dryness of oropharynx

META: Hyperglycemia

Contraindications: Hypersensitivity to sympathomimetics, narrow-angle glaucoma

Precautions: Pregnancy category C, cardiac disorders, hyperthyroidism, diabetes mellitus, prostatic hypertrophy

Pharmacokinetics:

INH/SL: Onset 1-2 hr

SC: Onset 2 hr

REC: Onset 2-4 hr

Metabolized in liver, lungs, GI tract

⚘ Drug interactions of concern to dentistry:

• Hypotension, tachycardia: haloperidol, loxapine, phenothiazines, thioxanthenes

• Increased dysrhythmia: halogenated-hydrocarbon anesthetics

DENTAL CONSIDERATIONS

General:

• Monitor vital signs every appointment due to cardiovascular and respiratory side effects.

• Assess salivary flow as a factor in caries, periodontal disease, and candidiasis.

• Consider semisupine chair position for patients with respiratory disease.

• Short appointments and a stress reduction protocol may be required for anxious patients.

• Acute asthmatic episodes may be precipitated in the dental office. Sympathomimetic inhalants should be available for emergency use.

Teach patient/family:

• For inhalation dosage forms, rinse mouth with water after each dose to prevent dryness

When chronic dry mouth occurs, advise patient:

• To avoid mouth rinses with high alcohol content due to drying effects

• To use sugarless gum, frequent sips of water, or saliva substitutes

• To use daily home fluoride products for anticaries effect

isosorbide dinitrate

(eye´soe-sor-bide)

Dilatrate-SR, Isordil, Isordil Tembids, Isordil Titradose, Sorbitrate ♣ Apo-ISDN, Coronex, Novosorbide, Sorbitrate SA

Drug class.: Nitrate antianginal

Action: Decreases preload/afterload, which decreases left ventricular end-diastolic pressure, systemic vascular resistance

Uses: Chronic stable angina pectoris, prophylaxis of angina pain

Dosage and routes:

• *Adult:* PO 5-40 mg qid; SL 2.5-10 mg, may repeat q2-3h; chew tabs 5-10 mg prn or q2-3h as prophylaxis; sus rel 40-80 mg q8-12h

Available forms include: Sus rel caps 40 mg; tabs 5, 10, 20, 30, 40 mg; chew tabs 5, 10 mg; sus rel tabs 40 mg; SL tabs 2.5, 5, 10 mg

Side effects/adverse reactions:

▼ *ORAL:* Dry mouth, burning sensation to mucosa (SL tabs)

CNS: Vascular headache, flushing, dizziness, weakness, faintness

CV: Postural hypotension, **collapse,** tachycardia, syncope

GI: Nausea, vomiting

INTEG: Pallor, sweating, rash

MISC: **Methemoglobinemia,** twitching, hemolytic anemia

Contraindications: Hypersensitivity to this drug or nitrites, severe anemia, increased intracranial pressure, cerebral hemorrhage, acute MI

Precautions: Postural hypotension, pregnancy category C, lactation, children

Pharmacokinetics:

SUS ACTION: Duration 6-8 hr

PO: Onset 15-30 min, duration 4-6 hr

SL: Onset 2-5 min, duration 1-4 hr

▼ *ORAL:* Onset 3 min, duration 0.5-3 hr

Metabolized by liver, excreted in urine as metabolites (80%-100%)

⚕ Drug interactions of concern to dentistry:

• Increased effects: alcohol and other drugs that can lower blood pressure

DENTAL CONSIDERATIONS

General:

• Monitor vital signs every appointment due to cardiovascular side effects.

• After supine positioning, have patient sit upright for at least 2 min before standing to avoid orthostatic hypotension.

• Assess salivary flow as a factor in caries, periodontal disease, and candidiasis.

• Stress from dental procedures may compromise cardiovascular function; determine patient risk.

• Use vasoconstrictors with caution, in low doses, and with careful aspiration. Avoid use of gingival retraction cord with epinephrine.

• Short appointments and a stress reduction protocol may be required for anxious patients.

• Nitroglycerin should be available in case of acute anginal episode.

Consultations:

• Medical consult may be required to assess disease control and patient's ability to tolerate stress.

Teach patient/family:

• Importance of good oral hygiene to prevent soft tissue inflammation

When chronic dry mouth occurs, advise patient:
• To avoid mouth rinses with high alcohol content due to drying effects
• To use sugarless gum, frequent sips of water, or saliva substitutes
• To use daily home fluoride products for anticaries effect

---

isosorbide mononitrate
(eye'soe-sor-bide)
Imdur, ISMO, Monoket
Drug class.: Antianginal, organic nitrate

Action: Decreases preload/afterload, which decreases left ventricular end-diastolic pressure, systemic vascular resistance; arterial and venous dilation
Uses: Prevention of angina pectoris due to coronary artery disease
Dosage and routes:
• *Adult:* PO 20 mg bid, 7 hr apart
Available forms include: Tabs 10, 20 mg; ext rel 30, 60, 120 mg
Side effects/adverse reactions:
▼ *ORAL:* Dry mouth
CNS: Vascular headache, flushing, dizziness, weakness, faintness
CV: **Collapse,** postural hypotension, tachycardia, syncope
GI: Nausea, vomiting
INTEG: Pallor, sweating, rash
MISC: **Hemolytic anemia, methemoglobinemia,** twitching
Contraindications: Hypersensitivity to nitrites, severe anemia, increased intracranial pressure, cerebral hemorrhage, acute MI, closed-angle glaucoma
Precautions: Postural hypotension, pregnancy category C, lactation, children, glaucoma

Pharmacokinetics:
PO: Metabolized by the liver, excreted in urine as metabolites (80%-100%)
🦷 **Drug interactions of concern to dentistry:**
• Increased effects: alcohol and other vasodilator-type drugs
DENTAL CONSIDERATIONS
General:
• Monitor vital signs every appointment due to cardiovascular side effects.
• After supine positioning, have patient sit upright for at least 2 min before standing to avoid orthostatic hypotension.
• Stress from dental procedures may compromise cardiovascular function; determine patient risk.
• Assess salivary flow as a factor in caries, periodontal disease, and candidiasis.
• Short appointments and a stress reduction protocol may be required for anxious patients.
• Consider semisupine chair position for patients with respiratory distress.
• Use vasoconstrictors with caution, in low doses, and with careful aspiration. Avoid use of gingival retraction cord with epinephrine.
• Nitroglycerin should be available in case of an acute anginal episode.
Consultations:
• Medical consult may be required to assess disease control and patient's ability to tolerate stress.
Teach patient/family: *When chronic dry mouth occurs, advise patient:*
• To avoid mouth rinses with high alcohol content due to drying effects

---

- To use sugarless gum, frequent sips of water, or saliva substitutes
- To use daily home fluoride products for anticaries effect

---

isotretinoin

(eye-soe-tret′i-noyn)
Accutane
♣ Accutane-Roche
Drug class.: Retinoic acid isomer, vitamin A derivative

Action: Decreases sebum secretion; improves cystic acne
Uses: Severe recalcitrant cystic acne
Dosage and routes:
- *Adult:* PO 0.5-2 mg/kg/day in 2 divided doses × 15-20 wk
Available forms include: Caps 10, 20, 40 mg
Side effects/adverse reactions:
▼ *ORAL: Dry lips/mouth, angular cheilosis*
CNS: **Pseudotumor cerebri,** lethargy, fatigue, headache, depression
CV: Chest pain
GI: *Nausea, vomiting, anorexia, increased liver enzymes,* regional ileus, abdominal pain, weight loss
HEMA: **Thrombocytopenia,** decreased H & H, WBC, reticulocyte count
GU: **Hematuria, proteinuria,** hypouricemia
EENT: *Eye irritation, conjunctivitis, epistaxis, dry nose,* contact lens intolerance, optic neuritis
INTEG: *Dry skin, pruritus, joint/muscle pain, hair loss, photosensitivity,* urticaria, bruising, hirsutism, petechiae, hypopigmentation/hyperpigmentation, nail brittleness, onycholysis

MS: Hyperostosis, arthralgia, bone/joint/muscle pain
Contraindications: Hypersensitivity, inflamed skin, pregnancy
Precautions: Lactation, diabetes, photosensitivity, hepatic disease, depressive illness, pregnancy category X
Pharmacokinetics:
PO: Peak 2.9-3.2 hr, half-life 10-20 hr; metabolized in liver; excreted in urine, feces
🦷 Drug interactions of concern to dentistry:
- Additive photosensitization: tetracycline
- Pseudotumor cerebri, intracranial hypertension: minocycline, doxycycline or tetracycline
- Increased tissue drying: alcohol
DENTAL CONSIDERATIONS
General:
- Patients on chronic drug therapy may rarely have symptoms of blood dyscrasias, which can include infection, bleeding, and poor healing.
- Assess salivary flow as a factor in caries, periodontal disease, and candidiasis.
- An exaggerated healing response characterized by exuberant granulation tissue has been reported.
- Apply lubricant to dry lips for patient comfort before dental procedures.
Consultations:
- In a patient with symptoms of blood dyscrasias, request a medical consult for blood studies and postpone dental treatment until normal values are reestablished.
Teach patient/family:
- Importance of good oral hygiene to prevent soft tissue inflammation

---

When chronic dry mouth occurs, advise patient:
• To avoid mouth rinses with high alcohol content due to drying effects
• To use sugarless gum, frequent sips of water, or saliva substitutes
• To use daily home fluoride products for anticaries effect

---

isoxsuprine HCl
(eye-sox′syoo-preen)
Vasodilan, Voxsuprine
Drug class.: Peripheral vasodilator

Action: α-adrenoreceptor antagonist with β-adrenoreceptor-stimulating properties; may also act directly on vascular smooth muscle; causes cardiac stimulation, uterine relaxation
Uses: Symptoms of cerebrovascular insufficiency; peripheral vascular disease, including arteriosclerosis obliterans, thromboangiitis obliterans, Raynaud's disease
Dosage and routes:
• *Adult:* PO 10-20 mg tid or qid
Available forms include: Tabs 10, 20 mg
Side effects/adverse reactions:
CNS: Dizziness, weakness, tremors, anxiety
*CV: Hypotension, **tachycardia,*** palpitation, chest pain
GI: Nausea, vomiting, abdominal pain, distention
INTEG: Severe rash, flushing
Contraindications: Hypersensitivity, postpartum, arterial bleeding
Precautions: Pregnancy category C, tachycardia
Pharmacokinetics:
PO: Peak 1 hr, duration 3 hr, half-life 1.25 hr; excreted in urine; crosses placenta

⚕ Drug interactions of concern to dentistry:
• Increased effects: alcohol and drugs that also lower blood pressure
DENTAL CONSIDERATIONS
General:
• Monitor vital signs every appointment due to cardiovascular and respiratory side effects.
• After supine positioning, have patient sit upright for at least 2 min before standing to avoid orthostatic hypotension.
• Short appointments and a stress reduction protocol may be required for anxious patients.
• Drugs used for conscious sedation that lower blood pressure may potentiate the hypotensive effects.
• Use vasoconstrictors with caution, in low doses, and with careful aspiration. Avoid use of gingival retraction cord with epinephrine.
Consultations:
• Medical consult may be required to assess disease control and patient's ability to tolerate stress.

---

isradipine
(iz-ra′di-peen)
DynaCirc, DynaCirc CR
Drug class.: Calcium channel blocker

Action: Inhibits calcium ion influx across cell membrane during cardiac depolarization; produces relaxation of coronary vascular smooth muscle, peripheral vascular smooth muscle; dilates coronary vascular arteries; increases myocardial oxygen delivery in patients with vasospastic angina
Uses: Essential hypertension; un-

---

bold italic = life-threatening conditions

approved: angina, Raynaud's disease

Dosage and routes:
Hypertension
• *Adult:* PO 2.5 mg bid, increase at 3-4 wk intervals up to 10 mg bid
Angina
• *Adult:* PO 2.5-7.5 mg tid, maximum 20 mg/d
Available forms include: Caps 2.5, 5 mg; sus rel tabs 5, 10 mg

Side effects/adverse reactions:
▼ *ORAL:* Dry mouth (gingival overgrowth has not been documented with this drug)
CNS: Headache, fatigue, dizziness, fainting, sleep disturbances
CV: Peripheral edema, tachycardia, hypotension, chest pain
GI: Nausea, vomiting, diarrhea, gastric upset, constipation, hepatitis
HEMA: Thrombocytopenia, leukopenia, anemia
GU: Acute renal failure, nocturia, polyuria
INTEG: Rash, pruritus, urticaria, photosensitivity, hair loss
MISC: Flushing

Contraindications: Sick sinus syndrome, second- or third-degree heart block, hypotension <90 mm Hg systolic, hypersensitivity

Precautions: CHF, hypotension, hepatic disease, pregnancy category C, lactation, children, renal disease, elderly

Pharmacokinetics:
PO: Peak plasma levels at 2-3 hr; metabolized in liver; metabolites excreted in urine, feces; excreted in breast milk

🦷 **Drug interactions of concern to dentistry:**
• Decreased effect: indomethacin, possibly other NSAIDs, phenobarbital

• Increased effect: parenteral and inhalational general anesthetics or other drugs with hypotensive actions
• Increased effects of carbamazepine

DENTAL CONSIDERATIONS
General:
• Monitor cardiac status; take vital signs at each appointment because of CV side effects. Consider a stress reduction protocol to prevent stress-induced angina during the dental appointment.
• After supine positioning, have patient sit upright for at least 2 min before standing to avoid orthostatic hypotension.
• Place on frequent recall to monitor gingival condition.
• Limit use of sodium-containing products such as saline IV fluids for patients with a dietary salt restriction.
• Assess salivary flow as a factor in caries, periodontal disease, and candidiasis.
• Use vasoconstrictors with caution, in low doses, and with careful aspiration. Avoid use of gingival retraction cord with epinephrine.
• Patients on chronic drug therapy may rarely have symptoms of blood dyscrasias, which can include infection, bleeding, and poor healing.

Consultations:
• In a patient with symptoms of blood dyscrasias, request a medical consult for blood studies and postpone dental treatment until normal values are reestablished.
• Medical consult may be required to assess disease control and stress tolerance of patient.

Teach patient/family:
• Importance of good oral hygiene

to prevent soft tissue inflammation and minimize gingival overgrowth
• Need for frequent oral prophylaxis if overgrowth occurs

When chronic dry mouth occurs, advise patient:
• To avoid mouth rinses with high alcohol content due to drying effects
• To use sugarless gum, frequent sips of water, or saliva substitutes
• To use daily home fluoride products for anticaries effect

---

itraconazole
(i-tra-koe'na-zole)
Sporanox

Drug class.: Antifungal, systemic (triazole)

Action: Inhibits cytochrome P-450 enzymes and blocks synthesis of essential membrane sterols in fungal organism

Uses: Aspergillosis, blastomycosis, histoplasmosis (pulmonary and extrapulmonary); fungal infections of nails (onychomycosis); *Candida* infections of esophagus or mouth (oral sol only)

Dosage and routes:
Blastomycosis and histoplasmosis
• *Adult:* PO 200 mg qd after a full meal, 200 mg bid for immunocompromised; max 400 mg day

Aspergillosis
• *Adult:* PO 200-400 mg qd

Fungal nail infection (tinea unguium)
• *Adult:* PO 200 mg daily for 12 wk

Oral candidiasis
• *Adult:* PO swish and swallow 200 mg/daily for 1-2 wk

Pharyngeal candidiasis
• *Adult:* Swish and swallow 100 mg daily for a minimum of 3 wk

Available forms include: Caps 100 mg; oral sol 10 mg/ml in 150 ml volume; inj 10 mg/ml (IV infusion)

Side effects/adverse reactions:
CNS: Fatigue, headache, dizziness, anorexia, malaise
CV: Hypertension, edema, vertigo
*GI: **Hepatitis,** nausea, vomiting, diarrhea, abdominal pain,* hepatic dysfunction
GU: Impotence, albuminuria
*INTEG: Rash, pruritus, **Stevens-Johnson syndrome***
META: Hypokalemia, elevated liver enzymes
*MISC: Fever, myalgia, **anaphylaxis***

Contraindications: Hypersensitivity, triazolam, pimozide, quinidine, oral midazolam; avoid use in patients with CHF or who have a history of CHF

Precautions: Pregnancy category C, lactation, liver dysfunction, oral anticoagulants (monitor patient)

Pharmacokinetics:
PO: Peak plasma level 4 hr; highly protein bound (98.5%); take with food; metabolized by liver; 3%-18% excreted in feces, 40% in urine as metabolites

⚕ Drug interactions of concern to dentistry:
• Increased risk of rhabdomyolysis: lovastatin and simvastatin
• Increased risk of hypoglycemia: oral antidiabetics
• Increased metabolism: phenobarbital, carbamazepine
• Increased risk of toxicity: cyclosporine
• Contraindicated with triazolam, midazolam
• Inhibits metabolism of certain benzodiazepines: alprazolam, chlordiazepoxide, clonazepam, chlorazepate, diazepam, estazolam,

---

flurazepam, halazepam, midazolam, quazepam, triazolam, buspirone, zyloprim, felodipine
• Decreased effects: didanosine
• Increased plasma levels: saquinavir, nisoldipine, haloperidol, carbamazepine
• Avoid itraconazole use with HMG-CoA reductase inhibitors or lower their dose
• May inhibit the metabolism of warfarin

DENTAL CONSIDERATIONS
General:
• Monitor vital signs every appointment due to cardiovascular side effects.
• Determine why the patient is taking the drug.
• Consider semisupine chair position for patient comfort due to GI effects of drug.

Consultations:
• Medical consult may be required to assess patient's ability to tolerate stress.

---

ketoconazole

(kee-toe-koe′na-zole)
Nizoral, Nizoral Cream, Nizoral Shampoo

Drug class.: Imidazole antifungal

Action: Alters cell membranes and inhibits several fungal enzymes
Uses: Systemic candidiasis, chronic mucocutaneous candidiasis, cutaneous candidiasis, candiduria, coccidioidomycosis, histoplasmosis, chromomycosis, paracoccidioidomycosis, tinea cruris, tinea pedis; unlabeled use: prostate cancer

Dosage and routes:
• *Adult and child >40 kg:* PO 200 mg qd; may increase to 400 mg qd if needed; high doses up to 1200 mg/day used in CNS fungal infections
• *Child >2 yr:* 3.5-6.6 mg/kg/day in a single dose

Cutaneous candidiasis
• *Adult:* TOP apply cream once daily to affected area

Dandruff
• *Adult:* Shampoo twice weekly at 3-day intervals for 4 wk

Available forms include: Tabs 200 mg, cream 2% in 15, 30, and 60 g tubes, shampoo 2% in 120 ml

Side effects/adverse reactions:
Side effects and interactions for PO form only

▼ *ORAL:* Lichenoid reactions
CNS: Headache, dizziness, lethargy, anxiety, insomnia, dreams, paresthesia
GI: Nausea, vomiting, anorexia, severe hepatotoxicity, diarrhea, cramps, abdominal pain, constipation, flatulence, GI bleeding
GU: Gynecomastia, impotence
INTEG: Pruritus, fever, chills, photophobia, rash, dermatitis, purpura, urticaria
SYST: Anaphylaxis

Contraindications: Hypersensitivity, pregnancy category C, lactation, meningitis, loratadine, triazolam, dofetilide
Precautions: Renal disease, hepatic disease, achlorhydria (drug-induced)
Pharmacokinetics:
PO: Peak 1-2 hr, half-life 2 hr, terminal 8 hr; highly protein bound; metabolized in liver; ex-

creted in bile, feces; requires acid pH for absorption; distributed poorly to CSF

🦷 **Drug interactions of concern to dentistry:**

• Hepatotoxicity: alcohol, high-dose long-term use, acetaminophen, carbamazepine, sulfonamides

• Increased serum levels: indinavir, saquinavir, nisoldipine, haloperidol, carbamazepine, tricyclic antidepressants

• Decreased absorption: antacids (take 2 hr after ketoconazole)

• Leukocyte disorders: tacrolimus

• Contraindicated with triazolam, lovastatin, dofetilide

• Inhibits the metabolism of certain benzodiazepines: alprazolam, chlordiazepoxide, clonazepam, clorazepate, diazepam, estazolam, flurazepam, halazepam, midazolam, quazepam, triazolam, zolpidem

• May inhibit metabolism of warfarin

DENTAL CONSIDERATIONS
General:

• To prevent reinoculation of *Candida* infection, dispose of toothbrush or other contaminated oral hygiene devices used during period of infection.

• Determine if medication controls disease.

• Place on frequent recall to evaluate healing response.

• Assess salivary flow as a factor in caries, periodontal disease, and candidiasis.

Teach patient/family:

• To avoid mouth rinses with high alcohol content due to drying effects

ketoprofen

(kee-toe-proe'fen)

Orudis, Orudis KT (OTC), Oruvail ♣ Apo-Keto, Apo-Keto-E, Novo-Keto-EC, Orudis-E, Orudis-SR, Rhodis, Rhodis-E

Drug class.: Nonsteroidal antiinflammatory

Action: Inhibits prostaglandin synthesis by interfering with cyclooxygenase needed for biosynthesis; possesses analgesic, antiinflammatory, antipyretic properties

Uses: Osteoarthritis, rheumatoid arthritis, dysmenorrhea; unapproved: gouty arthritis, vascular headache

Dosage and routes:

• *Adult:* PO 150-300 mg in divided doses tid-qid, not to exceed 300 mg/day, or ext rel 200 mg/day; PO (OTC) 1 or 2 tabs q4-6h, limit 6 tabs/day or 75 mg

Available forms include: Tabs (OTC) 12.5 mg; caps 25, 50, 75 mg; sus rel caps 100, 150, 200 mg; supp 100 mg (Canada only)

Side effects/adverse reactions:

▼ *ORAL:* Stomatitis, bleeding, bitter taste, increased thirst, dry mouth, lichenoid reaction

CNS: Dizziness, drowsiness, fatigue, tremors, confusion, insomnia, anxiety, depression

CV: Tachycardia, peripheral edema, palpitation, dysrhythmias

GI: Cholestatic hepatitis, nausea, anorexia, vomiting, diarrhea, jaundice, constipation, flatulence, cramps, peptic ulcer

HEMA: Blood dyscrasias

---

*GU: **Nephrotoxicity: dysuria, hematuria, oliguria, azotemia***

EENT: Tinnitus, hearing loss, blurred vision

INTEG: Purpura, rash, pruritus, sweating

Contraindications: Hypersensitivity, asthma, severe renal disease, severe hepatic disease

Precautions: Pregnancy category B, lactation, children, bleeding disorders, GI disorders, cardiac disorders, hypersensitivity to other antiinflammatory agents, elderly

Pharmacokinetics:

PO: Peak 2 hr, half-life 3-3.5 hr; 99% plasma-protein binding; metabolized in liver; excreted in urine (metabolites), breast milk

⚘ Drug interactions of concern to dentistry:

• GI ulceration, bleeding: aspirin, other NSAIDs, alcohol, corticosteroids
• Nephrotoxicity: acetaminophen (prolonged use)
• Possible risk of decreased renal function: cyclosporine
• Increased photosensitizing effect: tetracycline

When prescribed for dental pain:
• Risk of increased effects: oral anticoagulants, oral antidiabetics, lithium, methotrexate
• Decreased effects of diuretics

DENTAL CONSIDERATIONS

General:
• Patients on chronic drug therapy may rarely have symptoms of blood dyscrasias, which can include infection, bleeding, and poor healing.
• Assess salivary flow as a factor in caries, periodontal disease, and candidiasis.

• Avoid prescribing for dental use in first and last trimester of pregnancy.
• Avoid prescribing aspirin-containing products.
• Consider semisupine chair position for patients with arthritic disease.

Consultations:
• In a patient with symptoms of blood dyscrasias, request a medical consult for blood studies and postpone dental treatment until normal values are reestablished.
• Medical consult may be required to assess disease control.

Teach patient/family:
• Importance of good oral hygiene to prevent soft tissue inflammation
• Caution to prevent injury when using oral hygiene aids

When chronic dry mouth occurs, advise patient:
• To avoid mouth rinses with high alcohol content due to drying effects
• To use sugarless gum, frequent sips of water, or saliva substitutes
• To use daily home fluoride products for anticaries effect

---

ketorolac/ketorolac tromethamine/ ketorolac tromethamine injection

(kee′toe-role-ak)

Toradol

Drug class.: Nonsteroidal antiinflammatory

Action: Inhibits prostaglandin synthesis by interfering with cyclooxygenase needed for biosynthesis; possesses analgesic, antiinflammatory, antipyretic properties

Uses: Acute mild-to-moderate pain, not for chronic pain use

Dosage and routes:
• *Adult <65 yr:* IM one 60 mg dose, or multiple doses of 30 mg q6h (120 mg/day limit); IV one 30 mg dose; PO (oral use is indicated only as continuation therapy to IV/IM doses) 20 mg first dose followed by 10 mg q4-6h (limit 40 mg/day), but only after 60 mg IM as a single dose, 30 mg IV as a single dose, or 30 mg multiple doses IV or IM, not to exceed 5 days
• *Adult >65 yr or weight <110 lb or renal impairment:* IM one 30 mg dose, or multiple doses of 15 mg q6h (60 mg/day limit); PO (indicated only as continuation therapy to IV/IM doses) 10 mg first dose followed by 10 mg q4-6h (40 mg/day limit), but only after 30 mg IM single dose, 15 mg IV single dose, or 15 mg multiple dose IV or IM, not to exceed 5 days
• *Adult >65 yr:* IV one 30 mg dose, or 15 mg with renal impairment

Available forms include: Inj 15, 30 mg (prefilled syringes); tabs 10 mg

Side effects/adverse reactions:
▼ *ORAL:* Dry mouth, lichenoid reaction
CNS: Dizziness, drowsiness, fatigue, tremors, confusion, insomnia, anxiety, depression
CV: Tachycardia, peripheral edema, palpitation, dysrhythmias
GI: **Cholestatic hepatitis,** nausea, anorexia, vomiting, diarrhea, jaundice, constipation, flatulence, cramps, peptic ulcer
HEMA: **Blood dyscrasias**
GU: **Nephrotoxicity: dysuria, hematuria, oliguria, azotemia**

EENT: Tinnitus, hearing loss, blurred vision
INTEG: Purpura, rash, pruritus, sweating

Contraindications: Hypersensitivity, asthma, severe renal disease, severe hepatic disease, probenecid

Precautions: Pregnancy category B, lactation, children, bleeding disorders, GI disorders, cardiac disorders, hypersensitivity to other antiinflammatory agents

Pharmacokinetics:
IM: Peak 50 min, half-life 6 hr

🦷 Drug interactions of concern to dentistry:
• GI ulceration, bleeding: aspirin, alcohol, corticosteroids
• Contraindicated with probenecid
• Possible risk of decreased renal function: cyclosporine
When prescribed for dental pain:
• Risk of increased effects: oral anticoagulants, oral antidiabetics, lithium, methotrexate
• Decreased antihypertensive effects of diuretics, β-blockers, ACE inhibitors

DENTAL CONSIDERATIONS
General:
• Assess salivary flow as a factor in caries, periodontal disease, and candidiasis.
• Avoid prescribing for dental use in pregnancy.
• Avoid prescribing aspirin-containing products.
• Avoid long-term use for chronic pain syndromes; combined use of IV/IM and oral doses must not exceed 5 days.

Consultations:
• Medical consult may be required to assess disease control.

K

---

bold italic = life-threatening conditions

Teach patient/family:
• To avoid mouth rinses with high alcohol content due to drying effects

---

ketotifen fumarate

(kee-toe-tye'-fen)

Zaditor

Drug class.: Antihistamine

Action: Noncompetitive antagonist for histamine (H_1) receptors, stabilizes mast cells

Uses: Temporary prevention of itching of the eyes due to allergic conjunctivitis

Dosage and routes:
• *Adult:* Ophth 1 drop in affected eye(s) q8-12h

Available forms include: Ophth sol 5, 7.5 ml bottle with dropper (0.025%)

Side effects/adverse reactions:

CNS: Headache

EENT: Conjunctival infection, rhinitis, burning, stinging, eye pain, dry eyes, photophobia

INTEG: Rash

Contraindications: Hypersensitivity

Precautions: Prevent contamination of ophthalmic solution by careful use, do not wear contact lens if eyes are red, delay inserting contacts up to 10 min after drops are placed in eyes; pregnancy category C, lactation, children <3 yr

Pharmacokinetics: Limited information

Drug interactions of concern to dentistry:
• None reported

DENTAL CONSIDERATIONS

General:
• Protect patient's eyes from accidental spatter during dental treatment.
• Avoid dental light in patient's eyes; offer dark glasses for patient comfort.

---

labetalol

(la-bet'a-lole)

Normodyne, Trandate

Drug class.: Nonselective adrenergic β-blocker and α-blocker

Action: Produces decreases in BP without reflex tachycardia or significant reduction in heart rate through mixture of α-blocking and β-blocking effects; elevated plasma renins are reduced

Uses: Mild-to-severe hypertension

Dosage and routes:

Hypertension
• *Adult:* PO 100 mg bid; may be given with a diuretic, may increase to 200 mg bid after 2 days, may continue to increase q1-3d; doses may reach 2.4 g/day

Hypertensive crisis
• *Adult:* IV inf 200 mg in 160 ml D5W, run at 2 ml/min, stop infusion after desired response obtained, repeat q6-8h as needed; IV bol 20 mg over 2 min, may repeat 40-80 mg q10min, not to exceed 300 mg

Available forms include: Tabs 100, 200, 300 mg; inj 5 mg/ml in 20, 40 ml amps

Side effects/adverse reactions:

▼ *ORAL:* Dry mouth, taste changes, lichenoid reaction

CNS: Dizziness, mental changes, drowsiness, fatigue, headache, catatonia, depression, anxiety, nightmares, paresthesias, lethargy

CV: Orthostatic hypotension, bradycardia, **CHF, ventricular dys-**

rhythmias, chest pain, AV block
GI: Nausea, vomiting, diarrhea
*RESP: **Bronchospasm,** dyspnea, wheezing*
*HEMA: **Agranulocytosis, thrombo-cytopenia***
GU: Impotence, dysuria, ejaculatory failure
EENT: Tinnitus, visual changes, sore throat, double vision, dry/burning eyes
INTEG: Rash, alopecia, urticaria, pruritus, fever
Contraindications: Hypersensitivity to β-blockers, cardiogenic shock, second- or third-degree heart block, sinus bradycardia, CHF, bronchial asthma
Precautions: Major surgery, pregnancy category C, lactation, diabetes mellitus, renal disease, thyroid disease, COPD, well-compensated heart failure, CAD, nonallergic bronchospasm
Pharmacokinetics:
PO: Onset 1-2 hr, peak 2-4 hr, duration 8-12 hr
IV: Peak 5 min; half-life 6-8 hr; metabolized by liver (metabolites inactive); excreted in urine, bile, breast milk; crosses placenta
🥄 Drug interactions of concern to dentistry:
• Decreased metabolism: lidocaine
• Decreased effect: sympathomimetics
• Decreased hypotensive effects: indomethacin and other NSAIDs
• Increased hypotension, myocardial depression: hydrocarbon-inhalation anesthetics
• Increased plasma levels: diphenhydramine
DENTAL CONSIDERATIONS
General:
• Monitor vital signs every ap-pointment due to cardiovascular side effects.
• Patients on chronic drug therapy may rarely have symptoms of blood dyscrasias, which can include infection, bleeding, and poor healing.
• Assess salivary flow as a factor in caries, periodontal disease, and candidiasis.
• After supine positioning, have patient sit upright for at least 2 min before standing to avoid orthostatic hypotension.
• Limit use of sodium-containing products, such as saline IV fluids, for patients with a dietary salt restriction.
• Stress from dental procedures may compromise cardiovascular function; determine patient risk.
• Short appointments and a stress reduction protocol may be required for anxious patients.
Consultations:
• Medical consult may be required to assess disease control and patient's ability to tolerate stress.
• In a patient with symptoms of blood dyscrasias, request a medical consult for blood studies and postpone dental treatment until normal values are reestablished.
Teach patient/family: *When chronic dry mouth occurs, advise patient:*
• To avoid mouth rinses with high alcohol content due to drying effects
• To use sugarless gum, frequent sips of water, or saliva substitutes
• To use daily home fluoride products for anticaries effect

lamivudine (3TC)

(la-mi'vyoo-deen)

Epivir, Epivir-HBV

Drug class.: Antiviral, nucleoside analog

Action: Inhibition of HIV reverse transcriptase (by active phosphorylated metabolite); also inhibits RNA- and DNA-dependent DNA polymerase

Uses: Used in combination with zidovudine for the treatment of HIV infection and to reduce disease progression and death in AIDS; chronic hepatitis B associated with evidence of hepatitis B viral replication and liver inflammation

Dosage and routes:

HIV infection

• *Adult and child 12-16 yr:* PO 150 mg bid (in combination with zidovudine); for adults with low body weight (<50 kg), the recommended dose is 2 mg/kg bid in combination with zidovudine

• *Child 3 mo-12 yr:* PO 4 mg/kg (limit 150 mg) bid in combination with zidovudine

Chronic hepatitis B

• *Adult:* 100 mg qd (Epivir-HBV dose forms)

Available forms include: Tabs 100, 150 mg; oral sol 5 mg/5 ml, 10 mg/ml in 240 ml volume

Side effects/adverse reactions:

CNS: Malaise, fatigue, headache, anorexia, neuropathy, dizziness, insomnia, depression

GI: Nausea, diarrhea, vomiting, abdominal pain, **pancreatitis**

RESP: Cough, nasal complaints

HEMA: **Neutropenia,** anemia

INTEG: Rash

MS: Pain, myalgia

MISC: Fever, chills, peripheral neuropathy, paresthesia

Contraindications: Hypersensitivity, history of pancreatitis as child

Precautions: Reduce dose in renal disease, pregnancy category C, lactation

Pharmacokinetics:

PO: Rapid absorption, wide tissue distribution, low plasma protein binding (36%), eliminated mostly unchanged in urine

🦷 **Drug interactions of concern to dentistry:**

• None reported

DENTAL CONSIDERATIONS

General:

• Patients on chronic drug therapy may rarely have symptoms of blood dyscrasias, which can include infection, bleeding, and poor healing.

• Examine for oral manifestation of opportunistic infections.

Consultations:

• In a patient with symptoms of blood dyscrasias, request a medical consult for blood studies and postpone dental treatment until normal values are reestablished.

• Medical consult may be required to assess disease control and patient's ability to tolerate stress.

Teach patient/family:

• Importance of good oral hygiene to prevent soft tissue inflammation

• Caution patient to prevent trauma when using oral hygiene aids

• That secondary oral infection may occur; must see dentist immediately if infection occurs

lamotrigine

(la-moe'tri-jeen)
Lamictal

Drug class.: Antiepileptic

Action: May be due to blockage of voltage-dependent sodium channels with inhibition of excitatory amino acids

Uses: Adjunctive treatment of refractive partial seizures in adults and adjunctive treatment for Lennox-Gastaut syndrome in pediatric and adult patients

Dosage and routes:

• *Adult and child >16 yr:* PO with enzyme-inducing anticonvulsant drugs (but not valproic acid), the initial dose is 50 mg/day × 2 wk, then 50 mg bid × 2 wk; may increase dose 100 mg/wk as needed, limit 500 mg/day

• *Adult and child >16 yr:* PO with enzyme-inducing anticonvulsant drugs and valproic acid, the initial dose is 25 mg qod × 2 wk, then 25 mg/day × 2 wk; may increase dose 25-50 mg/day q1-2wk as needed, limit 150 mg/day

Enzyme-inducing drugs include phenytoin, phenobarbital, and carbamazepine

Available forms include: Tabs 25, 150, 100, 200 mg; chew tabs 5, 25 mg

Side effects/adverse reactions:

▼ *ORAL:* Dry mouth, facial edema (rarely), halitosis, gingival overgrowth, stomatitis
CNS: Dizziness, headache, somnolence, fever, ataxia, insomnia, tremor, depression, anxiety, vertigo
CV: Hot flashes, palpitation, dysrhythmia
GI: Vomiting, nausea, abdominal pain, diarrhea

RESP: Respiratory complaints, cough
HEMA: Anemia, **leukopenia, leukocytosis**
GU: Dysmenorrhea, vaginitis
EENT: Pharyngitis, rhinitis, blurred vision, diplopia, ear pain
INTEG: Skin rash, **Stevens-Johnson syndrome, toxic epidermal necrolysis, angioedema,** pruritus, photosensitivity
MS: Hyperkinesia, neck pain, myasthenia symptoms, arthralgia

Contraindications: Hypersensitivity

Precautions: Pregnancy category C, lactation, elderly, children <16 yr, dose adjustment with other anticonvulsants, seizure risk with drug withdrawal, renal or hepatic impairment; can cause Stevens-Johnson syndrome, toxic epidermal necrolysis

Pharmacokinetics:

PO: Rapid absorption, peak plasma levels 1.3-4.2 hr; 55% plasma protein bound; liver metabolism; renal excretion

🦷 **Drug interactions of concern to dentistry:**

• Increased excretion: high-dose acetaminophen (900 mg tid), but significance is unclear; carbamazepine

• Increased blood levels of carbamazepine

DENTAL CONSIDERATIONS
General:

• Early morning appointments and a stress reduction protocol may be required for anxious patients.

• Determine type of epilepsy, seizure frequency, and quality of seizure control. A stress reduction protocol may be required.

• Evaluate respiration characteristics and rate.

• Assess salivary flow as factor in caries, periodontal disease, and candidiasis.

• Patients on chronic drug therapy may rarely have symptoms of blood dyscrasias, which can include infection, bleeding, and poor healing.

• Place on frequent recall due to oral side effects.

Consultations:

• Medical consult may be required to assess disease control and the patient's ability to tolerate stress.

• In a patient with symptoms of blood dyscrasias, request a medical consult for blood studies. and postpone dental treatment until normal values are reestablished.

Teach patient/family:

• Importance of good oral hygiene to prevent soft tissue inflammation

• Use of electric toothbrush if patient has difficulty holding conventional devices

When chronic dry mouth occurs, advise patient:

• To avoid mouth rinses with high alcohol content due to drying effects

• To use daily home fluoride products for anticaries effect

• To use sugarless gum, frequent sips of water, or saliva substitutes

---

lansoprazole

(lan-soe′pra-zole)
Prevacid

Drug class.: Antisecretory, proton pump inhibitor

Action: Suppresses gastric acid production by binding to the hydrogen/potassium ATPase enzyme system to inhibit the final step in gastric acid production

Uses: Short-term treatment for healing and symptomatic relief of active duodenal ulcer and benign gastric ulcer, erosive esophagitis, and GERD; maintenance of healing of duodenal ulcers; long-term treatment of pathologic hypersecretory syndromes; NSAID-associated gastric ulcers in patients who continue NSAID use

Dosage and routes:

Duodenal ulcers

• *Adult:* PO 15 mg/day ac × 4 wk

Erosive esophagitis

• *Adult:* PO 30 mg/day ac (up to 8 wk)

Hypersecretory syndromes

• *Adult:* PO 60 mg/day (up to 120 mg in divided doses)

H. pylori related

• *Adult:* PO lansoprazole 30 mg along with clarithromycin 500 mg and amoxicillin 1 g bid × 14 days; or in clarithromycin resistance, lansoprazole 30 mg and amoxicillin 1 g tid × 14 days

Gastric ulcer

• *Adult:* PO 30 mg qd × 8 wk

Available forms include: Caps 15, 30 mg

Side effects/adverse reactions:

▼ *ORAL:* Candidiasis, stomatitis, halitosis (all <1%), dry mouth, taste alteration

CNS: Headache, dizziness

GI: Abdominal pain, diarrhea, nausea, vomiting

RESP: Cough, asthma, bronchitis, dyspnea

HEMA: Anemia

GU: Abnormal menses, glycosuria, gynecomastia, breast tenderness

EENT: Tinnitus, amblyopia, eye pain
MS: Myalgia, musculoskeletal pain
Contraindications: Hypersensitivity
Precautions: Pregnancy category B, lactation, children <18 yr, elderly (limit doses to 30 mg/day), severe hepatic disease
Pharmacokinetics:
PO: Peak plasma levels 1.7 hr, half-life 1.5 hr; 97% plasma protein bound; extensive liver metabolism; metabolites mainly excreted in feces, less in urine

⚕ Drug interactions of concern to dentistry:
• Drug interactions not established but potentially can interfere with absorption of amoxicillin, ketoconazole

DENTAL CONSIDERATIONS
General:
• Consider semisupine chair position for patient comfort due to GI effects of disease.
• Question the patient about tolerance of NSAIDs or aspirin related to GI problem.
• Patients with gastroesophageal reflux may have oral symptoms, including burning mouth, secondary candidiasis, and oral signs of dental erosion.
• Assess salivary flow as factor in caries, periodontal disease, and candidiasis.
Teach patient/family:
• To avoid mouth rinses with high alcohol content due to drying effects
When chronic dry mouth occurs, advise patient:
• To avoid mouth rinses with high alcohol content due to drying effects

• To use daily home fluoride products for anticaries effect
• To use sugarless gum, frequent sips of water, or saliva substitutes

---

latanoprost
(la-ta′noe-prost)
Xalatan
Drug class.: Prostaglandin F_{2a} analogue

Action: A prostanoid F_2 alpha analog believed to reduce intraocular pressure by increasing uveoscleral outflow of aqueous humor
Uses: Open-angle glaucoma and ocular hypertension in patients intolerant to other intraocular pressure-lowering drugs
Dosage and routes:
• *Adult:* Instill 1 drop in affected eye(s) qd in PM
Available forms include: Ophthalmic sol 0.005% (50 μg/ml) in 2.5 ml
Side effects/adverse reactions:
RESP: Upper respiratory infection, cold, flu
EENT: Blurred vision, burning, stinging, itching, foreign body sensation, increased iris pigmentation, dry eye, pain, edema, retinal artery embolus, retinal detachment (rare)
INTEG: Rash
MS: Muscle pain, chest pain, angina pain
Contraindications: Hypersensitivity to latanoprost or other ingredients in the sterile ophthalmic solution
Precautions: Gradual change in eye color, avoid contamination of sterile solution, renal or hepatic impairment, remove contact lens before using, administer at least 5

---

bold italic = life-threatening conditions   *For periodic updates, visit* **www.mosby.com**

min apart if other ophthalmic drug is also used, pregnancy category C, nursing, pediatrics

Pharmacokinetics:

OPHTH: Absorbed through cornea, peak conc 2 hr, hydrolyzed by esterases in cornea to active acid, metabolized in liver, half-life 17 min, renal excretion; onset 3-4 hr, maximum effect 8-12 hr

🦷 Drug interactions of concern to dentistry:

• None reported at this time; avoid use of anticholinergic drugs, atropine-like drugs, propantheline, and diazepam (benzodiazepines)

DENTAL CONSIDERATIONS

General:

• Check compliance of patient with prescribed drug regimen for glaucoma.

• Avoid dental light in patient's eyes; offer dark glasses for patient comfort.

• Protect patient's eyes from accidental spatter during dental treatment.

Consultations:

• Medical consult may be required to assess disease control.

---

leflunomide

(le-flu′no-mide)

Arava

Drug class.: Antiarthritic, immunosuppressive

Action: Acts as an immunomodulating agent by blocking dihydroorotate dehydrogenase enzymes, which results in inhibition of pyrimidine synthesis. This results in antiproliferative effects on cells dependent on this pathway.

Uses: To reduce signs and symptoms and to retard structural damage in active rheumatoid arthritis as demonstrated by x-ray erosion and joint space narrowing

Dosage and routes:

• *Adult:* PO loading dose 100 mg × 3 days, maintenance dose 20 mg daily, higher doses not recommended

Available forms include: Tabs 10, 20, 100 mg

Side effects/adverse reactions:

▼ ORAL: Mouth ulceration, candidiasis, dry mouth, taste disturbances

CNS: Headache, asthenia, dizziness, paresthesia

CV: Hypertension, palpitation

GI: Diarrhea, abdominal pain, nausea, dyspepsia, colitis

RESP: Cough, URI, bronchitis

HEMA: Anemia

GU: UTI

EENT: Rhinitis, sinusitis

INTEG: Rash, pruritus

META: Elevation of liver enzymes ALT, AST

MS: Synovitis, tenosynovitis, joint discomfort

MISC: Alopecia, allergic reactions

Contraindications: Hypersensitivity, pregnancy, woman of childbearing age not using reliable contraception, significant hepatic impairment, hepatitis B or C, lactation

Precautions: Chronic renal or hepatic insufficiency, rifampin, pregnancy category X, child <18 yr

Pharmacokinetics:

PO: Loading dose required, converted to active metabolite, peak levels of metabolite 6-12 hr, half-life of metabolite (2 wk), highly protein bound (99%), metabolites removed by renal (43%) and fecal excretion (48%)

⚗ Drug interactions of concern to dentistry:
• None reported

DENTAL CONSIDERATIONS

General:
• Monitor vital signs every appointment due to cardiovascular side effects.
• Consider semisupine chair position for patient if GI side effects occur.
• Examine for oral manifestation of opportunistic infection.
• If acute oral infection occurs, inform physician.
• Assess salivary flow as a factor in caries, periodontal disease, and candidiasis.

Consultations:
• Consult if needed.

Teach patient/family:
• Importance of good oral hygiene to prevent soft tissue inflammation
• Use of electric toothbrush if patient has difficulty holding conventional devices

When chronic dry mouth occurs, advise patient:
• To avoid mouth rinses with high alcohol content due to drying effects
• To use daily home fluoride products for anticaries effect
• To use sugarless gum, frequent sips of water, or saliva substitutes

---

letrozole

(let′roe-zole)
Femara

Drug class.: Antineoplastic

Action: Acts as a nonsteroidal competitive inhibitor of aromatase enzyme and thereby interferes with the conversion of androgens to estrogens

Uses: Locally advanced or metastatic breast cancer in postmenopausal women either hormone receptor positive or hormone receptor unknown; advanced breast cancer in postmenopausal women with disease progression following antiestrogen therapy

Dosage and routes:
• *Adult:* PO 2.5 mg qd
Available forms include: Tabs 2.5 mg

Side effects/adverse reactions:
*CNS: **Hemorrhagic stroke, hemiparesis,** headache, insomnia, TIA
CV: Hot flushes, **MI, coronary heart disease,** leg edema, hypertension, angina
GI: Nausea, constipation, diarrhea, vomiting, abdominal pain
RESP: Dyspnea, coughing
HEMA: **Peripheral thromboembolic events**
INTEG: Rash, pruritus
ENDO: Hypercholesterolemia
META: Weight loss, elevated SGOT, SGPT and bilirubin
MS: Fatigue, weakness
MISC: Bone pain, back pain, arthralgia, chest pain, hair loss,* breast pain

Contraindications: Hypersensitivity

Precautions: Pregnancy category D, lactation, children (no studies), for postmenopausal women only, thrombocytopenia and decreased lymphocyte counts, liver impairment

Pharmacokinetics:
PO: Rapid, complete absorption; steady state plasma levels 2-6 wk; depression of serum estrogen levels in 24 hr; maximum suppression 2-3 days; weakly

---

bold italic = life-threatening conditions

bound to plasma protein; metabolized by CYP450 3A4 and CYP450 2A6; excreted mainly in urine

💊 Drug interactions of concern to dentistry:
• None reported

DENTAL CONSIDERATIONS
General:
• Patients taking opioids for acute or chronic pain should be given alternative analgesics for dental pain.
• Patient on chronic drug therapy may rarely present with symptoms of blood dyscrasias, which can include infection, bleeding, and poor healing.
• Palliative medication may be required for management of oral side effects.
• Examine for oral manifestation of opportunistic infection.
• Consider semisupine chair position for patient comfort if GI side effects occur.
• Monitor vital signs every appointment due to cardiovascular and respiratory side effects.

Consultations:
• In a patient with symptoms of blood dyscrasias, request a medical consult for blood studies and postpone treatment until normal values are reestablished.

Teach patient/family:
• Importance of good oral hygiene to prevent soft tissue inflammation
• Alert the patient to the possibility of secondary oral infection and the need to see dentist immediately if signs of infection occur

leucovorin calcium (citrovorum factor/folinic acid)
(loo-koe-vor′in)
Wellcovorin

Drug class.: Folic acid antagonist antidote, antineoplastic adjunct

Action: Chemically reduced derivative of folic acid; converted to tetrahydrofolate; counteracts folic acid antagonists

Uses: Megaloblastic or macrocytic anemia caused by folic acid deficiency, overdose of folic acid antagonist, methotrexate toxicity, toxicity caused by pyrimethamine or trimethoprim; used with fluorouracil in colorectal cancer

Dosage and routes:
Megaloblastic anemia caused by enzyme deficiency
• *Adult and child:* PO 1 mg for life
Megaloblastic anemia caused by deficiency of folate
• *Adult and child:* IM 1 mg or less qd, continued until adequate response
Methotrexate toxicity
• *Adult and child:* PO/IM/IV 10 mg/m^2 q6h until methotrexate levels fall
Pyrimethamine toxicity
• *Adult and child:* PO/IM 5 mg qd with each dose of antagonist
Trimethoprim toxicity
• *Adult and child:* PO/IM 400 µg qd

Available forms include: Tabs 5, 15, 25 mg; inj IM 3 mg/ml; powder for inj 50, 100, 350 mg/vial

Side effects/adverse reactions:
RESP: Wheezing
INTEG: Rash, pruritus, erythema

Contraindications: Hypersensitivity, anemias other than megaloblastic not associated with B_{12} deficiency

Precautions: Pregnancy category C

🦷 **Drug interactions of concern to dentistry:**
• None reported

DENTAL CONSIDERATIONS
General:
• Signs of folate deficiency may appear in oral tissues.
• Determine why the patient is taking the drug.
• Patients with severe anemia or cancer or those receiving cancer chemotherapy may have oral complaints. Palliative therapy may be required.

Consultations:
• Medical consult may be required to assess disease control.

Teach patient/family:
• Importance of good oral hygiene to prevent soft tissue inflammation
• Caution to prevent trauma when using oral hygiene aids
• To report oral lesions, soreness, or bleeding to dentist
• That secondary oral infection may occur; must see dentist immediately if infection occurs
• Importance of updating medical/drug record if physician makes any changes in evaluation or drug regimen

---

levalbuterol HCl
(lev'al-byoo-ter-ole)
Xopenex
Drug class.: Bronchodilator

Action: Selective β_2-adrenergic agonist; causes relaxation of smooth muscles of all airways

Uses: Treatment or prevention of bronchospasm in adults and children >12 yr with reversible obstructive airway disease

Dosage and routes:
• *Adult and child >12 yr:* Inh 0.63 mg tid by nebulizer

Severe asthma not responding to 0.63 mg
• *Adult and child >12 yr:* Inh 1.25 mg tid by nebulizer

Available forms include: Inh sol 0.63, 1.25 mg in 3 ml vials

Side effects/adverse reactions:
▼ *ORAL:* Dry mouth
CNS: Migraine, dizziness, nervousness, tremor, anxiety, insomnia, paresthesia
CV: Tachycardia, ECG changes
GI: Dyspepsia, diarrhea, nausea, gastroenteritis
RESP: Flulike syndrome, cough
EENT: Rhinitis, sinusitis, turbinate edema, dry throat
META: Increased plasma glucose, decreased serum K^+, eye itch
MS: Back pain, leg cramps
MISC: Pain

Contraindications: Hypersensitivity to this drug or racemic albuterol

Precautions: Paradoxic bronchospasm, cardiovascular disorders, seizures, diabetes, hyperthyroidism, coronary insufficiency, cardiac arrhythmias, hypertension, not to exceed recommended dose, β-adrenergic blockers, MAO inhibitors, tricyclic antidepressants, pregnancy category C, lactation, children <12 yr

L

Pharmacokinetics:
INH: Relief of bronchoconstriction 20 min, half-life 3-4 hr, low plasma levels

🦷 **Drug interactions of concern to dentistry:**
• Significant reduction of effects: β-adrenergic blockers
• Potentiation of CV effects: MAO inhibitors, tricyclic antidepressants
• No specific dental drug interactions reported

DENTAL CONSIDERATIONS
General:
• Monitor vital signs every appointment due to cardiovascular side effects.
• Assess salivary flow as a factor in caries, periodontal disease, and candidiasis.
• Consider semisupine chair position for patients with respiratory disease.
• Short, midday appointments and a stress reduction protocol may be required for anxious patients.
• Be aware that aspirin or sulfite preservatives in vasoconstrictor-containing products can exacerbate asthma.
• Acute asthmatic episodes may be precipitated in the dental office. Rapid-acting sympathomimetic inhalants should be available for emergency use. A stress reduction protocol may be required.

Consultations:
• Medical consult may be required to assess disease control and patient's ability to tolerate stress.

Teach patient/family:
• For inhalation dosage forms, rinse mouth with water after each dose to prevent dryness
When chronic dry mouth occurs, advise patient:
• To avoid mouth rinses with high alcohol content due to drying effects
• To use daily home fluoride products for anticaries effect
• To use sugarless gum, frequent sips of water, or saliva substitutes

---

levamisole HCl
(lee-vam′i-sol)
Ergamisol
Drug class.: Immunomodulator

Action: May increase the action of macrophages, monocytes, and T cells, which will restore immune function; complete action is unknown

Uses: Treatment of Dukes' stage C colon cancer, given with fluorouracil after surgical resection

Dosage and routes:
• *Adult:* PO 50 mg q8h × 3 days, begin treatment at least 1 wk but no more than 4 wk after resection, given with fluorouracil 450 mg/m²/day; IV given daily × 5 days beginning 21-34 days after resection, maintenance is 50 mg q8h × 3 days q2wk × 1 yr, given with fluorouracil 45 mg/m²/day by IV push qwk starting 28 days after the initial 5-day course × 1 yr

Available forms include: Tabs 50 mg (base)

Side effects/adverse reactions:
▼ *ORAL:* Stomatitis, altered taste, lichenoid drug reaction
CNS: Dizziness, headache, paresthesia, somnolence, depression, anxiety, fatigue, fever, mental changes, ataxia, insomnia
CV: Chest pain, edema
GI: Nausea, vomiting, anorexia, diarrhea, constipation, flatulence, dyspepsia, abdominal pain

HEMA: ***Granulocytopenia, leukopenia, thrombocytopenia, agranulocytosis***
EENT: Altered sense of smell, blurred vision, conjunctivitis
INTEG: Rash, pruritus, alopecia, dermatitis, urticaria
META: Hyperbilirubinemia
MISC: Rigors, infection, arthralgia, myalgia
Contraindications: Hypersensitivity
Precautions: Pregnancy category C, lactation, children, blood dyscrasias
Pharmacokinetics:
PO: Peak 1.5-2 hr, elimination half-life 3-4 hr; metabolized by liver

🦷 **Drug interactions of concern to dentistry:**
• Disulfiram-like reaction: alcohol
DENTAL CONSIDERATIONS
General:
• Patients on chronic drug therapy may rarely have symptoms of blood dyscrasias, which can include infection, bleeding, and poor healing.
• Palliative treatment may be required for oral side effects.
• Place on frequent recall to evaluate healing response.
• Consider semisupine chair position when GI side effects occur.
Consultations:
• In a patient with symptoms of blood dyscrasias, request a medical consult for blood studies and postpone dental treatment until normal values are reestablished.
• Medical consult may be required to assess disease control.
Teach patient/family:
• To call physician if sore throat, swollen lymph nodes, malaise, or fever occur because other infections may exist
• To avoid mouth rinses with high alcohol content
• Importance of good oral hygiene to prevent soft tissue inflammation
• Caution to prevent injury when using oral hygiene aids
• To report oral lesions, soreness, or bleeding to dentist

---

levetiracetam
(lev-tir-a′se-tam)
Keppra
Drug class: Antiepileptic

Action: Mechanism of action is unknown; however, drugs of this type have dopaminergic, cholinergic, and glutamatergic activity; reported to have antiepileptic, anxiolytic, and cognitive enhancing activity; other suggestions include disruption of epileptiform burst firing and seizure propagation.
Uses: Adjunctive therapy in adults with partial onset seizures
Dosage and routes:
• *Adult:* PO initial dose 1000 mg/day given as 500 mg bid; additional doses may be given every 2 wk (1000 mg/day increments); max daily dose 3000 mg; doses must be adjusted with renal impairment; has been used in combination with other antiepileptic drugs
Available forms include: Tabs 250, 500, 750 mg
Side effects/adverse reactions:
Based on limited information
▼ *ORAL:* Gingivitis (unspecified as to cause)
CNS: Drowsiness, somnolence, headache, dizziness, fatigue, amne-

---

sia, anxiety, ataxia, depression, emotional lability, hostility, vertigo
GI: Nausea, anorexia, abdominal pain, dyspepsia, diarrhea
RESP: Cough
HEMA: Decrease in mean RBC count, decrease in mean hemoglobin and mean hematocrit, leukopenia
GU: Increase in serum creatinine, UTI
EENT: Pharyngitis, rhinitis, sinusitis, diplopia
INTEG: Rash
MS: Arthralgia
MISC: Asthenia, coordination difficulties, infection
Contraindications: Hypersensitivity
Precautions: Renal impairment, hemodialysis, pregnancy category C, lactation, may increase phenytoin blood levels, risk of seizures on withdrawal, children <16 yr
Pharmacokinetics:
PO: Bioavailability 100%, onset 1 hr, peak plasma levels 20 min-2 hr, half-life 6-8 hr, <10% plasma protein bound, limited hepatic metabolism, renal excretion (66%)
⚕ Drug interactions of concern to dentistry:
• None reported
DENTAL CONSIDERATIONS
General:
• Short appointments and a stress reduction protocol may be required for anxious patients.
• Ask patient about type of epilepsy, seizure frequency, and quality of seizure control.
Consultation:
• Medical consult may be required to assess disease control and the patient's ability to tolerate stress.
• In patients with symptoms of blood dyscrasias, request a medical consult for blood studies and postpone treatment until normal values are reestablished.
Teach patient/family:
• Importance of updating health and drug history if physician makes changes in evaluation or drug regimens

---

levobunolol HCl

(lee-voe-byoo'noe-lole)
AKBeta, Betagan Liquifilm
Drug class.: β-adrenergic blocker

Action: Reduces production of aqueous humor by unknown mechanisms
Uses: Chronic open-angle glaucoma, ocular hypertension
Dosage and routes:
• *Adult:* Instill 1 gtt in affected eye(s) qd or bid
Available forms include: Sol 0.25%, 0.5%
Side effects/adverse reactions:
CNS: Ataxia, dizziness, lethargy
⚕ Drug interactions of concern to dentistry:
• Avoid use of anticholinergic drugs, atropine-like drugs, propantheline, and diazepam (benzodiazepines)
DENTAL CONSIDERATIONS
General:
• Check compliance of patient with prescribed drug regimen for glaucoma.
• Avoid dental light in patient's eyes; offer dark glasses for patient comfort.
Consultations:
• Consultation with physician may be needed if sedation or anesthesia is required.

levocabastine HCl

(lee've-kab-as-teen)

Livostin

Drug class.: Antihistamine, H_1-receptor antagonist

Action: Selective antagonist for histamine at H_1-receptors; little or no systemic absorption; intended for topical effect

Uses: Temporary relief of seasonal allergic conjunctivitis

Dosage and routes:

Ophthalmic

• *Adult and child >12 yr:* Instill 1 gtt in affected eye qid; may continue for up to 2 wk

Available forms include: Ophth susp 0.05% in 2.5, 5, 10 ml dropper bottles

Side effects/adverse reactions:

▼ *ORAL:* Dry mouth

CNS: Headache, fatigue, somnolence

GI: Nausea

RESP: Dyspnea, cough

EENT: Local stinging/burning, red eyes, eyelid edema, lacrimation

INTEG: Rash, erythema

Contraindications: Hypersensitivity; avoid while contact lenses are being used

Precautions: Pregnancy category C, lactation, children <12 yr

Pharmacokinetics:

OPHTH: Systemic absorption low; mean plasma concentration 1-2 ng/ml

🐾 Drug interactions of concern to dentistry:

• No documented interactions with dental drugs

DENTAL CONSIDERATIONS

General:

• Question patient about history of allergy to avoid using other potential allergens.

• Avoid dental light in patient's eyes; offer dark glasses for patient comfort.

• Evaluate respiration characteristics and rate.

• Using for less than 2 wk should not present a problem with dry mouth.

Teach patient/family: *When chronic dry mouth occurs, advise patient:*

• To avoid mouth rinses with high alcohol content due to drying effects

• To use daily home fluoride products for anticaries effect

• To use sugarless gum, frequent sips of water, or saliva substitutes

levodopa

(lee-voe-doe'pa)

Dopar, Larodopa

Drug class.: Antiparkinson agent

Action: Levodopa is decarboxylated to dopamine, which can interact with dopamine receptors

Uses: Parkinsonism or parkinsonian symptoms

Dosage and routes:

• *Adult:* PO 0.5-1 g qd either bid or qid with food; dose is titrated to tolerated side effects; may be increased by 0.75 g q3-7d, not to exceed 8 g/day

Available forms include: Caps 100, 250, 500 mg; tabs 100, 250, 500 mg

Side effects/adverse reactions:

▼ *ORAL: Dry mouth,* bitter taste

CNS: Involuntary choreiform movements, hand tremors, fatigue, headache, anxiety, twitching, numbness, weakness, confusion,

agitation, insomnia, nightmares, psychosis, hallucinations, hypomania, severe depression, dizziness
CV: Orthostatic hypotension, tachycardia, hypertension, palpitation
GI: Nausea, vomiting, anorexia, abdominal distress, flatulence, dysphagia, diarrhea, constipation
*HEMA: **Hemolytic anemia, leukopenia, agranulocytosis***
EENT: Blurred vision, diplopia, dilated pupils
INTEG: Rash, sweating, alopecia
MISC: Urinary retention, incontinence, weight change, dark urine
Contraindications: Hypersensitivity, narrow-angle glaucoma, undiagnosed skin lesions, MAO inhibitors
Precautions: Renal disease, cardiac disease, hepatic disease, respiratory disease, MI with dysrhythmia, convulsions, peptic ulcer, pregnancy category C, asthma, endocrine disease, affective disorders, psychosis, lactation, children <12 yr
Pharmacokinetics:
PO: Peak 1-3 hr, metabolites excreted in urine
☙ Drug interactions of concern to dentistry:
• Decreased absorption: anticholinergics
• Decreased therapeutic effect: benzodiazepines, pyridoxine (vitamin B_6)

DENTAL CONSIDERATIONS
General:
• Patients on chronic drug therapy may rarely have symptoms of blood dyscrasias, which can include infection, bleeding, and poor healing.

• Assess salivary flow as a factor in caries, periodontal disease, and candidiasis.
• After supine positioning, have patient sit upright for at least 2 min before standing to avoid orthostatic hypotension.
• Avoid dental light in patient's eyes; offer dark glasses for patient comfort.
Consultations:
• In a patient with symptoms of blood dyscrasias, request a medical consult for blood studies and postpone dental treatment until normal values are reestablished.
• Take precautions if dental surgery is anticipated and anesthesia is required.
• Medical consult may be required to assess disease control.
Teach patient/family:
• To use electric toothbrush if patient has difficulty holding conventional devices
When chronic dry mouth occurs, advise patient:
• To avoid mouth rinses with high alcohol content due to drying effects
• To use sugarless gum, frequent sips of water, or saliva substitutes
• To use daily home fluoride products for anticaries effect

---

levodopa-carbidopa
(lee-voe-doe'pa) (kar-bi-doe'pa)
Sinemet 10/100, Sinemet 25/100, Sinemet 25/250, Sinemet CR
Drug class.: Antiparkinson agent

Action: Decarboxylation of levodopa to periphery is inhibited by carbidopa; more levodopa is made available for transport to brain and conversion to dopamine in the brain

Uses: Treatment of idiopathic, symptomatic, or postencephalitic parkinsonism

Dosage and routes:
• *Adult:* PO 1 tab of 10 mg carbidopa/100 mg levodopa tid or qid in divided doses, not to exceed 8 tabs/day; dose ratio may require adjustments

Available forms include: Tabs 10/100, 25/100, 25/250, (carbidopa/levodopa); sus rel tabs 25/100 and 50/200 (carbidopa with 200 mg levodopa)

Side effects/adverse reactions:
▼ *ORAL: Dry mouth,* bitter taste
CNS: Involuntary choreiform movements, hand tremors, fatigue, headache, anxiety, twitching, numbness, weakness, confusion, agitation, insomnia, nightmares, psychosis, hallucinations, hypomania, severe depression, dizziness
CV: Orthostatic hypotension, tachycardia, hypertension, palpitation
GI: Nausea, vomiting, anorexia, abdominal distress, flatulence, dysphagia, diarrhea, constipation
*HEMA: **Hemolytic anemia, leukopenia, agranulocytosis***
EENT: Blurred vision, diplopia, dilated pupils
INTEG: Rash, sweating, alopecia
MISC: Urinary retention, incontinence, weight change, dark urine

Contraindications: Hypersensitivity, narrow-angle glaucoma, undiagnosed skin lesions

Precautions: Renal disease, cardiac disease, hepatic disease, respiratory disease, MI with dysrhythmias, convulsions, peptic ulcer, pregnancy category C

Pharmacokinetics:
PO: Peak 1-3 hr, excreted in urine (metabolites)

Drug interactions of concern to dentistry:
• Decreased absorption: anticholinergics
• Decreased therapeutic effect: benzodiazepines, pyridoxine (vitamin B_6)

DENTAL CONSIDERATIONS
General:
• Patients on chronic drug therapy may rarely have symptoms of blood dyscrasias, which can include infection, bleeding, and poor healing.
• Assess salivary flow as a factor in caries, periodontal disease, and candidiasis.
• After supine positioning, have patient sit upright for at least 2 min before standing to avoid orthostatic hypotension.
• Avoid dental light in patient's eyes; offer dark glasses for patient comfort.

Consultations:
• In a patient with symptoms of blood dyscrasias, request a medical consult for blood studies and postpone dental treatment until normal values are reestablished.
• Take precautions if dental surgery is anticipated and anesthesia is required.
• Medical consult may be required to assess disease control.

Teach patient/family:
• To use electric toothbrush if patient has difficulty holding conventional devices
When chronic dry mouth occurs, advise patient:
• To avoid mouth rinses with high alcohol content due to drying effects

---

bold italic = life-threatening conditions   *For periodic updates, visit* **www.mosby.com**

- To use sugarless gum, frequent sips of water, or saliva substitutes
- To use daily home fluoride products for anticaries effect

levofloxacin

(lee-voe-flox'a-sin)
Levaquin
Drug class.: Fluoroquinolone antiinfective

Action: A broad-spectrum bactericidal agent that inhibits the enzymes topoisomerase II (DNA gyrase) and topoisomerase IV required for bacterial DNA replication, transcription repair, and recombination

Uses: Acute infections due to susceptible bacterial strains causing acute maxillary sinusitis, acute bacterial exacerbation of chronic bronchitis, community-acquired pneumonia, complicated and uncomplicated skin and skin structure infections, uncomplicated UTI, and acute pyelonephritis

Dosage and routes:
- *Adult:* PO 250-750 mg q24h for 3-14 days depending on the type of infection
- *Adult:* IV 500 mg by slow infusion over 60 min q24h depending on type of infection

Reduce dose in renal impairment
Available forms include: Tabs 250, 500 mg; vials 500, 750 mg (25 mg/ml); Premix IV bags 250, 500, 750 mg in D5W (5 mg/ml)

Side effects/adverse reactions:

▼ *ORAL:* Taste alteration, dry mouth (<0.5%)
CNS: Headache, dizziness, insomnia, anorexia, anxiety, tremor
CV: Edema
GI: Abdominal pain, dyspepsia, diarrhea, nausea, flatulence, vomiting
HEMA: Hemolytic anemia
GU: Vaginitis
EENT: Rhinitis, pharyngitis
INTEG: Pruritus, rash, photosensitivity, **anaphylaxis,** increased sweating, urticaria, erythema multiforme, Stevens-Johnson syndrome
ENDO: Alteration of blood glucose levels
MS: Tendon rupture
MISC: Chest and back pain

Contraindications: Hypersensitivity to quinolone antiinfectives

Precautions: Children <18 yr; seizure disorders, renal insufficiency, excessive exposure to sunlight, alterations in blood glucose (diabetes), pregnancy category C, lactation, drink fluids liberally; tendon rupture of shoulder, hand, and Achilles tendon

Pharmacokinetics:

PO: Bioavailability 99%, peak plasma levels 1-2 hr; 24%-38% protein bound, limited metabolism, primarily excreted in urine as unchanged drug
IV: After 60 min infusion see peak plasma concentration 6.2 µg/ml; steady state in 48 hr with 500 mg/day

⚬ Drug interactions of concern to dentistry:
- Interference with absorption: solutions with multivalent cations (e.g., Mg^{2+})
- Increased seizure risk: NSAIDs
- May increase effects of warfarin (monitor bleeding)

DENTAL CONSIDERATIONS
General:
- Determine why patient is taking the drug.

• If dental drugs prescribed, advise patient of potential for photosensitivity.

Consultations:

• Consult with patient's physician if an acute dental infection occurs and another antiinfective is required.

Teach patient/family:

• To minimize exposure to sunlight and wear sunscreen if sun exposure is planned

• To discontinue treatment and inform dentist immediately if patient experiences pain or inflammation of a tendon, and to rest and refrain from exercise

---

levomethadyl acetate HCl

(lee-voe-meth'a-dil)

Orlaam

Drug class.: Synthetic opioid

Action: Mimics the action of opioid analgesics by interacting with CNS opioid receptors

Uses: Management of opioid dependence

Dosage and routes:

Opioid addiction

• *Adult:* PO initial 20-40 mg 3 × weekly (at 48-72 hr intervals); adjust dose in increments of 5-10 mg over 1 or 2 wk to reach steady state; dose adjustment required for each patient; maintenance 60-90 mg 3 × weekly, limit 140 mg/wk

Available forms include: Sol PO 10 mg/ml in 474 ml; available only from FDA, DEA, or state-approved treatment programs

Side effects/adverse reactions:

▼ *ORAL:* Dry mouth

CNS: Depression, weakness, postural hypotension, tachycardia

CV: Dysrhythmia

GI: Abdominal pain, constipation, nausea, vomiting

RESP: Coughing

GU: Decreased libido

INTEG: Skin rash, goose flesh

MS: Muscle cramps

MISC: Sweating, flulike symptoms

Contraindications: Hypersensitivity

Precautions: Pregnancy category C, lactation, increased intracranial pressure, MI (acute), severe heart disease, respiratory depression, hepatic disease, renal disease, child <18 yr, addictive personality

Pharmacokinetics:

PO: Onset 2-4 hr, cumulative 22-48 hr; metabolized by liver; excreted by kidneys; crosses placenta; excreted in breast milk

🖢 **Drug interactions of concern to dentistry:**

• Risk of opioid toxicity: opioid analgesics

• Risk of withdrawal symptoms: mixed agonist/antagonist opioids

• Increased CNS effects: alcohol, sedative-hypnotics, other CNS depressants

DENTAL CONSIDERATIONS

General:

• Monitor vital signs every appointment due to cardiovascular side effects.

• Patients using this drug are being treated for opioid dependence; avoid the use of any drug with abuse potential.

• Consider aspirin, acetaminophen, or NSAIDs for the management of dental-related pain.

• Take precautions if dental surgery is anticipated and general anesthesia is required.

• Assess salivary flow as a factor in caries, periodontal disease, and candidiasis.

• If opioid or sedative drugs are required for patient management and comfort, advise current drug abuse care facility or aftercare program as appropriate.

Consultations:

• Consults may be difficult to obtain where treatment confidentiality of drug dependence is followed.

• Medical consult may be required to assess disease control.

Teach patient/family:

• Importance of good oral hygiene to prevent soft tissue inflammation

When chronic dry mouth occurs, advise patient:

• To avoid mouth rinses with high alcohol content due to drying effects

• To use daily home fluoride products for anticaries effect

• To use sugarless gum, frequent sips of water, or saliva substitutes

---

levonorgestrel implant

(lee-voe-nor-jes'trel)
Norplant System
Drug class.: Contraceptive system

Action: As a progestin, transforms proliferative endometrium into secretory endometrium; inhibits secretion of pituitary gonadotropins, which prevents follicular maturation and ovulation

Uses: Prevention of pregnancy

Dosage and routes:

• *Adult:* 6 caps subdermally implanted in the upper arm during first 7 days of onset of menses; for long-term use up to 5 yr

Population Council's levonorgestrel

• *Adult:* Two-rod implant system for 3 years of contraception

Available forms include: Kit of 6 caps, 36 mg/cap

Side effects/adverse reactions:

CNS: Dizziness, headache, nervousness

GI: Nausea, abdominal discomfort

GU: Amenorrhea, cervical erosion, breakthrough bleeding, dysmenorrhea, vaginal candidiasis, breast changes, vaginitis

INTEG: Alopecia, dermatitis, hirsutism, acne, hypertrichosis, infection at site, pain/itching at site

MISC: Change in appetite, weight gain

Contraindications: Hypersensitivity, pregnancy category X, thrombophlebitis, undiagnosed genital bleeding, liver tumors, breast carcinoma, liver disease

Precautions: Depression, psychosis, lactation, fluid retention, contact lens wearers

Pharmacokinetics: Max concentration at 24 hr; plasma levels average 0.30 mg/ml over 5 yr as drug is slowly and continuously released

⚡ Drug interactions of concern to dentistry:

• Decreased contraception: carbamazepine

• Antibiotics have been shown to decrease effects of oral contraceptives, but no data have been reported on this system

DENTAL CONSIDERATIONS

General:

• Until more data are available,

---

advise patient to use additional contraception when antibiotics are prescribed.

Teach patient/family:

• Importance of good oral hygiene to prevent soft tissue inflammation

---

levothyroxine sodium (T₄, L-thyroxine sodium)

(lee-voe-thye-rox'een)

Euthyrox, Levo-T, Levothroid, Levoxyl, Synthroid, Unithroid ♣ Eltroxin, PMS-Levothyroxine

Drug class.: Thyroid hormone

Action: Increases metabolic rate, with increase in cardiac output, O_2 consumption, body temperature, blood volume, growth/development at cellular level

Uses: Hypothyroidism, myxedema coma, thyroid hormone replacement, cretinism

Dosage and routes:

• *Adult:* PO 0.025-0.1 mg qd, increased by 0.05-0.1 mg q1-4wk until desired response; maintenance 0.1-0.4 mg qd

• *Child:* PO 0.01-0.05 qd; may increase 0.025-0.05 mg q1-4wk until desired response

Cretinism

• *Child:* IV 0.025-0.05 mg qd; may increase by 0.05-0.1 mg PO q2-3wk

Myxedema coma

• *Adult:* IV 0.2-0.5 mg; may increase by 0.1-0.3 mg after 24 hr; place on oral medication asap

Available forms include: Inj IV 200, 500 μg/vial; tabs 0.025,

0.05, 0.075, 0.088, 0.1, 0.112, 0.125, 0.137, 0.15, 0.175, 0.2, 0.3 mg

Side effects/adverse reactions:

*CNS: Anxiety, insomnia, tremors, **thyroid storm,** headache*

*CV: Tachycardia, palpitation, angina, dysrhythmias, **cardiac arrest,** hypertension*

GI: Nausea, diarrhea, increased or decreased appetite, cramps

MISC: Menstrual irregularities, weight loss, sweating, heat intolerance, fever

Contraindications: Adrenal insufficiency, MI, thyrotoxicosis

Precautions: Elderly, angina pectoris, hypertension, ischemia, cardiac disease, pregnancy category A, lactation

Pharmacokinetics:

IV/PO: Peak 12-48 hr, half-life 6-7 days; distributed throughout body tissues

⚕ Drug interactions of concern to dentistry:

• Increased effects of sympathomimetics when thyroid doses are not carefully monitored or in patients with coronary artery disease

DENTAL CONSIDERATIONS

General:

• Uncontrolled hypothyroid patients may be more responsive to CNS depressants.

• Increased nervousness, excitability, sweating, or tachycardia may indicate a patient with uncontrolled hyperthyroidism or a dose of medication that is too high. Uncontrolled patients should be referred for medical treatment.

Consultations:

• Medical consult may be required to assess disease control.

---

lidocaine HCl (cardiac)

(lye'doe-kane)

Lidopen Auto-Injector, Xylocaine

Drug class.: Antidysrhythmic (class IB)

Action: Increases electrical stimulation threshold of ventricle and His-Purkinje system, which stabilizes cardiac membrane and decreases automaticity and excitability of ventricles

Uses: Ventricular tachycardia, ventricular dysrhythmias during cardiac surgery, MI, digitalis toxicity, cardiac catheterization

Dosage and routes:

• *Adult:* IV bol 50-100 mg over 2-3 min, repeat q3-5 min, not to exceed 300 mg in 1 hr, begin IV inf; IV inf 20-50 µg/kg/min; IM 200-300 mg in deltoid muscle (use 10% sol only for IM)

• *Elderly, CHF-reduced liver function:* IV bol give one-half adult dose

• *Child:* IV bol 1 mg/kg, then IV INF 30 µg/kg/min

Available forms include: IV inf 0.2%, 0.4%, 0.8%; IV Ad 4%, 10%, 20%; IV Dir 1%, 2%; IM 300 mg/ml, 10%

Side effects/adverse reactions:

CNS: Headache, dizziness, nervousness, convulsions, involuntary movement, confusion, tremor, drowsiness, euphoria

CV: Bradycardia, hypotension, heart block, cardiovascular collapse, arrest

GI: Nausea, vomiting, anorexia

RESP: Respiratory depression, dyspnea

EENT: Blurred vision, tinnitus

INTEG: Rash, urticaria, edema, swelling

MISC: Febrile response, phlebitis at injection site

Contraindications: Hypersensitivity to amides, severe heart block, supraventricular dysrhythmias, Adams-Stokes syndrome, Wolff-Parkinson-White syndrome

Precautions: Pregnancy category B, lactation, children, renal disease, liver disease, CHF, respiratory depression, malignant hyperthermia (questionable), elderly; need to monitor ECG

Pharmacokinetics:

IV: Onset immediate, duration 20 min

IM: Onset 5-15 min, duration 1-1.5 hr; half-life 1-2 hr; moderate-to-high protein binding; metabolized in liver; excreted in urine; crosses placenta

🦷 **Drug interactions of concern to dentistry:**

• Increased effects: cimetidine, β-blockers, other dysrhythmics

• Increased neuromuscular blockade of neuromuscular blockers, succinylcholine

DENTAL CONSIDERATIONS

General:

• Because this is an emergency drug used in ICUs, emergency departments, and hospitals, patients using it would not be having elective dental treatment.

• Use of lidocaine to control dysrhythmias requires immediate medical consult or removal of patient to emergency care facility.

• Monitor ECG when used; observe for lidocaine toxicity.

• Monitor patient's vital signs and support as required.

lidocaine HCl (local)
(lye'doe-kane)

Dilocaine, Duo-Trach Kit, Lidoject, Octocaine, Xylocaine, Xylocaine-MPF

With vasoconstrictor: Octocaine with Epinephrine, Xylocaine with Epinephrine

Drug class.: Amide local anesthetic

Action: Inhibits ion fluxes across membranes, particularly sodium transport across cell membrane; decreases rise of depolarization phase of action potential; blocks nerve action potential

Uses: Local dental anesthesia; peripheral nerve block; caudal anesthesia; epidural, spinal, surgical anesthesia

Dosage and routes:

Dental injection: infiltration or conduction block

• *Lidocaine 2% without vasoconstrictor:* Max dose 6.6 mg/kg or 300 mg per dental appointment* for healthy patients; doses must be adjusted downward for medically compromised, debilitated, or elderly and for each individual patient. **Always use the lowest effective dose, a slow injection rate, and a careful aspiration technique.**

Example calculations illustrating amount of drug administered per dental cartridge(s)

# of cartridges (1.8 ml)	mg of lidocaine (2%)
1	36
2	72
4	144

*Maximum dose is cited from *USP-DI*, ed 16, 1996, US Pharmacopeial Convention, Inc., and from the manufacturer's package insert. Doses may differ in other published reference resources.

Lidocaine 2% with 1:50,000 epinephrine: Epinephrine 3 µg/kg, with a limit of 0.2 mg/patient.

Manufacturer's package insert indicates that the max dose of lidocaine with vasoconstrictors is 500 mg. Adjust doses for each individual patient as previously indicated.

Example calculations illustrating amount of drug administered per dental cartridge(s)

# of cartridges (1.8 ml)	mg of lidocaine (2%)	mg (µg) of vasoconstrictor (1:50,000)
1	36	0.036 (36)
2	72	0.072 (72)
3	108	0.108 (108)
4	144	0.144 (144)
5	180	0.180 (180)
5.5	198	0.198 (198)

Lidocaine 2% with 1:100,000 epinephrine: The same doses and adjustments to doses apply as previously indicated.

---

bold italic = life-threatening conditions

Example calculations illustrating amount of drug administered per dental cartridge(s)

# of cartridges (1.8 ml)	mg of lidocaine (2%)	mg (µg) of vasoconstrictor (1:100,000)
1	36	0.018 (18)
2	72	0.036 (36)
3	108	0.054 (54)
6	216	0.108 (108)
8	288	0.144 (144)
10	360	0.180 (180)

Available forms include: Inj 0.5%, 1%, 1.5%, 2%, 4%, 5%; inj with epinephrine 0.5%, 1%, 1.5%, 2%; epinephrine concentrations range from 1:50,000 to 1:200,000; usual dental use is 2% conc with 1:100,000 epinephrine; other % sols are used in medical applications

Side effects/adverse reactions:

▼ *ORAL:* Numbness, tingling, trismus

CNS: **Convulsions, loss of consciousness,** drowsiness, disorientation, tremors, shivering, anxiety, restlessness

CV: **Myocardial depression, cardiac arrest, dysrhythmias,** bradycardia, hypotension, hypertension, fetal bradycardia

GI: Nausea, vomiting

RESP: **Status asthmaticus, respiratory arrest, anaphylaxis**

EENT: Blurred vision, tinnitus, pupil constriction

INTEG: Rash, urticaria, allergic reactions, edema, burning, skin discoloration at injection site, tissue necrosis

Contraindications: Hypersensitivity, cross-sensitivity among amides (rare), severe liver disease

Precautions: Elderly, severe drug allergies, pregnancy category B, large doses of local anesthetics in patients with myasthenia gravis

Pharmacokinetics: Onset 2-10 min, duration 20 min-4 hr; metabolized by liver, metabolites may contribute to toxicity in one dose; excreted in urine (metabolites)

⚕ Drug interactions of concern to dentistry:

• CNS depressants: increased risk of CNS depression with all CNS depressants, especially in children and when larger doses are used

• Avoid placing dental cartridges in disinfectant solutions with heavy metals or surface-active agents; may see release of metal ions into local anesthetic solutions with tissue irritation following injection

• Avoid excessive exposure of dental cartridges to light or heat, which hastens deterioration of vasoconstrictor; observe for color change in local anesthetic solution

• Risk of cardiovascular side effects: rapid intravascular administration of local anesthetic containing vasoconstrictor, either alone or in patients taking tricyclic antidepressants, MAO inhibitors, digitalis drugs, cocaine, phenothiazines, β-blockers, and in presence of halogenated hydrocarbon general anesthetics; use smallest effective vasoconstrictor dose and careful aspiration technique

• Avoid use of vasoconstrictors in patients with uncontrolled hyperthyroidism, diabetes, angina, or hypertension; refer these patients for medical treatment before elective dental procedures

DENTAL CONSIDERATIONS

General:

• Monitor vital signs every appointment due to cardiovascular and respiratory side effects.

• Drug is often used with vasoconstrictor for increased duration of action.

• Lubricate dry lips before injection or dental treatment as required.

Teach patient/family:

• To use care to prevent injury while numbness exists and to refrain from gum chewing and eating following dental anesthesia

• To report any signs of infection, muscle pain, or fever to dentist when feeling returns

• To report any unusual soft tissue reactions

---

lidocaine HCl (topical)

(lye'doe-kane)

generic, Xylocaine Liquid, Xylocaine Ointment, Xylocaine Spray, Xylocaine Viscous

Drug class.: Topically acting local anesthetic, amide

Action: Inhibits nerve impulses from sensory nerves, which produces anesthesia

Uses: Topical anesthesia of inflamed or irritated mucous membranes; to reduce gag reflex in dental radiologic examination or in dental impressions

Dosage and routes:

• *Adult and older child:* Rinse with 5-15 ml visc sol q4h, or rinse just before meals to reduce pain of aphthous ulcers; expectorate after rinsing

Available forms include: Visc sol 2% in 100, 450 ml bottles; spray 10% in 30 ml, oint 5% in 3.5, 35 g; sol 4% in 50 ml

Side effects/adverse reactions:

INTEG: Rash, irritation, sensitization

Contraindications: Hypersensitivity, application to large areas

Precautions: Sepsis, pregnancy category B, denuded skin

DENTAL CONSIDERATIONS

General:

• Do not overuse; use just before eating to reduce pain of aphthous ulcers.

• If affected area is infected, do not apply.

Teach patient/family:

• To report rash, irritation, redness, or swelling to dentist

---

lidocaine transoral delivery system

(lye'doe-kane)

DentiPatch

Drug class.: Amide local anesthetic

Action: Inhibits nerve impulses from sensory nerves, which produces anesthesia

Uses: Mild topical anesthesia of mucous membranes of the mouth before superficial dental procedures

Dosage and routes:

• *Adult:* TOP apply one patch to area of application after drying with gauze; leave in place until local anesthesia is produced, but *no longer than 15 min*

Available forms include: Patches 2 cm^2 (containing 46.1 mg); carton of 50, 100 patches

Side effects/adverse reactions:

▼ *ORAL: Taste alteration, stomatitis, erythema, mucosa irritation*
CNS: Headache, excitatory or depressor actions, dizziness, nervousness, confusion, tinnitus, twitching, tremors (associated with excessive systemic absorption)
CV: Bradycardia, hypotension, *cardiovascular collapse* (with excessive systemic absorption)
GI: Nausea
MISC: Allergic reactions to this agent or to other ingredients in the formulation (rare)

Contraindications: Hypersensitivity to amide-type local anesthetics

Precautions: Local anesthetic toxicity, no pediatric (child <12 yr) or geriatric studies have been made, liver dysfunction, onset longer for maxilla, pregnancy category B, lactation, contains phenylalanine (caution phenylketonurics)

Pharmacokinetics:

TOP: Onset 2.5 min, duration of approximately 30 min after removal; blood levels <0.1 ng/ml limited absorption; hepatic metabolism, urinary excretion

Drug interactions of concern to dentistry:
• None reported with dental drugs

DENTAL CONSIDERATIONS

General:
• Use no more than one patch per area, remove after 15 min to avoid toxicity.

Teach patient/family:
• Advise patient to prevent injury while numbness is present, to refrain from gum chewing and eating after dental treatment
• To report unresolved oral lesions to dentist

---

lincomycin HCl

(lin-koe-mye'sin)
Lincocin, Lincorex
Drug class.: Antibacterial

Action: Binds to 50S subunit of bacterial ribosomes; suppresses protein synthesis

Uses: Infections caused by group A β-hemolytic streptococci, pneumococci, staphylococci (respiratory tract, skin, soft tissue, urinary tract infections; osteomyelitis; septicemia), and anaerobes

Dosage and routes:
• *Adult:* PO 500 mg q6-8h, not to exceed 8 g/day; IM 600 mg/day or q12h; IV 600 mg-1 g q8-12h, dilute in 100 ml IV sol, infuse over 1 hr, not to exceed 8 g/day
• *Child >1 mo:* PO 30-60 mg/kg/day in divided doses q6-8h; IM 10 mg/kg/day q12h; IV 10-20 mg/kg/day in divided doses q8-12h, dilute to 100 ml IV sol, infuse over 1 hr

Available forms include: Caps 500 mg; inj IM/IV 300 mg/ml in 2 ml, 10 ml vials

Side effects/adverse reactions:

▼ *ORAL:* Candidiasis
GI: Nausea, vomiting, abdominal pain, diarrhea, pseudomembranous colitis
HEMA: Leukopenia, eosinophilia, agranulocytosis, thrombocytopenia
GU: Vaginitis, increased AST/ALT, bilirubin, alk phosphatase, jaundice, urinary frequency

italic = common side effects

INTEG: Rash, urticaria, pruritus, erythema, pain, abscess at injection site

Contraindications: Hypersensitivity, ulcerative colitis/enteritis, infants <1 mo

Precautions: Renal disease, liver disease, GI disease, elderly, pregnancy category not listed, lactation

Pharmacokinetics:
PO: Peak 2-4 hr, duration 6 hr
IM: Peak 30 min, duration 8-12 hr
Half-life 4-6 hr; metabolized in liver; excreted in urine, bile, feces as active/inactive metabolites; crosses placenta; excreted in breast milk

🦷 Drug interactions of concern to dentistry:
• Decreased action of erythromycin
• Oral contraceptives: Advise patient of a potential risk for decreased contraceptive action, to maintain compliance with oral contraceptive use while using antibiotics, and to consider the use of additional nonhormonal contraception

DENTAL CONSIDERATIONS
General:
• Determine why the patient is taking the drug.

Consultations:
• Medical consult may be required to assess disease control.

Teach patient/family:
• Importance of good oral hygiene to prevent soft tissue inflammation
• Caution to prevent injury when using oral hygiene aids
• To notify dentist if diarrhea occurs

When used for dental infection, advise patient:
• To report sore throat, oral burning sensation, fever, fatigue, any of which could indicate superinfection
• To take at prescribed intervals and complete dosage regimen
• To immediately notify the dentist if signs or symptoms of infection increase

---

linezolid
(li-ne′zoh-lid)
Zyvox
Drug class.: Antibiotic, oxazolidinone derivative

Action: Binds to the 50S subunit of bacterial ribosomal RNA, preventing the functions of the initiation complex essential to bacterial translation; has both bacteriostatic and bactericidal activity depending on the bacterial species; nonantibiotic action includes inhibition of monoamine oxidase enzymes

Uses: For vancomycin-resistant *E. faeceum* infections; nosocomial pneumonia due to *S. aureus* (methicillin-resistant and susceptible) and *S. pneumoniae* (penicillin susceptible); complicated skin and skin structure infections due to *S. aureus* (methicillin-resistant and susceptible), *S. Pyogenes,* or *S. agalactiae;* uncomplicated skin and skin structure infections due to *S. aureus* (methicillin-susceptible); and community-acquired pneumonia due to *S. pneumoniae* (penicillin-susceptible) or *S. aureus* (methicillin-susceptible).

Dosage and routes:
• *Adult:* PO/IV depending on type of infection 600 mg q12h for 10-28 days; for uncomplicated infection 400 mg orally q12h for 10-14 days
Available forms include: Tabs 400, 600 mg; oral susp 100 mg/5 ml in 150 ml vol; IV plastic infusion bags 200 (100 ml), 400 (200 ml), 600 mg (300 ml)

Side effects/adverse reactions:
▼ *ORAL:* Candidiasis, tongue discoloration
CNS: Headache, dizziness
CV: Hypotension
*GI: Diarrhea, nausea, **antibiotic associated pseudomembranous colitis,*** dyspepsia, GI pain
*HEMA: **Thrombocytopenia***
GU: Vaginal candidiasis
INTEG: Rash, pruritus
META: Altered liver function tests, decrease in lab HgB levels

Contraindications: Hypersensitivity

Precautions: May promote overgrowth of nonsusceptible bacterial strains, monitor platelet counts in patients at risk for bleeding, pregnancy category C, lactation, pediatric doses not established, use >28 days, selectively inhibits monoamine oxidase enzymes, potentiation of serotonergic drugs, hepatic disease, hemodialysis patients

Pharmacokinetics:
PO: Rapid absorption, peak plasma levels 1-2 hr, absolute bioavailability ~100%, well distributed, plasma protein binding 31%, hepatic metabolism, renal excretion

⚖ **Drug interactions of concern to dentistry:**
• Potential to increase pressor effects of indirect action sympathomimetic drugs and vasopressors, such as dopaminergic drugs, phenylephrine, phenylpropanolamine, and pseudoephedrine
• Interactions with vasoconstrictors in local anesthetics has not been studied

DENTAL CONSIDERATIONS
General:
• Determine why patient is taking the drug.
• Use vasoconstrictor with caution, in low doses and with careful aspiration. Avoid using gingival retraction cord containing epinephrine.
• Patient on chronic drug therapy may rarely present with symptoms of blood dyscrasias, which can include infection, bleeding, and poor healing.
• Examine for oral manifestation of opportunistic infection.
• In a patient with symptoms of blood dyscrasias, request a medical consult for blood studies and postpone treatment until normal values are reestablished.
• Consider semisupine chair position for patient comfort if GI side effects occur.

Consultations:
• Medical consult may be required to assess disease control and patient's ability to tolerate stress.
• Physician consult is advised in the presence of an acute dental infection requiring another antibiotic.

Teach patient/family:
• That secondary oral infection may occur; need to see dentist immediately if infection occurs
• To report sore throat, oral burning sensation, fever, fatigue, any of which could indicate presence of a superinfection

liothyronine sodium (T₃)

(lye-oh-thye'roe-neen)
Cytomel, Triostat
Drug class.: Thyroid hormone

Action: Increases metabolic rate with increase in cardiac output, O_2 consumption, body temperature, blood volume, growth/development at cellular level

Uses: Hypothyroidism, myxedema coma, thyroid hormone replacement, cretinism, nontoxic goiter, T_3 suppression test

Dosage and routes:
• *Adult:* PO 25 μg qd, increased by 12.5-25 μg q1-2wk until desired response; maintenance 25-75 μg qd

Available forms include: Tabs 5, 25, 50 μg; inj 10 μg/ml in 1 ml vial

Side effects/adverse reactions:
*CNS: Insomnia, tremors, **thyroid storm (overdose)**,* headache
*CV: **Tachycardia, palpitation, angina, dysrhythmias, cardiac arrest**,* hypertension
GI: Nausea, diarrhea, increased or decreased appetite, cramps
MISC: Menstrual irregularities, weight loss, sweating, heat intolerance, fever

Contraindications: Adrenal insufficiency, MI, thyrotoxicosis

Precautions: Elderly, angina pectoris, hypertension, ischemia, cardiac disease, pregnancy category A, lactation

Pharmacokinetics:
PO: Peak 12-48 hr, half-life 0.6-1.4 days

⚖ Drug interactions of concern to dentistry:
• Hypertension, tachycardia: ketamine

• Increased effects of sympathomimetics when thyroid doses are not carefully monitored or in patients with coronary artery disease

DENTAL CONSIDERATIONS
General:
• Patients with uncontrolled hypothyroidism may be more responsive to CNS depressants.
• Increased nervousness, excitability, sweating, or tachycardia may indicate a patient with uncontrolled hyperthyroidism or a dose of medication that is too high. Uncontrolled patients should be referred for medical treatment.

Consultations:
• Medical consult may be required to assess disease control.

---

liotrix

(lye'oh-trix)
Thyrolar
Drug class.: Thyroid hormone

Action: Increases metabolic rate, cardiac output, O_2 consumption, body temperature, blood volume, growth/development at cellular level

Uses: Hypothyroidism, thyroid hormone replacement

Dosage and routes:
• *Adult and child:* PO 15-30 mg qd, increased by 15-30 mg q1-2wk until desired response, may increase by 15-30 mg q2wk in child
• *Geriatric:* PO 15-30 mg, double dose q6-8wk until desired response

Available forms include: Tabs 15, 30, 60, 120, 180 mg as thyroid equivalent

Side effects/adverse reactions:
CNS: Insomnia, tremors, headache, ***thyroid storm***

L

---

bold italic = life-threatening conditions

CV: Tachycardia, palpitation, angina, dysrhythmias, hypertension, cardiac arrest

GI: Nausea, diarrhea, increased or decreased appetite, cramps

MISC: Menstrual irregularities, weight loss, sweating, heat intolerance, fever

Contraindications: Adrenal insufficiency, MI, thyrotoxicosis

Precautions: Elderly, angina pectoris, hypertension, ischemia, cardiac disease, pregnancy category A, lactation

Pharmacokinetics:

PO: Peak 12-48 hr, half-life 6-7 days

Drug interactions of concern to dentistry:

• Hypertension, tachycardia: ketamine

• Increased effects of sympathomimetics when thyroid doses are not carefully monitored or in patients with coronary artery disease

DENTAL CONSIDERATIONS

General:

• Patients with uncontrolled hypothyroidism may be more responsive to CNS depressants.

• Increased nervousness, excitability, sweating, or tachycardia may indicate a patient with uncontrolled hyperthyroidism or a dose of medication that is too high. Uncontrolled patients should be referred for medical treatment.

Consultations:

• Medical consult may be required to assess disease control.

Teach patient/family:

• Importance of good oral hygiene to prevent soft tissue inflammation

• To avoid mouth rinses with high alcohol content due to drying effects

lisinopril

(lyse-in'oh-pril)

Prinivil, Zestril

Drug class.: Angiotensin-converting enzyme (ACE) inhibitor

Action: Selectively suppresses renin-angiotensin-aldosterone system; inhibits ACE, which prevents conversion of angiotensin I to angiotensin II

Uses: Mild-to-moderate hypertension, post-MI if hemodynamically stable, heart failure

Dosage and routes:

• *Adult:* PO 10-40 mg qd; may increase to 80 mg qd if required; PO post-MI initial dose 5 mg, then 5 mg after 24 hr, 10 mg after 48 hr, and 10 mg/day for 6 wk

Heart failure

PO 5 mg/day with a diuretic, dose range 5-20 mg

Available forms include: Tabs 2.5, 5, 10, 20, 40 mg

Side effects/adverse reactions:

▼ *ORAL:* Dry mouth, angioedema

CNS: Vertigo, depression, stroke, insomnia, paresthesia, headache, fatigue, asthenia

CV: Hypotension, chest pain, palpitation, angina, dysrhythmia, syncope

GI: Nausea, vomiting, anorexia, constipation, flatulence, GI irritation

RESP: Cough, dyspnea

HEMA: Eosinophilia, leukopenia, decreased Hct/Hgb

GU: Proteinuria, renal insufficiency, sexual dysfunction, impotence

EENT: Blurred vision, nasal congestion

INTEG: Rash, pruritus

Contraindications: Hypersensitivity

Precautions: Pregnancy category C, lactation, renal disease, hyperkalemia

Pharmacokinetics: Peak 6-8 hr; excreted unchanged in urine

⚖ Drug interactions of concern to dentistry:

• Increased hypotension: alcohol, phenothiazines

• Decreased hypotensive effects: indomethacin and possibly other NSAIDs, sympathomimetics

DENTAL CONSIDERATIONS

General:

• Monitor vital signs every appointment due to cardiovascular and respiratory side effects.

• After supine positioning, have patient sit upright for at least 2 min before standing to avoid orthostatic hypotension.

• Patients on chronic drug therapy may rarely have symptoms of blood dyscrasias, which can include infection, bleeding, and poor healing.

• Assess salivary flow as a factor in caries, periodontal disease, and candidiasis.

• Limit use of sodium-containing products, such as saline IV fluids, for patients with a dietary salt restriction.

• Use vasoconstrictors with caution, in low doses, and with careful aspiration.

• Short appointments and a stress reduction protocol may be required for anxious patients.

Consultations:

• Medical consult may be required to assess disease control and patient's ability to tolerate stress.

• In a patient with symptoms of blood dyscrasias, request a medical consult for blood studies and postpone dental treatment until normal values are reestablished.

• Take precautions if dental surgery is anticipated and sedation or general anesthesia is required; there is a risk of a hypotensive episode.

Teach patient/family:

• Importance of good oral hygiene to prevent soft tissue inflammation

• Caution to prevent injury when using oral hygiene aids

When chronic dry mouth occurs, advise patient:

• To avoid mouth rinses with high alcohol content due to drying effects

• To use sugarless gum, frequent sips of water, or saliva substitutes

• To use daily home fluoride products for anticaries effect

---

lithium carbonate/ lithium citrate

(lith'ee-um)

Lithium carbonate: Eskalith, Eskalith CR, Lithonate

♣ Carbolith, Duralith, Lithizine, PMS-Lithium Carbonate

Lithium citrate:

♣ PMS-Lithium Citrate

Drug class.: Antimanic, inorganic salt

Action: May alter sodium and potassium ion transport across cell membrane in nerve, muscle cells; may affect norepinephrine and serotonin in the CNS

Uses: Manic-depressive illness (manic phase), prevention of bipolar manic depressive psychosis; unapproved: depression, vascular headache

Dosage and routes:

• *Adult:* PO 300-600 mg tid, maintenance 300 mg tid or qid; slow rel tabs 300 mg bid, dose should be individualized to maintain blood levels at 0.5-1.5 mEq/L; slow rel 900 mg bid

Available forms include: Caps 150, 300, 600 mg; tabs 300 mg; ext rel tabs 300, 450 mg; oral sol 8 mEq/5 ml

Side effects/adverse reactions:

▼ *ORAL: Increased thirst, dry mouth*

CNS: Headache, drowsiness, dizziness, tremors, twitching, ataxia, seizures, slurred speech, restlessness, confusion, stupor, memory loss, clonic movements

*CV: Hypotension, **circulatory collapse, edema,** ECG changes, dysrhythmias*

GI: Anorexia, nausea, vomiting, diarrhea, incontinence, abdominal pain

*HEMA: **Leukocytosis***

*GU: **Polyuria, glycosuria, proteinuria, albuminuria,** urinary incontinence,* polydipsia, edema

EENT: Tinnitus, blurred vision

INTEG: Drying of hair, alopecia, rash, pruritus, hyperkeratosis, follicular mycosis fungoides

ENDO: Hyponatremia

MS: Muscle weakness

Contraindications: Hepatic disease, renal disease, brain trauma, OBS, pregnancy category D, lactation, children <12 yr, schizophrenia, severe cardiac disease, severe renal disease, severe dehydration

Precautions: Elderly, thyroid disease, seizure disorders, diabetes mellitus, systemic infection, urinary retention

Pharmacokinetics:

PO: Onset rapid, peak 0.5-4 hr, half-life 18-36 hr, depending on age; well absorbed by oral method; 80% of filtered lithium is reabsorbed by the renal tubules; excreted in urine; crosses placenta, blood-brain barrier; excreted in breast milk

🦷 **Drug interactions of concern to dentistry:**

• Increased toxicity: aspirin, indomethacin, other NSAIDs, haloperidol, metronidazole

• Increased effects of neuromuscular blocking agents

DENTAL CONSIDERATIONS

General:

• Assess salivary flow as a factor in caries, periodontal disease, and candidiasis.

• After supine positioning, have patient sit upright for at least 2 min before standing to avoid orthostatic hypotension.

Consultations:

• Medical consult may be required to assess disease control.

Teach patient/family:

• Importance of good oral hygiene to prevent soft tissue inflammation

• Caution to prevent injury when using oral hygiene aids

When chronic dry mouth occurs, advise patient:

• To avoid mouth rinses with high alcohol content due to drying effects

• To use sugarless gum, frequent sips of water, or saliva substitutes

• To use daily home fluoride products for anticaries effect

Iodoxamide tromethamine

(loe-dox'a-mide)

Alomide Ophthalmic

Drug class.: Mast cell stabilizer

Action: Prevents release of mediators of inflammation from mast cells involved with type 1 immediate hypersensitivity reactions

Uses: Vernal keratoconjunctivitis, vernal conjunctivitis, keratitis

Dosage and routes:

Opthalmic

• *Adult and child >2 yr:* 1-2 gtt in each affected eye qid up to 3 mo

Available forms include: Sol 0.1%

Side effects/adverse reactions:

CNS: Headache, dizziness, somnolence

GI: Nausea

RESP: Sneezing

EENT: Burning/stinging eyes, itching, blurred vision, lacrimation, dry nose

INTEG: Rash

Contraindications: Hypersensitivity

Precautions: Pregnancy category B, child <2 yr, lactation, avoid contact lens use

Pharmacokinetics: Elimination half-life 8.5 hr, excreted in urine

Drug interactions of concern to dentistry:

• None reported

DENTAL CONSIDERATIONS

General:

• Question patient about history of allergy to avoid using other potential allergens.

• Avoid dental light in patient's eyes; offer dark glasses for patient comfort.

---

lomefloxacin HCl

(loe-me-flox′a-sin)

Maxaquin

Drug class.: Fluoroquinolone antiinfective

Action: A broad-spectrum bactericidal agent that inhibits the enzymes topoisomerase II (DNA gyrase) and topoisomerase IV required for bacterial DNA replication, transcription, repair, and recombination

Uses: Treatment of lower respiratory tract infections (pneumonia, bronchitis); genitourinary infections (prostatitis, UTIs); preoperatively to reduce UTIs in transurethral and transrectal surgical procedures due to susceptible gram-negative organisms

Dosage and routes:

• *Adult:* PO 400 mg/day × 7-14 days depending on type of infection

Renal impairment

• *Adult:* PO 200 mg/dose

Prophylaxis of UTI

• *Adult:* PO 400 mg 2-6 hr before surgery

Available forms include: Tabs 400

Side effects/adverse reactions:

▼ *ORAL:* Dry mouth, candidiasis, stomatitis, glossitis

CNS: Dizziness, headache, somnolence, depression, insomnia, nervousness, confusion, agitation

GI: Diarrhea, nausea, vomiting, anorexia, flatulence, heartburn, increased AST/ALT, constipation, abdominal pain, pseudomembranous colitis

EENT: Visual disturbances, phototoxicity

INTEG: Rash, pruritus, urticaria

MS: Tendinitis, tendon rupture

Contraindications: Hypersensitivity to quinolones

Precautions: Pregnancy category C, lactation, children, elderly, renal disease, seizure disorders, excessive sunlight; tendon rupture in shoulder, hand, and Achilles tendons

Pharmacokinetics:
PO: Peak 1-2 hr, half-life 6-8 hr; excreted in urine as active drug, metabolites

⚕ Drug interactions of concern to dentistry:
• Decreased effects: antacids
• Increased levels of cyclosporine, caffeine

DENTAL CONSIDERATIONS
General:
• Due to drug interactions, do not use ingestible sodium bicarbonate products such as the air polishing system (Prophy Jet) unless 2 hr have passed since lomefloxacin was taken.
• Use caution in prescribing caffeine-containing analgesics.
• Determine why the patient is taking the drug.
• Avoid dental light in patient's eyes; offer dark glasses for patient comfort.
• Ruptures of the shoulder, hand, and Achilles tendons that required surgical repair or resulted in prolonged disability have been reported with this drug.

Consultations:
• Consult with patient's physician if an acute dental infection occurs and another antiinfective is required.

Teach patient/family:
• Caution to prevent injury when using oral hygiene aids
• To avoid mouth rinses with high alcohol content due to drying effects
• To minimize exposure to sunlight and wear sunscreen if sun exposure is planned
• To discontinue treatment and inform dentist immediately if patient experiences pain or inflammation of a tendon, and to rest and refrain from exercise

---

lomustine (CCNU)
(loe-mus′teen)
CeeNU

Drug class.: Antineoplastic alkylating agent

Action: Interferes with RNA and DNA strands, which leads to cell death
Uses: Hodgkin's disease; lymphomas; melanomas; multiple myeloma; brain, lung, bladder, kidney, colon cancer

Dosage and routes:
• *Adult*: PO 130 mg/m^2 as a single dose q6wk; titrate dose to WBC level; do not give repeat dose unless WBC count is >4000/mm^3, platelet count >100,000/mm^3

Available forms include: Caps 10, 40, 100 mg; dosepak

Side effects/adverse reactions:
▼ *ORAL: Stomatitis*
GI: Nausea, vomiting, anorexia, hepatotoxicity
RESP: Fibrosis, pulmonary infiltrate
HEMA: Thrombocytopenia, leukopenia, myelosuppression, anemia
GU: Azotemia, renal failure
INTEG: Burning at injection site

Contraindications: Hypersensitivity, leukopenia, thrombocytopenia, pregnancy category D, lactation

Precautions: Radiation therapy, geriatric patient

Pharmacokinetics:
PO: Well absorbed, half-life 16-48 hr; 50% protein bound; metabo-

lized in liver; excreted in urine; crosses blood-brain barrier; excreted in breast milk

🦷 Drug interactions of concern to dentistry:
• This drug depresses bone marrow function, which may increase risk of bleeding; avoid drugs that can increase bleeding, such as aspirin, NSAIDs

DENTAL CONSIDERATIONS
General:
• Patients on chronic drug therapy may rarely have symptoms of blood dyscrasias, which can include infection, bleeding, and poor healing.
• Consider semisupine chair position for patient comfort if GI side effects occur.
• Palliative medication may be required for oral side effects.
• Consider local hemostasis measures to prevent excessive bleeding.
• Prophylactic antibiotics may be indicated to prevent infection if surgery or deep scaling is planned.
• Patients taking opioids for acute or chronic pain should be given alternative analgesics for dental pain.
• Avoid prescribing aspirin-containing products.

Consultations:
• In a patient with symptoms of blood dyscrasias, request a medical consult for blood studies and postpone dental treatment until normal values are reestablished.
• Patients on cancer chemotherapy should have an adequate WBC count before completing dental procedures that may produce a wound. Consult to determine blood count before appointment.

Teach patient/family:
• Importance of good oral hygiene to prevent soft tissue inflammation
• Caution to prevent trauma when using oral hygiene aids
• That secondary oral infection may occur; must see dentist immediately if infection occurs
• To report oral lesions, soreness, or bleeding to dentist
• To avoid mouth rinses with high alcohol content due to drying and irritating effects
• Importance of updating medical/drug record if physician makes any changes in evaluation or drug regimens

loperamide HCl
(loe-per'a-mide)
Imodium, Imodium A-D, Kaopectate II, Maalox Antidiarrheal, Pepto Diarrhea Control
🍁 APO-Loperamide, Nu-Loperamide, PMS-Loperamide Hydrochloride, Rho-Loperamide
Drug class.: Antidiarrheal (opioid)

Action: Direct action on intestinal muscles to decrease GI peristalsis
Uses: Diarrhea (cause undetermined), chronic diarrhea, ileostomy discharge
Dosage and routes:
• *Adult:* PO 4 mg, then 2 mg after each loose stool, not to exceed 16 mg/day
• *Child 2-5 yr:* PO 1 mg, not more than 3 times daily
• *Child 5-8 yr:* PO 2 mg bid on day 1, then 0.1 mg/kg after each loose stool
• *Child 8-12 yr:* PO 2 mg tid on day 1, then 0.1 mg/kg after each loose stool

---

bold italic = life-threatening conditions   *For periodic updates, visit* **www.mosby.com**

Available forms include: Tabs 2 mg; caps 2 mg; liq 1 mg/5 ml, 1 mg/ml

Side effects/adverse reactions:

▼ *ORAL: Dry mouth*

CNS: Dizziness, drowsiness, fatigue, fever

GI: Nausea, vomiting, constipation, **toxic megacolon,** abdominal pain, anorexia

RESP: Respiratory depression

INTEG: Rash

Contraindications: Hypersensitivity, severe ulcerative colitis, pseudomembranous colitis

Precautions: Pregnancy category B, lactation, children <2 yr, liver disease, dehydration, bacterial disease

Pharmacokinetics:

PO: Onset 0.5-1 hr, duration 4-5 hr; metabolized in liver; excreted in feces as unchanged drug; small amount in urine

🦷 **Drug interactions of concern to dentistry:**

• Increased action: opioid analgesics

DENTAL CONSIDERATIONS
General:

• Assess salivary flow as a factor in caries, periodontal disease, and candidiasis.

• Evaluate respiration characteristics and rate.

• Consider semisupine chair position for patient comfort due to GI effects of drug.

• This drug product is normally used only for a few doses for acute problems; however, some patients may have to take it for longer time periods as dictated by contributing disease.

Teach patient/family: *When chronic dry mouth occurs, advise patient:*

• To avoid mouth rinses with high alcohol content due to drying effects

• To use sugarless gum, frequent sips of water, or saliva substitutes

• To use daily home fluoride products for anticaries effect

---

loracarbef

(loe-ra-kar'bef)

Lorabid

Drug class.: Antibiotic, second-generation cephalosporin

Action: Inhibits bacterial cell wall synthesis, which renders cell wall osmotically unstable

Uses: Gram-negative organisms: *H. influenzae, E. coli, P. mirabilis, Klebsiella;* gram-positive organisms: *S. pneumoniae, S. pyogenes, S. aureus;* upper/lower respiratory tract, urinary tract, and skin infections; otitis media; some in vitro activity against anaerobes

Dosage and routes:

UTI

• *Adult:* PO 200-400 mg qd × 7-14 days depending on the infection

Acute otitis media

• *Child:* PO 15-30 mg/kg bid × 7 days

Available forms include: Caps 200, 400 mg; susp 100, 200 mg/5 ml

Side effects/adverse reactions:

▼ *ORAL:* Candidiasis, glossitis

CNS: Dizziness, headache, fatigue, paresthesia, fever, chills, confusion

GI: Diarrhea, nausea, vomiting, anorexia, dysgeusia, bleeding, increased AST/ALT, bilirubin, LDH, alk phosphatase, abdominal pain,

loose stools, flatulence, heartburn, stomach cramps, colitis, jaundice
RESP: Dyspnea
HEMA: Leukopenia, thrombocytopenia, agranulocytosis, neutropenia, lymphocytosis, eosinophilia, pancytopenia, hemolytic anemia, leukocytosis, granulocytopenia, anemia
GU: Nephrotoxicity, renal failure, pyuria, dysuria, reversible interstitial nephritis, vaginitis, pruritus, candidiasis, increased BUN
INTEG: Anaphylaxis, rash, urticaria, dermatitis
Contraindications: Hypersensitivity to cephalosporins or related antibiotics
Precautions: Pregnancy category B, lactation, children, renal disease
Pharmacokinetics:
PO: Peak 1 hr, half-life 1 hr; excreted in urine as unchanged drug
Drug interactions of concern to dentistry:
• Decreased effects: tetracyclines, erythromycins, lincomycins
When used for dental infection:
• May reduce effect of oral contraceptives
DENTAL CONSIDERATIONS
General:
• Take precautions regarding allergy to medication.
• Determine why the patient is taking the drug.
• Examine for evidence of oral manifestations of blood dyscrasias (infection, bleeding, poor healing).
Consultations:
• Medical consult may be required to assess disease control.
• Medical consult for blood studies (CBC); leukopenic or thrombocytopenic side effects may result in infection, delayed healing, and ex-

cessive bleeding. Postpone elective dental treatment until normal values are maintained.
Teach patient/family:
• Importance of good oral hygiene to prevent soft tissue inflammation

loratadine

(lor-at'a-deen)
Claritin, Claritin RediTabs, Claritin Syrup
Drug class.: Antihistamine, H$_1$ histamine antagonist

Action: Acts on blood vessels, GI system, respiratory system by competing with histamine for H$_1$-receptor site; decreases allergic response by blocking histamine
Uses: Seasonal allergic rhinitis, idiopathic chronic urticaria
Dosage and routes:
• *Adult and child <6 yr:* PO 10 mg qd
• *Child 2-11 yr:* PO 10 mg (10 ml) qd
• *Child 2-5 yr:* PO syr 5 mg qd
Available forms include: Tabs 10 mg; rapid disintegration tabs 10 mg; syr 1 mg/1 ml
Side effects/adverse reactions:
▼ *ORAL:* Dry mouth
CNS: Dizziness, drowsiness, poor coordination, fatigue, anxiety, euphoria, confusion, paresthesia, neuritis, low incidence of sedation
GI: Nausea, anorexia, diarrhea
RESP: Increased thick secretions, wheezing, chest tightness
GU: Retention, dysuria
EENT: Blurred vision, dilated pupils, tinnitus, nasal stuffiness, dry nose/throat

Contraindications: Hypersensitivity, ketoconazole

Precautions: Pregnancy category B, increased intraocular pressure, bronchial asthma, patients at risk for syncope or drowsiness, reduce dose in renal impairment to every other day

Pharmacokinetics:

PO: Peak 1.5 hr; metabolized in liver to active metabolites; excreted in urine

⚖ Drug interactions of concern to dentistry:

• Increased CNS depression: all CNS depressants, alcohol
• Increased anticholinergic effect: anticholinergics, antihistamines, antiparkinsonian drugs
• Increased plasma concentration: ketoconazole

DENTAL CONSIDERATIONS

General:

• Assess salivary flow as a factor in caries, periodontal disease, and candidiasis.
• Consider semisupine chair position for patients with respiratory disease.
• Conscious sedation drugs may produce synergistic, sedative action.

Teach patient/family:

• Importance of good oral hygiene to prevent soft tissue inflammation

When chronic dry mouth occurs, advise patient:

• To avoid mouth rinses with high alcohol content due to drying effects
• To use sugarless gum, frequent sips of water, or saliva substitutes
• To use daily home fluoride products for anticaries effect

lorazepam

(lor-a'ze-pam)
Ativan, Lorazepam Intensol
🍁 Apo-Lorazepam, Novo-Lorazem, Nu-Loraz

Drug class.: Benzodiazepine, antianxiety

Controlled Substance Schedule IV

Action: Depresses subcortical levels of CNS, including limbic system and reticular formation

Uses: Anxiety, preoperatively in sedation, acute alcohol withdrawal symptoms, muscle spasm; unapproved: insomnia

Dosage and routes:

Anxiety

• *Adult:* PO 2-6 mg/day in divided doses, not to exceed 10 mg/day

Insomnia

• *Adult:* PO 2-4 mg hs; only minimally effective after 2 wk continuous therapy

Preoperatively

• *Adult:* IM/IV 2-4 mg; PO 2-4 mg (4 mg maximum dose); IV initial dose not to exceed 2 mg

Available forms include: Tabs 0.5, 1, 2 mg; IM/IV inj 2, 4 mg/ml, conc oral sol 2 mg/ml

Side effects/adverse reactions:

▼ *ORAL:* Dry mouth

CNS: Dizziness, drowsiness, confusion, headache, anxiety, tremors, stimulation, fatigue, depression, insomnia, hallucinations, weakness, unsteadiness, anterograde amnesia

*CV: Orthostatic hypotension, **ECG changes, tachycardia,*** hypotension

GI: Constipation, nausea, vomiting, anorexia, diarrhea

EENT: Blurred vision, tinnitus, mydriasis

INTEG: Rash, dermatitis, itching

---

italic = common side effects

Contraindications: Hypersensitivity to benzodiazepines, narrow-angle glaucoma, psychosis, pregnancy category D, child <12 yr, history of drug abuse, COPD

Precautions: Elderly, debilitated, hepatic disease, renal disease

Pharmacokinetics:

PO: Peak 1-3 hr, duration 3-6 hr, half-life 14 hr; metabolized by liver; excreted by kidneys; crosses placenta, excreted in breast milk

☙ Drug interactions of concern to dentistry:

• Increased effects: alcohol, all CNS depressants

• Increased sedation, hallucination: scopolamine

DENTAL CONSIDERATIONS

General:

• After supine positioning, have patient sit upright for at least 2 min before standing to avoid orthostatic hypotension.

• Elderly persons are more prone to orthostatic hypotension and have increased sensitivity to anticholinergic and sedative effects; use lower dose.

• When administered with opioid analgesic, reduce dose of opioid by one third.

• Psychologic and physical dependence may occur with chronic administration.

• Have someone drive patient to and from dental office when used for conscious sedation.

Consultations:

• Medical consult may be required to assess disease control.

Teach patient/family:

• Importance of good oral hygiene to prevent soft tissue inflammation

• To avoid mouth rinses with high alcohol content due to drying effects

losartan potassium

(loe-sar´tan)
Cozaar

Drug class.: Angiotensin II receptor antagonist

Action: Blocks the vasoconstrictor and aldosterone-releasing effects of angiotensin II

Uses: Hypertension, as a single drug or in combination with other antihypertensives

Dosage and routes:

• *Adult:* PO initial 50 mg/day; can be given once or twice daily in total daily doses ranging from 25-100 mg

Available forms include: Tabs 25, 50, 100 mg

Side effects/adverse reactions:

▼ *ORAL:* Dry mouth (<1%), taste alteration (rare)

CNS: Dizziness, insomnia

CV: Low incidence, including palpitation, hypotension; *dysrhythmias*

GI: Diarrhea, dyspepsia, nausea

RESP: Cough, infection, dyspnea

GU: Urinary frequency

EENT: Nasal congestion, sinusitis, blurred vision, tinnitus

INTEG: Dry skin, rash, urticaria

MS: Pain, cramps

MISC: Fatigue

Contraindications: Hypersensitivity, second or third trimester of pregnancy

Precautions: Pregnancy category C (first trimester) and D (second or third trimester), lactation, children, sodium- and volume-depleted patients, renal impairment

Pharmacokinetics:

PO: Good oral absorption, peak levels 1 hr, metabolites 3-4 hr;

highly bound to plasma proteins; liver metabolism; partially converted to active metabolites (first-pass metabolism); excreted in urine, feces

⚖ Drug interactions of concern to dentistry:
• Potential for increased hypotensive effects with other hypotensive drugs and sedatives
• Use ketoconazole with caution because of a potential to inhibit metabolism of losartan

DENTAL CONSIDERATIONS
General:
• Monitor vital signs every appointment due to cardiovascular effects.
• Limit use of sodium-containing products, such as saline IV fluids, for those patients with a dietary salt restriction.
• Stress from dental procedures may compromise cardiovascular function; determine patient risk.
• Assess salivary flow as a factor in caries, periodontal disease, and candidiasis.
• Short appointments and a stress reduction protocol may be required for anxious patients.
• Consider semisupine chair position for patient comfort due to respiratory side effects of drug.
• Use precaution if sedation or general anesthesia is required; risk of hypotensive episode.
Consultations:
• Medical consult may be required to assess disease control and patient's ability to tolerate stress.
Teach patient/family:
• Importance of updating health and drug history if physician makes any changes in evaluation or drug regimens

When chronic dry mouth occurs, advise patient:
• To avoid mouth rinses with high alcohol content due to drying effects
• Of need for daily home fluoride to prevent caries
• To use sugarless gum, frequent sips of water, or saliva substitutes

loteprednol etabonate (optic)
(loe-te-pred′nol)
Alrex, Lotemax
Drug class.: Topical glucocorticoid

Action: Glucocorticoids have multiple actions that include anti-inflammatory and immunosuppressant effects. They inhibit phospholipase A_2, interfering with or reducing the synthesis of prostaglandins and leukotrienes. They also bind to cytoplasmic glucocorticoid receptors (GRs) and enter the cell nucleus to bind with DNA. This results in the synthesis of various enzymes such as collagenase, elastase, and cytokines that play important roles in inflammation and immunosuppression. They also suppress the production of lymphocytes, monocytes, and eosinophils.
Uses: For steroid-responsive inflammation of the conjunctiva, cornea, and anterior segments of the globe associated with allergic conjunctivitis, acne rosacea, iritis, superficial punctate keratitis, and so on when topical steroid use is acceptable to reduce inflammation and edema (Lotemax 0.5%); temporary relief of symptoms of seasonal allergic conjunctivitis (Alrex 0.2%)

italic = common side effects

Dosage and routes:
• *Adult:* TOP instill 1 or 2 gtt into the conjunctival sac of the affected eye qid; during initial treatment (first week) up to 1 gtt qh can be used if necessary; reevaluate if no response in 2 days; also used 24 hr after ocular surgery 1-2 gtt qid for up to 2 wk
Available forms include: Sterile ophthalmic suspension 0.2% and 0.5% in 2.5, 5, 10, 15 ml plastic bottles
Side effects/adverse reactions:
CNS: Headache
RESP: Pharyngitis
EENT: Abnormal vision, blurring, burning, discharge, dry eyes, itching, photophobia, rhinitis.
Contraindications: Hypersensitivity; viral diseases of cornea and conjunctiva, including herpes keratitis, vaccina, and varicella; mycobacteria and fungal eye infections
Precautions: Prolonged use may result in glaucoma, increased risk of secondary ocular infections, delayed healing after cataract surgery; avoid contamination of sterile container; pregnancy category C, lactation, use in children not established
Pharmacokinetics:
INSTILL: Absorbed amounts are believed to be rapidly metabolized, metabolites excreted in urine; systemic effects unknown or not evident
🦷 **Drug interactions of concern to dentistry:**
• None reported
DENTAL CONSIDERATIONS
General:
• Avoid dental light in patient's eyes; offer dark glasses for patient comfort.

• Determine why patient is taking the drug.

lovastatin
(loe'va-sta-tin)
Mevacor
Drug class.: Cholesterol-lowering agent

Action: Inhibits HMG-CoA reductase enzyme, which reduces cholesterol synthesis; reduced synthesis of VLDL; plasma triglyceride levels may also be decreased
Uses: As an adjunct in homozygous familial hypercholesterolemia, mixed hyperlipidemia, elevated serum triglyceride levels and type IV hyperproteinemia, also reduces total cholesterol LDL-C, apoB, and triglyceride levels; patient should first be placed on cholesterol-lowering diet
Dosage and routes:
• *Adult:* PO 20 mg qd with evening meal; may increase to 20-80 mg/day in single or divided doses, not to exceed 80 mg/day; dosage adjustments should be made qmo
Available forms include: Tabs 10, 20, 40 mg
Side effects/adverse reactions:
CNS: Dizziness, headache
*GI: Nausea, constipation, diarrhea, dyspepsia, flatus, abdominal pain, heartburn, **liver dysfunction***
EENT: Blurred vision, dysgeusia, lens opacities
INTEG: Rash, pruritus
*MS: Muscle cramps, myalgia, **myositis, rhabdomyolysis***
Contraindications: Pregnancy category X, lactation, active liver disease, drugs that inhibit the enzyme CYP3A4
Precautions: Past liver disease,

---

bold italic = life-threatening conditions

alcoholics, severe acute infections, trauma, hypotension, uncontrolled seizure disorders, severe metabolic disorders, electrolyte imbalances

Pharmacokinetics:

PO: Peak 2-4 hr; highly protein bound; metabolized in liver (metabolites); excreted in urine, feces, breast milk; crosses placenta

🦷 Drug interactions of concern to dentistry:

• Increased myalgia, myositis: erythromycin, cyclosporine

• Contraindicated with itraconazole, ketoconazole, erythromycin

DENTAL CONSIDERATIONS

General:

• Consider semisupine chair position for patient comfort due to GI side effects.

Teach patient/family:

• To avoid mouth rinses with high alcohol content due to drying effects

---

loxapine HCl/loxapine succinate

(lox'a-peen)

Loxitane, Loxitane-C, Loxitane IM

♣ Loxapac

Drug class.: Antipsychotic

Action: Depresses cerebral cortex, hypothalamus, limbic system, all of which control activity and aggression; blocks neurotransmission produced by dopamine at synapse; exhibits strong α-adrenergic, cholinergic-blocking action; mechanism for antipsychotic effects is unclear

Uses: Psychotic disorders

Dosage and routes:

• *Adult:* PO 10 mg bid-qid initially, may be rapidly increased depending on severity of condition, main-

tenance 60-100 mg/day; IM 12.5-50 mg q4-6h or more until desired response, then start PO form

Available forms include: Caps 5, 10, 25, 50 mg; conc 25 mg/ml; inj IM 50 mg/ml

Side effects/adverse reactions:

▼ *ORAL: Dry mouth*

*CNS: Extrapyramidal symptoms: pseudoparkinsonism, akathisia, dystonia, tardive dyskinesia, drowsiness, headache, **seizures**, confusion*

*CV: Orthostatic hypotension, **cardiac arrest**, ECG changes, tachycardia*

GI: Nausea, vomiting, anorexia, constipation, diarrhea, jaundice, weight gain

*RESP: **Laryngospasm, respiratory depression**, dyspnea*

*HEMA: **Anemia, leukopenia, leukocytosis, agranulocytosis***

GU: Urinary retention, urinary frequency, enuresis, impotence, amenorrhea, gynecomastia

EENT: Blurred vision, glaucoma

INTEG: Rash, photosensitivity, dermatitis

Contraindications: Hypersensitivity, blood dyscrasias, coma, child, brain damage, bone marrow depression, alcohol and barbiturate withdrawal states

Precautions: Pregnancy category C, lactation, seizure disorders, hepatic disease, cardiac disease, prostatic hypertrophy, cardiac conditions, child <16 yr

Pharmacokinetics:

PO: Onset 20-30 min, peak 2-4 hr, duration 12 hr

IM: Onset 15-30 min, peak 15-20 min, duration 12 hr

Initial half-life 5 hr, terminal half-life 19 hr; metabolized by liver;

excreted in urine; crosses placenta; excreted in breast milk

⚓ Drug interactions of concern to dentistry:
• Increased effects of both drugs: anticholinergics
• Increased CNS depression: alcohol, all CNS depressants
• Decreased effects of sympathomimetics, carbamazepine

DENTAL CONSIDERATIONS
General:
• Patients on chronic drug therapy may rarely have symptoms of blood dyscrasias, which can include infection, bleeding, and poor healing.
• Assess salivary flow as a factor in caries, periodontal disease, and candidiasis.
• Assess for presence of extrapyramidal motor symptoms, such as tardive dyskinesia and akathisia. Extrapyramidal motor activity may complicate dental treatment.
• After supine positioning, have patient sit upright for at least 2 min to avoid orthostatic hypotension.

Consultations:
• In a patient with symptoms of blood dyscrasias, request a medical consult for blood studies and postpone dental treatment until normal values are reestablished.
• If signs of tardive dyskinesia or akathisia are present, refer to physician.
• Physician should be informed if significant xerostomic side effects occur (increased caries, sore tongue, problems eating or swallowing, difficulty wearing prosthesis) so a medication change can be considered.

Teach patient/family:
• Importance of good oral hygiene to prevent soft tissue inflammation
• Caution to prevent injury when using oral hygiene aids
• To use electric toothbrush if patient has difficulty holding conventional devices
When chronic dry mouth occurs, advise patient:
• To avoid mouth rinses with high alcohol content due to drying effects
• To use sugarless gum, frequent sips of water, or saliva substitutes
• To use daily home fluoride products for anticaries effect

---

magaldrate (aluminum magnesium complex)
(mag'al-drate)
Iosopan, Riopan
Drug class.: Antacid/aluminum/magnesium hydroxide

Action: Neutralizes gastric acidity
Uses: Antacid for hyperacidity
Dosage and routes:
• *Adult:* Susp 5-10 ml (400-800 mg) with water between meals, hs, not to exceed 100 ml/day
Available forms include: Susp 540 mg/5 ml
Side effects/adverse reactions:
▼ *ORAL:* Chalky taste
GI: Constipation, diarrhea, nausea, vomiting, thirst, stomach cramps
META: Hypermagnesemia, hypophosphatemia, hypercalcemia
Contraindications: Hypersensitivity to this drug or aluminum products, intestinal obstruction
Precautions: Elderly, fluid restriction, decreased GI motility, GI obstruction, dehydration, renal disease, sodium-restricted diets, preg-

nancy category C, colitis, gastric outlet obstruction syndrome, colostomy

Pharmacokinetics:

PO: Onset 10-15 min, duration >3 hr

☙ Drug interactions of concern to dentistry:

• Decreased absorption of anticholinergics, corticosteroids, sodium fluoride, tetracycline, ketoconazole, chlordiazepoxide, ciprofloxacin, metronidazole

DENTAL CONSIDERATIONS

General:

• If prescribing oral form of a drug for which risk of decreased absorption is reported, advise taking doses at least 2 hr after or before antacid use.

• Avoid drugs that could exacerbate upper GI distress (aspirin and NSAIDs).

• Consider semisupine chair position for patient comfort due to GI effects of disease.

---

maprotiline HCl

(ma-proe'ti-leen)

generic

Drug class.: Tetracyclic antidepressant

Action: Blocks reuptake of norepinephrine and serotonin into nerve endings, increasing action of norepinephrine and serotonin at nerve cells

Uses: Depression, depression with anxiety; unapproved: neurogenic pain, tension headache

Dosage and routes:

• *Adult:* PO 25-75 mg/day in moderate depression; may increase to 150 mg/day, not to exceed 225 mg

in hospitalized patients; severely depressed patients who are hospitalized may be given 300 mg/day

• *Elderly:* 50-75 mg/day

Available forms include: Tabs 25, 50, 75 mg

Side effects/adverse reactions:

▼ *ORAL: Dry mouth*

CNS: Dizziness, vertigo, nervousness, drowsiness, **seizures,** confusion, headache, anxiety, tremors, stimulation, weakness, insomnia, nightmares, EPS (elderly), increased psychiatric symptoms, sedation, manic hallucinations

CV: Orthostatic hypotension, ECG changes, tachycardia, **hypertension** (rare), palpitation

GI: Diarrhea, nausea, vomiting, **hepatitis, paralytic ileus,** increased appetite, cramps, epigastric distress, jaundice

HEMA: **Agranulocytosis, thrombocytopenia, eosinophilia, leukopenia**

GU: Retention, **acute renal failure**

EENT: Blurred vision, tinnitus, mydriasis

INTEG: Rash, urticaria, sweating, pruritus, vasculitis, photosensitivity

Contraindications: Hypersensitivity to tricyclic antidepressants, recovery phase of MI, convulsive disorders, prostatic hypertrophy

Precautions: Suicidal patients, severe depression, increased intraocular pressure, narrow-angle glaucoma, urinary retention, cardiac disease, hepatic or renal disease, hypothyroidism, hyperthyroidism, electroshock therapy, elective surgery, elderly, pregnancy category B, lactation, prostate hypertrophy, schizophrenia, MAO inhibitors

---

Pharmacokinetics:

PO: Onset 15-30 min, peak 12 hr, duration up to 3 wk, half-life 27-58 hr, steady state 6-10 days; protein binding 80%, metabolized by liver; excreted by kidneys, feces; crosses placenta

🦷 Drug interactions of concern to dentistry:

• Increased effects of direct-acting sympathomimetics (epinephrine)

• Potential risk of increased CNS depression: alcohol, and all CNS depressants

• Decreased antihypertensive effect: clonidine, guanadrel, guanethidine

DENTAL CONSIDERATIONS
General:

• Monitor vital signs every appointment due to cardiovascular side effects.

• Patients on chronic drug therapy may rarely have symptoms of blood dyscrasias, which can include infection, bleeding, and poor healing.

• Assess salivary flow as a factor in caries, periodontal disease, and candidiasis.

• After supine positioning, have patient sit upright for at least 2 min before standing to avoid orthostatic hypotension.

• The use of epinephrine in gingival retraction cord is contraindicated. Use vasoconstrictors with caution, in low doses, and with careful aspiration.

Consultations:

• In a patient with symptoms of blood dyscrasias, request a medical consult for blood studies and postpone dental treatment until normal values are reestablished.

• Take precautions if dental surgery is anticipated and anesthesia is required.

• Medical consult may be required to assess disease control.

• Physician should be informed if significant xerostomic side effects occur (increased caries, sore tongue, problems eating or swallowing, difficulty wearing prosthesis) so a medication change can be considered.

Teach patient/family:

• Importance of good oral hygiene to prevent soft tissue inflammation

• Caution to prevent injury when using oral hygiene aids

When chronic dry mouth occurs, advise patient:

• To avoid mouth rinses with high alcohol content due to drying effects

• To use sugarless gum, frequent sips of water, or saliva substitutes

• To use daily home fluoride products for anticaries effect

---

mecamylamine HCl
(mek-a-mil′a-meen)
Inversine

Drug class.: Antihypertensive, ganglionic blocker

Action: Occupies receptor site, prevents acetylcholine from attaching to postsynaptic nerve ending in autonomic ganglia

Uses: Moderate-to-severe hypertension, malignant hypertension; unlabeled use: hyperreflexia, smoking cessation

Dosage and routes:

• *Adult:* PO 2.5 mg bid; may increase in increments of 2.5 mg × 2 days until desired response; main-

---

tenance 25 mg/day in 3 divided doses

Available forms include: Tabs 2.5 mg

Side effects/adverse reactions:

▼ *ORAL: Dry mouth,* glossitis, bitter taste

CNS: Drowsiness, sedation, dizziness, **convulsions,** headache, tremors, weakness, syncope, paresthesia, dizziness

CV: Postural hypotension, **CHF,** irregular heart rate

GI: Paralytic ileus, anorexia, nausea, vomiting, constipation

GU: Impotence, urinary retention, decreased libido

EENT: Blurred vision, nasal congestion, dilated pupils

Contraindications: Hypersensitivity, MI, coronary insufficiency, renal disease, glaucoma, organic pyloric stenosis, uremia, uncooperative patients, mild/labile hypertension

Precautions: CVA, prostatic hypertrophy, bladder neck obstruction, urethral stricture, renal dysfunction (elevated BUN), cerebral dysfunction, pregnancy category C, vigorous exercise, stress-related activity

Pharmacokinetics:

PO: Onset 0.5-2 hr, duration 6-12 hr; excreted unchanged in urine, feces, breast milk; crosses placenta

⚓ Drug interactions of concern to dentistry:

• Increased vasopressor response: sympathomimetics

• Decreased hypotensive effect: sympathomimetics, NSAIDs, especially indomethacin

• Increased hypotensive response: sedative drugs that may also lower blood pressure

DENTAL CONSIDERATIONS

General:

• Monitor vital signs every appointment due to cardiovascular side effects.

• After supine positioning, have patient sit upright for at least 2 min before standing to avoid orthostatic hypotension.

• Assess salivary flow as a factor in caries, periodontal disease, and candidiasis.

• Consider semisupine chair position for patient comfort due to GI effects of disease.

• Early-morning appointments and a stress reduction protocol may be required for anxious patients.

• Stress from dental procedures may compromise cardiovascular function; determine patient risk.

• Use vasoconstrictors with caution, in low doses, and with careful aspiration.

• Avoid use of gingival retraction cord with epinephrine.

• Limit use of sodium-containing products (e.g., air polishing system and IV fluids) for patients with a dietary salt restriction.

• Take precautions if dental surgery is anticipated and anesthesia is required.

Consultations:

• Medical consult may be required to assess disease control.

Teach patient/family:

• Importance of good oral hygiene to prevent soft tissue inflammation

When chronic dry mouth occurs, advise patient:

• To avoid mouth rinses with high alcohol content due to drying effects

• To use daily home fluoride products for anticaries effect

• To use sugarless gum, frequent sips of water, or saliva substitutes

---

meclizine HCl
(mek'li-zeen)

Antivert 25, Antivert 50, Bonine, Dramamine less Drowsy, Meni-D, Vergon

✦ Bonamine

Drug class.: Antihistamine

Action: A nonspecific CNS depressant with anticholinergic and antihistaminic activity
Uses: Vertigo, motion sickness
Dosage and routes:
• *Adult:* PO 25-100 mg qd in divided doses or 25-50 mg 1 hr before traveling
Available forms include: Tabs 12.5, 25, 50 mg; chew tabs 25 mg; film-coated tabs 25 mg; caps 25, 30 mg
Side effects/adverse reactions:
▼ *ORAL:* Dry mouth
CNS: Drowsiness, dizziness, sedation, fatigue, restlessness, headache, insomnia, extrapyramidal symptoms
GI: Nausea, anorexia, vomiting
EENT: Blurred vision
Contraindications: Hypersensitivity to cyclizines
Precautions: Children, narrow-angle glaucoma, urinary retention, lactation, prostatic hypertrophy, elderly, pregnancy category B, asthma
Pharmacokinetics:
PO: Onset 1 hr, duration 8-24 hr, half-life 6 hr
🍃 **Drug interactions of concern to dentistry:**
• Increased effect of alcohol, other CNS depressants, anticholinergics

DENTAL CONSIDERATIONS
General:
• Assess salivary flow as a factor in caries, periodontal disease, and candidiasis.
Teach patient/family: *When chronic dry mouth occurs, advise patient:*
• To avoid mouth rinses with high alcohol content due to drying effects
• To use daily home fluoride products for anticaries effect
• To use sugarless gum, frequent sips of water, or saliva substitutes

---

meclofenamate sodium
(me-kloe-fen-am'ate)

generic

Drug class.: Nonsteroidal antiinflammatory

Action: Inhibits prostaglandin synthesis by interfering with cyclooxygenase needed for biosynthesis; possesses analgesic, antiinflammatory, antipyretic properties
Uses: Mild-to-moderate pain, osteoarthritis, rheumatoid arthritis; unapproved: vascular headache, menorrhagia
Dosage and routes:
Analgesia, antirheumatic
• *Adult:* PO 50-100 mg every 4-6 hr not to exceed 400 mg daily
Primary dysmenorrhea
• *Adult:* PO 100 mg tid up to 6 days
Available forms include: Caps 50, 100 mg
Side effects/adverse reactions:
▼ *ORAL:* Stomatitis, bitter taste, dry mouth, lichenoid reaction
CNS: Dizziness, drowsiness, fa-

M

---

tigue, tremors, confusion, insomnia, anxiety, depression
CV: Tachycardia, peripheral edema, palpitation, dysrhythmias
*GI: **Cholestatic hepatitis,*** diarrhea, nausea, anorexia, vomiting, jaundice, constipation, flatulence, cramps, peptic ulcer
*HEMA: **Blood dyscrasias***
*GU: **Nephrotoxicity: dysuria, hematuria, oliguria, azotemia***
EENT: Tinnitus, hearing loss, blurred vision
INTEG: Purpura, rash, pruritus, sweating
Contraindications: Hypersensitivity, asthma induced by aspirin, severe renal disease, severe hepatic disease, allergy to other NSAIDs
Precautions: Pregnancy category not listed, lactation, children, bleeding disorders, upper GI disorders, cardiac disorders, hypersensitivity to other antiinflammatory agents
Pharmacokinetics:
PO: Peak serum levels 30 min, half-life 3-3.5 hr; metabolized in liver; excreted in urine (metabolites), less in feces and breast milk
🦷 **Drug interactions of concern to dentistry:**
• GI ulceration, bleeding: aspirin, alcohol, corticosteroids
• Nephrotoxicity: acetaminophen (prolonged use)
• Possible risk of decreased renal function: cyclosporine
When prescribed for dental pain:
• Risk of increased effects: oral anticoagulants, oral antidiabetics, lithium, methotrexate
• Decreased effects of diuretics, β-adrenergic blockers
DENTAL CONSIDERATIONS
General:
• Patients on chronic drug therapy

may rarely have symptoms of blood dyscrasias, which can include infection, bleeding, and poor healing.
• Assess salivary flow as a factor in caries, periodontal disease, and candidiasis.
• Avoid prescribing for dental use in last trimester of pregnancy.
• Avoid prescribing aspirin-containing products.
• Consider semisupine chair position for patients with rheumatic disease.
Consultations:
• In a patient with symptoms of blood dyscrasias, request a medical consult for blood studies and postpone dental treatment until normal values are reestablished.
• Medical consult may be required to assess disease control.
Teach patient/family:
• Importance of good oral hygiene to prevent soft tissue inflammation
• Caution to prevent injury when using oral hygiene aids
When chronic dry mouth occurs, advise patient:
• To avoid mouth rinses with high alcohol content due to drying effects
• To use sugarless gum, frequent sips of water, or saliva substitutes
• To use daily home fluoride products for anticaries effect

---

medroxyprogesterone acetate

(me-drox'ee-proe-jes'te-rone)
Amen, Curretab, Cycrin, Depo-Provera, Provera
Drug class.: Progestogen

Action: Inhibits secretion of pituitary gonadotropins, preventing follicular maturation and ovulation; stimulates growth of mammary tissue; antineoplastic action against endometrial cancer

Uses: Uterine bleeding (abnormal), secondary amenorrhea, endometrial cancer, metastatic renal cancer, contraceptive; with estrogens to reduce incidence of endometrial hyperplasia, cancer

Dosage and routes:
Secondary amenorrhea
• *Adult:* PO 5-10 mg qd × 5-10 days
Endometrial/renal cancer
• *Adult:* IM 400-1000 mg/wk
Uterine bleeding
• *Adult:* PO 5-10 mg qd × 5-10 days starting on 16th day of menstrual cycle
Available forms include: Tabs 2.5, 5, 10 mg; inj susp 100, 400 mg/ml

Side effects/adverse reactions:
▼ *ORAL:* Gingival bleeding, gingival overgrowth
CNS: Dizziness, headache, migraines, depression, fatigue
CV: **Thromboembolism, stroke, pulmonary embolism, MI,** hypotension, thrombophlebitis, edema
GI: Nausea, **cholestatic jaundice,** vomiting, anorexia, cramps, increased weight
GU: Gynecomastia, testicular atrophy, impotence, **spontaneous abortion,** endometriosis, amenorrhea, cervical erosion, breakthrough bleeding, dysmenorrhea, vaginal candidiasis, breast changes
EENT: Diplopia
INTEG: Rash, urticaria, acne, hirsutism, alopecia, oily skin, seborrhea, purpura, melasma, photosensitivity
META: Hyperglycemia

Contraindications: Breast cancer, hypersensitivity, thromboembolic disorders, reproductive cancer, genital bleeding (abnormal, undiagnosed), pregnancy category X

Precautions: Lactation, hypertension, asthma, blood dyscrasias, gallbladder disease, CHF, diabetes mellitus, bone disease, depression, migraine headache, convulsive disorders, hepatic disease, renal disease, family history of cancer of breast or reproductive tract

Pharmacokinetics:
PO: Peak levels 2-7 hr, duration 24 hr, depot injection active up to 3 mo; metabolized in liver; excreted in urine, feces

DENTAL CONSIDERATIONS
General:
• Place on frequent recall to evaluate inflammatory and healing response.
Teach patient/family:
• Importance of good oral hygiene to prevent soft tissue inflammation

M

---

mefenamic acid
(me-fe-nam′ik)
Ponstel

Drug class.: Nonsteroidal antiinflammatory

Action: Inhibits prostaglandin synthesis by interfering with cyclooxygenase needed for biosynthesis; possesses analgesic, antiinflammatory, antipyretic properties

Uses: Mild-to-moderate pain, dysmenorrhea, inflammatory disease

Dosage and routes:
• *Adult and child >14 yr:* PO 500 mg, then 250 mg q4h; use not to exceed 1 wk
Available forms include: Caps 250 mg

---

bold italic = life-threatening conditions　　*For periodic updates, visit* **www.mosby.com**

Side effects/adverse reactions:

▼ *ORAL:* Lichenoid reaction

CNS: Dizziness, drowsiness, fatigue, tremors, confusion, insomnia, anxiety, depression

CV: Tachycardia, peripheral edema, palpitation, dysrhythmias

*GI: **Cholestatic hepatitis,*** nausea, anorexia, vomiting, diarrhea, jaundice, constipation, flatulence, cramps, peptic ulcer

*HEMA: **Blood dyscrasias***

*GU: **Nephrotoxicity: dysuria, hematuria, oliguria, azotemia***

EENT: Tinnitus, hearing loss, blurred vision

INTEG: Purpura, rash, pruritus, sweating

Contraindications: Hypersensitivity, asthma, severe renal disease, severe hepatic disease

Precautions: Pregnancy category C, lactation, children, bleeding disorders, GI disorders, cardiac disorders, hypersensitivity to other antiinflammatory agents

Pharmacokinetics:

PO: Peak 2 hr, half-life 3-3.5 hr; extensive protein binding; metabolized in liver; excreted in urine (metabolites), breast milk

🦷 **Drug interactions of concern to dentistry:**

• GI bleeding, ulceration: aspirin, alcohol, corticosteroids

• Nephrotoxicity: acetaminophen (prolonged use and high doses)

• Possible risk of decreased renal function: cyclosporine

When prescribed for dental pain:

• Risk of increased effects of oral anticoagulants, oral antidiabetics, lithium, methotrexate

• Decreased effects of diuretics

DENTAL CONSIDERATIONS

General:

• Avoid prescribing for dental use in last trimester of pregnancy.

• Avoid prescribing aspirin-containing products.

Consultations:

• Medical consult may be required to assess disease control.

---

megestrol acetate

(me-jes'trole)

Megace

♣ Apo-Megestrol

Drug class.: Antineoplastic (progestin)

Action: Affects endometrium by antiluteinizing effect, which is thought to bring about cell death

Uses: Breast, endometrial cancer, renal cell cancer

Dosage and routes:

• *Adult:* PO 40-320 mg/day in divided doses

Available forms include: Tabs 20, 40 mg; oral susp 40 mg/5 ml

Side effects/adverse reactions:

▼ *ORAL:* Gingival bleeding, gingival overgrowth

CNS: Mood swings

*CV: **Thrombophlebitis***

GI: Nausea, vomiting, anorexia, diarrhea, abdominal cramps

*GU: **Hypercalcemia,*** gynecomastia, fluid retention

INTEG: Alopecia, rash, pruritus, purpura

Contraindications: Hypersensitivity, pregnancy category X

Pharmacokinetics:

PO: Duration 1-3 days, half-life 60 min; metabolized in liver; excreted in feces, breast milk

italic = common side effects

DENTAL CONSIDERATIONS

General:
• Place on frequent recall to evaluate inflammatory and healing response.
• Patients receiving chemotherapy may require palliative treatment for stomatitis.

Teach patient/family:
• Importance of good oral hygiene to prevent soft tissue inflammation

---

meloxicam
(mel-ox′i-cam)

Mobic

Drug class.: Nonsteroidal antiinflammatory

Action: May be related to a nonselective inhibition of cyclooxygenase isoenzymes preventing the synthesis of prostaglandins

Uses: Relief of signs and symptoms of osteoarthritis

Dosage and routes:
• *Adult:* PO 7.5 mg daily, max daily dose 15 mg

Available forms include: Tabs 7.5 mg

Side effects/adverse reactions:
▼ *ORAL:* Facial edema, dry mouth, ulcerative stomatitis, taste perversion

CNS: Headache, dizziness, anxiety, insomnia, fatigue, malaise, vertigo

CV: Peripheral edema, hot flashes, syncope, variation in blood pressure, arrhythmia

GI: Abdominal pain, diarrhea, dyspepsia, nausea, flatulence, ulcer, esophagitis, GERD

RESP: URI, cough, asthma, bronchospasm

HEMA: Agranulocytosis, thrombocytopenia, leukopenia, anemia

GU: Renal failure, hematuria, interstitial nephritis, pharyngitis

EENT: Abnormal vision, tinnitus

INTEG: Stevens-Johnson syndrome, toxic epidermal necrolysis, rash, pruritus, erythema multiforme

META: Liver failure; elevations of AST, ALT, GGT, BUN; hepatitis; dehydration

MS: Arthralgia, back pain

MISC: Anaphylaxis, flulike symptoms, falling, allergic reactions

Contraindications: Hypersensitivity; patients who have experienced asthma, urticaria, or allergic-type reactions after taking aspirin or other NSAIDs; advanced renal disease

Precautions: Preexisting asthma, anaphylactic reactions to NSAIDs, serious GI side effects may occur, GI ulcer or GI bleeding; avoid in late pregnancy, liver dysfunction, dehydration, long term use, edema, heart failure, hypertension, ACE inhibitors, pregnancy category C, lactation, elderly

Pharmacokinetics:
PO: Bioavailability 89%, max plasma levels in 4-5 hr, $T_{1/2}$ = 15-20 hr, plasma protein binding 99.4%, almost completely metabolized, CYP450 3A4 is a minor pathway for metabolism, equal excretion of metabolites in feces and urine

👆 Drug interactions of concern to dentistry:
• Increased risk of GI side effects: long duration NSAIDs, aspirin (except low dose form), oral glucocorticoids, alcoholism, smoking, older age, and generally poor health
• Increased blood levels: lithium
• Reduced natruretic effect: furosemide and other loop diuretics

---

bold italic = life-threatening conditions

DENTAL CONSIDERATIONS

General:

• Assess salivary flow as a factor in caries, periodontal disease, and candidiasis.

• Patient on chronic drug therapy may rarely present with symptoms of blood dyscrasias, which can include infection, bleeding, and poor healing.

• Consider semisupine chair position for patient comfort if GI side effects occur.

Consultations:

• In a patient with symptoms of blood dyscrasias, request a medical consult for blood studies and postpone treatment until normal values are reestablished.

Teach patient/family:

• Use of electric toothbrush if patient has difficulty holding conventional devices

• Importance of updating health and drug history if physician makes any changes in evaluation or drug regimens

• Importance of good oral hygiene to prevent soft tissue inflammation

• To prevent trauma when using oral hygiene aids

When chronic dry mouth occurs advise patient:

• To avoid mouth rinses with high alcohol content due to drying effects

• To use daily home fluoride products for anticaries effect

• To use sugarless gum, frequent sips of water or saliva substitutes

melphalan

(mel′fa-lan)

Alkeran

Drug class.: Antineoplastic

Action: Responsible for cross-linking DNA strands, which leads to cell death

Uses: Palliative treatment of multiple myeloma and nonresectable epithelial carcinoma of the ovary

Dosage and routes:

Multiple myeloma

• *Adult:* PO 6 mg daily for 2-3 wk while evaluating WBC counts; 2 mg maintenance doses may be used depending on blood cell count; IV 16 mg/m^2 as a single infusion at 2 wk intervals × 4 doses

Epithelial ovarian cancer

• *Adult:* PO 0.2 mg/kg daily for 5 days as a single course; repeat q4-5wk depending on blood cell count

Available forms include: Tabs 2 mg; powder for inj 50 mg

Side effects/adverse reactions:

▼ *ORAL:* Stomatitis, oral ulceration

GI: Nausea, vomiting

*RESP: **Fibrosis, dysplasia***

*HEMA: **Thrombocytopenia, neutropenia, myelosuppression,** anemia*

GU: Amenorrhea, hyperuricemia

INTEG: Rash, urticaria

Contraindications: Cancer with prior resistance to drug, lactation, hypersensitivity

Precautions: Pregnancy category D, bone marrow depression, renal impairment

Pharmacokinetics: Half-life 1.5 hr; first-pass hepatic metabolism;

plasma levels vary; metabolites excreted in urine

⚕ Drug interactions of concern to dentistry:
• Increased toxicity: antineoplastics, radiation

DENTAL CONSIDERATIONS
General:
• Patients receiving chemotherapy may be taking chronic opioids for pain. Consider NSAIDs for dental pain management.
• Patients receiving chemotherapy may require palliative therapy for stomatitis.
• Patients on chronic drug therapy may rarely have symptoms of blood dyscrasias, which can include infection, bleeding, and poor healing.

Consultations:
• Medical consult may be required to assess disease control.
• In a patient with symptoms of blood dyscrasias, request a medical consult for blood studies and postpone dental treatment until normal values are reestablished.

Teach family/patient:
• About the possibility of secondary oral infection; must see dentist immediately if infection occurs
When chronic dry mouth occurs, advise patient:
• To avoid mouth rinses with high alcohol content due to drying effects
• To use sugarless gum, frequent sips of water, or saliva substitutes
• To use daily home fluoride products for anticaries effect

mepenzolate bromide
(me-pen'zoe-late)
Cantil

Drug class.: Gastrointestinal anticholinergic

Action: Inhibits muscarinic actions of acetylcholine at postganglionic parasympathetic neuroeffector sites

Uses: Treatment of peptic ulcer disease, irritable bowel syndrome in combination with other drugs; other GI disorders

Dosage and routes:
• *Adult:* PO 25-50 mg qid with meals, hs; titrate to patient response

Available forms include: Tabs 25 mg

Side effects/adverse reactions:
▼ *ORAL: Dry mouth,* absence of taste

CNS: Confusion, stimulation in elderly, headache, insomnia, dizziness, drowsiness, anxiety, weakness, hallucination

CV: Palpitation, tachycardia

GI: Constipation, paralytic ileus, heartburn, nausea, vomiting, dysphagia

GU: Hesitancy, retention, impotence

EENT: Blurred vision, photophobia, mydriasis, cycloplegia, increased ocular tension

INTEG: Urticaria, rash, pruritus, anhidrosis, fever, allergic reactions

Contraindications: Hypersensitivity to anticholinergics, narrow-angle glaucoma, GI obstruction, myasthenia gravis, paralytic ileus, GI atony, toxic megacolon

Precautions: Hyperthyroidism, coronary artery disease, dysrhyth-

M

---

bold italic = life-threatening conditions

mias, CHF, ulcerative colitis, hypertension, hiatal hernia, hepatic disease, renal disease, pregnancy category C, elderly, urinary retention, prostatic hypertrophy

Pharmacokinetics:

PO: Onset 1 hr, duration 3-4 hr; metabolized by liver; excreted in urine

Drug interactions of concern to dentistry:
- Increased anticholinergic effect: other anticholinergic drugs
- Constipation, urinary retention: opioid analgesics
- Decreased absorption of ketoconazole; take doses 2 hr apart

DENTAL CONSIDERATIONS

General:
- Monitor vital signs every appointment due to cardiovascular side effects.
- Assess salivary flow as a factor in caries, periodontal disease, and candidiasis.
- Avoid dental light in patient's eyes; offer dark glasses for patient comfort.
- Consider semisupine chair position for patient comfort due to GI effects of disease.

Consultations:
- Physician should be informed if significant xerostomic side effects occur (increased caries, sore tongue, problems eating or swallowing, difficulty wearing prosthesis) so a medication change can be considered.

Teach patient/family: *When chronic dry mouth occurs, advise patient:*
- To avoid mouth rinses with high alcohol content due to drying effects
- To use sugarless gum, frequent sips of water, or saliva substitutes

- To use daily home fluoride products for anticaries effect

---

meperidine HCl
(me-per′i-deen)
Demerol
International generic name: pethidine

Drug class.: Synthetic narcotic analgesic

Controlled Substance Schedule II, Canada N

Action: Interacts with opioid receptors in the CNS to alter pain perception

Uses: Moderate-to-severe pain, preoperatively in sedation techniques

Dosage and routes:

Pain
- *Adult:* PO/SC/IM 50-150 mg q3-4h prn; dose should be decreased if given IV
- *Child:* PO/SC/IM 1 mg/kg q4-6h prn, not to exceed 100 mg q4h

Preoperatively
- *Adult:* IM/SC 50-100 mg q30-90 min before surgery; dose should be reduced if given IV
- *Child:* IM/SC 1-2.2 mg/kg 30-90 min before surgery

Available forms include: Inj SC/IM/IV 25, 50, 75, 100 mg/ml; tabs 50, 100 mg; syr 50 mg/5 ml

Side effects/adverse reactions:

▼ *ORAL:* Dry mouth

*CNS: Drowsiness, dizziness, confusion, headache, sedation, euphoria, **increased intracranial pressure***

CV: Palpitation, bradycardia, change in BP, tachycardia (IV)

GI: Nausea, vomiting, anorexia, constipation, cramps

*RESP: **Respiratory depression***

---

italic = common side effects

GU: Increased urinary output, dysuria, urinary retention

EENT: Tinnitus, blurred vision, miosis, diplopia, depressed corneal reflex

INTEG: Rash, urticaria, bruising, flushing, diaphoresis, pruritus

Contraindications: Hypersensitivity, addiction (narcotic), MAO inhibitors, ritonavir, sibutramine

Precautions: Addictive personality, pregnancy category B, lactation, increased intracranial pressure, MI (acute), severe heart disease, respiratory depression, hepatic disease, renal disease, child <18 yr

Pharmacokinetics:

PO: Onset 15 min, peak 1 hr, duration 4-5 hr

SC/IM: Onset 10 min, peak 1 hr, duration 2-4 hr

IV: Onset 5 min, duration 2 hr Half-life 3-4 hr; metabolized by liver (to active/inactive metabolites); excreted by kidneys; crosses placenta; excreted in breast milk; a toxic metabolite can result from regular use

🦷 Drug interactions of concern to dentistry:

• Increased effects with all CNS depressants

• Contraindication: MAO inhibitors, sibutramine

• Increased effects of anticholinergics

• Suspected increase in normeperidine levels: ritonavir

DENTAL CONSIDERATIONS

General:

• After supine positioning, have patient sit upright for at least 2 min to avoid orthostatic hypotension.

• Psychologic and physical dependence may occur with chronic administration.

Teach patient/family:

• To avoid mouth rinses with high alcohol content due to drying effects

---

mephenytoin

(me-fen'i-toyn)

Mesantoin

Drug class.: Hydantoin anticonvulsant

Action: Reduces electrical discharges in motor cortex, reducing seizures

Uses: Generalized tonic-clonic seizures, single or complex-partial seizures

Dosage and routes:

• *Adult:* PO 50-100 mg/day, may increase by 50-100 mg q7d, up to 200 mg tid with upper limit 800 mg/day

• *Child:* PO 50-100 mg/day or 100-450 mg/m²/day in 3 divided doses initially, then increase 50-100 mg q7d, up to 200 mg tid in divided doses q8h; pediatric limit 400 mg/day

Available forms include: Tabs 100 mg

Side effects/adverse reactions:

▼ *ORAL:* Gingival hyperplasia, oral ulceration (Stevens-Johnson syndrome)

CNS: Drowsiness, dizziness, fatigue, irritability, tremors, insomnia, depression

GI: Nausea, vomiting

*RESP: **Pulmonary fibrosis***

*HEMA: **Agranulocytosis, leukopenia, neutropenia, pancytopenia, eosinophilia, lymphadenopathy***

EENT: Photophobia, conjunctivitis, nystagmus, diplopia

INTEG: Rash, exfoliative dermatitis

---

bold italic = life-threatening conditions

Contraindications: Hypersensitivity to hydantoins, sinus bradycardia, heart block, Adams-Stokes syndrome

Precautions: Alcoholism, hepatic disease, renal disease, blood dyscrasias, CHF, elderly, pregnancy category not listed, lactation, respiratory depression, diabetes mellitus

Pharmacokinetics:

PO: Onset 30 min, duration 24-48 hr, half-life (including active metabolite) up to 144 hr; metabolized by liver; excreted by kidneys

Drug interactions of concern to dentistry:

• Decreased effects: chronic alcohol use, barbiturates, antihistamines, CNS depressants, haloperidol, loxapine, xanthines

• Increased effects: benzodiazepines, salicylates, halothane, fluconazole, ketoconazole, metronidazole

• Hepatotoxicity: acetaminophen

• Decreased effects of carbamazepine, acetaminophen, corticosteroids, doxycycline

DENTAL CONSIDERATIONS

General:

• Evaluate respiration characteristics and rate.

• Examine for evidence of oral manifestations of blood dyscrasias (infection, bleeding, poor healing).

• Place on frequent recall to evaluate self-care and healing response.

• Avoid dental light in patient's eyes; offer dark glasses for patient comfort.

• Determine type of epilepsy, seizure frequency, and quality of seizure control. A stress reduction protocol may be required.

• Early-morning appointments and a stress reduction protocol may be required for anxious patients.

Consultations:

• Medical consult for blood studies (CBC); leukopenic or thrombocytopenic side effects may result in infection, delayed healing, and excessive bleeding. Postpone dental treatment until normal values are maintained.

• Take precautions if dental surgery is anticipated and anesthesia is required.

Teach patient/family:

• Importance of good oral hygiene to prevent soft tissue inflammation

• Caution in use of oral hygiene aids to prevent injury

• To avoid mouth rinses with high alcohol content due to drying effects

---

mephobarbital

(me-foe-bar′bi-tal)

Mebaral

♣ Gemonil

Drug class.: Barbiturate anticonvulsant

Controlled Substance Schedule IV, Canada C

Action: A nonspecific depressant of the CNS; may enhance GABA activity in the brain

Uses: Generalized tonic-clonic (grand mal) or absence (petit mal) seizures

Dosage and routes:

• *Adult:* PO 400-600 mg/day or in divided doses

• *Child:* PO 6-12 mg/kg/day in divided doses q6-8h

Available forms include: Tabs 32, 50, 100 mg

Side effects/adverse reactions:
CNS: Dizziness, headache, hangover, paradoxic stimulation, drowsiness, increased pain
CV: Hypotension, bradycardia
GI: Nausea, vomiting, epigastric pain
RESP: Wheezing, hyperpnea
HEMA: **Thrombocytopenia, agranulocytosis, megaloblastic anemia**
EENT: Tinnitus, hearing loss
INTEG: Rash, urticaria, purpura, erythema multiforme, facial edema
ENDO: Hypoglycemia, hyponatremia, hypokalemia
Contraindications: Hypersensitivity to barbiturates, pregnancy category D
Precautions: Hepatic disease, renal disease, lactation, alcoholism, drug abuse, hyperthyroidism
Pharmacokinetics:
PO: Onset 20-60 min, duration 68 hr
REC: Onset slow, duration 4-6 hr, half-life 34 hr; metabolized by liver; excreted by kidneys
🥄 **Drug interactions of concern to dentistry:**
• Increased effects: alcohol, all CNS depressants
• Decreased effects of corticosteroids, doxycycline, carbamazepine
DENTAL CONSIDERATIONS
General:
• Determine type of epilepsy, seizure frequency, and quality of seizure control. A stress reduction protocol may be required.
• Monitor vital signs every appointment due to cardiovascular and respiratory side effects.
• Patients on chronic drug therapy may rarely have symptoms of

blood dyscrasias, which can include infection, bleeding, and poor healing.
• Barbiturates induce liver microsomal enzymes, which alters the metabolism of other drugs.
• Avoid drugs that may lower seizure threshold (phenothiazines).
• Be sure patient is regularly taking medication.
Consultations:
• In a patient with symptoms of blood dyscrasias, request a medical consult for blood studies and postpone dental treatment until normal values are reestablished.
• Medical consult may be required to assess disease control and patient's ability to tolerate stress.
Teach patient/family:
• Importance of good oral hygiene to prevent soft tissue inflammation
• Caution to prevent injury when using oral hygiene aids
• To avoid mouth rinses with high alcohol content due to drying effects

---

mepivacaine HCl (local)
(me-piv′a-kane)
Carbocaine, Carbocaine with Neo-Cobefrin, Isocaine, Polocaine, Polocaine MPF
With vasoconstrictor: Carbocaine with Neo-Cobefrin, Isocaine/Levonordefrin, Polocaine/Levonordefrin
Drug class.: Amide local anesthetic

Action: Inhibits ion fluxes across membranes, particularly sodium transport across cell membrane;

---

decreases rise of depolarization phase of action potential; blocks nerve action potential

Uses: Local dental anesthesia, nerve block, caudal anesthesia, epidural, pain relief, paracervical block, transvaginal block or infiltration

Dosage and routes:
Dental injection, infiltration, or conduction block
• *Mepivacaine 3% without vasoconstrictor:* Max dose 6.6 mg/kg, or limit of 300 mg per dental appointment* for healthy patients; doses must be adjusted downward for medically compromised, debilitated, or elderly and for each individual patient. **Always use lowest effective dose, a slow injection rate, and a careful aspiration technique.**

Example calculations illustrating amount of drug administered per dental cartridge(s)

# of cartridges (1.8 ml)	mg of mepivacaine (3%)
1	54
2	108
4	216

*Maximum dose cited from *USP-DI,* ed 16, 1996, US Pharmacopeial Convention, Inc.; drug package inserts indicate max dose of 400 mg. Doses may differ from other published reference resources.

Mepivacaine 2% with levonordefrin 1:20,000: The same considerations for dose adjustment apply as previously indicated. However, the max dose for a single dental appointment is listed at 400 mg.

Example calculations illustrating amount of drug administered per dental cartridge(s)

# of cartridges (1.8 ml)	mg of mepivacaine (2%)	mg (µg) of vasoconstrictor (1:20,000)
1	36	0.090 (90)
2	72	0.180 (180)
3	108	0.270 (270)
5	180	0.450 (450)
8	288	0.720 (720)
10	360	0.900 (900)

Available forms include: Inj 1%, 1.5%, 2%, 3%; inj 2% with levonordefrin 1:20,000

Side effects/adverse reactions:
▼ *ORAL:* Numbness, tingling, trismus

CNS: **Convulsions, loss of consciousness,** drowsiness, disorientation, tremors, shivering, anxiety, restlessness

CV: **Myocardial depression, cardiac arrest, dysrhythmias,** bradycardia, hypotension, hypertension, fetal bradycardia

GI: Nausea, vomiting

RESP: **Status asthmaticus, respiratory arrest, anaphylaxis**

EENT: Blurred vision, tinnitus, pupil constriction

INTEG: Rash, urticaria, allergic reactions, edema, burning, skin discoloration at injection site, tissue necrosis

Contraindications: Hypersensitivity, cross-sensitivity among amide local anesthetics (rare), elderly, severe liver disease

Precautions: Elderly, severe drug allergies, pregnancy category C

Pharmacokinetics:
INJ: Onset 2-10 min, duration 20

italic = common side effects

min to 4 hr; metabolized by liver; excreted in urine (metabolites)

Drug interactions of concern to dentistry:

• CNS depressants: may see increased risk of CNS depression with all CNS depressants, especially in children and when larger doses are used

• Avoid placing dental cartridges in disinfectant solutions with heavy metals or surface-active agents; may see release of metal ions into local anesthetic solutions with tissue irritation following injection

• Avoid excessive exposure of dental cartridges to light or heat, which hastens deterioration of vasoconstrictor; observe for color change in local anesthetic solution

• Risk of cardiovascular side effects: rapid intravascular administration of local anesthetic containing vasoconstrictor, either alone or in patients taking tricyclic antidepressants, MAO inhibitors, digitalis drugs, cocaine, phenothiazines, β-blockers, and in the presence of halogenated-hydrocarbon general anesthetics; use smallest effective vasoconstrictor dose and careful aspiration techniques

• Avoid use of vasoconstrictors in patients with uncontrolled hyperthyroidism, diabetes, angina, or hypertension; refer these patients for medical treatment before elective dental procedures

DENTAL CONSIDERATIONS
General:

• Drug is often used with a vasoconstrictor for increased duration of action.

• Monitor vital signs every appointment due to cardiovascular and respiratory side effects.

• Lubricate dry lips before injection.

Teach patient/family:

• To use care to prevent injury while numbness exists and to refrain from chewing gum and eating following dental anesthesia

• To report any signs of infection, muscle pain, or fever to dentist when feeling returns

• To report any unusual soft tissue reactions

---

meprobamate
(me-proe-ba′mate)
Equanil, Miltown
♣ Apo-Meprobamate
Drug class.: Sedative-hypnotic, anxiolytic

**Controlled Substance
Schedule IV**
Action: Nonspecific CNS depressant; acts in thalamus, limbic system, and spinal cord
Uses: Anxiety disorders
Dosage and routes:
• *Adult:* PO 1.2-1.6 g in 2-3 divided doses, not to exceed 2.4 g/day
• *Child 6-12 yr:* PO 100-200 mg bid-tid
Available forms include: Tabs 200, 400, 600 mg; caps 400 mg; susp rel caps 200, 400 mg
Side effects/adverse reactions:

▼ *ORAL:* Stomatitis, dry mouth
*CNS: Dizziness, drowsiness, **convulsions,** headache*
*CV: **Hyperthermia,** hypotension, tachycardia, palpitation*
GI: Nausea, vomiting, anorexia, diarrhea
*HEMA: **Thrombocytopenia, leukopenia, eosinophilia***

---

bold italic = life-threatening conditions

EENT: Blurred vision, tinnitus, mydriasis, slurred speech
INTEG: Urticaria, pruritus, maculopapular rash

Contraindications: Hypersensitivity, renal failure, porphyria, pregnancy category D, history of drug abuse or dependence

Precautions: Suicidal patients, severe depression, renal disease, hepatic disease, elderly

Pharmacokinetics:
PO: Onset 1 hr, half-life 6-16 hr; metabolized by liver; excreted by kidneys, in feces; crosses placenta, excreted in breast milk

🦷 Drug interactions of concern to dentistry
• Increased effects: CNS depressants, alcohol

DENTAL CONSIDERATIONS
General:
• Monitor vital signs every appointment due to cardiovascular side effects.
• Patients on chronic drug therapy may rarely have symptoms of blood dyscrasias, which can include infection, bleeding, and poor healing.
• Assess salivary flow as a factor in caries, periodontal disease, and candidiasis.
• Avoid dental light in patient's eyes; offer dark glasses for patient comfort.
• Determine why the patient is taking the drug.
• Psychologic and physical dependence may occur with chronic administration.

Consultations:
• In a patient with symptoms of blood dyscrasias, request a medical consult for blood studies and postpone dental treatment until normal values are reestablished.
• Medical consult may be required to assess disease control.

Teach patient/family:
• Importance of good oral hygiene to prevent soft tissue inflammation
• Caution to prevent injury when using oral hygiene aids
When chronic dry mouth occurs, advise patient:
• To avoid mouth rinses with high alcohol content due to drying effects
• To use sugarless gum, frequent sips of water, or saliva substitutes
• To use daily home fluoride products for anticaries effect

---

mercaptopurine (6-MP)
(mer-kap-toe-pyoor'een)
Purinethol
Drug class.: Antineoplastic-antimetabolite

Action: Inhibits purine metabolism at multiple sites, which inhibits DNA and RNA synthesis

Uses: Chronic myelocytic leukemia, acute lymphoblastic leukemia in children, acute myelogenous leukemia

Dosage and routes:
• *Adult and child:* PO 2.5 mg/kg/day, not to exceed 5 mg/kg/day; maintenance 1.5-2.5 mg/kg/day

Available forms include: Tabs 50 mg

Side effects/adverse reactions:
▼ *ORAL:* Gingivitis, stomatitis
CNS: Fever, headache, weakness
GI: Nausea, vomiting, anorexia, diarrhea, **hepatotoxicity** (with high doses), jaundice, gastritis

*HEMA: **Thrombocytopenia, leukopenia, myelosuppression, anemia***
*GU: **Renal failure, oliguria, hematuria,*** crystalluria, hyperuricemia
INTEG: Rash, dry skin, urticaria
Contraindications: Patients with prior drug resistance, leukopenia (<2500/mm³), thrombocytopenia (<100,000/mm³), anemia, pregnancy category D
Precautions: Renal disease
Pharmacokinetics:
PO: Incompletely absorbed when taken orally; metabolized in liver; excreted in urine
🦷 **Drug interactions of concern to dentistry:**
• Increased risk of hepatotoxicity: hepatotoxic drugs
DENTAL CONSIDERATIONS
General:
• Patients on chronic drug therapy may rarely have symptoms of blood dyscrasias, which can include infection, bleeding, and poor healing.
• Avoid prescribing aspirin-containing products.
• Prophylactic antibiotics may be indicated to prevent infection if surgery or deep scaling is planned.
• Patients receiving chemotherapy may require palliative treatment for stomatitis.
Consultations:
• In a patient with symptoms of blood dyscrasias, request a medical consult for blood studies and postpone dental treatment until normal values are reestablished.
Teach patient/family:
• Importance of good oral hygiene to prevent soft tissue inflammation
• Caution to prevent injury when using oral hygiene aids

• To avoid mouth rinses with high alcohol content

---

mesalamine
(me-sal′a-meen)
Asacol, Pentasa, Rowasa
🍁 Salofalk
Drug class.: Antiinflammatory

Action: Unknown, suggested to act topically in bowel to inhibit prostaglandin synthesis
Uses: Inflammatory bowel disease, ulcerative colitis, maintenance for remission of ulcerative colitis
Dosage and routes:
• *Adult:* PO 800 mg tid for up to 6 wk; rec 500 mg bid for 3-6 wk; retention enema 4 g hs for 3-6 wk
Available forms include: Del rel tabs 400 mg; con rel caps 250 mg; supp 500 mg; rec susp 4 g/60 ml
Side effects/adverse reactions:
▼ *ORAL:* Lichenoid reactions
CNS: Headache, fever, dizziness, insomnia, asthenia, weakness, fatigue
GI: Cramps, gas, nausea, diarrhea, rectal pain, constipation
EENT: Sore throat
INTEG: Rash, itching, alopecia
SYST: Flu, malaise, back pain, peripheral edema, leg and joint pain, UTI
Contraindications: Hypersensitivity
Precautions: Pregnancy category B, renal disease, lactation, children, sulfite sensitivity
Pharmacokinetics:
REC: Half-life 1 hr, metabolite half-life 5-10 hr; primarily excreted in feces but some in urine as metabolites

DENTAL CONSIDERATIONS
General:
• Consider semisupine chair position for patient comfort due to GI effects of disease.
Consultations
• To reduce any potential risk of antibiotic-associated pseudomembranous colitis, a consult is recommended before selecting an antibiotic for a dental infection.

---

mesoridazine besylate
(mez-oh-rid'a-zeen)
Serentil, Serentil Concentrate
Drug class.: Phenothiazine antipsychotic

Action: Blocks neurotransmission at dopaminergic synapses in the cerebral cortex, hypothalamus, and limbic system; exhibits strong peripheral α-adrenergic, cholinergic blocking action; mechanism for antipsychotic effects is unclear
Uses: Psychotic disorders, schizophrenia when inadequate response with other antipsychotic drugs
Dosage and routes:
Schizophrenia
• *Adult:* PO 50 mg tid, optimum dose 100-400 mg/day; IM 25 mg, may repeat 0.5-1 hr; dosage range 25-200 mg/day
Behavior problems
• *Adult:* PO 25 mg tid; optimum dose 75-300 mg/day
Alcoholism
• *Adult:* PO 25 mg bid; optimum dose 50-200 mg/day
Schizoaffective disorders
• *Adult:* PO 10 mg tid; optimum dose 30-150 mg/day
Available forms include: Tabs 10, 25, 50, 100 mg; conc 25 mg/ml; inj IM 25 mg/ml

Side effects/adverse reactions:
▼ *ORAL: Dry mouth,* lichenoid reaction
CNS: Extrapyramidal symptoms: pseudoparkinsonism, akathisia, dystonia, tardive dyskinesia, drowsiness, headache
CV: Orthostatic hypotension, ***cardiac arrest, torsades de pointes arrhythmias,*** hypertension, ECG changes, tachycardia
GI: Nausea, vomiting, anorexia, constipation, diarrhea, jaundice, weight gain
*RESP: **Laryngospasm, respiratory depression,** dyspnea*
*HEMA: **Anemia, leukopenia, leukocytosis, agranulocytosis***
GU: Urinary retention, urinary frequency, enuresis, impotence, amenorrhea, gynecomastia
EENT: Blurred vision, glaucoma
INTEG: Rash, photosensitivity, dermatitis
Contraindications: Hypersensitivity, circulatory collapse, liver damage, cerebral arteriosclerosis, coronary disease, severe hypertension/hypotension, blood dyscrasias, coma, brain damage, bone marrow depression, narrow-angle glaucoma, drugs known to prolong the QTc interval
Precautions: Pregnancy category C, lactation, seizure disorders, hypertension, hepatic disease, cardiac disease, prostatic hypertrophy, intestinal obstruction, respiratory conditions, dose related prolongation of QTc interval
Pharmacokinetics:
PO: Onset erratic, peak 2 hr, duration 4-6 hr
IM: Onset 15-30 min, peak 30 min, duration 6-8 hr
Metabolized by liver, excreted in

italic = common side effects

urine, crosses placenta, excreted in breast milk

Drug interactions of concern to dentistry:

• Increased sedation: other CNS depressants, alcohol, barbiturate anesthetics, opioid analgesics
• Hypotension, tachycardia: epinephrine
• Increased extrapyramidal effects: phenothiazines and related drugs (haloperidol, droperidol), metoclopramide
• Additive photosensitization: tetracyclines
• Increased anticholinergic effects: anticholinergics

DENTAL CONSIDERATIONS
General:

• Monitor vital signs every appointment due to cardiovascular side effects.
• Patients on chronic drug therapy may rarely have symptoms of blood dyscrasias, which can include infection, bleeding, and poor healing.
• After supine positioning, have patient sit upright for at least 2 min before standing to avoid orthostatic hypotension.
• Assess salivary flow as a factor in caries, periodontal disease, and candidiasis.
• Avoid dental light in patient's eyes; offer dark glasses for patient comfort.
• Assess for presence of extrapyramidal motor symptoms, such as tardive dyskinesia and akathisia. Extrapyramidal motor activity may complicate dental treatment.
• Geriatric patients are more susceptible to drug effects; use lower dose.
• Use vasoconstrictors with caution, in low doses, and with careful

aspiration. Avoid use of gingival retraction cord with epinephrine.

Consultations:

• In a patient with symptoms of blood dyscrasias, request a medical consult for blood studies and postpone dental treatment until normal values are reestablished.
• Take precautions if dental surgery is anticipated and anesthesia is required.
• Refer to physician if signs of tardive dyskinesia or akathisia are present.
• Physician should be informed if significant xerostomic side effects occur (increased caries, sore tongue, problems eating or swallowing, difficulty wearing prosthesis) so a medication change can be considered.

Teach patient/family:

• Importance of good oral hygiene to prevent soft tissue inflammation
• Caution to prevent injury when using oral hygiene aids
• To use electric toothbrush if patient has difficulty holding conventional devices

When chronic dry mouth occurs, advise patient:

• To avoid mouth rinses with high alcohol content due to drying effects
• To use sugarless gum, frequent sips of water, or saliva substitutes
• To use daily home fluoride products for anticaries effect

---

metaproterenol sulfate
(met-a-proe-ter´e-nol)
Alupent
Drug class.: Selective β_2-agonist

Action: Relaxes bronchial smooth

muscle by direct action on β₂-adrenergic receptors

Uses: Bronchial asthma, bronchospasm

Dosage and routes:

• *Adult and child >12 yr:* Inh 2-3 puffs; may repeat q3-4h, not to exceed 12 puffs/day

Asthma/bronchospasm

• *Adult:* PO 20 mg q6-8h

• *Child >9 yr or >27 kg:* PO 20 mg q6-8h or 0.4-0.9 mg/kg/dose tid

• *Child 6-9 yr or <27 kg:* PO 10 mg q6-8h or 0.4-0.9 mg/kg/dose tid

Available forms include: Tabs 10, 20 mg; aerosol 0.65 mg/dose; syr 10 mg/5 ml; sol nebuliz 0.4, 0.6%, 5%

Side effects/adverse reactions:

▼ *ORAL:* Dry mouth, taste changes

CNS: Tremors, anxiety, insomnia, headache, dizziness, stimulation

CV: Cardiac arrest, palpitation, tachycardia, hypertension

GI: Nausea

RESP: Cough, throat dryness/irritation, nasal congestion

Contraindications: Hypersensitivity to sympathomimetics, narrow-angle glaucoma

Precautions: Pregnancy category C, cardiac disorders, hyperthyroidism, diabetes mellitus, prostatic hypertrophy

Pharmacokinetics:

PO: Onset 15-30 min, peak 1 hr, duration 4 hr, excreted in urine as metabolites

 Drug interactions of concern to dentistry:

• Increased effects of both drugs: other sympathomimetics, CNS stimulants

• Increased dysrhythmias: halogenated hydrocarbon anesthetics

DENTAL CONSIDERATIONS

General:

• Assess salivary flow as a factor in caries, periodontal disease, and candidiasis.

• Consider semisupine chair position for patients with respiratory disease.

• Short appointments and a stress reduction protocol may be required for anxious patients.

• Be aware that aspirin or sulfite preservatives in vasoconstrictor-containing products can exacerbate asthma.

• Acute asthmatic episodes may be precipitated in the dental office. Sympathomimetic inhalants should be available for emergency use.

Consultations:

• Medical consult may be required to assess disease control and patient's ability to tolerate stress.

Teach patient/family:

• For inhalation dosage forms: rinse mouth with water after each dose to prevent dryness

When chronic dry mouth occurs, advise patient:

• To avoid mouth rinses with high alcohol content due to drying effects

• To use sugarless gum, frequent sips of water, or saliva substitutes

• To use daily home fluoride products for anticaries effect

---

metaxalone

(me-tax′a-lone)

Skelaxin

Drug class.: Muscle relaxant

Action: Mechanism of action unknown; may cause generalized CNS depression

Uses: Adjunct to rest, physical

therapy and other measures for relief of discomfort associated with acute, painful musculoskeletal conditions

Dosage and routes:
• *Adult and child >12 yr:* PO 800 mg tid to qid
Available forms include: Tabs 400 mg

Side effects/adverse reactions:
CNS: Drowsiness, dizziness, headache, nervousness, irritability
GI: Nausea, vomiting, upset stomach, jaundice
HEMA: Leukopenia, ***hemolytic anemia***
INTEG: Rash, pruritus

Contraindications: Hypersensitivity, patient with tendency to drug-induced hemolytic or other anemias, pregnancy, renal or hepatic impairment

Precautions: Preexisting hepatic impairment, lactation, children <12 yr, alcohol use

Pharmacokinetics:
PO: Onset ~1 hr, peak effect ~2 hr, duration ~4-6 hr; metabolites excreted in urine

👄 **Drug interactions of concern to dentistry:**
• No data reported; however, this drug does cause a nonspecific CNS depression: monitor patients if other CNS depressants are used

DENTAL CONSIDERATIONS
General:
• Determine why patient is taking the drug.
• Patient on chronic drug therapy may rarely present with symptoms of blood dyscrasias, which can include infection, bleeding, and poor healing.
• Consider semisupine chair position for patient comfort if GI side effects occur.

Consultations:
• In a patient with symptoms of blood dyscrasias, request a medical consult for blood studies and postpone treatment until normal values are reestablished.

Teach patient/family:
• Importance of updating health and drug history if physician makes any changes in evaluation or drug regimens

---

metformin HCl
(met-for′min)
Glucophage, Glucophage XR, Novo-Metformin

Drug class.: Oral hypoglycemic, biguanide derivative

Action: Exact mechanism unknown, requires insulin secretion to function properly; associated with a decrease in hepatic glucose production and a decrease in intestinal glucose absorption; improves insulin sensitivity through an increase in peripheral glucose uptake and utilization

Uses: Type 2 diabetes mellitus; polycystic ovary syndrome

Dosage and routes:
• *Adult:* Must be individualized; PO initial 500 mg bid with morning and evening meals, increase dose by 500 mg at weekly intervals, daily limit 2500 mg; or 850 mg once daily with morning meal, increase dose in increments of 850 mg every other week, administered in divided doses, max 2550 mg/day; EXT REL initial dose 500 mg/day with dinner, increase by 500 mg/day each week as needed up to 2000 mg/day

M

---

bold italic = life-threatening conditions

Maintenance dose
• *Adult:* PO 500 or 850 mg bid or tid taken with meals; EXT REL 500-2000 mg once daily
Available forms include: Tabs 500, 850 mg; ext rel tabs 500 mg
Side effects/adverse reactions:

▼ *ORAL:* Unpleasant taste, metallic taste
GI: Diarrhea, nausea, vomiting, abdominal bloating, flatulence
HEMA: **Megaloblastic anemia,** lower B_{12} levels
ENDO: Hypoglycemia
MISC: **Lactic acidosis** (incidence rare)
Contraindications: Hypersensitivity, renal or hepatic disease, patients receiving radiologic exam with parenteral iodinated contrast media, diabetic ketoacidosis, acute or chronic metabolic acidosis, conditions requiring close blood glucose control; CHF, especially those at risk for hypoperfusion and hypoxemia
Precautions: Elderly, pregnancy category B, lactation, children, interferes with B_{12} absorption
Pharmacokinetics:
PO: Slow absorption, peak concentrations 2-2.5 hr; little or no protein binding; not metabolized; excreted mainly in urine
Drug interactions of concern to dentistry:
• None reported
DENTAL CONSIDERATIONS
General:
• Short appointments and a stress reduction protocol may be required for anxious patients.
• Consider semisupine chair position for patient comfort if GI side effects occur.
• Question patient about self-mon-

itoring of drug's antidiabetic effect, including blood glucose values or finger-stick records.
• Ensure that patient is following prescribed diet and regularly takes medication.
• Patients with diabetes may be more susceptible to infection and have delayed wound healing.
• Place on frequent recall to evaluate healing response.
Consultations:
• Medical consult may be required to assess disease control and patient's ability to tolerate stress.
• Notify physician immediately if symptoms of lactic acidosis are observed (myalgia, respiratory distress, weakness, diarrhea, malaise, muscle cramps, somnolence).
• Medical consult may include data from patient's blood glucose monitoring, including glycosylated hemoglobin or HbA_{1c} testing.
• Oral and maxillofacial surgical procedures associated with significantly restricted food intake require a medical consult and temporary cessation of metformin use.
Teach patient/family:
• Importance of good oral hygiene to prevent soft tissue inflammation
• That alteration of taste may be due to drug side effects

---

methadone HCl
(meth'a-done)
Dolophine, Methadose
Drug class.: Synthetic narcotic analgesic

Controlled Substance Schedule II, Canada N
Action: Interacts with opioid re-

ceptors in the CNS to alter pain perception

Uses: Severe pain, opioid withdrawal program

Dosage and routes:

Pain

• *Adult:* PO/SC/IM 2.5-10 mg q4-12h prn

Narcotic withdrawal

• *Adult:* PO 15-40 mg/day individualized initially, then 20-120 mg/day titrated to patient response

Available forms include: Inj SC/IM 10 mg/ml; tabs 5, 10 mg; oral sol 5, 10 mg/5 ml; dispersible tabs 40 mg

Side effects/adverse reactions:

▼ *ORAL:* Dry mouth

CNS: Drowsiness, dizziness, confusion, headache, sedation, euphoria

CV: Palpitation, bradycardia, change in BP

GI: Nausea, vomiting, anorexia, constipation, cramps, biliary tract spasm

RESP: Respiratory depression

GU: Increased urinary output, dysuria, urinary retention

EENT: Tinnitus, blurred vision, miosis, diplopia

INTEG: Rash, urticaria, bruising, flushing, diaphoresis, pruritus

Contraindications: Hypersensitivity, addiction (narcotic), MAO inhibitors

Precautions: Addictive personality, pregnancy category B, lactation, increased intracranial pressure, MI (acute), severe heart disease, respiratory depression, hepatic disease, renal disease, child <18 yr

Pharmacokinetics:

PO: Onset 30-60 min, duration 6-8 hr, cumulative 22-48 hr

SC/IM: Onset 10-20 min, peak 1 hr, duration 6-8 hr, cumulative 22-48 hr

Half-life 1-1.5 days; 90% bound to plasma proteins; metabolized by liver; excreted by kidneys; crosses placenta; excreted in breast milk

Drug interactions of concern to dentistry:

• Increased CNS depression: alcohol, narcotics, sedative-hypnotics, skeletal muscle relaxants, benzodiazepines, and other CNS depressants

• Increased effects of anticholinergics

DENTAL CONSIDERATIONS

General:

• Assess salivary flow as a factor in caries, periodontal disease, and candidiasis.

• Psychologic and physical dependence may occur with chronic administration.

• Determine why the patient is taking the drug.

• Be aware of the needs of patients who are in recovery from substance abuse.

• In an opioid-dependent patient, NSAIDs are the drugs of choice for posttreatment pain control.

Consultations:

• Patients in the methadone maintenance program should not receive additional opioids or other controlled substances without a consult.

Teach patient/family: *When chronic dry mouth occurs, advise patient:*

• To avoid mouth rinses with high alcohol content due to drying effects

• To use sugarless gum, frequent sips of water, or saliva substitutes

• To use daily home fluoride products for anticaries effect

---

methamphetamine HCl

(meth-am-fet′a-meen)
Desoxyn, Desoxyn Gradumet
Drug class.: Amphetamine

Controlled Substance
Schedule II
Action: Increases release of norepinephrine and dopamine in cerebral cortex to reticular activating system
Uses: Exogenous obesity, minimal brain dysfunction, attention deficit disorder with hyperactivity
Dosage and routes:
Attention deficit disorder
• *Child >6 yr:* PO 2.5-5 mg qd or bid increasing by 5 mg/wk
Obesity
• *Adult:* PO 2.5-5 mg, 30 min ac, or 10-15 mg long-acting tabs qd in AM
Available forms include: Tabs 5 mg; long-acting tabs 5, 10, 15 mg
Side effects/adverse reactions:
▼ *ORAL:* Dry mouth, unpleasant taste
CNS: Hyperactivity, insomnia, restlessness, talkativeness, dizziness, headache, chills, stimulation, dysphoria, irritability, aggressiveness, tremor
CV: Palpitation, tachycardia, hypertension, decreased heart rate, dysrhythmia
GI: Anorexia, diarrhea, constipation, weight loss, cramps
GU: Impotence, change in libido
INTEG: Urticaria
Contraindications: Hypersensitivity to sympathomimetic amines, hyperthyroidism, hypertension, glaucoma hypertrophy, severe arteriosclerosis, drug abuse, cardiovascular disease, anxiety
Precautions: Gilles de la Tourette's syndrome, pregnancy category C, lactation, child <3 yr
Pharmacokinetics:
PO: Duration 3-6 hr; metabolized by liver; excreted by kidneys; crosses blood-brain barrier
🦷 **Drug interactions of concern to dentistry:**
• Increased effect of methamphetamine: CNS stimulants, sympathomimetics
• Decreased effects of both drugs: haloperidol, sedative-hypnotics
• Ventricular dysrhythmia: inhalation anesthetics

DENTAL CONSIDERATIONS
General:
• Assess salivary flow as a factor in caries, periodontal disease, and candidiasis.
Consultations:
• Physician should be informed if significant xerostomic side effects occur (increased caries, sore tongue, problems eating or swallowing, difficulty wearing prosthesis) so a medication change can be considered.
Teach patient/family: *When chronic dry mouth occurs, advise patient:*
• To avoid mouth rinses with high alcohol content due to drying effects
• To use sugarless gum, frequent sips of water, or saliva substitutes
• To use daily home fluoride products for anticaries effect

---

methazolamide
(meth-a-zoe'la-mide)
Neptazane

Drug class.: Carbonic anhydrase inhibitor

Action: Decreases production of aqueous humor in eye, which lowers intraocular pressure

Uses: Open-angle glaucoma or preoperatively in narrow-angle glaucoma; can be used with miotic, osmotic agents

Dosage and routes:
• *Adult:* PO 50-100 mg bid or tid
Available forms include: Tabs 25, 50 mg

Side effects/adverse reactions:
▼ *ORAL:* Taste alteration (tingling, burning, numbness has occurred with similar drugs)
CNS: Drowsiness, *paresthesia,* **convulsions,** *stimulation, fatigue,* anxiety, depression, headache, dizziness, confusion, sedation, nervousness
GI: Nausea, vomiting, anorexia, constipation, diarrhea, melena, weight loss, hepatic insufficiency
HEMA: **Aplastic anemia, hemolytic anemia, leukopenia, agranulocytosis, thrombocytopenia, purpura, pancytopenia**
GU: Frequency, hypokalemia, **glucosuria, hematuria,** dysuria, polyuria, uremia
EENT: Myopia, tinnitus
INTEG: Rash, **Stevens-Johnson syndrome,** pruritus, urticaria, fever, photosensitivity
ENDO: Hyperglycemia
Contraindications: Hypersensitivity to sulfonamides or thiazide diuretics, severe renal disease, severe hepatic disease, electrolyte imbalances (hyponatremia, hypokalemia), hyperchloremic acidosis, Addison's disease, COPD

Precautions: Hypercalciuria, pregnancy category C, lactation, children

Pharmacokinetics:
PO: Slow absorption, onset 2-4 hr, peak 6-8 hr, duration 10-18 hr, half-life 14 hr; excreted in urine; crosses placenta

Drug interactions of concern to dentistry:
• Exacerbation of glaucoma: anticholinergics
• Toxicity: salicylates in large doses

DENTAL CONSIDERATIONS
General:
• Patients on chronic drug therapy may rarely have symptoms of blood dyscrasias, which can include infection, bleeding, and poor healing.
• Avoid prescribing aspirin-containing products.
• Consider semisupine chair position for patient comfort if GI side effects occur.
• Avoid dental light in patient's eyes; offer dark glasses for patient comfort.
• Protect patient's eyes from accidental spatter during dental treatment.

Consultations:
• In a patient with symptoms of blood dyscrasias, request a medical consult for blood studies and postpone dental treatment until normal values are reestablished.

Teach patient/family:
• Importance of good oral hygiene to prevent soft tissue inflammation

---

• Caution to prevent trauma when using oral hygiene aids

---

methenamine hippurate/ methenamine mandelamine

(meth-en'a-meen) (hip'yoo-rate)
Methenamine hippurate: Hiprex, Urex
♣ Hip-Rex
Methenamine mandelate
Drug class.: Urinary antiinfective

Action: In acid urine, it is hydrolyzed to ammonia and formaldehyde, which are bactericidal
Uses: Prophylaxis and treatment of uncomplicated UTIs
Dosage and routes:
• *Adult and child >12 yr: PO* 1 g q12h, max 4 g/24 hr
• *Child 6-12 yr: PO* 500 mg-1 g q12h
Neurogenic bladder
• *Adult: PO* 1 g qid pc
• *Child 6-12 yr: PO* 500 mg qid pc
• *Child <6 yr: PO* 18 mg/kg in 4 divided doses pc
Available forms include: Tabs 1 g; oral susp 500 mg/5 ml; enteric-coated tabs 500 mg, 1 g
Side effects/adverse reactions:
▼ *ORAL:* Stomatitis
CNS: Headache
GI: Nausea, vomiting, anorexia, abdominal pain, increased AST/ALT
GU: Albuminuria, hematuria, dysuria, bladder irritation, crystalluria
EENT: Tinnitus
INTEG: Pruritus, rash, urticaria
Contraindications: Hypersensi-

tivity, severe dehydration, renal insufficiency
Precautions: Renal disease, pregnancy category C, lactation
Pharmacokinetics:
PO: Excreted in urine, half-life 4 hr
🦷 **Drug interactions of concern to dentistry:**
• None

DENTAL CONSIDERATIONS
General:
• Determine why the patient is taking the drug.
• Antibiotics for dental infections are not contraindicated, but a physician notification may be advisable.
• Palliative treatment may be required for oral side effects.
• Consider semisupine chair position for patient comfort due to GI effects of drug.

---

methimazole

(meth-im'a-zole)
Tapazole
Drug class.: Thyroid hormone antagonist

Action: Inhibits synthesis of thyroid hormones by decreasing iodine use in manufacture of thyroglobulin and iodothyronine; does not affect already formed hormones
Uses: Hyperthyroidism, preparation for thyroidectomy, thyrotoxic crisis, thyroid storm
Dosage and routes:
Hyperthyroidism
• *Adult: PO* 15-60 mg/day in divided doses depending on severity of condition; continue until euthyroid; maintenance 5-30 mg qd or in divided doses

---

italic = common side effects

• *Child:* PO 0.4 mg/kg/day in divided doses q12h; continue until euthyroid; maintenance dose 0.2 mg/kg/day in one dose or divided doses q12h

Preparation for thyroidectomy

• *Adult and child:* PO same as above; iodine may be added for 10 days before surgery

Thyrotoxic crisis

• *Adult and child:* PO same as hyperthyroidism with iodine and propranolol

Available forms include: Tabs 5, 10 mg

Side effects/adverse reactions:

▼ *ORAL:* Taste alteration

CNS: Drowsiness, headache, vertigo, fever, paresthesias, neuritis

*GI: Nausea, diarrhea, vomiting, **jaundice, hepatitis***

*HEMA: **Agranulocytosis, leukopenia, thrombocytopenia, hypothrombinemia, lymphadenopathy, aplastic anemia,** bleeding,* vasculitis

*GU: **Nephritis***

INTEG: Rash, urticaria, pruritus, alopecia, hyperpigmentation, lupus-like syndrome

ENDO: Enlarged thyroid

MS: Myalgia, arthralgia, nocturnal muscle cramps

Contraindications: Hypersensitivity, pregnancy category D (third trimester), lactation

Precautions: Infection, bone marrow depression, hepatic disease, pregnancy (first, second trimester)

Pharmacokinetics:

PO: Onset 30-40 min, duration 2-4 hr, half-life 1-2 hr; excreted in urine, bile, breast milk; crosses placenta

🥄 **Drug interactions of concern to dentistry:**

• Increased CV side effects in uncontrolled patients: anticholinergics and sympathomimetics

• Patients with uncontrolled hyperthyroidism are at risk when vasoconstrictors are used

• Patients with uncontrolled hypothyroidism may be more responsive to CNS depressants

DENTAL CONSIDERATIONS

General:

• Monitor vital signs every appointment due to cardiovascular effects of disease.

• Patients on chronic drug therapy may rarely have symptoms of blood dyscrasias; examine for evidence of oral manifestations of blood dyscrasias (infection, bleeding, poor healing).

• Evaluate for clotting ability during periodontal instrumentation.

• Evaluate for control of hyperthyroidism. Patients with uncontrolled condition should not be treated in the dental office until thyroid values are normalized.

• Patients with uncontrolled condition should be referred for medical evaluation and treatment.

Consultations:

• Medical consult may be required to assess disease control.

• Medical consult for blood studies (CBC); leukopenic or thrombocytopenic side effects may result in infection, delayed healing, and excessive bleeding. Postpone elective dental treatment until normal values are maintained.

Teach patient/family:

• Importance of good oral hygiene to prevent soft tissue inflammation

• Caution in use of oral hygiene aids to prevent injury

M

---

bold italic = life-threatening conditions

methocarbamol

(meth-oh-kar′ba-mole)

Robaxin, Robaxin 750

Drug class.: Skeletal muscle relaxant

Action: Depresses multisynaptic pathways in the spinal cord

Uses: Adjunct for relief of spasm and pain in musculoskeletal conditions

Dosage and routes:

Pain

• *Adult:* PO 1.5 g/day × 2-3 days, then 1 g qid; IM 500 mg in each gluteal region, may repeat q8h; IV bol 1-3 g/day at 3 ml/min; IV inf 1 g/250 ml D$_5$W or NS, not to exceed 3 g/day

Available forms include: Tabs 500, 750 mg; inj IM/IV 100 mg/ml

Side effects/adverse reactions:

▼ *ORAL:* Metallic taste

CNS: Dizziness, weakness, drowsiness, seizures, headache, tremor, depression, insomnia

CV: Postural hypotension, bradycardia

GI: Nausea, vomiting, hiccups, anorexia

HEMA: Hemolysis, increased hemoglobin (IV only)

GU: Brown, black, or green urine

EENT: Diplopia, temporary loss of vision, blurred vision, nystagmus

INTEG: Rash, pruritus, fever, facial flushing, urticaria

Contraindications: Hypersensitivity, child <12 yr, intermittent porphyria

Precautions: Renal disease, hepatic disease, addictive personalities, pregnancy category C, myasthenia gravis, epilepsy

Pharmacokinetics:

PO: Onset 0.5 hr, peak 1-2 hr, half-life 1-2 hr; metabolized in liver; excreted in urine (unchanged); crosses placenta

🦷 **Drug interactions of concern to dentistry:**

• Increased CNS depression: alcohol, narcotics, sedative-hypnotics

DENTAL CONSIDERATIONS

General:

• Determine why the patient is taking the drug.

• Consider semisupine chair position if back is involved.

Teach patient/family:

• Importance of good oral hygiene to prevent soft tissue inflammation

• Caution to prevent injury when using oral hygiene aids

• To avoid mouth rinses with high alcohol content due to drying effects

methotrexate/ methotrexate sodium (amethopterin, MTX)

(meth-oh-trex′ate)

Rheumatrex Dose Pak

Drug class.: Folic acid antagonist, antineoplastic

Action: Inhibits an enzyme that reduces folic acid, which is needed for nucleic acid synthesis in all cells

Uses: Acute lymphocytic leukemia; in combination for breast, lung, head, neck cancer; lymphosarcoma; psoriasis; gestational choriocarcinoma; hydatidiform mole; rheumatoid arthritis

Dosage and routes:
Leukemia
• *Adult and child:* PO 3.3 mg/m^2/day, maintenance 30 mg/m^2/day 2× weekly; IV 2.5 mg/kg q2wk
Choriocarcinoma
• *Adult and child:* PO 15-30 mg/m^2 qd × 5 days, then off 1 wk; may repeat
Psoriasis
• *Adult:* PO/IV/IM 10 mg to 25 mg/weekly single dose or PO 2.5 mg q12h × 3 doses; limit 30 mg/wk
Rheumatoid Arthritis
• *Adult:* PO initial 7.5 mg/wk as a single dose or 2.5 mg q12h × 3 doses
Available forms include: Tabs 2.5 mg; inj IV 25 mg/ml; powder for inj IV 20, 25, 50, 100, 250 mg; sodium inj IV 2.5, 25 mg/ml

Side effects/adverse reactions:
▼ *ORAL: Ulcerative stomatitis, gingivitis,* bleeding
CNS: **Convulsions,** dizziness, headache, confusion, hemiparesis, malaise, fatigue, chills, fever
*GI: Nausea, vomiting, anorexia, diarrhea, **hepatotoxicity, GI hemorrhage,** abdominal pain, cramps, ulcer, gastritis, hematemesis*
*HEMA: **Leukopenia, thrombocytopenia, myelosuppression, anemia***
*GU: **Renal failure, hematuria, azotemia, uric acid nephropathy,** urinary retention, menstrual irregularities, defective spermatogenesis*
INTEG: Rash, alopecia, dry skin, urticaria, photosensitivity, folliculitis, vasculitis, petechiae, ecchymosis, acne, alopecia, painful plaque lesions in psoriasis
MISC: Rare reports of bone and soft tissue necrosis after radiation therapy
Contraindications: Hypersensi-

tivity, leukopenia (<2500/mm^3), thrombocytopenia (<100,000/mm^3), anemia, patients with psoriasis and severe renal/hepatic disease, pregnancy category D
Precautions: Renal disease, lactation, other drugs with potential for hepatotoxicity
Pharmacokinetics:
PO: Readily absorbed when taken orally, peak 1-4 hr
IV/IM: Peak 0.5-2 hr
50% plasma protein bound; not metabolized; excreted in urine (unchanged); crosses placenta, blood-brain barrier

⚡ Drug interactions of concern to dentistry:
• Increased toxicity: aspirin, alcohol, NSAIDs
• Possible fatal interactions: NSAIDs, high-dose IV methotrexate
• Suspected increase in methotrexate toxicity: amoxicillin, tetracycline, doxycycline

DENTAL CONSIDERATIONS
General:
• Patients on chronic drug therapy may rarely have symptoms of blood dyscrasias, which can include infection, bleeding, and poor healing.
• Avoid prescribing aspirin- or NSAID-containing products.
• Place on frequent recall due to increased risk for infection and to evaluate healing response.
• Determine why the patient is taking the drug.
• Palliative treatment may be needed if stomatitis occurs.
Consultations:
• In a patient with symptoms of blood dyscrasias, request a medical

M

consult for blood studies and postpone dental treatment until normal values are reestablished.
• Medical consult may be required to assess disease control.

Teach patient/family:
• Importance of good oral hygiene to prevent soft tissue inflammation
• Caution to prevent injury when using oral hygiene aids
• About palliative therapy for sore mouth
• To avoid mouth rinses with high alcohol content due to drying effects

---

methsuximide

(meth-sux'i-mide)
Celontin
Drug class.: Anticonvulsant

Action: Inhibits spike wave formation in absence seizures (petit mal); decreases amplitude, frequency, duration, spread of discharge in minor motor seizures

Uses: Refractory absence seizures (petit mal)

Dosage and routes:
• *Adult and child:* PO 300 mg/day; may increase by 300 mg/wk, not to exceed 1.2 g/day in divided doses

Available forms include: Half-strength caps 150 mg; caps 300 mg

Side effects/adverse reactions:
▼ *ORAL:* Gingival overgrowth, glossitis, ulcers (Stevens-Johnson syndrome)

CNS: Drowsiness, dizziness, fatigue, euphoria, lethargy, irritability, depression, insomnia, anxiety, aggressiveness, ataxia, headache, confusion

GI: Nausea, vomiting, heartburn, anorexia, diarrhea, abdominal pain, cramps, constipation

HEMA: Agranulocytosis, aplastic anemia, thrombocytopenia, leukocytosis, eosinophilia, pancytopenia

GU: Hematuria, renal damage, vaginal bleeding

EENT: Myopia, blurred vision, photophobia

INTEG: Stevens-Johnson syndrome, urticaria, pruritic erythema, hirsutism

Contraindications: Hypersensitivity to succinimide derivatives

Precautions: Hepatic disease, renal disease, pregnancy category C, lactation

Pharmacokinetics:
PO: Onset 15-30 min, peak 1-2 hr, duration 4-6 hr
REC: Onset slow, duration 4-6 hr
Half-life 2.6-4 hr; metabolized by liver; excreted by kidneys

🥄 **Drug interactions of concern to dentistry:**
• Enhanced CNS depression: alcohol, CNS depressants
• Decreased effects: phenothiazines, thioxanthenes, barbiturates
• Changes in seizure pattern, frequency: haloperidol

DENTAL CONSIDERATIONS
General:
• Patients on chronic drug therapy may rarely have symptoms of blood dyscrasias, which can include infection, bleeding, and poor healing.
• Avoid dental light in patient's eyes; offer dark glasses for patient comfort.
• Determine type of epilepsy, seizure frequency, and quality of seizure control. A stress reduction protocol may be required.
• Place on frequent recall to monitor gingival condition.

Consultations:

• In a patient with symptoms of blood dyscrasias, request a medical consult for blood studies and postpone dental treatment until normal values are reestablished.

• Take precautions if dental surgery is anticipated and anesthesia is required.

• Medical consult may be required to assess disease control.

Teach patient/family:

• Importance of good oral hygiene to prevent soft tissue inflammation

• Caution to prevent injury when using oral hygiene aids

• To avoid mouth rinses with high alcohol content if oral side effects occur

---

methyldopa/ methyldopate

(meth-il-doe′pa)

Aldomet

🍁 Apo-Methyldopa, Dopamet, Novomedopa, Nu-Medopa

Drug class.: Centrally acting antihypertensive

Action: Stimulates central inhibitory α-adrenergic receptors or acts as false transmitter, resulting in reduction of arterial pressure

Uses:

Hypertension

Dosage and routes:

• *Adult:* PO 250 mg bid or tid, then adjusted q2d as needed, 0.5-3 g qd in 2-4 divided doses (maintenance), not to exceed 3 g/day; IV 250-500 mg in 100 ml D_5W q6h, run over 30-60 min, not to exceed 1 g q6h

• *Child:* PO 10 mg/kg/day in 2-4 divided doses, not to exceed 65 mg/kg or 3 g/day, whichever is less; IV 20-40 mg/kg/day in 4 divided doses, not to exceed 65 mg/kg

Available forms include: Tabs 125, 250, 500 mg; oral susp 250 mg/5 ml; inj IV 50 mg/ml

Side effects/adverse reactions:

▼ *ORAL:* Dry mouth, bleeding, lichenoid lesions

CNS: Drowsiness, weakness, dizziness, sedation, headache, depression, psychosis

CV: Bradycardia, myocarditis, orthostatic hypotension, angina, edema, weight gain

GI: Nausea, vomiting, diarrhea, constipation, hepatic dysfunction

HEMA: **Leukopenia, thrombocytopenia,** anemia, positive Coombs' test

GU: Impotence, failure to ejaculate

EENT: Nasal congestion, eczema

INTEG: Lupus-like syndrome

Contraindications: Active hepatic disease, hypersensitivity, blood dyscrasias

Precautions: Pregnancy category C, liver disease, eclampsia, severe cardiac disease

Pharmacokinetics:

PO: Peak 4-6 hr, duration 12-24 hr

IV: Peak 2 hr, duration 10-16 hr

Metabolized by liver, excreted in urine

👉 **Drug interactions of concern to dentistry:**

• Decreased effects: indomethacin and other NSAIDs

• Increased pressor response: epinephrine and other sympathomimetics

• Increased sedation: haloperidol, alcohol, CNS depressants

• Increased hypotensive action of general anesthetics

---

bold italic = life-threatening conditions   *For periodic updates, visit* **www.mosby.com**

DENTAL CONSIDERATIONS
General:
• Monitor vital signs every appointment due to cardiovascular side effects.
• Patients on chronic drug therapy may rarely have symptoms of blood dyscrasias, which can include infection, bleeding, and poor healing.
• Assess salivary flow as a factor in caries, periodontal disease, and candidiasis.
• Limit use of sodium-containing products such as saline IV fluids for patients with a dietary salt restriction.
• After supine positioning, have patient sit upright for at least 2 min before standing to avoid orthostatic hypotension.
• Stress from dental procedures may compromise cardiovascular function; determine patient risk.

Consultations:
• In a patient with symptoms of blood dyscrasias, request a medical consult for blood studies and postpone dental treatment until normal values are reestablished.
• Medical consult may be required to assess disease control and stress tolerance.

Teach patient/family:
• Importance of good oral hygiene to prevent soft tissue inflammation
• Caution to prevent injury when using oral hygiene aids
When chronic dry mouth occurs, advise patient:
• To avoid mouth rinses with high alcohol content due to drying effects
• To use sugarless gum, frequent sips of water, or saliva substitutes
• To use daily home fluoride products for anticaries effect

methylphenidate HCl
(meth-il-fen'i-date)
Concerta, Metadate CD, Metadate ER, Methylin, Methylin ER, Ritalin, Ritalin LA, Ritalin SR
♣ *PMS-Methylphenidate*
Drug class.: CNS stimulant, related to amphetamines

Controlled Substance Schedule II, Canada C
Action: Increases release of norepinephrine, dopamine in cerebral cortex to reticular activating system; exact mode of action not known
Uses: Attention deficit disorder with hyperactivity, narcolepsy
Dosage and routes:
Attention deficit disorder
• *Adult:* PO 20-30 mg/day in divided doses bid or tid, 45 min before meals
• *Child >6 yr:* 5 mg before breakfast and lunch, increasing by 5-10 mg/wk, not to exceed 60 mg/day; long acting form 18-36 mg qd in AM
Narcolepsy
• *Adult:* PO 10 mg bid-tid, 30-45 min before meals; may increase up to 40-50 mg/day
Available forms include: Tabs 5, 10, 20 mg; ext rel tabs 10, 18, 20, 36, 54 mg; ext rel caps 20 mg
Side effects/adverse reactions:
▼ *ORAL:* Dry mouth
CNS: Hyperactivity, insomnia, restlessness, talkativeness, dizziness, headache, akathisia, dyskinesia, Gilles de la Tourette's syndrome
CV: Palpitation, tachycardia, BP changes, angina, dysrhythmias

GI: Nausea, anorexia, diarrhea, constipation, weight loss, abdominal pain

HEMA: ***Thrombocytopenia***

GU: ***Uremia***

INTEG: ***Exfoliative dermatitis,*** urticaria, rash, erythema multiforme

ENDO: Growth retardation

Contraindications: Hypersensitivity, anxiety, history of Gilles de la Tourette's syndrome, history of seizures

Precautions: Hypertension, depression, pregnancy category C, seizures, lactation, drug abuse

Pharmacokinetics:

PO: Onset 0.5-1 hr, duration 4-6 hr; metabolized by liver; excreted by kidneys

🦷 Drug interactions of concern to dentistry:

• Increased effects of anticholinergics, CNS stimulants, tricyclic antidepressants, and sympathomimetics

DENTAL CONSIDERATIONS

General:

• Monitor vital signs often due to cardiovascular side effects.

• Patients on chronic drug therapy may rarely have symptoms of blood dyscrasias, which can include infection, bleeding, and poor healing.

• Assess salivary flow as a factor in caries, periodontal disease, and candidiasis.

• Use vasoconstrictors with caution, in low doses, and with careful aspiration.

• Determine why the patient is taking the drug.

Consultations:

• In a patient with symptoms of blood dyscrasias, request a medical consult for blood studies and postpone dental treatment until normal values are reestablished.

• Medical consult may be required to assess disease control.

Teach patient/family:

• Importance of good oral hygiene to prevent soft tissue inflammation

• Caution to prevent injury when using oral hygiene aids

When chronic dry mouth occurs, advise patient:

• To avoid mouth rinses with high alcohol content due to drying effects

• To use sugarless gum, frequent sips of water, or saliva substitutes

• To use daily home fluoride products for anticaries effect

---

methylprednisolone/ methylprednisolone acetate/ methylprednisolone sodium succinate

(meth-il-pred-nis'oh-lone)

Methylprednisolone: Medrol, Medrol Dosepak, Meprolone

Methylprednisolone acetate: depMedalone 40, depMedalone 80, Depoject, Depo-Medrol, Depopred 40, Depopred 80, Depo-Prodate, Duralone 40, Duralone 80, Medralone 40, Medralone 80, M-Prednisol 40, M-Prednisol 80, Rep-Pred 40, Rep-Pred 80

Methylprednisolone sodium succinate: A-MethaPred, Solu-Medrol

Drug class.: Glucocorticoid, immediate acting

Action: Glucocorticoids have multiple actions that include antiinflammatory and immunosuppres-

M

sant effects. They inhibit phospholipase A_2, interfering with or reducing the synthesis of prostaglandins and leukotrienes. They also bind to cytoplasmic glucocorticoid receptors (GRs) and enter the cell nucleus to bind with DNA. This results in the synthesis of various enzymes such as collagenase, elastase, and cytokines that play important roles in inflammation and immunosuppression. They also suppress the production of lymphocytes, monocytes, and eosinophils.

Uses: Severe inflammation, shock, adrenal insufficiency, collagen disorders

Dosage and routes:
Adrenal insufficiency/inflammation
• *Adult:* PO 2-60 mg in 4 divided doses; IM 40-80 mg (acetate); IM/IV 10-250 mg (succinate); intraarticular 4-30 mg (acetate)
• *Child:* IV 117 µg to 1.66 mg/kg in 3-4 divided doses (succinate)
Shock
• *Adult:* IV 100-250 mg q2-6h (succinate)
Available forms include: Tabs 2, 4, 6, 8, 16, 24, 32 mg; inj (acetate) 20, 40, 80 mg/ml

Caution: *Do not administer acetate preparations IV;* inj (succinate) 40, 125, 500, 1000, 2000 mg/vial

Side effects/adverse reactions:
▼ *ORAL:* **Candidiasis,** dry mouth, poor wound healing, petechiae
CNS: Depression, flushing, sweating, headache, mood changes
*CV: Hypertension, **circulatory collapse, thrombophlebitis, embolism,** tachycardia

GI: Diarrhea, nausea, abdominal distention, **GI hemorrhage, increased appetite, pancreatitis**
HEMA: **Thrombocytopenia**
EENT: Fungal infections, increased intraocular pressure, blurred vision
INTEG: Acne, poor wound healing, ecchymosis, petechiae
MS: Fractures, osteoporosis, weakness

Contraindications: Psychosis, hypersensitivity, idiopathic thrombocytopenia, acute glomerulonephritis, amebiasis, fungal infections, nonasthmatic bronchial disease, child <2 yr, AIDS, TB

Precautions: Pregnancy category C, diabetes mellitus, glaucoma, osteoporosis, seizure disorders, ulcerative colitis, CHF, myasthenia gravis, renal disease, esophagitis, peptic ulcer, rifampin

Pharmacokinetics:
PO: Peak 1-2 hr, duration 1.5 days
IM: Peak 4-8 days, duration 1-4 wk
INTRAARTICULAR: Peak 1 wk
Half-life >3.5 hr

⚕ Drug interactions of concern to dentistry:
• Decreased action: barbiturates, rifampin, rifabutin
• Increased GI side effects: alcohol, salicylates, NSAIDs
• Increased action: ketoconazole, macrolide antibiotics
• Hepatotoxicity: acetaminophen (chronic, high doses)

DENTAL CONSIDERATIONS
General:
• Patients on chronic drug therapy may rarely have symptoms of blood dyscrasias, which can include infection, bleeding, and poor healing.

italic = common side effects

• Assess salivary flow as a factor in caries, periodontal disease, and candidiasis.
• Symptoms of oral infections may be masked.
• Place on frequent recall to evaluate healing response.
• Prophylactic antibiotics may be indicated to prevent infection if surgery or deep scaling is planned.
• Avoid prescribing aspirin-containing products.
• Determine dose and duration of steroid therapy for each patient to assess risk for stress tolerance and immunosuppression.
• Patients who have been or are currently on chronic steroid therapy (>2 wk) may require supplemental steroids for dental treatment.

Consultations:
• In a patient with symptoms of blood dyscrasias, request a medical consult for blood studies and postpone dental treatment until normal values are reestablished.
• Medical consult may be required to assess disease control.
• Consult may be required to confirm steroid dose and duration of use.

Teach patient/family:
• Importance of good oral hygiene to prevent soft tissue inflammation
• Caution to prevent injury when using oral hygiene aids due to reduced healing response
When chronic dry mouth occurs, advise patient:
• To avoid mouth rinses with high alcohol content due to drying effects
• To use sugarless gum, frequent sips of water, or saliva substitutes

• To use daily home fluoride products for anticaries effect

---

methysergide maleate
(meth-i-ser′jide)
Sansert
Drug class.: Serotonin antagonist

Action: Competitively blocks serotonin HT receptors in CNS and periphery
Uses: Prophylaxis for migraine and other vascular headaches
Dosage and routes:
• *Adult:* PO 4-8 mg daily with meals
Available forms include: Tabs 2 mg
Side effects/adverse reactions:
CNS: Tremors, anxiety, insomnia, headache, dizziness, euphoria, confusion, depersonalization, hallucination, paresthesia, drowsiness
CV: Retroperitoneal fibrosis, cardiac fibrosis, valvular thickening, palpitation, tachycardia, postural hypertension, angina, thrombophlebitis, ECG changes
GI: Nausea, vomiting, weight gain
HEMA: Blood dyscrasias
INTEG: Flushing, rash, alopecia
MS: Arthralgia, myalgia
Contraindications: Hypersensitivity to ergot, tartrazine, pregnancy category X, occlusion (peripheral, vascular), CAD, hepatic disease, renal or liver disease, peptic ulcer, hypertension, connective tissue disease, fibrotic pulmonary disease, severe atherosclerosis, valvular heart disease
Precautions: Lactation, children

M

Pharmacokinetics:

PO: Half-life 10 hr; metabolized by liver; excreted in urine (metabolites/unchanged drug)

🐾 Drug interactions of concern to dentistry:

• Increased vasoconstriction: systemically administered sympathomimetics

DENTAL CONSIDERATIONS

General:

• Patients on chronic drug therapy may rarely have symptoms of blood dyscrasias, which can include infection, bleeding, and poor healing.

• After supine positioning, have patient sit upright for at least 2 min to avoid orthostatic hypotension.

• Use vasoconstrictors with caution, in low doses, and with careful aspiration.

• Avoid use of gingival retraction cord with epinephrine.

Consultations:

• In a patient with symptoms of blood dyscrasias, request a medical consult for blood studies and postpone dental treatment until normal values are reestablished.

• Medical consult may be required to assess disease control.

---

metoclopramide HCl

(met-oh-kloe-pra'mide)

Maxolon, Octamide, Reglan
♣ Apo-Metoclop, Maxeran, PMS-Metoclopramide

Drug class.: Central dopamine receptor antagonist

Action: Enhances response to acetylcholine of tissue in upper GI tract, which causes contraction of gastric muscle, relaxes pyloric and duodenal segments, increases peristalsis without stimulating secretions; antiemetic action occurs centrally, possibly by action on chemoreceptor trigger zone

Uses: Prevention of nausea, vomiting induced by chemotherapy, radiation, delayed gastric emptying, gastroesophageal reflux

Dosage and routes:

Nausea/vomiting

• *Adult:* IV 2 mg/kg 30 min before administration of chemotherapy, then q2h × 2 doses, and then q3h × 3 doses

Post op nausea/vomiting

• *Adult:* IM 10 mg-20 mg

Delayed gastric emptying

• *Adult:* PO 10 mg 30 min ac, hs × 2-8 wk

Gastroesophageal reflux

• *Adult:* PO 10-15 mg qid 30 min ac

Available forms include: Tabs 5, 10 mg; syr 5 mg/5 ml; inj IV 5 mg/ml

Side effects/adverse reactions:

▼ *ORAL:* Dry mouth

CNS: Sedation, fatigue, restlessness, headache, sleeplessness, dystonia, dizziness, drowsiness, tardive dyskinesia, Parkinson-like tremors

CV: Hypotension, supraventricular tachycardia, hypertension (IV)

GI: Constipation, nausea, anorexia, vomiting

*HEMA: **Agranulocytosis, neutropenia, leukopenia***

GU: Decreased libido, prolactin secretion, amenorrhea, galactorrhea

INTEG: Urticaria, rash

Contraindications: Hypersensitivity to this drug or procaine or procainamide, seizure disorder, pheochromocytoma, breast cancer, GI obstruction

---

Precautions: Pregnancy category B, lactation, GI hemorrhage, CHF, asthma, hypertension, Parkinson's disease, renal failure

Pharmacokinetics:

IV: Onset 1-3 min, duration 1-2 hr
PO: Onset 0.5-1 hr, duration 1-2 hr
IM: Onset 10-15 min, duration 1-2 hr

Half-life 4 hr, metabolized by liver, excreted in urine

🦷 Drug interactions of concern to dentistry:

• Decreased GI action: anticholinergics, opioids
• Increased sedation: alcohol, other CNS depressants
• Increased effects of succinylcholine

DENTAL CONSIDERATIONS

General:

• Assess salivary flow as a factor in caries, periodontal disease, and candidiasis.
• Assess for presence of extrapyramidal motor symptoms, such as tardive dyskinesia and akathisia. Extrapyramidal motor activity may complicate dental treatment.
• Determine why the patient is taking the drug.
• Consider semisupine chair position for patient comfort due to GI effects of disease.

Teach patient/family: *When chronic dry mouth occurs, advise patient:*

• To avoid mouth rinses with high alcohol content due to drying effects
• To use sugarless gum, frequent sips of water, or saliva substitutes
• To use daily home fluoride products for anticaries effect

metolazone

(me-tole′a-zone)

Mykrox, Zaroxolyn

Drug class.: Diuretic with thiazide-like effects

Action: Acts on distal tubule by increasing excretion of water, sodium, chloride, and potassium

Uses: Edema, hypertension, CHF

Dosage and routes:

Edema
• *Adult:* PO 5-20 mg/day

Hypertension
• *Adult:* PO 2.5-5 mg/day

Available forms include: Tabs 0.5, 2.5, 5, 10 mg

Side effects/adverse reactions:

▼ *ORAL: Dry mouth, increased thirst*

CNS: Dizziness, fatigue, weakness, drowsiness, paresthesia, anxiety, depression, headache

CV: Irregular pulse, orthostatic hypotension, palpitation, volume depletion

*GI: Nausea, vomiting, anorexia, **hepatitis,** constipation, diarrhea, cramps, pancreatitis, GI irritation*

*HEMA: **Aplastic anemia, hemolytic anemia, leukopenia, agranulocytosis, thrombocytopenia,** neutropenia*

*GU: Frequency, **uremia, glucosuria,** polyuria*

EENT: Blurred vision

*INTEG: **Rash,** urticaria, purpura, photosensitivity, fever*

META: Hyperglycemia, hyperuricemia, increased creatinine, BUN

ELECT: Hypokalemia, hypomagnesia, hypercalcemia, hyponatremia, hypochloremia

Contraindications: Hypersensitivity to thiazides or sulfonamides, anuria, pregnancy category D

---

bold italic = life-threatening conditions

Precautions: Hypokalemia, renal disease, hepatic disease, gout, COPD, lupus erythematosus, diabetes mellitus

Pharmacokinetics:

PO: Onset 1 hr, peak 2 hr, duration 12-24 hr, half-life 8 hr; excreted unchanged by kidneys; crosses placenta; enters breast milk

🦷 **Drug interactions of concern to dentistry:**

• Increased photosensitization: tetracycline

• Decreased hypotensive response: indomethacin and other NSAIDs

DENTAL CONSIDERATIONS

General:

• Patients on chronic drug therapy may rarely have symptoms of blood dyscrasias, which can include infection, bleeding, and poor healing.

• Assess salivary flow as a factor in caries, periodontal disease, and candidiasis.

• After supine positioning, have patient sit upright for at least 2 min before standing to avoid orthostatic hypotension.

• Short appointments and a stress reduction protocol may be required for anxious patients.

• Limit use of sodium-containing products, such as saline IV fluids, for those patients with a dietary salt restriction.

• Stress from dental procedures may compromise cardiovascular function; determine patient risk.

Consultations:

• In a patient with symptoms of blood dyscrasias, request a medical consult for blood studies and postpone dental treatment until normal values are reestablished.

• Medical consult may be required to assess disease control and patient's ability to tolerate stress.

Teach patient/family:

• Importance of good oral hygiene to prevent soft tissue inflammation

• Caution to prevent injury when using oral hygiene aids

When chronic dry mouth occurs, advise patient:

• To avoid mouth rinses with high alcohol content due to drying effects

• To use sugarless gum, frequent sips of water, or saliva substitutes

• To use daily home fluoride products for anticaries effect

---

metoprolol tartrate

(met-oh′proe-lol)

Lopressor, Toprol XL

🍁 Apo-Metoprolol, Lopresor SR, Novometoprol

Drug class.: Antihypertensive, selective β_1-blocker

Action: This is a selective β_1-adrenergic antagonist. At higher doses selectivity may be lost with antagonism of β_2-receptors as well. The antihypertensive mechanism of action is unclear but may include a reduction in cardiac output and inhibition of renin release by the renal juxtaglomerular apparatus. Peripheral resistance decreases with long-term use. The antianginal action (when indicated for this use) may be related to a decrease in myocardial oxygen demand and negative chronotropic and inotropic effects. The antiarrhythmic action (when indicated for this use) has been related to a reduction in spontaneous pacemaker firing and slowing of AV nodal conduction.

italic = common side effects

Uses: Mild-to-moderate hypertension, acute MI to reduce cardiovascular mortality, angina pectoris

Dosage and routes:

Hypertension
• *Adult:* PO 50 mg bid or 100 mg qd; may give up to 200-450 mg in divided doses

Myocardial infarction
• *Adult:* Early treatment, IV bol 5 mg q2min × 3, then 50 mg PO 15 min after last dose and q6h × 48 hr; late treatment, PO maintenance 100 mg bid × 3 mo

Available forms include: Tabs 50, 100 mg; ext rel 25, 50, 100, 200 mg; inj IV 1 mg/ml

Side effects/adverse reactions:

▼ *ORAL:* Dry mouth

CNS: Insomnia, dizziness, **depression,** mental changes, hallucinations, anxiety, headaches, nightmares, confusion, fatigue

CV: Bradycardia, CHF (palpitation), **cardiac arrest, AV block,** dysrhythmias, hypotension

GI: Nausea, vomiting, **diarrhea,** hiccups, constipation, flatulence, colitis, cramps

RESP: **Bronchospasm,** dyspnea, wheezing

HEMA: **Agranulocytosis, eosinophilia, thrombocytopenic purpura**

GU: Impotence

EENT: Sore throat, dry/burning eyes

INTEG: Rash, purpura, alopecia, dry skin, urticaria, pruritus

Contraindications: Hypersensitivity to β-blockers, cardiogenic shock, second- or third-degree heart block, sinus bradycardia, CHF, bronchial asthma

Precautions: Major surgery, pregnancy category C, lactation, diabetes mellitus, renal disease, thyroid disease, COPD, heart failure, CAD, nonallergic bronchospasm, hepatic disease

Pharmacokinetics:

PO: Peak 2-4 hr, duration 13-19 hr, half-life 3-4 hr; metabolized in liver (metabolites); excreted in urine; crosses placenta; excreted in breast milk

🦷 **Drug interactions of concern to dentistry:**
• Increased hypotension, bradycardia: fentanyl derivatives, inhalation anesthetics
• Decreased antihypertensive effects: indomethacin and possibly other NSAIDs, sympathomimetics
• May slow metabolism of lidocaine
• Decreased β-blocking effects (or decreased β-adrenergic effects) of epinephrine, levonordefrin, isoproterenol, and other sympathomimetics
• Increased plasma concentrations: diphenhydramine

DENTAL CONSIDERATIONS

General:
• Monitor vital signs every appointment due to cardiovascular and respiratory side effects.
• After supine positioning, have patient sit upright for at least 2 min before standing to avoid orthostatic hypotension.
• Patients on chronic drug therapy may rarely have symptoms of blood dyscrasias, which can include infection, bleeding, and poor healing.
• Assess salivary flow as a factor in caries, periodontal disease, and candidiasis.
• Stress from dental procedures may compromise cardiovascular function; determine patient risk.
• Short appointments and a stress

M

---

bold italic = life-threatening conditions

reduction protocol may be required for anxious patients.

• Use vasoconstrictors with caution, in low doses, and with careful aspiration. Avoid use of gingival retraction cord with epinephrine.

Consultations:

• In a patient with symptoms of blood dyscrasias, request a medical consult for blood studies and postpone dental treatment until normal values are reestablished.

• Medical consult may be required to assess disease control and patient's ability to tolerate stress.

• Take precautions if general anesthesia is required for dental surgery.

Teach patient/family:

• Importance of good oral hygiene to prevent soft tissue inflammation

• Caution to prevent injury when using oral hygiene aids

When chronic dry mouth occurs, advise patient:

• To avoid mouth rinses with high alcohol content due to drying effects

• To use sugarless gum, frequent sips of water, or saliva substitutes

• To use daily home fluoride products for anticaries effect

---

metronidazole/ metronidazole HCl

(me-troe-ni'da-zole)

Flagyl, Flagyl IV RTU, Flagyl 375, Flagyl ER, Helidac, Metric 21, Metro Gel-Vaginal, Metro IV, Protostat

✦ Apo-Metronidazole, Novonidazole, Trikacide

Drug class.: Trichomonacide, amebicide, antiinfective

Action: Direct-acting amebicide/

trichomonacide binds, degrades DNA in organism

Uses: Intestinal amebiasis, amebic abscess, trichomoniasis, refractory trichomoniasis, bacterial anaerobic infections, giardiasis; unapproved: refractory adult periodontitis

Dosage and routes:

Bacterial vaginosis

• *Adult:* TOP 1 applicator intravag qd or bid × 5 days

Trichomoniasis

• *Adult:* PO 250 mg tid × 7 days, or 2 g in single dose; do not repeat treatment for 2-3 wk

Refractory trichomoniasis

• *Adult:* PO 250 mg bid × 10 days

Amebic abscess

• *Adult:* PO 500-750 mg tid × 5-10 days

• *Child:* PO 35-50 mg/kg/day in 3 divided doses × 10 days

Intestinal amebiasis

• *Adult:* PO 750 mg tid × 5-10 days

• *Child:* PO 35-50 mg/kg/day in 3 divided doses × 10 days; then give oral iodoquinol

Anaerobic bacterial infections

• *Adult:* IV inf 15 mg/kg over 1 hr, then 7.5 mg/kg IV or PO q6h, not to exceed 4 g/day

Periodontitis

• *Adult:* PO 250 mg tid for 7-10 days

Giardiasis

• *Adult:* PO 250 mg tid × 5 days

• *Child:* PO 5 mg/kg tid × 5 days

H. pylori infection

• *Adult:* PO 250 mg 4× daily in combination with 262 mg of bismuth subsalicylate and 500 mg of tetracycline (Helidac), with meals and hs × 14 days, combine with H₂ histamine antagonist

Available forms include: Tabs 250, 500 mg; ext rel tabs 750 mg; HCl inj IV 500 mg

Side effects/adverse reactions:

▼ *ORAL:* Dry mouth, furry tongue, bitter taste, metallic taste, glossitis, stomatitis

CNS: Headache, dizziness, **convulsions,** confusion, depression, fatigue, drowsiness, insomnia, paresthesia, peripheral neuropathy, incoordination, depression

CV: Flat T waves

GI: Nausea, vomiting, ***pseudomembranous colitis,*** diarrhea, epigastric distress, anorexia, constipation, abdominal cramps

HEMA: Leukopenia, bone marrow aplasia

GU: ***Albuminuria, nephrotoxicity,*** dysuria, cystitis, decreased libido, polyuria, incontinence, dyspareunia

EENT: Blurred vision, sore throat, retinal edema

INTEG: Rash, pruritus, urticaria, flushing

Contraindications: Hypersensitivity to this drug, renal disease, hepatic disease, contracted visual or color fields, blood dyscrasias, pregnancy (first trimester), lactation, CNS disorders

Precautions: *Candida* infections, pregnancy category B (second, third trimesters); avoid unnecessary use because shown to be carcinogenic in rodents

Pharmacokinetics:

IV/PO: Peak 1-2 hr, half-life 6.2-11.5 hr; crosses placenta; excreted in feces

🐝 **Drug interactions of concern to dentistry:**

• Antabuse-like reaction: alcohol, alcohol-containing products

• Decreased action: phenobarbital

• Possible increase in blood levels of tacrolimus

DENTAL CONSIDERATIONS

General:

• Patients on chronic drug therapy may rarely have symptoms of blood dyscrasias, which can include infection, bleeding, and poor healing.

• Assess salivary flow as a factor in caries, periodontal disease, and candidiasis.

• Determine why the patient is taking the drug.

Consultations:

• In a patient with symptoms of blood dyscrasias, request a medical consult for blood studies and postpone dental treatment until normal values are reestablished.

• Medical consult may be required to assess disease control.

Teach patient/family:

• To avoid alcoholic beverages

• That taste alterations may occur

• Importance of good oral hygiene to prevent soft tissue inflammation

• Caution to prevent injury when using oral hygiene aids

When chronic dry mouth occurs, advise patient:

• To avoid mouth rinses with high alcohol content due to drying effects

• To use sugarless gum, frequent sips of water, or saliva substitutes

• To use daily home fluoride products for anticaries effect

---

mexiletine HCl

(mex´i-le-teen)

Mexitil

Drug class.: Antidysrhythmic (class IB, lidocaine analog)

Action: Blocks fast sodium channel in His-Purkinje system, decreasing the effective refractory period and shortening the duration of the action potential

Uses: Documented life-threatening ventricular dysrhythmias

Dosage and routes:
• *Adult:* PO 200-400 mg q8h

Available forms include: Caps 150, 200, 250 mg

Side effects/adverse reactions:

▼ *ORAL:* Dry mouth, altered taste, stomatitis

CNS: **Convulsions,** headache, dizziness, confusion, tremors, psychosis, nervousness, paresthesia, weakness, fatigue, coordination difficulties, change in sleep habits

CV: **Heart block, cardiovascular collapse, arrest, left ventricular failure, cardiogenic shock,** hypotension, bradycardia, angina, PVCs, sinus node slowing, syncope

GI: **Hepatitis,** nausea, vomiting, anorexia, diarrhea, abdominal pain, peptic ulcer, GI bleeding

RESP: **Fibrosis, embolism,** dyspnea, pneumonia

HEMA: **Thrombocytopenia, leukopenia, agranulocytosis, hypoplastic anemia,** SLE syndrome

GU: Urinary hesitancy, decreased libido

EENT: Blurred vision, hearing loss, tinnitus

INTEG: Rash, alopecia, dry skin

MISC: Edema, arthralgia, fever

Contraindications: Hypersensitivity to amides, cardiogenic shock, blood dyscrasias, severe heart block

Precautions: Pregnancy category C, lactation, children, renal disease, liver disease, CHF, respiratory depression, myasthenia gravis

Pharmacokinetics:
PO: Peak 2-3 hr, half-life 12 hr; metabolized by liver; excreted unchanged by kidneys (10%); excreted in breast milk

🦷 **Drug interactions of concern to dentistry:**
• No specific interactions are reported with dental drugs; however, any drug that could affect the cardiac action of mexiletine should be used in the least effective dose, such as other local anesthetics, vasoconstrictors, and anticholinergics

DENTAL CONSIDERATIONS
General:
• Monitor vital signs every appointment due to cardiovascular side effects.
• Patients on chronic drug therapy may rarely have symptoms of blood dyscrasias, which can include infection, bleeding, and poor healing.
• Assess salivary flow as a factor in caries, periodontal disease, and candidiasis.
• Stress from dental procedures may compromise cardiovascular function; determine patient risk.

Consultations:
• In a patient with symptoms of blood dyscrasias, request a medical consult for blood studies and postpone dental treatment until normal values are reestablished.
• Medical consult should be made to assess disease control.
• Medical consult may be required to assess patient's ability to tolerate stress.

Teach patient/family:
• Importance of good oral hygiene to prevent soft tissue inflammation

• Caution to prevent injury when using oral hygiene aids
When chronic dry mouth occurs, advise patient:
• To avoid mouth rinses with high alcohol content due to drying effects
• To use sugarless gum, frequent sips of water, or saliva substitutes
• To use daily home fluoride products for anticaries effect

---

miconazole nitrate (topical)
(mi-kon′a-zole)
Femizol-M, Micatin, Miconazole-7, Monistat Cream, Monistat-Derm, Monistat-7, Monistat 3, M-Zole 3
Drug class.: Antifungal

Action: Interferes with fungal cell membrane, increasing permeability and leading to leaking of nutrients
Uses: Tinea pedis, tinea cruris, tinea corporis, tinea versicolor, vaginal or vulvae *Candida albicans*
Dosage and routes:
• *Adult and child:* TOP apply to affected area bid × 2-4 wk
• *Adult:* Intravag give 1 applicator or supp × 7 days hs; 3-day treatment—intravag insert 200 mg supp qd with topical cream bid
Available forms include: Cream, lotion, powder, spray 2%; vag cream 2%; vag supp 100, 200 mg
Side effects/adverse reactions:
GU: Vulvovaginal burning, itching, pelvic cramps
INTEG: Rash, urticaria, stinging, burning, contact dermatitis
Contraindications: Hypersensitivity

Precautions: Child <2 yr, pregnancy category B, lactation
DENTAL CONSIDERATIONS
General:
• Examine oral mucous membranes for signs of fungal infection.
• Broad-spectrum antibiotics may evoke vaginal yeast infections.
Teach patient/family:
• To prevent reinoculation of *Candida* infection, dispose of toothbrush or other contaminated oral hygiene devices used during period of infection

---

midazolam HCl
(mid′ay-zoe-lam)
Versed
Drug class.: Benzodiazepine general anesthetic, anesthesia adjunct

Controlled Substance Schedule IV
Action: Depresses subcortical levels in CNS; may act on limbic system, reticular formation; may potentiate γ-aminobutyric acid (GABA) by binding to specific benzodiazepine receptors
Uses: Conscious sedation, general anesthesia induction, sedation for diagnostic endoscopic procedures, intubation, preoperative sedation, amnesia
Dosage and routes:
Warning: Midazolam should be administered by persons trained in the administration of general anesthesia/IV conscious sedation. Patients must be continuously monitored and facilities for the maintenance of a patent airway, ventilatory support, oxygen sup-

---

bold italic = life-threatening conditions

plementation, and circulatory resuscitation must be immediately available.

ALL DOSES MUST BE INDIVIDUALIZED

Preoperative sedation, ASA I and ASA II <60 yr
• *Adult:* IM 0.07-0.08 mg/kg (usually 5 mg for average adult) 0.5-1 hr before general anesthesia
• *Child:* IM 0.08-0.2 mg/kg 0.5-1 hr before general anesthesia

Induction of general anesthesia
• *Adult <55 yr:* Unpremedicated patients—IV 0.2-0.35 mg/kg over 30 sec, wait 2 min, follow with 25% of initial dose if needed; premedicated patients—0.15-0.35 mg/kg over 20-30 sec, allow 2 min for effect
• *Adult >55 yr:* ASA I or II, unpremedicated—IV 0.15-0.3 mg/kg administered over 20-30 sec; for ASA III or ASA IV, 0.15-0.25 mg/kg over 20-30 sec

Conscious sedation (use 1 mg/ml formulation)
• *Adult <60 yr:* Unpremedicated—IV titrate dose slowly, wait at least 2 min for response, titrate in small increments; doses of more than 5 mg are seldom required; dose may be as low as 1 mg but should not exceed 2.5 mg/min in the average healthy adult; allow at least 2 min to evaluate response; use of the more dilute solution, 1 mg/ml, allows for slower injection control; solutions can be diluted with 0.9% normal saline or dextrose 5% in water; avoid bolus doses; total dose of 5 mg is usually not necessary; patients with narcotic premedication or other CNS depressants: reduce midazolam dose by 30%
• *Adult >60 yr, debilitated:* Unpre-

medicated—IV (titrate doses) 1 mg or less slowly, wait at least 2 min; total dose of 3.5 mg usually unnecessary; doses must be carefully adjusted for this patient group; patients with other CNS depressant medication: reduce dose by 50%

IV sedation in children
• *Child 6 mo-5 yr:* Caution—IV administer dose over 2-3 min and allow an additional 2-3 min before treatment or giving an additional dose; titrate with small incremental doses; reduce dose if other CNS depressants are used; initial dose 0.05-0.1 mg/kg; do not exceed 6 mg total
• *Child 6-12 yr:* Follow same cautions as for younger children—IV initial dose 0.025-0.05 mg/kg, total dose up to 0.4 mg/kg may be required; do not exceed 10 mg
• *Child 12-16 yr:* IV same as adult dose

Available forms include: Vials 1, 5 mg/ml in 1, 2, 5, 10 ml; 1 mg/ml in 2, 5, 10 ml; syr 2 mg/ml in 118 ml

Side effects/adverse reactions:

▼ *ORAL:* Increased salivation (because drugs with anticholinergic action are often used in general anesthesia techniques, salivation is usually not observed), acidic taste

CNS: Retrograde amnesia, headache, oversedation, euphoria, confusion, anxiety, insomnia, slurred speech, paresthesia, weakness, chills, agitation

*CV: **Hypotension, cardiac arrest,*** PVCs, tachycardia, bigeminy, nodal rhythm

GI: Nausea, vomiting, hiccups, increased salivation

*RESP: **Apnea, bronchospasm, respiratory depression, laryngospasm,*** coughing, dyspnea

EENT: Blurred vision, nystagmus,

italic = common side effects

diplopia, blocked ears, loss of balance

INTEG: Pain, urticaria, swelling at injection site, rash, pruritus, phlebitis

MS: Involuntary movement, tremor

Contraindications: Hypersensitivity to benzodiazepines, shock, coma, alcohol intoxication, acute narrow-angle glaucoma, ritonavir, nelfinavir, indinavir

Precautions: COPD, CHF, chronic renal failure, chills, elderly, debilitated, pregnancy category D, children <18 yr; to be used only by health care professionals skilled in airway maintenance and ventilation and resuscitation techniques

Pharmacokinetics:

IM: Onset 15 min, peak 0.5-1 hr

IV: Onset 3-5 min, onset of anesthesia 1.5-2.5 min, half-life 1.2-12.3 hr; protein binding 97%; metabolized in liver; metabolites excreted in urine; crosses placenta, blood-brain barrier

☞ Drug interactions of concern to dentistry:

• Prolonged respiratory depression: all CNS depressants, including alcohol, barbiturates, narcotics. All doses of midazolam must be reduced when used in combination with any CNS depressant. Serious respiratory and cardiovascular depression, including death, has occurred when midazolam is used in combination with other CNS depressants or given too rapidly. Medically compromised and elderly patients are at greater risk.

• Increased serum levels and prolonged effect of benzodiazepines: erythromycin, ketoconazole, itraconazole, fluconazole, miconazole (systemic), diltiazem

• Contraindicated with nelfinavir, ritonavir, indinavir

DENTAL CONSIDERATIONS

General:

• Monitor vital signs every 5 min during general anesthesia due to cardiovascular and respiratory side effects. Monitor vital signs at regular intervals during recovery.

• Degree of CNS depression is dose dependent; titrate all doses.

• Drug produces amnesia, especially in the elderly patient.

• A longer recovery period could be observed in an obese patient because half-life may be extended.

• Assist patient with ambulation until drowsy period has passed.

Teach patient/family:

• Drug may impair reaction time; avoid driving or potentially hazardous activities until drowsiness or weakness subsides

• That amnesia occurs; events may not be remembered

Treatment of overdose:

• O_2, vasopressors, flumazenil, resuscitation measures as required

---

miglitol

(mig'li-tol)

Glyset

Drug class.: Oligosaccharide, glucosidase enzyme inhibitor

Action: Inhibits α-glucosidase enzyme in GI tract to slow breakdown of carbohydrates to glucose, which results in reduced plasma glucose levels

Uses: Type 2 diabetes when diet control is ineffective in controlling blood glucose levels, used as single agent or in combination with other oral hypoglycemics

---

Dosage and routes:
• *Adult:* PO individualize doses; initial dose 25 mg tid with first bite of each meal; max recommended dose 100 mg tid; increase initial dose based on side effects and postprandial plasma glucose; usual maintenance dose 50 mg tid
Available forms include: Tabs 25, 50, 100 mg
Side effects/adverse reactions:
GI: Diarrhea, flatulence, abdominal pain, soft stools
INTEG: Rash
MISC: Low serum iron
Contraindications: Hypersensitivity, diabetic ketoacidosis, inflammatory bowel disease, colonic ulceration, partial intestinal obstruction, chronic intestinal diseases associated with disorders of absorption and digestion
Precautions: Renal impairment, hypoglycemia, pregnancy category B, lactation, children
Pharmacokinetics:
PO: Peak plasma levels 2-3 hr; negligible plasma protein binding, not metabolized, urinary excretion
⚡ Drug interactions of concern to dentistry:
• None reported with dental drugs; information is lacking at this time
DENTAL CONSIDERATIONS
General:
• Ensure that patient is following prescribed diet and regularly takes medication.
• Type 2 patients may also be using insulin. Should symptomatic hypoglycemia occur while taking this drug, use dextrose rather than sucrose because of interference with sucrose metabolism.
• Place on frequent recall to evaluate healing response.
• Short appointments and a stress reduction protocol may be required for anxious patients.
• Diabetics may be more susceptible to infection and have delayed wound healing.
• Consider semisupine chair position for patient comfort if GI side effects occur.
• Question patient about self-monitoring of drug's antidiabetic effect, including blood glucose values or finger-stick records.
• Examine for oral manifestation of opportunistic infection.
Consultations:
• Medical consult may be required to assess disease control and patient's ability to tolerate stress.
• Medical consult may include data from patient's blood glucose monitoring, including glycosylated hemoglobin or HbA_{1c} testing.
Teach patient/family:
• Importance of updating health and drug history if physician makes any changes in evaluation or drug regimens
• Importance of good oral hygiene to prevent soft tissue inflammation

---

minocycline HCl
(mi-noe-sye'kleen)
Dyancin, Minocin, Vectrin
Drug class.: Tetracycline antiinfective

Action: Inhibits protein synthesis, phosphorylation in microorganisms by binding to 30S ribosomal subunits, reversibly binding to 50S ribosomal subunits; bacteriostatic
Uses: Syphilis, *C. trachomatis* infection, gonorrhea, lymphogranuloma venereum, rickettsial infections, inflammatory acne, *M.*

italic = common side effects

marinum, Neisseria meningitis carriers, actinomycosis, anthrax, ANUG, AA-induced periodontitis, and other susceptible infections; dental product is an adjunct to scaling and root planing in adult periodontitis

Dosage and routes:
• *Adult:* PO/IV 200 mg first day, then 100 mg q12h or 50 mg q6h, not to exceed 400 mg/24 hr IV
• *Child >8 yr, <45 kg:* PO/IV 4.4 mg/kg first day, then 2.2 mg/kg/day PO in divided doses q12h
Available forms include: Caps 50, 100 mg; caps pellet filled 50, 100 mg; oral susp 25 mg/5 ml in 60 ml; powder for inj IV 100, 200 mg/vial

Side effects/adverse reactions:
▼ *ORAL:* Candidiasis, tooth staining, discolored mucous membranes, discolored tongue, lichenoid reaction
CNS: Dizziness, fever, light-headedness, vertigo
CV: Pericarditis
GI: Nausea, abdominal pain, vomiting, diarrhea, hepatotoxicity, anorexia, enterocolitis, flatulence, abdominal cramps, epigastric burning
HEMA: Eosinophilia, neutropenia, thrombocytopenia, hemolytic anemia
GU: Increased BUN, renal failure, nephrotoxicity, polyuria, polydipsia
EENT: Dysphagia
INTEG: Rash, urticaria, photosensitivity, increased pigmentation, exfoliative dermatitis, pruritus, angioedema, bluish-gray color of skin
Contraindications: Hypersensitivity to tetracyclines, children <8 yr, pregnancy category D
Precautions: Hepatic disease, lactation

Pharmacokinetics:
PO: Peak 2-3 hr, half-life 11-17 hr; 55%-88% protein bound; excreted in urine, feces, breast milk; crosses placenta

🦷 **Drug interactions of concern to dentistry:**
• Decreased effect: antacids, milk, or other calcium- and aluminum-containing products
• Decreased effect of penicillins
• Oral contraceptives: advise patient of a potential risk for decreased contraceptive action, to maintain compliance with oral contraceptive use while using antibiotics, and to consider the use of additional nonhormonal contraception

DENTAL CONSIDERATIONS
General:
• This drug is reported to cause intrinsic staining in erupted permanent teeth not associated with the calcification stage.
• The drug readily distributes to gingival crevicular fluid.
• Do not prescribe drug during pregnancy or <8 yr due to tooth discoloration.
• Caution patients about driving or performing other tasks requiring alertness.
• Advise patient if dental drugs prescribed have a potential for photosensitivity.
• Do not use ingestible sodium bicarbonate products such as the air polishing system (Prophy Jet) at the same time dose is taken; take minocycline 2 hr later.
• Determine why the patient is taking the drug.
Consultations:
• Medical consult may be required to assess disease control.

M

---

bold italic = life-threatening conditions

Teach patient/family:
• Importance of good oral hygiene to prevent soft tissue inflammation
• Caution to prevent injury when using oral hygiene aids
• To avoid mouth rinses with high alcohol content due to drying effects

When used for dental infection, advise patient:
• To report sore throat, oral burning sensation, fever, fatigue, any of which could indicate superinfection
• To take at prescribed intervals and complete dosage regimen
• To immediately notify the dentist if signs or symptoms of infection increase

---

minocycline HCl (microspheres)
(mi-noe-sye′kleen)
Arestin

Drug class.: Tetracycline antiinfective

Action: Inhibits protein synthesis, phosphorylation in microorganisms by binding to 30S ribosomal subunits, bacteriostatic

Uses: Adjunctive therapy to scaling and root planning procedures for reduction of pocket depth in adult periodontitis; also used as part of a periodontal maintenance program, which includes good oral hygiene, scaling, and root planing

Dosage and routes:
• *Adult:* Connect cartridge to handle, remove tip and insert to base of periodontal pocket, express the powder while gradually withdrawing tip from pocket base

Available forms include: Box of 2 trays, each containing 12 cartridges (1 mg minocycline)

Side effects/adverse reactions:
▼ *ORAL: Dental pain,* stomatitis, ulceration
CNS: Headache
GI: Dyspepsia
RESP: Pharyngitis
MISC: Flulike syndrome, infection

Contraindications: Hypersensitivity

Precautions: Use in acute periodontal abscess has not been studied, has not been tested in immunocompromised patients, pregnant women or patient with implants, overgrowth of opportunistic organisms, predisposition to candidiasis, pregnancy category D, lactation, efficacy in children unknown

Pharmacokinetics: With exposure to crevicular fluid, minocycline is released from channels in the microspheres, therapeutic levels are said to last for 14 days, data not available on systemic absorption

⚗ Drug interactions of concern to dentistry:
• No dental drug interactions reported with this product

DENTAL CONSIDERATIONS
General:
• Follow all general precautions when using tetracyclines.

Teach patient/family:
• Avoid eating hard, crunchy foods for 1 week
• Postpone toothbrushing for 12 hours
• Postpone use of interproximal cleaning devices for 10 days
• Notify dentist immediately if pain, swelling or other unexpected symptoms occur

---

minoxidil

(mi-nox'i-dil)
Systemic: Loniten
Topical: Rogaine, Rogaine Extra Strength for Men, Rogaine for Men, Rogaine for Women
♣ Apo-gain, Gen-Minoxidil, Minoxigaine

Drug class.: Antihypertensive

Action: Directly relaxes arteriolar smooth muscle, reducing peripheral resistance

Uses: Severe hypertension not responsive to other therapy (used with a diuretic); topically to treat alopecia (mechanism unknown)

Dosage and routes:
• *Adult:* PO 5 mg/day, not to exceed 100 mg daily; usual range 10-40 mg/day in single doses
• *Child <12 yr:* Initial 0.2 mg/kg/day; effective range 0.25-1 mg/kg/day; max 50 mg/day

Alopecia
• *Adult:* Apply topically; rub 1 ml into scalp bid

Available forms include: Tabs 2.5, 10 mg; top 2%, 5%

Side effects/adverse reactions:
CNS: Drowsiness, dizziness, sedation, headache, depression, fatigue
CV: Severe rebound hypertension on withdrawal, CHF, pulmonary edema, pericardial effusion, tachycardia, angina, increased T wave, edema, sodium/water retention
GI: Nausea, vomiting
HEMA: Hct, Hgb, erythrocyte count may decrease initially
GU: Gynecomastia, breast tenderness
INTEG: Stevens-Johnson syndrome, pruritus, rash, hirsutism

Contraindications: Acute MI, dissecting aortic aneurysm, hypersensitivity, pheochromocytoma

Precautions: Pregnancy category C, lactation, children, renal disease, CAD, CHF

Pharmacokinetics:
PO: Onset 30 min, peak 2-3 hr, duration 75 hr, half-life 4.2 hr; metabolized in liver; metabolites excreted in urine, feces

⚡ Drug interactions of concern to dentistry:
• Decreased effects: NSAIDs, indomethacin, sympathomimetics
• Increased hypotension: CNS depressant drug used in conscious sedation technique may also lower blood pressure

DENTAL CONSIDERATIONS
General:
• Monitor vital signs every appointment due to cardiovascular side effects.
• Patients on chronic drug therapy may rarely have symptoms of blood dyscrasias, which can include infection, bleeding, and poor healing.
• Limit use of sodium-containing products, such as saline IV fluids, for patients with a dietary salt restriction.
• Short appointments and a stress reduction protocol may be required for anxious patients.
• After supine positioning, have patient sit upright for at least 2 min before standing to avoid orthostatic hypotension.

Consultations:
• In a patient with symptoms of blood dyscrasias, request a medical consult for blood studies and postpone dental treatment until normal values are reestablished.

M

---

bold italic = life-threatening conditions

• Medical consult may be required to assess disease control and stress tolerance.

---

mirtazapine

(mir-taz'a-peen)
Remeron, Remeron SolTab

Drug class.: Tetracyclic antidepressant

Action: Mechanism of antidepressant effect is unknown; acts in CNS as an antagonist for presynaptic α_2-adrenergic inhibitory receptors, antagonizes serotonin 5-HT$_2$ and 5-HT$_3$ receptors and histamine H$_1$ receptors

Uses: Depression

Dosage and routes:

• *Adult:* PO initial dose 15 mg qd in PM, effective dose range 15-45 mg/day, allow 1-2 wk between dose changes to evaluate response

Available forms include: Tabs 15, 30, 45 mg; tabs oral disintegrating 15, 30, 45 mg

Side effects/adverse reactions:

▼ *ORAL: Dry mouth (25%), thirst,* glossitis, gingival hemorrhage, stomatitis (rare), tongue discoloration, ulcerative stomatitis, salivary gland enlargement, increased salivation, aphthous stomatitis, candidiasis, tongue edema

CNS: Somnolence, dizziness, abnormal dreams, malaise, mania, hypomania, confusion, tremor, migraine

CV: Peripheral edema, hypertension, vasodilation, MI, angina pectoris, bradycardia, syncope, hypotension

GI: Nausea, constipation, vomiting, abdominal pain, anorexia, increased ALT

RESP: Cough, flulike syndrome, dyspnea

*HEMA: **Agranulocytosis, leukopenia, thrombocytopenia,*** lymphadenopathy, lymphocytosis, pancytopenia, petechia, anemia (all rare)

GU: Urinary frequency

EENT: Sinusitis, eye pain

INTEG: Rash, pruritus, dry skin, herpes simplex, herpes zoster, photosensitivity

MS: Asthenia, arthralgia, back pain, myalgia, neck pain, neck rigidity

MISC: Increased appetite, weight gain, increased cholesterol/triglycerides

Contraindications: Hypersensitivity, MAO inhibitors

Precautions: Hepatic impairment, renal impairment, elderly, pregnancy category C, nursing, pediatric, suicidal ideation, cardiovascular or cerebrovascular disease aggravated by hypotension, avoid alcohol use

Pharmacokinetics:

PO: Rapid absorption, half-life 20-40 hr; peak levels 2 hr, liver metabolism, bioavailability 50%, urinary excretion, 85% plasma protein binding

🥄 **Drug interactions of concern to dentistry:**

• Impairment of cognitive and motor performance with diazepam or other drugs used in conscious sedation

• Use opioid analgesics with caution due to impairment of cognitive or motor performance; NSAIDs may be a more appropriate choice

DENTAL CONSIDERATIONS

General:

• Patients on chronic drug therapy may rarely have symptoms of

---

blood dyscrasias, which can include infection, bleeding, and poor healing.

• Assess salivary flow as a factor in caries, periodontal disease, and candidiasis.

• Monitor vital signs every appointment due to cardiovascular side effects.

• Consider semisupine chair position when GI or MS side effects occur.

• Place on frequent recall if oral side effects are a problem.

Consultations:

• In a patient with symptoms of blood dyscrasias, request a medical consult for blood studies and postpone dental treatment until normal values are reestablished.

• Take precaution if dental surgery is anticipated and sedation or general anesthesia is required; there is risk of hypotensive episode.

• Medical consult may be required to assess disease control.

• Physician should be informed if significant xerostomic side effects occur (increased caries, sore tongue, problems eating or swallowing, difficulty wearing prosthesis) so a medication change can be considered.

Teach patient/family:

• Importance of good oral hygiene to prevent soft tissue inflammation

• Caution to prevent soft tissue trauma when using oral hygiene aids

• Importance of updating health history/drug record if physician makes any changes in evaluation or drug regimens

• Caution about driving or performing other tasks requiring alertness

When chronic dry mouth occurs, advise patient:

• To avoid mouth rinses with high alcohol content due to drying effects

• To use daily home fluoride products for anticaries effect

• To use sugarless gum, frequent sips of water, or saliva substitutes

---

misoprostol

(mye-soe-prost′ole)

Cytotec

Drug class.: Gastric mucosa protectant

Action: A prostaglandin E_1 analog that inhibits gastric acid secretion, may protect gastric mucosa; can increase bicarbonate, mucus production

Uses: Prevention of nonsteroidal, antiinflammatory, drug-induced gastric ulcers; unapproved: duodenal ulcers

Dosage and routes:

• *Adult:* PO 200 µg qid with food for duration of NSAID therapy; if 200 µg is not tolerated, 100 µg may be given

Available forms include: Tabs 100, 200 µg

Side effects/adverse reactions:

GI: Diarrhea, nausea, vomiting, flatulence, constipation, dyspepsia, abdominal pain

GU: Spotting, cramps, hypermenorrhea, menstrual disorders

Contraindications: Hypersensitivity, pregnancy category X

Precautions: Lactation, children, elderly, renal disease

Pharmacokinetics:

PO: Peak 12 min; plasma steady state achieved within 2 days; excreted in urine

DENTAL CONSIDERATIONS

General:

• Avoid NSAIDs and salicylates in patients with upper active GI disease; acetaminophen/opioids are more appropriate for pain control in these patients.

Consultations:

• Medical consult may be required to assess disease control.

---

mitotane

(mye′toe-tane)

Lysodren

Drug class.: Antineoplastic

Action: Acts on adrenal cortex to suppress activity and adrenal steroid production

Uses: Adrenocortical carcinoma; unapproved: Cushing's syndrome

Dosage and routes:

• *Adult:* PO 2-6 g/day in divided doses tid or qid; can increase to 10 g; may need to decrease dose if severe reactions occur

Available forms include: Tabs 500 mg

Side effects/adverse reactions:

CNS: Lethargy, somnolence, vertigo, dizziness, light-headedness, flushing, sedation

GI: Nausea, vomiting, anorexia, diarrhea

*GU: **Proteinuria, hematuria***

EENT: Blurring, retinopathy, double vision

INTEG: Rash

*ENDO: **Adrenal cortical insufficiency***

MS: Muscle ache

Contraindications: Hypersensitivity

Precautions: Lactation, hepatic disease, pregnancy category C, infection

Pharmacokinetics: Adequately absorbed orally (40%), half-life 18-159 days; hepatic metabolism; excreted in urine, bile

⚗ Drug interactions of concern to dentistry:

• Increased CNS depression: all CNS depressants

• Decreased effects of corticosteroids; if glucocorticoid replacement is needed, use hydrocortisone

DENTAL CONSIDERATIONS

General:

• Evaluate respiration characteristics and rate.

• Drug may cause adrenal hypofunction, especially under conditions of stress such as surgery, trauma, or acute illness. Patients should be carefully monitored and given hydrocortisone or mineralocorticoid as needed.

• Consider semisupine chair position for patient comfort if GI side effects occur.

• Patients taking opioids for acute or chronic pain should be given alternative analgesics for dental pain.

Consultations:

• Medical consult may be required to assess disease control and patient's ability to tolerate stress.

Teach patient/family:

• That secondary oral infection may occur; must see dentist immediately if infection occurs

---

- To report oral lesions, soreness, or bleeding to dentist
- Importance of updating medical/drug record if physician makes any changes in evaluation or drug regimen

---

modafinil
(mo-daf'i-nil)
Provigil
Drug class.: CNS stimulant (orphan drug status)

Action: Mechanism of action remains uncertain; has wake-promoting actions similar to amphetamine and other sympathomimetics; may have CNS α_1-receptor agonist activity; enhancement of dopamine has also been observed in animals
Uses: Improve wakefulness in narcolepsy
Dosage and routes:
- *Adult:* PO 200 mg qd, 400 mg/day doses have been used
Available forms include: Tabs 100, 200 mg
Side effects/adverse reactions:
▼ *ORAL:* Orofacial dyskinesia, dry mouth
CNS: Headache, nervousness, anxiety, insomnia, depression, cataplexy, confusion, amnesia
CV: Hypertension, hypotension
GI: Nausea, diarrhea, anorexia
RESP: Rhinitis, pharyngitis
EENT: Blurred vision
INTEG: Dry skin
META: Abnormal liver function
Contraindications: Hypersensitivity
Precautions: Ischemic heart disease, left ventricular hypertrophy, mitral valve prolapse, recent MI, unstable angina, renal impairment, hepatic impairment, pregnancy category C, lactation, children <16 yr, drug abuse
Pharmacokinetics:
PO: Absorption delayed by food, peak plasma levels 2-4 hr, plasma protein binding (60%), hepatic metabolism, excreted mostly in urine (81%), produces hepatic cytochrome P-450 enzymes (CYP3A4)
🦷 **Drug interactions of concern to dentistry:**
- No documented dental drug interactions reported; however, because it induces cytochrome P-450 enzymes, other P-450 enzyme inducers or inhibitors (antifungal agents, erythromycin) could result in a drug interaction
DENTAL CONSIDERATIONS
General:
- Monitor vital signs every appointment due to cardiovascular side effects.
- Assess salivary flow as a factor in caries, periodontal disease, and candidiasis.
- Consider semisupine chair position for patient comfort due to GI side effects of drug.
- Short appointments and a stress reduction protocol may be required for anxious patients.
Teach patient/family:
- To prevent trauma when using oral hygiene aids
When chronic dry mouth occurs, advise patient:
- To avoid mouth rinses with high alcohol content due to drying effects
- To use daily home fluoride products for anticaries effect
- To use sugarless gum, frequent sips of water, or saliva substitutes

---

moexipril hydrochloride

(moe'x-i-pril)

Univasc

Drug class.: Angiotensin-converting enzyme (ACE) inhibitor

Action: Selectively suppresses renin-angiotensin-aldosterone system; inhibits ACE; prevents conversion of angiotensin I to angiotensin II; results in dilation of arterial, venous vessels; decreased aldosterone secretion results in diuresis and natriuresis

Uses: Hypertension as a single drug or in combination with a thiazide diuretic

Dosage and routes:

As single drug (not taking diuretic)

• *Adult:* PO 7.5 mg 1 hr ac daily; range 7.5-39 mg/day in 1 or 2 divided doses 1 hr ac

With diuretic

• *Adult:* PO as single drug, but discontinue diuretic 2-3 days to avoid symptomatic hypotension; then restart diuretic carefully, if required; otherwise start with 3.75 mg under medical supervision

Renal impairment

• *Adult:* Dose limited to 15 mg/day

Available forms include: Tabs 7.5, 15 mg

Side effects/adverse reactions:

▼ *ORAL: Angioedema,* dry mouth (<1%)

CNS: Dizziness, fatigue

CV: Symptomatic hypotension, postural hypotension, hyperkalemia, peripheral edema, chest pain, palpitation

GI: Diarrhea, hepatic failure

RESP: Cough, pharyngitis

HEMA: Neutropenia, agranulocytosis

GU: Acute renal failure, oliguria, azotemia, urinary frequency

EENT: Tinnitus

INTEG: Flushing, rash, photosensitivity

MS: Myalgia

MISC: Anaphylactic reactions

Contraindications: Hypersensitivity, pregnancy (second or third trimester), angioedema history with other ACE inhibitors

Precautions: Food retards absorption, renal or hepatic impairment, CHF, SLE, scleroderma, renal artery stenosis, lactation, children, pregnancy categories C (first trimester) and D (second and third trimesters)

Pharmacokinetics:

PO: Peak plasma levels 1.5 hr; converted to active metabolite (moexiprilat); 50% plasma protein bound; excreted in urine, feces

🦷 **Drug interactions of concern to dentistry:**

• IV fluids containing potassium: risk of hyperkalemia

• Increased hypotension: other hypotensive drugs, alcohol, phenothiazines

• Decreased hypotensive effects: indomethacin, possibly other NSAIDs, sympathomimetics

DENTAL CONSIDERATIONS

General:

• Monitor vital signs every appointment due to cardiovascular side effects.

• After supine positioning, have patient sit upright for at least 2 min before standing to avoid orthostatic hypotension.

• Take precautions if dental surgery is anticipated and general anesthesia is required.

• Patients on chronic drug therapy may rarely have symptoms of blood dyscrasias, which can include infection, bleeding, and poor healing.
• Stress from dental procedures may compromise cardiovascular function; determine patient risk.
• Assess salivary flow as a factor in caries, periodontal disease, and candidiasis.
• Short appointments and a stress reduction protocol may be required for anxious patients.

Consultations:
• Medical consult may be required to assess disease control and patient's ability to tolerate stress.
• In a patient with symptoms of blood dyscrasias, request a medical consult for blood studies and postpone dental treatment until normal values are reestablished.

Teach patient/family:
• Importance of good oral hygiene to prevent soft tissue inflammation
• Caution to prevent trauma when using oral hygiene aids
• To report oral lesions, soreness, or bleeding to dentist

When chronic dry mouth occurs, advise patient:
• To avoid mouth rinses with high alcohol content due to drying effects
• Of need for daily home fluoride to prevent caries
• To use sugarless gum, frequent sips of water, or saliva substitutes

---

molindone HCl
(moe-lin′done)
Moban, Moban Concentrate
Drug class.: Antipsychotic

Action: Depresses cerebral cor-tex, hypothalamus, limbic system, which control activity, aggression; blocks neurotransmission produced by dopamine at synapse; exhibits strong α-adrenergic, anticholinergic blocking action; mechanism for antipsychotic effects is unclear

Uses: Psychotic disorders

Dosage and routes:
• *Adult:* PO 50-75 mg/day, increasing to 225 mg/day if needed

Available forms include: Tabs 5, 10, 25, 50, 100 mg; conc 20 mg/ml

Side effects/adverse reactions:
▼ *ORAL: Dry mouth*
CNS: Extrapyramidal symptoms: pseudoparkinsonism, akathisia, dystonia, tardive dyskinesia, drowsiness, headache, seizures
*CV: Orthostatic hypotension, **cardiac arrest, tachycardia,** ECG changes, hypertension*
GI: Nausea, vomiting, anorexia, constipation, diarrhea, jaundice, weight gain
*RESP: **Laryngospasm, respiratory depression,** dyspnea*
*HEMA: **Anemia, leukopenia, leukocytosis, agranulocytosis***
GU: Urinary retention, urinary frequency, enuresis, impotence, amenorrhea, gynecomastia, menstrual irregularities
EENT: Blurred vision, glaucoma
INTEG: Rash, photosensitivity, dermatitis

Contraindications: Hypersensitivity, coma, child

Precautions: Pregnancy category C, lactation, hypertension, hepatic disease, cardiac disease, Parkinson's disease, brain tumor, glaucoma, urinary retention, diabetes mellitus, respiratory disease, prostatic hypertrophy

---

Pharmacokinetics:

PO: Onset erratic, peak 1.5 hr, duration 24-36 hr, half-life 1.5 hr; metabolized by liver; excreted in urine, feces; may cross placenta; excreted in breast milk

🦷 **Drug interactions of concern to dentistry:**

• Increased sedation: alcohol, other CNS depressants

• Increased anticholinergic effect: anticholinergics, antihistamines

DENTAL CONSIDERATIONS

General:

• Patients on chronic drug therapy may rarely have symptoms of blood dyscrasias, which can include infection, bleeding, and poor healing.

• Assess salivary flow as a factor in caries, periodontal disease, and candidiasis.

• After supine positioning, have patient sit upright for at least 2 min before standing to avoid orthostatic hypotension.

• Assess for presence of extrapyramidal motor symptoms, such as tardive dyskinesia and akathisia. Extrapyramidal motor activity may complicate dental treatment.

• Geriatric patients are more susceptible to drug effects; use lower dose.

• Use vasoconstrictors with caution, in low doses, and with careful aspiration.

Consultations:

• In a patient with symptoms of blood dyscrasias, request a medical consult for blood studies and postpone dental treatment until normal values are reestablished.

• Medical consult may be required to assess disease control.

Teach patient/family:

• Importance of good oral hygiene to prevent soft tissue inflammation

• Caution to prevent injury when using oral hygiene aids

When chronic dry mouth occurs, advise patient:

• To avoid mouth rinses with high alcohol content due to drying effects

• To use sugarless gum, frequent sips of water, or saliva substitutes

• To use daily home fluoride products for anticaries effect

---

mometasone furoate monohydrate

(moe-met′a-sone)

Nasonex

Drug class.: Synthetic corticosteroid

Action: Glucocorticoids have multiple actions that include antiinflammatory and immunosuppressant effects. They inhibit phospholipase A_2 interfering with or reducing the synthesis of prostaglandins and leukotrienes. They also bind to cytoplasmic glucocorticoid receptors (GRs) and enter the cell nucleus to bind with DNA. This results in the synthesis of various enzymes such as collagenase, elastase, and cytokines that play important roles in inflammation and immunosuppression. They also suppress the production of lymphocytes, monocytes, and eosinophils.

Uses: Prophylaxis and treatment of seasonal allergic rhinitis; treatment of symptoms of perennial allergic rhinitis

Dosage and routes:
• *Adult and child >12 yr:* INH (nasal) 2 sprays in each nostril daily

Available forms include: Nasal spray 50 µg each actuation (120 sprays in bottle)

Side effects/adverse reactions:
CNS: Headache
RESP: Pharyngitis, coughing, URI
GU: Dysmenorrhea
EENT: Epistaxis, sinusitis
MS: Pain
MISC: Viral infection

Contraindications: Hypersensitivity

Precautions: Caution in transferring patient from systemic to inhalation steroids; active or quiescent tuberculosis, untreated fungal, bacterial or viral infections, pregnancy category C, lactation, safety and efficacy in child <12 yr not established

Pharmacokinetics:
INH: Virtually undetectable in plasma; if absorbed see extensive metabolism, any metabolites excreted in bile

🦷 Drug interactions of concern to dentistry:
• None reported

DENTAL CONSIDERATIONS
General:
• Allergic rhinitis may be a factor in mouth breathing and drying of oral tissues.
• Examine for oral manifestation of opportunistic infection.

Teach patient/family:
• Importance of gargling, rinsing mouth with water, and expectorating after each aerosol dose.

montelukast sodium
(mon-te-loo′kast)
Singulair
Drug class.: Selective leukotriene receptor antagonist

Action: Competitive and selective antagonist for cysteinyl leukotriene receptor ($CysLT_1$)

Uses: Prophylaxis and chronic treatment of asthma

Dosage and routes:
• *Adult and child >15 yr:* PO 10 mg hs
• *Child 6-14 yr:* PO 5 mg chewable tabs hs
• *Child 2-5 yr:* PO 4 mg chewable tabs hs

Available forms include: Chew tabs 4, 5, 10 mg

Side effects/adverse reactions:
▼ *ORAL: Unspecified dental pain*
CNS: Dizziness, headache
GI: Abdominal pain, dyspepsia, gastroenteritis
RESP: Cough, influenza
EENT: Nasal congestion
META: Increased ALT and AST
MS: Asthenia
MISC: Fatigue

Contraindications: Hypersensitivity

Precautions: Not for acute asthma attacks, not for treatment of exercise-induced bronchospasm or ASA-induced bronchospasm, chewable tablets contain aspartame, pregnancy category B, lactation

Pharmacokinetics:
PO: Rapidly absorbed, peak levels 3-4 hr, bioavailability 73%-64%, highly plasma protein bound (99%), extensive hepatic metabolism, excretion in bile

M

🐾 Drug interactions of concern to dentistry:
• None reported

DENTAL CONSIDERATIONS
General:
• Midday appointments and a stress reduction protocol may be required for anxious patients.
• Avoid prescribing aspirin-containing products.
• Acute asthmatic episodes may be precipitated in the dental office. Rapid-acting sympathomimetic inhalants should be available for emergency use. A stress reduction protocol may be required.
• Be aware that aspirin or sulfite preservatives in vasoconstrictor-containing products can exacerbate asthma.
• Consider semisupine chair position for patients with respiratory disease and when GI side effects are a problem.

Consultations:
• Medical consult may be required to assess disease control.

Teach patient/family:
• Importance of updating health and drug history if physician makes any changes in evaluation or drug regimens

---

moricizine

(mor-i′siz-een)
Ethmozine

Drug class.: Antidysrhythmic, type I

Action: Decreased rate of rise of action potential, which prolongs the refractory period and shortens the action potential duration; depression of inward influx if sodium mediates the effects; drug may slow atrial and AV nodal conduction

Uses: Documented life-threatening dysrhythmias

Dosage and routes:
• *Adult:* PO 600-900 mg/day in 3 divided doses; dose must be individualized

Available forms include: Film-coated tabs 200, 250, 300 mg

Side effects/adverse reactions:
▼ *ORAL:* Dry mouth, altered taste, stomatitis, swelling of lips and tongue
CNS: Dizziness, headache, fatigue, perioral numbness, euphoria, nervousness, sleep disorders, depression, tinnitus, fatigue
CV: **MI,** palpitation, chest pain, CHF, hypertension, syncope, dysrhythmias, bradycardia, thrombophlebitis
GI: Nausea, abdominal pain, vomiting, diarrhea
RESP: **Apnea,** dyspnea, hyperventilation, asthma, pharyngitis, cough
GU: Sexual dysfunction, difficult urination, dysuria, incontinence
MISC: Sweating, musculoskeletal pain

Contraindications: Second- and third-degree heart block, right bundle branch block, cardiogenic shock, hypersensitivity

Precautions: CHF, hypokalemia, hyperkalemia, sick sinus syndrome, pregnancy category B, lactation, children, impaired hepatic and renal function, cardiac dysfunction

Pharmacokinetics: Peak 0.5-2.2 hr, half-life 1.5-3.5 hr; protein binding >90%; metabolized by the liver; metabolites excreted in feces, urine

---

🦷 **Drug interactions of concern to dentistry:**
• No specific interactions are reported with dental drugs; however, any drug that could affect the cardiac action of moricizine (e.g., other local anesthetics, vasoconstrictors, anticholinergics) should be used in the least effective dose

DENTAL CONSIDERATIONS
General:
• Monitor vital signs every appointment due to cardiovascular side effects.
• Assess salivary flow as a factor in caries, periodontal disease, and candidiasis.
• Stress from dental procedures may compromise cardiovascular function; determine patient risk.

Consultations:
• Medical consult should be made to assess disease control and patient's ability to tolerate stress.

Teach patient/family:
• Importance of good oral hygiene to prevent soft tissue inflammation
• Caution to prevent injury when using oral hygiene aids
When chronic dry mouth occurs, advise patient:
• To avoid mouth rinses with high alcohol content due to drying effects
• To use sugarless gum, frequent sips of water, or saliva substitutes
• To use daily home fluoride products for anticaries effect

morphine sulfate
(mor′feen)
Astramorph PF, Duramorph PF, Infumorph 200, Kadian, MS Contin, MSIR, Oramorph SR, RMS, Roxanol, Roxanol 100, Roxanol SR, Roxanol T
🍁 MOS
Drug class.: Narcotic analgesic

Controlled Substance
Schedule II, Canada N
Action: Depresses pain impulse transmission at the CNS by interacting with opioid receptors
Uses: Severe pain
Dosage and routes:
• *Adult:* SC/IM 4-15 mg q4h prn; PO 10-30 mg q4h prn; ext rel q12-24h; rec 10-20 mg q4h prn; IV 4-10 mg diluted in 4-5 ml of water for injection, over 5 min
• *Child:* SC 0.1-0.2 mg/kg, not to exceed 15 mg
Available forms include: Inj SC/IM/IV 0.5, 1, 2, 4, 5, 8, 10, 15, 25, 50 mg/ml; tabs 15, 30 mg; con rel tabs 15, 30, 60, 100, 200 mg; ext rel tabs 15, 30, 60, 100 mg; soluble tabs 10, 15, 30 mg; caps 15, 30 mg; sus rel caps 20, 30, 50, 60, 100 mg; oral sol 10, 20 mg/5 ml, 20 mg/ml, 100 mg/5 ml; rec supp 5, 10, 20, 30 mg
Side effects/adverse reactions:
▼ *ORAL:* Dry mouth
CNS: Drowsiness, dizziness, confusion, headache, sedation, euphoria
CV: Palpitation, bradycardia, change in BP
GI: Nausea, vomiting, anorexia, constipation, cramps, biliary tract pressure
*RESP: **Respiratory depression***

GU: Increased urinary output, dysuria, urinary retention
EENT: Tinnitus, blurred vision, miosis, diplopia
INTEG: Rash, urticaria, bruising, flushing, diaphoresis, pruritus
Contraindications: Hypersensitivity, addiction (narcotic), hemorrhage, bronchial asthma, increased intracranial pressure, MAO inhibitors
Precautions: Addictive personality, pregnancy category C, lactation, MI (acute), severe heart disease, elderly, respiratory depression, hepatic disease, renal disease, child <18 yr
Pharmacokinetics:
PO: Onset variable, peak variable, duration variable
SC: Onset 15-30 min, peak 50-90 min, duration 3-5 hr
IV: Peak 20 min
Half-life 2.5-3 hr; metabolized by liver; excreted by kidneys; crosses placenta; excreted in breast milk
⚖ Drug interactions of concern to dentistry:
• Increased CNS depression: alcohol, all CNS depressants
• Contraindication: MAO inhibitors
• Increased effects of anticholinergics

DENTAL CONSIDERATIONS
General:
• Monitor vital signs every appointment due to cardiovascular and respiratory side effects.
• Assess salivary flow as a factor in caries, periodontal disease, and candidiasis.
• After supine positioning, have patient sit upright for at least 2 min before standing to avoid orthostatic hypotension.

• Psychologic and physical dependence may occur with chronic administration.
• Determine why the patient is taking the drug.
• Consider the use of NSAIDs when additional analgesia is required.
Teach patient/family: *When chronic dry mouth occurs, advise patient:*
• To use daily home fluoride products for anticaries effect
• To avoid mouth rinses with high alcohol content due to drying effects
• To use sugarless gum, frequent sips of water, or saliva substitutes

---

moxifloxacin HCl
(mox-i-flox′a-sin)
Avelox

Drug class.: Fluoroquinolone anti-infective

Action: A broad-spectrum bactericidal agent that inhibits the enzymes topoisomerase II (DNA gyrase) and topoisomerase IV required for bacterial DNA replication, transcription repair, and recombination
Uses: Acute bacterial sinusitis (*S. pneumoniae, H. influenzae,* or *M. catarrhalis*); acute bacterial exacerbation of chronic bronchitis (*S. pneumoniae, H. influenzae, H. parainfluenzae, K. pneumoniae, M. catarrhalis* or *S. aureus*); community acquired pneumonia (*S. pneumoniae, H. influenzae, M. catarrhalis, M. pneumoniae,* or *C. pneumoniae*)
Dosage and routes:
• *Adult and child >18 yr:* PO 400 mg qd, duration varies from 5-10

---

days depending on type of infection; take at least 4 hr before or 8 hr after antacids (Mg^{2+}, Al^{3+}), sucralfate, metal cations (Fe^{2+}, Zn^{2+}), or didanosine

• *Adult:* IV inf >60 min, 400 mg qd for 5-14 days depending on the infection

Available forms include: Tabs 400 mg

Side effects/adverse reactions:

▼ *ORAL: Taste perversion,* candidiasis, dry mouth, stomatitis (infrequent)

*CNS: Dizziness, lightheadedness, headache, **prolonged QT interval,** risk of seizures, malaise, insomnia, confusion, tremor, vertigo

CV: Palpitation, tachycardia, hypertension, vasodilation

GI: Nausea, diarrhea, vomiting, abdominal pain, dyspepsia, pseudomembranous colitis

RESP: Asthma, dyspnea

*HEMA: **Thrombocytopenia, eosinophilia, leukopenia***

GU: Vaginal candidiasis, vaginitis

EENT: Pharyngitis, rhinitis, coughing, sinusitis, tinnitus, amblyopia

INTEG: Photosensitivity (has not been shown with this drug), skin rash, pruritus, urticaria

META: Abnormal liver function tests, GGTP elevated, hyperlipidemia, hyperglycemia

MS: Tendon rupture, cartilage damage, leg pain, arthralgia, myalgia

*MISC: **Anaphylaxis** (rare),* allergic reactions

Contraindications: Hypersensitivity to fluoroquinolones

Precautions: Divalent cations, retard absorption, not for use with class 1A and III antiarrhythmics, use in children not studied, cross resistance with other fluoroquinolones, may prolong QT interval in some patients, seizures, use with NSAIDs, pregnancy category C, children <18 yr, lactation

Pharmacokinetics:

PO: Well absorbed, bioavailability 90%, steady state plasma levels in 3 days, plasma protein binding 50%, widely distributed even to saliva, hepatic metabolism, sulfate conjugates excreted in feces, glucuronide conjugates excreted in urine

🦷 Drug interactions of concern to dentistry:

• Increased risk of CNS stimulation and seizures: NSAIDs

• Decreased absorption: divalent and trivalent antacids, iron and zinc salts

• Caution when using erythromycin, tricyclic antidepressants (no data, risk of ↑ QT interval)

DENTAL CONSIDERATIONS
General:

• Determine why patient is taking the drug.

• Examine for oral manifestation of opportunistic infection.

• Advise patient if dental drugs prescribed have a potential for photosensitivity.

• Ruptures of the shoulder, hand, and Achilles tendons that required surgical repair or resulted in prolonged disability have been reported with the use of fluoroquinolones. Question patient about history of side effects associated with fluoroquinolone use.

• Monitor vital signs every appointment due to cardiovascular side effects.

• Patient on chronic drug therapy may rarely present with symptoms

M

---

of blood dyscrasias, which can include infection, bleeding, and poor healing.

• Consider semisupine chair position for patient comfort if GI side effects occur.

Consultations:

• In a patient with symptoms of blood dyscrasias, request a medical consult for blood studies and postpone treatment until normal values are reestablished.

• Physician consult is advised in the presence of an acute dental infection requiring another antibiotic.

Teach patient/family: *If used for dental infection:*

• To minimize exposure to sunlight and wear sunscreen if sun exposure is planned

• To discontinue treatment and inform dentist immediately if patient experiences pain or inflammation of a tendon, and to rest and refrain from exercise

---

mupirocin/mupirocin calcium

(myoo-peer'o-sin)
Bactroban, Bactroban Cream, Bactroban Nasal 2%

Drug class.: Topical antiinfective, pseudomonic acid A

Action: Inhibits bacterial protein synthesis

Uses: Impetigo caused by *S. aureus,* β-hemolytic streptococci, *S. pyogenes;* nasal membranes: *S. aureus*

Dosage and routes:

• *TOP:* Apply small amount to affected area tid

• *CREAM:* For secondary infected, traumatic skin lesions; apply small amount to affected area tid × 10 days

• *NASAL:* Divide one half of the ointment from the single-use tube between the nostrils and apply bid for 5 days

Available forms include: Oint 2% (20 mg/g), 15, 30 g; nasal oint 2% single-use tube 1 g; cream 2% in 1 g

Side effects/adverse reactions:

INTEG: Burning, stinging, itching, rash, dry skin, swelling, contact dermatitis, erythema, tenderness, increased exudate

Contraindications: Hypersensitivity

Precautions: Pregnancy category B, lactation

DENTAL CONSIDERATIONS

General:

• The dentist may choose to avoid elective dental treatment if the infected site may be affected by dental treatment.

---

mycophenolate mofetil

(mye-koe-fen'oh-late moe'fe-til)
CellCept

Drug class.: Immunosuppressant

Action: Selective inhibitor of inosine monophosphate dehydrogenase, thereby preventing the synthesis of guanosine nucleotide and resulting in cytostatic effects on T and B lymphocytes

Uses: Prophylaxis of organ rejection in patients receiving allogenic renal transplants, cardiac transplants (in combination with cyclosporine and corticosteroids)

Dosage and routes:

• *Adult:* PO 1 g bid in combination with corticosteroids and cyclosporine in renal transplant (within 72 hr of transplant)

Available forms include: Tabs 500 mg; caps 250 mg; powder for inj 500 mg; powder oral susp 200 mg/ml in 225 ml

Side effects/adverse reactions:

▼ *ORAL: Candidiasis*

CNS: Fever, headache, tremor, insomnia, dizziness

CV: Hypertension, chest pain, peripheral edema

*GI: Diarrhea, abdominal pain, nausea, dyspepsia, vomiting, **ischemic colitis,** GI bleeding*

RESP: Infection, dyspnea, cough, pharyngitis

*HEMA: **Leukopenia, sepsis, anemia, thrombocytopenia***

*GU: Infection, hematuria, **renal tubular necrosis***

INTEG: Acne, rash

MS: Back pain, asthenia

Contraindications: Hypersensitivity

Precautions: Active GI diseases, pregnancy category C, lactation, reduce dose in severe chronic renal impairment, increased risk of development of lymphomas or other malignancies and susceptibility to infection

Pharmacokinetics:

PO: Rapidly absorbed; highly plasma bound (97%); metabolized to mycophenolic acid (MPA), the active form of the drug; primary excretion in urine (93%)

👉 **Drug interactions of concern to dentistry:**

• Increased plasma concentration: acyclovir

• Decreased availability of MPA: drugs that alter the GI flora

DENTAL CONSIDERATIONS

General:

• Determine why the patient is taking the drug.

• Short appointments and a stress reduction protocol may be required for anxious patients.

• Patients who have been or are currently on chronic steroid therapy (>2 wk) may require supplemental steroids for dental treatment.

• Patients on chronic drug therapy may rarely have symptoms of blood dyscrasias, which can include infection, bleeding, and poor healing.

• Place on frequent recall due to oral side effects.

• Determine dose and duration of steroid for patient to assess risk for stress tolerance and immunosuppression.

• Examine for oral manifestation of opportunistic infections.

• Monitor vital signs every appointment due to cardiovascular and respiratory side effects.

• Consider semisupine chair position for patient comfort if GI side effects occur.

• Antibiotic prophylaxis is usually recommended in patients with organ transplants and immunosuppression.

• Monitor time since organ/tissue transplant; note duration of transplant and status of renal function.

• Place on frequent recall due to possible blood dyscrasias and oral side effects.

Consultations:

• Medical consult may be required

to assess disease control and patient's ability to tolerate stress.

• In a patient with symptoms of blood dyscrasias, request a medical consult for blood studies and postpone dental treatment until normal values are reestablished.

• Request baseline blood pressure in renal transplant patients for patient evaluation before dental treatment.

Teach patient/family:

• That secondary oral infection may occur; must see dentist immediately if infection occurs

• Importance of good oral hygiene to prevent soft tissue inflammation

• Need for frequent recall due to possible blood dyscrasias and oral side effects

• To report oral lesions, soreness, or bleeding to dentist

---

nabumetone
(na-byoo'me-tone)
Relafen

Drug class.: Nonsteroidal antiinflammatory

Action: Inhibits prostaglandin synthesis by interfering with cyclooxygenase needed for biosynthesis; possesses analgesic, antiinflammatory, antipyretic properties

Uses: Osteoarthritis, rheumatoid arthritis, acute or chronic treatment

Dosage and routes:

• *Adult:* PO 1000 mg as a single dose; may increase to 1500-2000 mg/day if needed; may give qd or bid

Available forms include: Tabs 500, 750 mg

Side effects/adverse reactions:

▼ *ORAL:* Dry mouth, bleeding, stomatitis, lichenoid reactions

CNS: Dizziness, headache, drowsiness, fatigue, tremors, confusion, insomnia, anxiety, depression, nervousness

CV: Tachycardia, peripheral edema, palpitation, dysrhythmias, CHF

GI: Cholestatic hepatitis, constipation, flatulence, cramps, peptic ulcer, gastritis, nausea, anorexia, vomiting, diarrhea, jaundice

RESP: Bronchospasm, dyspnea, pharyngitis

HEMA: Blood dyscrasias

GU: Nephrotoxicity, dysuria, hematuria, oliguria, azotemia, cystitis

EENT: Tinnitus, hearing loss, blurred vision

INTEG: Purpura, rash, pruritus, sweating, photosensitivity

Contraindications: Hypersensitivity to this drug or aspirin, iodides, NSAIDs, asthma, severe renal disease

Precautions: Pregnancy category C, lactation, children, bleeding disorders, GI disorders, cardiac disorders, renal disorders, hepatic dysfunction, elderly

Pharmacokinetics:

PO: Peak 2.5-4 hr, half-life 22-30 hr; plasma protein binding >90%; metabolized in liver to active metabolite; excreted in urine (metabolites), breast milk

⚕ Drug interactions of concern to dentistry:

• GI ulceration, bleeding: aspirin, alcohol, corticosteroids

• May decrease effects of nabumetone: salicylates

• Nephrotoxicity: acetaminophen (prolonged use and high doses)

• Possible risk of decreased renal function: cyclosporine

DENTAL CONSIDERATIONS

General:

• Patients on chronic drug therapy may rarely have symptoms of blood dyscrasias, which can include infection, bleeding, and poor healing.

• Assess salivary flow as a factor in caries, periodontal disease, and candidiasis.

• Avoid prescribing for dental use in last trimester of pregnancy.

• Avoid prescribing aspirin-containing products.

• Consider semisupine chair position for patients with arthritic disease.

Consultations:

• In a patient with symptoms of blood dyscrasias, request a medical consult for blood studies and postpone dental treatment until normal values are reestablished.

• Medical consult may be required to assess disease control.

Teach patient/family:

• Importance of good oral hygiene to prevent soft tissue inflammation

• Caution to prevent injury when using oral hygiene aids

When chronic dry mouth occurs, advise patient:

• To avoid mouth rinses with high alcohol content due to drying effects

• Of need for daily use of home fluoride

• To use sugarless gum, frequent sips of water, or saliva substitutes

nadolol

(nay-doe′lole)

Corgard

♣ Syn-Nadolo

Drug class.: Nonselective β-adrenergic blocker

Action: This is a nonselective β_1- and β_2-adrenergic antagonist. The antihypertensive mechanism of action is unclear, but it may include a reduction in cardiac output and inhibition of renin release by the renal juxtaglomerular apparatus. Peripheral resistance decreases with long-term use. The antianginal action (when indicated for this use) may be related to a decrease in myocardial oxygen demand and negative chronotropic and inotropic effects. The antiarrhythmic action (when indicated for this use) has been related to a reduction in spontaneous pacemaker firing and slowing of AV nodal conduction.

Uses: Chronic stable angina pectoris, mild-to-moderate hypertension; unapproved: dysrhythmias, MI prophylaxis, vascular headache

Dosage and routes:

Hypertension

• *Adult:* PO 40 mg qd, increase by 40-80 mg q3-7d; dose range 40-320 mg/d

Angina

• *Adult:* PO 40 mg/day, can increase dose over 3-7 day intervals until desired clinical response or pronounced slowing of heart; maintenance dose 40-80 mg/day; upper dose 240 mg/d

Available forms include: Oral tabs 20, 40, 80, 120, 160 mg

Side effects/adverse reactions:

▼ *ORAL:* Dry mouth, taste disturbances

CNS: Depression, hallucinations, dizziness, fatigue, lethargy, paresthesia, headache

CV: *Bradycardia, hypotension,* ***CHF,*** palpitation, AV block

GI: Nausea, vomiting, diarrhea, colitis, constipation, cramps, flatulence, hepatomegaly, pancreatitis

RESP: ***Laryngospasm, bronchospasm,*** dyspnea, respiratory dysfunction, cough, wheezing, nasal stuffiness, pharyngitis

HEMA: ***Agranulocytosis, thrombocytopenia,*** chest pain, peripheral ischemia, flushing, edema, vasodilation, conduction disturbances

EENT: Sore throat

INTEG: Rash, pruritus, fever

Contraindications: Hypersensitivity to this drug, cardiac failure, cardiogenic shock, second- or third-degree heart block, bronchospastic disease, sinus bradycardia, CHF, COPD

Precautions: Diabetes mellitus, pregnancy category C, renal disease, lactation, hyperthyroidism, peripheral vascular disease, myasthenia gravis

Pharmacokinetics:

PO: Onset variable, peak 3-4 hr, duration 17-24 hr, half-life 16-20 hr; not metabolized; excreted in urine (unchanged), bile, breast milk

🐝 Drug interactions of concern to dentistry:

• Decreased effects: sympathomimetics (epinephrine, norepinephrine, isoproterenol)

• Slows metabolism of nadolol: lidocaine

• Increased hypotension, myocardial depression: fentanyl derivatives, hydrocarbon inhalation anesthetics

• Decreased hypotensive effect: indomethacin and other NSAIDs

DENTAL CONSIDERATIONS

General:

• Monitor vital signs every appointment due to cardiovascular side effects.

• Patients on chronic drug therapy may rarely have symptoms of blood dyscrasias, which can include infection, bleeding, and poor healing.

• After supine positioning, have patient sit upright for at least 2 min before standing to avoid orthostatic hypotension.

• Limit use of sodium-containing products, such as saline IV fluids, for patients with a dietary salt restriction.

• Assess salivary flow as a factor in caries, periodontal disease, and candidiasis.

• Stress from dental procedures may compromise cardiovascular function; determine patient risk.

• Short appointments and a stress reduction protocol may be required for anxious patients.

• Consider semisupine chair position for patients with respiratory distress.

Consultations:

• In a patient with symptoms of blood dyscrasias, request a medical consult for blood studies and postpone dental treatment until normal values are reestablished.

• Take precautions if dental surgery is anticipated and anesthesia is required.

• Medical consult may be required to assess disease control and patient's ability to tolerate stress.

Teach patient/family:

• Importance of good oral hygiene to prevent soft tissue inflammation

• Caution to prevent injury when using oral hygiene aids

When chronic dry mouth occurs, advise patient:

• To avoid mouth rinses with high alcohol content due to drying effects

• Of need for daily home fluoride to prevent caries

• To use sugarless gum, frequent sips of water, or saliva substitutes

---

naftifine HCl
(naf'ti-fin)

Naftin

Drug class.: Topical antifungal

Action: Interferes with cell membrane permeability in fungi such as *T. rubrum, T. mentagrophytes, T. tonsurans, E. floccosum, M. canis, M. audouinii, M. gypseum, Candida;* broad-spectrum antifungal

Uses: Tinea cruris, tinea corporis

Dosage and routes:

• Massage into affected area, surrounding area bid; continue for 7-14 days

Available forms include: Cream 1%; gel 1%

Side effects/adverse reactions:

INTEG: Burning, stinging, dryness, itching, local irritation

Contraindications: Hypersensitivity

Precautions: Pregnancy category B, lactation, children

---

nalmefene HCl
(nal'me-feen)

Revex

Drug class.: Opioid antagonist

Action: Reverses the effects of opioids by competitive antagonism of opioid receptors

Uses: Management of opioid over-

dose and complete or partial reversal of opioid drug effects, including respiratory depression

Dosage and routes:

Reversal of opioid depression

• *Adult:* IV use 100 µg/ml strength; initial dose 0.25 µg/kg followed by 0.25 µg/kg, incremental dose at 2-5 min intervals; cumulative doses over 1.0 µg/kg do not provide additional therapeutic effect; titrate all doses

Body weight (kg)	ml of 100 µg/ml solution
50	0.125
60	0.150
70	0.175
80	0.200
90	0.225
100	0.250

Known or suspected opioid overdose

• *Adult:* IV use 1 mg/ml strength; initial 0.5 mg/70 kg; if needed, a second dose of 1.0 mg/70 kg, 2-5 min later; doses over 1.5 mg/70 kg are unlikely to be beneficial

Available forms include: Ampule 100 µg/ml in 1 ml ampule; 1 mg/ml in 2 ml ampule

Side effects/adverse reactions:

▼ *ORAL:* Dry mouth (<1%)

CNS: Dizziness, headache, dysphoria, perception of pain, nervousness

CV: Tachycardia, hypertension, dysrhythmia, hypotension

GI: Nausea, abdominal cramps, vomiting, diarrhea

RESP: Pharyngitis, pulmonary edema

GU: Urinary retention

INTEG: Pruritus

N

---

bold italic = life-threatening conditions

MS: Myalgia, joint pain

MISC: Chills

Contraindications: Hypersensitivity

Precautions: Pregnancy category B, nursing, children, withdrawal symptoms in opioid addicts, renal impairment

Pharmacokinetics:

IV: Onset 2 min, peak plasma conc 1.1-2.3 hr; can also be given IM or SC; hepatic metabolism; excreted in urine

🦷 **Drug interactions of concern to dentistry:**

• None reported

DENTAL CONSIDERATIONS

General:

• This drug is intended for acute use only, but listed side effects can sometimes be seen.

• There is a risk of seizures reported in animal studies; be aware of this potential.

• Serious cardiovascular events have been associated with opioid reversal in postoperative patients; doses should be carefully titrated to reduce these events.

• Buprenorphine depression may not be completely reversed.

• In all cases, the establishment of a patent airway, ventilatory assistance, oxygen administration, and circulatory access should complement or precede opioid antagonist use.

• Significant opioid depression occurring in the dental office may require relocation of the patient to a medical facility for comprehensive management.

• Patients discharged from the office/emergency facility should be carefully observed for the return of opioid-induced depression.

naloxone HCl

(nal-ox'one)

Narcan

Drug class.: Narcotic antagonist

Action: Competes with narcotics at narcotic receptor sites

Uses: Respiratory depression induced by narcotics, to reverse postoperative opioid depression

Dosage and routes:

Narcotic-induced respiratory depression

• *Adult and adolescent:* IV/SC/IM 0.4-2 mg; repeat q2-3 min, if needed

Postoperative respiratory depression

• *Adult:* IV 0.1-0.2 mg q2-3min prn

• *Child:* IV/IM/SC 0.01 mg/kg q2-3min prn

Asphyxia neonatorum

• *Neonates:* IV 0.01 mg/kg given into umbilical vein after delivery; may repeat in q2-3min × 3 doses

Available forms include: Inj IV/IM/SC 0.02, 0.4 mg/ml in 1 ml ampules

Side effects/adverse reactions:

CNS: Drowsiness, nervousness, restlessness, excitement

CV: Rapid pulse, increased or decreased systolic BP high doses

GI: Nausea, vomiting

RESP: Hyperpnea

MISC: Sweating

Contraindications: Hypersensitivity, cardiac irritability

Precautions: Pregnancy category B, opioid dependence

Pharmacokinetics: Onset 1-2 min (IV), 2-5 min (IM), peak effect 5-15 min, duration variable up to 45 min, half-life 60-90 min; metabolized by liver; excreted by kidneys; crosses placenta; excreted in breast milk

🦷 **Drug interactions of concern to dentistry:**
• Antagonizes effects of opioid agonists and mixed agonist/antagonists

DENTAL CONSIDERATIONS
General:
• This drug is intended for acute use only, but listed side effects can sometimes be seen.
• There is a risk of seizures reported in animal studies; be aware of this potential.
• Serious cardiovascular events have been associated with opioid reversal in postoperative patients; doses should be carefully titrated to reduce these events.
• Buprenorphine depression may not be completely reversed.
• In all cases, the establishment of a patent airway, ventilatory assistance, oxygen administration, and circulatory access should complement or precede opioid antagonist use.
• Significant opioid depression occurring in the dental office may require relocation of the patient to a medical facility for comprehensive management.
• Patients discharged from the office/emergency facility should be carefully observed for the return of opioid-induced depression.

---

naltrexone HCl
(nal-trex'one)
Depade, ReVia, Trexan
Drug class.: Narcotic antagonist

Action: Competes with opioids at opioid receptor sites

Uses: Used in treatment of opioid addiction following detoxification, alcoholism

Dosage and routes:
Use after patient is opioid free for at least 7-10 days
• *Adult:* PO 25 mg, may give 25 mg after 1 hr if there are no withdrawal symptoms; 50-150 mg may be given qd depending on patient need; maintenance 50 mg q24h
Alcoholism
• *Adult:* PO 50 mg/day
Available forms include: Tabs 50 mg

Side effects/adverse reactions:
▼ *ORAL:* Increased thirst
CNS: Stimulation, drowsiness, dizziness, confusion, convulsion, headache, flushing, hallucinations
CV: Rapid pulse, pulmonary edema, hypertension
GI: Nausea, vomiting, diarrhea, heartburn, **hepatitis,** anorexia
RESP: Wheezing, hyperpnea
HEMA: **Thrombocytopenia, agranulocytosis, leukopenia, neutropenia, hemolytic anemia,** increased pro-time
EENT: Tinnitus, hearing loss
INTEG: Rash, urticaria, bruising
Contraindications: Hypersensitivity, opioid dependence, hepatic failure, hepatitis
Precautions: Pregnancy category C
Pharmacokinetics:
PO: Onset 15-30 min, peak 1-2 hr, duration is dose dependent, half-life 4 hr; extensive first-pass metabolism; metabolized by liver; excreted by kidneys; crosses placenta; excreted in breast milk

N

⚕ Drug interactions of concern to dentistry:
• Decreased effects of opioid narcotics

DENTAL CONSIDERATIONS
General:
• Monitor vital signs every appointment due to cardiovascular and respiratory side effects.
• Patients on chronic drug therapy may rarely have symptoms of blood dyscrasias, which can include infection, bleeding, and poor healing.
• Patients should not be given opioid analgesics for dental pain management. Substitute with NSAID and long-acting local anesthetics.
• The dental professional must be aware of the patient's disease, and the patient must be active in treatment for chemical dependency.

Consultations:
• In a patient with symptoms of blood dyscrasias, request a medical consult for blood studies and postpone dental treatment until normal values are reestablished.
• Medical consult may be required to assess disease control.
• Inform aftercare provider or counselor if sedative medications are required for proper management.

Teach patient/family:
• Importance of good oral hygiene to prevent soft tissue inflammation
• Caution to prevent injury when using oral hygiene aids

naphazoline HCl
(naf-az'oh-leen)
AK-Con Ophthalmic, Albalon, Allerest Eye Drops, Allergy Drops, Clear Eyes, Comfort Eye Drops, Digest 2, 20/20 Eye Drops, Maximum Strength Eye Drops, Nafazair, Naphcon, Naphcon Forte, VasoClear, Vasocon

Drug class.: Ophthalmic vasoconstrictor

Action: Vasoconstriction of eye arterioles; decreases eye engorgement by stimulation of α-adrenergic receptors
Uses: Relieves hyperemia, irritation in superficial corneal vascularity

Dosage and routes:
• *Adult:* Instill 1-2 gtt up to tid or qid as needed
Available forms include: Sol 0.012%, 0.02%, 0.03%

Side effects/adverse reactions:
CNS: Headache, dizziness, sedation, anxiety, weakness, sweating (systemic absorption)
CV: CV collapse (systemic absorption), hypertension, dysrhythmias, tachycardia
EENT: Pupil dilation, increased intraocular pressure, photophobia
Contraindications: Hypersensitivity, glaucoma (narrow-angle)
Precautions: Hypertension, hyperthyroidism, elderly, severe arteriosclerosis, cardiac disease, pregnancy category C

Pharmacokinetics:
INSTILL: Duration 2-3 hr
⚕ Drug interactions of concern to dentistry:
• Increased pressor effects: tricyclic antidepressants

DENTAL CONSIDERATIONS
General:
• Monitor vital signs every appointment due to cardiovascular side effects.
• Avoid dental light in patient's eyes; offer dark glasses for patient comfort.
• Protect patient's eyes from accidental spatter during dental treatment.

---

naproxen/naproxen sodium
(na-prox'en)

Naproxen: EC Naprosyn, Naprosyn, Naprosyn Oral Suspension

♣ Apo-Naproxen, Naprosyn-E, Naprosyn SR, Naxen, Novo-Naprox, Nu-Prox

Naproxen sodium: Anaprox, Anaprox DS; *OTC:* Aleve

♣ Apo-Napro-Na, Apo-Napro-Na DS, Novo-Naprox Sodium, Novo-Naprox Sodium DS, Synflex, Synflex DS

Drug class.: Nonsteroidal antiinflammatory

Action: Inhibits prostaglandin synthesis by interfering with cyclooxygenase needed for biosynthesis; possesses analgesic, antiinflammatory, antipyretic properties

Uses: Mild-to-moderate pain, osteoarthritis, rheumatoid, juvenile, gouty arthritis, ankylosing spondylitis, primary dysmenorrhea; unapproved: migraine, PMS, fever

Dosage and routes:
• *Adult:* PO 500 mg q12h or 250 mg q6-8 hr, not to exceed 1 g/day (base); 550 mg, then 275 mg q6-8h prn, not to exceed 1475 mg (sodium); sus rel: 1000 mg once daily

Available forms include: Tabs 200 mg (OTC), 250, 275, 375, 500 550 mg; sus rel tabs 375, 500 mg; susp 125 mg/5 ml

Side effects/adverse reactions:
▼ *ORAL:* Stomatitis, bleeding, dry mouth, lichenoid reactions
CNS: Dizziness, drowsiness, fatigue, tremors, confusion, insomnia, anxiety, depression
CV: Tachycardia, peripheral edema, palpitation, dysrhythmias
GI: **Cholestatic hepatitis,** nausea, anorexia, vomiting, diarrhea, jaundice, constipation, flatulence, cramps, peptic ulcer
HEMA: **Blood dyscrasias**
GU: **Nephrotoxicity: dysuria, hematuria, oliguria, azotemia**
EENT: Tinnitus, hearing loss, blurred vision
INTEG: Purpura, rash, pruritus, sweating
Contraindications: Hypersensitivity, asthma, severe renal disease, severe hepatic disease
Precautions: Pregnancy category B, lactation, children, bleeding disorders, GI disorders, cardiac disorders, hypersensitivity to other antiinflammatory agents, elderly, >2 alcohol drinks daily
Pharmacokinetics:
PO: Peak 2-4 hr, half-life 3-3.5 hr; 99% protein binding; metabolized in liver; excreted in urine (metabolites), breast milk
🥄 **Drug interactions of concern to dentistry:**
• GI ulceration, bleeding: aspirin, alcohol, corticosteroids

• Nephrotoxicity: acetaminophen (chronic use and high doses)
• Possible risk of decreased renal function: cyclosporine
• Increased photosensitization: tetracycline

When prescribed for dental pain:
• Risk of increased effects: oral anticoagulants, oral antidiabetics, lithium, methotrexate
• Decreased antihypertensive effects of diuretics, β-adrenergic blockers, and ACE inhibitors

DENTAL CONSIDERATIONS
General:
• Patients on chronic drug therapy may rarely have symptoms of blood dyscrasias, which can include infection, bleeding, and poor healing.
• Assess salivary flow as a factor in caries, periodontal disease, and candidiasis.
• Avoid prescribing for dental use in last trimester of pregnancy.
• Avoid prescribing aspirin-containing products.
• Consider semisupine chair position for patients with arthritic disease.

Consultations:
• In a patient with symptoms of blood dyscrasias, request a medical consult for blood studies and postpone dental treatment until normal values are reestablished.
• Medical consult may be required to assess disease control.

Teach patient/family:
• Importance of good oral hygiene to prevent soft tissue inflammation
• Caution to prevent injury when using oral hygiene aids
When chronic dry mouth occurs, advise patient:
• To avoid mouth rinses with high alcohol content due to drying effects
• Of need for daily use of home fluoride products to prevent caries
• To use sugarless gum, frequent sips of water, or saliva substitutes

---

naratriptan HCl
(nar´a-trip-tan)
Amerge
Drug class.: Serotonin agonist

Action: A selective agonist for 5-HT_{1D} and 5-HT_{1B} receptors located on intracranial blood vessels leading to vasoconstriction and possibly inhibition of proinflammatory neuropeptide release

Uses: Acute treatment of migraine attacks with or without aura in adults

Dosage and routes:
• *Adult:* PO 1-2.5 mg with fluids; dose can be repeated once after 4 hr; max dose 5 mg/24 hr
Available forms include: Tabs 1, 2.5 mg

Side effects/adverse reactions:
▼ *ORAL:* Dry mouth
CNS: Paresthesias, dizziness, drowsiness, malaise, fatigue
CV: Palpitation, hypertension, tachyarrhythmias
GI: Nausea, vomiting, discomfort, dyspepsia
RESP: Bronchitis, cough
HEMA: Leukocytosis
GU: Bladder inflammation, polyuria
EENT: Throat/neck symptoms, photophobia, sinusitis, tinnitus, blurred vision, vertigo
INTEG: Sweating, rash
ENDO: Polydipsia, thirst
MS: Muscle pain, arthralgia

Contraindications: Hypersensitivity, ischemic heart disease, vasospastic coronary artery disease, cerebrovascular or periperipheral vascular disease, uncontrolled hypertension, severe renal or hepatic impairment, hemiplegic or basilar migraine, ergot-containing drugs

Precautions: Risk of serious cardiovascular events, renal/hepatic dysfunction, SSRI antidepressants, pregnancy category C, lactation, use in children not established, not recommended in elderly

Pharmacokinetics:
PO: Bioavailability 70%, peak levels 2-3 hr, protein binding 28%-31%, metabolized by cytochrome P-450 enzymes; 50% of dose excreted in urine unchanged; 30% as metabolite

⚡ Drug interactions of concern to dentistry:
• No specific interactions with dental drugs reported
• Should not be used within 24 hr of another $5HT_1$ agonist

DENTAL CONSIDERATIONS
General:
• This is an acute-use drug, thus it is doubtful that patients will come to the office if acute migraine is present.
• Be aware of patient's disease, its severity, and frequency when known.

Consultations:
• If treating chronic orofacial pain, consult with physician of record.
• Medical consult may be required to assess disease control and patient's ability to tolerate stress.

Teach patient/family:
• Importance of updating health and drug history if physician makes any changes in evaluation or drug regimens

• That dryness of the mouth may occur when taking this drug; avoid mouth rinses with high alcohol content due to additional drying effects.

---

nateglinide
(na-teg′lin-ide)
Starlix
Drug class.: Oral antidiabetic, meglitinide class

Action: Lowers blood glucose by stimulation of insulin release from the pancreatic β-cells; binds to ATP-dependent potassium channels in functioning β-cells with opening of calcium channels and subsequent insulin release

Uses: Type 2 diabetes mellitus when hyperglycemia cannot be controlled by diet and exercise, can be used in combination with metformin, not for patients who have been chronically treated with other antidiabetic drugs

Dosage and routes:
• *Adult:* PO 120 mg tid before meals as a single drug or in combination with metformin

Patients near HbA1C goal
• *Adult:* PO Treatment can be initiated with 60-mg dose as a single drug or in combination with metformin

Available forms include: Tabs 60, 120 mg

Side effects/adverse reactions:
CNS: Dizziness, tremor
GI: Diarrhea, upset stomach
RESP: URI, flu symptoms, bronchitis, coughing
INTEG: Increased sweating

Contraindications: Hypersensitivity, Type 1 diabetes, diabetic ketoacidosis

---

Precautions: Hypoglycemia (geriatric, malnourished, adrenal insufficiency or pituitary insufficiency more susceptible to hypoglycemia), β blocker may mask hypoglycemia, administer before meals, infection, hepatic dysfunction, pregnancy category C, lactation, children

Pharmacokinetics:

PO: Rapid absorption, peak plasma levels 1 hr, bioavailability 73%, plasma protein binding 98%, hepatic metabolism (CYP450 2C9 [70%] and CYP450 3A4 [30%]); excretion renal (83%), feces (10%)

⚕ Drug interactions of concern to dentistry:

• Most drug interactions not clearly identified; may act as an inhibitor of CYP450 2C9 enzymes but not CYP450 3A4

• Does not appear to interact with highly protein bound drugs

• Potential potentiation of hypoglycemic effects: NSAIDs, salicylates, nonselective β-blockers

DENTAL CONSIDERATIONS

General:

• If dentist prescribes any of the drugs listed in the drug interaction section, monitor patient blood sugar levels.

• Consider semisupine chair position for patient comfort if GI side effects occur.

• Ensure that patient is following prescribed diet and regularly takes medication.

• Place on frequent recall to evaluate healing response.

• Short appointments and a stress reduction protocol may be required.

• Diabetics may be more susceptible to infection and have delayed wound healing.

Consultations:

• Medical consult may include data from patient's blood glucose monitoring, including glycosylated hemoglobin or HbA1c testing.

• Medical consult may be required to assess disease control and patient's ability to tolerate stress.

Teach patient/family:

• To prevent trauma when using oral hygiene aids

• Importance of updating health and drug history if physician makes any changes in evaluation or drug regimens

---

nedocromil sodium

(ne-doe-kroe′mill)

Tilade (inhalation)

♣ Alocril (ophthalmic solution)

Drug class.: Antiasthmatic, mast cell stabilizer

Action: Stabilizes the membrane of the sensitized mast cell, preventing release of chemical mediators after an antigen-IgE interaction

Uses: Prophylaxis only in reversible obstructive airway diseases (ROADs) such as asthma; ophthalmic solution for allergic conjunctivitis

Dosage and routes:

• *Adult and child >12 yr:* Inh 4 mg bid-qid

Allergic conjunctivitis

• *Adult:* Ophth 1 or 2 gtt in each eye bid

Available forms include: Inhaler spray unit 1.75 mg per actuation; ophthalmic sol 2%

Side effects/adverse reactions:

▼ *ORAL:* Dry/burning mouth, bitter taste (aerosol)

CNS: Headache, dizziness, neuritis

GI: Nausea, vomiting, anorexia

GU: Frequency, dysuria

EENT: Throat irritation, cough, nasal congestion, burning eyes

INTEG: Rash, urticaria, angioedema

MS: Joint pain/swelling

Contraindications: Hypersensitivity to this drug or lactose, status asthmaticus

Precautions: Pregnancy category B, lactation, renal disease, hepatic disease, child <12 yr

Pharmacokinetics:

INH: Peak 15 min, duration 4-6 hr, half-life 80 min; excreted unchanged in feces

DENTAL CONSIDERATIONS

General:

• Assess salivary flow as a factor in caries, periodontal disease, and candidiasis.

• Consider semisupine chair position for patients with respiratory disease.

• Short appointments and a stress reduction protocol may be required for anxious patients.

• Be aware that aspirin or sulfite preservatives in vasoconstrictor-containing products can exacerbate asthma.

Consultations:

• Medical consult may be required to assess disease control.

Teach patient/family:

• To avoid mouth rinses with high alcohol content due to drying effects

• For inhalation dosage forms, rinse mouth with water after each dose to prevent dryness

---

nefazodone HCl

(nef-ay′zoe-done)

Serzone

Drug class.: Antidepressant

Action: Inhibits neuronal uptake of serotonin and norepinephrine; the exact mechanism of antidepressant activity remains unknown

Uses: Major depressive disorders

Dosage and routes:

• *Adult:* PO initial dose 200 mg/day in 2 divided doses bid; gradually increase dose in increments of 100-200 mg/day, depending on response and need (all doses are given bid); dose range in clinical trials was 300-600 mg/day; initial doses in elderly should be reduced by one half

Available forms include: Tabs 50, 100, 150, 200, 250 mg

Side effects/adverse reactions:

▼ *ORAL: Dry mouth,* taste alteration, candidiasis (rare), stomatitis

CNS: Somnolence, dizziness, insomnia, confusion, light-headedness, headache, memory impairment, abnormal dreams, mania

CV: Postural hypotension, hypotension, dysrhythmias (rare), peripheral edema, *life-threatening liver failure*

GI: Constipation, nausea, dyspepsia, diarrhea, increased appetite, gastroenteritis

RESP: Pharyngitis, cough, bronchitis

GU: Urinary frequency, UTI, vaginitis, urinary retention, impotence

EENT: Blurred vision, abnormal vision, visual field defect, eye pain, tinnitus

INTEG: Rash, pruritus, dry skin, urticaria

---

bold italic = life-threatening conditions

MS: Neck rigidity

MISC: Flulike syndrome, chills, fever

Contraindications: Hypersensitivity, coadministration of MAO inhibitors

Precautions: Mania, hypomania, suicidal tendencies, seizures, history of MI or unstable heart conditions, hepatic impairment, pregnancy category C, lactation, child <18 yr, elderly (requires dose adjustment), priapism history, alcohol use

Pharmacokinetics: Bioavailability 20% with PO doses, peak plasma levels 1 hr, half-life 2-4 hr; highly protein bound 99%; extensive hepatic metabolism; metabolites excreted in urine

👙 **Drug interactions of concern to dentistry:**

• Must *not* be used with MAO inhibitors

• Risk of significant adverse drug interaction with triazolam, alprazolam, alcohol-containing products

• No information available on use of this drug in patients who are candidates for conscious sedation or general anesthesia

DENTAL CONSIDERATIONS

General:

• Assess salivary flow as a factor in caries, periodontal disease, and candidiasis.

• Take vital signs every appointment due to cardiovascular side effects.

• After supine positioning, have patient sit upright for at least 2 min before standing to avoid postural hypotension.

• There is no information concerning the use of vasoconstrictors in patients taking this drug.

Consultations:

• Medical consult may be required to assess disease control.

• Physician should be informed if significant xerostomic side effects occur (increased caries, sore tongue, problems eating or swallowing, difficulty wearing prosthesis) so a medication change can be considered.

• Because there is no experience with the use of conscious sedation or general anesthesia in patients taking this drug, a medical consult is recommended for risk evaluation.

Teach patient/family: *When chronic dry mouth occurs, advise patient:*

• To avoid mouth rinses with high alcohol content due to drying effects

• Of need for daily use of home fluoride products to prevent caries

• To use sugarless gum, frequent sips of water, or saliva substitutes

---

nelfinavir mesylate

(nel-fin′a-veer)

Viracept

Drug class.: Antiviral

Action: Inhibits HIV-I protease enzymes leading to the production of immature, noninfectious virus

Uses: HIV infection when indicated by surrogate marker changes in patients receiving nelfinavir in combination with nucleoside analogues or alone for up to 24 wk

Dosage and routes:

• *Adult:* PO tabs 750 mg tid or 1250 mg bid with meals or light snack

• *Child 2-13 yr:* PO 20-30 mg/kg per dose tid with meals or light snack. Oral powder may be used for children unable to take tablets. Oral powder can be mixed with a small amount of water, milk formula, soy formula, soy milk, or dietary supplement. Do not use acidic juices or applesauce.

Available forms include: Tabs 250 mg; oral powder 50 mg/g (as free base nelfinavir)

Side effects/adverse reactions:

▼ *ORAL:* Oral ulceration (<2%)

CNS: Anxiety, depression, dizziness, sleep disorder, migraine, insomnia

GI: Diarrhea, nausea, anorexia, dyspepsia, vomiting, hepatitis, pancreatitis, GI bleeding

RESP: Pharyngitis, dyspnea, sinusitis

HEMA: Anemia, leukopenia, thrombocytopenia, abnormal laboratory values

GU: Kidney calculus, sexual dysfunction

EENT: Rhinitis

INTEG: Rash, pruritus, urticaria

META: Increased alk phosphatase, creatine phosphokinase, hyperlipidemia, abnormal liver function tests

MS: Arthralgia, asthenia, myalgia, myopathy, cramps

Contraindications: Hypersensitivity, concurrent use with triazolam, midazolam, ergot derivatives, rifampin, amiodarone, or quinidine

Precautions: Pediatric use, phenylketonuria (powder contains phenylalanine), diabetes mellitus, hyperglycemia, hepatic impairment, development of resistance, hemophilia, pregnancy category B, lactation, child <2 yr

Pharmacokinetics:

PO: Peak plasma levels 2-4 hr with food; peak plasma levels 3-4 µg/ml, plasma protein bound (98%), hepatic metabolism, active metabolite, excreted mostly in feces (87%), minor urinary excretion (1%-2%)

⚕ Drug interactions of concern to dentistry:

• Contraindicated with triazolam, midazolam

• Increased plasma concentrations of fentanyl

DENTAL CONSIDERATIONS

General:

• Examine for oral manifestation of opportunistic infection.

• Patient on chronic drug therapy may rarely have symptoms of blood dyscrasias, which can include infection, bleeding, and poor healing.

• Palliative medication may be required for management of oral side effects.

Consultations:

• In a patient with symptoms of blood dyscrasias, request a medical consult for blood studies and postpone treatment until normal values are reestablished.

• Medical consult may be required to assess disease control.

Teach patient/family:

• Importance of good oral hygiene to prevent soft tissue inflammation

• Caution to prevent trauma when using oral hygiene aids

• Importance of updating health and drug history if physician makes any changes in evaluation or drug regimens

• That secondary oral infection may occur; must see dentist immediately if infection occurs

N

---

bold italic = life-threatening conditions   *For periodic updates, visit* **www.mosby.com**

neostigmine bromide/ neostigmine methylsulfate

(nee-oh-stig'meen)

Prostigmin Bromide/Prostigmin

Drug class.: Cholinesterase inhibitor

Action: Inhibits destruction of acetylcholine, increasing its concentration at sites where acetylcholine is released; this facilitates transmission of impulses across myoneural junction

Uses: Myasthenia gravis, nondepolarizing neuromuscular blocker, antagonist, bladder distention, postoperative ileus

Dosage and routes:

Myasthenia gravis

• *Adult:* PO 15-375 mg/day; IM/IV 0.5-2 mg q1-3h

• *Child:* PO 2 mg/kg/day q3-4h

Tubocurarine antagonist

• *Adult:* IV 0.5-2 mg slowly, may repeat if needed (give 0.6-1.2 mg atropine before this drug)

Abdominal distention/postoperative ileus

• *Adult:* IM/SC 0.25-1 mg q4-6h, depending on condition

Available forms include: Tabs 15 mg; inj IM/SC/IV 1:1000, 1:2000, 1:4000

Side effects/adverse reactions:

▼ *ORAL: Increased salivation*

CNS: ***Paralysis, convulsions,*** dizziness, headache, sweating, confusion, weakness, incoordination

CV: ***Cardiac arrest,*** tachycardia, dysrhythmias, bradycardia, hypotension, AV block, ECG changes

GI: *Nausea, diarrhea, vomiting, cramps,* increased secretions

RESP: ***Respiratory depression, bronchospasm, constriction, laryngospasm, respiratory arrest***

GU: Frequency, incontinence

EENT: Miosis, blurred vision, lacrimation

INTEG: Rash, urticaria, flushing

Contraindications: Obstruction of intestine, renal system, pregnancy category C, bromide sensitivity

Precautions: Bradycardia, hypotension, seizure disorders, bronchial asthma, coronary occlusion, hyperthyroidism, dysrhythmias, peptic ulcer, megacolon, poor GI motility, lactation, children

Pharmacokinetics:

PO: Onset 45-75 min, duration 2.5-4 hr

IM/SC: Onset 10-30 min, duration 2.5-4 hr

IV: Onset 4-8 min, duration 2-4 hr Metabolized in liver, excreted in urine

♣ Drug interactions of concern to dentistry:

• Decreased action: hydrocarbon inhalation anesthetics, corticosteroids

• Decreased action of anticholinergics (may be contraindicated)

• Increased action of succinylcholine

• Increased toxicity of ester-type local anesthetics

DENTAL CONSIDERATIONS

General:

• Monitor vital signs every appointment due to cardiovascular and respiratory side effects.

• Use amide-type local anesthetic agent.

• Early-morning and brief appointments preferred due to effects of disease on oral musculature.

Consultations:
• Take precautions if dental surgery is anticipated and anesthesia is required.
• Medical consult may be required to assess disease control and patient's tolerance for stress.

---

nevirapine (NVP)
(ne-vye′ra-peen)
Viramune
Drug class.: Antiviral

Action: A nonnucleoside reverse transcriptase inhibitor for HIV-1, results in blockade of RNA-dependent and DNA-dependent polymerase

Uses: Used in combination with nucleoside analogs for HIV-1 infection in adults who have demonstrated clinical or immunologic deterioration

Dosage and routes:
• *Adult:* PO 200 mg qd × 14 days; then 200 mg bid in combination with nucleoside analog retroviral agent

Available forms include: Tabs 200 mg

Side effects/adverse reactions:
▼ *ORAL:* Oral ulceration (Stevens-Johnson syndrome)
CNS: Headache, fever, fatigue, somnolence
GI: Nausea, diarrhea
INTEG: Rash (Stevens-Johnson syndrome)
ENDO: Hepatitis
MS: Myalgias, paresthesia
META: Abnormal liver function tests

Contraindications: Hypersensitivity, protease inhibitors

Precautions: Severe life-threatening skin reactions (Stevens-Johnson syndrome), fatal hepatotoxicity has occurred, renal dysfunction, pregnancy category C, lactation, children

Pharmacokinetics:
PO: Absorption 90%, peak plasma levels 4 hr, plasma protein binding 60%, hepatic metabolism, fecal excretion mainly, urinary excretion also

⚡ Drug interactions of concern to dentistry:
• Should not be given with ketoconazole

DENTAL CONSIDERATIONS
General:
• Determine why patient is taking the drug.
• Examine for oral manifestation of opportunistic infection.

Consultations:
• Medical consult may be required to assess disease control.

Teach patient/family:
• Importance of good oral hygiene to prevent soft tissue inflammation
• To report oral lesions, soreness, or bleeding to dentist
• Importance of updating health history/drug record if physician makes any changes in evaluation or drug regimens
• That secondary oral infection may occur; must see dentist immediately if infection occurs

---

niacin (vitamin B₃/ nicotinic acid)/ niacinamide (nicotinamide)

(nye'a-sin) (nye-a-sin'a-mide)

Niacin (nicotinic acid): generic, Niacor, Niaspan, Nicolar, Nicotinex, Slo-Niacin

♣ Novo-Niacin

Niacinamide: generic

Drug class.: Vitamin B₃

Action: Needed for conversion of fats, protein, carbohydrates by oxidation-reduction; acts directly on vascular smooth muscle, causing vasodilation; high doses decrease serum lipids

Uses: Pellagra, hyperlipidemias (niacin), peripheral vascular disease (niacin)

Dosage and routes:

Adjunct in hyperlipidemia

• *Adult:* PO 1.5-3 g qd in 3 divided doses after meals, may be increased to 6 g/day; ext rel 500 or 1000 mg for 1 mo, increasing to 1.5 or 2 g hs if inadequate response, daily dose should not be increased >500 mg in 4 wk period

Pellagra

• *Adult:* IM/SC/PO/IV inf 10-20 mg, not to exceed 500 mg total dose

• *Child:* IM/SC/PO/IV inf 300 mg until desired response

Peripheral vascular disease

• *Adult:* PO 250-800 mg qd in divided doses

Available forms include: Nicotinic acid—tabs 50, 100, 250, 500 mg; time rel caps 125, 250, 400, 500 mg; time rel tabs 150, 250, 500, 750, 1000 mg; elix 50 mg/5 ml; niacinamide—tabs 100, 500 mg

Side effects/adverse reactions:

▼ *ORAL:* Dry mouth

CNS: Paresthesia, headache, dizziness, anxiety

CV: Postural hypotension, vasovagal attacks, dysrhythmias, vasodilation

GI: ***Jaundice,*** nausea, vomiting, anorexia, flatulence, diarrhea, peptic ulcer

RESP: Wheezing

GU: ***Glycosuria, hypoalbuminemia,*** hyperuricemia

EENT: Blurred vision, ptosis

INTEG: Flushing, dry skin, rash, pruritus

Contraindications: Hypersensitivity, peptic ulcer, hepatic disease, lactation, hemorrhage, severe hypotension

Precautions: Glaucoma, cardiovascular disease, CAD, diabetes mellitus, gout, schizophrenia, pregnancy category A

Pharmacokinetics:

PO: Peak 30-70 min, half-life 45 min; metabolized in liver; 30% excreted unchanged in urine

🥄 **Drug interactions of concern to dentistry:**

• None reported

DENTAL CONSIDERATIONS

General:

• Take vital signs every appointment due to cardiovascular side effects.

• After supine positioning, have patient sit upright for at least 2 min before standing to avoid postural hypotension.

• Assess salivary flow as a factor in caries, periodontal disease, and candidiasis.

Teach patient/family: *When*

italic = common side effects

chronic dry mouth occurs, advise patient:

• To avoid mouth rinses with high alcohol content due to drying effects

• Of need for daily use of home fluoride products to prevent caries

• To use sugarless gum, frequent sips of water, or saliva substitutes

---

nicardipine HCl

(nye-kar′de-peen)

Cardene, Cardene IV, Cardene SR

Drug class.: Calcium channel blocker

Action: Inhibits calcium ion influx across cell membrane during cardiac depolarization; produces relaxation of coronary vascular smooth muscle, peripheral vascular smooth muscle; dilates coronary vascular arteries; decreases SA/AV node conduction

Uses: Chronic stable angina pectoris, hypertension

Dosage and routes:

Angina

• *Adult:* PO 20 mg tid initially; may increase after 3 days (range 20-40 mg tid)

Hypertension

• *Adult:* PO 20 mg tid initially, then increase after 3 days (range 20-40 mg tid)

Available forms include: Caps 20, 30 mg; sus rel caps 30, 45, 60 mg; IV 2.5 mg/ml in 10 ml amps

Side effects/adverse reactions:

▼ *ORAL:* Dry mouth, sore throat (gingival overgrowth has been reported with other calcium channel blockers)

CNS: Headache, fatigue, drowsiness, dizziness, anxiety, depression, weakness, insomnia, confusion, paresthesia, somnolence

*CV: **MI, pulmonary edema,** dysrhythmia, edema, CHF, bradycardia, hypotension, palpitation

*GI: **Hepatitis,** nausea, vomiting, diarrhea, gastric upset, constipation, abdominal cramps

*GU: **Acute renal failure,** nocturia, polyuria

INTEG: Rash, pruritus, urticaria, photosensitivity, hair loss

MISC: Blurred vision, flushing, nasal congestion, sweating, shortness of breath, gynecomastia, hyperglycemia, sexual difficulties

Contraindications: Sick sinus syndrome, second- or third-degree heart block, hypotension <90 mm Hg systolic, hypersensitivity

Precautions: CHF, hypotension, hepatic injury, pregnancy category C, lactation, children, renal disease, elderly

Pharmacokinetics:

PO: Onset 10 min, peak 1-2 hr, half-life 2-5 hr; metabolized by liver; excreted in urine (98% as metabolites)

🦷 **Drug interactions of concern to dentistry:**

• Decreased effect: indomethacin, possibly other NSAIDs, phenobarbital

• Increased effect: parenteral and inhalational general anesthetics or other drugs with hypotensive actions

• Increased effects of nondepolarizing muscle relaxants

• Increased effects of carbamazepine

DENTAL CONSIDERATIONS

General:

• Monitor cardiac status; take vital signs at each appointment because

---

of CV side effects. Consider a stress reduction protocol to prevent stress-induced angina during the dental appointment.
• After supine positioning, have patient sit upright for at least 2 min to avoid orthostatic hypotension.
• Place on frequent recall to monitor gingival condition.
• Limit use of sodium-containing products, such as saline IV fluids, for patients with a dietary salt restriction.
• Assess salivary flow as a factor in caries, periodontal disease, and candidiasis.
• Use vasoconstrictors with caution, in low doses, and with careful aspiration. Avoid use of gingival retraction cord with epinephrine.

Consultations:
• Medical consult may be required to assess disease control and tolerance for stress.

Teach patient/family:
• Importance of good oral hygiene to prevent soft tissue inflammation and minimize gingival overgrowth
• Need for frequent oral prophylaxis if hyperplasia occurs
When chronic dry mouth occurs, advise patient:
• To avoid mouth rinses with high alcohol content due to drying effects
• Of need for daily use of home fluoride products to prevent caries
• To use sugarless gum, frequent sips of water, or saliva substitutes

nicotine inhalation/ nicotine spray/nicotine transdermal system

(nik'oh-teen)
Inhalation: Nicotrol Inhaler
Spray: Nicotrol NS
Transdermal: Habitrol, Nicoderm CQ, Nicotrol
Drug class.: Smoking deterrent

Action: Binds to acetylcholine receptors at autonomic ganglia in the adrenal medulla, at neuromuscular junctions, and in the brain
Uses: Cigarette smoking cessation program

Dosage and routes:
• *Inhalation:* Individualize dose, range 6-16 cartridges/day for 3 mo; individual use will vary, gradually reduce dose over time
• *Nasal spray:* One spray in each nostril (1 mg total); adjust dose to individual of 1 or 2 doses/hr not to exceed 5 doses/hr or 40 doses/day and for no longer than 3 mo
• *Adult:* TRANS dose varies with 24- or 16-hr system selected; one example is 21 mg/day for 6 wk, then 14 mg/day for 2 wk, then 7 mg/day for 2 wk; for 16-hr system: 15 mg per 16-hr day for 6 wk

Available forms include: Transderm patch delivering 7, 14, 21 mg/day for 24-hr system and 15 mg for 16-hr system; spray pump 0.5 mg of nicotine per actuation; INH 4 mg per actuation in cartridges

Side effects/adverse reactions:
▼ *ORAL:* Dry mouth
CNS: Abnormal dreams, insomnia, nervousness, headache, dizziness, paresthesia

GI: Diarrhea, dyspepsia, constipation, nausea, abdominal pain, vomiting
INTEG: Erythema, pruritus, rash, burning at application site, cutaneous hypersensitivity, sweating
MS: Arthralgia, myalgia
Contraindications: Hypersensitivity, children, pregnancy, lactation, nonsmokers, during immediate post-MI period, life-threatening dysrhythmias, severe or worsening angina pectoris, hypertension
Precautions: Skin disease, angina pectoris, MI, renal or hepatic insufficiency, peptic ulcer, serious cardiac dysrhythmias, hyperthyroidism, pheochromocytoma, insulin-dependent diabetes, elderly, pregnancy category D
Pharmacokinetics:
TRANS: Half-life 3-4 hr; protein binding <5%; 30% is excreted unchanged in urine
⚑ Drug interactions of concern to dentistry:
• Decreased dose at cessation of smoking: acetaminophen, caffeine, oxazepam, pentazocine
• Decreased metabolism of propoxyphene
DENTAL CONSIDERATIONS
General:
• Assess salivary flow as a factor in caries, periodontal disease, and candidiasis.
Teach patient/family: *When chronic dry mouth occurs, advise patient:*
• To avoid mouth rinses with high alcohol content due to drying effects
• Of need for daily use of home fluoride products to prevent caries
• To use sugarless gum, frequent sips of water, or saliva substitutes

When used in conjunction with a smoking cessation program in the dental office, teach:
• All aspects of product drug; give package insert to patient and explain
• That patch is to be used only to deter smoking
• Not to use during pregnancy; birth defects may occur
• To keep used and unused system out of reach of children and pets; potentially toxic if chewed or swallowed
• To apply once a day to a non-hairy, clean, dry area of skin on upper body or upper outer arm
• To stop smoking immediately when beginning treatment with patch
• To apply promptly after removing from protective covering; system may lose strength

---

nicotine polacrilex
(nik′o-teen)
Nicorette, Nicorette DS
Drug class.: Smoking deterrent

Action: Agonist at nicotinic receptors in the peripheral and central nervous systems; acts at sympathetic ganglia; on chemoreceptors of the aorta and carotid bodies; also affects adrenal-releasing catecholamines
Uses: Deters cigarette smoking when combined with a program of smoking cessation
Dosage and routes:
• *Adult (<25 cigarettes/day):* Gum initial start with 2 mg gum; slowly chew gum until it tingles; place gum between cheek and gum; when tingle is gone chew again;

use up to 9 pieces/day but no more than 24 pieces/day

• *Adult (>25 cigarettes/day):* Wk 1-6: chew 1 piece q1-2h; wk 7-9 chew 1 piece q2-4h; wk 10-12 chew 1 piece q4-8h

Available forms include: Gum 2, 4 mg/piece of gum

Side effects/adverse reactions:

▼ *ORAL:* Burning in mucosa, occlusal stress, unpleasant taste, increased salivation, dry mouth (rare), sore throat

CNS: Dizziness, vertigo, insomnia, headache, confusion, convulsions, depression, euphoria, numbness, tinnitus

CV: Dysrhythmias, tachycardia, palpitation

GI: Nausea, vomiting, anorexia, indigestion, diarrhea, abdominal pain, constipation, eructation

RESP: Breathing difficulty, cough, hoarseness, sneezing, wheezing

Contraindications: Hypersensitivity, immediate post-MI recovery period, severe angina pectoris, pregnancy category X, nicotine patch therapy

Precautions: Vasospastic disease, dysrhythmias, uncontrolled hypertension, diabetes mellitus, pregnancy, children, hyperthyroidism, pheochromocytoma, coronary disease, esophagitis, peptic ulcer, insulin or prescription medications for asthma or depression

Pharmacokinetics:

PO: Onset 15-30 min, half-life 2-3 hr, 30-120 hr (terminal); metabolized in liver; excreted in urine

⚕ Drug interactions of concern to dentistry:

• Increased blood levels with cessation of smoking: propoxyphene

DENTAL CONSIDERATIONS
General:

• Take vital signs every appointment due to cardiovascular side effects.

• TMJ disorder may be aggravated by chewing due to heavier viscosity of gum.

Teach patient/family:

• Need for good oral hygiene to prevent periodontal inflammation

When chronic dry mouth occurs, advise patient:

• To avoid mouth rinses with high alcohol content due to drying effects

• Of need for daily use of home fluoride products to prevent caries

• To use sugarless gum, frequent sips of water, or saliva substitutes

When used in conjunction with a smoking cessation program in the dental office, teach:

• All aspects of product use; give package insert to patient and explain

• That gum is to be used only to deter smoking

• To avoid use in pregnancy; birth defects may occur

• To stop smoking when beginning treatment with gum

• To dispose of gum carefully as nicotine will still be present; to protect from children

nifedipine

(nye-fed'i-peen)
Procardia, Procardia SL, Procardia XL
♣ Adalat, Adalat CC, Adalat PA, Apo-Nifed, Novo-Nifedin, Nu-Nifed

Drug class.: Calcium channel blocker

Action: Inhibits calcium ion influx across cell membrane during cardiac depolarization; produces relaxation of coronary vascular smooth muscle, dilates coronary arteries; increases myocardial oxygen delivery in patients with vasospastic angina; dilates peripheral arteries

Uses: Chronic stable angina pectoris, vasospastic angina, hypertension (sustained release only)

Dosage and routes:
• *Adult:* PO (immed rel) 10 mg tid, increase in 10 mg increments q4-6h, not to exceed 180 mg or single dose of 30 mg; PO (sus rel) 30-60 mg qd, may increase q7-14 days, doses >120 mg not recommended
Available forms include: Caps 10, 20 mg; sus rel tabs 30, 60, 90 mg

Side effects/adverse reactions:
▼ *ORAL: Gingival overgrowth,* dry mouth
CNS: Giddiness, headache, fatigue, drowsiness, dizziness, anxiety, depression, weakness, insomnia, light-headedness, paresthesia, tinnitus, blurred vision
CV: Dysrhythmia, edema, CHF, **MI,** hypotension, palpitation, pulmonary edema, tachycardia
GI: Nausea, vomiting, diarrhea, gastric upset, constipation, increased liver function studies

GU: Nocturia, polyuria
INTEG: Rash, pruritus, flushing, photosensitivity, hair loss
MISC: Flushing, sexual difficulties, cough, fever, chills

Contraindications: Hypersensitivity

Precautions: CHF, hypotension, sick sinus syndrome, second- or third-degree heart block, hypotension <90 mm Hg systolic, hepatic injury, pregnancy category C, lactation, children, renal disease

Pharmacokinetics:
PO: Onset 20 min, peak 0.5-6 hr, half-life 2-5 hr; metabolized by liver; excreted in urine (98% as metabolites)

⚡ Drug interactions of concern to dentistry:
• Decreased effect: indomethacin, possibly other NSAIDs, phenobarbital
• Increased effect: parenteral and inhalational general anesthetics or other drugs with hypotensive actions
• Increased effects of nondepolarizing muscle relaxants
• Increased effects of carbamazepine

DENTAL CONSIDERATIONS
General:
• Monitor cardiac status; take vital signs at each appointment because of CV side effects. Consider a stress reduction protocol to prevent stress-induced angina during the dental appointment.
• After supine positioning, have patient sit upright for at least 2 min before standing to avoid orthostatic hypotension at dismissal.
• Place on frequent recall to monitor gingival condition.
• Limit use of sodium-containing

N

---

bold italic = life-threatening conditions

products, such as saline IV fluids, for patients with a dietary salt restriction.

• Assess salivary flow as a factor in caries, periodontal disease, and candidiasis.

• Use vasoconstrictors with caution, in low doses, and with careful aspiration. Avoid use of gingival retraction cord with epinephrine.

Consultations:

• Medical consult may be required to assess disease control and stress tolerance.

Teach patient/family:

• Importance of good oral hygiene to prevent soft tissue inflammation and minimize gingival overgrowth

• Need for frequent oral prophylaxis if hyperplasia occurs

When chronic dry mouth occurs, advise patient:

• To avoid mouth rinses with high alcohol content due to drying effects

• Of need for daily use of home fluoride products to prevent caries

• To use sugarless gum, frequent sips of water, or saliva substitutes

---

nisoldipine

(nye′sol-di-peen)
Sular

Drug class.: Calcium channel antagonist (dihydropyridine group)

Action: Inhibits calcium ion influx across cell membrane during cardiac depolarization; produces relaxation of coronary vascular smooth muscle; dilates coronary arteries; decreases SA/AV node conduction; dilates peripheral vessels

Uses: Hypertension as a single agent or in combination with other antihypertensive medications

Dosage and routes:

• *Adult <65 yr:* PO initial dose 20 mg daily; can increase dose by 10 mg weekly or at longer intervals depending on patient response and blood pressure control

• *Maintenance dose:* 20-40 mg daily; doses above 60 mg daily are not recommended; do not take with high-fat meals

• *Adult >65 yr or in renal impairment:* PO reduce initial dose to 10 mg daily

Available forms include: Tabs 10, 20, 30, 40 mg

Side effects/adverse reactions:

▼ *ORAL:* Dry mouth, facial edema, gingival overgrowth, glossitis, mouth ulcers

CNS: Headache, dizziness, migraine, abnormal dreams

CV: Peripheral edema, vasodilation, palpitation, CHF, CVA, chest pain, postural hypotension

GI: Anorexia, diarrhea, colitis, dyspepsia, flatulence

HEMA: Anemia, ecchymosis, leukopenia, petechiae

GU: Dysuria, impotence, urinary frequency

EENT: Pharyngitis, sinusitis, abnormal vision, watery eyes

INTEG: Rash, dry skin, pruritus

MS: Arthralgia, leg cramps, myalgia

MISC: Flulike syndrome, malaise

Contraindications: Hypersensitivity

Precautions: Avoid high-fat meals, severe coronary artery disease, monitor blood pressure, CHF, severe hepatic impairment, do not break or crush tablets, pregnancy category C, lactation, geriatric patients

Pharmacokinetics:

PO: Low bioavailability 5%, presystemic metabolism in intestinal wall, peak plasma levels 6-12 hr, highly metabolized, urinary excretion 60%-90%

🦷 **Drug interactions of concern to dentistry:**

• Possible increase in serum levels: fluconazole, ketoconazole, itraconazole

• Decreased antihypertensive effect: indomethacin, possibly other NSAIDs, phenobarbital

• Increased effect: parenteral and inhalational general anesthetics or other drugs with hypotensive actions

• Increased effects of carbamazepine

DENTAL CONSIDERATIONS:

General:

• Stress from dental procedures may compromise cardiovascular function; determine patient risk.

• Monitor vital signs every appointment due to cardiovascular side effects.

• Short appointments and a stress reduction protocol may be required for anxious patients.

• When taken with grapefruit juice may see increased plasma levels.

• Limit use of sodium-containing products such as saline IV fluids for those patients with a dietary salt restriction.

• After supine positioning, have patient sit upright for at least 2 min before standing to avoid orthostatic hypotension.

• Assess salivary flow as a factor in caries, periodontal disease, and candidiasis.

Consultations:

• Medical consult may be required to assess disease control and patient's ability to tolerate stress.

Teach patient/family:

• Need for frequent oral prophylaxis if gingival overgrowth should occur

When chronic dry mouth occurs, advise patient:

• To avoid mouth rinses with high alcohol content due to drying effects

• To use daily home fluoride products for anticaries effect

• To use sugarless gum, frequent sips of water, or saliva substitutes

---

nitrofurantoin/ nitrofurantoin macrocrystals

(nye-troe-fyoor'an-toyn)

Furadantin, Macrobid, Macrodantin

🍁 Apo-Nitrofurantoin

Drug class.: Urinary tract antiinfective

Action: Appears to inhibit bacterial enzymes

Uses: UTIs caused by *E. coli, Klebsiella, Pseudomonas, P. vulgaris, P. morganii, Serratia, Citrobacter, S. aureus*

Dosage and routes:

• *Adult and child >12 yr:* PO 50-100 mg qid pc or 50-100 mg hs for long-term treatment

• *Child 1 mo-3 yr:* PO 5-7 mg/kg/day in 4 divided doses; 1-3 mg/kg/day for long-term treatment

Available forms include: Caps 25, 50, 100 mg; susp 25 mg/5 ml

---

bold italic = life-threatening conditions

Side effects/adverse reactions:

▼ *ORAL:* Angioedema, brown discoloration of saliva, tooth staining, tingling or burning of mouth

CNS: Dizziness, headache, drowsiness, peripheral neuropathy

GI: Nausea, vomiting, abdominal pain, diarrhea, **cholestatic jaundice**

INTEG: Pruritus, rash, urticaria, angioedema, alopecia, tooth staining

Contraindications: Hypersensitivity, anuria, severe renal disease

Precautions: Pregnancy category not listed (pregnant women at term), lactation

Pharmacokinetics:

PO: Half-life 20-60 min; crosses blood-brain barrier, placenta; excreted in breast milk; excreted as inactive metabolites in liver

🦷 **Drug interactions of concern to dentistry:**

• Increased effects: anticholinergic drugs

DENTAL CONSIDERATIONS
General:

• Determine why the patient is taking the drug.

Consultations:

• Medical consult may be required to assess disease control and to select an antiinfective if a dental infection is diagnosed.

nitroglycerin
(nye-troe-gli´ser-in)

Nitroglycerin transmucosal tab: Nitrogard

Nitroglycerin lingual aerosol: Nitrolingual

Nitroglycerin extended release cap: Nitroglyn, Nitro-Time

Nitroglycerin extended release tab: Nitrong

🍁 Nitrong SR

Nitroglycerin injection: Nitro-Bid IV, Tridil

Nitroglycerin sublingual tab: NitroQuick, Nitrostat

Topical dose forms: Nitro-Bid, Nitrol

Nitroglycerin transdermal patch: Deponit, Minitran, Nitrek, Nitrodisc, Nitro-Dur, Transderm-Nitro

Drug class.: Inorganic nitrate, vasodilator

Action: Decreases preload/afterload, decreasing left ventricular end-diastolic pressure, systemic vascular resistance; arterial and venous dilation

Uses: Chronic stable angina pectoris, prophylaxis of angina pain, CHF associated with acute MI, controlled hypotension in surgical procedures

Dosage and routes:

• *Adult:* SL dissolve tablet under tongue when pain begins; may repeat q5min until relief occurs; take no more than 3 tabs/15 min; use 1 tab prophylactically 5-10 min before activities; sus rel caps q6-12h on empty stomach; top 1-2 q8h, increase to 4 q4h as needed; IV 5 µg/min, then increase by 5 µg/min q3-5min, if no response after 20 µg/min, increase by 10-20 µg/min until desired response; trans apply 1 pad qd to a hair-free site

Available forms include: Buccal tabs 1, 2, 3 mg; spray 0.4 mg/meter spray; sus rel caps 2.5, 6.5, 9, 13 mg; sus rel tabs 2.6, 6.5, 9 mg; inj 0.5, 5 mg/ml; SL tabs 0.15, 0.3, 0.4, 0.6 mg; top oint 2%; trans derm syst 0.1, 0.2, 0.3, 0.4, 0.6, 0.8 mg/hr

Side effects/adverse reactions:

▼ *ORAL:* Dry mouth, burning sensation

CNS: Headache, flushing, dizziness

CV: Postural hypotension, ***collapse,*** tachycardia, syncope

GI: Nausea, vomiting

INTEG: Pallor, sweating, rash

Contraindications: Hypersensitivity to this drug or nitrites, severe anemia, increased intracranial pressure, cerebral hemorrhage

Precautions: Postural hypotension, pregnancy category C, lactation

Pharmacokinetics:

SUS REL: Onset 20-45 min, duration 3-8 hr

SL: Onset 1-3 min, duration 30 min

TRANSDERM: Onset 0.5-1 hr, duration 12-24 hr

IV: Onset immediate, duration variable

TRANSMUC: Onset 3 min, duration 10-30 min

AEROSOL: Onset 2 min, duration 30-60 min

TOP OINT: Onset 30-60 min, duration 2-12 hr

Metabolized by liver, excreted in urine

🐾 **Drug interactions of concern to dentistry:**

• Increased hypotensive effects: alcohol, opioids, aspirin in 1 g single doses, benzodiazepines, phenothiazines, and other drugs used in conscious sedation techniques

DENTAL CONSIDERATIONS

General:

• Take vital signs every appointment due to cardiovascular side effects.

• After supine positioning, have patient sit upright for at least 2 min before standing to avoid orthostatic hypotension.

• Assess salivary flow as a factor in caries, periodontal disease, and candidiasis.

• Ensure that patient's drug is easily available if angina occurs.

• A benzodiazepine or nitrous oxide/oxygen may be prescribed to allay anxiety.

• Check expiration date on prescription to ensure drug activity. If bottle has been opened, there is a 3-month shelf life.

• Stress from dental procedures may compromise cardiovascular function; determine patient risk.

• Talk with patient about disease control (frequency of angina episodes).

• Use vasoconstrictors with caution, in low doses, and with careful aspiration. Avoid gingival retraction cord with epinephrine.

• Short appointments and a stress reduction protocol may be required for anxious patients.

• Consider semisupine chair position for patients with cardiovascular disease.

Consultations:

• Medical consult may be required to assess disease control and patient's ability to tolerate stress.

Teach patient/family:

• Importance of good oral hygiene to prevent soft tissue inflammation

N

• Caution to prevent injury when using oral hygiene aids

When chronic dry mouth occurs, advise patient:

• To avoid mouth rinses with high alcohol content due to drying effects

• Of need for daily use of home fluoride products to prevent caries

• To use sugarless gum, frequent sips of water, or saliva substitutes

---

nizatidine

(ni-za′ti-deen)

Axid, Axid AR

♣ Apo-Nizatidine

Drug class.: H$_2$ histamine receptor antagonist

Action: Inhibits histamine at H$_2$ receptor site in parietal cells, inhibiting gastric acid secretion

Uses: Duodenal ulcer, Zollinger-Ellison syndrome, gastric ulcers, hypersecretory conditions, gastroesophageal reflux disease, stress ulcers; unapproved: GI symptoms associated with NSAID use in rheumatoid arthritis

Dosage and routes:

Duodenal ulcer

• *Adult:* PO 300 mg daily hs or 150 mg bid

Maintenance

• *Adult:* PO 150 mg daily hs; gastroesophageal reflux 150 mg bid

Available forms include: Caps 150, 300 mg; tabs 75 mg

Side effects/adverse reactions:

CNS: Somnolence, fatigue, insomnia, headache

GI: Nausea, vomiting, abdominal discomfort, diarrhea, constipation

GU: Impotence, decreased libido

INTEG: Pruritus, urticaria, rash, increased sweating

Contraindications: Hypersensitivity

Precautions: Pregnancy category C, hepatic disease, renal disease, lactation, children <16 yr

Pharmacokinetics: Peak plasma levels 0.5-3 hr, half-life 2.5-3.5 hr, duration up to 12 hr; primary renal excretion

♣ **Drug interactions of concern to dentistry:**

• Increased serum salicylate when administered with high doses of aspirin

• Decreased absorption of ketoconazole (take doses 2 hr apart)

DENTAL CONSIDERATIONS

General:

• Avoid prescribing aspirin-containing products in patients with active GI disease.

Teach patient/family:

• To avoid mouth rinses with high alcohol content due to drying effects

---

norethindrone/ norethindrone acetate

(nor-eth-in′drone)

Aygestin

Drug class.: Progesterone derivative

Action: Inhibits secretion of pituitary gonadotropins, preventing follicular maturation, ovulation

Uses: Uterine bleeding (abnormal), amenorrhea, endometriosis, contraceptive

Dosage and routes:

• *Adult:* PO 5-20 mg qd on days 5-25 of menstrual cycle

Amenorrhea:
• *Adult:* PO 2.5-10 mg qd × 5-10/day, during second half of cycle

Endometriosis
• *Adult:* PO 5 mg qd × 2 wk, then increased by 2.5 mg qd × 2 wk, up to 15 mg qd

Available forms include: Tabs 5 mg

Side effects/adverse reactions:
▼ *ORAL:* Gingival bleeding, gingival overgrowth
CNS: Dizziness, headache, migraines, depression, fatigue
CV: **Thromboembolism, stroke, pulmonary embolism, MI,** hypotension, thrombophlebitis, edema
*GI: Nausea, **cholestatic jaundice,** vomiting, anorexia, cramps, increased weight
*GU: Gynecomastia, testicular atrophy, impotence, **spontaneous abortion,** amenorrhea, endometriosis, cervical erosion, breakthrough bleeding, dysmenorrhea, vaginal candidiasis, breast changes
EENT: Diplopia
INTEG: Rash, urticaria, acne, hirsutism, alopecia, oily skin, seborrhea, purpura, melasma
META: Hyperglycemia

Contraindications: Breast cancer, hypersensitivity, thromboembolic disorders, reproductive cancer, genital bleeding (abnormal, undiagnosed), cerebral hemorrhage, pregnancy category X

Precautions: Lactation, hypertension, asthma, blood dyscrasias, gallbladder disease, CHF, diabetes mellitus, bone disease, depression, migraine headache, convulsive disorders, hepatic disease, renal disease, family history of breast or reproductive tract cancer

Pharmacokinetics:
PO: Duration 24 hr; metabolized in liver; excreted in urine, feces

🦷 **Drug interactions of concern to dentistry:**
• Decreased effectiveness of oral contraceptives: antibiotics, barbiturates

DENTAL CONSIDERATIONS
General:
• Place on frequent recall to evaluate gingival inflammation, if present.
• An increased incidence of dry socket has been reported after extraction.
• Monitor vital signs at each appointment.

Teach patient/family:
• Need for good oral hygiene to prevent periodontal inflammation
• That smoking cessation decreases risk of serious adverse cardiovascular effects
• Need for additional method of birth control while undergoing antibiotic therapy

---

norfloxacin
(nor-flox′-a-sin)
Noroxin

Drug class.: Fluoroquinolone antiinfective

Action: A broad-spectrum bactericidal agent that inhibits the enzymes topoisomerase II (DNA gyrase) and topoisomerase IV required for bacterial DNA replication, transcription repair, and recombination

Uses: Adult UTIs (including complicated) caused by *E. coli, E. cloacae, P. mirabilis, K. pneumoniae,* group D strep, indole-positive *Proteus, C. freundii, S. aureus*

Dosage and routes:
Uncomplicated
• *Adult:* PO 400 mg bid × 7-10 days 1 hr before or 2 hr after meals, for prostatitis give for 28 days
Complicated
• *Adult:* PO 400 mg bid × 10-21 days; 400 mg qd × 7-10 days in impaired renal function
Available forms include: Tabs 400 mg
Side effects/adverse reactions:
▼ *ORAL:* Dry mouth, stomatitis
CNS: Headache, dizziness, fatigue, somnolence, depression, insomnia
GI: Nausea, constipation, increased ALT/AST, flatulence, heartburn, vomiting, diarrhea
EENT: Visual disturbances, phototoxicity
INTEG: Rash, blue-black discoloration
MS: Tendinitis, tendon rupture
Contraindications: Hypersensitivity to quinolones
Precautions: Pregnancy category C, lactation, children, renal disease, seizure disorders, tendon rupture in shoulder, hand, and Achilles tendons
Pharmacokinetics:
PO: Peak 1 hr, steady state 2 days, half-life 3-4 hr; excreted in urine as active drug, metabolites
⚘ Drug interactions of concern to dentistry:
• Decreased absorption: sodium bicarbonate
DENTAL CONSIDERATIONS
General:
• Assess salivary flow as a factor in caries, periodontal disease, and candidiasis.
• Determine why the patient is taking the drug.
• Due to drug interaction, do not

use ingestible sodium bicarbonate products such as the air polishing system (Prophy Jet) unless at least 2 hr have passed since norfloxacin was taken.
• Avoid dental light in patient's eyes; offer dark glasses for patient comfort.
• Ruptures of the shoulder, hand, and Achilles tendons that required surgical repair or resulted in prolonged disability have been reported with this drug.
Consultations:
• Consult with patient's physician if an acute dental infection occurs and another antiinfective is required.
Teach patient/family:
• To avoid mouth rinses with high alcohol content due to drying effects
• To discontinue treatment and inform dentist immediately if patient experiences pain or inflammation of a tendon, and to rest and refrain from exercise

---

norgestrel
(nor-jess'trel)
Ovrette
Drug class.: Progesterone derivative

Action: Inhibits secretion of pituitary gonadotropins, preventing follicular maturation, ovulation
Uses: Oral contraception
Dosage and routes:
• *Adult:* PO 1 tablet qd beginning on day 1 of cycle and continuing
Available forms include: Tabs 0.075 mg

Side effects/adverse reactions:

▼ *ORAL:* Gingival bleeding, dry socket

CNS: Dizziness, headache, migraines, depression, fatigue

CV: ***Thromboembolism, stroke, pulmonary embolism, MI,*** hypotension, thrombophlebitis, edema

GI: Nausea, ***cholestatic jaundice,*** vomiting, anorexia, cramps, increased weight

GU: Gynecomastia, testicular atrophy, impotence, endometriosis, ***spontaneous abortion,*** amenorrhea, cervical erosion, breakthrough bleeding, dysmenorrhea, vaginal candidiasis, breast changes

EENT: Diplopia

INTEG: Rash, urticaria, acne, hirsutism, alopecia, oily skin, seborrhea, purpura, melasma

META: Hyperglycemia

Contraindications: Breast cancer, hypersensitivity, thromboembolic disorders, reproductive cancer, genital bleeding (abnormal, undiagnosed), cerebral hemorrhage, pregnancy category X

Precautions: Lactation, hypertension, asthma, blood dyscrasias, gallbladder disease, CHF, diabetes mellitus, bone disease, depression, migraine headache, convulsive disorders, hepatic disease, renal disease, family history of breast or reproductive tract cancer

Pharmacokinetics:

PO: Duration 24 hr, excreted in urine and feces, metabolized in liver

⚕ Drug interactions of concern to dentistry:

• Decreased effectiveness of oral contraceptives: antibiotics, barbiturates

DENTAL CONSIDERATIONS

General:

• Place on frequent recall to evaluate gingival inflammation, if present.

• An increased incidence of dry socket has been reported after extraction.

• Monitor vital signs at each appointment.

Teach patient/family:

• Need for good oral hygiene to prevent periodontal inflammation

• That smoking cessation decreases risk of serious and adverse cardiovascular side effects

• Need for additional method of birth control while undergoing antibiotic therapy

---

nortriptyline HCl

(nor-trip′ti-leen)
Aventyl, Pamelor

Drug class.: Antidepressant—tricyclic

Action: Blocks reuptake of norepinephrine, serotonin into nerve endings, increasing action of norepinephrine, serotonin in nerve cells

Uses: Major depression

Dosage and routes:

• *Adult:* PO 25 mg tid or qid; may increase to max of 150 mg/day; may give daily dose hs

Available forms include: Caps 10, 25, 75 mg; sol 10 mg/5 ml

Side effects/adverse reactions:

▼ *ORAL: Dry mouth, unpleasant taste,* bleeding, sublingual adenitis

CNS: Dizziness, drowsiness, confusion, headache, anxiety, tremors, stimulation, weakness, insomnia, nightmares, EPS (elderly), increased psychiatric symptoms

---

bold italic = life-threatening conditions

CV: Orthostatic hypotension, ECG changes, tachycardia, **hypertension,** palpitation
GI: Constipation, **hepatitis, paralytic ileus,** *increased appetite, nausea, vomiting, cramps, epigastric distress, jaundice*
HEMA: **Agranulocytosis, thrombocytopenia, eosinophilia, leukopenia**
GU: Retention, **acute renal failure**
EENT: Blurred vision, tinnitus, mydriasis
INTEG: Rash, urticaria, sweating, pruritus, photosensitivity
Contraindications: Hypersensitivity to tricyclic antidepressants, recovery phase of MI, convulsive disorders, prostatic hypertrophy
Precautions: Suicidal patients, severe depression, increased intraocular pressure, narrow-angle glaucoma, urinary retention, cardiac disease, hepatic disease, hyperthyroidism, electroshock therapy, elective surgery, pregnancy category C, MAO inhibitors
Pharmacokinetics:
PO: Steady state 4-19 days, half-life 18-28 hr; metabolized by liver; excreted by kidneys; crosses placenta; excreted in breast milk
⚕ Drug interactions of concern to dentistry:
• Increased anticholinergic effects: muscarinic blockers, antihistamines, phenothiazines
• Increased effects of direct-acting sympathomimetics (epinephrine, levonordefrin)
• Potential risk of increased CNS depression: alcohol, barbiturates, benzodiazepines, and other CNS depressants
• Decreased antihypertensive effect: clonidine, guanadrel, guanethidine

DENTAL CONSIDERATIONS
General:
• Take vital signs every appointment due to cardiovascular side effects.
• Assess salivary flow as a factor in caries, periodontal disease, and candidiasis.
• Patients on chronic drug therapy may rarely have symptoms of blood dyscrasias, which can include infection, bleeding, and poor healing.
• After supine positioning, have patient sit upright for at least 2 min before standing to avoid orthostatic hypotension.
• Use vasoconstrictors with caution, in low doses, and with careful aspiration. Avoid use of gingival retraction cord with epinephrine.
• Place on frequent recall due to oral side effects.
Consultations:
• In a patient with symptoms of blood dyscrasias, request a medical consult for blood studies and postpone dental treatment until normal values are reestablished.
• Medical consult may be required to assess disease control.
• Physician should be informed if significant xerostomic side effects occur (increased caries, sore tongue, problems eating or swallowing, difficulty wearing prosthesis) so a medication change can be considered.
Teach patient/family:
• Importance of good oral hygiene to prevent soft tissue inflammation
• Caution to prevent injury when using oral hygiene aids

italic = common side effects

When chronic dry mouth occurs, advise patient:

• To avoid mouth rinses with high alcohol content due to drying effects

• Of need for daily use of home fluoride products to prevent caries

• To use sugarless gum, frequent sips of water, or saliva substitutes

---

nystatin
(nye-sta′tin)

Mycostatin, Nilstat, Nystex, Pedi-Dri

♣ Nadostine, Nyaderm

Drug class.: Antifungal

Action: Interferes with fungal DNA replication; binds sterols in fungal cell membrane, increasing permeability and leaking of cell nutrients

Uses: *Candida* species causing oral, vaginal, intestinal infections

Dosage and routes:
Oral infection
• *Adult:* Susp 400,000-600,000 U qid × 14 days
• *Adult and child:* TOP apply to affected area bid-tid × 14 days; loz 200,000 up to 400,000 U, dissolve slowly in mouth 4-5 ×/day up to 14 days
• *Child and infant >3 mo:* Susp 250,000-500,000 U qid
• *Newborn and premature infant:* Susp 100,000 U qid

Extemporaneous powder: 1/8 tsp powder (500,000 units) in 1/2 cup of water (120 ml); use as an oral rinse tid or qid

GI infection
• *Adult:* PO 500,000-1,000,000 U tid

Vaginal infection
• *Adult:* Vag tabs 100,000 U inserted high into vagina qd-bid × 2 wk

Available forms include: Tabs 500,000 U; vag tabs 100,000 U; powder 50 million, 150 million, 500 million, 1 billion, 2 billion, 5 billion U; susp 100,000 U in 60 ml and 473 ml units; top cream, oint, powder 100,000 U/g in 15 mg and 60 g units; loz 200,000 U

Side effects/adverse reactions:
GI: Nausea, vomiting, anorexia, diarrhea, cramps
INTEG: Rash, urticaria (rare)

Contraindications: Hypersensitivity

Precautions: Pregnancy category not listed

Pharmacokinetics:
PO: Little absorption, excreted in feces

DENTAL CONSIDERATIONS
General:
• Determine why the patient is taking the drug.
• Broad-spectrum antibiotic may contribute to oral *Candida* infections.

Teach patient/family:
• That long-term therapy may be needed to clear infection; to complete entire course of medication
• Not to use commercial mouthwashes for mouth infection unless prescribed by dentist
• To soak full or partial dentures in a suitable antifungal solution nightly
• To prevent reinoculation of *Candida* infection by disposing of toothbrush or other contaminated oral hygiene devices used during period of infection

---

ofloxacin

(oh-flocks'a-sin)

Floxin, Floxin IV

Drug class.: Fluoroquinolone anti-infective

Action: A broad-spectrum bactericidal agent that inhibits the enzymes topoisomerase II (DNA gyrase) and topoisomerase IV required for bacterial DNA replication, transcription repair, and recombination

Uses: Treatment of lower respiratory tract infections (pneumonia, bronchitis), genitourinary infections (prostatitis, UTIs) caused by *E. coli, K. pneumoniae, C. trachomatis, N. gonorrhoeae;* skin and skin structure infections

Dosage and routes:

Lower respiratory tract infections/ skin and skin structure infections

• *Adult:* PO 400 mg q12h × 10 days

Cervicitis, urethritis

• *Adult:* PO 300 mg q12h × 7 days

Prostatitis

• *Adult:* PO 300 mg q12h × 6 wk

Acute, uncomplicated gonorrhea

• *Adult:* PO 400 mg as a single dose

Pneumonia

• *Adult:* 400 mg by IV infusion given over 60 min q12h × 10 days

Available forms include: Tabs 200, 300, 400 mg; inj 200 mg/50 ml D_5W, 400 mg in 10, 20 ml vials or 100 ml (D_5W) bottles

Side effects/adverse reactions:

▼ *ORAL:* Candidiasis, dry mouth, dysgeusia

CNS: Dizziness, headache, fatigue, somnolence, depression, insomnia, lethargy, malaise, nervousness, anxiety

GI: Diarrhea, nausea, vomiting, anorexia, flatulence, heartburn, increased AST/ALT, abdominal pain/cramps, constipation, decreased appetite, dyspepsia

EENT: Visual disturbances, phototoxicity

INTEG: Rash, pruritus

MS: Tendinitis, tendon rupture

Contraindications: Hypersensitivity to quinolones

Precautions: Pregnancy category C, lactation, children <18 yr, elderly, renal disease, seizure disorders, excessive sunlight, tendon rupture in shoulder, hand, and Achilles tendons

Pharmacokinetics:

PO: Peak 1-2 hr, steady state 2 days, half-life 9 hr; excreted in urine as active drug, metabolites; 0.9% bioavailability

🦷 **Drug interactions of concern to dentistry:**

• Decreased effects: antacids

DENTAL CONSIDERATIONS

General:

• Due to drug interaction, do not use ingestible sodium bicarbonate products such as the air polishing system (Prophy Jet) unless 2 hr have passed since ofloxacin was taken.

• Examine for oral manifestation of opportunistic infections.

• Avoid dental light in patient's eyes; offer dark glasses for patient comfort.

• Minimize exposure to sunlight and wear sunscreen if sun exposure is planned.

• Ruptures of the shoulder, hand, and Achilles tendons that required surgical repair or resulted in prolonged disability have been reported with this drug.

Consultations:

• Consult with patient's physician

if an acute dental infection occurs and another antiinfective is required.

Teach patient/family:
• Importance of good oral hygiene to prevent soft tissue inflammation
• To avoid mouth rinses with high alcohol content due to drying effects
• To discontinue treatment and inform dentist immediately if patient experiences pain or inflammation of a tendon, and to rest and refrain from exercise

---

ofloxacin (optic)
(oh-flocks'a-sin)
Ocuflox Ophthalmic Solution
Drug class.: Fluoroquinolone antiinfective, topical

Action: A broad-spectrum bactericidal agent that inhibits the enzyme DNA gyrase needed for the replication of DNA
Uses: Treatment of bacterial conjunctivitis caused by susceptible organisms, corneal ulcers
Dosage and routes:
• *Adult and child:* Instill 1 gtt in each eye q2-4h × 2 days; then 1 gtt qid up to 5 days
Available forms include: Sol 0.3% in 5 ml
Side effects/adverse reactions:
CNS: Dizziness
EENT: Burning sensation in eye, photophobia, redness
Contraindications: Hypersensitivity
Precautions: Pregnancy category C, children <1 yr
Pharmacokinetics:
TOP: Low systemic absorption, renal excretion of metabolites

DENTAL CONSIDERATIONS
General:
• Avoid dental light in patient's eyes; offer dark glasses for patient comfort and safety protection during dental treatment.

---

olanzapine
(oh lan'za-peen)
Zyprexa, Zyprexa Zydis
Drug class.: Antipsychotic

Action: Antipsychotic mechanism is unknown; acts as an antagonist for serotonin, dopamine, muscarinic, histamine, and α_1-adrenergic receptors
Uses: Psychotic disorders, schizophrenia, bipolar disorder
Dosage and routes:
• *Adult:* PO initial dose 5-10 mg qd, target dose is 10 mg/day; use 5-mg dose for patients at higher risk for orthostatic hypotension and nonsmoking women >65 yr
Bipolar mania
• *Adult:* PO 10-15 mg/day; can adjust dose in 5 mg increments q24h up to 20 mg/day
Available forms include: Tabs 2.5, 5, 7.5, 10, 15, 20 mg, orally-disintegrating tabs 5, 10 mg
Side effects/adverse reactions:
▼ *ORAL:* Dry mouth (7%)
CNS: Extrapyramidal events, somnolence, agitation, dizziness, personality disorder, insomnia, nervousness, hostility, headache, anxiety
CV: Orthostatic hypotension, tachycardia
GI: Constipation, increased appetite, abdominal pain
RESP: Rhinitis, cough, pharyngitis
GU: Premenstrual syndrome
INTEG: Vesiculobullous rash

MS: Joint pain, extremity pain, twitching

META: Weight gain, edema, fever

Contraindications: Hypersensitivity

Precautions: Pregnancy category C, lactation, paralytic ileus, elderly; combination of age, smoking, and gender (female) may increase clearance rate; neuroleptic malignant syndrome, CV disease, cerebrovascular disease, seizures, orthostatic hypotension, Alzheimer's dementia, prostate hypertrophy, glaucoma

Pharmacokinetics:

PO: Well absorbed, peak plasma levels 6 hr, hepatic metabolism, half-life 21-54 hr; renal and fecal excretion

♣ Drug interactions of concern to dentistry:

• Potentiation of orthostatic hypotension: diazepam, alcohol

DENTAL CONSIDERATIONS

General:

• Consider semisupine chair position for patient comfort due to GI effects of drug.

• Assess salivary flow as factor in caries, periodontal disease, and candidiasis.

• Monitor vital signs every appointment due to cardiovascular side effects.

• After supine positioning have patient sit upright for at least 2 min to avoid orthostatic hypotension.

• Patients on chronic drug therapy may rarely have symptoms of blood dyscrasias, which can include infection, bleeding, and poor healing.

• Assess for presence of extrapyramidal motor symptoms, such as tardive dyskinesia and akathisia. Extrapyramidal motor activity may complicate dental treatment.

Consultations:

• In a patient with symptoms of blood dyscrasias, request a medical consult for blood studies and postpone dental treatment until normal values are reestablished.

• Medical consult may be required to assess disease control.

• Physician should be informed if significant xerostomic side effects occur (increased caries, sore tongue, problems eating or swallowing, difficulty wearing prosthesis) so a medication change can be considered.

Teach patient/family:

• Importance of good oral hygiene to prevent soft tissue inflammation

• Use of electric toothbrush if patient has difficulty holding conventional devices

• Caution patients about driving or performing other tasks requiring alertness

When chronic dry mouth occurs, advise patient:

• To avoid mouth rinses with high alcohol content due to drying effects

• To use daily home fluoride products for anticaries effect

• To use sugarless gum, frequent sips of water, or saliva substitutes

---

olopatadine HCl
(oh-loe-pa-ta'deen)
Patanol
Drug class.: Ophthalmic antihistamine

Action: Selective H_1-receptor antagonist and inhibitor of histamine release from mast cells

Uses: Temporary prevention of itching of eye due to allergic conjunctivitis

Dosage and routes:
• *Adult:* TOP 1 or 2 gtt in each affected eye bid at 6- to 8-hr intervals

Available forms include: Sol 0.1% in 5-ml drop dispenser

Side effects/adverse reactions:

▼ *ORAL: Taste alteration*

EENT: Burning, dry eye, keratitis, lid edema, pruritus, foreign body reaction

MISC: Cold syndrome

Contraindications: Hypersensitivity

Precautions: Topical use only, do not use while wearing contact lenses, pregnancy category C, lactation, children <3 yr

Pharmacokinetics:

TOP: Low to nondetectable plasma levels, peak in 2 hr, renal excretion

🦷 **Drug interactions of concern to dentistry:**
• None reported

DENTAL CONSIDERATIONS

General: Protect patient's eyes from accidental spatter during dental treatment.

---

olsalazine sodium

(ole-sal'a-zeen)

Dipentum

Drug class.: Antiinflammatory, salicylate derivative

Action: Bioconverted to 5-aminosalicylic acid, which decreases inflammation in the colon

Uses: Maintenance of remission of ulcerative colitis in patients intolerant to sulfasalazine

Dosage and routes:
• *Adult:* PO 1 g/day in 2 divided doses with meals

Available forms include: Caps 250 mg

Side effects/adverse reactions:

▼ *ORAL:* Stomatitis

CNS: Headache, insomnia, hallucinations, depression, vertigo, fatigue, drug fever, chills, dizziness, drowsiness, tremors

CV: Allergic myocarditis, second-degree heart block, hypertension, peripheral edema, chest pain, palpitation

GI: Nausea, vomiting, abdominal pain, hepatitis, pancreatitis, diarrhea, bloating

RESP: **Bronchospasm,** shortness of breath

HEMA: **Leukopenia, neutropenia, thrombocytopenia, agranulocytosis, anemia**

GU: Frequency, dysuria, hematuria, impotence

INTEG: **Stevens-Johnson syndrome,** erythema, photosensitivity, rash, dermatitis, urticaria, alopecia

SYST: **Anaphylaxis**

Contraindications: Hypersensitivity to salicylates, child <14 yr

Precautions: Pregnancy category C, lactation, impaired hepatic function, severe allergy, bronchial asthma, renal disease

Pharmacokinetics:

PO: Partially absorbed, peak 1.5 hr, half-life 5-10 hr; excreted in urine as 5-aminosalicylic acid and metabolites; crosses placenta

DENTAL CONSIDERATIONS

General:
• Consider semisupine chair position for patient comfort due to GI effects of disease.

Consultations:
• Avoid drugs that could aggravate

---

bold italic = life-threatening conditions

an inflammatory colon disease; consult is recommended before selection of an antibiotic.

Teach patient/family:
• Importance of good oral hygiene to prevent soft tissue inflammation
• Caution to prevent injury when using oral hygiene aids
• To avoid mouth rinses with high alcohol content due to drying effects

---

omeprazole

(oh-me'pray-zol)
Prilosec
♣ Losec

Drug class.: Antisecretory, proton pump inhibitor

Action: Suppresses gastric acid production by binding to the hydrogen/potassium ATPase enzyme system to inhibit the final step in gastric acid production

Uses: Gastroesophageal reflux disease (GERD), severe erosive esophagitis, poorly responsive systemic GERD, pathologic hypersecretory conditions (Zollinger-Ellison syndrome, systemic mastocytosis, multiple endocrine adenomas), with clarithromycin, short-term treatment of gastric ulcers; not approved for long-term ulcer maintenance therapy

Dosage and routes:
Severe erosive esophagitis/poorly responsive gastroesophageal reflux disease
• *Adult:* PO 20 mg qd × 4-8 wk; take before eating

Gastric ulcers
• *Adult:* PO 40 mg qd × 2 wk, then 20 mg qd × 2 wk

Duodenal ulcer
• *Adult:* PO 40 mg in am × 14 days with clarithromycin 500 mg tid; on days 15-28, 20 mg day; 20 mg with clarithromycin 500 mg and amoxicillin 1000 mg each bid × 10 days

Pathologic hypersecretory conditions
• *Adult:* PO 60 mg/day; may increase to 120 mg tid; daily doses >80 mg in divided doses

Available forms include: Caps (del rel) 10, 20, 40 mg

Side effects/adverse reactions:
▼ *ORAL:* Dry mouth, mucosal atrophy of tongue, taste perversion, candidiasis

CNS: Headache, dizziness, asthenia, nervousness, anxiety disorders

CV: Chest pain, angina, tachycardia, bradycardia, palpitation, peripheral edema

GI: Diarrhea, abdominal pain, vomiting, nausea, constipation, flatulence, acid regurgitation, abdominal swelling, anorexia, irritable colon, esophageal candidiasis

RESP: Upper respiratory infections, cough, epistaxis

HEMA: Pancytopenia, thrombocytopenia, neutropenia, leukocytosis, anemia

GU: Proteinuria, hematuria, UTI, frequency, increased creatinine, testicular pain, glycosuria

EENT: Tinnitus

INTEG: Rash, dry skin, urticaria, pruritus, alopecia

META: Hypoglycemia, increased hepatic enzymes, weight gain

MISC: Back pain, fever, fatigue, malaise

Contraindications: Hypersensitivity

Precautions: Pregnancy category C, lactation, children

Pharmacokinetics:

PO: Peak 30 min-3.5 hr, half-life 30 min-1 hr; protein binding 95%; eliminated in urine as metabolites and in feces; in the elderly the elimination rate is decreased, bioavailability is increased

👄 Drug interactions of concern to dentistry:

• Increased serum levels: diazepam

DENTAL CONSIDERATIONS

General:

• Question the patient about tolerance of NSAIDs or aspirin related to GI problem.

• Consider semisupine chair position for patient comfort due to GI effects of disease.

• Assess salivary flow as a factor in caries, periodontal disease, and candidiasis.

Teach patient/family:

• Caution to prevent injury when using oral hygiene aids

When chronic dry mouth occurs, advise patient:

• To avoid mouth rinses with high alcohol content due to drying effects

• Of need for daily use of home fluoride products to prevent caries

• To use sugarless gum, frequent sips of water, or saliva substitutes

---

ondansetron HCl

(on-dan-see′tron)
Zofran, Zofran ODT
Drug class.: Antiemetic

Action: A selective 5-HT$_3$ antagonist; antiemetic effect may be mediated centrally, peripherally, or both

Uses: Prevention of nausea/vomit-ing associated with cancer chemotherapy, radiotherapy, and postoperative nausea and vomiting

Dosage and routes:

• *Adult and child >12 yr:* PO 8 mg tid, administer first dose 30 min before chemotherapy and then at 4- and 8-hr intervals, continue 1-2 days after chemotherapy; IV 0.15 mg/kg, give first dose over 15 min and 30 min before chemotherapy and at 4- and 8-hr intervals

Prevention nausea/vomiting due to radiotherapy

• *Adult:* PO 8 mg 1-2 hr prior to each fraction of radiotherapy

Prevention post op nausea/vomiting

• *Adult:* IV prior to or after surgery 4 mg over 2-5 min or IM 4 mg PO 16 mg 1 hr before induction of anesthesia

Available forms include: Tabs 4, 8, 24 mg; oral disintegrating tabs 4, 8 mg; IV 2 mg/ml in 20 ml vials; sol 4 mg/5 ml in 50 ml

Side effects/adverse reactions:

▼ *ORAL:* Dry mouth (1%-2%)

CNS: Headache, weakness, possible EPS, grand mal seizures

CV: Hypokalemia, ECG alterations, vascular occlusive events

GI: Constipation, abdominal pain

RESP: Bronchospasm

EENT: Transient blurred vision

INTEG: Rash

MISC: Anaphylaxis

Contraindications: Hypersensitivity

Precautions: Pregnancy category B, lactation, children <12 yr, elderly

Pharmacokinetics:

PO: Well absorbed, peak plasma levels 1.9 hr, food increases absorption; extensive metabolism

---

***bold italic** = life-threatening conditions*

IV: Rapid peak levels; protein binding 70%-76%; extensively metabolized

⚓ Drug interactions of concern to dentistry:
• None reported

DENTAL CONSIDERATIONS
General:
• Be aware that patient is receiving active chemotherapy.
• Avoid procedures or drugs that could promote nausea/vomiting.
• Patients with cancer may be taking chronic opioids for pain. Consider NSAID for dental pain management.
• Patients receiving chemotherapy may require palliative therapy for stomatitis.
• An increased gag reflex may make dental procedures, such as obtaining radiographs or impressions, difficult.
Consultations:
• Medical consult may be required to assess disease control.
Teach patient/family: *When chronic dry mouth occurs, advise patient:*
• To avoid mouth rinses with high alcohol content due to drying effects
• Of need for daily use of home fluoride products to prevent caries
• To use sugarless gum, frequent sips of water, or saliva substitutes

oral contraceptives

Estrogens: ethinyl estradiol, mestranol
Progestins: desogestrel, ethynodiol diacetate, levonorgestrel, medroxyprogesterone acetate, norethindrone, norgestimate, norgestrel
Many products are available. Examples:
Monophasic products: Alesse, Apri, Avione 28, Brevicon, Cyclessa, Demulen 1/35, Demulen 1/50, Desogen, Levite, Levlen, Levora, Loestrin 21, Loestrin Fe, Lo/Ovral, Modicon, Necon 0.5/35, Necon 1/35, Necon 1/50, Nelova 0.5/35E, Nelova 1/35E, Nelova 1/50, Nordette, Norethin 1/35E, Norinyl 1+50, Ortho-Cept, Ortho-Cyclen, Ortho-Novum 1/35, Ortho-Novum 1/50, Ovcon 35, Ovcon-50, Ovral-28, Zovia 1/35E, Zovia 1/50E, others
Biphasic products: Janest-28, Mircette, Necon 10/11, Nelova 10/11, Ortho-Novum 10/11
Triphasic products: Berlex, Estrostep-21, Estrostep Fe, Ortho-Novum 7/7/7, Ortho Tri-Cyclen, Tri-Levlen, Tri-Norinyl, Triphasil, Trivora, Trivora-28, Yasmin
Injectable once monthly: Lunelle
Patch: OrthoEvra Patch
Vaginal ring: Nuva Ring (etonorgestrel and ethinyl estradiol)
Drug class.: Estrogen/progestin combinations

Action: Prevents ovulation by suppressing follicle-stimulating hormone, luteinizing hormone
Uses: To prevent pregnancy, endo-

metriosis, hypermenorrhea, hypogonadism; acne (Tri-Cyclen)

Dosage and routes:

• *Adult:* PO 1 qd starting on day 5 of menstrual cycle (day 1 is first day of period)

• *INJ:* 0.5 ml IM inj every month, not to exceed 33 days

• *PATCH:* Wear 1 patch each week (7 days) × 3 wk; skip week 4

20/21-tablet packs

• *Adult:* PO 1 qd starting on day 7 of menstrual cycle (day 1 is first day of period); then on for 20 or 21 days, off 7 days

28-tablet packs

• *Adult:* PO 1 qd continuously

Biphasic

• *Adult:* PO 1 qd × 10 days, then next color 1 qd × 11 days

Triphasic

• *Adult:* PO 1 qd; check package insert for each new brand

Endometriosis

• *Adult:* PO 1 qd × 20 days from day 5-24 of cycle; check package insert for specific instructions

Available forms include: Check specific brand

Side effects/adverse reactions:

▼ *ORAL:* Gingival bleeding, dry socket

CNS: Depression, fatigue, dizziness, nervousness, anxiety, headache

CV: Increased BP, thromboembolic conditions, fluid retention, edema

GI: Nausea, vomiting, cramps, diarrhea, bloating, constipation, change in appetite, ***cholestatic jaundice***

HEMA: Increased fibrinogen, clotting factor

GU: Breakthrough bleeding, amenorrhea, spotting, dysmenorrhea, galactorrhea, endocervical hyperplasia, vaginitis, cystitis-like syndrome, breast change

EENT: Optic neuritis, retinal thrombosis, cataracts

INTEG: Melasma, acne, rash, urticaria, erythema multiforme or nodosum, pruritus, hirsutism, alopecia, photosensitivity

ENDO: Decreased glucose tolerance, increased TBG, PBI, T_4, T_3

Contraindications: Pregnancy category X, lactation, reproductive cancer, thrombophlebitis, MI, hepatic tumors, hepatic disease, CAD, women 40 yr and over, CVA

Precautions: Depression, hypertension, renal disease, seizure disorders, lupus erythematosus, rheumatic disease, migraine headache, amenorrhea, irregular menses, breast cancer (fibrocystic), gallbladder disease, diabetes mellitus, heavy smoking, acute mononucleosis, sickle cell disease

Pharmacokinetics:

PO: Excreted in breast milk

🦷 **Drug interactions of concern to dentistry:**

• Decreased effectiveness of oral contraceptives: rifampin, barbiturates, antibiotics: Advise patient of a potential risk for decreased contraceptive action, to maintain compliance with oral contraceptive use while using antibiotics, and to consider the use of additional nonhormonal contraception

DENTAL CONSIDERATIONS:

General:

• Monitor vital signs every appointment due to cardiovascular side effects.

• Place on frequent recall to evaluate gingival inflammation, if present.

---

bold italic = life-threatening conditions   *For periodic updates, visit* **www.mosby.com**

• An increased incidence of dry socket has been reported after extraction.

• Consider semisupine chair position for patient comfort if GI side effects occur.

Teach patient/family:

• Need for good oral hygiene to prevent periodontal inflammation

• That smoking cessation decreases risk of serious adverse cardiovascular effects

---

orlistat

(or′li-stat)

Xenical

Drug class.: Antiobesity

Action: A reversible inhibitor of lipases; acts in the intestinal lumen to inhibit both gastric and pancreatic lipases, thereby preventing the metabolism of fats into absorbable fatty acids

Uses: Obesity management, including weight loss and maintenance in conjunction with a reduced-calorie diet; used in patients with a defined body mass index with other risk factors for cardiovascular disease

Dosage and routes:

• *Adult:* PO 120 mg tid with each meal containing fat; give during meal or up to 1 hr after meal

Available forms include: Caps 120 mg

Side effects/adverse reactions:

▼ *ORAL:* Gingiva and tooth disorder (not defined)

CNS: Headache, dizziness, sleep disruption, anxiety

GI: Oily spotting, flatus with discharge, fecal urgency, oily or fatty stool, increased defecation, fecal

incontinence, abdominal pain, *liver failure,* vomiting

RESP: Influenza, URI, LRI

GU: Menstrual irregularity, UTI

EENT: Otitis

INTEG: Rash, dry skin

MS: Back pain, myalgia, joint discomfort

MISC: Fatigue

Contraindications: Chronic malabsorption syndrome, cholestasis or hypersensitivity reactions to this product, lactation; organic causes of obesity should first be identified

Precautions: Adherence to dietary guidelines, supplemental fat-soluble vitamins may be required along with betacarotene, nephrolithiasis, pregnancy category B, use in children not established

Pharmacokinetics:

PO: Poor oral absorption (minimal), low plasma levels, highly plasma protein bound (99%), metabolized in intestinal wall, majority of dose passes through GI tract for fecal excretion.

🐾 **Drug interactions of concern to dentistry:**

• None reported

DENTAL CONSIDERATIONS

General:

• Although no dental drug interactions are reported, observe expected outcomes of systemically administered drugs.

• Severely obese patients may have type 2 diabetes or cardiovascular diseases.

• Consider semisupine chair position for patient comfort if GI side effects occur.

• Ensure that patient is following prescribed diet and regularly takes medication.

Consultations:
• Medical consult may be required to assess disease control.

Teach patient/family:
• Importance of updating health and drug history if physician makes any changes in evaluation or drug regimens

---

orphenadrine citrate

(or-fen'a-dreen)

Norflex

♣ Antiflex, Banflex, Flexoject, Myolin, Myotrol

Drug class.: Skeletal muscle relaxant, central acting

Action: Acts centrally to depress polysynaptic pathways to relax skeletal muscle, inhibit muscle spasm

Uses: Pain in musculoskeletal conditions

Dosage and routes:
• *Adult:* PO 100 mg bid; IM/IV 60 mg q12h

Available forms include: Tabs 100 mg; sus rel tabs 100 mg; inj IM/IV 30 mg/ml

Side effects/adverse reactions:

▼ *ORAL:* Dry mouth

CNS: Dizziness, weakness, drowsiness, headache, disorientation, insomnia, stimulation, hallucination, agitation, syncope

CV: Tachycardia, palpitation

GI: Nausea, vomiting, constipation

HEMA: Aplastic anemia

GU: Urinary hesitancy, retention

EENT: Pupil dilation, blurred vision, increased intraocular pressure, mydriasis

INTEG: Rash, pruritus, urticaria

Contraindications: Hypersensitivity, narrow-angle glaucoma, GI obstruction, myasthenia gravis, stenosing peptic ulcer, bladder neck obstruction, cardiospasm

Precautions: Pregnancy category not listed, children, cardiac disease, tachycardia, caution in lactation

Pharmacokinetics:
PO: Peak 2 hr, duration 4-6 hr, half-life 14 hr; metabolized in liver; excreted in urine (unchanged)

🦷 **Drug interactions of concern to dentistry:**
• Increased CNS effects: propoxyphene, CNS depressants, alcohol
• Increased anticholinergic effect: other anticholinergics

DENTAL CONSIDERATIONS
General:
• Consider semisupine chair position for patients with back pain.
• Patients on chronic drug therapy may rarely have symptoms of blood dyscrasias, which can include infection, bleeding, and poor healing.
• Assess salivary flow as a factor in caries, periodontal disease, and candidiasis.

Consultations:
• In a patient with symptoms of blood dyscrasias, request a medical consult for blood studies and postpone dental treatment until normal values are reestablished.
• Medical consult may be required to assess disease control.

Teach patient/family:
• Importance of good oral hygiene to prevent soft tissue inflammation
• Caution to prevent injury when using oral hygiene aids

When chronic dry mouth occurs, advise patient:

• To avoid mouth rinses with high alcohol content due to drying effects
• Of need for daily use of home fluoride products to prevent caries
• To use sugarless gum, frequent sips of water, or saliva substitutes

oseltamivir phosphate
(oh-sel′ta-me-veer)
Tamiflu
Drug class.: Antiviral

Action: Inhibits neuraminidase, which is essential for replication of influenza type A and B viruses
Uses: Uncomplicated acute illness due to influenza infection in adults who have been symptomatic for no more than 2 days; more effective against influenza type A virus; prophylaxis for adults and child >13 yr
Dosage and routes:
• *Adult and child >13 yr:* PO 75 mg bid × 5 days; initiate treatment within 2 days of onset of symptoms
• *Child >1 yr:* PO oral susp 30 mg bid if <15 kg (33 lb); 45 mg bid if >15 kg to 23 kg (>31 to 51 lb); 60 mg bid if >23 kg to 40 kg (>57 to 88 lb); 75 mg bid if >40 kg (>88 lb)
Prophylaxis (after exposure or close contact to flu)
• *Adult and child >13 yr:* PO 75 mg/day × 7 days (no doses approved for <13 yr)
Available forms include: Caps 75 mg; powder for oral susp 12 mg/ml in 100 ml
Side effects/adverse reactions:
CNS: Insomnia, vertigo, headache
GI: Nausea, vomiting, abdominal pain
RESP: Bronchitis, cough
MISC: Fatigue

Contraindications: Hypersensitivity
Precautions: Renal impairment, pregnancy category C, lactation
Pharmacokinetics:
PO: Readily absorbed, hepatic conversion to oseltamivir carboxylate, low plasma protein binding (3%), half-life 1-3 hr, excreted in urine (99%)
🦷 **Drug interactions of concern to dentistry:**
• None reported
DENTAL CONSIDERATIONS
General:
• Acute influenza patients are unlikely to be seen in the dental office except for dental emergencies.
• Consider semisupine chair position for patient comfort due to respiratory effects of disease.

oxandrolone
(ox-an′droe-lone)
Oxandrin
Drug class.: Androgenic anabolic steroid

Controlled Substance Schedule III
Action: Reverses catabolic tissue processes; promotes buildup of protein; increases erythropoietin production
Uses: Catabolic or tissue wasting processes, such as extensive surgery, burns, infection, or trauma; HIV wasting syndrome; Turner's syndrome
Dosage and routes:
• *Adult:* PO 2.5 mg bid-qid, not to exceed 20 mg qd × 2-3 wk
• *Child:* PO 0.25 mg/kg/day × 2-4 wk, not to exceed 3 mo

Available forms include: Tabs 2.5 mg

Side effects/adverse reactions:

CNS: Dizziness, headache, fatigue, tremors, paresthesia, flushing, sweating, anxiety, lability, insomnia

CV: Increased BP, *edema* (in cardiac patients)

GI: ***Cholestatic jaundice, peliosis hepatitis, liver cell tumors,*** nausea, vomiting, constipation, weight gain

HEMA: ***Increased prothrombin time,*** iron deficiency anemia

GU: ***Hematuria,*** amenorrhea, vaginitis, decreased libido, decreased breast size, clitoral hypertrophy, testicular atrophy, gynecomastia (males), priapism

EENT: Conjunctional edema, nasal congestion

INTEG: Rash, acneiform lesions, oily hair/skin, flushing, sweating, acne vulgaris, alopecia, hirsutism

ENDO: Abnormal GTT, decreased glucose tolerance, increased LDL

MS: Cramps, spasms

Contraindications: Severe renal disease, severe cardiac disease, severe hepatic disease, hypersensitivity, pregnancy category X, lactation, genital bleeding (abnormal), prostate or breast carcinoma in males, breast cancer in females with hypercalcemia

Precautions: Diabetes mellitus, CV disease, MI, increased risk of prostatic hypertrophy, prostatic carcinoma, virilization (women), increased prothrombin time

Pharmacokinetics:

PO: Metabolized in liver; excreted in urine; crosses placenta; excreted in breast milk

Drug interactions of concern to dentistry:

- Increased risk of bleeding: aspirin
- Edema: ACTH, adrenal steroids

DENTAL CONSIDERATIONS

General:

- Monitor vital signs every appointment due to cardiovascular side effects.
- Determine why the patient is taking the drug.
- Consider local hemostasis measures to prevent excessive bleeding.
- Short appointments and a stress reduction protocol may be required for anxious patients.
- If signs of anemia are observed in oral tissues, physician consult may be required.
- Avoid prescribing aspirin-containing products.

Consultations:

- Medical consult may be required to assess disease control and patient's ability to tolerate stress.
- Medical consult should include partial prothrombin or prothrombin times.

Teach patient/family:

- Importance of good oral hygiene to prevent soft tissue inflammation
- That secondary oral infection may occur; must see dentist immediately if infection occurs

---

oxaprozin

(ox'a-proe-zin)

Daypro

Drug class.: Nonsteroidal antiinflammatory

Action: Inhibits prostaglandin synthesis by interfering with cyclooxygenase needed for bio-

---

synthesis; possesses analgesic, antiinflammatory, antipyretic properties

Uses: Rheumatoid arthritis, osteoarthritis, and ankylosing spondylitis

Dosage and routes:
• *Adult:* PO 600-1200 mg daily; max dose 1800 mg/day

Available forms include: Tabs 600 mg

Side effects/adverse reactions:
▼ *ORAL:* Dry mouth, stomatitis, lichenoid reaction, oral ulceration
CNS: Dizziness, drowsiness, fatigue, tremors, confusion, insomnia, anxiety, depression
CV: Tachycardia, peripheral edema, palpitation, dysrhythmias
GI: ***Cholestatic hepatitis,*** nausea, anorexia, vomiting, diarrhea, jaundice, constipation, flatulence, cramps, peptic ulcer
HEMA: ***Blood dyscrasias***
GU: ***Nephrotoxicity: dysuria, hematuria, oliguria, azotemia***
EENT: Tinnitus, hearing loss, blurred vision
INTEG: Purpura, rash, pruritus, sweating, photosensitivity

Contraindications: Hypersensitivity, asthma, severe renal disease, severe hepatic disease

Precautions: Pregnancy category not established, lactation, children, bleeding disorders, GI disorders, cardiac disorders, hypersensitivity to other antiinflammatory agents, diabetes

Pharmacokinetics:
PO: Peak 1-2 hr, half-life 2-4 hr; 90%-99% plasma protein binding; metabolized in liver (inactive metabolites); excreted in urine (inactive metabolites)

💊 Drug interactions of concern to dentistry:
• GI ulceration, bleeding: aspirin, alcohol, corticosteroids
• Decreased action: salicylates
• Nephrotoxicity: acetaminophen (prolonged use and high doses)
• Possible risk of decreased renal function: cyclosporine
When prescribed for dental pain:
• Risk of increased effects: oral anticoagulants, oral antidiabetics, lithium, methotrexate
• Decreased antihypertensive effects of diuretics, β-adrenergic blockers, and ACE inhibitors

DENTAL CONSIDERATIONS
General:
• Patients on chronic drug therapy may rarely have symptoms of blood dyscrasias, which can include infection, bleeding, and poor healing.
• Assess salivary flow as a factor in caries, periodontal disease, and candidiasis.
• Avoid prescribing for dental use in pregnancy.
• Consider semisupine chair position for patients with arthritic disease.

Consultations:
• Medical consult may be required to assess disease control.
• In a patient with symptoms of blood dyscrasias, request a medical consult for blood studies and postpone dental treatment until normal values are reestablished.

Teach patient/family:
• Importance of good oral hygiene to prevent soft tissue inflammation
• Caution to prevent injury when using oral hygiene aids

When chronic dry mouth occurs, advise patient:
- To avoid mouth rinses with high alcohol content due to drying effects
- Of need for daily use of home fluoride products to prevent caries
- To use sugarless gum, frequent sips of water, or saliva substitutes

---

oxazepam
(ox-a′ze-pam)
Serax
♣ Apo-Oxazepam, Novoxapam
Drug class.: Benzodiazepine

Controlled Substance Schedule IV
Action: Produces CNS depression by interacting with a benzodiazepine receptor to facilitate the action of the inhibitory neurotransmitter γ-aminobutyric acid (GABA)
Uses: Anxiety, alcohol withdrawal
Dosage and routes:
Anxiety
- *Adult:* PO 10-30 mg tid-qid
Alcohol withdrawal
- *Adult:* PO 15-30 mg tid-qid
Available forms include: Caps 10, 15, 30 mg; tabs 15 mg
Side effects/adverse reactions:
▼ *ORAL:* Dry mouth
CNS: Dizziness, drowsiness, confusion, headache, anxiety, tremors, fatigue, depression, insomnia, hallucinations, paradoxic excitement, transient amnesia, syncope, hangover
CV: Orthostatic hypotension, ECG changes, tachycardia, hypotension
GI: Nausea, vomiting, anorexia, abdominal discomfort
EENT: Blurred vision, tinnitus, mydriasis
INTEG: Rash, dermatitis, itching

Contraindications: Hypersensitivity to benzodiazepines, narrow-angle glaucoma, psychosis, pregnancy category D, child <12 yr
Precautions: Elderly, debilitated, hepatic disease, renal disease
Pharmacokinetics:
PO: Peak 2-4 hr, half-life 5-15 hr; metabolized by liver; excreted by kidneys
🦷 **Drug interactions of concern to dentistry:**
- Increased effects: CNS depressants, alcohol, and anticonvulsant medications

DENTAL CONSIDERATIONS
General:
- Monitor vital signs every appointment due to cardiovascular side effects.
- Psychologic and physical dependence may occur with chronic administration.
- Geriatric patients are more susceptible to drug effects; use lower dose.
- Assess salivary flow as a factor in caries, periodontal disease, and candidiasis.
Consultations:
- Medical consult may be required to assess disease control.
Teach patient/family:
- To avoid mouth rinses with high alcohol content due to drying effects

---

oxcarbazepine
(ox-carb′az-e-peen)
Trileptal
Drug class.: Anticonvulsant

Action: Mechanism of antiseizure effect is unknown; the 10-monohydroxy-carbamazepine metabolite accounts for pharmacologic activ-

---

ity. May block sodium channels; inhibits seizure propagation and affects potassium conductance and calcium channels

Uses: Monotherapy or adjunctive therapy of partial seizures in adults with epilepsy; adjunctive therapy for partial seizures in children (4-16 yr) with epilepsy

Dosage and routes:

• *Adult:* PO initial 600 mg/day using bid regimen, doses may be increased to max of 1200 mg/day; patients taking other anticonvulsant drugs must be observed and plasma levels of other anticonvulsants must be monitored; patients should also be observed closely when switching to monotherapy

• *Child 4-16 yr:* PO initial dose 8-10 mg/kg, not to exceed 600 mg/day; give doses in bid regimen; target maintenance dose over 2 wk; final dose depends on patient's weight.

Available forms include: Tabs 150, 300, 600 mg

Side effects/adverse reactions:

▼ *ORAL:* Dry mouth (high doses), gingival overgrowth (infrequent), taste alterations, stomatitis

CNS: Dizziness, headache, somnolence, fatigue, insomnia, tremor, nervousness, altered thinking (high dose)

CV: Hypotension (high dose), bradycardia, palpitation, syncope

GI: Nausea, vomiting, abdominal pain, diarrhea, dyspepsia, constipation, gastritis

RESP: UTI, coughing, bronchitis

HEMA: Purpura (high doses), ***leukopenia, thrombocytopenia***

GU: UTI, urination frequency

EENT: Diplopia, nystagmus, rhinitis, vertigo, pharyngitis

INTEG: Rash, **SLE,** *Stevens-*

Johnson syndrome, toxic epidermal necrolysis, erythema multiforme, acne, dermatitis

META: Weight increase, hyponatremia, hypocalcemia, hyperglycemia, elevated liver enzymes

MS: Muscle weakness

MISC: Ataxia, leg edema

Contraindications: Hypersensitivity to this drug or carbamazepine

Precautions: Development of hyponatremia, withdraw drug slowly to avoid seizures, cognitive CNS adverse effects, decreases effect of oral contraceptives, caution when used with other anticonvulsants, renal impairment, pregnancy category C, lactation

Pharmacokinetics:

PO: Complete absorption, extensive hepatic metabolism to the 10-monohydroxy metabolite, may induce CYP450 3A4/5 enzymes, $T_{1/2}$ of parent drug and metabolite is 9 hr; plasma protein binding 40%, renal excretion.

🦷 **Drug interactions of concern to dentistry:**

• Possible increase in CNS depression: all CNS depressants, alcohol

• No dental drug interactions reported; CYP 450 3A4/5 enzyme inducers may decrease plasma levels

DENTAL CONSIDERATIONS

General:

• Monitor vital signs every appointment due to cardiovascular side effects.

• Patient on chronic drug therapy may rarely present with symptoms of blood dyscrasias, which can include infection, bleeding, and poor healing.

• Assess salivary flow as a factor in caries, periodontal disease, and candidiasis

• Consider semisupine chair position for patient comfort if GI side effects occur.

• Short appointments and a stress reduction protocol may be required for anxious patients.

• Determine type of epilepsy, seizure frequency, and quality of seizure control.

Consultations:

• In a patient with symptoms of blood dyscrasias, request a medical consult for blood studies and postpone treatment until normal values are reestablished.

• Medical consult may be required to assess disease control and patient's ability to tolerate stress.

Teach patient/family:

• Importance of good oral hygiene to prevent soft tissue inflammation

• To prevent trauma when using oral hygiene aids

When chronic dry mouth occurs, advise patient:

• To avoid mouth rinses with high alcohol content due to drying effects

• To use daily home fluoride products for anticaries effect

• To use sugarless gum, frequent sips of water, or saliva substitutes

---

oxidized cellulose
Oxycel, Surgicel

Drug class.: Cellulose hemostatic

Action: Mechanism unclear; may act physically to absorb blood and promote an artificial clot

Uses: Hemostasis in surgery, oral surgery, exodontia

Dosage and routes:

• *Adult and child:* TOP apply using sterile technique as needed; remove after bleeding stops, if possible, or leave in place if needed

Available forms include: TOP knitted fabric in pads, pledgets, and strips of various sizes

Side effects/adverse reactions:

CNS: Headache in epistaxis

EENT: Sneezing, burning in epistaxis

INTEG: Burning, stinging, encapsulation of fluid, foreign bodies

Contraindications: Hypersensitivity, large artery hemorrhage, oozing surfaces, implantation in bone deficit, placement around optic nerve and optic chiasm

Precautions: Do not autoclave; inactivation of topical thrombin

DENTAL CONSIDERATIONS

General:

• Apply dry; use only amount needed to control bleeding.

• Place loosely and avoid packing; remove excess before closure in surgery; irrigate first, then remove using sterile technique.

• Ensure therapeutic response: decreased bleeding in surgery.

• Can be left in situ when necessary, but should be removed once bleeding is controlled.

• Application of topical thrombin solution to the cellulose gauze will inactivate thrombin because of acidity.

---

oxtriphylline
(ox-trye'fi-lin)
Choledyl SA
♣ Apo-Oxitriphylline, PMS-Oxtriphylline

Drug class.: Choline salt of theophylline, bronchodilator

Action: Relaxes smooth muscle of respiratory system by block-

---

ing phosphodiesterase, increasing cAMP

Uses: Acute bronchial asthma, reversible bronchospasm in chronic bronchitis and COPD

Dosage and routes:

• *Adult and child >12 yr:* PO 200 mg qid

• *Child 2-12 yr:* PO 4 mg/kg q6h; may be increased to desired response, therapeutic level

Available forms include: Elix 100 mg/5 ml; syr 50 mg/5 ml; tabs 100, 200; sus rel tabs 400, 600 mg

Side effects/adverse reactions:

▼ *ORAL:* Bitter taste

CNS: Anxiety, restlessness, insomnia, dizziness, **convulsions,** headache, light-headedness, muscle twitching

CV: Palpitation, sinus tachycardia, hypotension

GI: Nausea, vomiting, anorexia, diarrhea, dyspepsia

RESP: Increased rate

INTEG: Flushing, urticaria

Contraindications: Hypersensitivity to xanthines, tachydysrhythmias

Precautions: Elderly, CHF, cor pulmonale, hepatic disease, active peptic ulcer disease, diabetes mellitus, hyperthyroidism, hypertension, children, pregnancy category C, glaucoma, prostatic hypertrophy

Pharmacokinetics:

PO: Peak 1 hr; metabolized in liver; excreted in urine, breast milk; crosses placenta

🦷 Drug interactions of concern to dentistry:

• Increased action: erythromycin (macrolides), ephedrine, xanthines, fluoroquinolones

• Decreased therapeutic effects: barbiturates, β-adrenergic blockers, nicotine

DENTAL CONSIDERATIONS

General:

• Evaluate respiration characteristics and rate.

• Consider semisupine chair position for patient comfort due to GI effects of disease.

• Short appointments and a stress reduction protocol may be required for anxious patients.

• Be aware that aspirin or sulfite preservatives in vasoconstrictor-containing products can exacerbate asthma.

• Acute asthmatic episodes may be precipitated in the dental office. Sympathomimetic inhalants should be available for emergency use.

• Discuss tobacco cessation for patients using tobacco.

---

oxybutynin chloride

(ox-i-byoo'ti-nin)

Ditropan, Ditropan XL

Drug class.: Antispasmodic

Action: Relaxes smooth muscles in urinary tract

Uses: Antispasmodic for neurogenic bladder, overactive bladder

Dosage and routes:

• *Adult:* PO 5 mg bid-tid, not to exceed 5 mg qid; XL formulation once-daily dosage

• *Child >5 yr:* PO 5 mg bid, not to exceed 5 mg tid

Available forms include: Syr 5 mg/5 ml; tabs 5 mg; ext rel tabs 5, 10 mg

Side effects/adverse reactions:

▼ *ORAL:* Dry mouth

CNS: Restlessness, dizziness, drowsiness, **convulsions,** confusion, insomnia, weakness, hallucinations

CV: Palpitation, tachycardia, hypotension
GI: Nausea, vomiting, anorexia, abdominal pain, constipation
GU: Dysuria, retention, hesitancy
EENT: Blurred vision, increased intraocular tension
INTEG: Urticaria, dermatitis
Contraindications: Hypersensitivity, GI obstruction, GI hemorrhage, GU obstruction, glaucoma, severe colitis, myasthenia gravis, unstable CV status in acute hemorrhage
Precautions: Pregnancy category C, lactation, suspected glaucoma, children <12 yr, hiatal hernia, esophageal reflux, coronary heart disease, CHF, hypertension
Pharmacokinetics:
PO: Onset 0.5-1 hr, peak 3-4 hr, duration 6-10 hr; metabolized by liver; excreted in urine
Drug interactions of concern to dentistry:
• Increased anticholinergic effect: anticholinergic drugs
• Increased depressant effect of both drugs: CNS depressants, alcohol
DENTAL CONSIDERATIONS
General:
• Assess salivary flow as a factor in caries, periodontal disease, and candidiasis.
• Monitor vital signs every appointment due to cardiovascular side effects.
• Avoid dental light in patient's eyes; offer dark glasses for patient comfort.
• Consider semisupine chair position for patient comfort if GI side effects occur.
Consultations:
• Physician should be informed if significant xerostomic side effects

occur (increased caries, sore tongue, problems eating or swallowing, difficulty wearing prosthesis) so a medication change can be considered.
Teach patient/family:
• Importance of good oral hygiene to prevent soft tissue inflammation
When chronic dry mouth occurs, advise patient:
• To avoid mouth rinses with high alcohol content due to drying effects
• Of need for daily use of home fluoride products to prevent caries
• To use sugarless gum, frequent sips of water, or saliva substitutes

---

oxycodone
(ox-i-koe'done)
Endocodone, M-Oxy, OxyContin, OxyFast, OxyIR, Percolone, Roxicodone, Roxicodone Intensol
♣ Supeudol
Combinations: Codoxy, Percocet-Demi, Percodan, Tylox
♣ Endodan, Percocet, Roxiprin
Drug class.: Synthetic opioid analgesic

Controlled Substance Schedule II, Canada N
Action: Interacts with opioid receptors in the CNS to alter pain perception
Uses: Moderate-to-severe pain, normally used in combination with aspirin or acetaminophen
Dosage and routes:
• *Adult:* PO 1-2 tabs q6h prn (usually in combination with nonopioid analgesics)
Moderate to severe pain (around the clock analgesia)
• *Adult:* PO immed release 10-30 mg q4h; con rel tabs are for use

only in opioid-tolerant patients; these doses are generally intended for cancer patients and not for use in general dental pain management
Available forms include: Tabs 5 mg; oral sol 5 mg/5 ml; oral sol concentrate 20 mg/ml, con rel tabs 10, 20, 40, 80, 160 mg; caps immed rel 5 mg; tabs immed rel 15, 30 mg

Side effects/adverse reactions:
▼ *ORAL:* Dry mouth
CNS: Drowsiness, dizziness, confusion, headache, sedation, euphoria
CV: Palpitation, bradycardia, tachycardia
GI: Nausea, vomiting, anorexia, constipation, cramps
*RESP: **Respiratory depression***
GU: Decreased urinary output, oliguria, dysuria, urinary retention
EENT: Tinnitus, blurred vision, miosis, diplopia
INTEG: Rash, urticaria, bruising, flushing, diaphoresis, pruritus
Contraindications: Hypersensitivity, addiction (narcotic)
Precautions: Addictive personality, pregnancy category B, lactation, increased intracranial pressure, MI (acute), severe heart disease, respiratory depression, hepatic disease, renal disease, child <18 yr, physical dependence

Pharmacokinetics:
PO: Onset 10-15 min, peak 0.5-1 hr, duration 4-5 hr; detoxified by liver; excreted in urine, breast milk; crosses placenta

Drug interactions of concern to dentistry:
• Increased effects with other CNS depressants: alcohol, other narcotics, sedative-hypnotics, skeletal muscle relaxants, phenothiazines, benzodiazepines

• Contraindication: MAO inhibitors
• Increased effects of anticholinergics

DENTAL CONSIDERATIONS
General:
• Monitor vital signs every appointment due to cardiovascular and respiratory side effects.
• Assess salivary flow as a factor in caries, periodontal disease, and candidiasis.
• Psychologic and physical dependence may occur with chronic administration.
• Determine why the patient is taking the drug.
Teach patient/family:
• To avoid mouth rinses with high alcohol content due to drying effects

---

oxymetazoline HCl (nasal)
(ox-i-met-az'oh-leen)
Afrin, Afrin Children's Nose Drops, Afrin Sinus, Allerest 12 Hour Nasal, Cheracol Nasal, Dristan 12 Hour, Nostrilla, NTZ Long-Acting, Sinex Long-Lasting, and many others

Drug class.: Nasal decongestant, sympathomimetic amine

Action: Produces vasoconstriction (rapid, long acting) of arterioles, thereby decreasing fluid exudation, mucosal engorgement
Uses: Nasal congestion
Dosage and routes:
• *Adult and child >6 yr:* Instill 2-3 gtt or sprays to each nostril bid
• *Child 2-6 yr:* Instill 2-3 gtt or sprays 0.025% sol bid, not to exceed 5 days

Available forms include: Sol 0.025%, 0.05%

Side effects/adverse reactions:

CNS: Anxiety, restlessness, tremors, weakness, insomnia, dizziness, fever, headache

GI: Nausea, vomiting, anorexia

EENT: Irritation, burning, sneezing, stinging, dryness, rebound congestion

INTEG: Contact dermatitis

Contraindications: Hypersensitivity to sympathomimetic amines

Precautions: Child <6 yr, elderly, diabetes, cardiovascular disease, hypertension, hyperthyroidism, increased ICP, prostatic hypertrophy, pregnancy category C, glaucoma

🦷 **Drug interactions of concern to dentistry:**

• Increased risk of hypertension: tricyclic antidepressants, but it requires adequate systemic absorption of oxymetazoline

DENTAL CONSIDERATIONS

General:

• Excessive use can lead to rebound congestion and cardiovascular side effects; follow recommended dosing intervals.

• Extensive nasal swelling and congestion may interfere with optimal use of nitrous oxide/oxygen sedation.

---

oxymetholone

(ox-i-meth'oh-lone)

Anadrol-50

♣ Anapolon 50

Drug class.: Androgenic anabolic steroid

Controlled Substance Schedule III

Action: Reverses catabolic tissue processes; promotes buildup of protein; increases erythropoietin production

Uses: Anemia associated with bone marrow failure and red cell production deficiencies; aplastic anemia, myelofibrosis, and anemia due to myelotoxic drugs

Dosage and routes:

Aplastic anemia

• *Adult and child:* PO 1-5 mg/kg/day, titrated to patient response, with minimum trial period of 3-6 mo

Available forms include: Tabs 50 mg

Side effects/adverse reactions:

CNS: Dizziness, headache, fatigue, tremors, paresthesia, flushing, sweating, anxiety, lability, insomnia

CV: **Edema** (in cardiac patients), increased BP

GI: **Peliosis hepatitis, liver cell tumors, cholestatic jaundice,** nausea, vomiting, constipation, weight gain

HEMA: **Increased prothrombin time, iron deficiency anemia**

GU: **Hematuria,** amenorrhea, vaginitis, decreased libido, decreased breast size, clitoral hypertrophy, testicular atrophy, gynecomastia (male), priapism

EENT: Conjunctival edema, nasal congestion

INTEG: Rash, acneiform lesions, oily hair/skin, flushing, sweating, acne vulgaris, alopecia, hirsutism

ENDO: Abnormal GTT, decreased glucose tolerance, increased LDL

MS: Cramps, spasms

Contraindications: Severe renal disease, severe cardiac disease, severe hepatic disease, hypersensitivity, pregnancy category X, lactation, genital bleeding (abnormal), prostate or breast carcinoma (males), breast cancer in females with hypercalcemia

Precautions: Diabetes mellitus, CV disease, MI, increased risk of prostatic hypertrophy, prostatic carcinoma, virilization (women), increased prothrombin time

Pharmacokinetics:

PO: Metabolized in liver, excreted in urine, crosses placenta, excreted in breast milk

Drug interactions of concern to dentistry:
• Increased risk of bleeding: aspirin
• Edema: ACTH, adrenal steroids

DENTAL CONSIDERATIONS

General:
• Monitor vital signs every appointment due to cardiovascular side effects.
• Determine why the patient is taking the drug.
• Consider local hemostasis measures to prevent excessive bleeding.
• Short appointments and a stress reduction protocol may be required for anxious patients.
• Avoid prescribing aspirin-containing products.

Consultations:
• Physician consult may be required if signs of anemia are observed in oral tissues.
• Medical consult may be required to assess disease control and patient's ability to tolerate stress.
• Medical consult should include partial prothrombin or prothrombin times.

Teach patient/family:
• Importance of good oral hygiene to prevent soft tissue inflammation
• That secondary oral infection may occur; must see dentist immediately if infection occurs

paclitaxel

(pac-li-tax′el)
Onxol, Taxol

Drug class.: Antineoplastic

Action: Obtained from Western Yew tree; unique action inhibits microtubule network reorganization essential for cell division

Uses: Metastatic ovarian cancer, non–small cell lung cancer; second-line treatment for AIDS-related Kaposi's sarcoma; adjuvant treatment of node-positive breast cancer sequential to a course of standard doxorubicin-containing combination chemotherapy

Dosage and routes:
• *Adult:* IV only, after oral premedication with PO dexamethasone, diphenhydramine, and H_2 antagonist, 135 mg/m^2 over 24 hr q3wk, depending on development of neutropenia; or IV 175 mg/m^2 over 3 hr q3wk

Available forms include: Inj 6 mg/ml in multiple-dose vials

Side effects/adverse reactions:

▼ *ORAL: Mucositis*

CV: Bradycardia, hypotension, abnormal ECG

GI: Nausea, vomiting, diarrhea, hepatic function impairment, ischemic colitis

RESP: Allergic dyspnea, infection

HEMA: Bone marrow depression, thrombocytopenia, anemia, bleeding

GU: UTIs

INTEG: Flushing, rash

METAB: Increased bilirubin, increased alk phosphatase, AST

MS: Myalgia, arthralgia

MISC: Alopecia, peripheral neuropathy, fever

Contraindications: Hypersensitivity, other products containing polyethylated castor oil, neutropenia <1500/mm^3

Precautions: Pregnancy category D, bone marrow depression, AV block, hepatic impairment, lactation, children, recent MI, angina pectoris, CHF history, current use of drug with effect on cardiac conduction system

Pharmacokinetics:

IV: Terminal half-life 5-17 hr; plasma protein binding 88%-98%, hepatic metabolism, excreted in bile

DENTAL CONSIDERATIONS

General:

• Consider semisupine chair position for patient comfort if GI side effects occur.

• Patients receiving chemotherapy may require palliative therapy for stomatitis.

• Patients on chronic drug therapy may rarely have symptoms of blood dyscrasias, which can include infection, bleeding, and poor healing.

Consultations:

• Medical consult may be required to assess disease control.

Teach patient/family:

• Importance of good oral hygiene to prevent soft tissue inflammation

• Caution to prevent trauma when using oral hygiene aids

pancrelipase

(pan-kre-li′pase)

Cotazym, Cotazyme-S, Creon-10, Creon-20, Creon-25, Ku-Zyme HP, Lipram, Pancrease, Pancrease MT 4, Ultrase MT, Viokase, Zymase

Drug class.: Digestant

Action: Pancreatic enzyme needed for proper pancreatic functioning in metabolizing lipids, proteins, and carbohydrates

Uses: Exocrine pancreatic secretion insufficiency, cystic fibrosis (digestive aid), steatorrhea, pancreatic enzyme deficiency, chronic pancreatitis

Dosage and routes:

• *Adult and child:* PO 1-3 caps/tabs ac or with meals, or 1 cap/tab with snack or 1-2 pdr pkt ac

Available forms include: Tabs 8000, 11,000, 30,000 U; caps 8000, 10,000, 12,000, 16,000 U; enteric-coated caps 4000, 4500, 5000, 10,000, 20,000, 25,000 U; powder 16,800 U

Side effects/adverse reactions:

▼ *ORAL:* Irritation to mucous membranes

GI: Anorexia, nausea, vomiting, diarrhea, cramps

RESP: Asthma attack

GU: Hyperuricuria, hyperuricemia

Contraindications: Allergy to pork

Precautions: Pregnancy category C

DENTAL CONSIDERATIONS

General:

• Consider semisupine chair position for patient comfort due to GI effects of disease.

• To avoid oral irritation, mouth should be rinsed or drug taken with liquid.

pantoprazole sodium
(pan-toe′pra-zole)
Protonix

Drug class.: Antisecretory, proton pump inhibitor

Action: Suppresses gastric acid production by binding to the hydrogen/potassium ATPase enzyme system to inhibit the final step in gastric acid production

Uses: Short-term treatment of erosive esophagitis associated with gastroesophageal reflux disease (GERD)

Dosage and routes:
• *Adult:* PO 40 mg day for up to 8 wk; for patients who have not healed, an additional 8 wk may be considered

Available forms include: Del rel tabs 40 mg

Side effects/adverse reactions:
▼ *ORAL:* Aphthous stomatitis, candidiasis, dry mouth, dysphagia (all <1%)
CNS: Headache, migraine, anxiety
CV: Arrhythmias, chest pain, palpitation (all <1%)
GI: Diarrhea, flatulence, abdominal pain, constipation, dyspepsia, gastroenteritis, nausea
RESP: Bronchitis, cough, URI
GU: Urinary frequency, UTI
EENT: Rhinitis, sinusitis
INTEG: Rash
META: Hyperglycemia, hyperlipidemia, abnormal liver function tests
MS: Back pain, asthenia, neck pain
MISC: Flu syndrome

Contraindications: Hypersensitivity

Precautions: Do not split, crush, or chew tablets; no data on children <18 yr, severe hepatic impairment, pregnancy category B, lactation

Pharmacokinetics:
PO (ENTERIC COATED TAB): Peak plasma levels 2.5 hr, bioavailability ~77%, plasma protein binding 98%, extensive hepatic metabolism (CYP450 2C19 enzyme system), excreted mainly in urine 71%, feces 18%

🦷 **Drug interactions of concern to dentistry:**
• No relevant drug interactions with other drugs metabolized by CYP450 2C19 enzymes
• No dental drug interactions reported; however with profound inhibition of gastric acid production, absorption of ketoconazole and amoxicillin could be affected

DENTAL CONSIDERATIONS
General:
• Consider semisupine chair position for patient comfort due to GI effects of disease.
• Question the patient about tolerance of NSAIDs or aspirin related to GI problem.
• Patients with gastroesophageal reflux disease may have oral symptoms, including burning mouth, secondary candidiasis, and signs of enamel erosion.
• Assess salivary flow as factor in caries, periodontal disease, and candidiasis.

Teach patient/family: *When chronic dry mouth occurs, advise patient:*
• To avoid mouth rinses with high alcohol content due to drying effects
• To use sugarless gum, frequent sips of water, or saliva substitutes
• To use daily home fluoride products for anticaries effect

papaverine HCl

(pa-pav′er-een)

Pavabid, Pavagen

Drug class.: Peripheral vasodilator

Action: Relaxes all smooth muscle, inhibits cyclic nucleotide phosphodiesterase, increasing intracellular cAMP and causing vasodilation

Uses: Arterial spasm resulting in cerebral and peripheral ischemia; myocardial ischemia associated with vascular spasm or dysrhythmias; angina pectoris; peripheral pulmonary embolism; visceral spasm as in ureteral, biliary, GI colic PVD; unapproved: with phentolamine or alprostadil for intracavernous injection for impotence

Dosage and routes:

• *Adult:* PO sus rel 150-300 mg q8-12h; IM/IV 30-120 mg q3h prn

Available forms include: Time rel caps 150 mg; inj IM/IV 30 mg/ml

Side effects/adverse reactions:

CNS: Headache, dizziness, drowsiness, sedation, vertigo, malaise, depression

*CV: **Tachycardia,*** increased BP

*GI: **Hepatotoxicity,*** nausea, anorexia, abdominal pain, constipation, diarrhea, jaundice, altered liver enzymes

RESP: Increased depth of respirations

INTEG: Flushing, sweating, rash, pruritus

Contraindications: Hypersensitivity, complete AV heart block

Precautions: Cardiac dysrhythmias, glaucoma, pregnancy category C, lactation, drug dependency, children, hepatic hypersensitivity, Parkinson's disease

Pharmacokinetics:

PO: Onset 30 sec, peak 1-2 hr, duration 3-4 hr

SUS REL: Onset erratic; 90% bound to plasma proteins; metabolized in liver; excreted in urine (inactive metabolites)

🥄 Drug interactions of concern to dentistry:

• Increased hypotension: alcohol, other drugs that may also lower blood pressure

DENTAL CONSIDERATIONS

General:

• Monitor vital signs every appointment due to cardiovascular and respiratory side effects.

• Short appointments and a stress reduction protocol may be required for anxious patients.

Consultations:

• Stress from dental procedures may compromise cardiovascular function; determine patient risk.

• Medical consult may be required to assess disease control.

Teach patient/family:

• To avoid mouth rinses with high alcohol content

• Importance of good oral hygiene to prevent soft tissue inflammation

paroxetine

(pa-rox′e-teen)

Paxil, Paxil CR

Drug class.: Antidepressant

Action: Selectively inhibits the uptake of serotonin in the brain

Uses: Depression, panic disorder, obsessive compulsive disorder, social anxiety disorder; unapproved: anxiety

---

bold italic = life-threatening conditions

Dosage and routes:
• *Adult:* PO initially 20 mg/day; increase 10 mg weekly to effect; not to exceed 50 mg/day
Panic disorder
• *Adult:* PO 10 mg qd
Available forms include: Tabs 10, 20, 30, 40 mg; caps modified rel 10, 20, 30, 40 mg; con rel tabs 12.5, 25 mg; oral susp 10 mg/5 ml

Side effects/adverse reactions:
▼ *ORAL: Dry mouth,* glossitis, aphthous stomatitis, (<0.1%), salivary gland enlargement (<0.1%), taste perversion
CNS: Somnolence, tremor, sweating, asthenia, insomnia, dizziness
CV: Palpitation, vasodilation, postural hypotension, syncope, tachycardia
GI: Constipation, nausea, diarrhea, anorexia, vomiting, flatulence, weight gain
RESP: Pharyngitis, yawning, respiratory complaints, coughing, rhinitis
GU: Decreased libido, sexual dysfunction, urinary frequency
EENT: Blurred vision, photophobia
SYST: Headache, myopathy, malaise, fever
METAB: Increased serum albumin, blood glucose, alk phosphatase

Contraindications: Hypersensitivity, MAO inhibitors

Precautions: Pregnancy category B, lactation, elderly, oral anticoagulants, renal or hepatic impairment, children, other serotonergic drugs

Pharmacokinetics:
PO: Peak plasma levels 5 hr (0.5-11 hr range), half-life 21 hr; highly protein bound; extensive first-pass metabolism; renal excretion

🦷 **Drug interactions of concern to dentistry:**
• Possible increased side effects: highly protein-bound drugs (aspirin), other antidepressants, alcohol
• Possible inhibition of fluoxetine metabolism: erythromycin, clarithromycin
• Increased half-life of diazepam

DENTAL CONSIDERATIONS
General:
• After supine positioning, have patient sit upright for at least 2 min to avoid orthostatic hypotension.
• Assess salivary flow as a factor in caries, periodontal disease, and candidiasis.
• Avoid dental light in patient's eyes; offer dark glasses for patient comfort.

Consultations:
• Medical consult may be required to assess disease control and patient's ability to tolerate stress.
• Physician should be informed if significant xerostomic side effects occur (increased caries, sore tongue, problems eating or swallowing, difficulty wearing prosthesis) so a medication change can be considered.

Teach patient/family: *When chronic dry mouth occurs, advise patient:*
• To avoid mouth rinses with high alcohol content due to drying effects
• Of need for daily use of home fluoride products to prevent caries
• To use sugarless gum, frequent sips of water, or saliva substitutes

pemirolast

(pe-mir'oh-last)

Alamast

Drug class.: Mast cell stabilizer

Action: Prevents release of mediators of inflammation from mast cells involved with type 1 immediate hypersensitivity reactions

Uses: Symptomatic treatment of ocular itching in allergic conjunctivitis

Dosage and routes:
• *Adult:* TOP 1-2 gtt in affected eye(s) qid

Available forms include: Sol 0.1%

Side effects/adverse reactions:

CNS: Headache

RESP: Bronchitis, cough

EENT: Rhinitis, burning eyes, dry eyes, ocular pain, sneezing, sinusitis, nasal congestion

ENDO: Dysmenorrhea

META: Increase in aminotransferases

MS: Back pain

MISC: Cold and flu symptoms

Contraindications: Hypersensitivity

Precautions: Pregnancy category C, lactation, children, do not wear contact lens if eyes are red, may affect soft contact lens, if no red eyes wait 10 min after using to place soft contacts

Pharmacokinetics:

TOP: Some systemic absorption occurs, detectable plasma levels noted, $T_{1/2}$ = 4.5 hr, hepatic metabolism, excreted in urine

🦷 Drug interactions of concern to dentistry:
• No dental drug interactions reported

DENTAL CONSIDERATIONS

General:
• Question patient about history of allergies to avoid using other potential allergens.
• Avoid dental light in patient's eyes; offer dark glasses for patient comfort.
• Protect patient's eyes from accidental spatter during dental treatment.

---

pemoline

(pem'oh-leen)

Cylert, Cylert Chewable

Drug class.: CNS stimulant

Controlled Substance Schedule IV

Action: Exact mechanism unknown; may act through dopaminergic mechanisms

Uses: Attention deficit disorder with hyperactivity

Dosage and routes:
• *Child >6 yr:* 37.5 mg in AM, increasing by 18.75 mg/wk, not to exceed 112.5 mg/day

Available forms include: Tabs 18.75, 37.5, 75 mg; chew tabs 37.5 mg

Side effects/adverse reactions:

CNS: Hyperactivity, insomnia, restlessness, dizziness, mild depression, headache, stimulation, irritability, aggressiveness, hallucinations, seizures, Tourette's syndrome, drowsiness, dyskinetic movements, fatigue, malaise

GI: Hepatic failure, nausea, anorexia, diarrhea, abdominal pain

MISC: Rashes, growth suppression in children, increased liver enzymes, hepatitis, jaundice

---

Contraindications: Hypersensitivity, hepatic insufficiency

Precautions: Renal disease, pregnancy category B, lactation, drug abuse, child <6 yr; liver function monitoring recommended

Pharmacokinetics:

PO: Peak 2-4 hr, duration 8 hr, half-life 12 hr; metabolized (50%) by liver; excreted (40%) by kidneys

⚗ Drug interactions of concern to dentistry: Increased irritability, stimulation: caffeine-containing products and food

DENTAL CONSIDERATIONS

General: Keep dental appointments short due to effects of disease.

Teach patient/family: Use of electric toothbrush for effective plaque control

---

penbutolol

(pen-byoo'toe-lole)

Levatol

Drug class.: Nonselective β-adrenergic blocker

Action: This is a nonselective β₁- and β₂-adrenergic antagonist. The antihypertensive mechanism of action is unclear, but it may include a reduction in cardiac output and inhibition of renin release by the renal juxtaglomerular apparatus. Peripheral resistance decreases with long-term use. The antianginal action (when indicated for this use) may be related to a decrease in myocardial oxygen demand and negative chronotropic and inotropic effects. The antiarrhythmic action (when indicated for this use) has been related to a reduction in spontaneous pacemaker firing and slowing of AV nodal conduction.

Uses: Hypertension alone or with thiazide diuretics

Dosage and routes:

• *Adult:* PO 20 mg qd, dose can be increased to 40-80 mg

Available forms include: Tabs 20 mg

Side effects/adverse reactions:

▼ *ORAL:* Dry mouth, taste alteration

CNS: Depression, hallucinations, dizziness, fatigue, lethargy, paresthesia, bizarre dreams, disorientation, syncope, vertigo, headache, sleep disturbances, nervousness, lethargy, behavior change, memory loss

CV: Bradycardia, hypotension, CHF, palpitation, AV block intensification, peripheral vascular insufficiency, vasodilation, chest pain, tachycardia

GI: Nausea, vomiting, diarrhea, colitis, constipation, cramps, hepatomegaly, gastric pain, acute pancreatitis, heartburn, anorexia

RESP: Dyspnea, respiratory dysfunction, *bronchospasm,* laryngospasm

HEMA: Agranulocytosis, thrombocytopenia, eosinophilia, leukopenia, pulmonary emboli, hyperlipidemia

GU: Impotence, decreased libido, UTIs, renal failure, urinary frequency or retention, dysuria, nocturia

EENT: Sore throat, *laryngospasm,* blurred vision, dry eyes

INTEG: Rash, pruritus, fever, photosensitivity

MS: Joint pain, arthralgia, muscle cramps, pain

META: Hyperglycemia, hypoglycemia

MISC: Facial swelling, weight change, Raynaud's phenomenon, lupus syndrome

Contraindications: Hypersensitivity to this drug, cardiac failure, cardiogenic shock, second- or third-degree heart block, bronchospastic disease, sinus bradycardia, CHF

Precautions: Diabetes mellitus, pregnancy category C, renal disease, lactation, hyperthyroidism, COPD, hepatic disease, children, myasthenia gravis, peripheral vascular disease, hypotension

Pharmacokinetics:

PO: Peak levels 1-1.5, half-life 3-5 hr; highly protein bound; hepatic metabolism

⚖ Drug interactions of concern to dentistry:

• Decreased hypotensive effect: indomethacin, NSAIDs

• Increased hypotension, myocardial depression: hydrocarbon inhalation anesthetics

• Hypertension, bradycardia: sympathomimetics (epinephrine, ephedrine)

• Slow metabolism of lidocaine

DENTAL CONSIDERATIONS

General:

• Monitor vital signs every appointment due to cardiovascular side effects.

• Patients on chronic drug therapy may rarely have symptoms of blood dyscrasias, which can include infection, bleeding, and poor healing.

• Limit use of sodium-containing products, such as saline IV fluids, for patients with a dietary salt restriction.

• Assess salivary flow as a factor in caries, periodontal disease, and candidiasis.

• After supine positioning, have patient sit upright for at least 2 min before standing to avoid orthostatic hypotension.

• Stress from dental procedures may compromise cardiovascular function; determine patient risk.

• Short appointments and a stress reduction protocol may be required for anxious patients.

• Use vasoconstrictor with caution, in low doses, and with careful aspiration.

• Avoid using gingival retraction cord containing epinephrine.

Consultations:

• In a patient with symptoms of blood dyscrasias, request a medical consult for blood studies and postpone dental treatment until normal values are reestablished.

• Medical consult may be required to assess disease control and patient's ability to tolerate stress.

Teach patient/family:

• Caution to prevent injury when using oral hygiene aids

• Importance of good oral hygiene to prevent soft tissue inflammation

• If taste alterations occur, consider drug effects

When chronic dry mouth occurs, advise patient:

• To avoid mouth rinses with high alcohol content due to drying effects

• Of need for daily use of home fluoride products to prevent caries

• To use sugarless gum, frequent sips of water, or saliva substitutes

penciclovir cream
(pen-sye'kloe-veer)
Denavir
Drug class.: Antiviral

Action: Inhibits viral DNA synthesis needed for viral replication in herpes simplex virus (HSV-1, HSV-2) following cellular kinase conversion to penciclovir triphosphate

Uses: Recurrent herpes labialis (cold sores)

Dosage and routes:
• *Adult:* TOP apply q2h while awake × 4 days; start treatment early in prodrome or when lesions first appear

Available forms include: Cream 1%, 2 g tube

Side effects/adverse reactions:
▼ *ORAL:* Taste alteration
CNS: Headache
INTEG: Hyperthesia, local anesthesia, pruritus, rash
MISC: Allergic reaction, pain

Contraindications: Hypersensitivity

Precautions: Acyclovir-resistant herpes viruses, patients <18 yr, use on mucous membranes not recommended, avoid applications near the eye, pregnancy category B, lactation

Pharmacokinetics:
TOP: Not detected in plasma or urine

DENTAL CONSIDERATIONS
General:
• Use in immunocompromised patients not established.
• Postpone dental treatment when oral herpetic lesions are present.

Teach patient/family:
• To dispose of toothbrush or other contaminated oral hygiene devices used during period of infection to prevent reinoculation of herpetic infection
• To apply with a finger cot or latex glove to prevent herpes infection on fingers

penicillin G benzathine
(pen-i-sill'in)
Bicillin L-A, Permapen
✚ Megacillin
Drug class.: Benzathine salt of natural penicillin

Action: Interferes with cell wall replication of susceptible organisms; osmotically unstable cell wall swells and bursts from osmotic pressure

Uses: Respiratory infections, scarlet fever, erysipelas, otitis media, pneumonia, skin and soft tissue infections, bejel, pinta, yaws; effective for gram-positive cocci *(Staphylococcus, S. pyogenes, S. viridans, S. faecalis, S. bovis, S. pneumoniae),* gram-negative cocci *(N. gonorrhoeae),* gram-positive bacilli *(B. anthracis, C. perfringens, C. tetani, C. diphtheriae, L. monocytogenes),* gram-negative bacilli *(E. coli, P. mirabilis, Salmonella, Shigella, Enterobacter, S. moniliformis),* spirochetes *(T. pallidum),* Actinomyces

Dosage and routes:
Early syphilis
• *Adult:* IM 2.4 million U in single dose

Prophylaxis of rheumatic fever, glomerulonephritis
• *Adult and child >60 lb:* IM 1.2 million U in single dose q2-3wk
• *Child <60 lb:* IM 600,000 U in single dose

italic = common side effects

Upper respiratory infections (group A streptococcal)
• *Adult:* IM 1.2 million U in single dose
• *Child >27 kg:* IM 900,000 U in single dose
• *Child <27 kg:* IM 50,000 U/kg in single dose
Available forms include: Inj IM 300,000, 600,000 U/ml; 1,200,000; 2,400,000, 3,000,000 U/dose
Side effects/adverse reactions:
▼ *ORAL: Candidiasis,* glossitis
*CNS: **Coma, convulsions,** lethargy, hallucinations, anxiety, depression, twitching
GI: Nausea, vomiting, diarrhea, increased AST/ALT, abdominal pain, colitis
*HEMA: **Bone marrow depression, granulocytopenia,** anemia, increased bleeding time
*GU: **Oliguria, proteinuria, hematuria, vaginal moniliasis, glomerulonephritis***
*INTEG: **Exfoliative dermatitis,** rash, urticaria, hives
META: Hyperkalemia, hypokalemia, alkalosis, hypernatremia
*MISC: **Anaphylaxis***
Contraindications: Hypersensitivity to penicillins; neonates
Precautions: Hypersensitivity to cephalosporins, pregnancy category B
Pharmacokinetics:
IM: Very slow absorption, hydrolyzed to penicillin G, duration 21-28 days, half-life 30-60 min; excreted in urine, breast milk; crosses placenta
🦷 **Drug interactions of concern to dentistry:**
• Decreased antimicrobial effect of penicillin: tetracyclines, erythromycins, lincomycins
• Increased penicillin concentrations: aspirin, probenecid
• Suspected increased risk of methotrexate toxicity
• Oral contraceptives: advise patient of a potential risk for decreased contraceptive action, to maintain compliance with oral contraceptive use while using antibiotics, and to consider the use of additional nonhormonal contraception

DENTAL CONSIDERATIONS
General:
• Take precautions regarding allergy to medication.
• Determine why the patient is taking the drug.
• Place on frequent recall to evaluate healing response.
Consultations:
• Medical consult may be required to assess disease control.
Teach patient/family: *When used for dental infection, advise patient:*
• To report sore throat, oral burning sensation, fever, fatigue, any of which could indicate superinfection
• To take at prescribed intervals and complete dosage regimen
• To immediately notify the dentist if signs or symptoms of infection increase

penicillin V potassium/ penicillin V
Beepen-K, Veetids
♣ Apo-Pen-VK, Nadopen-VK, NovoPen-VK, Nu-Pen-VK, Pen-Vee K, PVFK

Drug class.: Semisynthetic penicillin

Action: Interferes with cell wall

replication of susceptible organisms; the cell wall, rendered osmotically unstable, swells and bursts from osmotic pressure

Uses: Effective for gram-positive cocci *(S. aureus, S. viridans, S. faecalis, S. bovis, S. pneumoniae),* gram-negative cocci *(N. gonorrhoeae, N. meningitidis),* gram-positive bacilli *(B. anthracis, C. perfringens, C. tetani, C. diphtheriae),* gram-negative bacilli *(S. moniliformis),* spirochetes *(T. pallidum), Actinomyces, Peptococcus,* and *Peptostreptococcus* species

Dosage and routes:
Pneumococcal/staphylococcal infections
• *Adult:* PO 250-500 mg q6h
• *Child <12 yr:* PO 25,000-90,000 U/kg/day in 3-6 divided doses (125 mg = 200,000 U)

Streptococcal infections
• *Adult:* PO 250-500 mg q6-8h × 10 days

Prevention of recurrence of rheumatic fever/chorea
• *Adult:* PO 125-250 mg bid continuously

Vincent's infection of oropharynx
• *Adult:* PO 250-500 mg q6-8h

Available forms include: Tabs 250, 500 mg; film-coated tabs 250, 500 mg; powder for oral susp 125, 250 mg/5 ml

Side effects/adverse reactions:
▼ *ORAL:* Candidiasis, glossitis, stomatitis, black hairy tongue, dry mouth, altered taste
*CNS: **Depression, coma, convulsions,** lethargy, hallucinations, anxiety, twitching*
GI: Nausea, vomiting, diarrhea, abdominal pain, colitis, anorexia
*HEMA: **Bone marrow depression, granulocytopenia,*** eosinophilia, anemia, increased bleeding time

*GU: **Oliguria, proteinuria, hematuria, vaginitis, moniliasis, glomerulonephritis***
META: Hyperkalemia, hypokalemia, alkalosis; allergy symptoms: pruritus, urticaria, angioedema, bronchospasm, anaphylaxis

Contraindications: Hypersensitivity to penicillins; neonates

Precautions: Hypersensitivity to cephalosporins, pregnancy category B, lactation

Pharmacokinetics:
PO: Peak 30-60 min, duration 6-8 hr, half-life 30 min; excreted in urine, breast milk

🦷 Drug interactions of concern to dentistry:
• Decreased antimicrobial effectiveness of penicillin: tetracyclines, erythromycins, lincomycins
• Increased penicillin concentrations: probenecid
• Oral contraceptives: advise patient of a potential risk for decreased contraceptive action, to maintain compliance with oral contraceptive use while using antibiotics, and to consider the use of additional nonhormonal contraception

DENTAL CONSIDERATIONS
General:
• Take precautions regarding allergy to medication.
• Determine why the patient is taking the drug.
• If used for dental infection, place on frequent recall to evaluate healing response.

Consultations:
• Medical consult may be required to assess disease control.

Teach patient/family: *When used for dental infection, advise patient:*
• To report sore throat, oral burning

sensation, fever, fatigue, any of which could indicate superinfection
• To take at prescribed intervals and complete dosage regimen
• To immediately notify the dentist if signs or symptoms of infection increase

---

pentamidine/ pentamidine isethionate

(pen-tam'i-deen)

NebuPent, Pentam 300

♣ Pentacarinat, Pneumopent

Drug class.: Antiprotozoal

Action: Interferes with DNA/RNA synthesis in protozoa

Uses: *P. carinii* infections in immunocompromised patients

Dosage and routes:
• *Adult and child:* IV/IM 4 mg/kg/day × 2 wk; nebuliz 600 mg/6 ml NS via specific nebulizer

Available forms include: Inj IV/IM 300 mg/vial; aerosol 300 mg/vial

Side effects/adverse reactions:

▼ *ORAL:* Bad taste (metallic), dry mouth, gingivitis, ulcerations or abscess, hypersalivation

CNS: Disorientation, hallucinations, dizziness

CV: Hypotension, ventricular tachycardia, ECG abnormalities

*GI: Nausea, vomiting, anorexia, **acute pancreatitis,** increased AST/ALT*

*HEMA: **Leukopenia, thrombocytopenia,** anemia*

*GU: **Acute renal failure***

INTEG: Sterile abscess, pain at injection site, pruritus, urticaria, rash

META: Hyperkalemia, hypocalcemia, hypoglycemia

Precautions: Blood dyscrasias, hepatic disease, renal disease, diabetes mellitus, cardiac disease, hypocalcemia, pregnancy category C

Pharmacokinetics:

IV/IM: Excreted unchanged in urine (66%)

🦷 **Drug interactions of concern to dentistry:**
• Nephrotoxicity: aminoglycosides, polymyxin B, vancomycin

DENTAL CONSIDERATIONS

General:
• Monitor vital signs every appointment due to cardiovascular side effects.
• Patients on chronic drug therapy may rarely have symptoms of blood dyscrasias, which can include infection, bleeding, and poor healing.
• Place on frequent recall to evaluate healing response.
• Assess salivary flow as a factor in caries, periodontal disease, and candidiasis.
• Consider semisupine chair position for patients with respiratory disease.
• For inhalation dosage forms, rinse mouth with water after each dose to prevent dryness.
• Place on frequent recall due to oral side effects.

Consultations:
• In a patient with symptoms of blood dyscrasias, request a medical consult for blood studies and postpone dental treatment until normal values are reestablished.
• Medical consult may be required to assess disease control.

Teach patient/family:
• That secondary oral infection may occur; must see dentist immediately if infection occurs

---

bold italic = life-threatening conditions   *For periodic updates, visit* **www.mosby.com**

• Importance of good oral hygiene to prevent soft tissue inflammation
• Caution to prevent injury when using oral hygiene aids
• Importance of dietary suggestions to maintain oral and systemic health

When chronic dry mouth occurs, advise patient:

• To avoid mouth rinses with high alcohol content due to drying effects
• Of need for daily use of home fluoride products to prevent caries
• To use sugarless gum, frequent sips of water, or saliva substitutes

---

pentazocine HCl/ pentazocine lactate

(pen-taz′oh-seen)

Talwin, Talwin NX

Drug class.: Synthetic opioid/ mixed agonist/antagonist

Controlled Substance Schedule IV

Action: Interacts with opioid receptors in the CNS to alter pain perception

Uses: Moderate-to-severe pain alone or in combination with aspirin or acetaminophen

Dosage and routes:
• *Adult:* PO 50-100 mg q3-4h prn, not to exceed 600 mg/day; IV/ IM/SC 30 mg q3-4h prn, not to exceed 360 mg/day

Available forms include: SC/IM/ IV 30 mg/ml; tabs (NX) 50 mg in combination with 0.5 mg naloxone

Side effects/adverse reactions:

▼ *ORAL:* Dry mouth

CNS: Drowsiness, dizziness, confusion, headache, sedation, euphoria, hallucinations

CV: Palpitation, bradycardia, tachycardia, decreased BP (high doses)

GI: Nausea, vomiting, anorexia, constipation, cramps

*RESP: **Respiratory depression***

GU: Increased urinary output, dysuria

EENT: Tinnitus, blurred vision, miosis, diplopia

INTEG: Rash, urticaria, bruising, flushing, diaphoresis, pruritus

Contraindications: Hypersensitivity, addiction (narcotic)

Precautions: Addictive personality, pregnancy category B, lactation, increased intracranial pressure, head injury, MI (acute), severe heart disease, respiratory depression, hepatic disease, renal disease, children <18 yr, acute abdominal conditions, Addison's disease, prostatic hypertrophy

Pharmacokinetics:

SC/IM: Onset 15-30 min, peak 1-2 hr, duration 2-4 hr

IV: Onset 2-3 min, duration 4-6 hr Half-life 2-3 hr; extensive first-pass metabolism with less than 20% entering circulation; metabolized by liver; excreted by kidneys; crosses placenta

🦷 **Drug interactions of concern to dentistry:**
• Increased effects: all CNS depressants, alcohol
• Contraindication: MAO inhibitors
• Do not mix in solutions or syringe with barbiturates
• Additive side effects of opioid agonists
• Increased effects of anticholinergics
• Decreased effects of opioid agonists

---

italic = common side effects

DENTAL CONSIDERATIONS
General:
• Monitor vital signs every appointment due to cardiovascular and respiratory side effects.
• Assess salivary flow as a factor in caries, periodontal disease, and candidiasis.
• Consider semisupine chair position for patient comfort if GI side effects occur.
• Psychologic and physical dependence may occur with chronic administration.

Teach patient/family: *When chronic dry mouth occurs, advise patient:*
• To avoid mouth rinses with high alcohol content due to drying effects
• Of need for daily use of home fluoride products to prevent caries
• To use sugarless gum, frequent sips of water, or saliva substitutes

---

pentobarbital/ pentobarbital sodium
(pen-toe-bar′bi-tal)
Nembutal Sodium
✤ Nova-Rectal, Novopentobarb
Drug class.: Sedative-hypnotic barbiturate

Controlled Substance Schedule II, Canada C

Action: Depresses activity in brain cells, primarily in reticular activating system in brainstem; selectively depresses neurons in posterior hypothalamus, limbic structures
Uses: Insomnia, sedation, preoperative medication, increased intracranial pressure, dental anesthetic

Dosage and routes:
• *Adult:* PO 100-200 mg hs; IM 150-200 mg hs; IV 100 mg initially, then up to 500 mg; rec 120-200 mg hs
• *Child:* IM 3-5 mg/kg, not to exceed 100 mg
• *Child 2 mo-1 yr:* Rec 30 mg
• *Child 1-4 yr:* Rec 30-60 mg
• *Child 5-12 yr:* Rec 60 mg
• *Child 12-14 yr:* Rec 60-120 mg
Available forms include: Caps 50, 100 mg; elix 20 mg/5 ml; powder, rec supp 30, 60, 120, 200 mg; inj IM/IV 50 mg/ml
Side effects/adverse reactions:
CNS: Lethargy, drowsiness, hangover, **CNS depression,** dizziness, paradoxic stimulation in elderly and children, light-headedness, dependence, mental depression, slurred speech
CV: Hypotension, bradycardia, syncope
GI: Nausea, vomiting, diarrhea, constipation, epigastric pain, liver damage (long-term use)
RESP: **Depression, apnea, laryngospasm, bronchospasm,** circulatory collapse, hypoventilation
HEMA: **Agranulocytosis, thrombocytopenia, megaloblastic anemia** (long-term treatment)
INTEG: Rash, **Stevens-Johnson syndrome,** urticaria, pain, abscesses at injection site, angioedema, thrombophlebitis
Contraindications: Hypersensitivity to barbiturates, respiratory depression, addiction to barbiturates, severe liver/renal impairment, porphyria, uncontrolled pain
Precautions: Anemia, pregnancy category D, lactation, hepatic disease, renal disease, hypertension, elderly, acute/chronic pain

---

bold italic = life-threatening conditions *For periodic updates, visit* **www.mosby.com**

Pharmacokinetics:
PO: Onset 15-30 min, duration 4-6 hr
REC: Onset slow, duration 4-6 hr
Half-life 15-48 hr; metabolized by liver; excreted by kidneys (metabolites)

⚖ Drug interactions of concern to dentistry:
• Hepatotoxicity: halogenated-hydrocarbon anesthetics
• Increased CNS depression: alcohol, all other CNS depressants
• Increased metabolism of carbamazepine, tricyclic antidepressants, corticosteroids
• Decreased half-life of doxycycline

DENTAL CONSIDERATIONS
General:
• Determine why the patient is taking the drug.
• Monitor vital signs every appointment due to cardiovascular side effects. Evaluate respiration characteristics and rate.
• Patients on chronic drug therapy may rarely have symptoms of blood dyscrasias, which can include infection, bleeding, and poor healing.
When used for sedation in dentistry:
• Assess vital signs before use and q30min after use as sedative.
• Observe respiratory dysfunction: respiratory depression, character, rate, rhythm; hold drug if respirations <10/min or if pupils dilated.
• After supine positioning, have patient sit upright for at least 2 min before standing to avoid orthostatic hypotension.
• Have someone drive patient to and from dental office when used for conscious sedation.

• Barbiturates induce liver microsomal enzymes, which alter the metabolism of other drugs.
• Geriatric patients are more susceptible to drug effects; use lower dose.

Consultations:
• In a patient with symptoms of blood dyscrasias, request a medical consult for blood studies and postpone dental treatment until normal values are reestablished.

Teach patient/family:
• To avoid driving or other activities requiring alertness
• To avoid alcohol ingestion or CNS depressants; serious CNS depression may result
• To avoid OTC preparations (antihistamines, cold remedies) that contain CNS depressants

---

pentoxifylline
(pen-tox-i′fi-leen)
Trental
Drug class.: Hemorheologic agent

Action: Decreases blood viscosity, increases blood flow to affected microcirculation, and enhances tissue oxygenation in chronic peripheral arterial disease

Uses: Intermittent claudication related to chronic occlusive arterial disease of the limbs

Dosage and routes:
• *Adult:* PO 400 mg tid with meals
Available forms include: Con rel tabs 400 mg; tabs 400 mg

Side effects/adverse reactions:
▼ *ORAL:* Dry mouth, thirst, bad taste
CNS: Headache, anxiety, tremors, confusion, dizziness, drowsiness, nervousness, agitation, seizures
CV: Angina, dysrhythmias, palpita-

tion, hypotension, chest pain, dyspnea, edema

GI: Nausea, vomiting, anorexia, bloating, belching, constipation, dyspepsia, cholecystitis

EENT: Blurred vision, earache, sore throat, conjunctivitis

INTEG: Rash, pruritus, urticaria, brittle fingernails

MISC: Epistaxis, flulike symptoms: laryngitis, nasal congestion, leukopenia, malaise, weight changes, lymphedema

Contraindications: Hypersensitivity to this drug or xanthines

Precautions: Pregnancy category C, angina pectoris, cardiac disease, lactation, children, impaired renal function

Pharmacokinetics:

PO: Peak 1 hr, half-life 0.5-1 hr; degradation in liver; excreted in urine

DENTAL CONSIDERATIONS

General:

• Monitor vital signs every appointment due to cardiovascular side effects.

• Assess salivary flow as a factor in caries, periodontal disease, and candidiasis.

• Stress from dental procedures may compromise cardiovascular function; determine patient risk.

• Short appointments and a stress reduction protocol may be required for anxious patients.

• Talk with patient about potential systemic diseases (e.g., diabetes, CV disease) that may be associated with claudication.

Consultations:

• Medical consult may be required to assess disease control and patient's ability to tolerate stress.

Teach patient/family:

• Importance of good oral hygiene to prevent soft tissue inflammation

• Caution to prevent injury when using oral hygiene aids

When chronic dry mouth occurs, advise patient:

• To avoid mouth rinses with high alcohol content due to drying effects

• Of need for daily use of home fluoride products to prevent caries

• To use sugarless gum, frequent sips of water, or saliva substitutes

---

pergolide mesylate

(per′go-lide)

Permax

Drug class.: Antiparkinson agent

Action: Dopamine receptor agonist for D_1 and D_2 receptors

Uses: Adjunctive treatment of Parkinson's disease

Dosage and routes:

• *Adult:* PO initial 0.05 mg × 2 days; gradually increase by 0.1-0.15 mg/day q 3rd day over next 12 days. Doses can then be increased by 0.25 mg/day q 3rd day. Average dose 3 mg/day; max dose 5 mg/day usually in 3 divided doses/day.

Available forms include: Tabs 0.05, 0.25, 1 mg

Side effects/adverse reactions:

▼ *ORAL: Dry mouth,* sialadenitis, aphthous stomatitis

CNS: Dyskinesia, hallucinations, somnolence, confusion, dizziness, headache, insomnia, tremor, extrapyramidal syndrome, anxiety, psychosis

CV: Postural hypotension, syncope, palpitation, vasodilation

GI: Nausea, constipation, diarrhea, abdominal pain, dyspepsia

---

RESP: Dyspnea
HEMA: Anemia
GU: Frequency, UTI
EENT: Rhinitis, diplopia
INTEG: Sweating, rash
MS: Back pain, neck pain, myalgia, twitching, arthralgia
MISC: Flulike syndrome, fever, peripheral edema

Contraindications: Hypersensitivity to this drug or ergot derivatives

Precautions: Symptomatic hypotension, cardiac dysrhythmias, dose adjustment for patients on levodopa, discontinue drug slowly, pregnancy category B, lactation, children

Pharmacokinetics:
PO: Plasma protein binding 90%, metabolized, urinary excretion, half-life 27 hr

⚡ Drug interactions of concern to dentistry:
• Decreased action: phenothiazines, haloperidol, droperidol, thiothixenes, and metoclopramide

DENTAL CONSIDERATIONS
General:
• Monitor vital signs every appointment due to cardiovascular side effects.
• Short appointments may be required due to disease effects on musculature.
• Use precaution if sedation or general anesthesia is required; risk of hypotensive episode.
• After supine positioning have patient sit upright for at least 2 min before standing to avoid orthostatic hypotension.
• Assess salivary flow as a factor in caries, periodontal disease, and candidiasis.
• Assess for presence of extrapyramidal motor symptoms, such as tardive dyskinesia and akathisia. Extrapyramidal motor activity may complicate dental treatment.
• Consider semisupine chair position for patient comfort due to GI effects of drug.

Consultations:
• Medical consult may be required to assess disease control.

Teach patient/family:
• Use of electric toothbrush if patient has difficulty holding conventional devices
• Importance of updating health history/drug record if physician makes any changes in evaluation or drug regimens
When chronic dry mouth occurs, advise patient:
• To avoid mouth rinses with high alcohol content due to drying effects
• Of need for daily use of home fluoride products to prevent caries
• To use sugarless gum, frequent sips of water, or saliva substitutes

---

perindopril erbumine
(per-in'doe-pril)
Aceon

Drug class.: Angiotensin-converting enzyme (ACE) inhibitor

Action: Selectively suppresses renin-angiotensin-aldosterone system; inhibits ACE; prevents conversion of angiotensin I to angiotensin II; results in dilation of arterial and venous vessels

Uses: Essential hypertension as monotherapy or in combination with other antihypertensive medication

---

italic = common side effects

Dosage and routes:
Hypertension
• *Adult:* PO 4 mg qd; can be titrated upward to max of 16 mg/day; doses can be given bid if needed
• *Adult >65 yr:* PO 4 mg in 1 or 2 divided doses; daily dose limit 8 mg. Note: May have less efficacy in African-American patients
Available forms include: Tabs 2, 4, 8 mg

Side effects/adverse reactions:
▼ *ORAL:* **Angioedema (lips, tongue, mucous membranes),** dry mouth, taste disturbances
CNS: Orthostatic hypotension, headache, light-headedness, dizziness, nervousness
CV: Palpitation, edema
GI: Dyspepsia, nausea, diarrhea, abdominal pain, vomiting
RESP: Cough, URI
HEMA: **Agranulocytosis, neutropenia**
GU: Proteinuria, UTI, male sexual dysfunction
EENT: Sinusitis, ear infection, rhinitis, pharyngitis, tinnitus
INTEG: Rash
META: Hyperkalemia, ALT increase, triglyceride increase
MS: Asthenia, back pain, hypertonia, myalgia
MISC: **Anaphylaxis,** fever, upper extremity pain

Contraindications: Hypersensitivity to this drug or other ACE inhibitors, patients with a history of angioedema to other ACE inhibitors, pregnancy (second and third trimesters)

Precautions: Renal insufficiency, hypertension with CHF, severe CHF, renal artery stenosis, autoimmune disease, collagen vascular disease, pregnancy category C (first trimester); pregnancy category D (second and third trimesters), lactation

Pharmacokinetics:
PO: Absolute bioavailability 20%-30%, metabolized to active metabolite, perindoprilat, peak plasma levels 1 hr, active metabolite 3-4 hr; protein binding 10%-20%, hepatic metabolism, excreted mostly in urine (75%)

🦷 **Drug interactions of concern to dentistry:**
• Decreased hypotensive effects: NSAIDs, aspirin
• Increased hypotension: caution in use of other drugs that have hypotensive effects

DENTAL CONSIDERATIONS
General:
• Monitor vital signs every appointment due to cardiovascular side effects.
• Limit use of sodium-containing products such as saline IV fluids for those patients with a dietary salt restriction.
• Short appointments and a stress reduction protocol may be required for anxious patients.
• Stress from dental procedures may compromise cardiovascular function; determine patient risk.
• After supine positioning, have patient sit upright for at least 2 min to avoid orthostatic hypotension.
• Use precaution if sedation or general anesthesia is required; risk of hypotensive episode.
• Assess salivary flow as a factor in caries, periodontal disease, and candidiasis.
• Consider semisupine chair position for patient comfort if GI or respiratory side effects occur.

• Patients on chronic drug therapy may rarely have symptoms of blood dyscrasias, which can include infection, bleeding, and poor healing.

Consultations:

• In a patient with symptoms of blood dyscrasias, request a medical consult for blood studies and postpone treatment until normal values are reestablished.

• Medical consult may be required to assess disease control and patient's ability to tolerate stress.

Teach patient/family:

• Importance of updating health and drug history if physician makes any changes in evaluation or drug regimens

• Importance of good oral hygiene to prevent soft tissue inflammation

• To prevent trauma when using oral hygiene aids

When chronic dry mouth occurs, advise patient:

• To avoid mouth rinses with high alcohol content due to drying effects

• To use daily home fluoride products for anticaries effect

• To use sugarless gum, frequent sips of water, or saliva substitutes

---

perphenazine

(per-fen'a-zeen)

Trilafon

♣ APO-Perphenazine, PMS Perphenazine

Drug class.: Phenothiazine antipsychotic

Action: Blocks neurotransmission at dopaminergic synapses in the cerebral cortex, hypothalamus, and limbic system; exhibits strong peripheral α-adrenergic, anticholinergic blocking action; mechanism for antipsychotic effects is unclear

Uses: Psychotic disorders, schizophrenia, alcoholism, nausea, vomiting

Dosage and routes:

Nausea/vomiting/alcoholism/intractable hiccups

• *Adult:* IM 5-10 mg prn, max 15 mg in ambulatory patients, 30 mg in hospitalized patients; PO 8-16 mg/day in divided doses, up to 24 mg; IV not to exceed 5 mg, give diluted or slow IV drip

Psychiatric use in hospitalized patients

• *Adult:* PO 8-16 mg bid-qid, gradually increased to desired dose, not to exceed 64 mg/day; IM 5 mg q6h, not to exceed 30 mg/day

• *Child >12 yr:* PO 6-12 mg in divided doses

Nonhospitalized patients

• *Adult:* PO 4-8 mg tid; IM 5 mg q6h

Available forms include: Tabs 2, 4, 8, 16 mg; sol 16 mg/5 ml; inj IM 5 mg/ml; sus rel tabs 8 mg

Side effects/adverse reactions:

▼ *ORAL: Dry mouth,* enlarged parotid glands, lichenoid reaction

*CNS: Extrapyramidal symptoms: pseudoparkinsonism, akathisia, dystonia, tardive dyskinesia, **seizures,** headache*

*CV: Orthostatic hypotension, **cardiac arrest, tachycardia,** ECG changes, syncope*

GI: Nausea, vomiting, anorexia, constipation, diarrhea, jaundice, weight gain

*RESP: **Laryngospasm, respiratory depression,** dyspnea*

*HEMA: **Leukopenia, leukocytosis, agranulocytosis,** anemia*

---

italic = common side effects

GU: Urinary retention, urinary frequency, enuresis, impotence, amenorrhea, gynecomastia

EENT: Blurred vision, glaucoma

INTEG: Rash, photosensitivity, dermatitis

Contraindications: Hypersensitivity, blood dyscrasias, coma, child <12 yr, brain damage, bone marrow depression

Precautions: Pregnancy category C, lactation, seizure disorders, hypertension, hepatic disease, cardiac disease

Pharmacokinetics:

PO: Onset erratic, peak 2-4 hr

IM: Onset 10 min, peak 1-2 hr, duration 6 hr, occasionally 12-24 hr

Metabolized by liver, excreted in urine, crosses placenta, excreted in breast milk

Drug interactions of concern to dentistry:

• Increased sedation: other CNS depressants, alcohol, barbiturate anesthetics, opioid analgesics

• Hypotension, tachycardia: epinephrine

• Increased extrapyramidal effects: phenothiazines and related drugs (haloperidol, droperidol), metoclopramide

• Additive photosensitization: tetracyclines, fluoroquinolones

• Increased anticholinergic effects: anticholinergics

DENTAL CONSIDERATIONS

General:

• Monitor vital signs every appointment due to cardiovascular side effects.

• Patients on chronic drug therapy may rarely have symptoms of blood dyscrasias, which can include infection, bleeding, and poor healing.

• After supine positioning, have patient sit upright for at least 2 min before standing to avoid orthostatic hypotension.

• Assess salivary flow as a factor in caries, periodontal disease, and candidiasis.

• Avoid dental light in patient's eyes; offer dark glasses for patient comfort.

• Assess for presence of extrapyramidal motor symptoms, such as tardive dyskinesia and akathisia. Extrapyramidal motor activity may complicate dental treatment.

• Geriatric patients are more susceptible to drug effects; use lower dose.

• Use vasoconstrictors with caution, in low doses, and with careful aspiration. Avoid use of gingival retraction cord with epinephrine.

Consultations:

• In a patient with symptoms of blood dyscrasias, request a medical consult for blood studies and postpone dental treatment until normal values are reestablished.

• Take precautions if dental surgery is anticipated and anesthesia is required.

• If signs of tardive dyskinesia or akathisia are present, refer to physician.

• Physician should be informed if significant xerostomic side effects occur (increased caries, sore tongue, problems eating or swallowing, difficulty wearing prosthesis) so a medication change can be considered.

Teach patient/family:

• Importance of good oral hygiene to prevent soft tissue inflammation

• Caution to prevent injury when using oral hygiene aids

P

• To use electric toothbrush if patient has difficulty holding conventional devices

When chronic dry mouth occurs, advise patient:

• To avoid mouth rinses with high alcohol content due to drying effects

• Of need for daily use of home fluoride products to prevent caries

• To use sugarless gum, frequent sips of water, or saliva substitutes

---

phenazopyridine HCl

(fen-az-oh-peer'i-deen)
Azo-Standard, Baridium, Geridium, Prodium, Pyridium, Urodine, Urogesic, UTI Relief
♣ Phenazo

Drug class.: Urinary tract analgesic

Action: Exerts analgesic, anesthetic action on the urinary tract mucosa; exact mechanism of action unknown

Uses: Urinary tract irritation/infection

Dosage and routes:
• *Adult:* PO 100-200 mg tid
• *Child 6-12 yr:* PO 12 mg/kg/24 hr in 3 divided doses

Available forms include: Tabs 95, 97.2, 100, 200 mg

Side effects/adverse reactions:

CNS: Headache, vertigo

GI: Nausea, vomiting, GI bleeding, diarrhea, heartburn, hepatic toxicity

HEMA: Hemolytic anemia, methemoglobinemia (with overdose)

GU: Renal toxicity, orange-red urine

INTEG: Rash, urticaria, skin pigmentation

Contraindications: Hypersensitivity, hepatic disease

Precautions: Pregnancy category B, renal disease

Pharmacokinetics:

PO: Metabolized by liver, excreted by kidneys, crosses placenta, duration 6-8 hr

DENTAL CONSIDERATIONS

General:

• Consider semisupine chair position for patient comfort if GI side effects occur.

• Patients on chronic drug therapy may rarely have symptoms of blood dyscrasias, which can include infection, bleeding, and poor healing.

• Be aware that patient might have UTI; question if antiinfectives are also being used.

---

phendimetrazine tartrate

(fen-dye-me'tra-zeen)
Adipost, Bontril PDM, Dital, Dyrexan-OD, Melfiat-105, Plegine, Prelu-2, Rexigen Forte

Drug class.: Anorexiant, amphetamine-like

Controlled Substance Schedule III

Action: Exact mechanism of action of appetite suppression unknown, but may have an effect on satiety center of hypothalamus

Uses: Exogenous obesity

Dosage and routes:
• *Adult:* PO 35 mg bid-tid 1 hr ac, not to exceed 70 mg tid; sus rel 105 mg qd before breakfast

Available forms include: Tabs 35 mg; caps 35 mg; sus rel caps 105 mg

---

Side effects/adverse reactions:

▼ *ORAL:* Dry mouth, unpleasant taste

CNS: Hyperactivity, insomnia, restlessness, dizziness, tremors, headache

CV: Palpitation, tachycardia, hypertension

GI: Nausea, anorexia, diarrhea, constipation, cramps

HEMA: **Bone marrow depression, leukopenia, agranulocytosis**

GU: Dysuria

EENT: Blurred vision

INTEG: Urticaria

Contraindications: Hypersensitivity, hyperthyroidism, hypertension, glaucoma, severe arteriosclerosis, severe cardiovascular disease, children <12 yr, agitated states, MAO inhibitors

Precautions: Drug abuse, anxiety, pregnancy category C, lactation

Pharmacokinetics:

PO: Onset 30 min, peak 1-3 hr, duration 4-20 hr, half-life 2-10 hr; metabolized by liver; excreted by kidneys; crosses placenta; excreted in breast milk

🦷 Drug interactions of concern to dentistry:

• Hypertensive crisis: MAO inhibitors or within 14 days of MAO inhibitors

• Increased risk of dysrhythmia: hydrocarbon inhalation general anesthetics

• Decreased effect: tricyclic antidepressants, ascorbic acid, phenothiazines

• Caffeine or caffeine-containing products: may increase risk of insomnia and dry mouth

DENTAL CONSIDERATIONS

General:

• Monitor vital signs every appointment due to cardiovascular side effects.

• Assess salivary flow as a factor in caries, periodontal disease, and candidiasis.

• Determine why the patient is taking the drug.

• Psychologic and physical dependence may occur with chronic administration.

• Patients on chronic drug therapy may rarely have symptoms of blood dyscrasias, which can include infection, bleeding, and poor healing.

Consultations:

• In a patient with symptoms of blood dyscrasias, request a medical consult for blood studies and postpone dental treatment until normal values are reestablished.

Teach patient/family:

• Importance of good oral hygiene to prevent soft tissue inflammation

• To report oral lesions, soreness, or bleeding to dentist

• Caution to prevent injury when using oral hygiene aids

When chronic dry mouth occurs, advise patient:

• To avoid mouth rinses with high alcohol content due to drying effects

• Of need for daily use of home fluoride products to prevent caries

• To use sugarless gum, frequent sips of water, or saliva substitutes

---

phenelzine sulfate

(fen'el-zeen)

Nardil

Drug class.: Antidepressant, MAO inhibitor

Action: Increases concentrations

---

of endogenous epinephrine, norepinephrine, serotonin, dopamine in storage sites in CNS by inhibition of MAO; antidepressant mechanism uncertain

Uses: Depression when uncontrolled by other means

Dosage and routes:
• *Adult:* PO 45 mg/day in 3 divided doses; may increase to 60 mg/day; dose should be reduced to 15 mg/day for maintenance; not to exceed 90 mg/day

Available forms include: Tabs 15 mg

Side effects/adverse reactions:
▼ *ORAL:* Dry mouth
CNS: Dizziness, drowsiness, confusion, headache, anxiety, tremors, stimulation, weakness, hyperreflexia, mania, insomnia, fatigue, weight gain
CV: Orthostatic hypotension, hypertension, dysrhythmias, hypertensive crisis, peripheral edema
GI: Constipation, nausea, vomiting, *anorexia,* diarrhea, weight changes, abdominal pain
HEMA: Anemia
GU: Change in libido, frequency
EENT: Blurred vision
INTEG: Rash, flushing, increased perspiration
ENDO: SIADH-like syndrome

Contraindications: Hypersensitivity to MAO inhibitors, elderly, hypertension, CHF, severe hepatic disease, pheochromocytoma, severe renal disease, severe cardiac disease, fluoxetine, meperidine

Precautions: Suicidal patients, convulsive disorders, severe depression, schizophrenia, hyperactivity, diabetes mellitus, pregnancy category C

Pharmacokinetics: Metabolized by liver, excreted by kidneys

🦷 **Drug interactions of concern to dentistry:**
• Increased anticholinergic effect: anticholinergics, haloperidol, phenothiazines, antihistamines
• Hyperpyretic crisis, convulsions, hypertensive episode: meperidine, carbamazepine, cyclobenzaprine
• Cardiac dysrhythmia: caffeine-containing medications
• Increased risk of serotonin syndrome: tricyclic antidepressants, other serotonin reuptake inhibitors
• Increased sedative effects of alcohol, barbiturates, benzodiazepines, CNS depressants
• Increased pressor effects: indirect-acting sympathomimetics such as ephedrine, amphetamine

DENTAL CONSIDERATIONS
General:
• Monitor vital signs every appointment due to cardiovascular side effects.
• Assess salivary flow as a factor in caries, periodontal disease, and candidiasis.
• After supine positioning, have patient sit upright for at least 2 min before standing to avoid orthostatic hypotension.
• Hypertensive episodes are possible even though there are no specific contraindications to vasoconstrictor use in local anesthetics.
• Avoid prescribing caffeine-containing products.
• Take precautions if dental surgery is anticipated and general anesthesia is required.

Consultations:
• Medical consult may be required to assess disease control and patient's ability to tolerate stress.

Teach patient/family:
• To use electric toothbrush if pa-

italic = common side effects

tient has difficulty holding conventional devices

When chronic dry mouth occurs, advise patient:

• To avoid mouth rinses with high alcohol content due to drying effects

• Of need for daily use of home fluoride products to prevent caries

• To use sugarless gum, frequent sips of water, or saliva substitutes

---

phenobarbital/ phenobarbital sodium

(fee-noe-bar′bi-tal)

Bellatal, Luminal Sodium, Solfoton

Drug class.: Barbiturate anticonvulsant

**Controlled Substance
Schedule IV**

Action: A nonspecific depressant of the CNS; may enhance GABA activity in the brain

Uses: All forms of epilepsy, status epilepticus, febrile seizures in children, sedation, insomnia; unapproved: hyperbilirubinemia, chronic cholestasis

Dosage and routes:

Seizures

• *Adult:* PO 100-200 mg/day in divided doses tid or total dose hs

• *Child:* PO 4-6 mg/kg/day in divided doses q12h; may be given as single dose hs

Status epilepticus

• *Adult:* IV inf 10 mg/kg; run no faster than 50 mg/min; may give up to 20 mg/kg

• *Child:* IV inf 5-10 mg/kg; may repeat q10-15min, up to 20 mg/kg; run no faster than 50 mg/min

Sedation

• *Adult:* PO 30-120 mg/day in 2-3 divided doses

• *Child:* PO 6 mg/kg/day in 3 divided doses

Preoperative sedation

• *Adult:* IM 100-200 mg 1-1.5 hr before surgery

• *Child:* IM 1-3 mg/kg, 1-1.5 hr before surgery

Hyperbilirubinemia

• *Neonate:* PO 7 mg/kg/day from days 1-5 after birth; IM 5 mg/kg/day on day 1, then PO on days 2-7 after birth

Chronic cholestasis

• *Adult:* PO 90-180 mg/day in 2-3 divided doses

• *Child <12 yr:* PO 3-12 mg/kg/day in 2-3 divided doses

Available forms include: Caps 16 mg; elix 15, 20 mg/5 ml; tabs 15, 16, 16.2, 30, 60, 90, 100 mg; inj 30, 60, 65, 130 mg/ml

Side effects/adverse reactions:

CNS: Drowsiness, somnolence, paradoxic excitement (elderly), lethargy, hangover headache, flushing, hallucinations, coma, agitation, confusion, vertigo, insomnia, fever

CV: Bradycardia, hypotension, syncope

GI: Nausea, vomiting, diarrhea, constipation, liver damage (with chronic use)

RESP: Hypoventilation, apnea, respiratory depression, laryngospasm, bronchospasm, circulatory collapse

*INTEG: **Stevens-Johnson syndrome, angioedema,** rash,* urticaria, local pain, swelling, necrosis, thrombophlebitis, pemphigus-like reaction

Contraindications: Hypersensitivity to barbiturates, porphyria,

---

hepatic disease, respiratory disease, nephritis, hyperthyroidism, diabetes mellitus, elderly, lactation, pregnancy category D

Precautions: Anemia

Pharmacokinetics:

PO: Onset 2-60 min, peak 8-12 hr, duration 6-10 hr, half-life 53-118 hr; metabolized by liver; excreted by kidneys; crosses placenta; excreted in breast milk

⚖ Drug interactions of concern to dentistry:

• Increased effects: alcohol, all CNS depressants, saquinavir

• Decreased effects of corticosteroids, doxycycline, carbamazepine

DENTAL CONSIDERATIONS

General:

• Determine why the patient is taking the drug.

• Monitor vital signs every appointment due to cardiovascular side effects. Evaluate respiration characteristics and rate.

• Patients on chronic drug therapy may rarely have symptoms of blood dyscrasias, which can include infection, bleeding, and poor healing.

When used for sedation in dentistry:

• Assess vital signs before use and q30min after use as sedative.

• Observe respiratory dysfunction: respiratory depression, character, rate, rhythm; hold drug if respirations <10/min or if pupils are dilated.

• After supine positioning, have patient sit upright for at least 2 min to avoid orthostatic hypotension.

• Have someone drive patient to and from dental office when used for conscious sedation.

• Barbiturates induce liver microsomal enzymes, which alter the metabolism of other drugs.

• Geriatric patients are more susceptible to drug effects; use lower dose.

Consultations:

• In a patient with symptoms of blood dyscrasias, request a medical consult for blood studies and postpone dental treatment until normal values are reestablished.

Teach patient/family:

• To avoid driving or other activities requiring alertness

• To avoid alcohol ingestion or CNS depressants; serious CNS depression may result

• To use OTC preparations with caution because they may contain other CNS depressants (antihistamines, cold remedies)

---

phensuximide

(fen-sux′i-mide)

Milontin

Drug class.: Anticonvulsant, succinimide

Action: Suppresses spike, wave formation in absence seizures (petit mal); decreases amplitude, frequency, duration, spread of discharge in minor motor seizures

Uses: Absence (petit mal) seizures; unapproved: complex partial seizures

Dosage and routes:

• *Adult and child:* PO 500 mg-1 g bid or tid

Available forms include: Caps 500 mg

Side effects/adverse reactions:

▼ *ORAL:* Gingival bleeding, ulcerations (Stevens-Johnson syndrome); swelling of tongue and gingival enlargement (rare)

CNS: Drowsiness, dizziness, fatigue, euphoria, lethargy, anxiety, depression, irritability, insomnia, aggressiveness, weakness, headache

GI: Nausea, vomiting, heartburn, anorexia, diarrhea, abdominal pain, cramps, constipation

*HEMA: **Agranulocytosis, aplastic anemia, thrombocytopenia, leukocytosis, eosinophilia, pancytopenia***

*GU: **Hematuria, renal damage,*** urinary frequency, vaginal bleeding

EENT: Myopia, blurred vision

*INTEG: **Stevens-Johnson syndrome,*** urticaria, pruritic erythema, hirsutism

Contraindications: Hypersensitivity to succinimide derivatives

Precautions: Lactation, hepatic disease, pregnancy category D, renal disease, intermittent porphyria

Pharmacokinetics:

PO: Peak 1-4 hr, half-life 5-12 hr; metabolized by liver; excreted by kidneys

⚡ Drug interactions of concern to dentistry:

• Enhanced CNS depression: CNS depressants, alcohol

• Decreased effects: phenothiazines, thioxanthenes, barbiturates

DENTAL CONSIDERATIONS

General:

• Patients on chronic drug therapy may rarely have symptoms of blood dyscrasias, which can include infection, bleeding, and poor healing.

• Ask about type of epilepsy, seizure frequency, and quality of seizure control.

• A stress reduction protocol may be required for anxious patients.

• Consider semisupine chair position if GI side effects occur.

Consultations:

• In a patient with symptoms of blood dyscrasias, request a medical consult for blood studies and postpone dental treatment until normal values are reestablished.

• Medical consult may be required to assess disease control and patient's ability to tolerate stress.

Teach patient/family:

• Importance of good oral hygiene to prevent gingival inflammation

• To avoid mouth rinses with high alcohol content due to drying effects

• To prevent injury when using oral hygiene aids

• To report oral lesions, soreness, or bleeding to dentist

---

phentermine HCl/ phentermine resin

(fen'ter-meen)

Adipex-P, Fastin, Ionamin, Obe-Nix-30, Zantryl

Drug class.: Sympathomimetic, anorexiant

Controlled Substance Schedule IV

Action: Exact mechanism of action of appetite suppression unknown, but may have an effect on satiety center of hypothalamus

Uses: Exogenous obesity

Dosage and routes:

• *Adult:* PO 8 mg tid 30 min before meals or 15-37.5 mg qd

Available forms include: Tabs 8, 30, 37.5 mg; caps 15, 18.75, 30, 37.5 mg; time rel caps 15, 30 mg

Side effects/adverse reactions:

▼ *ORAL:* Dry mouth, unpleasant taste

CNS: Insomnia, restlessness, agitation, hyperactivity, dizziness, tremor, headache, anxiety, agitation, euphoria, dyskensia

CV: Palpitation, tachycardia, hypertension, ECG changes, dysrhythmias

GI: Nausea, anorexia, constipation, diarrhea

HEMA: Bone marrow depression, agranulocytosis, leukopenia

GU: Impotence, change in libido, dysuria, urinary frequency

EENT: Blurred vision, mydriasis

INTEG: Urticaria, rash

Contraindications: Hypersensitivity, hyperthyroidism, hypertension, glaucoma, severe arteriosclerosis, angina pectoris, cardiovascular disease, child <12 yr, MAO inhibitor–type medications

Precautions: Pregnancy category C, lactation, drug abuse, anxiety, tolerance

Pharmacokinetics:

SUS REL: Duration 10-14 hr; metabolized by liver; excreted by kidneys

PO (NOT CON REL DOSE FORMS): Rapid onset, duration 4 hr

⚕ Drug interactions of concern to dentistry:

• Hypertensive crisis: MAO inhibitors or within 14 days of MAO inhibitors

• Increased risk of dysrhythmia: hydrocarbon inhalation general anesthetics

• Decreased effect: tricyclic antidepressants, ascorbic acid, phenothiazines

• Caffeine or caffeine-containing products may increase risk of insomnia

DENTAL CONSIDERATIONS

General:

• Monitor vital signs every appointment due to cardiovascular side effects.

• Assess salivary flow as a factor in caries, periodontal disease, and candidiasis.

• Determine why the patient is taking the drug.

• Psychologic and physical dependence may occur with chronic administration.

• Patients on chronic drug therapy may rarely have symptoms of blood dyscrasias, which can include infection, bleeding, and poor healing.

Consultations:

• In a patient with symptoms of blood dyscrasias, request a medical consult for blood studies and postpone dental treatment until normal values are reestablished.

Teach patient/family:

• Importance of good oral hygiene to prevent soft tissue inflammation

• To prevent injury when using oral hygiene aids

• To report oral lesions, soreness, or bleeding to dentist

When chronic dry mouth occurs, advise patient:

• To avoid mouth rinses with high alcohol content due to drying effects

• Of need for daily use of home fluoride products to prevent caries

• To use sugarless gum, frequent sips of water, or saliva substitutes

phentolamine mesylate

(fen-tole'a-meen)
Regitine
♣ Rogitine

Drug class.: Antihypertensive

Action: α-adrenergic blocker; binds to α-adrenergic receptors, dilating peripheral blood vessels, lowering peripheral resistances, lowering blood pressure
Uses: Hypertension, pheochromocytoma, prevention and treatment of dermal necrosis following extravasation of norepinephrine or dopamine; unapproved: with papaverine for intracavernous injection for impotence
Dosage and routes:
Treatment of hypertensive episodes in pheochromocytoma
• *Adult: IV/IM* 5 mg 1-2 hr before surgery; repeat if necessary
• *Child:* IV/IM 1 mg 1-2 hr before surgery; repeat if necessary
Prevention/treatment of necrosis
• *Adult:* 5-10 mg/10 ml NS injected into area of norepinephrine extravasation within 12 hr; preventive dose 10 mg to each 1000 ml norepinephrine solution
Available forms include: Inj IM/IV 5 mg/ml
Side effects/adverse reactions:
▼ *ORAL:* Dry mouth
CNS: *Dizziness,* flushing, weakness
CV: *Hypotension, tachycardia, angina, dysrhythmias,* **MI**
GI: *Nausea, vomiting, diarrhea, abdominal pain*
EENT: Nasal congestion
Contraindications: Hypersensitivity, MI, coronary insufficiency, angina, peptic ulcer
Precautions: Pregnancy category C, lactation
Pharmacokinetics:
IV: Peak 2 min, duration 10-15 min
IM: Peak 15-20 min, duration 3-4 hr
Metabolized in liver, excreted in urine
⚡ Drug interactions of concern to dentistry:
• Hypotension, tachycardia: epinephrine
• Decreased pressor effects of epinephrine, ephedrine
DENTAL CONSIDERATIONS
General:
• This is an acute-use drug; hypertension and pheochromocytoma are the immediate concerns.
• Patients with untreated pheochromocytoma or with extreme, uncontrolled hypertension are not candidates for elective dental treatment. Physician consult is required.
• Short appointments and a stress reduction protocol may be required for anxious patients.
• Stress from dental procedures may compromise cardiovascular function; determine patient risk.
• Use vasoconstrictors with caution, in low doses, and with careful aspiration. Avoid use of gingival retraction cord with epinephrine.
• Assess vital signs at each appointment due to nature of disease.
Consultations:
• Medical consult may be required to assess disease control and patient's ability to tolerate stress.

P

---

bold italic = life-threatening conditions   *For periodic updates, visit* **www.mosby.com**

phenylephrine HCl (nasal)

(fen-ill-ef'rin)

Ah Chew, Alconefrin, Neo-Synephrine, Nostril, Rhinall, Sinex

Drug class.: Nasal decongestant, sympathomimetic

Action: Produces rapid and long-acting vasoconstriction of arterioles, thereby decreasing fluid exudation, mucosal engorgement

Uses: Nasal congestion (temporary relief)

Dosage and routes:
• *Adult:* Instill 2-3 gtt or sprays to nasal mucosa bid (0.25%-1%) q3-4h
• *Child 6-12 yr:* Instill 1-2 gtt or sprays (0.25%) q3-4h
• *Child <6 yr:* Instill 2-3 gtt or sprays (0.125%) q3-4h

Available forms include: Sol 0.125%, 0.16%, 0.25%, 0.5%, 1%; chew tabs 10 mg

Side effects/adverse reactions:
▼ *ORAL: Dry mouth,* bitter taste
CNS: Anxiety, restlessness, tremors, weakness, insomnia, dizziness, fever, headache
GI: Nausea, vomiting, anorexia
EENT: Irritation, burning, sneezing, stinging, dryness, rebound congestion
INTEG: Contact dermatitis

Contraindications: Hypersensitivity to sympathomimetic amines, MAO inhibitors

Precautions: Child <6 yr, elderly, diabetes, cardiovascular disease, hypertension, hyperthyroidism, increased IOP, prostatic hypertrophy, pregnancy category C, glaucoma, ischemic heart disease, excessive use

🐝 Drug interactions of concern to dentistry:
• None reported with normal topical use
With systemic absorption, see risk of:
• Bradycardia: β-adrenergic blockers
• Increased dysrhythmias and hypertension: tricyclic antidepressants

DENTAL CONSIDERATIONS
General:
• Consider semisupine chair position for patient comfort due to respiratory effects of disease.
• Assess salivary flow as a factor in caries, periodontal disease, and candidiasis.
• Patients with significant nasal congestion may complicate nasal administration of nitrous oxide/oxygen sedation.

Teach patient/family:
• That this product is not indicated for prolonged use because of congestion rebound; however, this may not always be the case

phenytoin sodium/ phenytoin sodium extended/phenytoin sodium prompt

(fen'i-toyn)

Dilantin, Dilantin Infatabs, Dilantin Kapseals, Dilantin-125

Drug class.: Hydantoin anticonvulsant

Action: Inhibits spread of seizure activity in motor cortex
Uses: Generalized tonic-clonic (grand mal) seizures, status epilepticus, nonepileptic seizures, tri-

geminal neuralgia, cardiac dys-rhythmias (class Ib) caused by digitalis-type drugs

Dosage and routes:

Seizures

• *Adult:* IV loading dose 900 mg-1.5 g run at 50 mg/min; if patient has received phenytoin, 100-300 mg run at 50 mg/min; PO loading dose 900 mg-1.5 g divided tid, then 300 mg/day (extended) or divided tid (extended/prompt)

• *Child:* IV loading dose 15 mg/kg run at 50 mg/min; if patient has received phenytoin, 5-7 mg/kg run at 50 mg/min, may repeat in 30 min; PO loading dose 15 mg/kg divided q8-12h, then 5-7 mg/kg in divided doses q12h

Ventricular dysrhythmias

• *Adult:* PO loading dose 1 g divided over 24 hr, then 500 mg/day for 2 days, maintenance 300 mg PO daily; IV 250 mg given over 5 min until dysrhythmias subside or 1 g is given, or 100 mg q15min until dysrhythmias subside or 1 g is given

• *Child:* PO 3-8 mg/kg or 250 mg/m^2/day as single dose or divided in 2 doses; IV 3-8 mg/kg given over several min, or 250 mg/m^2/day as single dose or divided in 2 doses

Available forms include: Susp 125 mg/5 ml; chew tabs 50 mg; inj 50 mg/ml; caps 30, 100 mg; caps prompt rel 100 mg

Side effects/adverse reactions:

▼ *ORAL: Gingival overgrowth,* oral ulceration (Stevens-Johnson syndrome), taste loss

CNS: Drowsiness, dizziness, insomnia, paresthesia, depression, headache, confusion, slurred speech, ataxia, numbness

CV: Hypotension, ventricular fibrillation

GI: Nausea, vomiting, constipation, hepatitis, anorexia, weight loss, jaundice, epigastric pain

HEMA: Agranulocytosis, leukopenia, aplastic anemia, thrombocytopenia, megaloblastic anemia

GU: Nephritis, albuminuria

EENT: Nystagmus, diplopia, blurred vision

INTEG: Rash, Stevens-Johnson syndrome, lupus erythematosus, hirsutism

MISC: Lymphadenopathy, hyperglycemia

Contraindications: Hypersensitivity, psychiatric condition, pregnancy category D, bradycardia, SA and AV block, Stokes-Adams syndrome

Precautions: Allergies, hepatic disease, renal disease

Pharmacokinetics:

PO: Duration 5 hr; metabolized by liver; excreted by kidneys

⚓ Drug interactions of concern to dentistry:

• Increased serum levels by: ketoconazole, fluconazole, fluoxetine, metronidazole

• Decreased effects: barbiturates, carbamazepine, chloral hydrate

• Hepatotoxicity: acetaminophen (chronic use and high doses only)

• Decreased effects of corticosteroids, doxycycline

DENTAL CONSIDERATIONS

General:

• Patients on chronic drug therapy may rarely have symptoms of blood dyscrasias, which can include infection, bleeding, and poor healing.

• Place on frequent recall to evaluate gingival condition and self-care.

---

bold italic = life-threatening conditions   *For periodic updates, visit* **www.mosby.com**

- Short appointments and a stress reduction protocol may be required for anxious patients.
- Ask about type of epilepsy, seizure frequency, and quality of seizure control.

Consultations:
- In a patient with symptoms of blood dyscrasias, request a medical consult for blood studies and postpone dental treatment until normal values are reestablished.
- Medical consult may be required to assess disease control and the patient's ability to tolerate stress.

Teach patient/family:
- Importance of good oral hygiene to prevent soft tissue inflammation and minimize gingival overgrowth
- Caution to prevent injury when using oral hygiene aids

---

phytonadione (vitamin K₁)

(fye-toe-na-dye′one)
AquaMEPHYTON, Mephyton

Drug class.: Vitamin K₁, fat-soluble vitamin

Action: Needed for adequate blood clotting (factors II, VII, IX, X)

Uses: Vitamin K malabsorption, hypoprothrombinemia, prevention of hypoprothrombinemia caused by oral anticoagulants

Dosage and routes:

Hypoprothrombinemia caused by vitamin K malabsorption
- *Adult:* PO/IM 2-25 mg; may repeat or increase to 50 mg
- *Child:* PO/IM 5-10 mg
- *Infants:* PO/IM 2 mg

Prevention of hemorrhagic disease of the newborn
- *Neonate:* SC/IM 0.5-1 mg after birth; repeat in 6-8 hr if required

Hypoprothrombinemia caused by oral anticoagulants
- *Adult:* PO/SC/IM 2.5-10 mg; may repeat 12-48 hr after PO dose or 6-8 hr after SC/IM dose, based on PT

Available forms include: Tabs 5 mg; inj aqueous colloidal IM/IV 2 mg/ml; inj aqueous dispersion 10 mg/ml (IM only)

Side effects/adverse reactions:

▼ *ORAL:* Unusual taste
CNS: Headache, **brain damage** (large doses)
CV: Cardiac irregularities
GI: Nausea, vomiting
HEMA: **Hemolytic anemia, hemoglobinuria, hyperbilirubinemia**
INTEG: Rash, urticaria, flushing, erythema, sweating
MISC: Bronchospasms, dyspnea, cramplike pain

Contraindications: Hypersensitivity, severe hepatic disease, last few weeks of pregnancy

Precautions: Pregnancy category C

Pharmacokinetics:
PO/INJ: Readily absorbed from duodenum and requires bile salts, rapid hepatic metabolism, onset of action 6-12 hr, normal PT in 12-24 hr, crosses placenta, renal and biliary excretion

🦷 **Drug interactions of concern to dentistry:**
- Decreased action: broad-spectrum antibiotics, salicylates (high doses)
- Antagonist to oral anticoagulants

DENTAL CONSIDERATIONS

General:
- Determine why the patient is taking this drug. Medical consult should be made before dental treatment.
- Patients on chronic drug therapy

may rarely have symptoms of blood dyscrasias, which can include infection, bleeding, and poor healing.

Consultations:
• Medical consultation to determine coagulation stability.

---

pilocarpine HCl/ pilocarpine nitrate (optic)

(pye-loe-kar′peen)

Adsorbocarpine, Akarpine, Isopto Carpine, Pilagan, Pilocar, Piloptic, Pilostat

✦ Miocarpine

Drug class.: Miotic, cholinergic agonist

Action: Acts directly on cholinergic receptor sites; induces miosis, spasm of accommodation, fall in intraocular pressure caused by stimulation of ciliary, pupillary sphincter muscles, leading to pulling of iris from filtration angle and resulting in increased outflow of aqueous humor

Uses: Primary glaucoma, early stages of wide-angle glaucoma (less useful in advanced stages), chronic open-angle glaucoma, acute narrow-angle glaucoma before emergency surgery; also used to neutralize mydriatics used during eye exam; may be used alternately with mydriatics to break adhesions between iris and lens

Dosage and routes:
• *Adult and child:* Instill sol 1-2 gtt of 1% or 2% solution in eye q6-8h; instill 20-40 µg/hr (Ocusert Pilo) in cul-de-sac of eye

Available forms include: Sol 0.25%-10%

Side effects/adverse reactions:
▼ *ORAL:* Excessive salivation
CV: Hypotension, tachycardia
GI: Nausea, vomiting, abdominal cramps, diarrhea
RESP: **Bronchospasm**
EENT: Blurred vision, browache, twitching of eyelids, eye pain with change in focus

Contraindications: Bradycardia, hyperthyroidism, coronary artery disease, hypertension, obstruction of GI/urinary tracts, epilepsy, parkinsonism, asthma

Precautions: Bronchial asthma, hypertension, pregnancy category C

DENTAL CONSIDERATIONS
General:
• Avoid drugs with anticholinergic activity, such as antihistamines, opioids, benzodiazepines, propantheline, atropine, and scopolamine.
• Avoid dental light in patient's eyes; offer dark glasses for patient comfort.
• Monitor vital signs every appointment due to cardiovascular and respiratory side effects.

Consultations:
• Medical consult may be required to assess disease control.

---

pilocarpine HCl (oral)

(pye-loe-kar′peen)

Salagen

Drug class.: Cholinergic agonist (parasympathomimetic)

Action: Mimics the action of acetylcholine on muscarinic receptors

Uses: Treatment of symptoms of xerostomia from salivary gland hypofunction caused by radiotherapy for cancer of the head and neck and Sjögren's syndrome

---

bold italic = life-threatening conditions

Dosage and routes:
• *Adult:* PO initially 5 mg tid; 10 mg tid may be considered for patients who are not responding adequately and who can tolerate the lower doses

Available forms include: Tabs 5 mg

Side effects/adverse reactions:
▼ *ORAL:* Taste alteration
CNS: Dizziness, headache, nervousness, anxiety
CV: Flushing, edema, tachycardia, palpitation, hypotension, hypertension, bradycardia
GI: Nausea, dyspepsia, diarrhea, abdominal pain, vomiting, diarrhea
HEMA: Leukopenia, lymphadenopathy
GU: Urinary frequency
EENT: Rhinitis, lacrimation, pharyngitis, amblyopia, conjunctivitis, sinusitis
INTEG: Rash
MS: Asthenia
MISC: Sweating (high doses)

Contraindications: Uncontrolled asthma, hypersensitivity, when miosis is undesirable (acute iritis, narrow-angle glaucoma)

Precautions: Pregnancy category C, children, lactation, cardiovascular disease, retinal diseases, pulmonary diseases (asthma, chronic bronchitis, COPD), biliary tract disease, history of renal colic, psychiatric disorders

Pharmacokinetics:
PO: Onset 20 min, peak effect 1 hr, duration 3-5 hr; renal excretion

⚛ Drug interactions of concern to dentistry
• With β-adrenergic agonists: use with caution; possibility of conduction disturbances

• Reduced effect: anticholinergic drugs
• Enhanced effects: other cholinergic agonists

DENTAL CONSIDERATIONS
General:
• Patients receiving chemotherapy may require palliative treatment for stomatitis.
• Assess salivary flow as a factor in caries, periodontal disease, and candidiasis.
• Monitor vital signs every appointment due to cardiovascular side effects.
• Place on frequent recall due to oral effects of head and neck radiation.

Consultations:
• Medical consult may be required to assess disease control.
• Medical consult may be necessary before prescribing for those patients with cardiovascular, retinal, or respiratory disease.

Teach patient/family:
• To use caution when driving at night or performing hazardous activities in reduced lighting (visual blurring)
• That sweating can become extensive with high dose; have patient take plenty of fluids, observe for dehydration, or discontinue drug

When chronic dry mouth occurs, advise patient:
• To avoid mouth rinses with high alcohol content due to drying effects
• Of need for daily use of home fluoride products to prevent caries
• To use sugarless gum, frequent sips of water, or saliva substitutes

---

italic = common side effects

pimozide

(pi'moe-zide)

Orap

Drug class.: Antipsychotic, antidyskinetic

Action: Blocks dopamine effects in the CNS

Uses: Motor and phonic tics in Gilles de la Tourette's syndrome; unapproved: psychotic disorders

Dosage and routes:

• *Adult and child >12 yr:* PO 1-2 mg qd in divided doses, usual dose 10 mg/day

Available forms include: Tabs 2, 4 mg

Side effects/adverse reactions:

▼ *ORAL: Dry mouth,* thirst, altered taste

CNS: Extrapyramidal symptoms: pseudoparkinsonism, akathisia, dystonia, tardive dyskinesia, drowsiness, headache, neuroleptic malignant syndrome, seizures, lethargy, sedation, muscle tightness

*CV: Orthostatic hypotension, **cardiac arrest, tachycardia,*** hypertension, ECG changes

GI: Nausea, vomiting, anorexia, constipation, diarrhea, jaundice, weight gain

GU: Urinary retention, urinary frequency, enuresis, impotence, amenorrhea, gynecomastia

EENT: Blurred vision, cataracts

INTEG: Rash, photosensitivity, dermatitis, hyperpyrexia

Contraindications: Hypersensitivity, CNS depression/coma, parkinsonism, liver disease, blood dyscrasias, renal disease, tics other than syndrome, cardiac dysrhythmias, macrolide antiinfectives, itraconazole

Precautions: Child <12 yr, pregnancy category C, lactation, hypertension, hepatic disease, cardiac disease, renal disease, breast cancer, hypokalemia

Pharmacokinetics:

PO: Onset erratic, peak 6-8 hr, half-life 50-55 hr; metabolized by liver; excreted in urine, feces

🦷 **Drug interactions of concern to dentistry:**

• Increased CNS depression: alcohol, CNS depressants

• Increased effects of both drugs: phenothiazines

• Increased effects of anticholinergic drugs

• Prolonged QT interval, fatal cardiac arrhythmia, contraindicated: clarithromycin, erythromycin, azithromycin, dirithromycin, itraconazole

DENTAL CONSIDERATIONS

General:

• Assess salivary flow as a factor in caries, periodontal disease, and candidiasis.

• Monitor vital signs every appointment due to cardiovascular side effects.

• Assess for presence of extrapyramidal motor symptoms, such as tardive dyskinesia and akathisia. Extrapyramidal motor activity may complicate dental treatment.

• After supine positioning, have patient sit upright for at least 2 min to avoid orthostatic hypotension.

• Consider action of drug in assessment of altered taste.

Consultations:

• Medical consult may be required to assess disease control.

---

bold italic = life-threatening conditions   *For periodic updates, visit* **www.mosby.com**

• If signs of tardive dyskinesia or akathisia are present, refer to physician.

Teach patient/family:
• Importance of good oral hygiene to prevent soft tissue inflammation
• Caution to prevent injury when using oral hygiene aids
When chronic dry mouth occurs, advise patient:
• To avoid mouth rinses with high alcohol content due to drying effects
• Of need for daily use of home fluoride products to prevent caries
• To use sugarless gum, frequent sips of water, or saliva substitutes

---

pindolol
(pin'doe-lole)
Visken
♣ Novo-Pindol, Syn-Pindolol
Drug class.: Nonselective β-adrenergic blocker

Action: This is a nonselective β_1- and β_2-adrenergic antagonist. The antihypertensive mechanism of action is unclear, but it may include a reduction in cardiac output and inhibition of renin release by the renal juxtaglomerular apparatus. Peripheral resistance decreases with long-term use. The antianginal action (when indicated for this use) may be related to a decrease in myocardial oxygen demand and negative chronotropic and inotropic effects. The antiarrhythmic action (when indicated for this use) has been related to a reduction in spontaneous pacemaker firing and slowing of AV nodal conduction.
Uses: Mild-to-moderate hypertension

Dosage and routes:
• *Adult:* PO 5 mg bid, usual dose 15 mg/day (5 mg tid); may increase by 10 mg/day q3-4wk to a max of 60 mg/day
Available forms include: Tabs 5, 10 mg

Side effects/adverse reactions:
▼ *ORAL:* Dry mouth, taste changes
CNS: Insomnia, dizziness, hallucinations, anxiety, fatigue
*CV: **CHF, AV block,** edema, chest pain, palpitation, claudication, tachycardia, **cardiac arrest,** hypertension, syncope
*GI: Nausea, abdominal pain, **mesenteric arterial thrombosis, ischemic colitis,** vomiting, diarrhea
*RESP: Dyspnea, **bronchospasm,** cough, rales
*HEMA: **Agranulocytosis, thrombocytopenia, purpura**
GU: Impotence, pollakiuria
EENT: Visual changes, double vision, sore throat, dry burning eyes
INTEG: Rash, alopecia, pruritus, fever
MISC: Joint pain, muscle pain, hypoglycemia

Contraindications: Hypersensitivity to β-blockers, cardiogenic shock, heart block (second or third degree), sinus bradycardia, CHF, cardiac failure, bronchial asthma, lactation

Precautions: Major surgery, pregnancy category B, diabetes mellitus, renal disease, thyroid disease, COPD, well-compensated heart failure, CAD, nonallergic bronchospasm, impaired hepatic function, children

Pharmacokinetics:
PO: Peak 1-2 hr, half-life 3-4 hr; 60%-65% is metabolized by liver;

---

excreted 35%-50% unchanged; excreted in breast milk

🦷 Drug interactions of concern to dentistry:
• Increased hypotension, bradycardia: anticholinergics, hydrocarbon inhalation anesthetics, fentanyl derivatives
• Decreased antihypertensive effects: indomethacin, sympathomimetics
• Increased effect of both drugs: phenothiazines, xanthines
• Decreased bronchodilation: theophyllines
• Hypertension, bradycardia: epinephrine, ephedrine
• Slow metabolism of drug: lidocaine

DENTAL CONSIDERATIONS
General:
• Monitor vital signs every appointment due to cardiovascular side effects.
• Patients on chronic drug therapy may rarely have symptoms of blood dyscrasias, which can include infection, bleeding, and poor healing.
• Stress from dental procedures may compromise cardiovascular function; determine patient risk.
• Use vasoconstrictors with caution, in low doses, and with careful aspiration. Avoid use of gingival retraction cord with epinephrine.
• Consider semisupine chair position for patient comfort if GI side effects occur.
• Assess salivary flow as a factor in caries, periodontal disease, and candidiasis.
• Consider drug effects if taste alteration occurs.

Consultations:
• In a patient with symptoms of blood dyscrasias, request a medical consult for blood studies and postpone dental treatment until normal values are reestablished.
• Medical consult may be required to assess disease control and patient's ability to tolerate stress.

Teach patient/family:
• Need for good oral hygiene to prevent soft tissue inflammation
• Caution to prevent injury when using oral hygiene aids
When chronic dry mouth occurs, advise patient:
• To avoid mouth rinses with high alcohol content due to drying effects
• Of need for daily use of home fluoride products to prevent caries
• To use sugarless gum, frequent sips of water, or saliva substitutes

---

pioglitazone
(pye-oh-gli'ta-zone)
Actos
Drug class.: Antidiabetic, oral

Action: An agonist for peroxisome proliferator-activated receptor gamma (PPAR-γ); improves target cell response to insulin without increasing insulin secretion; insulin must be present for this drug to act
Uses: Monotherapy, as an adjunct to diet and exercise in patients with type 2 diabetes mellitus; may also be used with metformin when metformin, diet, and exercise are not adequate for control

Dosage and routes:
• *Adult (monotherapy):* PO 15-30 mg qd, if response is inadequate can increase to 45 mg in increments

---

• *Adult (in combination/sulfonylurea, metformin):* PO 15-30 mg qd, adjust dose of sulfonylurea downward as required; max dose 45 mg/d

Available forms include: Tabs 15, 30, 45 mg

Side effects/adverse reactions:

▼ *ORAL:* Undefined tooth disorder

CNS: Paresthesias, headache

CV: Edema

GI: Abdominal pain

RESP: URI

EENT: Sinusitis, pharyngitis

HEMA: Anemia

ENDO: Hypoglycemia, ↑LDL cholesterol, ↑CPK, ↑ALT

MISC: Weight gain, myalgia

Contraindications: Hypersensitivity to pioglitazone or hypersensitivity to other glitazone oral antidiabetics

Precautions: Hepatic dysfunction (reduce dose), renal impairment, pregnancy category C, lactation, children <18 yr

Pharmacokinetics:

PO: Data lacking; some metabolism by cytochrome P-450 3A4 enzymes; highly plasma protein bound (98%), hepatic metabolism, some renal excretion

🦷 **Drug interactions of concern to dentistry:**

• None reported

DENTAL CONSIDERATIONS
General:

• Ensure that patient is following prescribed diet and regularly takes medication.

• Place on frequent recall to evaluate healing response.

• Short appointments and a stress reduction protocol may be required for anxious patients.

• Diabetics may be more susceptible to infection and have delayed wound healing.

• Question patient about self-monitoring of drug's antidiabetic effect, including blood glucose values or finger-stick records.

• Consider semisupine chair position for patient comfort if GI side effects occur.

Consultations:

• Medical consult may be required to assess disease control and patient's ability to tolerate stress.

• Medical consult may include data from patient's blood glucose monitoring, including glycosylated hemoglobin or HbA$_{1c}$ testing.

Teach patient/family:

• To prevent trauma when using oral hygiene aids

• Importance of updating health and drug history if physician makes any changes in evaluation or drug regimens

---

pirbuterol acetate

(perr-byoo′ter-ole)
Maxair

Drug class.: Bronchodilator

Action: Causes bronchodilation with little effect on heart rate by acting on β-receptors, causing increased cAMP and relaxation of smooth muscle

Uses: Reversible bronchospasm (prevention, treatment), including asthma; may be given with theophylline or steroids

Dosage and routes:

• *Adult and child >12 yr:* Aerosol 1-2 inh (0.4 mg) q4-6h; do not exceed 12 inh/day

Available forms include: Aerosol delivers 0.2 mg pirbuterol/actuation

Side effects/adverse reactions:
▼ *ORAL:* Taste changes, dry mouth

CNS: Tremors, anxiety, insomnia, headache, dizziness, stimulation, restlessness, hallucinations, drowsiness, irritability

CV: Palpitation, tachycardia, hypertension, angina, hypotension, dysrhythmias

GI: Heartburn, nausea, vomiting, anorexia

RESP: **Bronchospasm,** dyspnea, coughing

EENT: Dry nose, irritation of nose/throat

MS: Muscle cramps

Contraindications: Hypersensitivity to sympathomimetics, tachycardia

Precautions: Lactation, pregnancy category C, cardiac disorders, hyperthyroidism, diabetes mellitus, prostatic hypertrophy

Pharmacokinetics:
INH: Onset 3 min, peak 0.5-1 hr, duration 5 hr

DENTAL CONSIDERATIONS
General:
• Acute asthmatic episodes may be precipitated in the dental office. Sympathomimetic inhalants should be available for emergency use.

• Be aware that aspirin or sulfite preservatives in vasoconstrictor-containing products can exacerbate asthma.

• Monitor vital signs every appointment due to cardiovascular and respiratory side effects.

• Assess salivary flow as a factor in caries, periodontal disease, and candidiasis.

• Consider semisupine chair position for patients with respiratory disease.

• Short appointments and a stress reduction protocol may be required for anxious patients.

Consultations:
• Medical consult may be required to assess disease control and patient's ability to tolerate stress.

Teach patient/family:
• For inhalation dosage forms: rinse mouth with water after each dose to prevent dryness

When chronic dry mouth occurs, advise patient:

• To avoid mouth rinses with high alcohol content due to drying effects

• Of need for daily use of home fluoride products to prevent caries

• To use sugarless gum, frequent sips of water, or saliva substitutes

---

piroxicam
(peer-ox'i-kam)
Feldene
♣ Apo-Piroxicam, Novo-Pirocam, Nu-Pirox, PMS-Piroxicam

Drug class.: Nonsteroidal antiinflammatory

Action: Inhibits prostaglandin synthesis by interfering with cyclooxygenase needed for biosynthesis; possesses analgesic, antiinflammatory, antipyretic properties

Uses: Osteoarthritis, rheumatoid arthritis; unapproved: gouty arthritis

Dosage and routes:
• *Adult:* PO 20 mg qd or 10 mg bid

Available forms include: Caps 10, 20 mg; supp 10, 20 mg

Side effects/adverse reactions:
▼ *ORAL:* Stomatitis, bleeding, dry mouth, lichenoid reaction

---

CNS: Dizziness, drowsiness, head-ache, insomnia, depression, mal-aise, somnolence, nervousness, vertigo
CV: Peripheral edema
GI: Nausea, anorexia, vomiting, diarrhea, **cholestatic hepatitis,** jaundice, constipation, flatulence, cramps, peptic ulcer, epigastric distress, bleeding
*HEMA: **Blood dyscrasias***
*GU: **Nephrotoxicity: hematuria, oliguria, azotemia***
EENT: Tinnitus, hearing loss, blurred vision
INTEG: Purpura, rash, pruritus, sweating, photosensitivity, pemphigus-like reaction
META: Elevated ALT/AST, hypoglycemia
Contraindications: Hypersensitivity, asthma, severe renal disease, severe hepatic disease, ritonavir
Precautions: Pregnancy category C, lactation, children, bleeding disorders, GI disorders, cardiac disorders, hypersensitivity to other antiinflammatory agents, hypertension
Pharmacokinetics:
PO: Peak 2 hr, half-life 3-3.5 hr; 99% protein binding; metabolized in liver; excreted in urine (metabolites), breast milk
Drug interactions of concern to dentistry:
• GI ulceration, bleeding: aspirin, alcohol, corticosteroids
• Nephrotoxicity: acetaminophen (prolonged use and high doses)
• Possible risk of decreased renal function: cyclosporine
• Decreased action: salicylates
When prescribed for dental pain:
• Risk of increased effects of oral anticoagulants, oral antidiabetics, lithium, methotrexate

• Decreased antihypertensive effects of diuretics, β-adrenergic blockers, ACE inhibitors

DENTAL CONSIDERATIONS
General:
• Patients on chronic drug therapy may rarely have symptoms of blood dyscrasias, which can include infection, bleeding, and poor healing.
• Assess salivary flow as a factor in caries, periodontal disease, and candidiasis.
• Avoid prescribing for dental use during pregnancy.
• Minimize use of aspirin-containing products.
• Consider semisupine chair position for patients with arthritic disease or if GI side effects occur.
Consultations:
• In a patient with symptoms of blood dyscrasias, request a medical consult for blood studies and postpone dental treatment until normal values are reestablished.
• Medical consult may be required to assess disease control.
Teach patient/family:
• Importance of good oral hygiene to prevent soft tissue inflammation
• Caution to prevent injury when using oral hygiene aids
• To report oral lesions, soreness, or bleeding to dentist
When chronic dry mouth occurs, advise patient:
• To avoid mouth rinses with high alcohol content due to drying effects
• Of need for daily use of home fluoride products to prevent caries
• To use sugarless gum, frequent sips of water, or saliva substitutes

polymyxin B sulfate (ophthalmic)

(pol-i-mix′in)

Aerosporin

Drug class.: Antiinfective (ophthalmic)

Action: Inhibits cell wall permeability in susceptible organism

Uses: Superficial external ocular infections

Dosage and routes:
• *Adult and child:* Instill 1-2 gtt of 0.1%-0.25% sol bid-qid × 7-10 days

Available forms include: Powder for sol 500,000 U

Side effects/adverse reactions:
EENT: Poor corneal wound healing, temporary visual haze, overgrowth of nonsusceptible organisms, photosensitivity

Contraindications: Hypersensitivity; viral, mycobacterial, or fungal ocular infection

Precautions: Antibiotic hypersensitivity, pregnancy category B

DENTAL CONSIDERATIONS
General:
• Avoid dental light in patient's eyes; offer dark glasses for patient comfort and safety during dental treatment.

---

polythiazide

(pol-i-thye′azide)

Renese

Drug class.: Thiazide diuretic

Action: Acts on distal tubule by increasing excretion of water, sodium, chloride, potassium

Uses: Edema, hypertension, diuresis

Dosage and routes:
• *Adult:* PO 1-4 mg/day

Available forms include: Tabs 1, 2, 4 mg

Side effects/adverse reactions:
▼ *ORAL:* Dry mouth, increased thirst, bitter taste, lichenoid reaction

CNS: Drowsiness, paresthesia, anxiety, depression, headache, dizziness, fatigue, weakness, restlessness, syncope

CV: Irregular pulse, orthostatic hypotension, palpitation, volume depletion, dehydration

GI: Nausea, vomiting, anorexia, constipation, diarrhea, cramps, pancreatitis, GI irritation, hepatitis

HEMA: **Aplastic anemia, hemolytic anemia, leukopenia, agranulocytosis, thrombocytopenia,** neutropenia

GU: Frequency, polyuria, uremia, glucosuria, impotence, reduced libido

EENT: Blurred vision

INTEG: Rash, urticaria, purpura, photosensitivity, fever

META: Hyperglycemia, hyperuricemia, increased creatinine, BUN

ELECT: Hypokalemia, hypercalcemia, hyponatremia, hypochloremia

Contraindications: Hypersensitivity to thiazides or sulfonamides, anuria, renal decompensation, pregnancy category D

Precautions: Hypokalemia, renal disease, hepatic disease, gout, COPD, lupus erythematosus, diabetes mellitus

Pharmacokinetics:
PO: Onset 2 hr, peak 6 hr, duration 24-48 hr, half-life 26 hr; excreted

P

---

unchanged by kidneys; crosses placenta; excreted in breast milk

♣ Drug interactions of concern to dentistry:
• Decreased hypotensive response: indomethacin, NSAIDs, sympathomimetics
• Increased toxicity of nondepolarizing skeletal muscle relaxants

DENTAL CONSIDERATIONS
General:
• Take vital signs every appointment due to cardiovascular side effects.
• Patients on chronic drug therapy may rarely have symptoms of blood dyscrasias, which can include infection, bleeding, and poor healing.
• After supine positioning, have patient sit upright for at least 2 min before standing to avoid orthostatic hypotension.
• Assess salivary flow as a factor in caries, periodontal disease, and candidiasis.

Consultations:
• In a patient with symptoms of blood dyscrasias, request a medical consult for blood studies and postpone dental treatment until normal values are reestablished.
• Medical consult may be required to assess disease control.

Teach patient/family:
• Need for good oral hygiene to prevent periodontal inflammation
• Caution to prevent injury when using oral hygiene aids

When chronic dry mouth occurs, advise patient:
• To avoid mouth rinses with high alcohol content due to drying effects
• Of need for daily use of home fluoride products to prevent caries
• To use sugarless gum, frequent sips of water, or saliva substitutes

potassium acetate/ potassium bicarbonate/ potassium chloride/ potassium gluconate/ potassium phosphate

Potassium bicarbonate effervescent: Effer-K, K⁺ Care ET, K-Electrolyte, K-Ide, Klor-Con/EF, Klorvess, K-Lyte, Vesant

Potassium chloride: Cena-K, K⁺ 10, Kaochlor, Kaochlor-SF, Kaon-Cl, KayCiel, K-Dur, K-Lease, K-Lor, Klor-Con 8, Klor-Con 10, Klorvess, Klotrix, K-Norm, K-Tab, Micro-K, Rum-K, Slow-K, Ten-K, Tri-K

♣ Apo-K, Kalium, Novolente-K

Potassium gluconate: Kaon, Kayelixir, K-G Elixir

Drug class.: Potassium electrolyte

Action: Needed for adequate transmission of nerve impulses and cardiac contraction, renal function, intracellular ion maintenance

Uses: Prevention and treatment of hypokalemia

Dosage and routes:
Potassium bicarbonate
• *Adult:* PO dissolve 25-50 mEq in water qd-qid

Potassium acetate–hypokalemia
• *Adult and child:* PO 40-100 mEq/ day in divided doses 2-4 days

Hypokalemia (prevention)
• *Adult and child:* PO 20 mEq/day in 2-4 divided doses

Potassium chloride
• *Adult:* PO 40-100 mEq in divided doses tid-qid; IV 20 mEq/hr when diluted as 40 mEq/1000 ml, not to exceed 150 mEq/day

italic = common side effects

Potassium gluconate
• *Adult:* PO 40-100 mEq in divided doses tid-qid
Potassium phosphate
• *Adult:* IV 1 mEq/hr in sol of 60 mEq/L, not to exceed 150 mEq/day; PO 40-100 mEq/day in divided doses
Available forms include: Liq 20, 30, 40, 45 mEq per 15 ml; powder 15, 20, 25 mEq per packet; effervescent tabs 20, 25, 50 mEq per tablet; con rel tabs 6.7, 8.0, 10 mEq per tab; ext rel tabs 10, 20 mEq per tab; con rel caps 8, 10 mEq per capsule; IV preps 10 mEq/g, 40 mEq/ml in 10, 20 ml vials
Side effects/adverse reactions:
CNS: Confusion, hyperkalemia
*CV: **Cardiac depression, dysrhythmias, arrest, peaking T waves, lowered R and depressed RST, prolonged P-R interval, widened QRS complex,*** bradycardia
GI: Nausea, vomiting, cramps, pain, diarrhea, ulceration of small bowel
GU: Oliguria
INTEG: Cold extremities, rash
Contraindications: Renal disease (severe), severe hemolytic disease, Addison's disease, hyperkalemia, acute dehydration, extensive tissue breakdown
Precautions: Cardiac disease, potassium-sparing diuretic therapy, systemic acidosis, pregnancy category A, renal impairment
Pharmacokinetics:
PO: Excreted by kidneys and in feces
IV: Immediate onset of action
Drug interactions of concern to dentistry:
• Decreased potassium requirement: corticosteroids

• Increased GI side effects: anticholinergic drugs, NSAIDs
• Increased serum potassium: NSAIDs, cyclosporine
DENTAL CONSIDERATIONS
General:
• Patients taking potassium supplements will normally be taking a diuretic. Compliance with potassium supplements can be a problem. Verify serum potassium levels as required.
• Consider semisupine chair position for patient comfort if GI side effects occur.

---

povidone iodine
(poe'vi-done)
ACU-dyne, Aerodine, Betadine, Betagen, Biodine, Efodine, Iodex-P, Mallisol, Minidyne, Operand, Polydine
♣ Proviodine

Drug class.: Iodophor disinfectant

Action: Destroys a wide variety of microorganisms by local irritation, germicidal action
Uses: Cleansing wounds, disinfection, preoperative skin preparation removal
Dosage and routes:
• *Adult and child:* Sol use as needed, topical only
Available forms include: TOP—a variety of solutions, ointments, aerosols, foams, creams, gels, and pads
Side effects/adverse reactions:
*GU: **Renal damage***
META: Metabolic acidosis
INTEG: Irritation
Contraindications: Hypersensitivity to iodine, pregnancy category D (vaginal antiseptic)

Precautions: Extensive burns

🦷 **Drug interactions of concern to dentistry:**
• Do not use with alcohol or hydrogen peroxide

DENTAL CONSIDERATIONS
General:
• Assess for allergies to seafood; if present, drug should not be used.
• Store in tight, light-resistant container.
• Evaluate area of the body involved for irritation, rash, breaks, dryness, and scales.

Teach patient/family:
• To discontinue use if rash, irritation, or redness occurs

---

pramipexole dihydrochloride
(pra-mi-pex′ole)
Mirapex
Drug class.: Antiparkinson agent

Action: Acts as a dopamine agonist at D_2 receptor sites
Uses: Idiopathic Parkinson's disease
Dosage and routes:
• *Adult:* PO all doses should be titrated gradually beginning with an initial dose of 0.125 mg tid for 5-7 days; doses can be increased by increments each week to a tolerated range of 1.5-4.5 mg/day in 3 divided doses; dose must be reduced in renal impairment
Available forms include: Tabs 0.125, 0.25, 1, 1.5 mg
Side effects/adverse reactions:
▼ *ORAL:* Dry mouth, taste perversion
CNS: Hallucinations, dizziness, somnolence, insomnia, headache, malaise
CV: Postural hypotension, edema

GI: Nausea, constipation, dyspepsia, anorexia
GU: Impotence, urinary frequency
EENT: Vision abnormalities
INTEG: Rash
MS: Extrapyramidal syndrome
MISC: Asthenia, accidental injury
Contraindications: Hypersensitivity
Precautions: Orthostatic hypotension, hallucination risk higher >65 yr, renal insufficiency, caution in driving a car (somnolence), risk of falling asleep while performing daily activities, pregnancy category C, lactation, use not established in children
Pharmacokinetics:
PO: Rapid absorption, peak levels in 2 hr, bioavailability 90%, low plasma protein binding (15%), 90% of dose excreted unchanged in urine

🦷 **Drug interactions of concern to dentistry:**
• Increased CNS depression: all CNS depressants
• Possible decreased effects: dopamine antagonists (phenothiazines, butyrophenones, or thioxanthenes) and metoclopramide

DENTAL CONSIDERATIONS
General:
• Monitor vital signs every appointment due to cardiovascular side effects.
• Assess salivary flow as factor in caries, periodontal disease, and candidiasis.
• Consider semisupine chair position for patient comfort if GI side effects occur.
• After supine positioning, have patient sit upright for at least 2 min to avoid orthostatic hypotension.

Consultations:
• Medical consult may be required to assess disease control and patient's ability to tolerate stress.

Teach patient/family:
• Importance of good oral hygiene to prevent soft tissue inflammation
• Caution to prevent trauma when using oral hygiene aids
• Use of electric toothbrush if patient has difficulty holding conventional devices
• Importance of updating health and drug history if physician makes any changes in evaluation or drug regimens

When chronic dry mouth occurs, advise patient:
• To avoid mouth rinses with high alcohol content due to drying effects
• To use daily home fluoride products for anticaries effect
• To use sugarless gum, frequent sips of water, or saliva substitutes

---

pravastatin sodium
(pra'va-sta-tin)
Pravachol
Drug class.: Antihyperlipidemic

Action: Inhibits HMG-CoA reductase enzyme, reducing cholesterol synthesis; reduced synthesis of VLDL; plasma triglyceride levels may also be decreased

Uses: As an adjunct in homozygous familial hypercholesterolemia, mixed hyperlipidemia, elevated serum triglyceride levels and type IV hyperproteinemia, also reduces total cholesterol LDL-C, apo B, and triglyceride levels; patient should first be placed on cholesterol-lowering diet

Dosage and routes:
• *Adult:* PO 10-20 mg qd at hs (range 10-40 mg qd)
Available forms include: Tabs 10, 20, 40 mg

Side effects/adverse reactions:
CNS: Headache, dizziness, psychic disturbances, fatigue
CV: Chest pain
GI: ***Liver dysfunction, hepatitis,*** pancreatitis, nausea, constipation, diarrhea, dyspepsia, flatus, abdominal pain, heartburn, vomiting
GU: Gynecomastia, libido loss
EENT: Lens opacities, common cold, rhinitis, cough, cataracts
INTEG: Rash, pruritus
MS: ***Myositis, rhabdomyolysis,*** muscle cramps, myalgia
MISC: Alopecia, edema

Contraindications: Hypersensitivity, pregnancy category X, lactation, active liver disease

Precautions: Past liver disease, alcoholics, severe acute infections, trauma, hypotension, uncontrolled seizure disorders, severe metabolic disorders, electrolyte imbalances

Pharmacokinetics
PO: Peak 1-1.5 hr; highly protein bound; metabolized by liver; excreted in urine, feces, breast milk; crosses placenta

🦷 **Drug interactions of concern to dentistry:**
• Increased risk of myopathy or rhabdomyolysis: erythromycin, itraconazole

DENTAL CONSIDERATIONS
General:
• Monitor vital signs every appointment due to possible cardiovascular disease.
• Consider semisupine chair position for patient comfort if GI side effects occur.

P

---

prazosin HCl
(pra'zoe-sin)
Minipress

Drug class.: Antihypertensive, α-adrenergic antagonist

Action: Reduction in blood pressure results from blockage of α-adrenergic receptors and reduced peripheral resistance

Uses: Hypertension; unapproved: CHF, urinary retention in prostatic hypertrophy, pheochromocytoma

Dosage and routes:
• *Adult:* PO 1 mg bid or tid, increasing to 20 mg qd in divided doses if required; usual range 6-15 mg/day, not to exceed 1 mg initially

Available forms include: Caps 1, 2, 5 mg; tabs 1, 2, 5 mg

Side effects/adverse reactions:
▼ *ORAL:* Dry mouth, lichenoid drug reaction
CNS: Dizziness, headache, drowsiness, anxiety, depression, vertigo, weakness, fatigue, light-headedness, lethargy, syncope
CV: Palpitation, orthostatic hypotension, tachycardia, edema, dyspnea, angina
GI: Nausea, vomiting, diarrhea, constipation, abdominal pain
GU: Urinary frequency, incontinence, impotence, priapism
EENT: Blurred vision, epistaxis, tinnitus, red sclera

Contraindications: Hypersensitivity, severe CHF

Precautions: Pregnancy category C, children

Pharmacokinetics:
PO: Onset 2 hr, peak 1-3 hr, duration 6-12 hr, half-life 2-4 hr; metabolized in liver; excreted via bile, feces (>90%), in urine (<10%)

🐾 **Drug interactions of concern to dentistry:**
• Increased effects: epinephrine
• Decreased effect: indomethacin, NSAIDs

DENTAL CONSIDERATIONS
General:
• Monitor vital signs every appointment due to cardiovascular side effects.
• After supine positioning, have patient sit upright for at least 2 min before standing to avoid orthostatic hypotension.
• Assess salivary flow as a factor in caries, periodontal disease, and candidiasis.
• Limit use of sodium-containing products, such as saline IV fluids, for patients with a dietary salt restriction.
• Stress from dental procedures may compromise cardiovascular function; determine patient risk.
• Short appointments and a stress reduction protocol may be required for anxious patients.

Consultations:
• Medical consult may be required to assess disease control.

Teach patient/family: *When chronic dry mouth occurs, advise patient:*
• To avoid mouth rinses with high alcohol content due to drying effects
• Of need for daily use of home fluoride products to prevent caries
• To use sugarless gum, frequent sips of water, or saliva substitutes

prednicarbate

(pred'ni-kar-bate)

Dermatop Emollient Cream

Drug class.: Topical corticosteroid, group III potency

Action: Glucocorticoids have multiple actions that include antiinflammatory and immunosuppressant effects. They inhibit phospholipase A$_2$, interfering with or reducing the synthesis of prostaglandins and leukotrienes. They also bind to cytoplasmic glucocorticoid receptors (GRs) and enter the cell nucleus to bind with DNA. This results in the synthesis of various enzymes such as collagenase, elastase, and cytokines that play important roles in inflammation and immunosuppression. They also suppress the production of lymphocytes, monocytes, and eosinophils.

Uses: Relief of inflammatory and pruritic manifestations of corticosteroid-responsive dermatoses

Dosage and routes:
• *Adult:* TOP apply a thin film to affected area bid

Available forms include: Cream 0.1% in 15, 60 g

Side effects/adverse reactions:

INTEG: Skin atrophy, pruritus, burning, urticaria, edema, rash

Contraindications: Hypersensitivity

Precautions: Pregnancy category C, lactation, children <18 yr, occlusive dressings; bacterial, viral, or fungal skin infections

 Drug interactions of concern to dentistry:
• None reported

DENTAL CONSIDERATIONS
General:
• Determine why the patient is taking the drug.
• Use on oral herpetic ulcerations is contraindicated.

prednisolone/ prednisolone acetate/ prednisolone phosphate/ prednisolone tebutate

(pred-niss'oh-lone)

Prednisolone: Delta-Cortef, Prelone

Prednisolone acetate (not for IV use): Key-Pred 25 and 50, Predalone-50, Predcor-50

Prednisolone tebutate: Prednisol TBA

Prednisolone sodium phosphate: Hydeltrasol, Key-Pred-SP, Pediapred

Drug class.: Glucocorticoid, immediate acting

Action: Glucocorticoids have multiple actions that include antiinflammatory and immunosuppressant effects. They inhibit phospholipase A$_2$, interfering with or reducing the synthesis of prostaglandins and leukotrienes. They also bind to cytoplasmic glucocorticoid receptors (GRs) and enter the cell nucleus to bind with DNA. This results in the synthesis of various enzymes such as collagenase, elastase, and cytokines that play important roles in inflammation and immunosuppression. They also suppress the production of lymphocytes, monocytes, and eosinophils.

Uses: Severe inflammation, immunosuppression, neoplasms, adrenal insufficiency

Dosage and routes:
• *Adult:* PO 5-60 mg/day; IM 4-60 mg/day (acetate, phosphate); IV 4-60 mg (phosphate); 4-5 mg in small joints, 10-20 mg in large joints (phosphate); 8-20 mg in joint lesion (tebutate); 40 mg intralesional (acetate); 10-30 mg soft tissue (phosphate); syr 15 mg/5 ml

Available forms include: Tabs 5 mg; syr 5 mg/5 ml and 15 mg/5 ml; inj 25, 50 mg/ml (acetate); inj 20 mg/ml (terbutate); inj 20 mg/ml (phosphate); PO liq 5 mg/5 ml

Side effects/adverse reactions:
▼ *ORAL: Candidiasis,* dry mouth, delayed wound healing, petechiae
CNS: Depression, flushing, sweating, headache, mood changes
CV: Hypertension, **circulatory collapse, thrombophlebitis, embolism,** tachycardia
GI: Diarrhea, nausea, abdominal distention, **GI hemorrhage, pancreatitis,** increased appetite
HEMA: **Thrombocytopenia**
EENT: Fungal infections, increased intraocular pressure, blurred vision
INTEG: Acne, delayed wound healing, ecchymosis, petechiae, striae
MS: Fractures, osteoporosis, muscle weakness

Contraindications: Psychosis, hypersensitivity, idiopathic thrombocytopenia, acute glomerulonephritis, amebiasis, fungal infections, nonasthmatic bronchial disease, child <2 yr

Precautions: Pregnancy category C, diabetes mellitus, glaucoma, osteoporosis, seizure disorders, ulcerative colitis, CHF, myasthenia gravis, ulcerative GI disease, rifampin

Pharmacokinetics:
PO: Peak 1-2 hr, duration 2 days
IM: Peak 3-45 hr

⚖ Drug interactions of concern to dentistry:
• Decreased action: barbiturates, rifampin, rifabutin
• Increased side effects: alcohol, salicylates, NSAIDs
• Increased action: ketoconazole, macrolide antibiotics (erythromycin, clarithromycin, azithromycin)
• Hepatotoxicity: acetaminophen (chronic use, high doses)

DENTAL CONSIDERATIONS
General:
• Take vital signs every appointment due to cardiovascular side effects.
• Patients on chronic drug therapy may rarely have symptoms of blood dyscrasias, which can include infection, bleeding, and poor healing.
• Assess salivary flow as a factor in caries, periodontal disease, and candidiasis.
• Avoid prescribing aspirin-containing products.
• Place on frequent recall to evaluate healing response.
• Prophylactic antibiotics may be indicated to prevent infection if surgery or deep scaling is planned.
• Symptoms of oral infections may be masked.
• Determine dose and duration of steroid therapy for each patient to assess risk for stress tolerance and immunosuppression.
• Patients who have been or are currently on chronic steroid therapy (>2 wk) require supplemental steroids for dental treatment.
• Determine why the patient is taking the drug.

italic = common side effects

Consultations:
• In a patient with symptoms of blood dyscrasias, request a medical consult for blood studies and postpone dental treatment until normal values are reestablished.
• Medical consult may be required to assess disease control.
• Consult may be required to confirm steroid dose and duration of use.

Teach patient/family:
• Importance of good oral hygiene to prevent soft tissue inflammation
• Caution to prevent injury when using oral hygiene aids
When chronic dry mouth occurs, advise patient:
• To avoid mouth rinses with high alcohol content due to drying effects
• Of need for daily use of home fluoride products to prevent caries
• To use sugarless gum, frequent sips of water, or saliva substitutes

---

prednisone
(pred'ni-sone)
Deltasone, Liquid Pred, Meticorten, Orasone, Prednicen-M, Prednisone Intensol, Sterapred ❧ Apo-Prednisone, Winpred
Drug class.: Glucocorticoid, intermediate acting

Action: Glucocorticoids have multiple actions that include antiinflammatory and immunosuppressant effects. They inhibit phospholipase A_2, interfering with or reducing the synthesis of prostaglandins and leukotrienes. They also bind to cytoplasmic glucocorticoid receptors (GRs) and enter the cell nucleus to bind with DNA. This results in the synthesis of various enzymes such as collagenase, elastase, and cytokines that play important roles in inflammation and immunosuppression. They also suppress the production of lymphocytes, monocytes, and eosinophils.

Uses: Severe inflammation, immunosuppression, neoplasms, multiple sclerosis, collagen disorders, dermatologic disorders

Dosage and routes:
• *Adult:* PO 2.5-15 mg bid-qid, then qd or qod; maintenance up to 250 mg/day
Available forms include: Tabs 1, 2.5, 5, 10, 20, 25, 50 mg; oral sol 5 mg/5 ml; syr 5 mg/5 ml

Side effects/adverse reactions:
▼ *ORAL: Candidiasis,* dry mouth, poor wound healing, petechiae
CNS: Depression, flushing, sweating, headache, mood changes
*CV: Hypertension, **circulatory collapse, thrombophlebitis, embolism,** tachycardia*
*GI: Diarrhea, nausea, abdominal distention, **GI hemorrhage, pancreatitis,** increased appetite*
*HEMA: **Thrombocytopenia***
EENT: Fungal infections, increased intraocular pressure, blurred vision
INTEG: Acne, poor wound healing, ecchymosis, petechiae
MS: Fractures, osteoporosis, weakness

Contraindications: Psychosis, hypersensitivity, idiopathic thrombocytopenia, acute glomerulonephritis, amebiasis, fungal infections, nonasthmatic bronchial disease, child <2 yr, AIDS, TB

Precautions: Pregnancy category C, diabetes mellitus, glaucoma, osteoporosis, seizure disorders, ulcer-

---

ative colitis, CHF, myasthenia gravis, renal disease, esophagitis, peptic ulcer, rifampin

Pharmacokinetics:

PO: Peak 1-2 hr, duration 1-1.5 days, half-life 3.5-4 hr

🦷 **Drug interactions of concern to dentistry:**

• Decreased action: barbiturates, rifampin, rifabutin

• Increased side effects: alcohol, salicylates, NSAIDs

• Increased action: ketoconazole, macrolide antibiotics

• Hepatotoxicity: acetaminophen (chronic, high doses)

DENTAL CONSIDERATIONS

General:

• Monitor vital signs every appointment due to cardiovascular side effects.

• Patients on chronic drug therapy may rarely have symptoms of blood dyscrasias, which can include infection, bleeding, and poor healing.

• Avoid aspirin-containing products.

• Assess salivary flow as a factor in caries, periodontal disease, and candidiasis.

• Symptoms of oral infections may be masked.

• Place on frequent recall to evaluate healing response.

• Prophylactic antibiotics may be indicated to prevent infection if surgery or deep scaling is planned.

• Determine dose and duration of steroid therapy for each patient to assess risk for stress tolerance and immunosuppression.

• Patients who have been or are currently on chronic steroid ther-

apy (>2 wk) may require supplemental steroids for dental treatment.

• Determine why the patient is taking the drug.

Consultations:

• In a patient with symptoms of blood dyscrasias, request a medical consult for blood studies and postpone dental treatment until normal values are reestablished.

• Medical consult may be required to assess disease control.

• Consult may be required to confirm steroid dose and duration of use.

Teach patient/family:

• Importance of good oral hygiene to prevent soft tissue inflammation

• Caution to prevent injury when using oral hygiene aids

When chronic dry mouth occurs, advise patient:

• To avoid mouth rinses with high alcohol content due to drying effects

• Of need for daily use of home fluoride products to prevent caries

• To use sugarless gum, frequent sips of water, or saliva substitutes

---

prilocaine hydrochloride (local)

(pry'lo-kane)

Citanest

With vasoconstrictor: Citanest Forte with epinephrine

Drug class.: Amide local anesthetic

Action: Inhibits ion fluxes across membranes, particularly sodium transport across cell membrane; decreases rise of depolarization phase of action potential; blocks nerve action potential

Uses: Local dental anesthesia

Dosage and routes:

Dental injection: infiltration or conduction block

• *Prilocaine 4% without vasoconstrictor:* Max dose of 400 mg over a 2-hr period per dental appointment for healthy adult patient*; doses must be adjusted for medically compromised, debilitated, or elderly and for each individual patient. Doses in excess of 400 mg have caused methemoglobinemia. **Always use the lowest effective dose, a slow injection rate, and a careful aspiration technique.**

Example calculations illustrating amount of drug administered per dental cartridge(s)

# of dental cartridges (1.8 ml)	mg of prilocaine (4%)
1	72
2	144
3	216
4	288

*Max dose cited from *USP-DI*, ed 16, 1996, US Pharmacopeial Convention, Inc, as well as manufacturer's package insert. Doses may differ in other published reference resources.

• *Prilocaine 4% with epinephrine 1:200,000:* Recommended doses are the same; adjust doses for each individual as previously indicated

Example calculations illustrating amount of drug administered per dental cartridge(s)

# of cartridges (1.8 ml)	mg of prilocaine (4%)	mg (µg) vasoconstrictor (1:200,000)
1	72	0.009 (9)
2	144	0.018 (18)
4	288	0.036 (36)

Available forms include: 4% sol, 4% sol with epinephrine 1:200,000

Side effects/adverse reactions:

▼ *ORAL: Numbness, tingling,* trismus

*CNS: **Convulsions, loss of consciousness,** drowsiness, disorientation, tremors, shivering, anxiety, restlessness*

*CV: **Myocardial depression, cardiac arrest, dysrhythmias,** bradycardia, hypotension, hypertension*

GI: Nausea, vomiting

*RESP: **Status asthmaticus, respiratory arrest, anaphylaxis***

*HEMA: **Methemoglobinemia***

INTEG: Rash, urticaria, allergic reactions

Contraindications: Hypersensitivity, cross-sensitivity among amides (rare), severe liver disease

Precautions: Elderly, pregnancy category B, large doses of local anesthetic in myasthenia gravis, risk of methemoglobinemia

Pharmacokinetics:

INJ: Onset 2-10 min, duration 2-4 hr; metabolized in liver; excreted in urine

🦷 **Drug interactions of concern to dentistry:**

• CNS depressants: increased risk of CNS depression with all CNS

---

bold italic = life-threatening conditions

depressants, especially in children and when larger doses are used
• Avoid placing dental cartridges in disinfection solutions with heavy metals or surface-active agents; may see release of ions into local anesthetic solutions with tissue irritation following injection
• Avoid excessive exposure of dental cartridges to light or heat; hastens deterioration of vasoconstrictor; observe for color change in local anesthetic solution
• Risk of cardiovascular side effects; rapid intravascular administration of local anesthetic containing vasoconstrictor, either alone or in patients taking tricyclic antidepressants, MAO inhibitors, digitalis drugs, cocaine, phenothiazines, β-blockers, and in the presence of halogenated-hydrocarbon general anesthetics; use smallest effective vasoconstrictor dose and careful aspiration technique
• Avoid use of vasoconstrictors in patients with uncontrolled hyperthyroidism, diabetes, angina, or hypertension; refer these patients for medical treatment before elective dental treatment
DENTAL CONSIDERATIONS
General:
• Monitor vital signs every appointment due to cardiovascular side effects.
• Often used with vasoconstrictor for increased duration of action.
• Lubricate dry lips before injection or dental treatment as required.
Teach patient/family:
• To use care to prevent injury while numbness exists and to refrain from chewing gum and eating following dental anesthesia

• To report any signs of infection, muscle pain, or fever to dentist when feeling returns
• To report any unusual soft tissue reactions

---

primaquine phosphate
(prim'a-kween)
generic
Drug class.: Antiprotozoal

Action: Action is unknown; thought to destroy exoerythrocytic forms by gametocidal action
Uses: Malaria caused by *P. vivax;* unapproved: with clindamycin in the treatment of *P. carinii* in AIDS
Dosage and routes:
• *Adult:* PO 15 mg base qd × 2 wk
• *Child:* PO 0.9 mg/kg base daily × 2 wk
Available forms include: Tabs 26.3 mg (equivalent to 15 mg base)
Side effects/adverse reactions:
CNS: Headache
CV: Hypertension
GI: Nausea, vomiting, anorexia, cramps
*HEMA: **Agranulocytosis, granulocytopenia, leukopenia, hemolytic anemia, leukocytosis,** mild anemia, **methemoglobinemia***
EENT: Blurred vision, difficulty focusing
INTEG: Pruritus, skin eruptions
Contraindications: Hypersensitivity, anemia, lupus erythematosus, methemoglobinemia, porphyria, rheumatoid arthritis, methemoglobin reductase deficiency, G6PD deficiency
Precautions: Pregnancy category C

Pharmacokinetics:

PO: Half-life 3.7-9.6 hr; metabolized by liver (metabolites)

Drug interactions of concern to dentistry:

• None

DENTAL CONSIDERATIONS
General:

• Patients on chronic drug therapy may rarely have symptoms of blood dyscrasias, which can include infection, bleeding, and poor healing.

• Avoid dental light in patient's eyes; offer dark glasses for patient comfort.

Consultations:

• In a patient with symptoms of blood dyscrasias, request a medical consult for blood studies and postpone dental treatment until normal values are reestablished.

Teach patient/family:

• Importance of good oral hygiene to prevent soft tissue inflammation
• Caution to prevent injury when using oral hygiene aids

---

primidone

(pri'mi-done)

Mysoline

♣ APO-Primidone, PMS-Primidone, Sertan

Drug class.: Anticonvulsant, barbiturate derivative

Action: Raises seizure threshold by unknown mechanism; may be related to facilitation of GABA; metabolized to phenobarbital

Uses: Generalized tonic-clonic (grand mal), complex-partial psychomotor seizures

Dosage and routes:

• *Adult and child >8 yr (no prior treatment):* PO 100-125 mg hs, days 1-3; 100-125 mg bid, days 4-6; 100-125 mg tid, days 7-9; then 250 mg tid to qid, not to exceed 500 mg qid

• *Adult and child >8 yr (taking other anticonvulsants):* PO 100-125 mg hs, increase gradually as other drug is decreased

• *Child <8 yr (no prior treatment):* PO 50 mg hs, days 1-3; 50 mg bid, days 4-6; 100 mg bid, days 7-9; then maintenance dose of 125-250 mg tid

Available forms include: Tabs 50, 250 mg; susp 250 mg/5 ml

Side effects/adverse reactions:

CNS: Stimulation, drowsiness, dizziness, confusion, sedation, headache, flushing, hallucinations, coma, psychosis, ataxia, vertigo

GI: Nausea, vomiting, anorexia

HEMA: **Thrombocytopenia, leukopenia, neutropenia, eosinophilia, megaloblastic anemia,** reduces serum folate level, lymphadenopathy

GU: Impotence, polyuria

EENT: Diplopia, nystagmus, edema of eyelids

INTEG: Rash, edema, alopecia, lupus-like syndrome

Contraindications: Hypersensitivity, porphyria, pregnancy category D

Precautions: COPD, hepatic disease, renal disease, hyperactive children

Pharmacokinetics:

PO: Peak 4 hr, half-life 3-24 hr; excreted by kidneys, in breast milk

---

bold italic = life-threatening conditions

♣ Drug interactions of concern to dentistry:
• Increased CNS depression: alcohol, other CNS depressants
• Increased metabolism/hepatotoxicity: halothane, halogenated-hydrocarbon inhalation anesthetics
• Increased seizure threshold: haloperidol, phenothiazines
• Decreased effects of acetaminophen, corticosteroids, doxycycline, fenoprofen

DENTAL CONSIDERATIONS
General:
• Ask about type of epilepsy, seizure frequency, and quality of seizure control.
• After supine positioning, have patient sit upright for at least 2 min before standing to avoid orthostatic hypotension.
• Patients on chronic drug therapy may rarely have symptoms of blood dyscrasias, which can include infection, bleeding, and poor healing.
• Short appointments and a stress reduction protocol may be required for anxious patients.
Consultations:
• Medical consult may be required to assess disease control and patient's ability to tolerate stress.
• In a patient with symptoms of blood dyscrasias, request a medical consult for blood studies and postpone dental treatment until normal values are reestablished.
Teach patient/family:
• Importance of good oral hygiene to prevent soft tissue inflammation
• Caution to prevent injury when using oral hygiene aids
• To avoid mouth rinses with high alcohol content due to drying effects

probenecid
(proe-ben'e-sid)
generic
♣ Benuryl
Drug class.: Uricosuric

Action: Inhibits tubular reabsorption of urates, with increased excretion of uric acids
Uses: Hyperuricemia in gout, gouty arthritis, adjunct to cephalosporin or penicillin treatment by reducing excretion and maintaining high blood levels
Dosage and routes:
Gout/gouty arthritis
• *Adult:* PO 250 mg bid for 1 wk, then 500 mg bid, not to exceed 2 g/day; maintenance 500 mg/day for 6 mo
Adjunct in penicillin/cephalosporin treatment
• *Adult and child >50 kg:* PO 500 mg qid with antibiotic
• *Child <50 kg:* PO 25 mg/kg, then 40 mg/kg in divided doses qid
Available forms include: Tabs 500 mg
Side effects/adverse reactions:
▼ *ORAL:* Painful gingivae, increased thirst
CNS: Drowsiness, headache
CV: Bradycardia
GI: Gastric irritation, nausea, vomiting, anorexia, **hepatic necrosis**
RESP: **Apnea,** irregular respirations
GU: **Nephrotic syndrome,** glycosuria, frequency
INTEG: Rash, dermatitis, pruritus, fever
META: Acidosis, hypokalemia, hyperchloremia, hyperglycemia
Contraindications: Hypersensitivity, severe hepatic disease, blood

dyscrasias, severe renal disease, CrCl <50 mg/min, history of uric acid calculus, ketorolac

Precautions: Pregnancy category B, severe respiratory disease, lactation, cardiac edema, child <2 yr

Pharmacokinetics:

PO: Peak 2-4 hr, duration 8 hr, half-life 8-10 hr; metabolized by liver; excreted in urine; crosses placenta

🦷 Drug interactions of concern to dentistry:

• Increased toxicity: dapsone, indomethacin, other NSAIDs, acyclovir
• Increased sedation: benzodiazepines
• Decreased action: alcohol, salicylates
• Increased duration of action: penicillins, cephalosporins
• Contraindicated: ketorolac

DENTAL CONSIDERATIONS

General:

• Avoid prescribing aspirin-containing products.

Teach patient/family:

• Importance of good oral hygiene to prevent soft tissue inflammation
• Caution to prevent injury when using oral hygiene aids
• To avoid mouth rinses with high alcohol content due to drying effects

---

procainamide HCl

(proe-kane-a'mide)

Procanbid, Pronestyl, Pronestyl SR

Drug class.: Antidysrhythmic (class Ia)

Action: Depresses excitability of cardiac muscle to electrical stimulation and slows conduction in atrium, bundle of His, and ventricle

Uses: PVCs, atrial fibrillation, PAT, atrial dysrhythmias, ventricular tachycardia

Dosage and routes:

Atrial fibrillation/PAT

• *Adult:* PO 1-1.25 g, may give another 750 mg if needed; if no response then 500 mg-1 g q2h until desired response; maintenance 50 mg/kg in divided doses q6h

Ventricular tachycardia

• *Adult:* PO 1 g; maintenance 50 mg/kg/day given in 3 hr intervals; sus rel tabs 500 mg-1.25 g q6h

Other dysrhythmias

• *Adult:* IV bol 100 mg q5min, given 25-50 mg/min, not to exceed 500 mg; then IV inf 2-6 mg/min

Available forms include: Caps 250, 375, 500 mg; tabs 250, 375, 500 mg; sus rel tabs 250, 500, 750, 1000 mg; inj IV 100, 500 mg/ml

Side effects/adverse reactions:

▼ *ORAL:* Dry mouth

CNS: Headache, dizziness, confusion, psychosis, restlessness, irritability, weakness

*CV: Hypotension, **heart block, cardiovascular collapse, arrest***

GI: Nausea, vomiting, anorexia, diarrhea, hepatomegaly

*HEMA: **Agranulocytosis, thrombocytopenia, neutropenia, hemolytic anemia,** SLE syndrome*

INTEG: Rash, urticaria, edema, swelling, pruritus

Contraindications: Hypersensitivity, myasthenia gravis, severe heart block

Precautions: Pregnancy category C, lactation, children, renal disease, liver disease, CHF, respiratory depression, elderly

Pharmacokinetics:

PO: Peak 1-2 hr, duration 3 hr (8 hr extended)

IM: Peak 10-60 min, duration 3 hr

---

bold italic = life-threatening conditions

Half-life 3 hr; metabolized in liver to active metabolites; excreted unchanged by kidneys (60%)

🦷 Drug interactions of concern to dentistry:

• Decreased effects: barbiturates
• Increased effects of neuromuscular blockers, anticholinergics

DENTAL CONSIDERATIONS

General:

• Monitor vital signs every appointment due to cardiovascular side effects.
• Patients on chronic drug therapy may rarely have symptoms of blood dyscrasias, which can include infection, bleeding, and poor healing.
• After supine positioning, have patient sit upright for at least 2 min before standing to avoid orthostatic hypotension.
• Assess salivary flow as a factor in caries, periodontal disease, and candidiasis.
• Stress from dental procedures may compromise cardiovascular function; determine patient risk.

Consultations:

• In a patient with symptoms of blood dyscrasias, request a medical consult for blood studies and postpone dental treatment until normal values are reestablished.
• Medical consult may be required to assess disease control and patient's ability to tolerate stress.

Teach patient/family:

• Importance of good oral hygiene to prevent soft tissue inflammation
• Caution to prevent injury when using oral hygiene aids

When chronic dry mouth occurs, advise patient:

• To avoid mouth rinses with high alcohol content due to drying effects

• Of need for daily use of home fluoride products to prevent caries
• To use sugarless gum, frequent sips of water, or saliva substitutes

---

procarbazine HCl

(proe-kar′ba-zeen)

Matulane

♣ Natulan

Drug class.: Antineoplastic, miscellaneous

Action: Inhibits DNA, RNA, protein synthesis; has multiple sites of action; a nonvesicant, also inhibits monoamine oxidase enzymes

Uses: Lymphoma, Hodgkin's disease, cancers resistant to other therapy

Dosage and routes:

• *Adult:* PO 2-4 mg/kg/day for first wk; maintain dosage of 4-6 mg/kg/day until platelets and WBC count fall; after recovery: 1-2 mg/kg/day
• *Child:* PO 50 mg/day for 7 days, then 100 mg/m^2 until desired response, leukopenia, or thrombocytopenia occurs; 50 mg/day is maintenance after bone marrow recovery

Available forms include: Caps 50 mg

Side effects/adverse reactions:

▼ *ORAL:* Petechiae, bleeding, dry mouth, stomatitis

CNS: Headache, dizziness, insomnia, hallucinations, confusion, coma, pain, chills, fever, sweating, paresthesia

CV: Orthostatic hypotension, fast or slow heartbeat

GI: Nausea, vomiting, anorexia, diarrhea, constipation

RESP: Cough, pneumonitis

*HEMA: **Thrombocytopenia, anemia, leukopenia, myelosuppres-***

sion, bleeding tendencies, purpura, petechiae, epistaxis

GU: Azoospermia, cessation of menses

EENT: Retinal hemorrhage, nystagmus, photophobia, diplopia

INTEG: Rash, pruritus, dermatitis, alopecia, herpes, hyperpigmentation

Contraindications: Hypersensitivity, thrombocytopenia, bone marrow depression

Precautions: Renal disease, hepatic disease, pregnancy category D, radiation therapy

Pharmacokinetics:

PO: Peak levels 1 hr; concentrates in liver, kidney, skin; metabolized in liver, excreted in urine

🦷 Drug interactions of concern to dentistry:

• Increased CNS depression: barbiturates, antihistamines, narcotics
• Disulfiram-like reaction: ethyl alcohol
• Hypertension: indirect-acting sympathomimetics
• Increased anticholinergic effect: anticholinergic drugs, antihistamines
• Increased risk of severe toxic reactions: tricyclic antidepressants, meperidine and other opioids, tyramine-containing foods and other MAO inhibitors; may also include cyclobenzaprine and carbamazepine

DENTAL CONSIDERATIONS

General:

• Patients on chronic drug therapy may rarely have symptoms of blood dyscrasias, which can include infection, bleeding, and poor healing.
• Monitor vital signs every appointment due to cardiovascular side effects.

• Consider semisupine chair position when GI side effects occur.
• Assess salivary flow as a factor in caries, periodontal disease, and candidiasis.
• After supine positioning, have patient sit upright for at least 2 min before standing to avoid orthostatic hypotension.
• Avoid dental light in patient's eyes; offer dark glasses for patient comfort.
• Avoid aspirin-containing products because of bleeding risk.
• Avoid use of gingival retraction cord with epinephrine.
• Patients receiving chemotherapy may require palliative treatment for stomatitis.

Consultations:

• In a patient with symptoms of blood dyscrasias, request a medical consult for blood studies and postpone dental treatment until normal values are reestablished.
• Take precautions if dental surgery is anticipated and sedation or general anesthesia is required; there is risk of hypotensive episode.

Teach patient/family:

• Importance of good oral hygiene to prevent soft tissue inflammation
• Caution to prevent injury when using oral hygiene aids
• To report oral lesions, soreness, or bleeding to dentist

When chronic dry mouth occurs, advise patient:

• To avoid mouth rinses with high alcohol content due to drying effects
• Of need for daily use of home fluoride products to prevent caries
• To use sugarless gum, frequent sips of water, or saliva substitutes

P

prochlorperazine edisylate/ prochlorperazine maleate

(proe-klor-per′a-zeen)

Compazine

♣ PMS Prochlorperazine, Prorazin, Stemetil

Drug class.: Phenothiazine antipsychotic

Action: Blocks neurotransmission at dopaminergic synapses in the cerebral cortex, hypothalamus, and limbic system; exhibits strong peripheral α-adrenergic, anticholinergic blocking action; mechanism for antipsychotic effects is unclear

Uses: Antipsychotic; for nausea, vomiting

Dosage and routes:

Psychiatry

• *PO:* 5-10 mg tid-qid, increasing dosage every 2-3 days; more severe cases start 10 mg tid-qid; patients may tolerate 100-150 mg/day

Postoperative nausea/vomiting

• *Adult:* IM 5-10 mg 1-2 hr before anesthesia, may repeat in 30 min; IV 5-10 mg 15-30 min before anesthesia; IV inf 20 mg/L D_5W or NS 15-30 min before anesthesia, not to exceed 40 mg/day

Severe nausea/vomiting

• *Adult:* PO 5-10 mg tid-qid; sus rel 15 mg qd in AM or 10 mg q12h; rec 25 mg/bid; IM 5-10 mg; may repeat q4h, not to exceed 40 mg/day

• *Child 18-39 kg:* PO 2.5 mg tid or 5 mg bid, not to exceed 15 mg/day; IM 0.132 mg/kg

• *Child 14-17 kg:* PO/rec 2.5 mg bid-tid, not to exceed 10 mg/day; IM 0.132 mg/kg

• *Child 9-13 kg:* PO/rec 2.5 mg qd-bid, not to exceed 7.5 mg/day; IM 0.132 mg/kg

Available forms include: Oral syr 5 mg/ml; inj 5 mg/ml; tabs 5, 10, 25 mg; ext rel caps 10, 15, 30 mg; supp 2.5, 5, 25 mg

Side effects/adverse reactions:

▼ *ORAL:* Dry mouth, metallic taste, lichenoid reaction

CNS: Euphoria, **depression, extrapyramidal symptoms,** restlessness, tremor, dizziness

CV: **Circulatory failure, tachycardia**

GI: Nausea, vomiting, anorexia, diarrhea, constipation, weight loss, cramps

RESP: **Respiratory depression**

Contraindications: Hypersensitivity to phenothiazines, coma, seizure, encephalopathy, bone marrow depression

Precautions: Children <2 yr, pregnancy category C, elderly

Pharmacokinetics:

PO: Onset 30-40 min, duration 3-4 hr

SUS REL: Onset 30-40 min, duration 10-12 hr

REC: Onset 60 min, duration 3-4 hr

IM: Onset 10-20 min, duration 12 hr

Metabolized by liver, excreted by kidneys, crosses placenta, excreted in breast milk

🦷 Drug interactions of concern to dentistry:

• Increased sedation: other CNS depressants, alcohol, barbiturate anesthetics, opioid analgesics

• Hypotension, tachycardia: epinephrine

• Increased extrapyramidal effects: phenothiazines and related drugs (haloperidol, droperidol), metoclopramide
• Additive photosensitization: tetracyclines
• Increased anticholinergic effects: anticholinergics

DENTAL CONSIDERATIONS
General:
• Monitor vital signs every appointment due to cardiovascular side effects.
• Patients on chronic drug therapy may rarely have symptoms of blood dyscrasias, which can include infection, bleeding, and poor healing.
• After supine positioning, have patient sit upright for at least 2 min before standing to avoid orthostatic hypotension.
• Assess salivary flow as a factor in caries, periodontal disease, and candidiasis.
• Avoid dental light in patient's eyes; offer dark glasses for patient comfort.
• Assess for presence of extrapyramidal motor symptoms, such as tardive dyskinesia and akathisia. Extrapyramidal motor activity may complicate dental treatment.
• Geriatric patients are more susceptible to drug effects; use lower dose.
• Use vasoconstrictors with caution, in low doses, and with careful aspiration.

Consultations:
• In a patient with symptoms of blood dyscrasias, request a medical consult for blood studies and postpone dental treatment until normal values are reestablished.
• Take precautions if dental surgery is anticipated and anesthesia is required.
• If signs of tardive dyskinesia or akathisia are present, refer to physician.

Teach patient/family:
• Importance of good oral hygiene to prevent soft tissue inflammation
• Caution to prevent injury when using oral hygiene aids
• To use electric toothbrush if patient has difficulty holding conventional devices

When chronic dry mouth occurs, advise patient:
• To avoid mouth rinses with high alcohol content due to drying effects
• Of need for daily use of home fluoride products to prevent caries
• To use sugarless gum, frequent sips of water, or saliva substitutes

---

procyclidine HCl
(proe-sye′kli-deen)
Kemadrin
♣ PMS-Procyclidine, Procyclid
Drug class.: Anticholinergic, antidyskinetic

Action: Blockade of central acetylcholine receptors
Uses: Parkinson symptoms, extrapyramidal symptoms associated with neuroleptic drugs

Dosage and routes:
• *Adult:* PO 2.5 mg tid pc, titrated to patient response up to 5 mg tid
Available forms include: Tabs 5 mg; elixir 2.5 mg/5 ml

Side effects/adverse reactions:
▼ *ORAL: Dry mouth,* glossitis
CNS: Confusion, anxiety, restlessness, irritability, delusions, hallucinations, headache, sedation, de-

pression, incoherence, dizziness, light-headedness, memory loss

CV: Palpitation, tachycardia, postural hypotension, bradycardia

GI: Constipation, nausea, vomiting, abdominal distress, paralytic ileus, *epigastric distress*

GU: Hesitancy, retention

EENT: Blurred vision, photophobia, dilated pupils, difficulty swallowing, mydriasis

INTEG: Rash, urticaria, dermatoses

MS: Weakness, cramping

MISC: Increased temperature, flushing, decreased sweating, hyperthermia, heatstroke, numbness of fingers

Contraindications: Hypersensitivity, narrow-angle glaucoma, myasthenia gravis, GI/GU obstruction, child <3 yr, megacolon, stenosing peptic ulcer

Precautions: Pregnancy category C, elderly, lactation, tachycardia, prostatic hypertrophy, children, kidney or liver disease, drug abuse, hypotension, hypertension, psychiatric patients

Pharmacokinetics:

PO: Onset 30-45 min, duration 4-6 hr

🦷 **Drug interactions of concern to dentistry:**

• Increased anticholinergic effect: antihistamines, anticholinergics, meperidine

• Increased CNS depression: alcohol, CNS depressants

DENTAL CONSIDERATIONS

General:

• Monitor vital signs every appointment due to cardiovascular side effects.

• Assess salivary flow as a factor in caries, periodontal disease, and candidiasis.

• After supine positioning, have patient sit upright for at least 2 min before standing to avoid orthostatic hypotension.

• Avoid dental light in patient's eyes; offer dark glasses for patient comfort.

• Do not ingest sodium bicarbonate products, such as the air polishing system (Prophy Jet), within 1 hr of taking procyclidine.

• Place on frequent recall due to oral side effects.

Consultations:

• Medical consult may be required to assess disease control.

• Medical consult may be required to assess patient's ability to tolerate stress.

Teach patient/family:

• Use of electric toothbrush if patient has difficulty holding conventional devices

• Importance of good oral hygiene to prevent soft tissue inflammation

• Caution to prevent injury when using oral hygiene aids

When chronic dry mouth occurs, advise patient:

• To avoid mouth rinses with high alcohol content due to drying effects

• To use daily home fluoride products for anticaries effect

• To use sugarless gum, frequent sips of water, or saliva substitutes

---

promethazine HCl

(proe-meth'a-zeen)

Phenergan, Phenergan Fortis, Phenergan Plain

♣ Anergan, Histanil, Pentazine, Phencen-50, Prorex, V-Gan

Drug class.: Antihistamine, H_1-receptor antagonist

Action: Acts on blood vessels, GI,

respiratory system by competing with histamine for H_1-receptor site; decreases allergic response by blocking histamine

Uses: Motion sickness, rhinitis, allergy symptoms, sedation, nausea, preoperative or postoperative sedation

Dosage and routes:

Nausea
• *Adult:* PO/IM 25 mg, may repeat 12.5-25 mg q4-6h; rec 12.5-25 mg q4-6h
• *Child:* PO/IM/rec 0.5 mg/lb q4-6h

Motion sickness
• *Adult:* PO 25 mg bid
• *Child:* PO/IM/rec 12.5-25 mg bid

Allergy/rhinitis
• *Adult:* PO 12.5 mg qid or 25 mg hs
• *Child:* PO 6.25-12.5 mg tid or 25 mg hs

Sedation
• *Adult:* PO/IM 25-50 mg hs
• *Child:* PO/IM/rec 12.5-25 mg hs

Sedation (preoperative/postoperative)
• *Adult:* PO/IM/IV 25-50 mg
• *Child:* PO/IM/IV 12.5-25 mg

Available forms include: Tabs 12.5, 25, 50 mg; syr 6.25, 25 mg/5 ml; supp 12.5, 25, 50 mg; inj 25, 50 mg/ml

Side effects/adverse reactions:

▼ *ORAL:* Dry mouth

CNS: Dizziness, drowsiness, poor coordination, fatigue, anxiety, euphoria, confusion, paresthesia, neuritis

CV: Hypotension, palpitation, tachycardia

GI: Constipation, nausea, vomiting, anorexia, diarrhea

RESP: Increased thick secretions, wheezing, chest tightness

HEMA: **Thrombocytopenia, agranulocytosis, hemolytic anemia**

GU: Retention, dysuria, frequency

EENT: Blurred vision, dilated pupils, tinnitus, nasal stuffiness, dry nose/throat, photosensitivity

INTEG: Rash, urticaria, photosensitivity

Contraindications: Hypersensitivity to H_1-receptor antagonist, acute asthma attack, lower respiratory tract disease

Precautions: Increased intraocular pressure, renal disease, cardiac disease, hypertension, bronchial asthma, seizure disorder, stenosed peptic ulcers, hyperthyroidism, prostatic hypertrophy, bladder neck obstruction, pregnancy category C

Pharmacokinetics:

PO: Onset 20 min, duration 4-6 hr; metabolized in liver; excreted by kidneys, GI tract (inactive metabolites)

Drug interactions of concern to dentistry:
• Increased CNS depression: alcohol, all CNS depressants
• Hypotension: general anesthetics
• Increased effect of anticholinergic drugs

DENTAL CONSIDERATIONS
General:
• Determine why the patient is taking the drug.
• Patients on chronic drug therapy may rarely have symptoms of blood dyscrasias, which can include infection, bleeding, and poor healing.
• Monitor vital signs every appointment due to cardiovascular side effects.
• Assess salivary flow as a factor in caries, periodontal disease, and candidiasis.

• Assess vital signs q30min after use as sedative.

Teach patient/family: *When chronic dry mouth occurs, advise patient:*

• To avoid mouth rinses with high alcohol content due to drying effects

• Of need for daily use of home fluoride products to prevent caries

• To use sugarless gum, frequent sips of water, or saliva substitutes

---

propafenone
(proe-pa-fen′one)
Rythmol

Drug class.: Antidysrhythmic (class Ic)

Action: Able to slow conduction velocity; reduces cardiac muscle membrane responsiveness; inhibits automaticity; increases ratio of effective refractory period to action potential duration; β-blocking activity

Uses: Documented life-threatening dysrhythmias; unapproved: sustained ventricular tachycardia

Dosage and routes:

• *Adult:* PO initial doses 150 mg q8h; allow a 3-4 day interval before increasing dose; 900 mg max daily dose

Available forms include: Tabs 150, 225, 300 mg

Side effects/adverse reactions:

▼ *ORAL:* Dry mouth, altered taste, stomatitis

CNS: Seizures, headache, dizziness, abnormal dreams, syncope, confusion

CV: Sudden death, dysrhythmias, palpitation, AV block, intraventricular conduction delay, AV dissociation, CHF, atrial flutter

GI: Nausea, vomiting, hepatitis, constipation, dyspepsia, cholestasis, abnormal liver function studies

RESP: Dyspnea

HEMA: Leukopenia, agranulocytosis, granulocytopenia, thrombocytopenia, anemia

EENT: Blurred vision, tinnitus

INTEG: Rash

Contraindications: Second- and third-degree heart block, right bundle branch block, cardiogenic shock, hypersensitivity, bradycardia, uncontrolled CHF, sick sinus node syndrome, marked hypotension, bronchospastic disorders

Precautions: CHF, hypokalemia, hyperkalemia, recent MI, nonallergic bronchospasm, pregnancy category C, lactation, children, hepatic or renal disease

Pharmacokinetics: Peak 3-5 hr, half-life 2-10 hr; metabolized in liver; excreted in urine (metabolite)

⚕ Drug interactions of concern to dentistry:

• No specific interactions are reported; however, any drug that could affect the cardiac action of propafenone (other local anesthetics, vasoconstrictors, anticholinergics) should be used in the least effective dose

DENTAL CONSIDERATIONS

General:

• Monitor vital signs every appointment due to cardiovascular side effects.

• Patients on chronic drug therapy may rarely have symptoms of blood dyscrasias, which can include infection, bleeding, and poor healing.

- Assess salivary flow as a factor in caries, periodontal disease, and candidiasis.
- Stress from dental procedures may compromise cardiovascular function; determine patient risk.
- Consider semisupine chair position for patients with respiratory distress.

Consultations:
- In a patient with symptoms of blood dyscrasias, request a medical consult for blood studies and postpone dental treatment until normal values are reestablished.
- Medical consult may be required to assess disease control and patient's ability to tolerate stress.

Teach patient/family:
- Importance of good oral hygiene to prevent soft tissue inflammation
- Caution to prevent injury when using oral hygiene aids

When chronic dry mouth occurs, advise patient:
- To avoid mouth rinses with high alcohol content due to drying effects
- Of need for daily use of home fluoride products to prevent caries
- To use sugarless gum, frequent sips of water, or saliva substitutes

---

propantheline bromide
(proe-pan'the-leen)
Pro-Banthine
♣ Propanthel
Drug class.: Anticholinergic

Action: Inhibits muscarinic actions of acetylcholine at postganglionic parasympathetic neuroeffector sites
Uses: Treatment of peptic ulcer disease, irritable bowel syndrome,

duodenography, urinary incontinence; unapproved: reduction in salivary flow

Dosage and routes:
- *Adult:* PO 15 mg tid ac, 30 mg hs
- *Elderly:* PO 7.5 mg tid ac

Antisialagogue
- *Adult:* 7.5-15 mg 45-60 min before dental appointment

Available forms include: Tabs 7.5, 15 mg

Side effects/adverse reactions:
▼ *ORAL: Dry mouth,* absence of taste
CNS: Confusion, stimulation in elderly, headache, insomnia, dizziness, drowsiness, anxiety, weakness, hallucinations
CV: Palpitation, tachycardia
GI: Constipation, paralytic ileus, heartburn, nausea, vomiting, dysphagia
GU: Hesitancy, retention, impotence
EENT: Blurred vision, photophobia, mydriasis, cycloplegia, increased ocular tension
INTEG: Urticaria, rash, pruritus, anhidrosis, fever, allergic reactions

Contraindications: Hypersensitivity to anticholinergics, narrow-angle glaucoma, GI obstruction, myasthenia gravis, paralytic ileus, GI atony, toxic megacolon
Precautions: Hyperthyroidism, CAD, dysrhythmias, CHF, ulcerative colitis, hypertension, hiatal hernia, hepatic disease, renal disease, pregnancy category C, urinary retention, prostatic hypertrophy

Pharmacokinetics:
PO: Onset 30-45 min, duration 6

hr; metabolized by liver, GI system; excreted in urine, bile

🦷 Drug interactions of concern to dentistry:
• Increased anticholinergic effect: other anticholinergic drugs
• Constipation, urinary retention: opioid analgesics
• Decreased absorption of ketoconazole; take doses 2 hr apart

DENTAL CONSIDERATIONS
General:
• Assess salivary flow as a factor in caries, periodontal disease, and candidiasis.
• Avoid dental light in patient's eyes; offer dark glasses for patient comfort.
• Place on frequent recall due to oral side effects.
• Avoid prescribing aspirin-containing products.
• Consider semisupine chair position for patient comfort due to GI effects of disease.

Consultations:
• Physician should be informed if significant xerostomic side effects occur (increased caries, sore tongue, problems eating or swallowing, difficulty wearing prosthesis) so a medication change can be considered.

Teach patient/family: *When chronic dry mouth occurs, advise patient:*
• To avoid mouth rinses with high alcohol content due to drying effects
• Of need for daily use of home fluoride products to prevent caries
• To use sugarless gum, frequent sips of water, or saliva substitutes

propofol
(proe-po'fole)
Diprivan

Drug class.: General anesthetic

Action: Produces dose-dependent CNS depression; mechanism of action is unknown

Uses: Induction or maintenance of anesthesia as part of balanced anesthetic technique

Dosage and routes:

Warning: Propofol should be administered by persons trained in the administration of general anesthesia. Patients must be continuously monitored, and facilities for maintenance of a patent airway, ventilatory support, oxygen supplementation, and circulatory resuscitation must be immediately available. Strict aseptic technique must be followed in handling propofol.

Induction of general anesthesia
• *Adult <55 yr:* IV 2-2.5 mg/kg, approximately 40 mg q10sec until induction onset
• *Child >3 yr:* IV 2.5-3.5 mg/kg over 20-30 sec
• *Elderly or ASA III or IV patients:* IV: 1-1.5 mg/kg, approximately 20 mg q10sec until induction onset

Maintenance
• *Adult <55 yr:* IV 0.1-0.2 mg/kg/min (6-12 mg/kg/hr)
• *Child >3 yr:* IV 125-300 µg/kg/min (7.5-18 mg/kg/hr)
• *Elderly or ASAIII or IV patients:* IV 0.05-0.1 mg/kg/min (3-6 mg/kg/hr)

Intermittent bolus (maintenance)
• *Adult:* IV increments of 25-50 mg as needed

• Only general dose information is listed because all doses should be individualized and carefully adjusted for each patient.

Available forms include: Inj 10 mg/ml in 20 ml amp, 50, 100 ml inf vials

Side effects/adverse reactions:

▼ *ORAL:* Dry mouth, strange taste

CNS: Movement, headache, jerking, fever, dizziness, shivering, tremor, confusion, somnolence, paresthesia, agitation, abnormal dreams, euphoria, fatigue, dystonia

CV: Bradycardia, hypotension, hypertension, PVC, PAC, tachycardia, abnormal ECG, ST segment depression

GI: Nausea, vomiting, abdominal cramping, swallowing

RESP: **Apnea, cough, hiccups,** dyspnea, hypoventilation, sneezing, wheezing, tachypnea, hypoxia

GU: Urine retention, green urine

EENT: Blurred vision, tinnitus, eye pain

INTEG: Flushing, phlebitis, hives, burning/stinging at injection site

MS: Myalgia

META: Hyperlipidemia

MISC: Anaphylaxis

Contraindications: Hypersensitivity

Precautions: Elderly, debilitated, respiratory depression, severe respiratory disorders, cardiac dysrhythmias, pregnancy category B, labor and delivery, lactation, children <3 yr, epilepsy

Pharmacokinetics:

IV: Onset 40 sec, rapid distribution, half-life 1-8 min, terminal elimination half-life 5-10 hr; metabolized in liver by conjugation to inactivate metabolites; 70% excreted in urine

🖐 **Drug interactions of concern to dentistry:**

• Increased CNS depression: alcohol, narcotics, sedative-hypnotics, antipsychotics, skeletal muscle relaxants, inhalational anesthetics

DENTAL CONSIDERATIONS

General:

• Monitor vital signs at regular intervals during recovery after use as anesthetic.

• Have someone drive patient to and from dental office if used for general anesthesia.

• Geriatric patients more susceptible to drug effects; use lower dose.

• Use only with resuscitative equipment available and only by qualified persons trained in anesthesia.

Monitor:

• Injection site: phlebitis, burning/stinging.

• ECG for changes: PVC, PAC, ST segment changes.

• Allergic reactions: hives.

Administer:

• After diluting with D_5W, use only glass containers when mixing; not stable in plastic.

• By injection (IV only).

• Alone; do not mix with other agents before using.

Perform/provide:

• Storage in light-resistant area at room temperature.

• Coughing, turning, deep breathing for postoperative patients.

• Safety measures: siderails, night light, call bell within reach.

Evaluate:

• CNS changes: movement, jerking, tremors, dizziness, LOC, pupil reaction.

P

---

bold italic = life-threatening conditions

• Respiratory dysfunction: respiratory depression, character, rate, rhythm; notify physician if respirations are <10/min.

Treatment of overdose:

• Discontinue drug, artificial ventilation, administer vasopressor agents or anticholinergics.

---

propoxyphene HCl/ propoxyphene napsylate

(proe-pox'i-feen)

Darvon-N, Darvon Pulvules

Drug class.: Synthetic opioid narcotic analgesic

Controlled Substance Schedule IV

Action: Depresses pain impulse transmission in the CNS by interacting with opioid receptors

Uses: Mild-to-moderate pain

Dosage and routes:

• *Adult:* PO 65 mg q4h prn (HCl); PO 100 mg q4h prn (napsylate)

Available forms include: Caps HCl—65 mg; napsylate—tabs 100 mg

Side effects/adverse reactions:

▼ *ORAL:* Dry mouth

CNS: Drowsiness, dizziness, confusion, headache, sedation, **convulsions, hyperthermia,** euphoria

CV: **Dysrhythmias,** palpitation, bradycardia, change in BP

GI: Nausea, vomiting, anorexia, constipation, cramps

RESP: **Respiratory depression**

GU: Increased urinary output, dysuria

EENT: Tinnitus, blurred vision, miosis, diplopia

INTEG: **Rash,** urticaria, bruising, flushing, diaphoresis, pruritus

Contraindications: Hypersensitivity to ASA products (some preparations), addiction (narcotic), ritonavir

Precautions: Addictive personality, pregnancy category C, lactation, increased intracranial pressure, MI (acute), severe heart disease, respiratory depression, hepatic disease, renal disease, child <18 yr, alcoholism

Pharmacokinetics:

PO: Onset 15-30 min, peak 2-3 hr, duration 4-6 hr; metabolized by liver; half-life 6-12 hr; excreted by kidneys (as metabolites); equimolar doses of HCl or napsylate provide similar plasma levels

Drug interactions of concern to dentistry:

• Increased effects with other CNS depressants: alcohol, narcotics, sedative-hypnotics, skeletal muscle relaxants

• Contraindication: MAO inhibitors

• Increased effects of anticholinergics, antihypertensives, carbamazepine

DENTAL CONSIDERATIONS

General:

• Monitor vital signs due to cardiovascular and respiratory side effects.

• Consider semisupine chair position for patient comfort if GI side effects occur.

• Assess salivary flow as a factor in caries, periodontal disease, and candidiasis.

• Psychologic and physical dependence may occur with chronic administration.

• When combined with nonopioid analgesics (aspirin, NSAIDs, acetaminophen), permits better-quality pain relief.

Teach patient/family: *When chronic dry mouth occurs, advise patient:*

• To avoid mouth rinses with high alcohol content due to drying effects

• Of need for daily use of home fluoride products to prevent caries

• To use sugarless gum, frequent sips of water, or artificial saliva substitutes

---

propranolol HCl

(proe-pran′oh-lole)

Inderal, Inderal LA

♣ Apo-Propranolol, Detensol, Novo-Pranol, PMS-Propranolol

Drug class.: Nonselective β-adrenergic blocker

Action: This is a nonselective β_1- and β_2-adrenergic antagonist. The antihypertensive mechanism of action is unclear, but it may include a reduction in cardiac output and inhibition of renin release by the renal juxtaglomerular apparatus. Peripheral resistance decreases with long-term use. The antianginal action (when indicated for this use) may be related to a decrease in myocardial oxygen demand and negative chronotropic and inotropic effects. The antiarrhythmic action (when indicated for this use) has been related to a reduction in spontaneous pacemaker firing and slowing of AV nodal conduction.

Uses: Chronic stable angina pectoris, hypertension, supraventricular dysrhythmias (class II), migraine, MI prophylaxis, pheochromocytoma, essential tremor, hypertrophic cardiomyopathy, anxiety

Dosage and routes:
Dysrhythmias
• *Adult:* PO 10-30 mg tid-qid; IV bol 0.5-3 mg over 1 mg/min; may repeat in 2 min

Hypertension
• *Adult:* PO sus rel 40 mg bid or 80 mg qd initially; usual dose 120-240 mg/day bid-tid or 120-160 mg qd

Angina
• *Adult:* PO sus rel 80-320 mg in divided doses bid-qid or 80 mg qd; usual dose 160 mg qd

MI
• *Adult:* PO 180-240 mg/day tid-qid

Migraine
• *Adult:* PO sus rel 80 mg/day or in divided doses; may increase to 160-240 mg/day in divided doses

Available forms include: Sus rel caps 60, 80, 120, 160 mg; tabs 10, 20, 40, 60, 80, 90 mg; inj 1 mg/ml; oral sol 4 mg, 8 mg/ml; conc oral sol 80 mg/ml

Side effects/adverse reactions:

▼ *ORAL:* Dry mouth, lichenoid reaction

CNS: Depression, hallucinations, dizziness, fatigue, lethargy, paresthesias, bizarre dreams, disorientation

CV: Bradycardia, hypotension, CHF, palpitation, AV block, peripheral vascular insufficiency, vasodilation

GI: Nausea, vomiting, diarrhea, colitis, constipation, cramps, hepatomegaly, gastric pain, acute pancreatitis

RESP: Bronchospasm, dyspnea, respiratory dysfunction

HEMA: Agranulocytosis, thrombocytopenia

GU: Impotence, decreased libido, UTIs

P

---

bold italic = life-threatening conditions

EENT: ***Laryngospasm,*** blurred vision, sore throat, dry eyes

INTEG: Rash, pruritus, fever

MS: Joint pain, arthralgia, muscle cramps, pain

META: Hypoglycemia

MISC: Facial swelling, weight change, Raynaud's disease

Contraindications: Hypersensitivity to this drug, cardiac failure, cardiogenic shock, second- and third-degree heart block, bronchospastic disease, sinus bradycardia, CHF

Precautions: Diabetes mellitus, pregnancy category C, renal disease, lactation, hyperthyroidism, COPD, hepatic disease, children, myasthenia gravis, peripheral vascular disease, hypotension

Pharmacokinetics:

PO: Onset 30 min, peak 1-1.5 hr

IV: Onset 2 min, peak 15 min, duration 3-6 hr, half-life 3-5 hr (immed rel), 8-11 hr (sus rel); metabolized by liver; crosses placenta, blood-brain barrier; excreted in breast milk

🦷 Drug interactions of concern to dentistry:

• Decreased hypotensive effect: indomethacin, NSAIDs

• Increased hypotension, myocardial depression: hydrocarbon inhalation anesthetics

• Hypertension, bradycardia: sympathomimetics (epinephrine, ephedrine)

• Suspected increase in plasma levels: diphenhydramine

• Slow metabolism of lidocaine

DENTAL CONSIDERATIONS

General:

• Monitor vital signs every appointment due to cardiovascular side effects.

• Patients on chronic drug therapy may rarely have symptoms of blood dyscrasias, which can include infection, bleeding, and poor healing.

• Limit use of sodium-containing products, such as saline IV fluids, for patients with a dietary salt restriction.

• Assess salivary flow as a factor in caries, periodontal disease, and candidiasis.

• After supine positioning, have patient sit upright for at least 2 min before standing to avoid orthostatic hypotension.

• Stress from dental procedures may compromise cardiovascular function; determine patient risk.

• Short appointments and a stress reduction protocol may be required for anxious patients.

• Consider semisupine chair position for patients with respiratory distress.

• Use vasoconstrictors with caution, in low doses, and with careful aspiration. Avoid use of gingival retraction cord with epinephrine.

Consultations:

• In a patient with symptoms of blood dyscrasias, request a medical consult for blood studies and postpone dental treatment until normal values are reestablished.

• Medical consult may be required to assess disease control and patient's ability to tolerate stress.

Teach patient/family:

• Caution to prevent injury when using oral hygiene aids

• Importance of good oral hygiene to prevent soft tissue inflammation

When chronic dry mouth occurs, advise patient:

• To avoid mouth rinses with high alcohol content due to drying effects

• Of need for daily use of home fluoride products to prevent caries
• To use sugarless gum, frequent sips of water, or saliva substitutes

---

propylthiouracil (ptu)
(proe-pil-thye-oh-yoor′a-sil)
generic
♣ Propyl-Thyracil
Drug class.: Thyroid hormone antagonist

Action: Blocks synthesis of thyroid hormones T_3, T_4 (triiodothyronine), and T_4 (thyroxine)
Uses: Preparation for thyroidectomy, thyrotoxic crisis, hyperthyroidism, thyroid storm
Dosage and routes:
Hyperthyroidism
• *Adult:* PO 100 mg tid, increasing to 300 mg q8h if condition is severe; continue to euthyroid state, then 100 mg qd-tid
• *Child >10 yr:* PO 100 mg tid; continue to euthyroid state, then 25 mg tid to 100 mg bid
• *Child 6-10 yr:* PO 50-150 mg in divided doses q8h
Available forms include: Tabs 50 mg
Side effects/adverse reactions:
▼ *ORAL:* Loss of taste, bleeding (rare)
CNS: Drowsiness, headache, vertigo, fever, paresthesias, neuritis
GI: Nausea, diarrhea, vomiting, **jaundice, hepatitis**
HEMA: **Agranulocytosis, leukopenia, thrombocytopenia, hypothrombinemia, lymphadenopathy,** bleeding, vasculitis, periarteritis
GU: **Nephritis**
INTEG: Rash, urticaria, pruritus, alopecia, hyperpigmentation, lupus-like syndrome

MS: Myalgia, arthralgia, nocturnal muscle cramps
Contraindications: Hypersensitivity, pregnancy category D, lactation
Precautions: Infection, bone marrow depression, hepatic disease
Pharmacokinetics:
PO: Onset 30-40 min, duration 2-4 hr, half-life 1-2 hr; excreted in urine, bile, breast milk; crosses placenta
⚕ Drug interactions of concern to dentistry:
• Increased CV side effects in uncontrolled patients: anticholinergics and sympathomimetics
• Patients with uncontrolled hyperthyroidism are at risk when vasoconstrictors are used
• Patients with uncontrolled hypothyroidism may be more responsive to CNS depressants
DENTAL CONSIDERATIONS
General:
• Patients on chronic drug therapy may rarely have symptoms of blood dyscrasias, which can include infection, bleeding, and poor healing.
• Patients with uncontrolled hyperthyroidism should not be treated in the dental office until thyroid values are normalized.
• Uncontrolled patients should be referred for medical evaluation and treatment.
• Monitor vital signs every appointment due to cardiovascular side effects.
• Consider semisupine chair position for patient comfort if GI side effects occur.
Consultations:
• Medical consult may be required to assess disease control and patient's ability to tolerate stress.

---

bold italic = life-threatening conditions

protriptyline HCl

(proe-trip'te-leen)

Vivactil

♣ Triptil

Drug class.: Tricyclic antidepressant

Action: Inhibits both norepinephrine and serotonin (5-HT) uptake in the brain, although the precise antidepressant mechanism remains unclear

Uses: Depression; unapproved use: adjunctive use in narcolepsy and attention-deficit disorders

Dosage and routes:

• *Adult:* PO 15-40 mg/day in divided doses; may increase to 60 mg/day

• *Adolescent and elderly:* PO 5 mg tid

Available forms include: Tabs 5, 10 mg

Side effects/adverse reactions:

▼ *ORAL: Dry mouth, unpleasant taste,* bleeding, stomatitis

CNS: Dizziness, drowsiness, confusion, headache, anxiety, tremors, stimulation, weakness, insomnia, nightmares, EPS (elderly), increased psychiatric symptoms, paresthesia

CV: Orthostatic hypotension, ECG changes, tachycardia, **hypertension,** palpitation

GI: Diarrhea, **paralytic ileus, hepatitis,** increased appetite, nausea, vomiting, cramps, epigastric distress, jaundice

HEMA: **Agranulocytosis, thrombocytopenia, eosinophilia, leukopenia**

GU: Retention, **acute renal failure**

EENT: Blurred vision, tinnitus, mydriasis

INTEG: Rash, urticaria, sweating, pruritus, photosensitivity

Contraindications: Hypersensitivity to tricyclic antidepressants, recovery phase of MI, convulsive disorders, prostatic hypertrophy

Precautions: Suicidal patients, severe depression, increased intraocular pressure, narrow-angle glaucoma, urinary retention, cardiac disease, hepatic disease, hyperthyroidism, electroshock therapy, elective surgery, pregnancy category not established, MAO inhibitors

Pharmacokinetics:

PO: Onset 15-30 min, peak 24-30 hr, duration 4-6 hr, therapeutic effect 2-3 wk, half-life 67-89 hr; metabolized by liver; excreted by kidneys; crosses placenta

🐾 **Drug interactions of concern to dentistry:**

• Increased anticholinergic effects: muscarinic blockers, antihistamines, phenothiazines

• Increased effects of direct-acting sympathomimetics (epinephrine, levonordefrin)

• Possible risk of increased CNS depression: alcohol, barbiturates, benzodiazepines, and other CNS depressants

• Decreased antihypertensive effects of: clonidine, guanadrel, guanethidine

DENTAL CONSIDERATIONS

General:

• Take vital signs every appointment due to cardiovascular side effects.

• Assess salivary flow as a factor in caries, periodontal disease, and candidiasis.

italic = common side effects

• Patients on chronic drug therapy may rarely have symptoms of blood dyscrasias, which can include infection, bleeding, and poor healing.

• After supine positioning, have patient sit upright for at least 2 min before standing to avoid orthostatic hypotension.

• Use vasoconstrictors with caution, in low doses, and with careful aspiration. Avoid use of gingival retraction cord with epinephrine.

• Place on frequent recall due to oral side effects.

Consultations:

• In a patient with symptoms of blood dyscrasias, request a medical consult for blood studies and postpone dental treatment until normal values are reestablished.

• Medical consult may be required to assess disease control.

• Physician should be informed if significant xerostomic side effects occur (increased caries, sore tongue, problems eating or swallowing, difficulty wearing prosthesis) so a medication change can be considered.

Teach patient/family:

• Importance of good oral hygiene to prevent soft tissue inflammation

• Caution to prevent injury when using oral hygiene aids

When chronic dry mouth occurs, advise patient:

• To avoid mouth rinses with high alcohol content due to drying effects

• Of need for daily use of home fluoride products to prevent caries

• To use sugarless gum, frequent sips of water, or saliva substitutes

pseudoephedrine HCl/ pseudoephedrine sulfate

(soo-doe-e-fed'rin)

Afrin, Allermed, Cenafed, Congestion Relief, De-Fed-60, Dorcol, Drixoral Non-Drowsy Formula, Effidac24, Genaphed, Halofed, PediaCare Infant's, Pseudogest, Sudafed, Sudafed 12 Hour, Sudafed Liquid, Sudex, Seudotabs, and others

❧ Eltor 120, Robidrine

Drug class.: α-adrenergic agonist

Action: Acts primarily on α-receptors, causing vasoconstriction in blood vessels; has some beta activity and to a lesser degree CNS stimulant effects

Uses: Decongestant, nasal congestion

Dosage and routes:

• *Adult:* PO 60 mg q6h; ext rel 60-120 mg q12h

• *Child 6-12 yr:* PO 30 mg q6h, not to exceed 120 mg/day

• *Child 2-6 yr:* PO 15 mg q6h, not to exceed 60 mg/day

Available forms include: Caps 60 mg; ext rel caps 120 mg; sol 15 mg, 30 mg/5 ml drops; 7.5 mg/0.8 ml drops; tabs 30, 60 mg; ext rel tabs 120, 240 mg

Side effects/adverse reactions:

▼ *ORAL:* Dry mouth

CNS: Tremors, anxiety, **seizures,** insomnia, headache, dizziness, anxiety, hallucinations

CV: **Dysrhythmias,** palpitation, tachycardia, hypertension, chest pain

GI: Anorexia, nausea, vomiting

GU: Dysuria

P

EENT: Dry nose, irritation of nose and throat

Contraindications: Hypersensitivity to sympathomimetics, narrow-angle glaucoma, lactation

Precautions: Pregnancy category B, cardiac disorders, hyperthyroidism, diabetes mellitus, prostatic hypertrophy

Pharmacokinetics:

PO: Onset 15-30 min, duration 4-6 hr, 8-12 hr (ext rel); metabolized in liver; excreted in feces, breast milk

🦷 **Drug interactions of concern to dentistry:**

• Dysrhythmia: hydrocarbon inhalation anesthetics

• Increased CNS, CV effects: sympathomimetics

DENTAL CONSIDERATIONS
General:

• Assess salivary flow as a factor in caries, periodontal disease, and candidiasis.

• Monitor vital signs every appointment due to cardiovascular side effects.

• Consider semisupine chair position for patient comfort if GI side effects occur.

Teach patient/family:

• Use of electric toothbrush if patient has difficulty holding conventional devices

When chronic dry mouth occurs, advise patient:

• To avoid mouth rinses with high alcohol content due to drying effects

• Of need for daily use of home fluoride products to prevent caries

• To use sugarless gum, frequent sips of water, or saliva substitutes

pyrazinamide

(peer-a-zin′a-mide)
generic

♣ PMS-Pyrazinamide,   Tebrazid

Drug class.: Antitubercular

Action: Bactericidal interference with lipid, nucleic acid biosynthesis

Uses: TB, as an adjunct with other drugs

Dosage and routes:

• *Adult:* PO 20-35 mg/kg/day in 3-4 divided doses, not to exceed 3 g/day

Available forms include: Tabs 500 mg

Side effects/adverse reactions:

CNS: Headache

*GI: **Hepatotoxicity,*** abnormal liver function tests, peptic ulcer

*HEMA: **Hemolytic anemia***

GU: Urinary difficulty, increased uric acid

INTEG: Photosensitivity, urticaria

Contraindications: Hypersensitivity

Precautions: Pregnancy category C, child <13 yr

Pharmacokinetics:

PO: Peak 2 hr, half-life 9-10 hr; metabolized in liver, excreted in urine (metabolites/unchanged drug)

DENTAL CONSIDERATIONS
General:

• Determine why the patient is taking the drug (for prophylaxis or active therapy).

• Determine that noninfectious status exists by ensuring that (1) anti-TB drugs have been taken >3 wk, (2) culture has confirmed TB susceptibility to antiinfectives, (3) patient has had three consecutive negative sputum smears, and (4) patient is not in the coughing stage.

Consultations:

• Medical consult may be required to assess disease control.

Teach patient/family:

• Importance of taking medications for full length of regimen to ensure effectiveness of treatment and to prevent the emergence of resistant strains

---

pyridostigmine bromide

(peer-id-oh-stig′meen)

Mestinon, Mestinon SR, Regonol

Drug class.: Cholinergic

Action: Inhibits destruction of acetylcholine, increasing its concentration at sites where acetylcholine is released; this facilitates transmission of impulses across myoneural junction

Uses: Nondepolarizing muscle relaxant antagonist, myasthenia gravis

Dosage and routes:

Myasthenia gravis

• *Adult:* PO initial 30-60 mg q3-4h, titrate as required, not to exceed 1.5 g/day; IM/IV 1/30 of PO dose q2-3h; sus rel 180-540 mg 1-2 × daily at intervals of at least 6 hr

Tubocurarine antagonist

• *Adult:* 0.6-1.2 mg IV atropine, then 10-20 mg

Available forms include: Tabs 60 mg; sus rel tabs 180 mg; syr 60 mg/5 ml; inj IM/IV 5 mg/ml

Side effects/adverse reactions:

▼ *ORAL: Salivation, tongue weakness*

CNS: **Convulsions,** dizziness, headache, sweating, confusion, incoordination, paralysis

CV: Bradycardia, **cardiac arrest,** tachycardia, dysrhythmias, AV block, hypotension, ECG changes

GI: Nausea, diarrhea, vomiting, cramps

RESP: Increased bronchial secretions, **respiratory depression, bronchospasm, constriction, laryngospasm, respiratory arrest,** SOB

GU: Frequency, incontinence

EENT: Miosis, blurred vision, lacrimation

INTEG: Rash, urticaria, flushing

MS: Weakness (arms, neck), cramps, twitching

Contraindications: Bradycardia, hypotension, obstruction of intestine, renal system, sensitivity to bromides

Precautions: Seizure disorders, bronchial asthma, coronary occlusion, hyperthyroidism, dysrhythmias, peptic ulcer, megacolon, poor GI motility, pregnancy category C, elderly, lactation

Pharmacokinetics:

PO: Onset 20-30 min, duration 3-6 hr

IM/IV/SC: Onset 2-15 min, duration 2.5-4 hr; metabolized in liver, excreted in urine

⚕ Drug interactions of concern to dentistry:

• Decreased effects: atropine, scopolamine, and other anticholinergic drugs; methocarbamol

• Reduced rate of metabolism of ester local anesthetics

• Avoid anticholinergic drugs to control excessive salivation

DENTAL CONSIDERATIONS

General:

• Monitor vital signs every ap-

P

---

pointment due to cardiovascular and respiratory side effects.

• After supine positioning, have patient sit upright for at least 2 min before standing to avoid orthostatic hypotension.

• Schedule short appointments due to effects of disease on oral musculature.

• Avoid dental light in patient's eyes; offer dark glasses for patient comfort.

• Place on frequent recall due to oral side effects.

• Consider semisupine chair position if GI side effects occur.

Consultations:

• Medical consult may be required to assess disease control.

• Consult with physician about adjusting dose if excessive salivation becomes a problem.

Teach patient/family:

• Use of electric toothbrush or other oral hygiene aids if patient has difficulty in maintaining oral hygiene

• Importance of good oral hygiene to prevent soft tissue inflammation

• To prevent injury when using oral hygiene aids

---

pyridoxine HCl/ vitamin B$_6$

(peer-i-dox'een)

Aminolin, generic, Nestrex

Drug class.: Vitamin B$_6$, water soluble

Action: Needed for fat, protein, and carbohydrate metabolism as a coenzyme

Uses: Vitamin B$_6$ deficiency associated with inborn errors of metabolism, inadequate diet; unapproved: drug-induced deficiencies

Dosage and routes:

Vitamin B$_6$ deficiency (dietary deficiency)

• *Adult:* PO 10-20 mg qd × 3 wk, then 2-5 mg qd (large doses ranging from 50-200 mg daily are usually required for drug-induced deficiency)

• *Child:* PO 2-10 mg qd × 3 wk, then 2-5 mg qd

Available forms include: Tabs 25, 50, 100, 250, 500 mg; inj IM/IV 100 mg/ml

Side effects/adverse reactions:

CNS: Paresthesia, flushing, warmth, lethargy ataxia (rare with normal renal function)

INTEG: Pain at injection site

Contraindications: Hypersensitivity

Precautions: Pregnancy category A, lactation, children, Parkinson's disease

Pharmacokinetics:

PO/INJ: Half-life 2-3 wk; metabolized in liver; excreted in urine

⚡ **Drug interactions of concern to dentistry:**

• Decreased effectiveness: levodopa

• Decreased serum levels of phenytoin, phenobarbital

DENTAL CONSIDERATIONS

General:

• Vitamin B deficiency and peripheral neuropathy may manifest with oral symptoms of glossitis and cheilosis.

---

quazepam
(kway´ze-pam)
Doral

Drug class.: Benzodiazepine, sedative-hypnotic

Controlled Substance
Schedule IV

Action: Produces CNS depression by interacting with a benzodiazepine receptor to facilitate the action of the inhibitory neurotransmitter γ-aminobutyric acid (GABA)

Uses: Insomnia

Dosage and routes:
• *Adult:* PO 15 mg hs; may decrease if needed

Available forms include: Tabs 7.5, 15 mg

Side effects/adverse reactions:

▼ *ORAL:* Dry mouth, taste alteration

CNS: Lethargy, drowsiness, daytime sedation, dizziness, confusion, light-headedness, headache, anxiety, irritability, weakness, tremor, depression

CV: Chest pain, pulse changes, palpitation, tachycardia

GI: Nausea, vomiting, diarrhea, heartburn, abdominal pain, constipation, anorexia

HEMA: **Leukopenia, granulocytopenia** (rare)

MISC: Joint pain, congestion, dermatitis, sweating

Contraindications: Hypersensitivity to benzodiazepines, pregnancy category X, lactation, ritonavir

Precautions: Hepatic disease, renal disease, suicidal individuals, drug abuse, elderly, psychosis, child <18 yr, lactation, depression, pulmonary insufficiency

Pharmacokinetics:
PO: Onset 15-45 min, duration 7-8 hr; metabolized by liver; excreted by kidneys (inactive/active metabolites); crosses placenta; excreted in breast milk

🥄 Drug interactions of concern to dentistry:
• Increased effects of diazepam: CNS depressants, alcohol
• Delayed elimination: erythromycin

DENTAL CONSIDERATIONS
General:
• Assess salivary flow as a factor in caries, periodontal disease, and candidiasis.
• Psychologic and physical dependence may occur with chronic administration.
• Geriatric patients are more susceptible to drug effects; use a lower dose.
• Avoid using this drug in a patient with a history of drug abuse or alcoholism.
• Increased serum levels and prolonged effect of benzodiazepines: erythromycin, ketoconazole, itraconazole, fluconazole, miconazole (systemic).

Consultations:
• Medical consult may be required to assess disease control.

Teach patient/family:
When chronic dry mouth occurs, advise patient:
• To avoid mouth rinses with high alcohol content due to drying effects
• Of need for daily use of home fluoride products to prevent caries
• To use sugarless gum, frequent sips of water, or saliva substitutes

---

bold italic = life-threatening conditions *For periodic updates, visit* **www.mosby.com**

quetiapine fumarate
(kwe-tye'a-peen)
Seroquel

Drug class.: Antipsychotic, atypical

Action: Acts as an agonist at serotonin (5-HT$_2$) receptors and to a lesser extent at dopamine (D$_2$) receptors

Uses: Schizophrenia

Dosage and routes:
• *Adult:* PO initial dose 25 mg bid, on second day increase dose by 25 mg bid or tid, as tolerated, to target range of 300-400 mg daily by the fourth day; doses of 75 mg daily have been used

Available forms include: Tabs 25, 100, 200, 300 mg

Side effects/adverse reactions:

▼ *ORAL: Dry mouth* (8%-17%), taste perversion

CNS: Somnolence, headache, agitation, insomnia, dizziness, extrapyramidal symptoms, anorexia

CV: Orthostatic hypotension, tachycardia, palpitation, peripheral edema

GI: Abdominal pain, constipation, dyspepsia

RESP: Cough, dyspnea

HEMA: Leukopenia

EENT: Rhinitis, ear pain, pharyngitis, dry eyes, conjunctivitis

INTEG: Rash, sweating, pruritus

META: Elevation of liver enzymes, cholesterol, triglycerides

MS: Asthenia, dysarthia, hypertonia

MISC: Weight gain, flulike syndrome

Contraindications: Hypersensitivity, severe CNS depression

Precautions: Renal impairment, hepatic impairment, CV disease, thyroid disease, hyperprolactinemia, neuromalignant syndrome, tardive dyskinesia, seizure disorders, cataracts, dementia, suicide tendency, pregnancy category C, lactation

Pharmacokinetics:
PO: Peak serum levels 1.5 hr; hepatic metabolism, renal excretion (70% as unchanged drug)

🦷 **Drug interactions of concern to dentistry:**
• Risk of increased CNS depression: CNS depressants

DENTAL CONSIDERATIONS
General:
• Monitor vital signs every appointment due to cardiovascular and respiratory side effects.
• Assess salivary flow as factor in caries, periodontal disease, and candidiasis.
• Assess for presence of extrapyramidal motor symptoms, such as tardive dyskinesia and akathisia. Extrapyramidal motor activity may complicate dental treatment.
• After supine positioning, have patient sit upright for at least 2 min before standing to avoid orthostatic hypotension.
• Consider semisupine chair position for patient comfort if GI side effects occur.
• Patients on chronic drug therapy may rarely have symptoms of blood dyscrasias, which can include infection, bleeding, and poor healing.
• Place on frequent recall due to oral side effects.

Consultations:
• In a patient with symptoms of blood dyscrasias, request a medical

consult for blood studies and post-pone treatment until normal values are reestablished.

• Medical consult may be required to assess disease control and patient's ability to tolerate stress.

• If signs of tardive dyskinesia or akathisia are present, refer to physician.

• Consultation with physician may be needed if sedation or general anesthesia is required.

• Physician should be informed if significant xerostomic side effects occur (increased caries, sore tongue, problems eating or swallowing, difficulty wearing prosthesis) so a medication change can be considered.

Teach patient/family:

• Caution to prevent trauma when using oral hygiene aids

• Use of electric toothbrush if patient has difficulty holding conventional devices

• Importance of good oral hygiene to prevent soft tissue inflammation

• Importance of updating health and drug history if physician makes any changes in evaluation or drug regimens

• To be aware of oral side effects and potential sequelae

When chronic dry mouth occurs, advise patient:

• To avoid mouth rinses with high alcohol content due to drying effects

• To use daily home fluoride products for anticaries effect

• To use sugarless gum, frequent sips of water, or saliva substitutes

quinapril

(kwyn′a-pril)

Accupril

Drug class.: Angiotension-converting enzyme (ACE) inhibitor

Action: Selectively suppresses renin-angiotensin-aldosterone system; inhibits ACE; prevents conversion of angiotensin I to angiotensin II; results in dilation of arterial, venous vessels

Uses: Hypertension, alone or in combination with thiazide diuretics

Dosage and routes:

• *Adult:* PO 10 mg qd initially, then 20-80 mg/day divided bid or qd

• *Elderly >65 yr:* PO initial 10 mg qd, then titration to optimal response

Available forms include: Tabs 5, 10, 20, 40 mg

Side effects/adverse reactions:

▼ *ORAL:* Dry mouth

CNS: Headache, dizziness, fatigue, somnolence, depression, malaise, nervousness, vertigo

CV: Hypotension, postural hypotension, syncope, palpitation, angina pectoris, MI, tachycardia, vasodilation

GI: Nausea, constipation, vomiting, gastritis, GI hemorrhage

RESP: Cough, bronchitis

HEMA: **Thrombocytopenia, agranulocytosis**

GU: Increased BUN, creatinine, decreased libido, impotence

INTEG: **Angioedema,** rash, sweating, photosensitivity, pruritus

MS: Arthralgia, arthritis, myalgia, back pain

META: Hyperkalemia

MISC: Amblyopia

Contraindications: Hypersensitivity, children

Precautions: Pregnancy category D, impaired renal/liver function, dialysis patients, hypovolemia, blood dyscrasias, CHF, COPD, asthma, elderly, lactation

Pharmacokinetics:
PO: Peak 0.5-1 hr, half-life 2 hr; serum protein binding 97%; metabolized by liver (metabolites); metabolites excreted in urine

⚘ Drug interactions of concern to dentistry:
• Increased hypotension: alcohol, phenothiazines
• Decreased hypotensive effects: indomethacin and possibly other NSAIDs, sympathomimetics

DENTAL CONSIDERATIONS
General:
• Monitor vital signs every appointment due to cardiovascular side effects.
• After supine positioning, have patient sit upright for at least 2 min before standing to avoid orthostatic hypotension.
• Patients on chronic drug therapy may rarely have symptoms of blood dyscrasias, which can include infection, bleeding, and poor healing.
• Assess salivary flow as a factor in caries, periodontal disease, and candidiasis.
• Limit use of sodium-containing products, such as saline IV fluids, for patients with a dietary salt restriction.
• Use vasoconstrictors with caution, in low doses, and with careful aspiration.
• Stress from dental procedures may compromise cardiovascular function; determine patient risk.

• Short appointments and a stress reduction protocol may be required for anxious patients.

Consultations:
• Medical consult may be required to assess disease control and patient's ability to tolerate stress.
• In a patient with symptoms of blood dyscrasias, request a medical consult for blood studies and postpone dental treatment until normal values are reestablished.
• Take precautions if dental surgery is anticipated and sedation or general anesthesia is required; there is risk of a hypotensive episode.

Teach patient/family:
• Importance of good oral hygiene to prevent soft tissue inflammation
• Caution to prevent injury when using oral hygiene aids
When chronic dry mouth occurs, advise patient:
• To avoid mouth rinses with high alcohol content due to drying effects
• Of need for daily use of home fluoride products to prevent caries
• To use sugarless gum, frequent sips of water, or saliva substitutes

---

quinidine gluconate/ quinidine sulfate
(kwin'i-deen)
Quinaglute, Quinalan, Quinidex Extentabs, Quinora
♣ Apo-Quinidine, Novoquindin, Quinate
Drug class.: Antidysrhythmic (class Ia)

Action: Prolongs effective refractory period; decreases myocardial excitability, conduction velocity, and contractility; indirect anticholinergic properties

Uses: PVCs, atrial flutter and fibrillation, PAT, ventricular tachycardia

Dosage and routes:
Atrial fibrillation/flutter
• *Adult:* PO 200 mg q2-3h × 5-8 doses; may increase qd until sinus rhythm is restored; max 4 g/day given only after digitalization
Paroxysmal supraventricular tachycardia
• *Adult:* PO 400-600 mg q2-3h
All other dysrhythmias
• *Adult:* PO 50-200 mg as a test dose, then 200-400 mg q4-6h
Available forms include: Gluconate—sus rel tabs 324 mg; inj 80 mg/ml in 10-ml vials; sulfate—tabs 100, 200, 300 mg; caps 200, 300 mg; sus rel tabs 300 mg

Side effects/adverse reactions:
▼ *ORAL: Bitter taste, lichenoid drug reaction, pigmentation*
CNS: Headache, dizziness, involuntary movement, confusion, psychosis, restlessness, irritability, syncope, excitement
CV: Hypotension, bradycardia, **heart block, cardiovascular collapse, arrest,** PVCs
GI: Diarrhea, **hepatotoxicity,** nausea, vomiting, anorexia
RESP: Dyspnea, **respiratory depression**
HEMA: **Thrombocytopenia,** hemolytic anemia, agranulocytosis, hypoprothrombinemia
EENT: Cinchonism: tinnitus, blurred vision, hearing loss, mydriasis, disturbed color vision
INTEG: Rash, urticaria, angioedema, swelling, photosensitivity
Contraindications: Hypersensitivity, blood dyscrasias, severe heart block, myasthenia gravis, itraconazole
Precautions: Pregnancy category C, lactation, children, renal disease, potassium imbalance, liver disease, CHF, respiratory depression

Pharmacokinetics:
PO: Peak 0.5-6 hr (depending on form given), duration 6-8 hr, half-life 6-7 hr; metabolized in liver; excreted unchanged by kidneys

🦷 Drug interactions of concern to dentistry:
• May decrease effects of quinidine: barbiturates
• Increased anticholinergic effect: anticholinergic drugs
• Increased effects of neuromuscular blockers
• Contraindicated with: itraconazole

DENTAL CONSIDERATIONS
General:
• Monitor vital signs every appointment due to cardiovascular and respiratory side effects.
• Patients on chronic drug therapy may rarely have symptoms of blood dyscrasias, which can include infection, bleeding, and poor healing.
• After supine positioning, have patient sit upright for at least 2 min before standing to avoid orthostatic hypotension.
• Use vasoconstrictors with caution, in low doses, and with careful aspiration. Avoid use of gingival retraction cord with epinephrine.
• Consider semisupine chair position for patient comfort if GI side effects occur.

Consultations:
• In a patient with symptoms of blood dyscrasias, request a medical consult for blood studies and postpone dental treatment until normal values are reestablished.

---

bold italic = life-threatening conditions   *For periodic updates, visit* **www.mosby.com**

• Medical consult may be required to assess patient's ability to tolerate stress.

Teach patient/family:
• Importance of good oral hygiene to prevent soft tissue inflammation

---

quinine sulfate
(kwye'nine)
generic
Drug class.: Antimalarial

Action: Schizonticidal, but mechanism is unclear; increases refractory period in skeletal muscle

Uses: *P. falciparum* malaria, nocturnal leg cramps

Dosage and routes:
• *Adult:* PO 650 mg q8h over 3-7 days, given with concurrent antiinfective drugs

Available forms include: Caps 200, 260, 325 mg; tabs 260

Side effects/adverse reactions:
▼ *ORAL:* Lichenoid drug reaction
CNS: Convulsion, headache, stimulation, fatigue, irritability, bad dreams, dizziness, fever, confusion, anxiety
CV: Acute circulatory failure, angina, dysrhythmias, tachycardia, hypotension
GI: Nausea, vomiting, anorexia, diarrhea, epigastric pain
HEMA: Thrombocytopenia, purpura, hypothrombinemia, hemolysis
GU: Dysuria
EENT: Blurred vision, corneal changes, retinal changes, difficulty focusing, tinnitus, vertigo, deafness, photophobia, diplopia, night blindness
INTEG: Pruritus, pigment changes, skin eruptions, lichen planus–like

eruptions, flushing, facial edema, sweating
ENDO: Hypoglycemia

Contraindications: Hypersensitivity, G6PD deficiency, retinal field changes, pregnancy category X

Precautions: Blood dyscrasias, severe GI disease, neurologic disease, severe hepatic disease, psoriasis, cardiac dysrhythmias, tinnitus

Pharmacokinetics:
PO: Peak 1-3 hr, half-life 4-5 hr; metabolized in liver; excreted in urine

🦷 **Drug interactions of concern to dentistry:**
• Decreased absorption: magnesium or aluminum salts
• Prolonged duration of neuromuscular blocking drugs

DENTAL CONSIDERATIONS

General:
• Patients on chronic drug therapy may rarely have symptoms of blood dyscrasias, which can include infection, bleeding, and poor healing.
• Avoid dental light in patient's eyes; offer dark glasses for patient comfort.
• Monitor vital signs every appointment due to cardiovascular side effects.
• Consider semisupine chair position for patient comfort if GI side effects occur.

Consultations:
• Medical consult may be required to assess disease control.
• In a patient with symptoms of blood dyscrasias, request a medical consult for blood studies and postpone dental treatment until normal values are reestablished.

Teach patient/family:
• Importance of good oral hygiene to prevent soft tissue inflammation

---

quinupristin/dalfo-pristin
(qwen'nyoo-pris-ten) (dal'foe-pristen)
Synercid I.V.

Drug class.: Antiinfective, streptogramin

Action: Combination of quinupristin (30%) with dalfopristin (70%); inhibition of the synthesis of bacterial protein by irreversible binding to 50S ribosomal subunits

Uses: Serious or life-threatening infections due to vancomycin-resistant *Enterococcus faecium;* skin and skin structure infections caused by *Streptococcus pyogenes* or methicillin-susceptible *Staphylococcus aureus*

Dosage and routes:
• *Adult:* IV inf in D$_5$W over 60 min; for vancomycin-resistant *E. faecium,* 7.5 mg/kg q8h; for complicated skin and skin structure infections, 7.5 mg/kg q12h with minimum dose duration of 7 days
• *Child <16 yr:* Limited data available; no dose adjustment required

Available forms include: Single-dose vial: quinupristin 150 mg and dalfopristin 350 mg/10 ml vials

Side effects/adverse reactions:
▼ *ORAL:* Candidiasis
CNS: Headache, chest pain
CV: Infusion site reactions (pain, inflammation), peripheral edema
*GI: Nausea, vomiting, **pseudomembranous colitis,*** diarrhea, abdominal pain, dyspepsia, pancreatitis

GU: UTI
INTEG: Rash, pruritus
META: Hyperbilirubinemia, elevation of ALT, AST
MS: Arthralgia, myalgia, leg cramps
MISC: Asthenia, allergic reaction

Contraindications: Known hypersensitivity or prior hypersensitivity to other streptogramins, heparin flush

Precautions: Venous irritation, inhibits cytochrome P-450 3A4 enzymes, pregnancy category B, lactation

Pharmacokinetics:
IV: Both constituents are converted to active metabolites, short half-life but prolonged postantibiotic effect on *S. aureus* and *S. pneumoniae,* peak concentration 1 hr, protein-binding quinupristin (55%-78%), dalfopristin (11%-26%), extensive metabolism in liver and blood, renal excretion 20%, mostly fecal excretion

⚕ Drug interactions of concern to dentistry:
• Patients with serious, life-threatening systemic infections will not be candidates for dental care except for extreme emergencies

DENTAL CONSIDERATIONS
General:
• Examine for oral manifestation of opportunistic candida infection.

---

rabeprazole sodium
(ra-be'pray-zole)
Aciphex

Drug class.: Antisecretory

Action: Suppresses gastric acid production by binding to the hydrogen/potassium ATPase enzyme system to inhibit the final step in gastric acid production.

Uses: Gastroesophageal reflux disease (GERD), duodenal ulcers, and hypersecretory conditions (Zollinger-Ellison disease)

Dosage and routes:

GERD and duodenal ulcer

• *Adult:* PO 20 mg qd × 4-8 wk; if healing is not evident can continue 8 wk more

Hypersecretory conditions

• *Adult:* PO 60 mg qd; higher dose of 60 mg bid has been used

Available forms include: Del rel tabs 20 mg

Side effects/adverse reactions:

▼ *ORAL:* Dry mouth, mouth ulceration

CNS: Headache, insomnia, anxiety, abnormal dreams

CV: Hypertension, ECG abnormalities, syncope, palpitation, bundle branch block

GI: Diarrhea, nausea, abdominal pain

RESP: Dyspnea, asthma, hiccups

HEMA: Anemia, abnormal blood cell counts

EENT: Dry eyes, eye pain

INTEG: Photosensitivity, rash, pruritus, sweating

ENDO: Alteration in thyroid function

META: Weight gain, gout, abnormal liver function tests

MS: Asthenia, chest pain, neck rigidity, myalgia

MISC: Fever

Contraindications: Hypersensitivity

Precautions: Do not break, crush, or chew tablets, pregnancy category B, avoid nursing, pediatric use not studied

Pharmacokinetics:

PO: Del rel tabs: bioavailability 52%, peak plasma levels 2-5 hr, half-life 1-2 hr, highly plasma protein bound (96.3%), extensive hepatic metabolism (CYP450 3A), about 90% excreted in urine

👄 **Drug interactions of concern to dentistry:**

• None documented

DENTAL CONSIDERATIONS

General:

• Assess salivary flow as a factor in caries, periodontal disease, and candidiasis.

• Consider semisupine chair position for patient comfort due to GI side effects of disease.

• Patients with gastroesophageal reflux may present with oral symptoms including burning mouth, secondary candidiasis, and signs of tooth erosion.

• Question the patient about tolerance of NSAIDs or aspirin related to GI problems.

Teach patient/family:

• To prevent trauma when using oral hygiene aids

When chronic dry mouth occurs, advise patient:

• To avoid mouth rinses with high alcohol content due to drying effects

• To use daily home fluoride products for anticaries effect

• To use sugarless gum, frequent sips of water, or saliva substitutes

---

raloxifene hydrochloride

(ral-ox'i-feen)

Evista

Drug class.: Synthetic estrogen

Action: Acts as a selective estrogen receptor modulator (SERM) to reduce resorption of bone and decrease overall bone turnover; may act as an estrogen antagonist in uterine and breast tissues

Uses: Prevention and treatment of osteoporosis in postmenopausal women, supplemented with calcium as based on need

Dosages and routes:
• *Adult:* PO 60 mg daily
Available forms include: Tabs 60 mg

Side effects/adverse reactions:
CNS: Insomnia, depression
CV: Chest pain, *hot flashes*
GI: Nausea, vomiting, dyspepsia, flatulence
RESP: Cough
GU: Vaginitis, UTI, cystitis, leukorrhea, vaginal bleeding
EENT: Sinusitis, pharyngitis
INTEG: Rash, sweating
ENDO: Weight gain
MS: Leg cramps, arthralgia, myalgia
MISC: Flulike syndrome, infection

Contraindications: Hypersensitivity, pregnancy, prior history of venous thromboembolic events, premenopausal use, lactation, children

Precautions: Hepatic impairment, risk of thromboembolitic events, pregnancy category X, lactation

Pharmacokinetics:
PO: Rapidly absorbed, bioavailability 2%, plasma levels depend on systemic interconversion and enterohepatic cycling, highly bound to plasma proteins, extensive first-pass metabolism, glucuronide metabolites, mainly excreted in feces, urinary excretion is minor

Drug interactions of concern to dentistry:
• Reduced absorption: ampicillin
• Risk of potential drug interactions with other highly plasma protein-bound drugs is unknown, such as NSAIDs, aspirin, and diazepam

DENTAL CONSIDERATIONS
General:
• This drug should be discontinued 72 hr before prolonged immobilization such as hospitalization, post-surgical recovery, and bed rest.
• Consider short appointments and dental chair position if needed for patient comfort.

Consultations:
• Medical consult may be required to assess disease control and patient's ability to tolerate stress.

---

ramipril
(ra-mi′pril)
Altace

Drug class.: Angiotensin-converting enzyme (ACE) inhibitor

Action: Selectively suppresses renin-angiotensin-aldosterone system; inhibits ACE; prevents conversion of angiotensin I to angiotensin II; results in dilation of arterial, venous vessels

Uses: Hypertension; alone or in combination with thiazide diuretics; CHF immediately after MI; reduce risk of MI, stroke, and death due to cardiovascular causes

Dosage and routes:
• *Adult:* PO 2.5 mg qd initially, then 2.5-20 mg/day divided bid or qd; renal impairment: 1.25 mg qd with CrCl <40 ml/min/1.73 m², increase as needed to max of 5 mg/day

---

R

bold italic = life-threatening conditions

Reduction in risk of MI, stroke and death due to CV causes
• *Adult:* PO 2.5 mg/day × 1 wk initially; 5 mg/day × 3 wk, then increase dose as tolerated to 10 mg/day

Available forms include: Caps 1.25, 2.5, 5, 10 mg

Side effects/adverse reactions:
▼ *ORAL:* Angioedema (lips, tongue, mucous membranes), dry mouth

CNS: Headache, dizziness, **convulsions,** anxiety, insomnia, paresthesia, fatigue, depression, malaise, vertigo, hearing loss

CV: Hypotension, chest pain, palpitation, angina, syncope, dysrhythmia

GI: Nausea, constipation, vomiting, dyspepsia, dysphagia, anorexia, diarrhea, abdominal pain

RESP: Cough, dyspnea

HEMA: Eosinophilia, leukopenia, decreased Hct/Hgb

GU: Proteinuria, increased BUN, creatinine, impotence

INTEG: Angioedema, rash, sweating, photosensitivity, pruritus

MS: Arthralgia, arthritis, myalgia

META: Hyperkalemia

Contraindications: Hypersensitivity to ACE inhibitors, pregnancy category D, lactation, children

Precautions: Impaired renal/liver function, dialysis patients, hypovolemia, blood dyscrasias, CHF, COPD, asthma, elderly

Pharmacokinetics:
PO: Peak 1 hr, half-life 5 hr, duration 24 hr; high serum protein binding; metabolized by liver; metabolites excreted in urine, feces

🦷 **Drug interactions of concern to dentistry:**
• Increased hypotension: alcohol, phenothiazines
• Decreased hypotensive effects: indomethacin and possibly other NSAIDs, sympathomimetics

DENTAL CONSIDERATIONS
General:
• Monitor vital signs every appointment due to cardiovascular and respiratory side effects.
• After supine positioning, have patient sit upright for at least 2 min before standing to avoid orthostatic hypotension.
• Patients on chronic drug therapy may rarely have symptoms of blood dyscrasias, which can include infection, bleeding, and poor healing.
• Assess salivary flow as a factor in caries, periodontal disease, and candidiasis.
• Limit use of sodium-containing products, such as saline IV fluids, for patients with a dietary salt restriction.
• Use vasoconstrictors with caution, in low doses, and with careful aspiration.
• Stress from dental procedures may compromise cardiovascular function; determine patient risk.
• Short appointments and a stress reduction protocol may be required for anxious patients.

Consultations:
• Medical consult may be required to assess patient's ability to tolerate stress.
• In a patient with symptoms of blood dyscrasias, request a medical consult for blood studies and postpone dental treatment until normal values are reestablished.

• Take precautions if dental surgery is anticipated and sedation or general anesthesia is required; there is risk of a hypotensive episode.

Teach patient/family:

• Importance of good oral hygiene to prevent soft tissue inflammation

• Caution to prevent injury when using oral hygiene aids

When chronic dry mouth occurs, advise patient:

• To avoid mouth rinses with high alcohol content due to drying effects

• Of need for daily use of home fluoride products to prevent caries

• To use sugarless gum, frequent sips of water, or saliva substitutes

---

ranitidine

(ra-nye'te-deen)

Zantac, Zantac EFFERdose, Zantac 150 GELdose; *OTC:* Zantac 75

♣ Apo-Ranitidine, Gen-Ranitidine, Novo-Ranitidine, Nu-Ranit, Zantac-C

Drug class.: H_2 histamine receptor antagonist

Action: Inhibits histamine at H_2-receptor site in parietal cells, thus inhibiting gastric acid secretion

Uses: Duodenal ulcer, Zollinger-Ellison syndrome, gastric ulcers, hypersecretory conditions, gastroesophageal reflux disease, stress ulcers; unapproved: GI symptoms associated with NSAID use in rheumatoid arthritis

Dosage and routes:

• *Adult:* PO 150 mg bid or 300 mg hs; IM 50 mg q6-8h; IV bol 50 mg diluted to 20 ml over 5 min q6-8h;

IV int inf 50 mg/100 ml D_5 over 15-20 min q6-8h; PO (OTC dose) 75 mg qd-bid

Available forms include: Tabs (OTC) 75 mg; tabs 150, 300 mg; syr 15 mg/ml; inj IM/IV 0.5, 25 mg/ml; effervescent tabs 150 mg; effervescent granules 150 mg

Side effects/adverse reactions:

CNS: Headache, sleeplessness, dizziness, confusion, agitation, depression, hallucination

CV: Tachycardia, bradycardia, PVCs

GI: **Hepatotoxicity,** constipation, abdominal pain, diarrhea, nausea, vomiting

GU: Impotence, gynecomastia

EENT: Blurred vision, increased intraocular pressure

INTEG: Urticaria, rash, fever

Contraindications: Hypersensitivity

Precautions: Pregnancy category B, lactation, child <12 yr, hepatic disease, renal disease

Pharmacokinetics:

PO: Peak 2-3 hr, duration 8-12 hr, half-life 2-3 hr; less than 10% metabolized by liver; excreted in urine, breast milk

🦷 Drug interactions of concern to dentistry:

• Decreased absorption of diazepam, ketoconazole (take doses 2 hr apart)

DENTAL CONSIDERATIONS

General:

• Avoid prescribing aspirin-containing products in patients with active GI disease.

• Consider semisupine chair position for patient comfort due to GI effects of disease.

---

bold italic = life-threatening conditions   *For periodic updates, visit* **www.mosby.com**

repaglinide

(re-pag'lin-ide)

Prandin

Drug class.: Oral antidiabetic, meglitinide class

Action: Lowers blood glucose by stimulation of insulin release from the pancreatic β-cells; binds to ATP-dependent potassium channels in functioning β-cells with opening of calcium channels and subsequent insulin release

Uses: Type 2 diabetes mellitus when hyperglycemia cannot be controlled by diet and exercise; may also be used in combination with metformin

Dosage and routes:

Adult not previously treated or whose HbA$_{1c}$ is <8%

• *Adult:* PO initial dose 0.5 mg before meals; doses can be given 2, 3, or 4 times/day depending on blood glucose control; dose range 0.5-4.0 mg with limit of 16 mg/day

Adult previously treated with blood glucose-lowering drugs and whose HbA$_{1c}$ is ≥8%

• *Adult:* PO initial dose 1 or 2 mg before meals

Available forms include: Tabs 0.5, 1, 2 mg

Side effects/adverse reactions:

CNS: Headache, paresthesia

CV: Chest pain, angina, palpitation, hypertension, ECG changes

GI: Diarrhea, nausea, vomiting, constipation, dyspepsia

RESP: URI, bronchitis

EENT: Sinusitis, rhinitis

META: Hypoglycemia

MS: Arthralgia, back pain

Contraindications: Hypersensitivity, diabetic ketoacidosis, type 1 diabetes

Precautions: Increased cardiac mortality, hypoglycemia, hypoglycemia in patients taking β-adrenergic blockers, monitor laboratory values, pregnancy category C, lactation, pediatric patients

Pharmacokinetics:

PO: Rapid absorption, bioavailability 56%, peak plasma levels 1 hr; half-life 1 hr; plasma protein binding 98%, hepatic metabolism, metabolites excreted mainly in feces, small amount in urine

⚕ Drug interactions of concern to dentistry:

• Clinical studies have not been completed; metabolism may be inhibited by ketoconazole, miconazole, erythromycin

• Risk of increased hypoglycemia: NSAIDs, salicylates

DENTAL CONSIDERATIONS

General:

• If dentist prescribes any of the drugs listed in the drug interactions section, monitor patient blood sugar levels.

• Consider semisupine chair position for patient comfort due to GI side effects of drug.

• Ensure that patient is following prescribed diet and regularly takes medication.

• Place on frequent recall to evaluate healing response.

• Short appointments and a stress reduction protocol may be required.

• Diabetics may be more susceptible to infection and have delayed wound healing.

Consultations:

• Medical consult may include data from patient's blood glucose monitoring, including glycosylated hemoglobin or HbA_{1c} testing.

• Medical consult may be required to assess disease control and patient's ability to tolerate stress.

Teach patient/family:

• To prevent trauma when using oral hygiene aids

• Importance of updating health and drug history if physician makes any changes in evaluation or drug regimens

reserpine

(re-ser'peen)

♣ Novoreserpine, Reserfia

Drug class.: Antiadrenergic agent, antihypertensive

Action: Depletes catecholamine stores in CNS and in adrenergic nerve endings

Uses: Hypertension

Dosage and routes:

Hypertension

• *Adult:* PO 0.25-0.5 mg qd for 1-2 wk, then 0.1-0.25 mg qd maintenance

Available forms include: Tabs 0.1, 0.25, 1 mg

Side effects/adverse reactions:

▼ *ORAL: Dry mouth,* bleeding

CNS: Drowsiness, fatigue, lethargy, dizziness, depression, anxiety, headache, increased dreaming, nightmares, convulsions, parkinsonism, EPS (high doses)

CV: Thrombocytopenic purpura, bradycardia, chest pain, dysrhythmias, prolonged bleeding time

GI: Nausea, vomiting, cramps, peptic ulcer, increased appetite, anorexia

RESP: Bronchospasm, dyspnea, cough, rales

GU: Impotence, dysuria, nocturia,

sodium, water retention, edema, breast engorgement, galactorrhea, gynecomastia

EENT: Lacrimation, miosis, blurred vision, ptosis, epistaxis

INTEG: Rash, purpura, alopecia, flushing, warm feeling, pruritus, ecchymosis

Contraindications: Hypersensitivity, depression, suicidal patients, active peptic ulcer disease, ulcerative colitis, pregnancy category C

Precautions: Pregnancy, lactation, seizure disorders, renal disease

Pharmacokinetics:

PO: Peak 4 hr, duration 2-6 wk, half-life 50-100 hr; metabolized by liver; excreted in urine, feces, breast milk; crosses placenta, blood-brain barrier

⚡ Drug interactions of concern to dentistry:

• Increased CNS depression: barbiturates, alcohol, opioids

• Increased pressor effects: epinephrine

• Decreased pressor effects: ephedrine

• Decreased hypotensive effect: indomethacin and possibly other NSAIDs

DENTAL CONSIDERATIONS

General:

• Monitor vital signs every appointment due to cardiovascular side effects.

• Patients on chronic drug therapy may rarely have symptoms of blood dyscrasias, which can include infection, bleeding, and poor healing.

• Assess salivary flow as a factor in caries, periodontal disease, and candidiasis.

• After supine positioning, have

patient sit upright for at least 2 min before standing to avoid orthostatic hypotension.

• Limit use of sodium-containing products, such as saline IV fluids, for patients with a dietary salt restriction.

Consultations:

• Medical consult may be required to assess disease control.

Teach patient/family:

• Importance of good oral hygiene to prevent soft tissue inflammation

When chronic dry mouth occurs, advise patient:

• To avoid mouth rinses with high alcohol content due to drying effects

• Of need for daily use of home fluoride products to prevent caries

• To use sugarless gum, frequent sips of water, or saliva substitutes

---

riboflavin (vitamin B$_2$)

(rey'boo-flay-vin)

Various generic sources

Drug class.: Vitamin B$_2$, water soluble

Action: Needed for normal tissue respiratory reactions; functions as a coenzyme

Uses: Vitamin B$_2$ deficiency

Dosage and routes:

• *Adult and child >12 yr:* PO 5-50 mg qd

• *Child <12 yr:* PO 2-10 mg qd

Available forms include: Tabs 5, 10, 25, 50, 100 mg

Side effects/adverse reactions:

GU: Yellow discoloration of urine (large doses)

Contraindications: Child <12 yr

Precautions: Pregnancy category A, lactation

Pharmacokinetics:

PO: Readily absorbed, half-life 65-85 min; 60% protein bound; unused amounts excreted in urine (unchanged)

🦷 Drug interactions of concern to dentistry:

• Chronic alcohol use impairs absorption

• Patients taking tricyclic antidepressants or phenothiazines may require supplement

DENTAL CONSIDERATIONS

General:

• Patients deficient in B vitamins, including riboflavin, may have cheilosis, bald tongue, beefy red tongue, glossitis, or anemia.

• Determine why the patient is taking the drug.

Teach patient/family:

• About addition of needed foods that are rich in riboflavin

---

rifabutin

(rif'a-byoo-ten)

Mycobutin

Drug class.: Antimycobacterial agent

Action: Inhibits DNA-dependent RNA polymerase synthesis of bacterial RNA

Uses: Prevention of disseminated *M. avium* complex (MAC) disease with advanced HIV infection

Dosage and routes:

• *Adult:* PO 300 mg qd

Available forms include: Caps 150 mg

Side effects/adverse reactions:

▼ *ORAL:* Altered taste, colored saliva (brownish-orange)

CNS: Asthenia, headache, anorexia, insomnia

---

italic = common side effects

GI: Abdominal pain, flatulence, nausea, vomiting, diarrhea
HEMA: **Leukopenia, neutropenia, thrombocytopenia**
GU: Discolored urine
INTEG: Rash
MS: Myalgia
MISC: Fever
Contraindications: Hypersensitivity, active TB
Precautions: Pregnancy category B, lactation, concurrent corticosteroid therapy
Pharmacokinetics:
PO: Peak 2-4 hr, terminal half-life average 45 hr; moderately protein bound; hepatic metabolism; both renal and fecal excretion

🦷 **Drug interactions of concern to dentistry:**
• Decreases plasma concentrations of corticosteriods; may be significant
DENTAL CONSIDERATIONS
General:
• Examine for evidence of oral signs of opportunistic disease.
• Determine why the patient is taking the drug.
• Patients on chronic drug therapy may rarely have symptoms of blood dyscrasias, which can include infection, bleeding, and poor healing.
Consultations:
• Medical consult may be required to assess patient's ability to tolerate stress.
• In a patient with symptoms of blood dyscrasias, request a medical consult for blood studies and postpone dental treatment until normal values are reestablished.
Teach patient/family:
• To avoid mouth rinses with high alcohol content due to drying effects

• Importance of good oral hygiene to prevent soft tissue inflammation

---

rifampin

(rif'am-pin)
Rifadin, Rifadin IV, Rimactane
🍁 Rofact
Drug class.: Antitubercular antiinfective

Action: Inhibits DNA-dependent RNA polymerase synthesis of bacterial RNA
Uses: Pulmonary TB, meningococcal carriers (prevention); unapproved: leprosy and atypical mycobacterial infections
Dosage and routes:
• *Adult:* PO 600 mg/day as single dose 1 hr ac or 2 hr pc
• *Child >5 yr:* PO 10-20 mg/kg/day as single dose 1 hr ac or 2 hr pc; not to exceed 600 mg/day, with other antituberculars
Meningococcal carriers
• *Adult:* PO 600 mg bid × 2 days
• *Child >5 yr:* PO 10 mg/kg bid × 2 days, not to exceed 600 mg/dose
Available forms include: Caps 150, 300 mg; powder for inj 600 mg
Side effects/adverse reactions:
▼ *ORAL:* Stomatitis, glossitis, candidiasis, bleeding, discolored saliva
CNS: Headache, fatigue, anxiety, drowsiness, confusion
GI: **Pseudomembranous colitis,** nausea, vomiting, anorexia, diarrhea, heartburn, pancreatitis
HEMA: **Hemolytic anemia, eosinophilia, thrombocytopenia, leukopenia**
GU: **Hematuria, acute renal failure, hemoglobinuria**
EENT: Visual disturbances

R

---

bold italic = life-threatening conditions

INTEG: Rash, pruritus, urticaria, pemphigus-like reaction
MS: Ataxia, weakness
MISC: Flulike symptoms, menstrual disturbances, edema, shortness of breath

Contraindications: Hypersensitivity

Precautions: Pregnancy category C, lactation, hepatic disease, blood dyscrasias, concurrent therapy with corticosteroids

Pharmacokinetics:
PO: Peak 2-3 hr, duration >24 hr, half-life 3 hr; metabolized in liver (active/inactive metabolites); excreted in urine as free drug (30% crosses placenta); excreted in breast milk

Drug interactions of concern to dentistry:
• Increased risk of hepatotoxicity: acetaminophen (chronic use and high doses), alcohol, hydrocarbon inhalation anesthetics (except isoflurane)
• Decreased effects of corticosteroids, dapsone, diazepam, ketoconazole, fluconazole, itraconazole, oral contraceptives

DENTAL CONSIDERATIONS
General:
• Examine for oral manifestation of opportunistic infections.
• Patients on chronic drug therapy may rarely have symptoms of blood dyscrasias, which can include infection, bleeding, and poor healing.
• Determine why the patient is taking the drug (prophylaxis or active therapy).
• Determine that noninfectious status exists by ensuring that (1) anti-TB drugs have been taken >3 wk, (2) culture has confirmed TB susceptibility to antiinfectives, (3)

patient has had three consecutive negative sputum smears, and (4) patient is not in the coughing stage.

Consultations:
• Medical consult may be required to assess patient's ability to tolerate stress.
• In a patient with symptoms of blood dyscrasias, request a medical consult for blood studies and postpone dental treatment until normal values are reestablished.

Teach patient/family:
• To avoid mouth rinses with high alcohol content due to drying effects
• Importance of good oral hygiene to prevent soft tissue inflammation
• Importance of taking medications for full length of regimen to ensure effectiveness of treatment and to prevent the emergence of resistant strains

---

rifapentine
(rif′a-pen-teen)
Priftin

Drug class.: Antimycobacterial agent

Action: Inhibits DNA-dependent RNA polymerase; bactericidal for *Mycobacterium tuberculosis*

Uses: Pulmonary tuberculosis in combination with other antituberculosis drugs; unlabeled use includes prophylaxis of *Mycobacterium avium* complex in patients with AIDS

Dosage and routes:
• *Adult:* PO in combination with other anti-TB drugs; intensive phase 600 mg twice weekly at an interval of not less than 3 days for 2 mo, then continue once weekly for 4 mo in combination with

another anti-TB drug; concomitant use of pyridoxine (B$_6$) is recommended for malnourished patients, patients predisposed to neuropathy, and adolescents; can give with food

Available forms include: Tabs 150 mg

Side effects/adverse reactions: Note: Adverse effects are reported for combination drug therapy only and may or may not be due solely to rifapentine.

▼ *ORAL:* Reddish discoloration of saliva

CNS: Anorexia, headache, dizziness

CV: Hypertension

*GI: Nausea, vomiting, dyspepsia, diarrhea, **pseudomembranous colitis,** hyperbilirubinemia*

*HEMA: Anemia, lymphopenia, thrombocytosis, **leukopenia, neutropenia***

GU: Hyperuricemia, pyuria, proteinuria, hematuria

EENT: Hemoptysis

INTEG: Rash, pruritus, acne, urticaria

META: Increased ALT, AST

MS: Arthralgia, gout

MISC: Fatigue, reddish discoloration of urine, sweat, tears

Contraindications: Hypersensitivity to rifampin, rifabutin

Precautions: Significant hepatic dysfunction, induces hepatic microsomal enzymes, pregnancy category C, lactation, children <12 yr

Pharmacokinetics:

PO: Slow absorption, peak levels 5-6 hr, highly plasma protein bound (97%-93%), hepatic metabolism, 25-desacetylrifapentine is active metabolite, hepatic metabolism, excreted in feces (70%) and urine (17%)

💊 Drug interactions of concern to dentistry:

• May accelerate metabolism of clarithromycin, doxycycline, ciprofloxacin, fluconazole, ketoconazole, itraconazole, diazepam, barbiturates, corticosteroids, methadone, sildenafil, tricyclic antidepressants

DENTAL CONSIDERATIONS

General:

• Determine why patient is taking the drug (prophylaxis or active therapy).

• Examine for oral manifestation of opportunistic infections.

• Patients on chronic drug therapy may rarely have symptoms of blood dyscrasias, which can include infection, bleeding, and poor healing.

• Determine that noninfectious status exists by ensuring that (1) anti-TB drugs have been taken >3 wk, (2) culture has confirmed TB susceptibility to antiinfectives, (3) patient has had three consecutive negative sputum smears, and (4) patient is not in the coughing stage.

• Consider semisupine chair position for patient comfort due to GI side effects of drug.

Consultations:

• Medical consult may be required to assess disease control and patient's ability to tolerate stress.

• In a patient with symptoms of blood dyscrasias, request a medical consult for blood studies and postpone treatment until normal values are reestablished.

Teach patient/family:

• To avoid mouth rinses with high alcohol content due to drying effects

• To prevent trauma when using oral hygiene aids

---

bold italic = life-threatening conditions

• Importance of good oral hygiene to prevent soft tissue inflammation
• Importance of taking medication for full length of regimen to ensure effectiveness of treatment and prevent emergence of resistant strains
• Of potential for extrinsic oral staining side effect

---

riluzole
(ril'yoo-zole)
Rilutek
Drug class.: Glutamate antagonist

Action: Inhibits presynaptic release of glutamate in CNS; may also interfere with effects of excitatory amino acids and inactivation of voltage-dependent sodium channels

Uses: Treatment of amyotrophic lateral sclerosis (Lou Gehrig's disease)

Dosage and routes:
• *Adult:* PO 50 mg bid 1 hr before morning and evening meals or 2 hr after meals

Available forms include: Tabs 50 mg

Side effects/adverse reactions:
▼ *ORAL: Dry mouth* (3%), stomatitis (1%), candidiasis (0.5%), circumoral paresthesia (1.3%), glossitis
CNS: Asthenia, dizziness, depression, headache, hypertonia, insomnia, incoordination, anorexia
CV: Hypertension, peripheral edema, tachycardia, palpitation, postural hypotension
GI: Nausea, vomiting, dyspepsia, anorexia, diarrhea, flatulence
RESP: Cough, sinusitis
HEMA: Neutropenia
GU: UTI
EENT: Rhinitis

INTEG: Pruritus, eczema
META: Weight loss, liver enzyme abnormalities
MS: Stiffness, worsening of spasticity, fasciculation
Contraindications: Hypersensitivity
Precautions: Hepatic impairment, renal impairment, hypertension, other CNS disorders, pregnancy category C, lactation, children
Pharmacokinetics:
PO: Well absorbed, extensively metabolized by liver, excreted in urine/feces
🦷 Drug interactions of concern to dentistry:
• Unknown

DENTAL CONSIDERATIONS
General:
• Short appointments may be required due to nature of disease process.
• Monitor vital signs every appointment due to cardiovascular and respiratory side effects.
• Consider semisupine chair position for patient comfort.
• Assess salivary flow as factor in caries, periodontal disease, and candidiasis.
• Examine for oral manifestation of opportunistic infection.
• Patients on chronic drug therapy may rarely have symptoms of blood dyscrasias, which can include infection, bleeding, and poor healing.
• After supine positioning, have patient sit upright for at least 2 min before standing to avoid orthostatic hypotension.
Consultations:
• Medical consult may be required to assess disease control.
• In a patient with symptoms of blood dyscrasias, request a medical

consult for blood studies and postpone treatment until normal values are reestablished.

Teach patient/family:
• Instructions for management of oral hygiene, including use of electric toothbrush or directions to caregiver
• That professional oral hygiene home care may be needed
• Caution to prevent trauma when using oral hygiene aids

When chronic dry mouth occurs, advise patient:
• To avoid mouth rinses with high alcohol content due to drying effects
• To use daily home fluoride products for anticaries effect
• To use sugarless gum, frequent sips of water, or saliva substitutes

---

rimantadine HCl
(ri-man′ta-deen)
Flumadine
Drug class.: Antiviral

Action: May inhibit viral uncoating

Uses: Adult—prophylaxis and treatment of illnesses caused by strains of influenza A virus; child—prophylaxis against influenza A virus

Dosage and routes
Prophylaxis
• *Adult:* PO 100 mg bid; patients with severe hepatic dysfunction, renal failure, and elderly nursing home patients 100 mg/day
• *Child >10 yr:* PO use adult dose
• *Child <10 yr:* PO 5 mg/kg once daily, not to exceed 150 mg
Treatment
• *Adult:* PO 100 mg bid; 100 mg/day recommended for patients with

severe hepatic dysfunction, patients with renal failure, and elderly nursing home patients; continue therapy for 7 days from initial onset of symptoms

Available forms include: Tabs 100 mg; syr 50 mg/5 ml in 240 ml

Side effects/adverse reactions:
▼ *ORAL: Dry mouth,* stomatitis, altered taste
CNS: Insomnia, dizziness, headache, fatigue, nervousness, anorexia, depression
CV: Palpitation, hypertension, tachycardia, syncope
GI: Nausea, vomiting, diarrhea, dyspepsia
RESP: Dyspnea
EENT: Tinnitus, eye pain
INTEG: Rash
MS: Asthenia

Contraindications: Hypersensitivity, hypersensitivity to amantadine, nursing mothers, children <1 yr

Precautions: Pregnancy category C, elderly, epilepsy, hepatic or renal impairment, emergence of resistant viral strains

Pharmacokinetics:
PO: Peak plasma levels 6 hr; 40% plasma protein binding; hepatic metabolism; renal excretion

Drug interactions of concern to dentistry:
• Reduced peak plasma levels: aspirin, acetaminophen

DENTAL CONSIDERATIONS
General:
• Monitor vital signs at each appointment due to cardiovascular side effects.
• Determine why the patient is taking the drug (will probably be used only during peak seasons for influenza).

• Assess salivary flow as a factor in caries, periodontal disease, and candidiasis.

Teach patient/family:
• Importance of good oral hygiene to prevent soft tissue inflammation

When chronic dry mouth occurs, advise patient:
• To avoid mouth rinses with high alcohol content due to drying effects
• Of need for daily use of home fluoride products to prevent caries
• To use sugarless gum, frequent sips of water, or saliva substitutes

---

rimexolone
(re-mex′oh-lone)
Vexol

Drug class.: Corticosteroid

Action: Glucocorticoids have multiple actions that include antiinflammatory and immunosuppressant effects. They inhibit phospholipase A_2, interfering with or reducing the synthesis of prostaglandins and leukotrienes. They also bind to cytoplasmic glucocorticoid receptors (GRs) and enter the cell nucleus to bind with DNA. This results in the synthesis of various enzymes such as collagenase, elastase, and cytokines that play important roles in inflammation and immunosuppression. They also suppress the production of lymphocytes, monocytes, and eosinophils.

Uses: Inflammation of the eye associated with ocular surgery and uveitis

Dosage and routes:
Ocular surgery
• *Adult:* Ophth top after postoperative inflammation, instill 1 or 2 gtt qid beginning 24 hr after surgery; continue up to 2 wk

Uveitis
• *Adult:* Ophth top use 1 or 2 gtt in affected eye qh while awake × 1 wk; then 1 or 2 gtt q2h while awake × 1 wk; then reduce dose according to need

Available forms include: Susp 1% in 2.5, 5, 10 ml droptainers

Side effects/adverse reactions:
▼ *ORAL:* Alteration of taste (rare)
CNS: Headache (rare)
CV: Hypotension (rare)
EENT: Blurred vision, ocular pain, corneal edema, ulceration, increased ocular pressure
INTEG: Pruritus

Contraindications: Hypersensitivity, fungal or herpetic infections of eye

Precautions: Increased intraocular pressure, pregnancy category C, lactation, children, secondary ocular infections

Pharmacokinetics:
OPHTH TOP: Immediate onset, systemic absorption, extensive metabolism, excretion in feces

🦷 **Drug interactions of concern to dentistry:**
• None reported

DENTAL CONSIDERATIONS
General:
• Determine why the patient is taking the drug.
• Protect patient's eyes from accidental spatter during dental treatment.
• Avoid dental light in patient's eyes; offer dark glasses for patient comfort.

---

risedronate sodium

(ris-ed'roe-nate)

Actonel

Drug class.: Bisphosphonate

Action: Binds to bone hydroxyapatite, inhibits osteoclast-mediated bone resorption, and modulates bone metabolism

Uses: Paget's disease of bone; treatment and prevention of osteoporosis in postmenopausal women and glucocorticoid induced osteoporosis

Dosage and routes:

• *Adult:* PO 30 mg daily × 2 mo, take at least 30 min before first food or drink of the day (other than water), take in upright position with 6-8 oz water, avoid lying down for 30 min after dose is taken; patient should also take supplemental calcium and vitamin D if dietary intake is inadequate

Prevention/treatment osteoporosis

• *Adult:* PO 5 mg/day

Available forms include: Tabs 5, 30 mg

Side effects/adverse reactions:

CNS: Headache, dizziness

CV: Chest pain, peripheral edema

GI: Diarrhea, abdominal pain, nausea, constipation, belching, colic

RESP: Bronchitis, sinusitis

EENT: Amblyopia, tinnitus, dryness

INTEG: Rash

MS: Asthenia, arthralgia, bone pain, leg cramps, myasthenia

MISC: Flulike symptoms

Contraindications: Hypersensitivity, hypocalcemia

Precautions: Upper GI disease, avoid use in significant renal impairment, pregnancy category C, lactation, pediatric patients

Pharmacokinetics:

PO: Rapid oral absorption, food decreases bioavailability, bisphosphonates are not metabolized, renal excretion, unabsorbed drug excreted in feces

🦷 **Drug interactions of concern to dentistry:**

• Retarded absorption: calcium, antacids, medications with divalent cations

• Increased GI side effects: NSAIDs, aspirin

DENTAL CONSIDERATIONS

General:

• Be aware of the oral manifestations of Paget's disease (macrognathia, alveolar pain).

• Consider semisupine chair position for patient comfort due to GI side effects of drug.

• Short appointments may be required for patient comfort.

Consultations:

• Medical consult may be required to assess disease control.

Teach patient/family:

• Use of electric toothbrush if patient has difficulty holding conventional devices

risperidone

(ris-per'i-done)

Risperdal

Drug class: Antipsychotic (benzisoxazole derivative)

Action: Unclear, but may be related to antagonism for dopamine (D_2) and serotonin ($5\text{-}HT_2$) receptors; also has affinity for alpha

---

receptors and histamine (H$_1$) receptors

Uses: Psychotic disorders

Dosage and routes:

• *Adult:* PO initial 1 mg bid; increase by 1 mg bid on second and third day to 3 mg bid (target dose); further dose increase at 1 wk intervals; dose range 4-16 mg/day; reduce doses for elderly or debilitated patients or for those with severe renal or hepatic impairment (limit 3 mg/day)

Available forms include: Tabs 0.25, 0.5, 1, 2, 3, 4 mg; oral sol 1 mg/ml

Side effects/adverse reactions:

▼ *ORAL: Dry mouth,* stomatitis, taste alteration (rare)

CNS: Anxiety, **neuromalignant syndrome,** *EPS, dystonia, somnolence, hyperkinesia, dizziness,* tardive dyskinesia, syncope, motor impairment, insomnia

CV: Dysrhythmias, orthostatic hypotension, *tachycardia*

GI: Nausea, constipation, dyspepsia

RESP: Cough, dyspnea

HEMA: **Thrombocytopenia,** purpura, anemia, leukocytosis, leukopenia (all rare)

GU: Decreased libido, sexual dysfunction (male), menorrhagia, priapism, amenorrhea

EENT: Rhinitis, sinusitis, visual changes

INTEG: Rash, dry skin, photosensitivity

MS: Arthralgia

MISC: Hyperprolactinemia, akathisia

Contraindications: Hypersensitivity

Precautions: Pregnancy category C, lactation, seizures, suicidal patients, cardiac diseases, renal or hepatic impairment, elderly

Pharmacokinetics:

PO: Good absorption, peak plasma levels 1-2 hr; high plasma protein binding; extensive hepatic metabolism (active metabolite); renal excretion

Drug interactions of concern to dentistry:

• Increased excretion: chronic use of carbamazepine

• Increased sedation: other CNS depressants, alcohol, barbiturate anesthesia, opioid analgesics

• Increased extrapyramidal effects: phenothiazines and related drugs (haloperidol, droperidol), metoclopramide

• Additive photosensitization: tetracyclines

• Increased anticholinergic effects: anticholinergics such as atropine and scopolamine

DENTAL CONSIDERATIONS

General:

• Monitor vital signs every appointment due to cardiovascular side effects.

• Patients on chronic drug therapy may rarely have symptoms of blood dyscrasias, which can include infection, bleeding, and poor healing.

• After supine positioning, have patient sit upright for at least 2 min before standing to avoid orthostatic hypotension.

• Assess salivary flow as a factor in caries, periodontal disease, and candidiasis.

• Consider semisupine chair position for patient comfort due to GI effects of drug.

• Assess for presence of extrapyramidal motor symptoms, such as tardive dyskinesia and akathisia. Extrapyramidal motor activity may complicate dental treatment.

• Use vasoconstrictors with caution, in low doses, and with careful aspiration; avoid use of gingival retraction cord with epinephrine.

Consultations:

• In a patient with symptoms of blood dyscrasias, request a medical consult for blood studies and postpone dental treatment until normal values are reestablished.

• Take precautions if dental surgery is anticipated and anesthesia is required.

• If signs of tardive dyskinesia or other extrapyramidal symptoms are present, refer to physician.

• Physician should be informed if significant xerostomic side effects occur (increased caries, sore tongue, problems eating or swallowing, difficulty wearing prosthesis) so a medication change can be considered.

Teach patient/family:

• Importance of good oral hygiene to prevent soft tissue inflammation

• Caution to prevent injury when using oral hygiene aids

• Use of electric toothbrush if patient has difficulty holding conventional devices

When chronic dry mouth occurs, advise patient:

• To avoid mouth rinses with high alcohol content due to drying effects

• To use daily home fluoride products for anticaries effect

• To use sugarless gum, frequent sips of water, or saliva substitutes

ritonavir

(ri-toe′na-veer)

Norvir

Drug class.: Antiviral protease inhibitor

Action: Inhibits HIV-1 and HIV-2 proteases essential for production of HIV virion particles

Uses: Treatment of HIV infection in adults and children as single-drug therapy or in combination with nucleoside analogues

Dosage and routes:

• *Adult:* PO 600 mg bid with food; start with lower doses if nausea is a problem at outset

Available forms include: Caps 100 mg; oral sol 80 mg/ml in 240 ml

Side effects/adverse reactions:

▼ *ORAL: Circumoral paresthesia,* taste alteration, dry mouth

CNS: Headache, dizziness, somnolence, insomnia, anorexia

CV: Hypotension, palpitation, syncope

GI: Nausea, vomiting, abdominal pain, diarrhea

RESP: Cough, asthma, hiccough

HEMA: Anemia

GU: Dysuria

EENT: Pharyngitis

INTEG: Rash, urticaria, acne

MS: Asthenia, arthralgia, weakness

MISC: Peripheral paresthesia, weight loss

Contraindications: Hypersensitivity; **note multiple drug interactions with potential adverse effects**

Precautions: Hepatic impairment, pregnancy category B, lactation, children <12 yr, alters lab chemistry values (triglycerides, ALT, AST, GGT, CPK, uric acid)

Pharmacokinetics:

PO: Peak plasma levels with food 2 hr, hepatic metabolism, active metabolite excreted in feces, highly plasma protein bound (98%), half-life 3-5 hr

🦷 Drug interactions of concern to dentistry:

• Contraindicated with alprazolam, clorazepate, diazepam, bupropion, estazolam, flurazepam, midazolam, triazolam, zolpidem, meperidine, piroxicam, propoxyphene, chlordiazepoxide, halazepam, quazepam
• Increased plasma levels: clarithromycin, fluconazole, fluoxetine, desipramine, theophylline
• Possible alcohol-disulfiram reaction: metronidazole, disulfiram
• Decreased plasma levels with carbamazepine, dexamethasone, phenobarbital
• Increased plasma levels of fentanyl

Multiple drug interactions are reported; check before prescribing dental drugs.

DENTAL CONSIDERATIONS

General:

• Monitor vital signs every appointment due to cardiovascular side effects.
• Examine for oral manifestation of opportunistic infection.
• Place on frequent recall to evaluate healing response.
• Assess salivary flow as a factor in caries, periodontal disease, and candidiasis.
• Consider semisupine chair position for patient comfort due to GI effects of drug.

Consultations:

• Medical consult may be required to assess disease control.

Teach patient/family:

• Importance of good oral hygiene to prevent soft tissue inflammation
• That secondary oral infection may occur; must see dentist immediately if infection occurs

When chronic dry mouth occurs, advise patient:

• To avoid mouth rinses with high alcohol content due to drying effects
• To use daily home fluoride products for anticaries effect
• To use sugarless gum, frequent sips of water, or saliva substitutes

---

rivastigmine tartrate

(riv-a-stig'meen)

Exelon

Drug class.: Reversible cholinesterase inhibitor

Action: Inhibits destruction of acetylcholine; its role in Alzheimer's dementia is unknown, but may enhance cholinergic function

Uses: Mild to moderate Alzheimer's-type dementia

Dosage and routes:

• *Adult:* PO initial 1.5 mg bid; after 2 wk if this dose is tolerated increase to 3 mg bid; with 2-wk intervals between dose increases 4.5 mg bid then 6.0 mg bid may be attempted; max dose is 6 mg bid

Available forms include: Caps 1.5, 3.0, 4.5, 6 mg

Side effects/adverse reactions:

▼ *ORAL:* Dry mouth, alteration of taste, ulcerative stomatitis, increased salivation, facial edema (infrequent)

CNS: Dizziness, syncope, fatigue, malaise, headache, somnolence, tremor

italic = common side effects

CV: Hypertension, bradycardia, palpitation

GI: Nausea, vomiting, anorexia, dyspepsia, abdominal pain, flatulence

HEMA: (rare) ***Thrombocytopenic purpura,*** anemia, leukocytosis, hematoma

GU: UTI, impotence, atrophic vaginitis, hematuria

EENT: Rhinitis, tinnitus, epistaxis, diplopia

INTEG: Sweating

META: Weight loss, dehydration, hypokalemia

MS: Asthenia, myalgia, leg cramps

MISC: Accidental trauma, flulike syndrome

Contraindications: Hypersensitivity to this drug or other carbamate derivatives

Precautions: Significant GI reactions, nausea, vomiting, and weight-loss occur; history of GI ulcers or GI bleeding, patients taking NSAIDs, seizures, asthma, COPD, pregnancy category B, lactation, pediatric patients (no studies); smoking increases renal clearance

Pharmacokinetics:

PO: Well absorbed, bioavailability 40%, peak plasma levels 1 hr, widely distributed, plasma protein binding 40%, metabolized by cholinesterases, renal excretion

🦷 **Drug interactions of concern to dentistry:**

• Caution in use of NSAIDs if GI side effects are significant

• Decreased response to neuromuscular blocking agents used in general anesthesia

• Increased cholinergic response: other cholinergic drugs

• Decreased cholinergic response: anticholinergics or other drugs with anticholinergic actions

DENTAL CONSIDERATIONS

General:

• Determine why patient is taking the drug.

• Monitor vital signs every appointment due to cardiovascular side effects.

• Drug is used early in the disease; ensure that patient or caregiver understands informed consent.

• Place on frequent recall because early attention to dental health is important for Alzheimer's patients.

• Assess salivary flow as a factor in caries, periodontal disease, and candidiasis.

• Use precaution if sedation or general anesthesia is required; risk of hypotensive episode.

• Consider semisupine chair position for patient comfort if GI side effects occur.

• Patient on chronic drug therapy may rarely present with symptoms of blood dyscrasias, which can include infection, bleeding, and poor healing.

Consultations:

• Consultation with physician may be needed if sedation or general anesthesia is required.

• In a patient with symptoms of blood dyscrasias, request a medical consult for blood studies and postpone treatment until normal values are reestablished.

• Medical consult may be required to assess disease control and patient's ability to tolerate stress.

Teach patient/family:

• Use of electric toothbrush if patient has difficulty holding conventional devices

R

---

bold italic = life-threatening conditions   *For periodic updates, visit* **www.mosby.com**

- To prevent trauma when using oral hygiene aids
- Importance of good oral hygiene to prevent soft tissue inflammation

---

rizatriptan benzoate
(rye-za-trip'tan)

Maxalt, Maxalt-MLT

Drug class.: Serotonin agonist

Action: A selective agonist for 5-HT$_{1D}$ and 5-HT$_{1B}$ receptors on intracranial vessels leading to vasoconstriction and possibly inhibition of proinflammatory neuropeptide release

Uses: Acute treatment of migraine attacks with or without aura

Dosage and routes:

• *Adult:* PO initial dose 5-10 mg, can repeat dose in 2 hr, limit 30 mg/24 hr

Orally disintegrating tablet (MLT)

• *Adult:* PO remove tablet from sealed pouch immediately before use; place tablet on tongue, allow it to dissolve, and swallow with saliva; 5-10 mg initial dose, can repeat in 2 hr, limit 30 mg/24 hr

Available forms include: Tabs 5, 10 mg; orally disintegrating tabs 5, 10 mg

Side effects/adverse reactions:

▼ *ORAL:* Dry mouth

CNS: Fatigue, somnolence, dizziness, paresthesia, euphoria

CV: Palpitation, syncope, orthostatic hypotension

GI: Nausea, diarrhea, vomiting

RESP: Dyspnea, URI

GU: Hot flashes

EENT: Dry throat, nasal congestion, blurred vision, eye dryness

INTEG: Flushing

MS: Muscle weakness, arthralgia

MISC: Asthenia, pain or pressure (chest, neck, throat)

Contraindications: Hypersensitivity, MAO inhibitors, uncontrolled hypertension, ischemic heart disease, cerebrovascular or peripheral vascular disease, ergot-type drugs

Precautions: Risk of serious cardiovascular events, renal/hepatic impairment, SSRI antidepressants, pregnancy category C, lactation, use in children not established

Pharmacokinetics:

PO: Bioavailability 45%, mean peak plasma levels 1-1.5 hr for oral tablet, MLT tablets slower rate of absorption, peak levels 1.6-2.5 hr, metabolized by MAO type A, metabolites excreted in urine (82%) and feces (12%), plasma protein binding (14%)

🦷 **Drug interactions of concern to dentistry:**

• Increased plasma levels: propranolol

• No specific interactions with dental drugs reported

• Should not be used within 24 hr of another 5-HT agonist

DENTAL CONSIDERATIONS

General:

• This is an acute-use drug, thus it is doubtful that patients will be treated in the office if acute migraine is present.

• Be aware of patient's disease, its severity, and frequency, when known.

• Avoid dental light in patient's eyes; offer dark glasses for patient comfort.

• Short appointments and a stress reduction protocol may be required for anxious patients.

• After supine positioning, have

---

patient sit upright for at least 2 min to avoid orthostatic hypotension.
Consultations:
• If treating chronic orofacial pain, consult with physician of record.
• Medical consult may be required to assess disease control and patient's ability to tolerate stress.
Teach patient/family:
• Importance of updating health and drug history if physician makes any changes in evaluation or drug regimens

---

rofecoxib

(ro-fe-kox'ib)
Vioxx
Drug class.: Nonsteroidal antiinflammatory analgesic

Action: May be related to a selective inhibition of inducible cyclooxygenase 2 (COX 2) enzymes preventing the synthesis of prostaglandins
Uses: Relief of signs and symptoms of osteoarthritis; acute pain in adults, including dental pain; and primary dysmenorrhea
Dosage and routes:
Osteoarthritis
• *Adult:* PO initial dose 12.5 mg daily; max recommended dose 25 mg daily
Acute pain and primary dysmenorrhea
• *Adult:* PO 50 mg qd; use for more than 5 days for acute pain has not been studied
Available forms include: Tabs 12.5, 25, 50 mg; oral susp 12.5 mg/5 ml and 25 mg/5 ml in 150 ml volumes

Side effects/adverse reactions:
▼ *ORAL:* Dry mouth, aphthous stomatitis (low incidence)
CNS: Dizziness, fatigue, headache
CV: Hypertension (high dose), edema, PVC, tachycardia, palpitation
GI: Abdominal pain, diarrhea, dyspepsia, heartburn, epigastric discomfort, nausea
RESP: URI, bronchitis
HEMA: Anemia
GU: UTI
EENT: Sinusitis
INTEG: Rash, urticaria
MS: Back pain
MISC: Asthenia, influenza-like disease
Contraindications: Hypersensitivity; patients who have experienced asthma, urticaria, or allergic-type reactions to aspirin or other NSAIDs
Precautions: Serious GI toxicity including ulceration and bleeding; prior history of GI disease (ulcer or bleeding); preexisting asthma, severe renal impairment, severe hepatic impairment, dehydrated patients, fluid retention, CHF, hypertension, pregnancy category C, lactation, children <18 yr; patients should be made aware of potential GI and hepatic side effects
Pharmacokinetics:
PO: Bioavailability 93%, peak plasma levels 2-3 hr; high-fat meal delays peak plasma time; highly plasma protein bound (87%), hepatic metabolism, renal excretion (72%), minor fecal excretion
🦷 **Drug interactions of concern to dentistry:**
• Possible increased GI symptoms: aspirin

• As with other NSAIDs: reduced effectiveness of diuretics, ACE inhibitors

• Decreased plasma levels: rifampin

• Increased plasma levels of lithium, methotrexate, warfarin

• Monitor INR, small risk of bleeding: warfarin

DENTAL CONSIDERATIONS

General:

• Assess salivary flow as a factor in caries, periodontal disease, and candidiasis.

• Update health and drug history if physician makes changes in evaluation or drug regimens.

• Monitor vital signs every appointment due to cardiovascular side effects.

• Consider semisupine chair position for patient comfort if GI side effects occur.

Teach patient/family:

• Importance of good oral hygiene to prevent soft tissue inflammation

• Use of electric toothbrush if patient has difficulty holding conventional devices

When chronic dry mouth occurs, advise patient:

• To avoid mouth rinses with high alcohol content due to drying effects

• To use daily home fluoride products for anticaries effect

• To use sugarless gum, frequent sips of water, or saliva substitutes

---

ropinirole HCl

(roe-pin'i-role)

ReQuip

Drug class.: Antiparkinson agent

Action: Acts as a dopamine (D_2 and D_3) receptor agonist in the caudate-putamen region of the brain

Uses: Parkinson's disease

Dosage and routes:

• *Adult:* PO initial 0.25 mg tid with weekly incremental dose increase based on patient response

Dose schedule

Week	Dose	Total daily dose
1	0.25 mg tid	0.75 mg
2	0.5 mg tid	1.5 mg
3	0.75 mg tid	2.25 mg
4	1.0 mg tid	3.0 mg

Available forms include: Tabs 0.25, 0.5, 1, 2, 5 mg

Side effects/adverse reactions:

▼ *ORAL: Dry mouth*

CNS: Confusion, hallucination, drowsiness, somnolence, euphoria, dyskinesia, dizziness, headache

CV: Supraventricular ectopy, postural hypotension, syncope, fatigue, bradycardia

GI: Nausea, vomiting, dyspepsia, constipation

RESP: Bronchitis, URI

HEMA: **Thrombocytopenia** (rare), B_{12} deficiency, hypochromic anemia

GU: UTI

EENT: Pharyngitis, blurred vision, rhinitis

INTEG: Sweating

ENDO: Decrease in prolactin levels

META: Increased alk phosphatase, increased BUN

MS: Asthenia, leg cramps

MISC: Viral infection

Contraindications: Hypersensitivity

Precautions: Cardiovascular disease, severely impaired renal or hepatic function, lactation, pregnancy category C, syncope, hypotension

Pharmacokinetics:

PO: Peak plasma levels 1-2 hr, good oral absorption, bioavailability 55%, hepatic metabolism, 40% plasma protein binding, urinary excretion of metabolites

⚕ Drug interactions of concern to dentistry:

• Possible increase in sedation with all CNS depressants
• Possible diminished effects: dopamine antagonists, phenothiazines, haloperidol, droperidol, and metoclopramide

DENTAL CONSIDERATIONS

General:

• Monitor vital signs every appointment due to cardiovascular side effects.
• Assess salivary flow as factor in caries, periodontal disease, and candidiasis.
• After supine positioning, have patient sit upright for at least 2 min before standing to avoid orthostatic hypotension.
• Patients on chronic drug therapy may rarely have symptoms of blood dyscrasias, which can include infection, bleeding, and poor healing.
• Consider semisupine chair position for patient comfort if GI side effects occur.

Consultations:

• In a patient with symptoms of blood dyscrasias, request a medical consult for blood studies and postpone treatment until normal values are reestablished.
• Medical consult may be required to assess disease control and patient's ability to tolerate stress.

Teach patient/family:

• Caution to prevent trauma when using oral hygiene aids
• Use of electric toothbrush if patient has difficulty holding conventional devices
• Importance of good oral hygiene to prevent soft tissue inflammation
• Importance of updating health and drug history if physician makes any changes in evaluation or drug regimens

When chronic dry mouth occurs, advise patient:

• To avoid mouth rinses with high alcohol content due to drying effects
• To use daily home fluoride products for anticaries effect
• To use sugarless gum, frequent sips of water, or saliva substitutes

---

rosiglitazone maleate

(ros-i-gli′ta-zone)

Avandia

Drug class.: Oral antidiabetic

Action: An agonist for peroxisome proliferator-activated receptor gamma (PPAR-γ); improves target cell response to insulin without increasing insulin secretion; insulin must be present for this drug to act

Uses: Monotherapy, as an adjunct to diet and exercise in patients with type 2 diabetes mellitus; may also be used with metformin when metformin, diet, and exercise are not adequate for control

Dosage and routes:

• *Adult:* PO initial dose 4 mg in a single dose or 2 equal doses daily; after evaluation (12 wk) can increase to 8 mg daily

With metformin
• *Adult:* PO 4 mg daily as a single dose or 2 equal doses; after evaluation (12 wk) can increase dose to 8 mg daily
Available forms include: Tabs 2, 4, 8 mg
Side effects/adverse reactions:
CNS: Headache
CV: Edema
GI: Diarrhea
RESP: URI
HEMA: Anemia, decrease hemoglobin/hematocrit
EENT: Sinusitis
META: Hyperglycemia, hypoglycemia, hyperbilirubinemia
MISC: Fatigue
Contraindications: Hypersensitivity, patients with jaundice associated with use of troglitazone, type 1 diabetes
Precautions: May cause resumption of ovulation in premenopausal anovulatory women (risk of pregnancy), patients with edema, advanced heart failure, hepatic impairment, monitor liver enzymes, pregnancy category C, lactation
Pharmacokinetics:
PO: Absolute bioavailability 99%, peak plasma levels approximately 1 hr, half-life 3-4 hr; highly bound to plasma proteins (99.8%), extensive metabolism (CYP450 2C8), excreted mostly in urine (64%)
Drug interactions of concern to dentistry:
• None reported
DENTAL CONSIDERATIONS
General:
• Ensure that patient is following prescribed diet and regularly takes medication.
• Place on frequent recall to evaluate healing response.

• Short appointments and a stress reduction protocol may be required for anxious patients.
• Diabetics may be more susceptible to infection and have delayed wound healing.
• Question patient about self-monitoring of drug's antidiabetic effect, including blood glucose values or finger-stick records.
Consultations:
• Medical consult may include data from patient's blood glucose monitoring, including glycosylated hemoglobin or HbA_{1c} testing.
• Medical consult may be required to assess disease control and patient's ability to tolerate stress.
Teach patient/family:
• To prevent trauma when using oral hygiene aids
• Importance of updating health and drug history if physician makes any changes in evaluation or drug regimens

---

salmeterol xinafoate
(sal-me′te-role)
Serevent, Serevent Diskus
Drug class.: Long-acting selective β_2-agonist

Action: Relaxes bronchial smooth muscle by directly acting on β_2-adrenergic receptors; also inhibits release of mast cell mediators
Uses: Bronchospasm associated with COPD, maintenance treatment of asthma and exercise-induced bronchospasm
Dosage and routes:
Bronchospasm and asthma
• *Adult and child >12 yr:* PO inh 2 puffs bid (12 hr apart); avoid higher doses and more frequent

use; inh (powder) 1 inhalation of 50 µg bid

Exercise-induced bronchospasm (prevention)

• *Adult and child >12 yr:* 2 puffs 30-60 min before exercise, not more than once q12h and not in patients using the drug on a regular basis

Available forms include: Canisters 13 g containing 120 actuations, 6.5 g containing 60 actuations; inh powder 50 µg/disk

Side effects/adverse reactions:

▼ *ORAL: Dry throat,* dental pain (1%-3%, type or origin not defined)

CNS: Headache, tremors, anxiety, dizziness, vertigo, nervousness, fatigue

CV: Tachycardia, palpitation

GI: Stomachache, nausea, vomiting, diarrhea

RESP: Upper/lower respiratory infections, cough, **bronchospasm**

GU: Dysmenorrhea

EENT: Ear/nose/throat infections, nasopharyngitis, sinus headache

INTEG: Rash, urticaria

MS: Tremor, joint pain, muscular soreness, myalgia, back pain, muscle cramps, myositis

MISC: Immediate hypersensitivity reactions

Contraindications: Hypersensitivity

Precautions: Pregnancy category C, lactation, children <12 yr, hepatic impairment, coronary insufficiency, dysrhythmias, hypertension, convulsive disorders; **not for acute symptoms,** not to exceed recommended dose, paradoxic bronchospasm may occur with use;

not recommended for use with a spacer or other aerosol device

Pharmacokinetics:

PO/INH: Rapid onset 5-15 min, peak 4 hr, duration 12 hr; plasma levels are not used to predict local effects in the lung; 94%-98% plasma protein bound; metabolized in liver; excreted mainly in feces, to a lesser degree in urine

🐾 **Drug interactions of concern to dentistry:**

• Increased cardiovascular effects: tricyclic antidepressants

DENTAL CONSIDERATIONS
General:

• Monitor vital signs every appointment due to cardiovascular and respiratory side effects.

• Be aware that aspirin or sulfite preservatives in vasoconstrictor-containing products can exacerbate asthma.

• Acute asthmatic episodes may be precipitated in the dental office. Rapid-acting sympathomimetic inhalants should be available for emergency use. Salmeterol is not a rapid-acting drug and is not intended for use in acute asthmatic attacks.

• Consider semisupine chair position for patients with respiratory disease.

• Midmorning appointments and a stress reduction protocol may be required for anxious patients.

Consultations:

• Medical consult may be required to assess disease control and stress tolerance.

Teach patient/family:

• Importance of good oral hygiene to prevent soft tissue inflammation

---

salsalate

(sal'sa-late)

Amigesic, Argesic-SA, Artha-G, Disalcid, Marthritic, Mono-Gesic, Salflex, Salsitab

Drug class.: Salicylate, nonnarcotic analgesic

Action: Blocks formation of peripheral prostaglandins, which cause pain and inflammation; antipyretic action results from inhibition of hypothalamic heat-regulating center; does not inhibit platelet aggregation

Uses: Mild-to-moderate pain or fever, including arthritis, juvenile rheumatoid arthritis

Dosage and routes:

• *Adult:* PO 500-1000 mg in 2 or 3 doses/day

Available forms include: Caps 500 mg; tabs 500, 750 mg

Side effects/adverse reactions:

CNS: Stimulation, drowsiness, dizziness, confusion, ***convulsions,*** headache, flushing, hallucinations, coma

CV: Rapid pulse, ***pulmonary edema***

GI: *Nausea, vomiting, GI bleeding, diarrhea, heartburn,* anorexia, ***hepatotoxicity***

RESP: Wheezing, hyperpnea

HEMA: ***Thrombocytopenia, agranulocytosis, leukopenia, neutropenia, hemolytic anemia,*** increased prothrombin time

EENT: Tinnitus, hearing loss

INTEG: Rash, urticaria, bruising

ENDO: Hypoglycemia, hyponatremia, hypokalemia, alteration in acid-base balance

Contraindications: Hypersensitivity to salicylates, NSAIDs, GI bleeding, bleeding disorders, children <3 yr, vitamin K deficiency

Precautions: Anemia, hepatic disease, renal disease, Hodgkin's disease, pregnancy category C, lactation

Pharmacokinetics:

PO: Half-life 1 hr; highly protein bound; metabolized by liver; excreted by kidneys; slowly crosses blood-brain barrier and placenta

🥄 Drug interactions of concern to dentistry:

• Increased risk of GI complaints and occult blood loss: alcohol, NSAIDs, corticosteroids

• Increased risk of bleeding: oral anticoagulants, valproic acid, dipyridamole

• Avoid prolonged or concurrent use with NSAIDs, corticosteroids, acetaminophen

• Increased risk of hypoglycemia: oral antidiabetics

• Increased risk of toxicity: methotrexate, lithium, zidovudine

• Decreased effects of probenecid, sulfinpyrazone

DENTAL CONSIDERATIONS

General:

• Patients on chronic drug therapy rarely have symptoms of blood dyscrasias, which can include infection, bleeding, and poor healing.

• Potential cross-allergies with other salicylates such as aspirin.

• Consider semisupine chair position for patients with inflammatory joint diseases.

• Avoid prescribing aspirin-containing products because this drug is a salicylate.

• If used for dental patients, take with food or milk to decrease GI complaints; give 30 min before meals or 2 hr after meals; take with a full glass of water.

italic = common side effects

Consultations:
• In a patient with symptoms of blood dyscrasias, request a medical consult for blood studies and postpone dental treatment until normal values are reestablished.
• Medical consult may be required to assess disease control.

Teach patient/family:
• That salicylates should not be placed directly on a tooth or oral mucosa due to risk of chemical burns
• Not to exceed recommended dosage; acute toxicity may result
• To read label on other OTC drugs; many contain aspirin
• To avoid alcohol ingestion; GI bleeding may occur
• Importance of good oral hygiene to prevent soft tissue inflammation
• Caution to prevent injury when using oral hygiene aids

---

saquinavir mesylate
(sa-kwin'a-veer)
Invirase, Fotovase
Drug class.: Antiviral

Action: Inhibits HIV protease important for viral replication
Uses: Used in combination with nucleoside analogs, zidovudine, or zalcitabine in the treatment of AIDS

Dosage and routes:
Invirase
• *Adult:* PO 600 mg tid; take within 2 hr after eating with a nucleoside analog
Fotovase
• *Adult:* PO 1200 mg tid; take within 2 hr after eating with a nucleoside analog
Available forms include: Caps 200 mg

Side effects/adverse reactions:
▼ *ORAL:* Buccal mucosal ulceration (<2%), dry mouth, taste alteration, stomatitis
CNS: Headache, paresthesia, extremity numbness, dizziness, peripheral neuropathy
CV: Hypotension, syncope (infrequent)
GI: Diarrhea, abdominal discomfort, nausea, dyspepsia
RESP: Cough, dyspnea, pharyngitis, rhinitis, sinusitis
HEMA: Anemia, ***thrombocytopenia, pancytopenia***
GU: UTI
EENT: Blepharitis, earache, eye irritation, tinnitus
INTEG: Rash, pruritus, photosensitivity
ENDO: Dry eyes
MS: Musculoskeletal pain, myalgia
Contraindications: Hypersensitivity, rifampin
Precautions: Hepatic impairment, child <16 yr, pregnancy category B, lactation (unknown), bone marrow suppression, renal impairment

Pharmacokinetics:
PO: Peak serum levels 3 hr, serum levels decrease by 8 hr; hepatic metabolism; renal excretion

🦷 Drug interactions of concern to dentistry:
• Increased plasma levels of clindamycin, troleandomycin, ketoconazole, itraconazole, fentanyl
• Increased metabolism of carbamazepine, dexamethasone, phenobarbital

DENTAL CONSIDERATIONS
General:
• Examine for oral manifestations of opportunistic infections.
• Patients on chronic drug therapy may rarely have symptoms of

---

blood dyscrasias, which can include infection, bleeding, and poor healing.

• Palliative medication may be required for management of oral side effects.

Consultations:

• Medical consult may be required to assess disease control.

• In a patient with symptoms of blood dyscrasias, request a medical consult for blood studies and postpone dental treatment until normal values are reestablished.

Teach patient/family:

• Importance of good oral hygiene to prevent soft tissue inflammation

• Caution to prevent trauma when using oral hygiene aids

• That secondary oral infection may occur; must see dentist immediately if infection occurs

• Importance of updating medical/drug history if physician makes any changes in evaluation or drug regimen

---

scopolamine (transdermal)

(skoe-pol'a-meen)

Transderm Scop

♣ Transderm-V

Drug class.: Antiemetic, anticholinergic

Action: Competitive antagonism of acetylcholine at receptor sites in the eye, smooth muscle, cardiac muscle, glandular cells; inhibition of vestibular input to the CNS, resulting in inhibition of vomiting reflex

Uses: Prevention of motion sickness; prevent nausea, vomiting associated with anesthesia or opiate analgesia

Dosage and routes:

• *Adult:* Patch 1 placed behind ear 4-5 hr before travel

Not recommended for children

Available forms include: Patch 1.5 mg

Side effects/adverse reactions:

▼ *ORAL: Dry mouth*

CNS: Dizziness, drowsiness, confusion, disorientation, memory disturbances, hallucinations

GU: Difficult urination

EENT: Blurred vision, dilated pupils, altered depth perception, photophobia, dry/itchy/red eyes, acute narrow-angle glaucoma

INTEG: Rash, erythema

Contraindications: Hypersensitivity, glaucoma

Precautions: Children, elderly, pregnancy category C; pyloric, urinary, bladder neck, intestinal obstruction; liver, kidney disease

Pharmacokinetics:

PATCH: Onset 4-5 hr, duration 72 hr

🦷 **Drug interactions of concern to dentistry:**

• Increased anticholinergic effects: propantheline and other anticholinergic drugs

• Increased risk of CNS depression: alcohol, all CNS depressants

DENTAL CONSIDERATIONS

General:

• Avoid dental light in patient's eyes; offer dark glasses for patient comfort.

Teach patient/family:

• To avoid mouth rinses with high alcohol content due to drying effects

---

secobarbital/seco-barbital sodium

(see-koe-bar′bi-tal)

Seconal

♣ Novosecobarb

Drug class.: Sedative-hypnotic barbiturate

Controlled Substance Schedule II, Canada G

Action: Nonselective depression of the CNS, ranging from sedation to hypnosis to anesthesia to coma, depending on the dose administered

Uses: Insomnia, sedation, preoperative medication, status epilepticus, acute tetanus convulsions

Dosage and routes:

Insomnia

• *Adult:* PO 100-200 mg hs

Sedation (preoperatively)

• *Adult:* PO 100-200 mg 1-2 hr preoperatively

• *Child:* PO 2-6 mg/kg 1-2 hr preoperatively; rectal up to a max of 100 mg

Available forms include: Caps 100 mg

Side effects/adverse reactions:

▼ *ORAL:* Oral ulcerations (rare), bleeding (rare)

CNS: Lethargy, drowsiness, hangover, dizziness, paradoxic stimulation in the elderly and children, light-headedness, dependence, CNS depression, mental depression, slurred speech

CV: Hypotension, bradycardia

GI: Nausea, vomiting, diarrhea, constipation

RESP: **Apnea, laryngospasm, bronchospasm,** depression

HEMA: **Agranulocytosis, thrombocytopenia, megaloblastic anemia** (long-term treatment)

INTEG: Rash, **Stevens-Johnson syndrome,** urticaria, pain, abscesses at injection site, angioedema, thrombophlebitis

Contraindications: Hypersensitivity to barbiturates, respiratory depression, addiction to barbiturates, severe liver impairment, porphyria, uncontrolled severe pain

Precautions: Anemia, pregnancy category D, lactation, hepatic disease, renal disease, hypertension, elderly, acute/chronic pain

Pharmacokinetics:

IM: Onset 10-15 min, duration 3-6 hr

REC: Onset slow, duration 3-6 hr Half-life 15-40 hr; metabolized by liver; excreted by kidneys (metabolites)

🦷 Drug interactions of concern to dentistry:

• Hepatotoxicity: halogenated hydrocarbon anesthetics

• Increased CNS depression: alcohol, all CNS depressants

• Increased metabolism of carbamazepine, tricyclic antidepressants, corticosteroids

• Decreased half-life of doxycycline

DENTAL CONSIDERATIONS

General:

• Determine why the patient is taking the drug.

• Monitor vital signs every appointment due to cardiovascular side effects. Evaluate respiration characteristics and rate.

• Patients on chronic drug therapy may rarely have symptoms of

---

blood dyscrasias, which can include infection, bleeding, and poor healing.

When used for sedation in dentistry:

• Assess vital signs before and q30min after use as sedative.

• Observe respiratory dysfunction: respiratory depression, character, rate, rhythm; hold drug if respirations <10/min or if pupils are dilated.

• After supine positioning, have patient sit upright for at least 2 min before standing to avoid orthostatic hypotension.

• Have someone drive patient to and from dental office when used for conscious sedation.

• Barbiturates induce liver microsomal enzymes, which alter the metabolism of other drugs.

• Geriatric patients are more susceptible to drug effects; use a lower dose.

Consultations:

• In a patient with symptoms of blood dyscrasias, request a medical consult for blood studies and postpone dental treatment until normal values are reestablished.

Teach patient/family:

• To avoid driving or other activities requiring alertness

• To avoid alcohol ingestion and CNS depressants; serious CNS depression may result

• Caution when using OTC preparations (antihistamines, cold remedies) that contain CNS depressants

---

selegiline HCl (l-deprenyl)

(se-le'ji-leen)

Carbex, Eldepryl

♦ Apo-Selegiline, Gen-Selegiline, Novo-Selegiline, Nu-Selegiline, SD Deprenyl

Drug class.: Antiparkinson agent

Action: Increased dopaminergic activity by inhibiting MAO type B activity

Uses: Adjunct management of Parkinson's disease in patients being treated with levodopa/carbidopa

Dosage and routes:

• *Adult:* PO 10 mg/day in divided doses of 5 mg at breakfast and lunch; doses of 20 mg/day increase the risk of side effects/drug interactions

Available forms include: Tabs 5 mg, caps 5 mg

Side effects/adverse reactions:

▼ *ORAL:* Dry mouth

CNS: Increased tremors, chorea, restlessness, blepharospasm, increased bradykinesia, grimacing, tardive dyskinesia, dystonic symptoms, involuntary movements, increased apraxia, hallucinations, dizziness, mood changes, nightmares, delusions, lethargy, apathy, overstimulation, sleep disturbances, headache, migraine, numbness, muscle cramps, confusion, anxiety, tiredness, vertigo, personality change, back/leg pain

CV: Orthostatic hypotension, hypertension, dysrhythmia, palpitation, angina pectoris, hypotension, tachycardia, edema, sinus bradycardia, syncope

GI: Nausea, vomiting, constipation, weight loss, anorexia, diar-

rhea, heartburn, rectal bleeding, poor appetite, dysphagia
RESP: Asthma, shortness of breath
GU: Slow urination, nocturia, prostatic hypertrophy, hesitation, retention, frequency, sexual dysfunction
EENT: Diplopia, blurred vision, tinnitus
INTEG: Increased sweating, alopecia, hematoma, rash, photosensitivity, facial hair
Contraindications: Hypersensitivity; fluoxetine, meperidine
Precautions: Pregnancy category C, lactation, children
Pharmacokinetics:
PO: Rapidly absorbed, peak 0.5-2 hr; rapidly metabolized (active metabolites: *N*-desmethyldeprenyl, l-amphetamine, l-methamphetamine); metabolites excreted in urine

⚒ Drug interactions of concern to dentistry:
• *Fatal interaction:* opioids (especially meperidine); do not administer together
• Risk of serotonin syndrome: serotonin uptake inhibitors (fluoxetine, sertraline, paroxetine)

DENTAL CONSIDERATIONS
General:
• Monitor vital signs every appointment due to cardiovascular side effects.
• After supine positioning, have patient sit upright for at least 2 min before standing to avoid orthostatic hypotension.
• Assess for presence of extrapyramidal motor symptoms, such as tardive dyskinesia and akathisia. Extrapyramidal motor activity may complicate dental treatment.
• Assess salivary flow as a factor in caries, periodontal disease, and candidiasis.

Consultations:
• Medical consult may be required to assess disease control and patient's ability to tolerate stress.
• If signs of tardive dyskinesia or akathisia are present, refer to physician.

Teach patient/family:
• To use electric toothbrush if patient has difficulty holding conventional devices
When chronic dry mouth occurs, advise patient:
• To avoid mouth rinses with high alcohol content due to drying effects
• Of need for daily use of home fluoride products to prevent caries
• To use sugarless gum, frequent sips of water, or saliva substitutes

---

sertraline
(ser'tra-leen)
Zoloft
Drug class.: Antidepressant

Action: Selectively inhibits the uptake of serotonin in the brain
Uses: Major depression, obsessive-compulsive disorder, panic disorder; posttraumatic stress disorder
Dosage and routes:
• *Adult:* PO 50 mg qd; may increase to a max of 200 mg/day; do not change dose at intervals of <1 wk; administer qd in AM or PM
Posttraumatic stress disorder/panic disorder
• *Adult:* PO 25 mg/day; can increase to 50 mg/day after 1 wk
Available forms include: Tabs 25, 50, 100 mg; oral conc 20 mg/ml in 60 ml; (Canada) caps 25, 50, 100, 150, 200 mg

---

bold italic = life-threatening conditions

Side effects/adverse reactions:

▼ *ORAL: Dry mouth,* aphthous stomatitis (<0.1%), taste alteration, lichenoid reaction

CNS: Insomnia, headache, dizziness, somnolence, tremor, fatigue, twitching, confusion

CV: Palpitation, chest pain, postural hypotension, syncope

GI: Diarrhea, nausea, dyspepsia, constipation, anorexia, vomiting, flatulence

RESP: Rhinitis, pharyngitis, coughing

GU: Male sexual dysfunction, micturition disorder

EENT: Vision abnormalities, tinnitus

INTEG: Sweating, rash

MS: Myalgia

Contraindications: Hypersensitivity, MAOIs

Precautions: Pregnancy category B, lactation, elderly, hepatic/renal disease, epilepsy

Pharmacokinetics:

PO: Peak 6-10 hr, elimination half-life 25 hr; plasma protein binding 99%; extensively metabolized; metabolites excreted in urine

⚑ Drug interactions of concern to dentistry:

• Increased CNS depression: alcohol, CNS depressants

• Increased side effects: highly protein-bound drugs (aspirin)

• Increased half-life of diazepam

• Possible inhibition of sertraline metabolism: erythromycin, clarithromycin

DENTAL CONSIDERATIONS

General:

• Monitor vital signs every appointment due to cardiovascular side effects.

• After supine positioning, have patient sit upright for at least 2 min to avoid orthostatic hypotension.

• Assess salivary flow as a factor in caries, periodontal disease, and candidiasis.

• Avoid dental light in patient's eyes; offer dark glasses for patient comfort.

• Consider semisupine chair position for patient comfort if GI side effects occur.

Consultations:

• Medical consult may be required to assess patient's ability to tolerate stress.

• Physician should be informed if significant xerostomic side effects occur (increased caries, sore tongue, problems eating or swallowing, difficulty wearing prosthesis) so a medication change can be considered.

Teach patient/family:

• To use electric toothbrush if patient has difficulty holding conventional devices

When chronic dry mouth occurs, advise patient:

• To avoid mouth rinses with high alcohol content due to drying effects

• Of need for daily use of home fluoride products to prevent caries

• To use sugarless gum, frequent sips of water, or saliva substitutes

---

sibutramine

(si-byoo′tra-meen)

Meridia

Drug class.: Amphetamine analog anorexiant

Controlled Substance Schedule IV

Action: Anoretic action unclear, blocks the reuptake of norepineph-

italic = common side effects

rine, serotonin, and dopamine; action depends on formation of two active metabolites, M_1 and M_2

Uses: Obesity

Dosage and routes:

• *Adult:* PO initial dose 10 mg/day; after 4 wk can titrate dose to 15 mg/day; doses >15 mg/day are not recommended

Available forms include: Caps 5, 10, 15 mg

Side effects/adverse reactions:

▼ *ORAL: Dry mouth,* taste prevention

CNS: Headache, insomnia, irritability, asthenia, migraine

CV: Tachycardia, hypertension, palpitation

GI: Abdominal pain, dyspepsia, nausea

GU: Dysmenorrhea, UTI

EENT: Rhinitis, pharyngitis

MS: Back pain, arthralgia

MISC: Flu syndrome

INTEG: Skin rash, dry skin

META: Elevated ALT, AST, alk phosphatase

Contraindications: Hypersensitivity, MAO inhibitor, anorexia nervosa, severe hepatic or renal impairment, CAD, CHF, arrhythmias, stroke, other CNS appetite suppressants, meperidine

Precautions: Requires monitoring of BP, risk of serotonin syndrome with other serotonin reuptake inhibitors, glaucoma, pregnancy category C, lactation, children <16 yr, elderly, seizures

Pharmacokinetics:

PO: Rapid absorption, extensive first-pass metabolism, two active metabolites (M_1 and M_2), highly protein bound (94%-97%), hepatic metabolism; excreted mostly in urine, less in feces

⚖ Drug interactions of concern to dentistry:

• Avoid use of meperidine: risk of serotonin syndrome

DENTAL CONSIDERATIONS

General:

• Monitor vital signs every appointment due to cardiovascular side effects.

• Assess salivary flow as factor in caries, periodontal disease, and candidiasis.

• Information on any abuse liability is unknown.

• Determine why patient is taking the drug.

Teach patient/family:

When chronic dry mouth occurs, advise patient:

• To avoid mouth rinses with high alcohol content due to drying effects

• Of need for daily use of home fluoride products to prevent caries

• To use sugarless gum, frequent sips of water, or saliva substitutes

---

sildenafil citrate

(sil-den′a-fil)

Viagra

Drug class.: Impotence therapy

Action: A selective inhibitor of cyclic guanosine monophosphate (cGMP)–specific phosphodiesterase type 5 (PDE5). It enhances the effect of nitric oxide (produced by sexual stimulation) that is involved in increased production of cGMP, both of which are involved in the physiologic processes leading to penile erection. cGMP is required for smooth muscle relaxation in the corpus cavernosum that allows inflow of blood.

Uses: Male erectile dysfunction

Dosage and routes:
• *Adult:* PO (male only) 50 mg taken as needed approximately 1 hr before sexual activity with once-a-day dosing at a maximum. The dosage range is 25-100 mg based on tolerance and effectiveness. It can be taken anywhere from 0.5-4 hr before sexual activity. Sexual activity is required for effective response.

Available forms include: Tabs 25, 50, 100 mg

Side effects/adverse reactions:

▼ *ORAL:* Dry mouth, glossitis (very low incidence)

CNS: Headache, dizziness, insomnia, somnolence, abnormal dreams

CV: Flushing, syncope, palpitation, hemorrhoidal hemorrhage

GI: Dyspepsia, diarrhea, vomiting, dysphagia, gastritis

RESP: Dyspnea, increased cough, asthma

GU: UTI, cystitis, nocturia, urinary frequency, abnormal ejaculation

EENT: Nasal congestion, sinusitis

INTEG: Rash, urticaria, pruritus, contact dermatitis

MS: Musculoskeletal pain, synovitis

Contraindications: Hypersensitivity, patients who are currently using organic nitrates

Precautions: Complete medical and physical exam to determine cause of erectile dysfunction; because of cardiac risk associated with sexual activity, cardiovascular status should be evaluated; anatomic deformation of penis, conditions predisposing to priapism (sickle cell anemia, anemia, multiple myeloma, leukemia), retinitis pigmentosa, not indicated for women, children, or newborns, pregnancy category B; hepatic or renal impairment, men >65 yr

Pharmacokinetics:
PO: Rapid oral absorption, bioavailability 40%, peak plasma levels 30 min-2 hr, hepatic metabolism by cytochrome P-450 enzymes, active metabolite, highly plasma protein bound (96%), major excretion route in feces, lesser route in urine

🦷 Drug interactions of concern to dentistry:
• Avoid use of nitroglycerin within 24 hr
• Increased plasma levels due to interference with metabolism: cimetidine, erythromycin, ketoconazole, itraconazole

DENTAL CONSIDERATIONS
General:
• This is an acute-use drug intended to be taken just before sexual activity, and the reported incidence of oral side effects does not differ from a placebo. However, the potential interacting drugs should be avoided.

---

simvastatin
(sim′va-sta-tin)
Zocor

Drug class.: Antihyperlipidemic

Action: Inhibits HMG-CoA reductase enzyme, thus reducing cholesterol synthesis; reduced synthesis of VLDL; plasma triglyceride levels may also be decreased

Uses: As an adjunct in homozygous familial hypercholesterolemia, mixed hyperlipidemia, elevated serum triglyceride levels and type IV hyperproteinemia, also reduces total cholesterol LDL-C, apo B, and triglyceride levels; patient should first be placed on cholesterol-lowering diet

Dosage and routes:

• *Adult:* PO 5-10 mg qd with evening meal; may increase to 5-40 mg/day in single or divided doses; not to exceed 40 mg/day; dosage adjustments should be made qmo

Available forms include: Tabs 5, 10, 20, 40, 80 mg

Side effects/adverse reactions:

CNS: Dizziness, headache

*GI: Nausea, constipation, diarrhea, dyspepsia, flatulence, abdominal pain, heartburn, **liver dysfunction***

EENT: Blurred vision, dysgeusia, lens opacities

INTEG: Rash, pruritus

*MS: Muscle cramps, myalgia, **myositis, rhabdomyolysis***

Contraindications: Pregnancy category X, lactation, active liver disease

Precautions: Past liver disease, alcoholics, severe acute infections, trauma, hypotension, uncontrolled seizure disorders, severe metabolic disorders, electrolyte imbalances

Pharmacokinetics:

PO: Peak 1-2.5 hr; highly protein bound; metabolized in liver (active metabolites); excreted in bile, feces

⚕ Drug interactions of concern to dentistry:

• Increased myalgia, myositis: erythromycin, cyclosporin, itraconazole

DENTAL CONSIDERATIONS

General:

• Consider semisupine chair position for patient comfort due to GI side effects.

sodium fluoride

Fluoritabs, Flura-Drops, Flurodex Karidium, Luride Lozi-Tabs, Pediaflor, Pedi-Dent, Solu-Flur; also found in pediatric vitamin formulas

🍁 Fluor-A-Day, Fluotic

Drug class.: Fluoride ion

Action: Interacts with tooth structure to increase resistance to acid dissolution; promotes enamel remineralization and inhibits dental plaque microorganisms

Uses: Prevention of dental caries, osteoporosis

Dosage and routes:

• *Adult and child >12 yr:* TOP 10 ml 0.2% sol qd after brushing teeth; rinse mouth for >1 min with sol

• *Child 6-12 yr:* TOP 5 ml 0.2% sol

Revised fluoride supplement schedules (infants and children—ADA, American Academy of Pediatric Dentistry, American Academy of Pediatrics)

• Must ascertain fluoride concentration in patient's drinking water before prescribing, as shown in the following tables:

USA—fluoride supplementation schedule

Child's age	<0.3 ppm	0.3-0.6 ppm	>0.6 ppm
birth-6 mo	0.0	0.0	0.0
6 mo-3 yr	0.25 mg/day	0.0	0.0
3-6 yr	0.50 mg/day	0.25 mg/day	0.0
6-16 yr	1.0 mg/day	0.50 mg/day	0.0

S

Canada—fluoride supplementation schedule

Age	Canadian Paediatric Society (applies to all children)	Canadian Dental Association (applies to children with high risk of caries)
6 mo-2 yr	0.25 mg/day	0
3-5 yr	0.50 mg/day	0.25 mg/day (0.5 mg/day if fluoridated toothpaste is not used regularly)
6-12 yr	Not applicable	1.00 mg/day
6-16 yr	1.0 mg/day	Not applicable

Reference: Kowalchuk I: *CMAJ* 154(7): 1007, 1996.

Available forms include: Chew tabs 0.25 mg; tabs 0.5, 1 mg; effervescent tabs 10 mg; drops 0.125, 0.25, 0.5 mg/ml; rinse supplements 0.2 mg/ml; rinse 0.01%, 0.02%, 0.09%; gel 0.1%, 0.5%, 1.23%

Side effects/adverse reactions:

▼ *ORAL:* Mottled enamel (chronic use), stomatitis

ACUTE OVERDOSE: Black tarry stools, bloody vomit, diarrhea, decreased respiration, increased salivation, watery eyes

CHRONIC OVERDOSE: Hypocalcemia, tetany, respiratory arrest, constipation, loss of appetite, nausea, vomiting, weight loss

Contraindications: Hypersensitivity, renal insufficiency, GI ulcerations

Precautions: Child <6 yr (must evaluate total fluoride ingestion), pregnancy category not established

Pharmacokinetics:

PO: Efficient oral absorption; distributed to calcified tissues (bones and teeth); excreted in urine, feces; crosses placenta, excreted in breast milk

Drug interactions of concern to dentistry:
• Avoid use with dairy products and gastric alkalinizers

DENTAL CONSIDERATIONS

General:
• Determine fluoride concentration in water supply, then calculate dosage.
• In the United states, the use of fluoride supplements is not recommended when community drinking water contains at least 0.6 ppm fluoride or after age 16.
• Recommended dose should not be exceeded or dental fluorosis and osseous changes may occur.
• To reduce risk of accidental ingestion and overdosage, ADA recommends that a limit of 264 mg sodium fluoride be dispensed in prepackaged containers.
• Give drops after meals with fluids or undiluted tablets; may be chewed; do not swallow whole; may be given with water or juice; avoid milk.
• Systemic fluoride use during pregnancy has not been shown to prevent tooth decay in children.

Teach patient/family:
• To monitor children using gel or rinse; not to be swallowed
• Not to drink, eat, or rinse mouth for at least 0.5 hr after topical use
• To apply after brushing and flossing hs

• To store out of children's reach
Treatment of acute overdose:
• Gastric lavage with calcium chloride or calcium hydroxide solution to precipitate fluoride
• Maintenance of high urine output
• Refer to hospital emergency facility

---

sodium fluoride (topical)

Sodium fluoride (topical) non-abrasive: Karigel, Neutracare, Prevident
Sodium fluoride (topical) with abrasive: PreviDent 5000 Plus
Drug class.: Fluoride ion

Action: Interacts with enamel surface to increase resistance to acid dissolution; promotes enamel remineralization and inhibits dental plaque microorganisms
Uses: Prevention of dental caries, hypersensitive root surfaces
Dosage and routes:
• *Adult and child >6 yr:* Nonabrasive gels—use daily; apply thin ribbon to toothbrush for at least 1 min after regular brushing, preferably at bedtime; expectorate and refrain from eating, drinking, and rinsing; children should use under parental supervision.
Available forms include: Gel or cream 2 oz (56 g) squeeze tube 0.5% (as 1.1% sodium fluoride) with and without mild abrasive
Other fluoride topical products include the following daily-use gels: 1.1% APF (Thera-Flur); 0.4% SnF_2 (Control, Easy-Gel, Flocare, Flo-Gel, Florentine, Gel-Kam, Gel-Pro, Gel-Tin, Perfect Choice, Quick-Gel, Stan-Gard, Stop Gel)
Rinses: 0.05% APF daily use (NaF-rinse, Phos-Flur) and 0.2% NaF weekly use (NaFrinse, Point-Two, Preventive, Prevident)

Product strength	F⁻ ion (%)	ppm F equivalence
1.1% NaF	0.5	4950
0.4% SnF_2	0.10	970
0.2% NaF	0.10	910
0.05% NaF	0.02	230

Contraindications: Hypersensitivity; may be used in areas of fluoridated drinking water
Precautions: Child <6 yr (repeated swallowing of agent could cause dental fluorosis); do not use in pediatric patients <6 yr, infants. Supervise children <6 yr. A 2-oz tube of 1.1% NaF contains 250 mg fluoride, more than twice the amount that the ADA recommends to be dispensed in 1 container. Ingestion of as little as 0.29 oz could cause acute toxicity in a 1-year-old child. Repeated swallowing could cause fluorosis.

DENTAL CONSIDERATIONS
General:
• Neutral sodium fluoride preparations are recommended for patients with exposed root surfaces, which may be hypersensitive.
Teach patient/family:
• To apply daily a thin ribbon of dental cream or gel to toothbrush and brush thoroughly for 2 min, preferably at bedtime
• Expectorate after use and do not eat, drink, or rinse for 30 min
• Children should use under parental supervision

---

sotalol HCl

(soe'ta-lole)

Betapace, Betapace AF

♣ Sotacor

Drug class.: Nonselective β-adrenergic blocker

Action: This is a nonselective β_1- and β_2-adrenergic antagonist. The antihypertensive mechanism of action is unclear, but it may include a reduction in cardiac output and inhibition of renin release by the renal juxtaglomerular apparatus. Peripheral resistance decreases with long-term use. The antianginal action (when indicated for this use) may be related to a decrease in myocardial oxygen demand and negative chronotropic and inotropic effects. The antiarrhythmic action (when indicated for this use) has been related to a reduction in spontaneous pacemaker firing and slowing of AV nodal conduction.

Uses: Life-threatening ventricular dysrhythmias (class II), atrial fibrillation (Betapace AF only)

Dosage and routes:

• *Adult:* PO initial 80 mg bid; may be increased gradually to 240 or 320 mg/day; some patients may require 480-640 mg/day

Available forms include: Tabs 80, 120, 160, 240 mg; AF tabs 80, 120, 160 mg

Side effects/adverse reactions:

CNS: Fatigue, dizziness, asthenia, light-headedness, headache, insomnia, sedation

*CV: **Bradycardia, dysrhythmia, hypotension, CHF, syncope,** chest pain, palpitation*

GI: Nausea, vomiting, dyspepsia

*RESP: **Asthma, dyspnea***

GU: Sexual dysfunction

EENT: Visual problems

INTEG: Rash

Contraindications: Hypersensitivity to this drug, cardiac failure, cardiogenic shock, second- or third-degree heart block, bronchospastic disease, sinus bradycardia, CHF

Precautions: Pregnancy category B, lactation, diabetes mellitus, renal disease

Pharmacokinetics:

PO: Peak plasma levels 2.5-4 hr, half-life 12 hr; low protein binding; excreted in urine unchanged

🦷 Drug interactions of concern to dentistry:

• Decreased hypotensive effect: NSAIDs, indomethacin

• Increased hypotension, myocardial depression: hydrocarbon inhalation anesthetics

• Hypertension, bradycardia: sympathomimetics

• Slow metabolism of lidocaine

DENTAL CONSIDERATIONS

General:

• Monitor vital signs every appointment due to cardiovascular side effects.

• After supine positioning, have patient sit upright for at least 2 min before standing to avoid orthostatic hypotension.

• Stress from dental procedures may compromise cardiovascular function; determine patient risk.

• Use vasoconstrictors with caution, in low doses, and with careful aspiration. Avoid use of gingival retraction cord with epinephrine.

• Short appointments and a stress reduction protocol may be required for anxious patients.

Consultations:
• Medical consult should be made to assess disease control and patient's ability to tolerate stress.

---

sparfloxacin

(spar-flox'a-sin)
Zagam
Drug class.: Fluoroquinolone antiinfective

Action: A broad-spectrum bactericidal agent that inhibits the enzymes topoisomerase II (DNA gyrase) and topoisomerase IV required for bacterial DNA replication, transcription repair, and recombination

Uses: Community-acquired pneumonia and acute bacterial exacerbations of chronic bronchitis caused by susceptible microorganisms (*C. pneumoniae, H. influenza, M. pneumonia, S. pneumoniae, K. pneumoniae, M. catarrhalis, S. aureus, E. cloacae*)

Dosage and routes:
• *Adult >18 yr:* PO 400 mg first day, then 200 mg qd for total of 10 days therapy (total 11 tabs)
Renal impairment
• *Adult >18 yr:* PO 400 mg first day; then 200 mg q48h for total of 9 days therapy (6 tabs)
Available forms include: Tabs 200 mg

Side effects/adverse reactions:
▼ *ORAL: Taste alteration,* dry mouth
CNS: Headache, insomnia, convulsions, toxic psychoses, dizziness, light-headedness
CV: Prolonged QT interval, vasodilation, palpitation, postural hypotension
*GI: Diarrhea, nausea, dyspepsia, abdominal pain, vomiting, flatulence, **pseudomembranous colitis***
RESP: Pharyngitis, epistaxis, cough, sinusitis
HEMA: Cyanosis, ecchymosis
GU: Vaginitis, dysuria
EENT: Ear pain, tinnitus, diplopia, eye pain
INTEG: Photosensitization, pruritus
MS: Rupture of Achilles tendon, tendons in shoulder or hand
*MISC: **Anaphylaxis***

Contraindications: Hypersensitivity, photosensitivity, disopyramide, amiodarone, and class Ia and III antiarrhythmics, bepridil; patients with prolonged QT$_c$ interval, hypokalemia, significant bradycardia

Precautions: Antacids retard absorption, renal impairment, avoid exposure to sun, artificial ultraviolet light, patients <18 yr, seizures, CV arrhythmics, MI, congestive heart failure, pregnancy category C, lactation

Pharmacokinetics:
PO: Oral bioavailability 92%, peak plasma levels 3-6 hr, hepatic metabolism, equally excreted in urine and feces

☙ Drug interactions of concern to dentistry:
• Avoid concurrent use with erythromycin, pentamidine, tricyclic antidepressants, phenothiazines
• Concurrent administration with antacids greatly reduces oral absorption, can increase warfarin levels

DENTAL CONSIDERATIONS
General:
• Contraindicated for patients whose lifestyle or employment will not permit compliance with photosensitivity precautions.

S

---

bold italic = life-threatening conditions

• Determine why patient is taking the drug.
• Assess salivary flow as factor in caries, periodontal disease, and candidiasis.
• Consider semisupine chair position for patient comfort if GI side effects occur.
• Avoid dental light in patient's eyes; offer dark glasses for patient comfort.

Consultations:
• Consult with patient's physician if an acute dental infection occurs and another antiinfective is required.

Teach patient/family:
• To avoid exposure to sunlight and wear sunscreen if sun exposure is planned during treatment and for 5 days after treatment is stopped

---

spironolactone

(speer-on-oh-lak'tone)

Aldactone
♣ Novospiroton

Drug class.: Potassium-sparing diuretic

Action: Competes with aldosterone at receptor sites in distal tubule, resulting in excretion of sodium chloride, water, retention of potassium and phosphate
Uses: Edema, hypertension, diuretic-induced hypokalemia, primary hyperaldosteronism (diagnosis, short-term treatment, long-term treatment), nephrotic syndrome, cirrhosis of the liver with ascites
Dosage and routes:
Edema/hypertension
• *Adult:* PO 25-200 mg qd in single or divided doses
• *Child:* PO 3.3 mg/kg/day in single or divided doses

Hypokalemia
• *Adult:* PO 25-100 mg/day; if PO, K supplements must not be used
Primary hyperaldosteronism diagnosis
• *Adult:* PO 400 mg/day for 4 days or 4 wk depending on test, then 100-400 mg/day maintenance
Available forms include: Tabs 25, 50, 100 mg
Side effects/adverse reactions:
▼ *ORAL:* Gingival bleeding (rare); dry mouth may be a symptom of hyponatremia, lichenoid drug reaction
CNS: Headache, confusion, drowsiness, lethargy, ataxia
*GI: Diarrhea, **bleeding** (rare), gastritis, cramps, vomiting
HEMA: Decreased WBCs, platelets
INTEG: Rash, pruritus, urticaria
ENDO: Impotence, gynecomastia, irregular menses, amenorrhea, postmenopausal bleeding, hirsutism, deepening voice
ELECT: **Hyperkalemia,** hyperchloremic metabolic acidosis, hyponatremia
Contraindications: Hypersensitivity, anuria, severe renal disease, hyperkalemia, pregnancy category not established
Precautions: Dehydration, hepatic disease, lactation
Pharmacokinetics:
PO: Onset 24-48 hr, peak 48-72 hr; metabolized in liver; excreted in urine; crosses placenta
👈 **Drug interactions of concern to dentistry:**
• Nephrotoxicity: indomethacin and possibly other NSAIDs
• Decreased antihypertensive effect: indomethacin and possibly other NSAIDs

DENTAL CONSIDERATIONS
General:
• Monitor vital signs every appointment due to cardiovascular side effects.
• Assess salivary flow as a factor in caries, periodontal disease, and candidiasis.
• If dry mouth occurs, follow usual preventive and palliative measures, but consider hyponatremia as a contributing factor.
• Consider semisupine chair position for patient comfort if GI side effects occur.
Consultations:
• Medical consult may be required to assess disease control and patient's ability to tolerate stress.
Teach patient/family:
When chronic dry mouth occurs, advise patient:
• To avoid mouth rinses with high alcohol content due to drying effects
• Of need for daily use of home fluoride products to prevent caries
• To use sugarless gum, frequent sips of water, or saliva substitutes

---

stanozolol
(stan-oh'zoe-lole)
Winstrol
Drug class.: Androgenic anabolic steroid

Controlled Substance Schedule III
Action: Reverses catabolic tissue processes; promotes buildup of protein; increases erythropoietin production
Uses: Hereditary angioedema prophylaxis

Dosage and routes:
Angioedema
• *Adult:* PO 2 mg tid, then decrease q1-3mo, down to 2 mg qd or q2d
• *Child 6-12 yr:* PO up to 2 mg/day only during the attack
• *Child <6 yr:* PO 1 mg/day only during the attack
Available forms include: Tabs 2 mg
Side effects/adverse reactions:
CNS: Dizziness, headache, fatigue, tremors, paresthesia, flushing, sweating, anxiety, lability, insomnia
CV: ***Edema*** (in cardiac patients), increased BP
GI: ***Peliosis hepatitis, liver cell tumors, cholestatic jaundice,*** nausea, vomiting, constipation, weight gain
HEMA: Increased prothrombin time, iron deficiency anemia
GU: ***Hematuria,*** amenorrhea, vaginitis, decreased libido, decreased breast size, clitoral hypertrophy, testicular atrophy, gynecomastia (males), priapism
EENT: Conjunctival edema, nasal congestion
INTEG: Rash, acneiform lesions, oily hair/skin, flushing, sweating, acne vulgaris, alopecia, hirsutism
ENDO: Abnormal GTT, decreased glucose tolerance, increased LDL
MS: Cramps, spasms
Contraindications: Severe renal disease, severe cardiac disease, severe hepatic disease, hypersensitivity, pregnancy category X, lactation, genital bleeding (abnormal), prostate or breast carcinoma in males, breast cancer in females with hypercalcemia, nephrosis
Precautions: Diabetes mellitus, CV disease, MI, increased risk of

---

bold italic = life-threatening conditions

prostatic hypertrophy, prostatic carcinoma, virilization (women), increased prothrombin time

Pharmacokinetics:

PO: Metabolized in liver, excreted in urine, crosses placenta, excreted in breast milk

🦷 **Drug interactions of concern to dentistry:**

• Increased risk of bleeding: aspirin
• Edema: ACTH, adrenal steroids

DENTAL CONSIDERATIONS

General:

• Determine why the patient is taking the drug.
• Consider local hemostasis measures to prevent excessive bleeding.
• Psychologic and physical dependence may occur with chronic administration.
• Short appointments and a stress reduction protocol may be required for anxious patients.
• Monitor vital signs every appointment due to cardiovascular side effects.
• Avoid prescribing aspirin-containing products.

Consultations:

• If signs of anemia are observed in oral tissues, physician consult may be required.
• Medical consult may be required to assess disease control and patient's ability to tolerate stress.
• Medical consult should include partial prothrombin time, prothrombin time, or INR.

Teach patient/family:

• Importance of good oral hygiene to prevent soft tissue inflammation
• That secondary oral infection may occur; must see dentist immediately if infection occurs

---

stavudine (d4T)

(stav′yoo-deen)

Zerit

Drug class.: Antiviral, nucleoside analog

Action: A nucleoside analog that undergoes phosphorylation by cellular enzymes and inhibits HIV replication by termination of DNA elongation and inhibition of HIV reverse transcriptase

Uses: Treatment of advanced HIV infection when intolerant of other therapies or if significant deterioration occurs while receiving other therapies

Dosage and routes:

• *Adult:* PO 40 mg bid for patients >60 kg; 30 mg bid for patients <60 kg; dose interval 12 hr apart; doses must be adjusted to creatinine clearance and appearance of peripheral neuropathy
• *Child:* PO child <30 kg, 1 mg/kg/dose q 12 hr; child >30 kg receive adult dose

Available forms include: Caps 15, 20, 30, 40 mg; powder after reconstitution 1 mg/ml sol in 200 ml

Side effects/adverse reactions:

▼ *ORAL:* Ulcerative stomatitis, aphthous stomatitis

CNS: Headache, asthenia, malaise, anorexia, neuropathy, insomnia, anxiety, depression, nervousness

CV: Chest pain

*GI: Abdominal pain, diarrhea, nausea, vomiting, **pancreatitis, lactic acidosis, severe hepatomegaly with steatosis***

RESP: Dyspnea

*HEMA: **Neutropenia, thrombocytopenia,** lymphadenopathy*

GU: Dysuria

EENT: Conjunctivitis, abnormal vision
INTEG: Rash, pruritus
MS: Myalgia, arthralgia
MISC: Chills, fever, peripheral neurologic symptoms, sweating
Contraindications: Hypersensitivity
Precautions: Pregnancy category C, lactation, children, alcoholism, hepatic or renal impairment; monitor for peripheral neuropathy
Pharmacokinetics:
PO: Rapid absorption, peak plasma levels <1 hr; renal excretion
🦷 **Drug interactions of concern to dentistry:**
• None reported at this time
DENTAL CONSIDERATIONS
General:
• Examine for oral disease.
• Palliative treatment of oral ulcers may be required if they occur.
• Patients on chronic drug therapy may rarely have symptoms of blood dyscrasias, which can include infection, bleeding, and poor healing.
• Consider semisupine chair position for patient comfort due to GI effects of drug.
• Place on frequent recall due to oral side effects and immunocompromised condition.
Consultations:
• Refer to physician if signs of peripheral neuropathy occur.
• In a patient with symptoms of blood dyscrasias, request a medical consult for blood studies and postpone dental treatment until normal values are reestablished.
• Medical consult may be required to assess disease control.
Teach patient/family:
• Importance of good oral hygiene to prevent soft tissue inflammation

• To prevent injury when using oral hygiene aids
• To see dentist if secondary oral infection occurs
• To report oral lesions, soreness, or bleeding to dentist

sucralfate
(soo-kral′fate)
Carafate
♣ Apo-Sucralfate, Sulcrate
Drug class.: Protectant, aluminum salt of a sulfated sucrose

Action: Forms an ulcer-adherent complex that covers and protects the ulcer site
Uses: Duodenal ulcer
Dosage and routes:
• *Adult:* PO 1 g qid 1 hr ac, hs
Available forms include: Tabs 1 g; susp 1 g/10 ml in 420 ml
Side effects/adverse reactions:
▼ *ORAL:* Metallic taste, dry mouth
CNS: Drowsiness, dizziness
GI: Constipation, nausea, gastric pain, vomiting
INTEG: Urticaria, rash, pruritus
Contraindications: Hypersensitivity
Precautions: Pregnancy category B, lactation, children
Pharmacokinetics:
PO: Duration up to 5 hr
🦷 **Drug interactions of concern to dentistry:**
• Gastric irritation: chloral hydrate
• Decreased absorption of tetracyclines, fluoroquinolones
DENTAL CONSIDERATIONS
General:
• Prescribe acetaminophen for analgesia if needed. ASA and NSAIDs are contraindicated in active upper GI disease.

S

• Consider semisupine chair position for patient comfort due to GI effects of disease.
• Tetracycline doses should be given 2 hr before or after the sucralfate dose.

Teach patient/family:
• To avoid mouth rinses with high alcohol content due to drying effects

---

sulconazole nitrate

(sul-kon'a-zole)
Exelderm
Drug class.: Topical antifungal

Action: Interferes with fungal cell membrane, increasing permeability and leaking of nutrients

Uses: Treatment of tinea pedis, tinea corporis, tinea cruris, tinea versicolor; unapproved: cutaneous candidiasis

Dosage and routes:
• *Adult:* TOP apply once or twice daily × 3 wk, except tinea pedis use × 4 wk

Available forms include: Cream 1%; sol 1%

Side effects/adverse reactions:
INTEG: Stinging, burning, itching, redness

Contraindications: Hypersensitivity

Precautions: Pregnancy category C

DENTAL CONSIDERATIONS
General:
• There are no significant dental considerations. One possible concern will be those few patients with topical candidiasis, in whom broad-spectrum antiinfectives could potentially contribute to a superinfection.

---

sulfacetamide sodium (ophthalmic)

(sul-fa-see'ta-mide)
AK-Sulf, Bleph-10, Cetamide, Isopto Cetamide, Ocusulf-10, Sodium Sulamyd, Sulster
✤ Sulfex

Drug class.: Antibacterial sulfonamide

Action: Inhibits folic acid synthesis by preventing PABA use, which is necessary for bacterial growth

Uses: Conjunctivitis, superficial eye infections, corneal ulcers

Dosage and routes:
• *Adult and child:* Instill 1-2 gtt q2-3h; top apply 0.5-1 inch oint into conjunctival sac qid-tid and hs

Available forms include: Sterile ophth sol 1%, 10%, 15%, 30%; sterile ophth oint 10%

Side effects/adverse reactions:
EENT: Burning, stinging, swelling

Contraindications: Hypersensitivity

Precautions: Cross-sensitivity with other sulfas; pregnancy category C

🦷 **Drug interactions of concern to dentistry:**
• No specific interactions listed

DENTAL CONSIDERATIONS
General:
• Protect patient's eye from accidental spatter during dental treatment.

• Avoid dental light in patient's eyes; offer dark glasses for patient comfort.

sulfamethoxazole/ trimethoprim (SMZ/ TMP) (co-trimazole)

(sulf-a-meth-ox'a-zole)/(tri-meth'o-prim)

Bactrim, Cofatrim Forte, Cotrim, Septra (also all DS and pediatric brands)

♣ Apo-Sulfatrim,   Novo-Trimel, Nu-Cotrimox, Roubac

Drug class.: Sulfonamide and folic acid antagonist

Action: Sulfamethoxazole interferes with bacterial biosynthesis of proteins by competitive antagonism of PABA when adequate levels are maintained; trimethoprim blocks synthesis of tetrahydrofolic acid; this combination blocks two consecutive steps in bacterial synthesis of essential nucleic acids/ protein

Uses: UTIs, otitis media, acute and chronic prostatitis, shigellosis, *P. carinii* pneumonitis, chronic bronchitis, chancroid

Dosage and routes:

Urinary tract infections
• *Adult:* PO 160 mg TMP/800 mg SMZ q12h × 10-14 days
• *Child:* PO 8 mg/kg TMP/40 mg/kg SMZ qd in 2 divided doses q12h

Otitis media
• *Child:* PO 8 mg/kg TMP/40 mg/kg SMZ qd in 2 divided doses q12h × 10 days

Chronic bronchitis
• *Adult:* PO 160 mg TMP/800 mg SMZ q12h × 14 days

Pneumocystis carinii pneumonitis
• *Adult and child:* PO 20 mg/kg TMP/100 mg/kg SMZ qd in 4 divided doses q6h × 14 days; IV 15-20 mg/kg/day (based on TMP) in 3-4 divided doses for up to 14 days
Dosage reduction necessary in moderate-to-severe renal impairment (CrCl <30 ml/min)

Available forms include: Tabs 80 mg TMP/400 mg SMZ; DS (double strength): 160 mg TMP/ 800 mg SMZ; susp 40 mg/200 mg/5 ml; IV inj 16 mg TMP/80 mg SMZ/ml, 80 mg TMP/400 mg SMZ/5 ml

Side effects/adverse reactions:

▼ *ORAL:* Candidiasis, glossitis, stomatitis (Stevens-Johnson syndrome), salivary gland pain
CNS: Headache, insomnia, hallucinations, depression, vertigo, fatigue, anxiety, convulsions, drug fever, chills, aseptic meningitis
CV: Allergic myocarditis
*GI: Nausea, vomiting, abdominal pain, **hepatitis, enterocolitis,** pancreatitis, diarrhea, anorexia*
RESP: Cough, shortness of breath
*HEMA: **Leukopenia, neutropenia, thrombocytopenia, agranulocytosis, hemolytic anemia, hypoprothrombinemia, Henoch-Schönlein purpura, methemoglobinemia, eosinophilia***
*GU: **Renal failure, toxic nephrosis,** increased BUN, creatinine, crystalluria*
*INTEG: **Stevens-Johnson syndrome,** rash, dermatitis, urticaria, erythema, photosensitivity, pain, inflammation at injection site*

*SYST: **Anaphylaxis, SLE***

Contraindications: Hypersensitivity to trimethoprim or sulfonamides, pregnancy at term, megaloblastic anemia, infants <2 mo, CrCl <15 ml/min, lactation

Precautions: Pregnancy category C, renal disease, elderly, G6PD deficiency, impaired hepatic function, possible folate deficiency, severe allergy, bronchial asthma

Pharmacokinetics:

PO: Rapidly absorbed, peak 1-4 hr, half-life 8-13 hr; highly bound to plasma proteins; excreted in urine (metabolites and unchanged), breast milk; crosses placenta; TMP achieves high levels in prostatic tissue and fluid

⚖ Drug interactions of concern to dentistry:

• None identified

DENTAL CONSIDERATIONS

General:

• Determine why the patient is taking the drug.

• Patients on chronic drug therapy may rarely have symptoms of blood dyscrasias, which can include infection, bleeding, and poor healing.

• Ensure that dental therapy does not interfere with fluid intake.

Consultations:

• In a patient with symptoms of blood dyscrasias, request a medical consult for blood studies and postpone dental treatment until normal values are reestablished.

• Inform physician if antibiotics are required for dental infection.

Teach patient/family:

• Importance of good oral hygiene to prevent soft tissue inflammation

• Caution to prevent injury when using oral hygiene aids

sulfasalazine

(sul-fa-sal'a-zeen)

Asulfidine-En-Tabs, Azulfidine EN-tabs

♣ PMS-Sulfasalazine, Salazopyrin EN-Tab, SAS-500

Drug class.: Sulfonamide derivative with antiinflammatory action

Action: Acts as prodrug to deliver sulfapyridine and mesalamine (5-aminosalicylic acid) to the colon

Uses: Ulcerative colitis, Crohn's disease, rheumatoid arthritis, juvenile rheumatoid arthritis

Dosage and routes:

• *Adult:* PO 3-4 g/day in divided doses; maintenance 1.5-2 g/day in divided doses q6h

• *Child >2 yr:* PO 40-60 mg/kg/day in 4-6 divided doses, then 20-30 mg/kg/day in 4 doses; max 2 g/day

Available forms include: Tabs 500 mg; oral susp 250 mg/5 ml; del rel tabs 500 mg

Side effects/adverse reactions:

▼ *ORAL:* Stomatitis, glossitis, ulcers (Stevens-Johnson syndrome), bleeding, lichenoid reaction

*CNS: Headache, **convulsions,** confusion, insomnia, hallucinations, depression, vertigo, fatigue, anxiety, drug fever, chills*

*CV: **Allergic myocarditis***

*GI: Nausea, vomiting, abdominal pain, anorexia, **hepatitis,** pancreatitis, diarrhea*

*HEMA: **Leukopenia, neutropenia, thrombocytopenia, agranulocytosis, hemolytic anemia***

*GU: Reversible low sperm count, **renal failure, toxic nephrosis,** increased BUN, creatinine, crystalluria*

INTEG: ***Stevens-Johnson syndrome,*** rash, dermatitis, urticaria, erythema, photosensitivity
SYST: ***Anaphylaxis***

Contraindications: Hypersensitivity to sulfonamides or salicylates, pregnancy at term, child <2 yr, intestinal or urinary obstruction

Precautions: Pregnancy category B, lactation, impaired hepatic function, severe allergy, bronchial asthma, impaired renal function, intolerance to aspirin

Pharmacokinetics:
PO: Partially absorbed, peak 1.5-6 hr, half-life 5-10 hr; excreted in urine as sulfasalazine (15%), sulfapyridine (60%), 5-aminosalicylic acid, and metabolites (20%-33%); excreted in breast milk; crosses placenta

🦷 Drug interactions of concern to dentistry:
• Increased photosensitizing effects: tetracycline
• Decreased absorption: folic acid

DENTAL CONSIDERATIONS
General:
• Patients on chronic drug therapy may rarely have symptoms of blood dyscrasias, which can include infection, bleeding, and poor healing.
• Question patient about response to antibiotics to avoid responses that might provoke pseudomembranous colitis.
• Palliative medication may be required for management of oral side effects.
• Consider semisupine chair position for patient comfort due to GI effects of disease.

Consultations:
• Medical consult may be required to assess disease control and patient's ability to tolerate stress.
• In a patient with symptoms of blood dyscrasias, request a medical consult for blood studies and postpone dental treatment until normal values are reestablished.

Teach patient/family:
• Caution to prevent injury when using oral hygiene aids

---

sulfinpyrazone
(sul-fin-peer′a-zone)
Anturane
♣ Anturan, Apo-Sulfinpyrazone, Novopyrazone
Drug class.: Uricosuric

Action: Inhibits tubular reabsorption of urates and increases excretion of uric acid; inhibits prostaglandin synthesis, decreasing platelet aggregation

Uses: Chronic gouty arthritis

Dosage and routes:
Gout/gouty arthritis
• *Adult:* PO 100-200 mg bid for 1 wk, then 200-400 mg bid, not to exceed 800 mg/day

Available forms include: Tabs 100 mg; caps 200 mg

Side effects/adverse reactions:
▼ *ORAL:* Bleeding (rare)
CNS: ***Convulsions, coma,*** dizziness
GI: Gastric irritation, nausea, vomiting, anorexia, ***hepatic necrosis,*** GI bleeding
RESP: ***Apnea,*** irregular respirations
HEMA: ***Agranulocytosis*** (rare)
GU: Renal calculi, hypoglycemia
EENT: Tinnitus

S

INTEG: Rash, dermatitis, pruritus, fever, photosensitivity

Contraindications: Hypersensitivity to pyrazolone derivatives, severe hepatic disease, blood dyscrasias, severe renal disease, CrCl <50 mg/min, active peptic ulcer, GI inflammation, renal calculi

Precautions: Pregnancy category C, lactation

Pharmacokinetics:

PO: Peak 1-2 hr, duration 4-6 hr, half-life 3 hr; metabolized by liver, excreted in urine

Drug interactions of concern to dentistry:

• Increased bleeding: NSAIDs, aspirin

• Decreased effects of salicylates

DENTAL CONSIDERATIONS
General:

• Consider local hemostasis measures to prevent excessive bleeding.

• Avoid prescribing aspirin-containing products.

• Patients on chronic drug therapy may rarely have symptoms of blood dyscrasias, which can include infection, bleeding, and poor healing.

• Consider semisupine chair position for patient comfort if GI side effects occur.

• Evaluate respiration characteristics and rate.

Consultations:

• In a patient with symptoms of blood dyscrasias, request a medical consult for blood studies and postpone dental treatment until normal values are reestablished.

Teach patient/family:

• Caution to prevent injury when using oral hygiene aids

sulfisoxazole

(sul-fi-sox′a-zole)

♣ Apo-Sulfisoxazole, Novo-Soxazole, Sulfizole

Drug class.: Sulfonamide, short acting; antiinfective

Action: Interferes with bacterial biosynthesis of proteins by competitive antagonism of PABA

Uses: Urinary tract, systemic infections; chancroid; trachoma; toxoplasmosis; acute otitis media; lymphogranuloma venereum; eye infections

Dosage and routes:

• *Adult:* PO 2-4 g loading dose, then 1-2 g qid × 7-10 days

• *Child >2 mo:* PO 75 mg/kg or 2 g/m² loading dose, then 120-150 mg/kg/day or 4 g/m²/day in divided doses q6h, not to exceed 6 g/day

Available forms include: Tabs 500 mg; syr/pediatric susp 500 mg/5 ml

Side effects/adverse reactions:

▼ *ORAL:* Stomatitis, ulcers (Stevens-Johnson syndrome)

CNS: **Convulsions,** headache, insomnia, hallucinations, depression, vertigo, fatigue, anxiety, drug fever, chills, drowsiness

CV: **Allergic myocarditis**

GI: *Nausea, vomiting, abdominal pain,* **hepatitis, enterocolitis,** pancreatitis, diarrhea, anorexia

HEMA: **Leukopenia, thrombocytopenia, agranulocytosis, hemolytic anemia, aplastic anemia**

GU: **Renal failure, toxic nephrosis,** increased BUN, creatinine, crystalluria, hematuria, proteinuria

INTEG: **Stevens-Johnson syndrome,** rash, dermatitis, urticaria, erythema, photosensitivity, alopecia

*SYST: **Anaphylaxis***

Contraindications: Hypersensitivity to sulfonamides, sulfonylureas, thiazide, loop diuretics, salicylates, pregnancy at term

Precautions: Pregnancy category C, lactation, impaired hepatic function, severe allergy, bronchial asthma

Pharmacokinetics:

PO: Rapidly absorbed, peak 2-4 hr, half-life 4-7 hr; 85% protein bound; excreted in urine; crosses placenta

⚗ Drug interactions of concern to dentistry:

• Decreased effect: ester-type local anesthetics (procaine, tetracaine)
• Increased photosensitizing effect: tetracycline
• Decreased effect of penicillins, cephalosporins

DENTAL CONSIDERATIONS
General:

• Patients on chronic drug therapy may rarely have symptoms of blood dyscrasias, which can include infection, bleeding, and poor healing.
• Determine why the patient is taking the drug.
• Palliative medication may be required for management of oral side effects.
• Consider semisupine chair position for patient comfort if GI side effects occur.

Consultations:

• Medical consult may be required to assess disease control.
• In a patient with symptoms of blood dyscrasias, request a medical consult for blood studies and postpone dental treatment until normal values are reestablished.

Teach patient/family:

• Importance of good oral hygiene to prevent soft tissue inflammation

---

sulindac

(sul-in'dak)
Clinoril
♣ Apo-Sulin, Novo-Sundac
Drug class.: Nonsteroidal antiinflammatory

Action: Inhibits prostaglandin synthesis by interfering with cyclooxygenase, an enzyme needed for biosynthesis; possesses analgesic, antiinflammatory, antipyretic properties

Uses: Osteoarthritis, rheumatoid arthritis, acute gouty arthritis, tendinitis, bursitis, ankylosing spondylitis

Dosage and routes:
Arthritis

• *Adult:* PO 150 mg bid with food, may increase to 200 mg bid; max dose 400 mg day

Bursitis/acute arthritis

• *Adult:* PO 200 mg bid × 1-2 wk, then reduce dose

Available forms include: Tabs 150, 200 mg

Side effects/adverse reactions:

▼ *ORAL:* Dry mouth, gingival bleeding, mucosal ulceration and soreness, white spots in mouth or lips, aphthous stomatitis, bitter taste, glossitis, lichenoid reaction

CNS: Dizziness, drowsiness, fatigue, tremors, confusion, insomnia, anxiety, depression

CV: Tachycardia, peripheral edema, palpitations, dysrhythmias

*GI: **Cholestatic hepatitis,*** constipation, flatulence, cramps, peptic ulcer, nausea, anorexia, vomiting, diarrhea, jaundice

S

---

*HEMA: **Blood dyscrasias***
*GU: **Nephrotoxicity: dysuria, hematuria, oliguria, azotemia***
EENT: Tinnitus, hearing loss, blurred vision
INTEG: Purpura, rash, pruritus, sweating
Contraindications: Hypersensitivity, asthma (provoked by aspirin or NSAIDs), severe renal disease, severe hepatic disease, systemic lupus erythematosus
Precautions: Pregnancy category not established, lactation, children, bleeding disorders, GI disorders, cardiac disorders, hypersensitivity to other NSAIDs, geriatric patients
Pharmacokinetics:
PO: Peak 2 hr, half-life 3-3.5 hr; 93% protein binding; metabolized in liver; excreted in urine (metabolites), breast milk

⚡ Drug interactions of concern to dentistry:
• Increased bleeding, GI effects: alcohol, aspirin, steroids, other NSAIDs
• Renal toxicity: acetaminophen (prolonged use)
• Possible risk of decreased renal function: cyclosporine
• Increased photosensitizing effect: tetracycline
• Increased toxicity of methotrexate, cyclosporine
• Decreased plasma levels: diflunisal
DENTAL CONSIDERATIONS
General:
• Patients on chronic drug therapy may rarely have symptoms of blood dyscrasias, which can include infection, bleeding, and poor healing.

• Assess salivary flow as a factor in caries, periodontal disease, and candidiasis.
• Avoid prescribing in last trimester of pregnancy.
• Should oral inflammation or lesions occur, refer to physician and consider palliative treatment for the lesions.
• Consider semisupine chair position due to GI side effects, if present.
Consultations:
• Medical consult may be required to assess disease control.
• In a patient with symptoms of blood dyscrasias, request a medical consult for blood studies and postpone dental treatment until normal values are reestablished.
Teach patient/family:
• To report oral lesions, soreness, or bleeding to dentist
• Caution to prevent injury in use of oral hygiene aids
• Importance of good oral hygiene to prevent soft tissue inflammation
When chronic dry mouth occurs, advise patient:
• To avoid mouth rinses with high alcohol content due to drying effects
• Of need for daily use of home fluoride products to prevent caries
• To use sugarless gum, frequent sips of water, or saliva substitutes

---

sumatriptan succinate
(soo-ma-trip′tan)
Imitrex
Drug class.: Serotonin agonist

Action: Selective agonist for the vascular 5-HT (serotonin) receptor in cranial arteries, causing vasodilation with little or no effect on peripheral pressure

Uses: Migraine headaches; cluster headaches

Dosage and routes:

• *Adult:* SC 6 mg; max 2 injections/24 hr; side effects may limit dose

• *Adult:* PO 25-100 mg as a single dose; then, if required, 100 mg q2h, not to exceed 300 mg/day. If migraine returns after injection, 1 tab q2h, not to exceed 200 mg/day

• *Adult:* Intranasal 5, 10, or 20 mg as a single dose given in one nostril; dose may be repeated once after 2 hr with a daily limit of 40 mg

Available forms include: Tabs 25, 50, 100 mg; inj 12 mg/ml self-use syringes/vial; nasal spray 5 and 20 mg in 100-μl nasal spray device

Side effects/adverse reactions:

▼ *ORAL:* Discomfort in jaw/mouth/tongue

CNS: Dizziness, vertigo, drowsiness, sedation, headache, anxiety, fatigue

CV: Hypertension, hypotension, bradycardia, palpitation, dysrhythmias, coronary vasospasm

GI: Abdominal discomfort, dysphagia, diarrhea, reflux

RESP: Chest tightness, pressure in chest, dyspnea

GU: Dysuria

EENT: Discomfort in throat/sinuses/nasal cavity, photophobia

INTEG: Redness at injection site, sweating, rashes

MS: Weakness, neck pain, cramps, myalgia

MISC: Tingling, hot or burning sensation, numbness

Contraindications: IV use, is-

chemic heart disease, MI, uncontrolled hypertension and ergot-containing drugs

Precautions: Pregnancy category C, hepatic and renal impairment, elderly, lactation, children

Pharmacokinetics:

PO: Rapid onset, peak serum levels 5-20 min, terminal half-life 115 min

🦷 **Drug interactions of concern to dentistry:**

• None reported; avoid ergot-containing medications

DENTAL CONSIDERATIONS

General:

• Be aware of the patient's disease, its severity, and frequency, when known.

• Monitor vital signs every appointment due to cardiovascular side effects.

• Avoid dental light in patient's eyes; offer dark glasses for patient comfort.

Consultations:

• If treating chronic orofacial pain, consult with physician of record.

Teach patient/family:

• That oral symptoms uncommonly occur and will disappear when drug is discontinued

---

tacrine HCl

(tak'reen)
Cognex

Drug class.: Cholinesterase inhibitor

Action: A centrally acting, reversible inhibitor of cholinesterase enzyme

Uses: Treatment of mild-to-moderate cognitive defects associated with Alzheimer's disease

---

Dosage and routes:
• *Adult:* PO initially 10 mg qid × 4 wk min; after 4 wk titrate dose to 20 mg qid; higher doses up to 120-160 mg/day in 4 equal doses; monitored every 4 wk, all doses depend on transaminase levels and patient responses

Available forms include: Caps 10, 20, 30, 40 mg

Side effects/adverse reactions:
▼ *ORAL:* Glossitis, dry mouth, stomatitis, increased salivation (variable, low incidence)

CNS: Dizziness, confusion, ataxia, agitation, headache, paresthesia, nervousness, EPS, Bell's palsy (rare)

CV: Hypertension, peripheral edema, bradycardia, hypotension

GI: Increase in serum transaminase levels, nausea, vomiting, diarrhea, hepatotoxicity

RESP: Dyspnea, upper respiratory infection, coughing

HEMA: Leukopenia, thrombocytopenia, lymphadenopathy, anemia

GU: Urinary frequency or incontinence, infection

EENT: Rhinitis, sinusitis

INTEG: Rash, flushing of skin

MS: Arthralgia, muscle hypertonia

Contraindications: Hypersensitivity; previously treated patients with jaundice associated with elevated total bilirubin >3 mg/dl

Precautions: Pregnancy category C, cardiovascular disease, GI ulcers, general anesthesia, smokers, liver disease, seizures, asthma, lactation, children, decrease in absolute neutrophil count; liver enzyme monitoring required

Pharmacokinetics:
PO: Peak plasma levels 1-2 hr; plasma levels are higher in females; hepatic metabolism; renal excretion

⚜ Drug interactions of concern to dentistry:
• Potential increase in GI complaints: NSAIDs
• Action inhibited by anticholinergic drugs
• Increased effects with succinylcholine and other cholinergic agonists

DENTAL CONSIDERATIONS
General:
• Patients on chronic drug therapy may rarely have symptoms of blood dyscrasias, which can include infection, bleeding, and poor healing.
• Monitor vital signs every appointment due to cardiovascular and respiratory side effects.
• After supine positioning, have patient sit upright for at least 2 min before standing to avoid orthostatic hypotension.
• Assess salivary flow as a factor in caries, periodontal disease, and candidiasis.
• Take precautions if dental surgery is anticipated and anesthesia is required.
• Consider semisupine chair position for patient comfort due to GI effects of drug.
• Place on frequent recall because early attention to dental health is important for Alzheimer's patients.

Consultations:
• Medical consult may be required to assess disease control.
• In a patient with symptoms of blood dyscrasias, request a medical consult for blood studies and postpone dental treatment until normal values are reestablished.

italic = common side effects

Teach patient/family:
- Importance of good oral hygiene to prevent soft tissue inflammation
- To prevent injury when using oral hygiene aids
- Use of electric toothbrush if patient has difficulty holding conventional devices

When chronic dry mouth occurs, advise patient:
- To avoid mouth rinses with high alcohol content due to drying effects
- Of need for daily use of home fluoride products to prevent caries
- To use sugarless gum, frequent sips of water, or saliva substitutes

---

tacrolimus (FK506)
(ta-kroe′li-mus)
Prograf, Protopic
Drug class.: Immunosuppressant

Action: Inhibits T-lymphocyte activation, leading to immunosuppression

Uses: Prophylaxis of organ rejection in patients receiving allogeneic liver or kidney transplants; used in conjunction with steroids; moderate to severe eczema; unapproved uses: other transplant tissues, including bone marrow, pancreas, small bowel, also severe recalcitrant psoriasis

Dosage and routes:
- *Adult:* PO initial 0.15-0.30 mg/kg/day in 2 divided doses 12 hr apart no sooner than 6 hr after transplant and 8-12 hr after discontinuing IV infusion dose; IV (if patient cannot take PO) initial 0.05-0.10 mg/kg/day by infusion no sooner than 6 hr after graft
- *Pediatric:* 0.1 mg/kg/day IV and 0.3 mg/kg/day PO; show increased tolerance for doses at high end of adult schedules

Available forms include: Caps 0.5, 1, 5 mg; inj 5 mg/ml in 1-mg ampule

Side effects/adverse reactions:
▼ *ORAL:* Candidiasis
CNS: Tremors, headache, insomnia, paresthesia, anorexia, neurotoxicity, seizures
CV: Hyperkalemia, hypertension
GI: Diarrhea, nausea, vomiting, constipation
RESP: Pleural effusion, dyspnea
HEMA: Anemia, leukocytosis, thrombocytopenia, lymphoproliferative disorders, lymphoma
GU: **Nephrotoxicity,** hyperuricemia, oliguria, UTI
INTEG: Rash, pruritus
MISC: Anaphylaxis, *hyperglycemia*

Contraindications: Hypersensitivity, simultaneous use with cyclosporine, castor oil derivative allergy, potassium-sparing diuretics, lactation

Precautions: Pregnancy category C, renal impairment, hepatic impairment; discontinue cyclosporine doses 24 hr before using this drug

Pharmacokinetics:
PO: Peak levels 1.5-3.5 hr; highly bound to plasma proteins, erythrocytes; liver metabolism; urinary excretion of metabolites

🦷 **Drug interactions of concern to dentistry:**
- No confirmed studies to date: avoid drugs with potential for renal impairment
- Risk of increased blood levels with clotrimazole, fluconazole, ketoconazole, clarithromycin, erythromycin, and methylprednisolone
- Risk of decreased blood levels with carbamazepine, phenobarbital

---

DENTAL CONSIDERATIONS
General:
• Patients on immunosuppressant therapy have an increased susceptibility to infection.
• Patients on chronic drug therapy may rarely have symptoms of blood dyscrasias, which can include infection, bleeding, and poor healing.
• Monitor vital signs every appointment due to cardiovascular side effects.
• Prophylactic antibiotics may be indicated to prevent infection if surgery or deep scaling is planned.
• Examine for evidence of oral candidiasis. Topically acting antifungals may be preferred.

Consultations:
• Medical consult may be required to assess disease control.
• In a patient with symptoms of blood dyscrasias, request a medical consult for blood studies and postpone dental treatment until normal values are reestablished.
• Consult with patient's physician for recommendations for possible antibiotic prophylaxis before dental treatment or when considering the use of systemic antifungals.

Teach patient/family:
• Importance of good oral hygiene to prevent soft tissue inflammation
• Caution to prevent injury when using oral hygiene aids
• Use of electric toothbrush if patient has difficulty holding conventional devices
• That secondary oral infection may occur; must see dentist immediately if infection occurs
• To report oral lesions, soreness, or bleeding to dentist

tacrolimus (topical)
(ta-kroe'li-mus)
Protopic

Drug class.: Immunosuppressant (a macrolide derivative)

Action: Mechanism of action unknown; however it does inhibit T-lymphocyte activation and also inhibits transcription of genes associated with cytokine production

Uses: Short and intermittent long-term treatment of moderate-to-severe atopic dermatitis in patients who are not able to use or do not respond to alternative, conventional therapies

Dosage and routes:
• *Adult:* TOP apply thin layer of either strength to affected areas bid; rub in gently and completely. Continue applications for 1 wk after clearing of signs and symptoms
• *Child 2-5 yr:* TOP use 0.03% strength only; apply thin layer to affected area bid; rub in gently and completely. Continue applications for 1 wk after clearing of signs and symptoms

Available forms include: Oint 0.03%, 0.1% in 30, 60 g

Side effects/adverse reactions:
▼ *ORAL:* Taste alteration
CV: Headache
INTEG: Skin burning, pruritus, rash, folliculitis, acne, contact allergy, varicella zoster lesion
EENT: Sinusitis
MS: Myalgia
MISC: Flulike symptoms, fever, alcohol intolerance

Contraindications: Hypersensitivity, Netherton's Syndrome

Precautions: Infections at treatment site; lymphadenopathy, acute infections, mononucleosis, reduce exposure to sun or artificial sunlight, pregnancy category C, lactation, children <2 yr use has not been established

Pharmacokinetics:

TOP: Some systemic absorption; low systemic levels

Drug interactions of concern to dentistry:

• Although no drug interactions are documented, use with caution in patients taking CYP3A4 inhibitors: erythromycin, itraconazole, ketoconazole, fluconazole

DENTAL CONSIDERATIONS
General:

• Advise patient if dental drugs prescribed have a potential for photosensitivity.

---

tamoxifen citrate

(ta-mox′i-fen)
Nolvadex

♣ Apo-Tamoxifen, Gen-Tamoxifen, Novo-Tamoxifen, Tamofen, Tamone, Tamoplex

Drug class.: Antineoplastic, antiestrogen hormone

Action: Inhibits cell division by binding to cytoplasmic receptors (estrogen receptors); resembles normal cell complex but inhibits DNA synthesis

Uses: Advanced breast carcinoma that has not responded to other therapy in estrogen receptor-positive patients (usually postmenopausal), to reduce the incidence of breast cancer in healthy women with high risk of developing the disease; ductal carcinoma in situ

Dosage and routes:

• *Adult:* PO 10-20 mg bid or 20 mg daily

Available forms include: Tabs 10, 20 mg

Side effects/adverse reactions:

▼ *ORAL:* Altered taste

CNS: Hot flashes, headache, lightheadedness, depression

CV: Chest pain

GI: Nausea, vomiting

HEMA: Thrombocytopenia, leukopenia

GU: Vaginal bleeding, pruritus vulvae

EENT: Ocular lesions, retinopathy, corneal opacity, blurred vision (high doses)

INTEG: Rash, alopecia

META: Hypercalcemia

Contraindications: Hypersensitivity, pregnancy category D

Precautions: Leukopenia, thrombocytopenia, lactation, cataracts

Pharmacokinetics:

PO: Peak 4-7 hr, half-life 7 days (1 wk terminal); excreted primarily in feces

DENTAL CONSIDERATIONS
General:

• Patients on chronic drug therapy may rarely have symptoms of blood dyscrasias, which can include infection, bleeding, and poor healing.

• Consider semisupine chair position for patient comfort if GI side effects occur.

Consultations:

• Medical consult may be required to assess disease control.

• In a patient with symptoms of blood dyscrasias, request a medical consult for blood studies and postpone dental treatment until normal values are reestablished.

Teach patient/family:
• Importance of good oral hygiene to prevent soft tissue inflammation

---

tamsulosin HCl

(tam-soo'loe-sin)
Flomax

Drug class.: Adrenoreceptor antagonist

Action: Acts as an antagonist for α-adrenoreceptors in the prostate
Uses: Benign prostatic hyperplasia (BPH)
Dosage and routes:
• *Adult:* PO 0.4 mg given 30 min after the same meal each day; patients failing to respond after 2-4 wk can be increased to 0.8 mg daily
Available forms include: Tabs 0.4 mg
Side effects/adverse reactions:
▼ *ORAL:* Tooth disorder (not defined)
CNS: Dizziness, vertigo, headache, somnolence, insomnia
CV: Orthostatic hypotension
GI: Nausea, diarrhea
RESP: Cough, pharyngitis
GU: Decreased libido, abnormal ejaculation
EENT: Rhinitis, amblyopia
MS: Asthenia, back pain, chest pain
MISC: Infection
Contraindications: Hypersensitivity
Precautions: Potential syncope risk due to hypotension, vertigo, dizziness, carcinoma of prostate, avoid use with other α-adrenoreceptor antagonists, not for use in women, pregnancy category B, lactation, children (not for use)

Pharmacokinetics:
PO: Good oral absorption, maximum plasma levels 4.5 hr (fasting), highly bound to plasma proteins (94%-99%), extensive liver metabolism, renal excretion

💊 Drug interactions of concern to dentistry:
• No interactions reported with usual dental drugs. It is possible but not known that risk of orthostatic hypotension could be increased with conscious sedation techniques.
• Opioids and anticholinergic drugs may enhance urinary retention; use alternative analgesics (NSAIDs)
• Caution in use or avoid concurrent use with other adrenergic antagonists

DENTAL CONSIDERATIONS
General:
• Monitor vital signs every appointment due to cardiovascular and respiratory side effects.
• Consider semisupine chair position for patient comfort when GI side effects occur.
• After supine positioning, have patient sit upright for at least 2 min before standing to avoid orthostatic hypotension.

---

tazarotene topical

(taz-ar'oh-teen)
Tazorac

Drug class.: Topical retinoid

Action: Unclear; binds to retinoid receptors and inhibits mouse ornithine decarboxylase activity associated with cell proliferation and hyperplasia; also inhibits corneocyte accumulation in rhino mouse skin

Uses: Topical treatment in stable plaque psoriasis, mild to moderate facial acne vulgaris

Dosage and routes:

Psoriasis

• *Adult:* TOP apply a thin film once daily in evening to psoriatic lesions to no more than 20% of body surface area; skin should be clean and dry before applying; avoid application to unaffected skin

Acne vulgaris

• *Adult:* TOP apply a thin film once daily in evening to skin area where acne lesions appear; skin should be dry and clean (0.1% gel only)

Available forms include: Top gel 0.05, 0.1% in 30 g and 100 g sizes; top cream 0.05, 0.1%

Side effects/adverse reactions:

INTEG: Pruritus, burning, stinging, erythema, worsening of psoriasis, rash, dermatitis, fissuring, dry skin, bleeding, desquamations

Contraindications: Pregnancy, hypersensitivity, eczematous skin

Precautions: Pregnancy category X, use birth control measures in women of childbearing age, avoid contact with eyes, eyelids, mouth; exposure to tanning (sun, sun lamps) or drugs that cause photosensitivity, lactation, children <12 yr

Pharmacokinetics:

TOP: After application converted to active metabolite by esterase hydrolysis, metabolite highly plasma protein bound (99%); half-life 18 hr; renal and fecal excretion; systemic absorption less than 1%, 4.5% found in stratum corneum layers of epidermis

🦷 **Drug interactions of concern to dentistry:**

• Increased risk of photosensitivity: tetracyclines, fluoroquinolones, phenothiazines

• Caution in use with systemic vitamin A

DENTAL CONSIDERATIONS

General:

• Apply lubricant to dry lips for patient comfort before dental procedures.

• Advise patient if dental drugs are prescribed that have a potential for photosensitivity.

Teach patient/family:

• Should not be used if pregnant

• Avoid application to oral mucous membranes or lips

---

telmisartan

(tel-mi-sar'tan)

Micardis

Drug class.: Angiotensin II (AT$_1$) receptor antagonist

Action: Blocks the vasoconstrictor and aldosterone releasing effects of angiotensin II

Uses: Hypertension, as a single drug or in combination with other antihypertensives

Dosage and routes:

• *Adult:* PO initial dose 40 mg qd, daily dosage range 20-80 mg

Available forms include: Tabs 40, 80 mg

Side effects/adverse reactions:

CNS: Headache, dizziness, fatigue

CV: Peripheral edema

GI: Diarrhea, dyspepsia, abdominal pain, nausea

RESP: URI, coughing

GU: UTI

EENT: Sinusitis, pharyngitis

---

bold italic = life-threatening conditions

MS: Myalgia

MISC: Back pain

Contraindications: Hypersensitivity

Precautions: Discontinue if pregnancy occurs, risk of fetal and neonatal injury, correct volume depletion if present, hepatic impairment, impaired renal function; pregnancy category C (first trimester) and D (second, third trimesters), lactation

Pharmacokinetics:

PO: Peak levels 0.5-1 hr, bioavailability is dose dependent at 40 mg (42%), excreted in feces (97%), some hepatic metabolism, highly plasma protein bound

🦷 Drug interactions of concern to dentistry:

• None reported

DENTAL CONSIDERATIONS

General:

• Monitor vital signs every appointment due to cardiovascular side effects.

• Stress from dental procedures may compromise cardiovascular function; determine patient risk.

• Use precaution if sedation or general anesthesia is required; risk of hypotensive episode.

• Short appointments and a stress reduction protocol may be required for anxious patients.

• Limit use of sodium-containing products such as saline IV fluids for those patients with a dietary salt restriction.

Consultations:

• Medical consult may be required to assess disease control and patient's ability to tolerate stress.

temazepam

(te-maz′e-pam)

Restoril

Drug class.: Benzodiazepine, sedative-hypnotic

Controlled Substance Schedule IV, Canada F

Action: Produces CNS depression at limbic, thalamic, hypothalamic levels of the CNS; interacts with benzodiazepine receptors to facilitate action of the inhibitory neurotransmitter γ-aminobutyric acid (GABA)

Uses: Sedative and hypnotic for insomnia

Dosage and routes:

• *Adult:* PO 15-30 mg hs

Available forms include: Caps 7.5, 15, 30 mg

Side effects/adverse reactions:

CNS: Lethargy, drowsiness, daytime sedation, dizziness, confusion, light-headedness, headache, anxiety, irritability

CV: Chest pain, pulse changes

GI: Nausea, vomiting, diarrhea, heartburn, abdominal pain, constipation, anorexia

*HEMA: **Leukopenia, granulocytopenia** (rare)*

Contraindications: Hypersensitivity to benzodiazepines, pregnancy category X, lactation, intermittent porphyria

Precautions: Anemia, hepatic disease, renal disease, suicidal individuals, drug abuse, elderly, psychosis, child <18 yr, acute narrow-angle glaucoma

Pharmacokinetics:

PO: Onset 30-45 min, duration 6-8 hr, half-life 8-14 hr; metabolized by liver; excreted by kidneys; crosses placenta; excreted in breast milk

Drug interactions of concern to dentistry:
• Increased action of both drugs: alcohol, all CNS depressants

DENTAL CONSIDERATIONS
General:
• Psychologic and physical dependence may occur with chronic administration.
• Geriatric patients are more susceptible to drug effects; use lower dose.

Teach patient/family:
• Importance of good oral hygiene to prevent soft tissue inflammation

---

tenofovir disoproxil fumarate

(te-noe′fo-veer)
Viread
Drug class.: Antiviral

Action: Following metabolic conversion to tenofovir diphosphate, it inhibits the activity of HIV reverse transcriptase
Uses: HIV-1 infection, in combination with other antiretroviral drugs
Dosage and routes:
• *Adult:* PO 300 mg/day with a meal
Available forms include: Tabs 300 mg
Side effects/adverse reactions:
CNS: Headache
GI: Nausea, diarrhea, vomiting, flatulence, anorexia, abdominal pain
HEMA: Neutropenia
GU: Proteinuria
META: Elevation in creatine ki-

nase, serum amylase, AST, ALT, serum glucose
MISC: Asthenia
Contraindications: Hypersensitivity; avoid breast feeding
Precautions: Obesity and prolonged nucleoside use–risk of lactic acidosis/severe hepatomegaly with steatosis; no data on hepatic impairment; redistribution of body fat, pregnancy category B
Pharmacokinetics:
PO: Bioavailability 5% (improves with meal); max serum levels 0.6-1.4 hr; low plasma protein binding, less than 7%; minimal systemic metabolism; excreted by glomerular filtration and active tubular secretion; use in children not evaluated

Drug interactions of concern to dentistry:
• Potential for competition for renal clearance: acyclovir, valacyclovir

DENTAL CONSIDERATIONS
General:
• Examine for oral manifestation of opportunistic infection.
Consultations:
• Medical consult may be required to assess disease control and patient's ability to tolerate stress.
Teach patient/family:
• Importance of good oral hygiene to prevent soft tissue inflammation/ infection

---

terazosin HCl

(ter-ay′zoe-sin)
Hytrin
Drug class.: Antihypertensive, antiadrenergic

Action: Decreases total vascular

resistance, leading to a decrease in BP; this occurs by blockade of α_1-adrenoreceptor

Uses: Hypertension as a single agent or in combination with diuretics or β-blockers; benign prostatic hypertrophy

Dosage and routes:
• *Adult:* PO 1 mg hs; usual dose range 1-5 mg daily; may increase dose slowly to desired response; not to exceed 20 mg/day

Benign prostatic hypertrophy
• *Adult:* PO initial dose 1 mg hs; increase dose by increasing daily to achieve the desired response; 10 mg/day may be required

Available forms include: Tabs 1, 2, 5, 10 mg

Side effects/adverse reactions:
▼ *ORAL:* Dry mouth
CNS: Dizziness, headache, drowsiness, anxiety, depression, vertigo, weakness, fatigue
CV: Orthostatic hypotension, palpitation, tachycardia, edema, rebound hypertension
GI: Nausea, vomiting, diarrhea, constipation, abdominal pain
RESP: Dyspnea, pharyngitis, rhinitis
GU: Urinary urgency, incontinence, impotence
EENT: Epistaxis, tinnitus, red sclera, nasal congestion, sinusitis

Contraindications: Hypersensitivity

Precautions: Pregnancy category C, children, lactation

Pharmacokinetics:
PO: Peak 1 hr, half-life 9-12 hr; highly bound to plasma proteins; metabolized in liver; excreted in urine, feces

🦷 Drug interactions of concern to dentistry:
• Decreased effects: NSAIDs, indomethacin

DENTAL CONSIDERATIONS
General:
• Monitor vital signs every appointment due to cardiovascular side effects.
• After supine positioning, have patient sit upright for at least 2 min before standing to avoid orthostatic hypotension.
• Assess salivary flow as a factor in caries, periodontal disease, and candidiasis.
• Limit use of sodium-containing products, such as saline IV fluids, for patients with a dietary salt restriction.
• Consider semisupine chair position for patient comfort if GI side effects occur.

Teach patient/family: *When chronic dry mouth occurs, advise patient:*
• To avoid mouth rinses with high alcohol content due to drying effects
• Of need for daily use of home fluoride products to prevent caries
• To use sugarless gum, frequent sips of water, or saliva substitutes

---

terbinafine HCl
(ter-bin'a-feen)
Lamisil

Drug class.: Antifungal, systemic

Action: Inhibits key enzyme, squalene epoxidase, involved with sterol synthesis with resultant fungal cell death
Uses: Treatment of onychomycosis

---

of the toenail or fingernail caused by dermatophytes (tinea unguium)

Dosage and routes:

Fingernail onychomycosis

• *Adult:* PO 250 mg qd × 6 wk

Toenail onychomycosis

• *Adult:* PO 250 mg qd × 12 wk

Available forms include: Tabs 250 mg

Side effects/adverse reactions:

▼ *ORAL: Taste disturbances*

GI: Diarrhea, dyspepsia, abdominal pain, nausea, flatulence, cholestatic hepatitis (rare)

HEMA: Severe neutropenia (rare), transient decrease in absolute lymphocyte counts

INTEG: Rash, urticaria, pruritus

META: Abnormal liver tests

MS: Arthralgia, myalgia

MISC: Malaise, fatigue

Contraindications: Hypersensitivity

Precautions: Preexisting liver or renal disease, pregnancy category B, use not recommended during nursing, pediatric patients

Pharmacokinetics:

PO: Bioavailability 40%, peak plasma levels approximately 2 hr; highly plasma protein bound (99%), extensive metabolism, excreted in urine (70%)

👥 **Drug interactions of concern to dentistry:**

• None reported

DENTAL CONSIDERATIONS

General:

• Determine why patient is taking the drug.

• Consider semisupine chair position for patient comfort if GI side effects occur.

• Patients on chronic drug therapy may rarely have symptoms of blood dyscrasias, which can include infection, bleeding, and poor healing.

Consultations:

• In a patient with symptoms of blood dyscrasias, request a medical consult for blood studies and postpone treatment until normal values are reestablished.

Teach patient/family:

• Importance of good oral hygiene to prevent soft tissue inflammation

• To prevent trauma when using oral hygiene aids

---

terbinafine HCl (topical)

(ter-bin'a-feen)

Lamisil, Lamisil DermaGel

Drug class.: Antifungal

Action: Inhibits squalene epoxidase, key enzyme, involved with sterol synthesis, resulting in fungal cell death

Uses: Tinea pedis, tinea cruris, tinea corporis; unapproved: cutaneous candidiasis, tinea versicolor

Dosage and routes:

• *Adult:* TOP apply to affected area bid until symptoms show significant improvement, usually 7-14 days; duration usually 7 days, but should not exceed 4 wk

Available forms include: Cream 1% in 15-, 30-g containers, gel 1% in 5, 15, 30 g

Side effects/adverse reactions:

INTEG: Irritation, burning, drying, itching

Contraindications: Hypersensitivity

Precautions: Pregnancy category B, lactation, children <12 yr

---

Drug interactions of concern to dentistry:
• None reported

---

terbutaline sulfate

(ter-byoo'ta-leen)

Brethaire, Brethine, Bricanyl

Drug class.: Selective β_2-agonist

Action: Relaxes bronchial smooth muscle by direct action on β_2-adrenergic receptors

Uses: Bronchospasm, asthma prophylaxis

Dosage and routes:

Bronchospasm

• *Adult and child >6 yr:* Inh 2 puffs qmin, then q4-6h; PO 2.5-5 mg q8h; SC 0.25 mg q8h

Available forms include: Tabs 2.5, 5 mg; aerosol 0.2 mg/actuation; inj 1 mg/ml in 2-ml ampules

Side effects/adverse reactions:

▼ *ORAL:* Dry mouth, unusual taste

CNS: Tremors, anxiety, insomnia, headache, dizziness, stimulation

CV: Palpitation, tachycardia, hypertension, *cardiac arrest*

GI: Nausea, vomiting

Contraindications: Hypersensitivity to sympathomimetics, narrow-angle glaucoma, tachydysrhythmias

Precautions: Pregnancy category B, cardiac disorders, hyperthyroidism, diabetes mellitus, prostatic hypertrophy, lactation, elderly, hypertension, glaucoma

Pharmacokinetics:

PO: Onset 0.5 hr, duration 4-8 hr

SC: Onset 6-15 min, duration 1.5 hr

INH: Onset 5-30 min, duration 3-6 hr

Drug interactions of concern to dentistry:
• Increased CNS side effects: other sympathomimetics
• Risk of dysrhythmias with halogenated-hydrocarbon anesthetics
• Increased vascular side effects: tricyclic antidepressants

DENTAL CONSIDERATIONS

General:

• Consider semisupine chair position for patients with respiratory disease.

• Monitor vital signs every appointment due to cardiovascular side effects.

• Assess salivary flow as a factor in caries, periodontal disease, and candidiasis.

• Be aware that aspirin or sulfite preservatives in vasoconstrictor-containing products can exacerbate asthma.

• Acute asthmatic episodes may be precipitated in the dental office. Sympathomimetic inhalants should be available for emergency use.

• Midday appointments and a stress reduction protocol may be required for anxious patients.

Teach patient/family:

• For inhalation dosage forms: to rinse mouth with water after each dose to help prevent dryness

• Use of electric toothbrush if patient has difficulty holding conventional devices

When chronic dry mouth occurs, advise patient:

• To avoid mouth rinses with high alcohol content due to drying effects

• Of need for daily use of home fluoride products to prevent caries

• To use sugarless gum, frequent sips of water, or saliva substitutes

terconazole
(ter-kone'a-zole)
Terazol 3, Terazol 7
Drug class.: Local antifungal

Action: Interferes with fungal DNA replication; binds sterols in fungal cell membranes, increasing permeability, leaking of nutrients
Uses: Vaginal, vulval, vulvovaginal candidiasis (moniliasis)
Dosage and routes:
• *Adult:* Vag 5 g (1 applicator full) hs × 7 days (0.4%); vag 5 g (1 applicator full) hs × 3 days (0.8%); supp 1 hs × 3 days
Available forms include: Vag cream 0.4%, 0.8%; vag supp 80 mg
Side effects/adverse reactions:
GU: Vulvovaginal burning, itching, pelvic cramps
INTEG: Rash, urticaria, stinging, burning
MISC: Headache, body pain
Contraindications: Hypersensitivity
Precautions: Children <2 yr, pregnancy, lactation
DENTAL CONSIDERATIONS
General:
• Be aware that broad-spectrum antibiotics can exacerbate vaginal candidiasis.

testosterone/ testosterone cypionate/ testosterone enanthate/testosterone propionate
(tess-toss'ter-one)
Testosterone Pellets: Testopel
Testosterone cypionate (IM use only, Canadian):
♣ Depo-Testosterone
Testosterone enanthate (IM use only): Delasteryl
♣ Delatestryl, Malogex
Testosterone transdermal: Androderm, Testoderm, Testoderm TTS
Testosterone gel: AndroGel
Drug class.: Androgen, anabolic steroid

Controlled Substance Schedule III
Action: In many tissues testosterone is converted to dihydrotestosterone, which interacts with cytoplasmic protein receptors to increase protein production; natural hormone that functions to regulate spermatogenesis and male secondary sex characteristics; also functions as an anabolic steroid
Uses: Treatment of androgen deficiency, delayed puberty, female breast cancer, certain anemias, gender changes, hypogonadism, cryptorchidism
Dosage and routes:
Replacement therapy
• *Adult (male):* IM 50-400 mg q2-4wk (cypionate or enanthate)
• *Adult (male):* Scrotal patch 1 patch (4 or 6 mg) q22-24h
Hypogonadotropic hypogonadism
• *Adult (gel):* TOP apply one (5-g packet) ~50 mg testosterone to

T

clean dry skin of shoulders or upper arms or abdomen (not to genitals) in AM; PELLETS dose varies from 150-400 mg q3-6 mo

Breast cancer
• *Adult (female):* IM 200-400 mg q2-4 wk (cypionate or enanthate)

Delayed puberty
• *Child (male):* IM l00 mg (max) per mo up to 4-6 mo (all forms)

Available forms include: Enanthate inj IM 200 mg/ml; cypionate inj IM 100, 200 mg/ml; scrotal patch 2.5, 4, 6 mg; gel 1%, pellets 75 mg

Side effects/adverse reactions:
CNS: Dizziness, headache, fatigue, tremors, paresthesias, flushing, sweating, anxiety, lability, insomnia

*CV: **Edema** (in cardiac patients),* increased BP

*GI: **Hepatic necrosis** (rare), **cholestatic jaundice,** nausea,* vomiting, constipation, weight gain

HEMA: Increased prothrombin time, iron deficiency anemia

GU: Amenorrhea, gynecomastia (males), hematuria, priapism, vaginitis, decreased libido, decreased breast size, clitoral hypertrophy, testicular atrophy

EENT: Conjunctival edema, nasal congestion

INTEG: Rash, acneiform lesions, oily hair/skin, flushing, sweating, acne vulgaris, alopecia, hirsutism

ENDO: Abnormal GTT

MS: Cramps, spasms, hypercalcification in breast

Contraindications: Severe renal disease, severe cardiac disease, severe hepatic disease, hypersensitivity, pregnancy category X, lactation, genital bleeding (abnormal), prostate or breast carcinoma (males), breast cancer in females with hypercalcemia

Precautions: Diabetes mellitus, CV disease, MI, increased risk of prostatic hypertrophy, prostatic carcinoma, virilization (women), increased prothrombin time

Pharmacokinetics:
IM: Highly protein bound, metabolized in liver, half-life 10-20 min; excreted in urine, breast milk; crosses placenta

PATCH: Absorption from scrotal skin much higher than other skin sites, half-life 10-100 min, peak levels 2-4 hr

🦷 Drug interactions of concern to dentistry:
• Increased risk of bleeding: aspirin
• Edema: ACTH, adrenal steroids

DENTAL CONSIDERATIONS
General:
• Avoid prescribing aspirin-containing products.
• Determine why the patient is taking the drug.
• Consider local hemostasis measures to prevent excessive bleeding.
• Short appointments and a stress reduction protocol may be required for anxious patients.
• Prophylactic antibiotics may be indicated to prevent infection if surgery or deep scaling is planned.
• Physician consult may be required if signs of anemia are observed in oral tissues.

Consultations:
• Medical consult may be required to assess disease control and patient's ability to tolerate stress.
• Medical consult should include partial prothrombin or prothrombin times.

italic = common side effects

Teach patient/family:
• Importance of good oral hygiene to prevent soft tissue inflammation
• Alert the patient to the possibility of secondary oral infection and the need to see dentist immediately if infection occurs

---

tetracaine/tetracaine HCl (topical)

(tet′ra-cane)

Pontocaine, Pontocaine Cream, Viractin

Drug class.: Topical anesthetic (ester group)

Action: Inhibits nerve impulses from sensory nerves, producing anesthesia

Uses: Local anesthesia of mucous membranes, pruritus, sunburn, sore throat, cold sores, oral pain, rectal pain and irritation, control of gagging

Dosage and routes:
• *Adult:* TOP apply to affected area using smallest effective amount at point of needle insertion

Available forms include: Oint 1%; cream 2%; gel 2%; sol 2%

Side effects/adverse reactions:
INTEG: Rash, irritation, sensitization, dermatitis

MISC: Hypersensitivity reactions (systemic), angioedema

More severe systemic reactions can be observed if excessive absorption leads to toxic doses

Contraindications: Hypersensitivity, infants <1 yr, application to large areas, PABA allergies

Precautions: Child <12 yr, sepsis, pregnancy category C, lactation, local infection, geriatric, debilitated patient

Pharmacokinetics:
TOP: Onset 3-10 min, duration up to 60 min; metabolized in plasma when absorbed; excreted in urine

🦷 **Drug interactions of concern to dentistry:**
• Specific drug interactions are not listed; it would be wise to use with caution in patients taking tocainide, mexiletine; significant systemic absorption could lead to synergistic and potentially toxic effects

DENTAL CONSIDERATIONS

General:
• Apply smallest effective dose; apply to small area because significant absorption can occur, especially from denuded areas.
• Absorption of excessive amounts of drug may lead to signs of local anesthetic toxicity; with correct use, toxicity is a rare event.
• Use for topical anesthesia or temporary relief of symptoms; reevaluate if symptoms persist.
• Toxic amounts can be absorbed from denuded mucosa or skin.
• Apply with cotton-tipped applicator by pressing, not rubbing, paste on lesion.

Teach patient/family:
• How to apply
• Not to chew gum or eat while numbness is present after dental treatment

Symptoms of systemic toxicity could include:
• Nervousness, nausea, excitement followed by drowsiness, convulsions, cardiac and respiratory depression
• Symptoms may vary because they depend on the amount of drug actually absorbed

---

tetracycline/tetracycline HCl

(tet-ra-sye'kleen)

Helidac Therapy, Panmycin, Sumycin, Tetracap, Tetracyn, Tetralan Syrup

♣ Apo-Tetra, Novotetra, Nu-Tetra

Drug class.: Tetracycline, broad-spectrum antibiotic

Action: Inhibits protein synthesis and phosphorylation in microorganisms; bacteriostatic

Uses: Syphilis, *C. trachomatis,* gonorrhea, lymphogranuloma venereum, *M. pneumoniae,* rickettsial infections, acne, actinomycosis, anthrax, bronchitis, GU infections, sinusitis, and many other infections produced by susceptible organisms; *H. pylori*–associated duodenal ulcer

Dosage and routes:

• *Adult:* PO 250-500 mg q6h 1 hr before or 2 hr after meals; IM 250 mg/day or 150 mg q12h; IV 250-500 mg q8-12h

• *Child >8 yr:* PO 25-50 mg/kg/day in divided doses q6h 1 hr before or 2 hr after meals; IM 15-25 mg/kg/day in divided doses q8-12h; IV 10-20 mg/kg/day in divided doses q12h

Gonorrhea

• *Adult:* PO 1.5 g, then 500 mg qid for a total of 9 g over 7 days

Chlamydia trachomatis

• *Adult:* PO 500 mg qid × 7 days

Syphilis

• *Adult:* PO 2-3 g in divided doses × 10-15 days; must treat 30 days if syphilis duration >1 yr

Urethral syndrome in women

• *Adult:* PO 500 mg qid × 7 days

Acne

• *Adult:* 1 g/day in divided doses; maintenance 125-500 mg/day

Available forms include: Oral susp 125 mg/5 ml; caps 100, 250, 500 mg; tabs 250, 500 mg

Side effects/adverse reactions:

▼ *ORAL: Tooth discoloration in children <8 yr, candidiasis, tongue discoloration and hypertrophy of papilla,* enamel hypoplasia, bleeding (long-term use), stomatitis, lichenoid drug reaction, erythema multiforme

CNS: Fever, headache, paresthesia

CV: Pericarditis

GI: Nausea, abdominal pain, vomiting, diarrhea, anorexia, *hepatotoxicity,* enterocolitis, flatulence, abdominal cramps, epigastric burning

HEMA: Eosinophilia, neutropenia, thrombocytopenia, leukocytosis, hemolytic anemia

GU: Increased BUN

EENT: Dysphagia

INTEG: Rash, urticaria, photosensitivity, increased pigmentation, exfoliative dermatitis, angioedema, pruritus

Contraindications: Hypersensitivity to tetracyclines, children <8 yr, pregnancy category D, lactation

Precautions: Renal disease, hepatic disease

Pharmacokinetics:

PO: Peak 2-3 hr, duration 6 hr, half-life 6-10 hr; 20%-60% protein bound; excreted in urine; crosses placenta; excreted in breast milk

🦷 **Drug interactions of concern to dentistry:**

• Decreased absorption: $NaHCO_3$, other antacids

• Decreased effect of penicillins, cephalosporins
• Possible increase in serum levels of methotrexate
• Oral contraceptives: advise patient of a potential risk for decreased contraceptive action, to maintain compliance with oral contraceptive use while using antibiotics, and to consider the use of additional nonhormonal contraception

DENTAL CONSIDERATIONS

General:
• Determine why the patient is taking tetracycline.
• Broad-spectrum antibiotics may be a factor in oral or vaginal *Candida* infections.
• Advise patient if dental drugs prescribed have a potential for photosensitivity.

Consultations:
• Medical consult may be required to assess disease control.

Teach patient/family:
• Importance of good oral hygiene to prevent soft tissue inflammation
• Caution to prevent injury when using oral hygiene aids
• To avoid milk products; to take with a full glass of water
• To take tetracycline doses 1 hr before or 2 hr after air polishing device (Prophy Jet), if used
When used for dental infection, advise patient:
• To report sore throat, oral burning sensation, fever, fatigue, any of which could indicate superinfection
• To take at prescribed intervals and complete dosage regimen
• To immediately notify the dentist if signs or symptoms of infection increase

tetracycline periodontal fiber
(tet-ra-sye′kleen)

Actisite

Drug class.: Tetracycline, broad-spectrum antiinfective

Action: Antimicrobial effect related to inhibition of protein synthesis; decreases incidence of post-surgical inflammation and edema; suppresses bacteria and acts as a barrier to bacterial entry; acts on cementum or fibroblasts to enhance periodontal ligament regeneration

Uses: Adjunctive treatment in adult periodontitis

Dosage and routes:
• *Fiber:* Adjust length to fit pocket depth and contour of teeth treated; fiber should contact base of pocket; apply cyanoacrylate adhesive to secure fiber for 10 days; replace if lost before 7 days; up to 11 teeth can be treated

Available forms include: Fiber supplied in boxes of 4 and 10 fibers, each 23 cm long and each with 12.7 mg tetracycline

Side effects/adverse reactions:
▼ *ORAL: Gingival inflammation and pain, glossitis,* local erythema, candidiasis, staining of tongue
EENT: Minor throat irritation
INTEG: Photosensitivity

Contraindications: Hypersensitivity, children <8 yr, acutely abscessed periodontal pocket

Precautions: Pregnancy category C, lactation, children, superinfection, patients with predisposition to candidiasis; must remove fibers after 10 days

T

---

bold italic = life-threatening conditions

Pharmacokinetics:

TOP: In vitro release rate 2 μg/cm/hr; gingival concentration maintained over 10 days; plasma levels below detectable limits

🦷 Drug interactions of concern to dentistry:

• It is not known if the tetracycline fiber will decrease the effectiveness of oral contraceptives; however, manufacturer recommends suggesting the use of an alternative form of contraception during the remaining cycle to female patients taking oral contraceptives

DENTAL CONSIDERATIONS
General:

• Take precautions regarding allergy to tetracyclines.

• Examine oral mucosa for candidiasis before placing fiber.

Teach patient/family:

• Do not chew hard, crusty, or sticky foods

• Do not brush or floss near treated area, but clean other teeth

• Avoid other oral hygienic practices that could dislodge fibers, such as the use of toothpicks

• Do not probe or pick at the treated area

• Notify dentist if fiber dislodges or falls out

• Notify dentist if pain, swelling, or other symptoms occur

---

theophylline

(thee-off′i-lin)

Accubron, Aquaphyllin, Asmalix, Broncodyl, Elixomin, Elixophyllin, Lanophyllin, Quibron-T, Respbid, Slo-Bid, Slo-Phyllin, Sustaire, Theo-24, Theobid, Theochron, Theoclear, Theolair, Theo-Sav, Theospan-SR, Theostat, Theovent, Theo-X, T-Phyl, Uni-Dur, Uniphyl

♣ Apo-Theo-LA, PMS-Theophylline

Drug class.: Xanthine

Action: Relaxes smooth muscle of respiratory system by blocking phosphodiesterase, thus increasing cAMP

Uses: Bronchial asthma, bronchospasm of COPD, chronic bronchitis; unapproved: apnea in the neonate

Dosage and routes:
Bronchospasm, bronchial asthma
• *Adult:* PO 100-200 mg q6h, dosage must be individualized
• *Child:* PO 50-100 mg q6h, not to exceed 12 mg/kg/24 hr

Available forms include: Caps 50, 100, 200, 250 mg; tabs 100, 125, 200, 225, 250, 300 mg; time rel tabs 100, 200, 250, 300, 400, 500, 600 mg; time rel caps 50, 65, 100, 125 mg; elix 80 mg/15 ml; sol 80 mg/15 ml; syr 150 mg/15 ml, 80 mg/15 ml

Side effects/adverse reactions:

▼ *ORAL:* Bitter taste, dry mouth
CNS: Anxiety, restlessness, insomnia, dizziness, convulsions, headache, light-headedness, muscle twitching
CV: Palpitation, sinus tachycardia, hypotension, other dysrhythmias

---

GI: Nausea, vomiting, anorexia, diarrhea, dyspepsia, gastric distress
RESP: Increased rate
INTEG: Flushing, urticaria
Contraindications: Hypersensitivity to xanthines, tachydysrhythmias
Precautions: Elderly, CHF, cor pulmonale, hepatic disease, active peptic ulcer disease, diabetes mellitus, hyperthyroidism, hypertension, children, pregnancy category C
Pharmacokinetics:
PO: Peak 1 hr; metabolized in liver; excreted in urine, breast milk; crosses placenta

🦷 **Drug interactions of concern to dentistry:**
• Increased action: erythromycin, ciprofloxacin
• Increased risk of cardiac dysrhythmia: halothane inhalation anesthesia, CNS stimulants
• Decreased effect: barbiturates, carbamazepine, ketoconazole
• May decrease sedative effects of benzodiazepines

DENTAL CONSIDERATIONS
General:
• Consider semisupine chair position for patients with respiratory disease.
• Monitor vital signs every appointment due to cardiovascular side effects.
• Assess salivary flow as a factor in caries, periodontal disease, and candidiasis.
• Be aware that aspirin or sulfite preservatives in vasoconstrictor-containing products can exacerbate asthma.
• Acute asthmatic episodes may be precipitated in the dental office. Sympathomimetic inhalants should be available for emergency use.

• Midday appointments and a stress reduction protocol may be required for anxious patients.
Consultations:
• Medical consult may be required to assess disease control.
Teach patient/family: *When chronic dry mouth occurs, advise patient:*
• To avoid mouth rinses with high alcohol content due to drying effects
• Of need for daily use of home fluoride products to prevent caries
• To use sugarless gum, frequent sips of water, or saliva substitutes

---

thiamine HCl (vitamin B$_1$)

(thye'a-min)
Thiamilate
🍁 Betaxin

Drug class.: Vitamin B$_1$, water soluble

Action: Needed for carbohydrate metabolism
Uses: Vitamin B$_1$ deficiency or prophylaxis, beriberi, Wernicke-Korsakoff syndrome
Dosage and routes:
Recommended dietary allowance (RDA)
• *Adult:* PO men 1.2-1.5 mg; women 1.0-1.1 mg; pregnant women 1.5 mg; lactating women 1.6 mg
• *Child:* PO 1-3 yr, 0.7 mg; 4-6 yr, 0.9 mg; 7-10 yr, 1 mg
Beriberi
• *Adult (critical):* IM or slow IV 5-100 mg tid; use injection only when necessary
• *Adult:* PO 5-10 mg tid with multivitamin, then RDA (dose recommendations are highly variable)

---

bold italic = life-threatening conditions

• *Infant (mild):* PO 10 mg qd
Alcohol-induced deficiency:
• *Adult:* PO 40 mg qd
Available forms include: Tabs 50, 100, 250 mg; enteric-coated tabs 20 mg; inj IM/IV 100 mg/ml
Side effects/adverse reactions:
Note: Parenteral doses are more likely to cause severe adverse reactions

▼ *ORAL: Angioedema*
CNS: Weakness, restlessness
CV: Collapse, pulmonary edema, hypotension
GI: Nausea, diarrhea, hemorrhage
EENT: Tightness of throat
INTEG: Cyanosis, sweating, warmth
SYST: Anaphylaxis (after parenteral doses)
Contraindications: None known
Precautions: Pregnancy category A, sensitivity to thiamine, Wernicke's encephalopathy
Pharmacokinetics:
PO/INJ: Unused amounts excreted in urine (unchanged)
DENTAL CONSIDERATIONS
General:
• Determine why the patient is taking this vitamin.
Teach patient/family:
• Food sources to be included in diet: yeast, whole grain, beef, liver, legumes

---

thiethylperazine maleate

(thye-eth-il-per'a-zeen)
Torecan
Drug class.: Phenothiazine-type, antiemetic

Action: Acts centrally by blocking chemoreceptor trigger zone, which in turn acts on vomiting center

Uses: Nausea, vomiting
Dosage and routes:
• *Adult:* PO/IM/rec 10 mg qd-tid
Available forms include: Tabs 10 mg; supp 10 mg; inj 5 mg/ml
Side effects/adverse reactions:

▼ *ORAL:* Dry mouth, metallic taste
CNS: Euphoria, depression, convulsions, restlessness, tremor, EPS, drowsiness
CV: Circulatory failure, tachycardia, postural hypotension, ECG changes
GI: Nausea, vomiting, anorexia, diarrhea, constipation, weight loss, cramps
RESP: Respiratory depression
GU: Urinary retention, dark urine
Contraindications: Hypersensitivity to phenothiazines, coma, seizure, encephalopathy, bone marrow depression
Precautions: Children <2 yr, pregnancy category C, elderly
Pharmacokinetics:
PO: Onset 45-60 min
REC: Onset 45-60 min
Metabolized by liver; excreted by kidneys; crosses placenta; excreted in breast milk
🦷 **Drug interactions of concern to dentistry:**
• Increased anticholinergic action: anticholinergics
• Increased CNS depression, hypotension: alcohol, CNS depressants
DENTAL CONSIDERATIONS
General:
• Defer elective dental treatment when symptoms are present.
Consultations:
• Medical consult may be required to assess disease control.

---

thioridazine HCl

(thye-oh-rid'a-zeen)

Mellaril

✤ Apo-Thioridazine,   Novo-Ridazine

Drug class.: Phenothiazine antipsychotic

Action: Blocks neurotransmission at dopaminergic synapses in the cerebral cortex, hypothalamus, and limbic system; exhibits strong peripheral α-adrenergic, anticholinergic blocking action; mechanism for antipsychotic effects is unclear

Uses: Psychotic disorders, schizophrenia, behavioral problems in children, alcohol withdrawal as adjunct, anxiety, major depressive disorders, organic brain syndrome

Dosage and routes:

Psychosis

• *Adult:* PO 25-100 mg tid; max dose 800 mg/day; dose is gradually increased to desired response, then reduced to minimum maintenance

Depression/behavioral problems/organic brain syndrome

• *Adult:* PO 25 tid; range from 10 mg bid-qid to 50 mg tid-qid

• *Child 2-12 yr:* PO 0.5-3 mg/kg/day in divided doses

Available forms include: Tabs 10, 15, 25, 50, 100, 150, 200, 300 mg; conc 30, 100 mg/ml; susp 25, 100 mg/5 ml

Side effects/adverse reactions:

▼ *ORAL: Dry mouth,* movements of lips and tongue (tardive dyskinesia), erythema multiforme, lichenoid reaction

*CNS: Extrapyramidal symptoms: pseudoparkinsonism, akathisia, dystonia, tardive dyskinesia, **seizures, headache,** confusion*

CV: Orthostatic hypotension, ***cardiac arrest,*** ECG changes, ***tachycardia***

GI: Nausea, vomiting, anorexia, constipation, diarrhea, jaundice, weight gain

*RESP: **Laryngospasm,** dyspnea, **respiratory depression***

HEMA: Anemia, ***leukopenia, leukocytosis, agranulocytosis***

GU: Urinary retention, enuresis, impotence, amenorrhea, gynecomastia

EENT: Blurred vision, glaucoma, dry eyes

INTEG: Rash, photosensitivity, dermatitis

Contraindications: Hypersensitivity, blood dyscrasias, coma, child <2 yr, brain damage, bone marrow depression

Precautions: Pregnancy category C, lactation, seizure disorders, hypertension, hepatic disease, cardiac disease

Pharmacokinetics:

PO: Onset erratic, peak 2-4 hr, half-life 26-36 hr; metabolized by liver; excreted in urine; crosses placenta; excreted in breast milk

🦷 **Drug interactions of concern to dentistry:**

• Increased sedation: other CNS depressants, alcohol, barbiturate anesthetics, opioid analgesics

• Hypotension, tachycardia: epinephrine (systemic)

• Increased extrapyramidal effects: phenothiazines and related drugs (haloperidol, droperidol), metoclopramide

• Additive photosensitization: tetracyclines

• Increased anticholinergic effects: anticholinergics

---

bold italic = life-threatening conditions

DENTAL CONSIDERATIONS
General:

• Monitor vital signs every appointment due to cardiovascular side effects.

• Patients on chronic drug therapy may rarely have symptoms of blood dyscrasias, which can include infection, bleeding, and poor healing.

• After supine positioning, have patient sit upright for at least 2 min before standing to avoid orthostatic hypotension.

• Assess salivary flow as a factor in caries, periodontal disease, and candidiasis.

• Avoid dental light in patient's eyes; offer dark glasses for patient comfort.

• Assess for presence of extrapyramidal motor symptoms, such as tardive dyskinesia and akathisia. Extrapyramidal motor activity may complicate dental treatment.

• Geriatric patients are more susceptible to drug effects; use lower dose.

• Use vasoconstrictors with caution, in low doses, and with careful aspiration.

Consultations:

• In a patient with symptoms of blood dyscrasias, request a medical consult for blood studies and postpone dental treatment until normal values are reestablished.

• Take precautions if dental surgery is anticipated and anesthesia is required.

• Refer to physician if signs of tardive dyskinesia or akathisia are present.

• Physician should be informed if significant xerostomic side effects occur (increased caries, sore tongue, problems eating or swallowing, difficulty wearing prosthesis) so a medication change can be considered.

Teach patient/family:

• Importance of good oral hygiene to prevent soft tissue inflammation

• Caution to prevent injury when using oral hygiene aids

• To use electric toothbrush if patient has difficulty holding conventional devices

When chronic dry mouth occurs, advise patient:

• To avoid mouth rinses with high alcohol content due to drying effects

• Of need for daily use of home fluoride products to prevent caries

• To use sugarless gum, frequent sips of water, or saliva substitutes

---

thiothixene
(thye-oh-thix'een)
Navane

Drug class.: Thioxanthene/antipsychotic

Action: Depresses cerebral cortex, hypothalamus, limbic system, which control activity, aggression; blocks neurotransmission produced by dopamine at the synapse; exhibits strong peripheral α-adrenergic blocking action; mechanism for antipsychotic effects is unclear

Uses: Psychotic disorders, schizophrenia, acute agitation

Dosage and routes:

• *Adult:* PO 2-5 mg bid-qid depending on severity of condition; dose is gradually increased to 15-30 mg/day if needed

Available forms include: Caps 1, 2, 5, 10, 20 mg; conc 5 mg/ml

---

Side effects/adverse reactions:

▼ *ORAL: Dry mouth,* uncontrolled tongue and lip movements

CNS: Extrapyramidal symptoms: pseudoparkinsonism, akathisia, dystonia, tardive dyskinesia, headache, seizures

CV: Orthostatic hypotension, **cardiac arrest, tachycardia,** hypertension, ECG changes

GI: Nausea, vomiting, anorexia, constipation, diarrhea, jaundice, weight gain

RESP: **Laryngospasm, respiratory depression,** dyspnea

HEMA: **Leukopenia, leukocytosis, agranulocytosis,** anemia

GU: Urinary retention, enuresis, impotence, amenorrhea, gynecomastia

EENT: Blurred vision, glaucoma

INTEG: Rash, photosensitivity, dermatitis

Contraindications: Hypersensitivity, blood dyscrasias, child <12 yr, bone marrow depression, circulatory collapse, CNS depression, coma, alcoholism, CV disease, hepatic disease, Reye's syndrome, narrow-angle glaucoma

Precautions: Pregnancy category C, lactation, seizure disorders, hypertension, hepatic disease

Pharmacokinetics:

PO: Onset slow, peak 2-8 hr, duration up to 12 hr

IM: Onset 15-30 min, peak 1-6 hr, duration up to 12 hr

Half-life 34 hr; metabolized by liver; excreted in urine; crosses placenta; excreted in breast milk

🥄 **Drug interactions of concern to dentistry:**

• Increased sedation: other CNS depressants, alcohol, barbiturate anesthetics, opioid analgesics

• Hypotension, tachycardia: epinephrine (systemic)

• Increased extrapyramidal effects: phenothiazines and related drugs (haloperidol, droperidol), metoclopramide

• Additive photosensitization: tetracyclines

• Increased anticholinergic effects: anticholinergics

DENTAL CONSIDERATIONS

General:

• Monitor vital signs every appointment due to cardiovascular side effects.

• Patients on chronic drug therapy may rarely have symptoms of blood dyscrasias, which can include infection, bleeding, and poor healing.

• After supine positioning, have patient sit upright for at least 2 min before standing to avoid orthostatic hypotension.

• Assess salivary flow as a factor in caries, periodontal disease, and candidiasis.

• Assess for presence of extrapyramidal motor symptoms, such as tardive dyskinesia and akathisia. Extrapyramidal motor activity may complicate dental treatment.

• Use vasoconstrictors with caution, in low doses, and with careful aspiration.

• Avoid dental light in patient's eyes; offer dark glasses for patient comfort.

• Geriatric patients are more susceptible to drug effects; use lower dose.

Consultations:

• In a patient with symptoms of blood dyscrasias, request a medical consult for blood studies and postpone dental treatment until normal values are reestablished.

---

bold italic = life-threatening conditions

• Take precautions if dental surgery is anticipated and anesthesia is required.
• If signs of tardive dyskinesia or akathisia are present, refer to physician.

Teach patient/family:
• Importance of good oral hygiene to prevent soft tissue inflammation
• Caution to prevent injury when using oral hygiene aids
• To use electric toothbrush if patient has difficulty holding conventional devices

When chronic dry mouth occurs, advise patient:
• To avoid mouth rinses with high alcohol content due to drying effects
• Of need for daily use of home fluoride products to prevent caries
• To use sugarless gum, frequent sips of water, or saliva substitutes

---

thyroid USP (desiccated)
(thye′roid)
Armour Thyroid, S-P-T, Thyrar Thyroid Strong
♣ Cholaxin

Drug class.: Thyroid hormone

Action: Increases metabolic rates; increases cardiac output, O_2 consumption, body temperature, blood volume, growth/development at cellular level
Uses: Hypothyroidism, cretinism, myxedema
Dosage and routes:
Hypothyroidism
• *Adult:* PO 65 mg qd, increased by 65 mg q30d until desired response; maintenance dose 65-195 mg qd
• *Geriatric:* PO 7.5-15 mg qd,

double dose q6-8wk until desired response
Creatinism/juvenile hypothyroidism
• *Child >1 yr:* PO up to 180 mg qd titrated to response
• *Child 4-12 mo:* PO 3-60 mg qd
• *Child 1-4 mo:* PO 15-30 mg qd, may increase q2wk, titrated to response; maintenance dose 30-45 mg qd
Myxedema
• *Adult:* PO 16 mg qd, double dose q2wk; maintenance 65-195 mg/day
Available forms include: Tabs 15, 30, 60, 90, 120, 180, 240, 300 mg; thyroid strong (each 60 mg = 90 mg USP) tabs 30, 60, 120, 180 mg; S-PT (pork thyroid in soybean oil) caps 120, 180, 300 mg
Side effects/adverse reactions:
CNS: Insomnia, tremors, headache, thyroid storm
CV: **Cardiac arrest,** tachycardia, palpitation, angina, dysrhythmias, hypertension
GI: Nausea, diarrhea, increased or decreased appetite, cramps
MISC: Menstrual irregularities, weight loss, sweating, heat intolerance, fever
Contraindications: Adrenal insufficiency, MI, thyrotoxicosis
Precautions: Elderly, angina pectoris, hypertension, ischemia, cardiac disease, pregnancy category A, lactation
Pharmacokinetics:
PO: Peak 12-48 hr, half-life 6-7 days
⚖ Drug interactions of concern to dentistry:
• Increased effects of sympathomimetics in those patients when thyroid doses are not carefully monitored or with coronary artery disease

---

italic = common side effects

DENTAL CONSIDERATIONS
General:
• Increased nervousness, excitability, sweating, or tachycardia may indicate uncontrolled hyperthyroidism or a dose of medication that is too high. Uncontrolled patients should be referred for medical treatment.

Consultations:
• Medical consult may be required to assess disease control.

---

tiagabine HCl
(tye-ag'a-been)
Gabitril
Drug class.: Anticonvulsant

Action: Antiseizure mechanism unknown; acts as an antagonist for γ-aminobutyric acid (GABA) uptake and may enhance the activity of GABA

Uses: Adjunctive therapy for partial seizures

Dosage and routes:
• *Adult and child >18 yr:* PO initial dose 4 mg; increase dose by 4-8 mg increments at weekly intervals until response or up to 32 mg/day
• *Child 12-18 yr:* PO initial dose 4 mg/day; after 1 wk can increase dose 2-8 mg/day; thereafter can be increased by 4-8 mg at weekly intervals up to total dose of 32 mg/day

Available forms include: Tabs 4, 12, 16, 20 mg

Side effects/adverse reactions:
▼ *ORAL:* Dry mouth (1%), gingivitis, stomatitis, gingival hyperplasia (uncommon)
CNS: Sedation, dizziness, headache, memory impairment, emotional state, nervousness, tremor, depression, confusion

CV: Hypertension, palpitation, tachycardia, edema
GI: Abdominal pain, nausea, diarrhea, vomiting, constipation, dyspepsia
RESP: Cough, bronchitis, dyspnea
HEMA: Lymphadenopathy
GU: UTI
EENT: Pharyngitis, amblyopia, ear pain
INTEG: Pruritus, rash, dry skin
MS: Asthenia, myalgia
MISC: Flulike syndrome, pain

Contraindications: Hypersensitivity

Precautions: Hepatic disease, Alzheimer's disease, dementia, organic brain disease, stroke

Pharmacokinetics:
PO: Rapid absorption, peak plasma levels 0.5-1 hr; highly plasma protein bound (95%), hepatic metabolism, some enterohepatic circulation

🥄 **Drug interactions of concern to dentistry:**
• Increased tiagabine clearance: carbamazepine, phenobarbital
• Use CNS depressants with caution because possible additional effects may occur

DENTAL CONSIDERATIONS
General:
• Monitor vital signs every appointment due to cardiovascular and respiratory side effects.
• Consider semisupine chair position for patient comfort when GI side effects occur.
• Short appointments and a stress reduction protocol may be required for anxious patients.
• Determine type of epilepsy, seizure frequency, and quality of seizure control.
• Assess salivary flow as factor in

---

caries, periodontal disease, and candidiasis.

• Place on frequent recall if oral side effects occur.

Consultations:

• Consultation with physician may be needed if sedation or general anesthesia is required.

Teach patient/family:

• Caution to prevent trauma when using oral hygiene aids

• Use of electric toothbrush if patient has difficulty holding conventional devices

• Importance of good oral hygiene to prevent soft tissue inflammation

• Importance of updating health and drug history if physician makes any changes in evaluation or drug regimens

• To be aware of oral side effects and potential sequelae

When chronic dry mouth occurs, advise patient:

• To avoid mouth rinses with high alcohol content due to drying effects

• To use daily home fluoride products for anticaries effect

• To use sugarless gum, frequent sips of water, or saliva substitutes

---

ticlopidine

(tye-chloe′pi-deen)

Ticlid

Drug class.: Platelet aggregation inhibitor

Action: Inhibits first and second phases of ADP-induced effects in platelet aggregation

Uses: Reducing the risk of stroke in high-risk patients

Dosage and routes:

• *Adult:* PO 250 mg bid with food

Available forms include: Tabs 250 mg

Side effects/adverse reactions:

*GI: **Cholestatic jaundice, hepatitis,*** increased cholesterol, LDL, VLDL, nausea, vomiting, diarrhea, GI discomfort

*HEMA: **Bleeding (epistaxis, hematuria, conjunctival hemorrhage, GI bleeding), agranulocytosis, neutropenia, thrombocytopenia, erythroleukemia, thrombotic thrombocytopenic purpura***

INTEG: Rash, pruritus

Contraindications: Hypersensitivity, active liver disease, blood dyscrasias

Precautions: Past liver disease, renal disease, elderly, pregnancy category B, lactation, children; increased bleeding risk requires hematologic monitoring every 2 wk for the first 3 mo of therapy

Pharmacokinetics: Peak 1-3 hr, half-life increases with repeated dosing; metabolized by the liver; excreted in urine, feces

Drug interactions of concern to dentistry:

• Increased bleeding tendencies: aspirin, NSAIDs

DENTAL CONSIDERATIONS

General:

• Patients on chronic drug therapy may rarely have symptoms of blood dyscrasias, which can include infection, bleeding, and poor healing.

• Consider local hemostatic measures to prevent excessive bleeding.

Consultations:

• Medical consult may be required to assess disease control and pa-

---

tient's ability to tolerate stress. Consult should include data on hematologic profile.

Teach patient/family:
• Caution to prevent injury when using oral hygiene aids

---

tiludronate disodium

(tye-loo′droe-nate)
Skelid

Drug class.: Biphosphonate derivative

Action: Acts to inhibit bone resorption by a mechanism that involves inhibition of osteoclastic activity

Uses: Paget's disease of bone in patients with twice normal upper limit values for serum alkaline phosphatase (SAP) and who are symptomatic and at risk for future complications

Dosage and routes:
• *Adult:* PO 400 mg/day taken with 6-8 oz of plain water only for 3 mo; do not take with other beverages; do not eat for 2 hr after dosing

Available forms include: Tabs 240 mg (equivalent to 200 mg tiludronic acid)

Side effects/adverse reactions:
▼ *ORAL:* Tooth disorder (not specified), dry mouth (<1%)
CNS: Headache, dizziness, paresthesia, nervousness, anxiety
CV: Peripheral edema, hypertension
GI: Nausea, diarrhea, dyspepsia, vomiting
RESP: URI, cough, pharyngitis
EENT: Rhinitis, sinusitis, cataract, conjunctivitis, glaucoma
INTEG: Rash, pruritus
ENDO: Hyperparathyroidism

META: Vitamin D deficiency
MS: Back pain, chest pain, arthralgia
MISC: Flulike symptoms

Contraindications: Hypersensitivity, severe renal failure

Precautions: Pregnancy category C, lactation, safety in children <18 yr not established

Pharmacokinetics:
PO: Rapid but incomplete absorption, bioavailability 6% (fasted), peak plasma levels 2 hr, little or no metabolism, excreted in urine

Drug interactions of concern to dentistry:
• Bioavailability decreased by calcium, food, aluminum or magnesium antacids
• Do not take indomethacin, aspirin, or calcium supplements 2 hr before or after tilundronate

DENTAL CONSIDERATIONS
General:
• Be aware of oral manifestations of Paget's disease (macrognathia, alveolar pain).
• Consider semisupine chair position for patient comfort when GI side effects occur.
• Consider short appointments for patient comfort.
• Assess salivary flow as a factor in caries, periodontal disease, and candidiasis.

Consultations:
• Medical consult may be required to assess disease control.

Teach patient/family:
• Caution to prevent trauma when using oral hygiene aids
• Importance of good oral hygiene to prevent soft tissue inflammation
• Importance of updating health and drug history if physician

---

makes any changes in evaluation or drug regimens

When chronic dry mouth occurs, advise patient:
• To avoid mouth rinses with high alcohol content due to drying effects
• To use daily home fluoride products for anticaries effect
• To use sugarless gum, frequent sips of water, or saliva substitutes

---

timolol maleate

(tye'moe-lole)
Blocadren
♣ Apo-Timol, Novo-Timol
Drug class.: Nonselective β-adrenergic blocker

Action: This is a nonselective β₁- and β₂-adrenergic antagonist. The antihypertensive mechanism of action is unclear, but it may include a reduction in cardiac output and inhibition of renin release by the renal juxtaglomerular apparatus. Peripheral resistance decreases with long-term use. The antianginal action (when indicated for this use) may be related to a decrease in myocardial oxygen demand and negative chronotropic and inotropic effects. The antiarrhythmic action (when indicated for this use) has been related to a reduction in spontaneous pacemaker firing and slowing of AV nodal conduction.

Uses: Mild-to-moderate hypertension, reduction of mortality risk after MI, migraine prophylaxis; unapproved: essential tremors, angina, cardiac dysrhythmias, anxiety

Dosage and routes:

Hypertension
• *Adult:* PO 10 mg bid, may increase by 10 mg q2-3d, not to exceed 60 mg/day

Myocardial infarction
• *Adult:* 10 mg bid

Available forms include: Tabs 5, 10, 20 mg

Side effects/adverse reactions:

▼ *ORAL:* Dry mouth
CNS: Insomnia, dizziness, hallucinations, anxiety
*CV: **CHF,** hypotension, bradycardia, edema, chest pain, claudication*
*GI: Nausea, vomiting, abdominal pain, **mesenteric arterial thrombosis, ischemic colitis,** diarrhea*
*RESP: **Bronchospasm, dyspnea,** cough, rales*
*HEMA: **Agranulocytosis, thrombocytopenia***
GU: Impotence, frequency
EENT: Visual changes, double vision, sore throat, dry/burning eyes
INTEG: Rash, alopecia, pruritus, fever
META: Hypoglycemia
MISC: Joint pain, muscle pain

Contraindications: Hypersensitivity to β-blockers, cardiogenic shock, second- or third-degree heart block, sinus bradycardia, CHF, cardiac failure

Precautions: Major surgery, pregnancy category C, lactation, diabetes mellitus, renal disease, thyroid disease, COPD, well-compensated heart failure, CAD, nonallergic bronchospasm

Pharmacokinetics:
PO: Peak 2-4 hr, half-life 3-4 hr; excreted 30%-45% unchanged; 60%-65% is metabolized by liver; excreted in breast milk

⚡ Drug interactions of concern to dentistry:
• Increased hypotension, bradycar-

dia: anticholinergics, sympathomimetics (epinephrine)
• Decreased antihypertensive effects: indomethacin and other NSAIDs
• Suspected increase in plasma levels: diphenhydramine
• May slow metabolism of lidocaine

DENTAL CONSIDERATIONS
General:
• Monitor vital signs every appointment due to cardiovascular side effects.
• Patients on chronic drug therapy may rarely have symptoms of blood dyscrasias, which can include infection, bleeding, and poor healing.
• Assess salivary flow as a factor in caries, periodontal disease, and candidiasis.
• Limit use of sodium-containing products, such as saline IV fluids, for patients with a dietary salt restriction.
• After supine positioning, have patient sit upright for at least 2 min before standing to avoid orthostatic hypotension.
• Stress from dental procedures may compromise cardiovascular function; determine patient risk.
• Short appointments and a stress reduction protocol may be required for anxious patients.
• Consider semisupine chair position for patients with nausea or respiratory distress.

Consultations:
• In a patient with symptoms of blood dyscrasias, request a medical consult for blood studies and postpone dental treatment until normal values are reestablished.
• Medical consult may be required to assess disease control and patient's ability to tolerate stress.

Teach patient/family:
• Importance of good oral hygiene to prevent soft tissue inflammation
• Caution to prevent injury when using oral hygiene aids
When chronic dry mouth occurs, advise patient:
• To avoid mouth rinses with high alcohol content due to drying effects
• Of need for daily use of home fluoride products to prevent caries
• To use sugarless gum, frequent sips of water, or saliva substitutes

---

timolol maleate (optic)
(tye'moe-lole)
Betimol, Timodal, Timoptic Solution, Timoptic-XE
♣ Apo-Timop, Gen-Timolol, Novo-Timolol, Nu-Timol
Drug class.: β-adrenergic blocker

Action: Reduces production of aqueous humor by unknown mechanism
Uses: Ocular hypertension, chronic open-angle glaucoma, secondary glaucoma, aphakic glaucoma
Dosage and routes:
• *Adult:* Instill 1 gtt of 0.25% sol in affected eye(s) bid, then 1 gtt for maintenance; may increase to 1 gtt of 0.5% sol bid if needed
Available forms include: Sol 0.25%, 0.5%, in 2.5, 5, 10, 15 ml; also unit dose container (Ocudose); gel forming sol 0.25%, 0.5% in 2.5, 5 ml
Side effects/adverse reactions:
CNS: Weakness, fatigue, depression, anxiety, headache, confusion
CV: Bradycardia, hypotension, dysrhythmias

---

bold italic = life-threatening conditions   *For periodic updates, visit* **www.mosby.com**

GI: Nausea
RESP: **Bronchospasm**
EENT: Eye irritation, conjunctivitis, keratitis
INTEG: Rash, urticaria

Contraindications: Hypersensitivity, asthma, second- or third-degree heart block, right ventricular failure, congenital glaucoma (infants), COPD

Precautions: May be absorbed systemically, can mask hypoglycemia in patients with diabetes, pregnancy category C, lactation, children

Pharmacokinetics:
INSTILL: Onset 15-30 min, peak 1-2 hr, duration 24 hr

Drug interactions of concern to dentistry:
• Avoid use of anticholinergic drugs, atropine-like drugs, propantheline, and diazepam (benzodiazepines)

DENTAL CONSIDERATIONS
General:
• Check compliance of patient with prescribed drug regimen for glaucoma.
• Avoid dental light in patient's eyes; offer dark glasses for patient comfort.

Consultations:
• Consultation with physician may be needed if sedation or anesthesia is required.

---

tizanidine HCl
(tye-zan'i-deen)
Zanaflex

Drug class.: Centrally acting α_2-adrenergic agonist

Action: Acts as an agonist at α_2-adrenoreceptor sites; believed to reduce spasticity by increasing presynaptic inhibition on motor neurons

Uses: Treatment of acute and intermittent management of increased muscle tone due to spasticity (multiple sclerosis, spinal cord injury)

Dosage and routes:
• *Adult:* PO initial 4 mg at 6-8 hr intervals; increase dose by 2-4 mg steps to satisfactory reduction of muscle tone; daily dose limit 36 mg

Available forms include: Tabs 4 mg

Side effects/adverse reactions:
▼ *ORAL: Dry mouth (3-10%)*
CNS: Light-headedness, dizziness, sedation, hallucination, drowsiness, psychosis, nervousness
CV: Hypotension, bradycardia, orthostatic hypotension, syncope
GI: Abdominal pain, diarrhea, dyspepsia, constipation
GU: UTI, candidiasis
EENT: Blurred vision, rhinitis, pharyngitis, ear pain
INTEG: Skin rash
META: Liver injury, liver enzymes elevated
MS: Asthenia, increased spasm, myasthenia

Contraindications: Hypersensitivity

Precautions: Long-term use, concurrent hypotensive drugs, renal impairment, oral contraceptives, pregnancy category C, lactation, elderly, children

Pharmacokinetics:
PO: Half-life 2.5 hr, peak levels 1.5 hr, first-pass metabolism, extensively metabolized, 30% plasma protein bound, excreted in urine and feces

---

🦷 Drug interactions of concern to dentistry:
- Additive CNS side effects: ethanol and other CNS depressants
- Orthostatic hypotension: drugs that lower blood pressure

DENTAL CONSIDERATIONS
General:
- Monitor vital signs every appointment due to cardiovascular side effects.
- Short appointments may be required due to effects of disease on musculature.
- Use precaution if sedation or general anesthesia is required; risk of hypotensive episode.
- Assess salivary flow as factor in caries, periodontal disease, and candidiasis.
- After supine positioning, have patient sit upright for at least 2 min before standing to avoid orthostatic hypotension.

Consultations:
- Medical consult may be required to assess disease control and patient's ability to tolerate stress.

Teach patient/family:
- Not to drive or perform other tasks requiring alertness
- Use of electric toothbrush if patient has difficulty holding conventional devices

When chronic dry mouth occurs, advise patient:
- To avoid mouth rinses with high alcohol content due to drying effects
- To use daily home fluoride products for anticaries effect
- To use sugarless gum, frequent sips of water, or saliva substitutes

tobramycin (ophthalmic)

(toe-bra-mye'sin)
Defy, Tobrex
🍁 AK-Tob

Drug class.: Antiinfective

Action: Inhibits bacterial protein synthesis
Uses: Infection of eye
Dosage and routes:
- *Adult and child:* Instill 1-2 gtt q1-4h depending on infection; oint 1 cm bid-tid
Available forms include: Oint 0.3%; sol 0.3%

Side effects/adverse reactions:
EENT: Poor corneal wound healing, visual haze (temporary), overgrowth of nonsusceptible organisms

Contraindications: Hypersensitivity

Precautions: Antibiotic hypersensitivity, pregnancy category D

DENTAL CONSIDERATIONS
General:
- Avoid directing dental light into patient's eyes; provide dark glasses during treatment to avoid irritation.
- Protect patient's eyes from accidental spatter during dental treatment.

tocainide HCl

(toe-kay'nide)
Tonocard

Drug class.: Antidysrhythmic (Class IB), lidocaine analog

Action: Decreases sodium and potassium conductance, decreasing myocardial excitability

---

bold italic = life-threatening conditions   *For periodic updates, visit* **www.mosby.com**

Uses: Documented life-threatening ventricular dysrhythmias

Dosage and routes:
• *Adult:* PO 400 mg q8h; range 1200-1800 mg/day

Available forms include: Tabs 400, 600 mg

Side effects/adverse reactions:

▼ *ORAL:* Dry mouth, oral ulcerations, erythema multiforme (rare)

CNS: Headache, dizziness, seizures, involuntary movement, confusion, psychosis, restlessness, irritability, paresthesia, tremors

CV: Hypotension, bradycardia, heart block, cardiovascular collapse, arrest, CHF, chest pain, angina, PVCs, tachycardia

GI: Nausea, vomiting, anorexia, diarrhea, hepatitis

RESP: Respiratory depression, pulmonary fibrosis, dyspnea

HEMA: Blood dyscrasias: leukopenia, agranulocytosis, hypoplastic anemia, thrombocytopenia

EENT: Tinnitus, blurred vision, hearing loss

INTEG: Rash, urticaria, edema, swelling

Contraindications: Hypersensitivity to amides, severe heart block

Precautions: Pregnancy category C, lactation, children, renal disease, liver disease, CHF, respiratory depression, myasthenia gravis, blood dyscrasias

Pharmacokinetics:

PO: Peak 0.5-3 hr; half-life 10-17 hr; metabolized by liver; excreted in urine

Drug interactions of concern to dentistry:
• No specific interactions are reported with dental drugs; however, any drug that could affect the cardiac action of tocainide (local anesthetics, vasoconstrictors, and anticholinergics) should be used in the least effective dose

DENTAL CONSIDERATIONS

General:
• Monitor vital signs every appointment due to cardiovascular and respiratory side effects.
• After supine positioning, have patient sit upright for at least 2 min before standing to avoid orthostatic hypotension.
• Patients on chronic drug therapy may rarely have symptoms of blood dyscrasias, which can include infection, bleeding, and poor healing.
• Assess salivary flow as a factor in caries, periodontal disease, and candidiasis.
• Stress from dental procedures may compromise cardiovascular function; determine patient risk.

Consultations:
• In a patient with symptoms of blood dyscrasias, request a medical consult for blood studies and postpone dental treatment until normal values are reestablished.
• Medical consult may be required to assess disease control and patient's ability to tolerate stress.

Teach patient/family:
• Importance of good oral hygiene to prevent soft tissue inflammation
• Caution to prevent injury when using oral hygiene aids

When chronic dry mouth occurs, advise patient:
• To avoid mouth rinses with high alcohol content due to drying effects
• Of need for daily use of home fluoride products to prevent caries
• To use sugarless gum, frequent sips of water, or saliva substitutes

tolazamide
(tole-az′a-mide)
Tolinase

Drug class.: Sulfonylurea (first-generation) oral antidiabetic

Action: Causes functioning β-cells in pancreas to release insulin, leading to drop in blood glucose levels; may improve binding to insulin receptors or increase the number of insulin receptors; this drug is not effective if patient lacks functioning β-cells

Uses: Type II (NIDDM) diabetes mellitus

Dosage and routes:
• *Adult:* PO 100 mg/day for FBS <200 mg/dl or 250 mg/day for FBS >200 mg/dl; dose should be titrated to patient response (1 g or less/day)
Available forms include: Tabs 100, 250, 500 mg

Side effects/adverse reactions:
▼ *ORAL:* Lichenoid reaction
CNS: Headache, weakness, fatigue, lethargy, dizziness, vertigo, tinnitus
GI: ***Hepatotoxicity, jaundice,*** heartburn, nausea, vomiting, diarrhea, constipation, gas
*HEMA: **Leukopenia, thrombocytopenia, agranulocytosis, aplastic anemia, pancytopenia, hemolytic anemia***
INTEG: Rash, (rare) allergic reactions, pruritus, urticaria, eczema, photosensitivity, erythema
*ENDO: **Hypoglycemia***

Contraindications: Hypersensitivity to sulfonylureas, juvenile or brittle diabetes

Precautions: Pregnancy category C, elderly, cardiac disease, thyroid disease, severe hypoglycemic reactions, renal disease, hepatic disease

Pharmacokinetics:
PO: Completely absorbed by GI route; onset 4-6 hr, peak 4-8 hr, duration 12-24 hr, half-life 7 hr; highly protein bound; metabolized in liver; excreted in urine (metabolites), breast milk

🦷 **Drug interactions of concern to dentistry:**
• Increased hypoglycemic reaction: NSAIDs, salicylates, ketoconazole, miconazole
• Decreased action of tolazamide: corticosteroids, sympathomimetics (epinephrine)

DENTAL CONSIDERATIONS
General:
• Patients on chronic drug therapy may rarely have symptoms of blood dyscrasias, which can include infection, bleeding, and poor healing.
• Place on frequent recall to evaluate healing response.
• Short appointments and a stress reduction protocol may be required for anxious patients.
• Patients with diabetes may be more susceptible to infection and have delayed wound healing.
• Ensure that patient is following prescribed diet and regularly takes medication.
• Question patient about self-monitoring of drug's antidiabetic effect.
• Avoid prescribing aspirin-containing products.

Consultations:
• In a patient with symptoms of blood dyscrasias, request a medical consult for blood studies and postpone dental treatment until normal values are reestablished.
• Medical consult may be required to assess disease control.

---

bold italic = life-threatening conditions

Teach patient/family:
• Importance of good oral hygiene to prevent soft tissue inflammation
• To avoid mouth rinses with high alcohol content due to drying effects

---

tolbutamide
(tole-byoo'ta-mide)
Orinase
✦ Apo-Tolbutamide,   Mobenol,
Novo-Butamide
Drug class.: Sulfonylurea (first-generation) oral antidiabetic

Action: Causes functioning β-cells in pancreas to release insulin, leading to drop in blood glucose levels; may improve binding to insulin receptors or increase the number of insulin receptors; this drug is not effective if patient lacks functioning β-cells
Uses: Type II diabetes mellitus
Dosage and routes:
• *Adult:* PO 1-2 g/day in divided doses, titrated to patient response
Available forms include: Tabs 500 mg
Side effects/adverse reactions:
▼ *ORAL:* Changes in taste sensation, lichenoid reaction
CNS: Headache, weakness, paresthesia, tinnitus, dizziness, vertigo
GI: Hepatotoxicity, cholestatic jaundice, nausea, fullness, heartburn, diarrhea
HEMA: Leukopenia, thrombocytopenia, agranulocytosis, aplastic anemia, increased AST/ALT, alk phosphatase
INTEG: Rash, allergic reactions, pruritus, urticaria, eczema, photosensitivity, erythema
ENDO: Hypoglycemia
MS: Joint pain

Contraindications: Hypersensitivity to sulfonylureas, juvenile or brittle diabetes
Precautions: Pregnancy category C, elderly, cardiac disease, thyroid disease, severe hypoglycemic reactions, renal disease, hepatic disease
Pharmacokinetics:
PO: Completely absorbed by GI route, onset 30-60 min, peak 3-5 hr, duration 6-12 hr, half-life 4-5 hr; 90%-95% is plasma protein bound; metabolized in liver; excreted in urine (metabolites), breast milk
🥄 **Drug interactions of concern to dentistry:**
• Increased hypoglycemic reactions: NSAIDs, salicylates, ketoconazole, miconazole
• Decreased effects: corticosteroids, sympathomimetics
DENTAL CONSIDERATIONS
General:
• Patients on chronic drug therapy may rarely have symptoms of blood dyscrasias, which can include infection, bleeding, and poor healing.
• Ensure that patient is following prescribed diet and regularly takes medication.
• Question patient about self-monitoring of drug's antidiabetic effect, including blood glucose values or finger-stick records.
• Place on frequent recall to evaluate healing response.
• Short appointments and a stress reduction protocol may be required for anxious patients.
• Patients with diabetes may be more susceptible to infection and have delayed wound healing.
• Avoid prescribing aspirin-containing products.
Consultations:
• In a patient with symptoms of

blood dyscrasias, request a medical consult for blood studies and postpone dental treatment until normal values are reestablished.

• Medical consult may be required to assess disease control.

• Medical consult may include data from patient's blood glucose monitoring, including glycosylated hemoglobin or HbA_{1c} testing.

Teach patient/family:

• Importance of good oral hygiene to prevent soft tissue inflammation

• To avoid mouth rinses with high alcohol content due to drying effects

---

tolcapone

(tole′ka-pone)

Tasmar

Drug class.: Antiparkinsonian

Action: Reversibly and selectively inhibits catechol-*O*-methyltransferase (COMT) and may alter the plasma pharmacokinetics of levodopa; levodopa (with carbidopa) plasma levels are more sustained

Uses: Adjunct to levodopa and carbidopa in the treatment of Parkinson's disease

Dosage and routes:

• *Adult:* PO initial 100 mg tid as an adjunct to levodopa/carbidopa therapy; use 200 mg tid with caution due to elevated ALT

Available forms include: Tabs 100, 200 mg

Side effects/adverse reactions:

▼ *ORAL: Xerostomia* (5%-6%)

CNS: Hallucinations, dyskinesia, sleep disorders, dystonia, anorexia, headache, dizziness, confusion, somnolence, excessive dreaming

CV: Orthostatic hypotension, chest pain

*GI: **Hepatocellular injury,*** diarrhea, nausea, anorexia, abdominal pain, constipation, vomiting

RESP: Pulmonary effusion, URI

GU: Hematuria, UTI, discolored urine

EENT: Sinus congestion

META: Elevation of SGT and AST

MS: Muscle cramps

MISC: Sweating, fatigue

Contraindications: Hypersensitivity, patients with SGPT/ALT and SGOT/AST exceeding upper limit of normal or other signs of hepatic impairment; informed consent required; history of nontraumatic rhabdomyolysis, hyperpyrexia, and confusion related to medication

Precautions: Discontinue drug with signs of hepatocellular injury, MAO inhibitors, hypotension, dyskinesia, pregnancy category C, lactation

Pharmacokinetics:

PO: Rapidly absorbed, bioavailability 65%, highly plasma protein bound (99.9%), hepatic metabolism, 60% excreted in urine, 40% in feces

💊 Drug interactions of concern to dentistry:

• Increased sedation: alcohol and all CNS depressants

• No other data for dental drugs reported

DENTAL CONSIDERATIONS

General:

• Notify physician immediately if symptoms of liver failure are observed (bleeding, jaundice, etc.).

• Assess salivary flow as a factor in caries, periodontal disease, and candidiasis.

• After supine positioning, have patient sit upright for at least 2 min to avoid orthostatic hypotension.

• Consider semisupine chair position for patient comfort due to GI side effects of drug.

Consultations:

• Medical consult may be required to assess disease control.

• Take precaution if dental surgery is anticipated; general anesthesia is required.

Teach patient/family:

• Use of electric toothbrush if patient has difficulty holding conventional devices

When chronic dry mouth occurs, advise patient:

• To avoid mouth rinses with high alcohol content due to drying effects

• To use daily home fluoride products for anticaries effect

• To use sugarless gum, frequent sips of water, or saliva substitutes

---

tolmetin sodium

(tole′met-in)

Tolectin, Tolectin DS

♣ Novo-Tolmetin

Drug class.: Nonsteroidal antiinflammatory

Action: Inhibits prostaglandin synthesis by interfering with cyclooxygenase needed for biosynthesis

Uses: Osteoarthritis, rheumatoid arthritis, juvenile rheumatoid arthritis

Dosage and routes:

• *Adult:* PO 400 mg tid, not to exceed 2 g/day

• *Child >2 yr:* PO 15-30 mg/kg/day in 3 or 4 divided doses

Available forms include: Tabs 200, 600 mg; caps 400 mg

Side effects/adverse reactions:

▼ *ORAL:* Dry mouth, gingival

bleeding, mucosal ulceration, lichenoid reaction

CNS: Dizziness, drowsiness, fatigue, tremors, confusion, insomnia, anxiety, depression

CV: Tachycardia, peripheral edema, palpitation, dysrhythmias

GI: ***Cholestatic hepatitis,*** nausea, anorexia, vomiting, diarrhea, jaundice, constipation, flatulence, cramps, peptic ulcer

HEMA: ***Blood dyscrasias***

GU: ***Nephrotoxicity: dysuria, hematuria, oliguria, azotemia***

EENT: Tinnitus, hearing loss, blurred vision

INTEG: Purpura, rash, pruritus, sweating

Contraindications: Hypersensitivity, asthma, severe renal disease, severe hepatic disease

Precautions: Pregnancy category C, lactation, children, bleeding disorders, GI disorders, cardiac disorders, hypersensitivity to aspirin, NSAIDs, peptic ulcer disease, geriatric patients

Pharmacokinetics:

PO: Peak 2 hr, half-life 3-3.5 hr; 99% protein binding; metabolized in liver; excreted in urine (metabolites), breast milk

🦷 Drug interactions of concern to dentistry:

• Increased risk of GI side effects: ASA, NSAIDs, ethanol (alcohol)

• Nephrotoxicity: acetaminophen (prolonged use and high doses)

• Possible risk of decreased renal function: cyclosporine

• Decreased antihypertensive effect of diuretics, β-adrenergic blockers, and ACE inhibitors

DENTAL CONSIDERATIONS

General:

• Patients on chronic drug therapy may rarely have symptoms of

blood dyscrasias, which can include infection, bleeding, and poor healing.

• Monitor vital signs every appointment due to cardiovascular side effects.

• Assess salivary flow as a factor in caries, periodontal disease, and candidiasis.

• Avoid prescribing for dental use in last trimester of pregnancy.

• Possibility of cross-allergenicity when patient is allergic to aspirin.

Consultations:

• Medical consult may be required to assess disease control.

• In a patient with symptoms of blood dyscrasias, request a medical consult for blood studies and postpone dental treatment until normal values are reestablished.

Teach patient/family:

• Importance of good oral hygiene to prevent soft tissue inflammation

• Caution to prevent injury when using oral hygiene aids

When chronic dry mouth occurs, advise patient:

• To avoid mouth rinses with high alcohol content due to drying effects

• Of need for daily use of home fluoride products to prevent caries

• To use sugarless gum, frequent sips of water, or saliva substitutes

---

tolterodine tartrate
(tole-ter′o-deen)
Detrol, Detrol LA
Drug class.: Antispasmodic

Action: Inhibits muscarinic actions of acetylcholine at postganglionic receptors
Uses: Overactive bladder, with symptoms of urinary frequency or incontinence

Dosage and routes:
• *Adult:* PO initial dose 2 mg bid; may be reduced to 1 mg bid based on individual response; ext rel 4 mg/day with liquids
With hepatic dysfunction or concurrent use with inhibitors of cytochrome P-450 3A4
• *Adult:* PO 1 mg bid
Available forms include: Tabs 1, 2 mg; ext rel caps 2, 4 mg
Side effects/adverse reactions:
▼ *ORAL: Dry mouth (39.5%)*
CNS: Headache, dizziness, fatigue, vertigo, somnolence, paresthesia, nervousness
GI: Dyspepsia, constipation, abdominal pain, nausea, diarrhea
RESP: URI, bronchitis, coughing
GU: Urinary retention, dysuria, UTI
EENT: Xerophthalmia, blurred vision, rhinitis
INTEG: Rash, erythema, pruritus, dry skin
MS: Arthralgia, back pain
MISC: Weight gain, flulike symptoms
Contraindications: Hypersensitivity, urinary retention, gastric retention, uncontrolled narrow-angle glaucoma
Precautions: Bladder obstruction, pyloric stenosis, GI obstructive disorders, treated narrow-angle glaucoma, significant hepatic dysfunction, renal impairment, pregnancy category C, lactation, pediatric use
Pharmacokinetics:
PO: Onset 1 hr, peak serum levels 1-2 hr, highly plasma protein bound (96%), hepatic metabolism, active metabolite, urinary excretion (77%)

Drug interactions of concern to dentistry:

• Studies not available; however, drugs that inhibit cytochrome P-450 3A4 enzymes, such as erythromycin, clarithromycin, ketoconazole, itraconazole, and fluoxetine, require a dose reduction to 1 mg bid
• Increased anticholinergic effects: possibly with other anticholinergic drugs

DENTAL CONSIDERATIONS
General:

• Assess salivary flow as a factor in caries, periodontal disease, and candidiasis.
• Consider semisupine chair position for patient comfort due to GI side effects of drug.
• Avoid dental light in patient's eyes; offer dark glasses for patient comfort.
• Avoid drugs with anticholinergic activity, such as antihistamines, opioids, benzodiazepines, propantheline, atropine, and scopolamine.

Consultations:

• Physician should be informed if significant xerostomic side effects occur (e.g., increased caries, sore tongue, problems eating or swallowing, difficulty wearing prosthesis) so a medication change can be considered.

Teach patient/family:

• Importance of good oral hygiene to prevent soft tissue inflammation
When chronic dry mouth occurs, advise patient:
• To avoid mouth rinses with high alcohol content due to drying effects
• To use daily home fluoride products for anticaries effect
• To use sugarless gum, frequent sips of water, or saliva substitutes

topiramate
(toe-pyre'a-mate)
Topamax
Drug class.: Anticonvulsant

Action: Anticonvulsant action is unclear; blocks repetitively elicited action potentials and enhances GABA activity along with antagonism of kainate activity on non-NMDA receptors

Uses: Adjunctive therapy for adult patients with partial-onset seizures or for primary generalized tonic-clonic seizures; Lennox-Gastaut syndrome

Dosage and routes:

• *Adult and child >17 yr:* PO 400 mg/day in 2 divided doses; initiate therapy at 50 mg/day and titrate to effective dose level
• *Child 2-16 yr:* PO total daily dose range 5-9 mg/kg/day in 2 equal doses; start at 25 mg hs × 1 wk, then increase at 1-2 wk intervals to achieve desired response

Available forms include: Tabs 25, 100, 200 mg; sprinkle caps 15, 25 mg

Side effects/adverse reactions:

▼ *ORAL:* Dry mouth (1.1%), gingival overgrowth (rare), taste alteration
CNS: Psychomotor slowing, somnolence, fatigue, ataxia, confusion, dizziness, memory problems, irritability, depression
CV: Palpitation, bradycardia
GI: Nausea, dyspepsia, abdominal pain
RESP: Coughing, bronchitis
HEMA: Epistaxis, *leukopenia, purpura, thrombocytopenia*
GU: Hematuria, UTI
EENT: Decreased hearing, eye

pain, photophobia, severe myopia, secondary angle closure glaucoma
INTEG: Dermatitis, acne
MS: Back pain, asthenia, leg pain, myalgia
MISC: Paresthesia
Contraindications: Hypersensitivity
Precautions: Renal impairment, hepatic impairment, rapid drug withdrawal, kidney stones, pregnancy category C, lactation, children
Pharmacokinetics:
PO: Rapid oral absorption, peak plasma levels 2 hr, low protein binding (13%-17%), 70% excreted in urine unchanged, little metabolism

⚡ Drug interactions of concern to dentistry:
• Increased CNS depression: opioids, sedatives, ethanol, and other CNS depressants

DENTAL CONSIDERATIONS
General:
• Patients on chronic drug therapy may rarely have symptoms of blood dyscrasias, which can include infection, bleeding, and poor healing.
• Short appointments and a stress reduction protocol may be required for anxious patients.
• Assess salivary flow as factor in caries, periodontal disease, and candidiasis.
• Avoid dental light in patient's eyes; offer dark glasses for patient comfort.
• Determine type of epilepsy, seizure frequency, and quality of seizure control. A stress reduction protocol may be required.
Consultations:
• In a patient with symptoms of blood dyscrasias, request a medical consult for blood studies and postpone dental treatment until normal values are reestablished.
• Medical consult may be required to assess disease control.

Teach patient/family:
• Importance of good oral hygiene to prevent soft tissue inflammation
• Caution to prevent trauma when using oral hygiene aids
• Use of electric toothbrush if patient has difficulty holding conventional devices
• Importance of updating health and drug history if physician makes any changes in evaluation or drug regimens
When chronic dry mouth occurs, advise patient:
• To avoid mouth rinses with high alcohol content due to drying effects
• To use daily home fluoride products for anticaries effect
• To use sugarless gum, frequent sips of water, or saliva substitutes

---

toremifene citrate
(tore'em-i-feen)
Fareston
Drug class.: Antineoplastic, antiestrogen agent

Action: Inhibits cell division by binding to cytoplasmic receptors (estrogen receptors); resembles normal cell complex but inhibits DNA synthesis
Uses: Metastatic breast cancer in postmenopausal women with estrogen receptor-positive or unknown tumors
Dosage and routes:
• *Adult:* PO 60 mg qd continued until disease progression is observed

---

Available forms include: Tabs 60 mg

Side effects/adverse reactions:

CNS: Dizziness
CV: Edema
GI: Nausea, vomiting
HEMA: Thrombophlebitis, thrombosis
GU: Vaginal discharge, vaginal bleeding
EENT: Cataracts, dry eyes, abnormal visual fields, glaucoma
INTEG: Sweating
ENDO: Hot flashes
META: Elevated SGOT, alk phosphatase, bilirubin, hypercalcemia

Contraindications: Hypersensitivity

Precautions: Thromboembolic diseases, endometrial hyperplasia, hypercalcemia with bone metastases, monitor leukocyte and platelet counts, pregnancy category D, tumor flare

Pharmacokinetics:

PO: Well absorbed, peak levels average 3 hr, extensive metabolism with active metabolite, enterohepatic circulation, highly protein bound (99.5%), excreted mainly in feces, 10% in urine

⚷ Drug interactions of concern to dentistry:
• None reported

DENTAL CONSIDERATIONS

General:
• Patients on chronic drug therapy may rarely have symptoms of blood dyscrasias, which can include infection, bleeding, and poor healing.
• Consider semisupine chair position for patient comfort due to GI side effects of drug.

Consultations:
• Medical consult may be required to assess disease control.

Teach patient/family:
• Importance of good oral hygiene to prevent soft tissue inflammation

---

torsemide

(tore′se-mide)
Demadex
Drug class.: Loop diuretic

Action: Acts on loop of Henle to decrease the reabsorption of chloride, sodium, and potassium with resultant diuresis

Uses: Hypertension and edema associated with CHF, liver disease, chronic renal failure

Dosage and routes:

Hypertension
• *Adult:* PO 5 mg/day; may increase to 10 mg after 4-6 wk if required

CHF, chronic renal failure
• *Adult:* PO or IV, 10-20 mg/day; may increase if inadequate response; no data for doses >200 mg

Hepatic cirrhosis
• *Adult:* PO or IV 5-10 mg/day

Available forms include: Tabs 5, 10, 20, 100 mg; inj IV 10 mg/ml in 2, 5 ml amps

Side effects/adverse reactions:

CNS: Dizziness, headache, fatigue, insomnia, nervousness, syncope
CV: Orthostatic hypotension, ECG abnormalities, chest pain, edema, dysrhythmias
GI: Diarrhea, nausea, dyspepsia, irritation, GI bleeding
RESP: Cough
GU: Excessive urination
EENT: Sore throat, rhinitis
INTEG: Rash, photosensitivity
MS: Asthenia, muscle cramps, arthralgia

italic = common side effects

Contraindications: Hypersensitivity, anuria, severe electrolyte depletion, hypersensitivity to sulfonylureas, hepatic coma

Precautions: Pregnancy category B, lactation, children <18 yr, dehydration, systemic lupus erythematosus, ototoxicity, electrolyte imbalance

Pharmacokinetics:

PO: Onset 1 hr, peak effects 1-2 hr, duration 6-8 hr; liver metabolism; renal excretion

IV: Onset 10 min, peak effect 1 hr, duration 6-8 hr

🦷 Drug interactions of concern to dentistry:

• Increased electrolyte imbalance: systemic corticosteroids

• Masked ototoxicity: phenothiazines

• Decreased antihypertensive effects: NSAIDs, especially indomethacin

• Increased sweating, hot flashes, weakness, CV symptoms: chloral hydrate (rare)

DENTAL CONSIDERATIONS

General:

• Monitor vital signs every appointment due to cardiovascular side effects.

• After supine positioning, have patient sit upright for at least 2 min before standing to avoid orthostatic hypotension.

• Patients on high-potency loop diuretics should be questioned about serum potassium levels or potassium supplement use.

• Short appointments and a stress reduction protocol may be required for anxious patients.

• Consider semisupine chair position if GI side effects occur.

Consultations:

• Medical consult may be required

to assess disease control and the patient's ability to tolerate stress.

Teach patient/family:

• Importance of updating health history/drug record if physician makes any changes in evaluation or drug regimen

---

tramadol HCl

(tra′ma-dole)

Ultram

Drug class.: Synthetic opioid analgesic

Action: Unknown, but it has been shown to bind to opioid receptors and inhibit the reuptake of norepinephrine and serotonin

Uses: Moderate-to-severe pain

Dosage and routes:

• *Adult:* PO 50-100 mg q4-6h, limit 400 mg/day (do not exceed limit); for moderately severe pain, 100 mg initial dose may be required

Moderate chronic pain not requiring rapid analgesic onset

• *Adult:* PO initial 25 mg/day, then titrate doses by 25 mg as separate doses q3d to max dose of 100 mg, then titrate doses by 50 mg q3d to max of 200 mg daily; max daily dose 400 mg

Renal/hepatic impairment or elderly >65 yr

• *Adult:* PO limit dose to 300 mg/day

Cirrhosis

• *Adult:* PO limit dose to 50 mg q12h

Available forms include: Tabs 50 mg

Side effects/adverse reactions:

▼ *ORAL:* Dry mouth (<5%), stomatitis

---

bold italic = life-threatening conditions

CNS: Dizziness, vertigo, headache, somnolence, seizures, anxiety, confusion, drug abuse risk

CV: Vasodilation, palpitation

GI: Constipation, vomiting, dyspepsia, diarrhea, flatulence

GU: Urinary retention, frequency

EENT: Visual disturbances

INTEG: Pruritus, sweating, rash

MS: Hypertonia

MISC: Malaise

Contraindications: Hypersensitivity to tramadol, codeine, or other opioids; acute alcohol, hypnotic, other opioid, or psychotropic drug intoxication, opioid addicts; pregnancy category C; lactation; child <16 yr; elderly; renal or hepatic impairment; risk of seizures in patients taking MAO inhibitors, tricyclic antidepressants, or other drugs that reduce the seizure threshold; increased intracranial pressure due to head injury

Precautions: Not a controlled substance, but dependence and abuse are possible

Pharmacokinetics:

PO: Rapid oral absorption, can be given with food, peak levels 2 hr, half-life 6-7 hr; hepatic metabolism; excreted in urine

🦷 Drug interactions of concern to dentistry:

• Increased risk of respiratory depression: anesthetics, alcohol

• Significant increase in metabolism: carbamazepine

• Increased serum concentrations: quinidine

• Increased risk of seizures: MAO inhibitors, tricyclic antidepressants, selective serotonin reuptake inhibitors

• Increased risk of sedation: other CNS depressant drugs, alcohol

DENTAL CONSIDERATIONS
General:

• Determine why the patient is taking the drug.

• Patients taking opioids for acute or chronic pain should be given alternative analgesics for dental pain.

• Geriatric patients are more susceptible to drug effects; use lower dose.

• Assess salivary flow as a factor in caries, periodontal disease, and candidiasis.

• Take precautions if dental surgery is anticipated and general anesthesia is required.

• Risk of cross-hypersensitivity to other opioid analgesics.

Teach patient/family:

• Caution to prevent trauma when using oral hygiene aids

• That opioid drugs may alter reaction time; caution patient about driving or operating complex equipment

When chronic dry mouth occurs, advise patient:

• To avoid mouth rinses with high alcohol content due to drying effects

• To use daily home fluoride products for anticaries effect

• To use sugarless gum, frequent sips of water, or saliva substitutes

---

trandolapril
(tran'dole-a-pril)
Mavik

Drug class.: Angiotensin-converting enzyme (ACE) inhibitor

Action: Selectively suppresses renin-angiotensin-aldosterone system; inhibits ACE; prevents conversion of angiotension I to angiotensin II; results in reduced peripheral resistance, decreased aldosterone secretion, and increase in plasma renin

Uses: Hypertension alone or in combination with other antihypertensive medications; maintenance therapy to prevent CHF after MI; ventricular dysfunction after MI

Dosage and routes:

Not taking diuretic
• *Adult:* PO initial dose 1 mg (non–African-American patient) and 2 mg (African-American patient) daily; adjust dose to BP response; usual dose 2-4 mg daily

Taking diuretic
• *Adult:* Discontinue diuretic for 2-3 days before initiating trandolapril therapy, add diuretic if BP is not controlled

When diuretic cannot be discontinued
• *Adult:* Initial dose is 0.5 mg with caution and medical supervision until BP is stabilized

Available forms include: Tabs 1, 2, 4 mg

Side effects/adverse reactions:

▼ *ORAL:* **Angioedema (lips, tongue, mucous membranes)**

CNS: Dizziness, drowsiness, insomnia, vertigo, headache, fatigue

CV: Hypotension, syncope, bradycardia, chest pain, palpitation, AV first-degree block, bradycardia, hyperkalemia

GI: Diarrhea, **pancreatitis,** cholestatic jaundice

RESP: Cough, URI, dyspnea

HEMA: **Neutropenia, leukopenia**

GU: Impotence, decreased libido

EENT: Throat inflammation, epistaxis

INTEG: Pruritus, rash, pemphigus

MS: Cramps, gout, extremity pain

MISC: **Anaphylactoid reactions**

Contraindications: Hypersensitivity or angioedema with prior use of ACE inhibitors, second or third trimester of pregnancy, lactation

Precautions: Angioedema (higher rate in African-American patients), congestive heart failure, ischemic heart disease, aortic stenosis, cerebrovascular disease, monitor WBC in SLE or scleroderma, impaired renal function, hyperkalemia, pregnancy category C (first trimester), pregnancy category D (second, third trimester), pediatric patients, potassium-sparing diuretics

Pharmacokinetics:

PO: Active metabolite trandolaprilat, peak levels trandolapril 1 hr, trandolaprilat 4-10 hr, excreted 66% in feces, 33% in urine, protein binding 80%

Drug interactions of concern to dentistry:
• Decreased absorption of tetracycline
• Drugs that lower blood pressure could possibly exaggerate hypotensive effects

DENTAL CONSIDERATIONS

General:
• Monitor vital signs every appointment due to cardiovascular disease.
• Limit use of sodium-containing products such as saline IV fluids for those patients with a dietary salt restriction.
• Stress from dental procedures may compromise cardiovascular function; determine patient risk.
• Short appointments and a stress reduction protocol may be required for anxious patients.
• Use precaution if sedation or general anesthesia is required; risk of hypotensive episode.
• After supine positioning, have

---

bold italic = life-threatening conditions

patient sit upright for at least 2 min before standing to avoid orthostatic hypotension.

• Consider semisupine chair position for patient comfort due to respiratory side effects of drug.

• Patients on chronic drug therapy may rarely have symptoms of blood dyscrasias, which can include infection, bleeding, and poor healing.

• Importance of updating health and drug history if physician makes any changes in evaluation or drug regimens.

Consultations:

• Medical consult may be required to assess disease control and patient's ability to tolerate stress.

Teach patient/family:

• Importance of good oral hygiene to prevent soft tissue inflammation

• Caution to prevent trauma when using oral hygiene aids

---

tranexamic acid

(tran-ex-am′ik)

Cyklokapron

Drug class.: Hemostatic, antithrombolytic

Action: Competitive inhibitor of plasminogen activation, decreases the conversion of plasminogen to plasmin; a much higher dose acts as a noncompetitive inhibitor of plasmin

Uses: Prophylaxis and treatment of hemophilia patients to reduce or prevent hemorrhage during and after extractions; unapproved: in hyperfibrinolysis-induced hemorrhage, angioedema; oral rinse (with systemic therapy) to reduce bleeding in oral surgery patients who are also taking anticoagulants

Dosage and routes:

Dental extraction in hemophilia patient

• *Adult and adolescent:* IV immediately before surgery, 10 mg/kg; after surgery give 25 mg/kg tid or qid for 2-8 days

• *Adult and adolescent:* PO beginning day before surgery, 25 mg/kg tid or qid; after surgery give 25 mg/kg tid or qid for 2-8 days; patients unable to take PO meds—IV, 10 mg/kg tid-qid

Note: Reduce dose with moderate to severe renal impairment

Unapproved: Dental procedures producing bleeding in patients taking oral anticoagulants (rinse)

Some reports suggest the use of tranexamic oral rinse for use in patients who cannot reduce their use of oral anticoagulants. One report (Ramstrom et al: *J Oral Maxillofac Surg* 51:1211-1216, 1963) used the following procedure:

• *Adult:* Before suturing, the area is irrigated with 10 ml of 4.8% tranexamic acid solution. Patients rinse for 2 min 4 times daily for the next 7 days. No food or drink is to be consumed within 1 hr of using mouthwash. Tranexamic acid mouthwash is not commercially available in Canada or the US. It could be extemporaneously prepared using the commercial tablets or injection. Because stability data for aqueous solutions are lacking, extemporaneous solutions should be freshly prepared.

In another report (Souto et al: *J Oral Maxillofac Surg* 54:27-32, 1996) a mouth rinse of 1 ampule of the antifibrinolytic agent for 2 min q6h for 2 days was used.

Available forms include: Tabs 500 mg; amps 100 mg/ml in 10 ml size

Side effects/adverse reactions:

CNS: Giddiness

CV: Hypotension (IV doses)

GI: Nausea, vomiting, diarrhea

EENT: Blurred vision

Contraindications: Patients with acquired defective color vision, subarachnoid hemorrhage

Precautions: Pregnancy category B, lactation, reduce dose in renal impairment, limited use experience in children

Pharmacokinetics:

PO: Bioavailability 30%-50%, low protein binding (<3%), peak plasma levels 3 hr, little metabolism, renal excretion

Drug interactions of concern to dentistry:

• Increased risk of bleeding: drugs that affect coagulation

• Factor IX complex: increased risk of thrombotic complications when used concurrently

DENTAL CONSIDERATIONS

General:

• Has been used as an antifibrinolytic mouthwash following oral surgery to prevent hemorrhage in patients taking oral anticoagulants.

Consultations:

• Hematologist consult is strongly recommended.

Teach patient/family:

• Importance of updating health and drug history if physician makes any changes in evaluation or drug regimens

• To report hemorrhage or bleeding not responding to postsurgical hemostasis

• Caution to prevent trauma when using oral hygiene aids

tranylcypromine sulfate

(tran-il-sip′roe-meen)

Parnate

Drug class.: Antidepressant, MAO inhibitor

Action: Increases concentrations of endogenous norepinephrine, serotonin, and dopamine in CNS storage sites by inhibiting MAO; the precise antidepressant mechanism is unknown

Uses: Depression (when uncontrolled by other means)

Dosage and routes:

• *Adult:* PO 10 mg bid; may increase to 30 mg/day after 2 wk; max 60 mg/day

Available forms include: Tabs 10 mg

Side effects/adverse reactions:

▼ *ORAL:* Dry mouth

CNS: Dizziness, drowsiness, confusion, headache, anxiety, tremors, stimulation, weakness, hyperreflexia, mania, insomnia, fatigue, weight gain

CV: Orthostatic hypotension, hypertension, dysrhythmias, hypertensive crisis

GI: Anorexia, constipation, nausea, vomiting, diarrhea, weight gain

HEMA: Anemia

GU: Change in libido, urinary retention

EENT: Blurred vision

INTEG: Rash, flushing, increased perspiration

ENDO: SIADH-like syndrome

Contraindications: Hypersensitivity to MAO inhibitors, elderly, hypertension, CHF, severe hepatic disease, pheochromocytoma, severe renal disease, severe cardiac disease

T

Precautions: Suicidal patients, convulsive disorders, severe depression, schizophrenia, hyperactivity, diabetes mellitus, pregnancy category C

Pharmacokinetics:

PO: Metabolized in liver, excreted by kidneys, crosses placenta, excreted in breast milk

🦷 Drug interactions of concern to dentistry:

• Increased pressor effects: indirect-acting sympathomimetics (ephedrine)
• Hyperpyretic crisis, convulsions, hypertensive episode, and death: carbamazepine, meperidine, and possibly other opioids
• Increased anticholinergic effects: anticholinergics and antihistamines
• Increased effects of alcohol, barbiturates, benzodiazepines, CNS depressants, fluoxetine, tricyclic antidepressants

DENTAL CONSIDERATIONS

General:

• After supine positioning, have patient sit upright for at least 2 min before standing to avoid orthostatic hypotension.
• Take vital signs every appointment due to cardiovascular side effects.
• Assess salivary flow as a factor in caries, periodontal disease, and candidiasis.
• Hypertensive episodes are possible even though there are no specific contraindications to vasoconstrictor use in local anesthetics.

Consultations:

• Medical consult may be required to assess patient's ability to tolerate stress.

Teach patient/family:

• To use electric toothbrush if patient has difficulty holding conventional devices

When chronic dry mouth occurs, advise patient:

• To avoid mouth rinses with high alcohol content due to drying effects
• Of need for daily home fluoride to prevent caries
• To use sugarless gum, frequent sips of water, or saliva substitutes

---

travoprost ophthalmic solution

(tra′voe-prost)

Travatan

Drug class.: A synthetic prostaglandin $F_{2\alpha}$ analogue

Action: Rapidly hydrolyzed to the biologically active, travoprost free acid that is a selective FP prostanoid receptor agonist; it reduces intraocular pressure (IOP) by increasing uveoscleral outflow

Uses: Reduction of elevated IOP in patients with open-angle glaucoma or ocular hypertension in patients who are intolerant to or who show insufficient response to other IOP-reducing drugs

Dosage and routes:

• *Adult:* TOP 1 gtt in affected eye(s) qd in PM

Available forms include: Sterile sol 0.004% in 2.5 ml

Side effects/adverse reactions:

CNS: Anxiety, depression, headache

CV: Angina pectoris, bradycardia, hypertension, hypotension

GI: Dyspepsia

RESP: Bronchitis, sinusitis

GU: UTI, incontinence

EENT: Ocular hyperemia, conjunc-

tival hyperemia, decreased visual acuity, eye discomfort, pain, pruritus, dry eyes, iris discoloration, keratitis, photophobia

META: Hypercholesterolemia

MISC: Back pain, arthritis

Contraindications: Hypersensitivity to this drug or benzalkonium chloride, pregnancy

Precautions: May cause changes in pigmented tissues (iris, eyelid) and growth of eyelashes (length, thickness, color); do not administer with contact lens in place; renal or hepatic impairment, pregnancy category C, lactation, pediatric use, macular edema

Pharmacokinetics:

TOP: Absorbed through cornea, peak plasma levels 30 min, free acid in cornea, free acid is further metabolized to inactive metabolite, rapid elimination

Drug interactions of concern to dentistry:

• None reported

DENTAL CONSIDERATIONS

General:

• Monitor vital signs every appointment due to cardiovascular and respiratory side effects and question patient about occurrence of CV side effects.

• Avoid drugs with anticholinergic activity such as antihistamines, opioids, benzodiazepines, propantheline, atropine, and scopolamine.

• Protect patient's eyes from accidental spatter during dental treatment.

• Avoid dental light in patient's eyes; offer dark glasses for patient comfort.

Consultations:

• Medical consult may be required to assess disease control.

Teach patient/family:

• Importance of updating health and drug history if physician makes any changes in evaluation or drug regimens

---

trazodone HCl

(traz'oh-done)

Desyrel

Drug class.: Antidepressant

Action: Selectively inhibits serotonin-specific reuptake in the brain

Uses: Depression; unapproved use: chronic pain, diabetes-associated painful neuropathy, burning mouth syndrome

Dosage and routes:

• *Adult:* PO 150 mg/day in divided doses; may be increased by 50 mg/day q3-4d, not to exceed 600 mg/day

Available forms include: Tabs 50, 100, 150, 300 mg

Side effects/adverse reactions:

▼ *ORAL: Dry mouth,* stomatitis

CNS: Dizziness, drowsiness, confusion, headache, anxiety, tremors, stimulation, weakness, insomnia, nightmares, EPS (elderly), increase in psychiatric symptoms

CV: Orthostatic hypotension, ECG changes, tachycardia, hypertension, palpitations

GI: Diarrhea, paralytic ileus, hepatitis, increased appetite, nausea, vomiting, cramps, epigastric distress, jaundice

HEMA: Agranulocytosis, thrombocytopenia, eosinophilia, leukopenia

GU: Retention, acute renal failure, priapism

EENT: Blurred vision, tinnitus, mydriasis

T

INTEG: Rash, urticaria, sweating, pruritus, photosensitivity

Contraindications: Hypersensitivity to tricyclic antidepressants, recovery phase of myocardial infarction, convulsive disorders, prostatic hypertrophy

Precautions: Suicidal patients, severe depression, increased intraocular pressure, narrow-angle glaucoma, urinary retention, cardiac disease, hepatic disease, hyperthyroidism, electroshock therapy, elective surgery, pregnancy category C

Pharmacokinetics:

PO: Half-life 4.4-7.5 hr; metabolized by liver; excreted by kidneys, feces

👄 **Drug interactions of concern to dentistry:**

• Increased anticholinergic effects: anticholinergic drugs

• Increased CNS depression: alcohol, all other CNS depressants

DENTAL CONSIDERATIONS

General:

• Take vital signs every appointment due to cardiovascular side effects.

• Patients on chronic drug therapy may rarely have symptoms of blood dyscrasias, which can include infection, bleeding, and poor healing.

• Assess salivary flow as a factor in caries, periodontal disease, and candidiasis.

• After supine positioning, have patient sit upright for at least 2 min before standing to avoid orthostatic hypotension.

Consultations:

• In a patient with symptoms of blood dyscrasias, request a medical consult for blood studies and postpone dental treatment until normal values are reestablished.

• Medical consult may be required to assess disease control.

• Physician should be informed if significant xerostomic side effects occur (increased caries, sore tongue, problems eating or swallowing, difficulty wearing prosthesis) so a medication change can be considered.

Teach patient/family:

• To report oral lesions, soreness, or bleeding to dentist

When chronic dry mouth occurs, advise patient:

• To avoid mouth rinses with high alcohol content due to drying effects

• Of need for daily use of home fluoride products to prevent caries

• To use sugarless gum, frequent sips of water, or saliva substitutes

---

tretinoin (vitamin A acid, retinoic acid)

(tre′ti-noyn)

Avita, Retin-A, Retin-A Micro, Retin-A Regimen Kit, Renova

🍁 Stieva-A, Stieva-A Forte

Drug class.: Vitamin A acid

Action: Decreases cohesiveness of follicular epithelium, decreases microcomedone formation

Uses: Acne vulgaris, reducing fine facial wrinkles associated with sun exposure and aging; unapproved: skin cancer, lichen planus

Dosage and routes:

• *Adult and child:* Topical; cleanse area, apply hs, cover lightly

Available forms include: TOP cream 0.025%, 0.05%, 0.1%; gel 0.01%, 0.025%, 0.1%; liq 0.05%

Side effects/adverse reactions:

INTEG: Rash, stinging, warmth, redness, erythema, blistering, crusting, peeling, contact dermatitis, hypopigmentation, hyperpigmentation

Contraindications: Hypersensitivity

Precautions: Pregnancy category C, lactation, eczema, sunburn

Pharmacokinetics:

TOP: Poor absorption, excreted in urine

🦷 **Drug interactions of concern to dentistry:**

• Increased peeling: medication-containing agents such as alcohol or astringents

• Avoid concurrent use with photosensitizing drugs: tetracycline, fluoroquinolones, sulfonamides

DENTAL CONSIDERATIONS

General:

• May cause dry, peeling skin if used around lips; provide lip lubricant for patient comfort during dental treatment.

• Advise patient if dental drugs prescribed have a potential for photosensitivity.

Teach patient/family:

• To avoid application on normal skin or getting cream in eyes, mouth, or other mucous membranes

---

triamcinolone acetonide

(trye-am-sin'oh-lone)

Azmacort Oral Inhaler, Nasacort AQ Nasal Spray, Nasacort Inhaler

Drug class.: Glucocorticoid, intermediate acting

Action: Glucocorticoids have multiple actions that include antiinflammatory and immunosuppressant effects. They inhibit phospholipase A_2, interfering with or reducing the synthesis of prostaglandins and leukotrienes. They also bind to cytoplasmic glucocorticoid receptors (GRs) and enter the cell nucleus to bind with DNA. This results in the synthesis of various enzymes such as collagenase, elastase, and cytokines that play important roles in inflammation and immunosuppression. They also suppress the production of lymphocytes, monocytes, and eosinophils.

Uses: Maintenance treatment of chronic asthma (Azmacort); seasonal and perennial allergic rhinitis (Nasacort)

Dosage and routes:

• *Adult:* Oral inh 2 inhalations tid or qid or 4 inhalations bid

• *Adult and child >12 yr:* Nasal spray initial 2 sprays in each nostril daily; may increase to bid after 4-7 days and patient response; maintenance dose 1 spray in each nostril daily

• *Child 6-12 yr:* Oral inh 1 or 2 inhalations tid or qid or 2-4 inhalations bid; max 12 inh/day

Available forms include: Oral inh 20 g inhaler 100 µg per actuation/240 metered dose container, (Nasacort) 10 g inhaler 55 µg per actuation; nasal spray 15 g container 55 µg per actuation/100 metered dose spray container

Side effects/adverse reactions:

▼ *ORAL: Candidiasis*

EENT: Dry throat, hoarseness, irritation

Contraindications: Acute asthma, status asthmaticus, nonasthmatic bronchitis, hypersensitivity

Precautions: TB; untreated fungal,

---

bold italic = life-threatening conditions

T

bacterial, or viral infections of respiratory tract; pregnancy category C, lactation, children <6 yr; different doses may be required for patients on systemic glucocorticoids or patients with chickenpox, measles

Pharmacokinetics:

INH ORAL: Little systemic absorption from lungs, hepatic metabolism

NASAL SPRAY: Little systemic absorption, peak plasma levels 1.5 hr

⚖ **Drug interactions of concern to dentistry:**

• None reported

DENTAL CONSIDERATIONS

General:

• Place on frequent recall due to oral side effects.

• Evaluate respiration characteristics, rate.

• Midday appointments and a stress reduction protocol may be required for anxious patients.

• Acute asthmatic episodes may be precipitated in the dental office. Rapid-acting sympathomimetic inhalants should be available for emergency use. Triamcinolone is not a rapid-acting drug and is not intended for use in acute asthmatic attacks.

• Be aware that aspirin or sulfite preservatives in vasoconstrictor-containing products can exacerbate asthma.

• Examine for oral manifestation of opportunistic infection.

Consultations:

• Medical consult may be required to assess disease control.

Teach patient/family:

• Importance of good oral hygiene to prevent soft tissue inflammation

• Importance of gargling, rinsing mouth with water, and expectorating after each aerosol dose

---

triamcinolone/ triamcinolone acetonide/ triamcinolone diacetate/triamcinolone hexacetonide

(trye-am-sin'oh-lone)

Triamcinolone (oral): Aristocort, Kenacort

Triamcinolone acetonide: Kenaject-40, Kenalog-10, Kenalog-40, Tac-3, Tac-40, Triam-A, Tri-Kort, Trilog

Triamcinolone diacetate (not for IV use): Amcort, Aristocort Forte, Clinacort, Triam Forte, Triamolone 40, Trilone

🍁 Tristoject

Triamcinolone diacetate syrup: Kenacort

Triamcinolone hexacetonide (not for IV use): Aristocort Intraarticular, Aristospan Intralesional

Drug class.: Glucocorticoid, intermediate-acting

Action: Glucocorticoids have multiple actions that include antiinflammatory and immunosuppressant effects. They inhibit phospholipase A_2, interfering with or reducing the synthesis of prostaglandins and leukotrienes. They also bind to cytoplasmic glucocorticoid receptors (GRs) and enter the cell nucleus to bind with DNA. This results in the synthesis of various enzymes such as collagenase, elastase, and cytokines that play important roles in inflammation and immunosuppression. They also suppress the production of lymphocytes, monocytes, and eosinophils.

Uses: Severe inflammation; immunosuppression; neoplasms; asthma (steroid dependent); collagen, respiratory, dermatologic disorders; seasonal and perennial allergic rhinitis

Dosage and routes:

• *Adult:* PO dose depends on disease to be treated with a range of 4-48 mg per day as a single dose or divided dose

• *Child:* PO dose depends on disease to be treated; suggested dose is 1.7 mg/kg as a single dose or divided dose

Parenteral doses

• *Adult:* Triamcinolone acetonide—IM, 40-80 mg at 4-wk intervals; intraarticular, 2.5-15 mg; intralesional, up to 1 mg per injection site; triamcinolone diacetate—IM, 40 mg once weekly; intraarticular, intralesional, or soft tissue 3-48 mg repeated at 1-8 wk intervals; triamcinolone hexacetonide—intraarticular, 2-20 mg at 3-4 wk intervals; intralesional up to 0.5 mg per square inch of skin, repeat as needed

Available forms include: Tabs 4, 8 mg; syr 4 mg/5 ml; inj 25, 40 mg/ml diacetate; inj 3, 10, 40 mg/ml acetonide; inj 20, 5 mg/ml hexacetonide

Side effects/adverse reactions:

▼ *ORAL:* Candidiasis, poor wound healing, petechiae, dry mouth

CNS: Depression, flushing, sweating, headache, mood changes

CV: Hypertension, circulatory collapse, thrombophlebitis, embolism, tachycardia, edema

GI: Diarrhea, nausea, abdominal distention, **GI hemorrhage, pancreatitis,** increased appetite

HEMA: **Thrombocytopenia**

EENT: Fungal infections, increased intraocular pressure, blurred vision

INTEG: Acne, poor wound healing, ecchymosis, petechiae

MS: Fractures, osteoporosis, weakness

Contraindications: Psychosis, hypersensitivity, idiopathic thrombocytopenia, acute glomerulonephritis, amebiasis, fungal and viral infections, nonasthmatic bronchial disease, child <2 yr, AIDS, TB

Precautions: Pregnancy category D, diabetes mellitus, glaucoma, osteoporosis, seizure disorders, ulcerative colitis, CHF, myasthenia gravis, renal disease, esophagitis, peptic ulcer, herpetic infections, rifampin

Pharmacokinetics:

PO/IM: Peak 1-2 hr, 2 days, 1-6 wk (IM), half-life 2-5 hr

⚘ Drug interactions of concern to dentistry:

• Decreased action: barbiturates, rifampin, rifabutin

• Increased GI side effects: alcohol, salicylates, NSAIDs

• Increased action: ketoconazole, macrolide antibiotics

DENTAL CONSIDERATIONS

General:

• Symptoms of oral infections may be masked.

• Examine for oral manifestation of opportunistic infections.

• Oral side effects may be more common with inhalation products;

significant steroid side effects are more likely to occur with chronic systemic doses.

• Acute asthmatic episodes may be precipitated in the dental office. Rapid-acting sympathomimetic inhalants should be available for emergency use. A stress reduction protocol may be required.

• Monitor vital signs every appointment due to cardiovascular side effects.

• Assess salivary flow as a factor in caries, periodontal disease, and candidiasis.

• Prophylactic antibiotics may be indicated to prevent infection.

• Place on frequent recall to monitor healing response.

• Determine dose and duration of steroid therapy for each patient to assess risk for stress tolerance and immunosuppression.

• Be aware that aspirin or sulfite preservatives in vasoconstrictor-containing products can exacerbate asthma.

• Patients who have been or are currently on chronic steroid therapy (>2 wk) may require supplemental steroids for dental treatment.

Consultations:

• Medical consult may be required to assess disease control.

• Consult may be required to confirm steroid dose and duration of use.

Teach patient/family:

• Importance of good oral hygiene to prevent soft tissue inflammation

• To report oral lesions, soreness, or bleeding to dentist

When chronic dry mouth occurs, advise patient:

• To avoid mouth rinses with high alcohol content due to drying effects

• To use daily home fluoride products for anticaries effect

• To use sugarless gum, frequent sips of water, or saliva substitutes

---

triamcinolone acetonide (topical)

(trye-am-sin'oh-lone)

Aristocort, Aristicort A, Delta-Tritex, Flutex, Kenalog, Kenalog-H, Kenonel, Triacet, Tri-derm

Dental products: Kenalog in Orabase, Oralone Dental

Drug class.: Topical corticosteroid, synthetic fluorinated agent, group II potency (0.5%), group III potency (0.1%), group IV potency (0.025%)

Action: Interacts with steroid cytoplasmic receptors to induce antiinflammatory effects; possesses antipruritic, antiinflammatory actions

Uses: Psoriasis, eczema, contact dermatitis, pruritus; topical dental paste used to treat nonviral inflammatory oral lesions, including aphthous stomatitis, lichen planus, and cicatricial pemphigoid

Dosage and routes:

• *Adult and child:* Apply to affected area bid-qid

Available forms include: Oint 0.025%, 0.1%, 0.5%; cream 0.025%, 0.1%, 0.5%; lotion 0.025%, 0.1%; aerosol 0.2 mg/2 sec; paste 0.1%, 0.5%

Side effects/adverse reactions:

▼ *ORAL:* Mucosal thinning and petechial hemorrhage (rare), stinging sensation (oral application)

INTEG: Burning, dryness, itching, irritation, acne, folliculitis, hypertrichosis, perioral dermatitis, hypopigmentation, atrophy, striae, allergic contact dermatitis, secondary infection

Contraindications: Hypersensitivity to corticosteroids, fungal or viral (herpetic) infections

Precautions: Pregnancy category C, lactation, viral infections, bacterial infections, diabetes mellitus, TB

DENTAL CONSIDERATIONS

General:

• Apply approximately 0.25 inch; measure with cotton-tipped applicator; press on lesion, do not rub. Use after brushing and eating and at bedtime for optimal effect.

• When used for oral lesions, return for oral evaluation if response of oral tissues has not occurred in 7-14 days.

Teach patient/family:

• To avoid sunlight on affected area; burns may occur

• Not to use on herpetic lesions

---

triamterene

(trye-am′ter-een)

Dyrenium

Drug class.: Potassium-sparing diuretic

Action: Acts on distal tubule to inhibit reabsorption of sodium and chloride; increases potassium retention

Uses: Edema; hypertension; more commonly used in combination with a thiazide diuretic

Dosage and routes:

• *Adult:* PO 100 mg bid pc, not to exceed 300 mg

Available forms include: Caps 50, 100 mg

Side effects/adverse reactions:

▼ *ORAL:* Dry mouth

CNS: Confusion, nervousness, numbness in hands or feet, weakness, headache, dizziness

GI: Nausea, diarrhea, vomiting, jaundice, liver disease

HEMA: Thrombocytopenia, megaloblastic anemia, low folic acid levels

GU: Azotemia, interstitial nephritis, increased BUN, creatinine, renal stones

INTEG: Photosensitivity, rash

ELECT: Hyperkalemia, hyponatremia, hypochloremia

Contraindications: Hypersensitivity, anuria, severe renal disease, severe hepatic disease, hyperkalemia, pregnancy category D

Precautions: Dehydration, hepatic disease, lactation, CHF, renal disease, cirrhosis

Pharmacokinetics:

PO: Onset 2 hr, peak 6-8 hr, duration 12-16 hr, half-life 3 hr; metabolized in liver; excreted in bile, urine

⚘ Drug interactions of concern to dentistry:

• Nephrotoxicity: possible risk with indomethacin, NSAIDs

• Decreased antihypertensive effect: possible risk with NSAIDs, indomethacin

• Decreased effect of folic acid

DENTAL CONSIDERATIONS
General:
• Limit use of sodium-containing products, such as saline IV fluids, for those patients with a dietary salt restriction.
• Assess salivary flow as a factor in caries, periodontal disease, and candidiasis.
• Take vital signs every appointment due to cardiovascular effects and possible hyperkalemia.
• Patients on chronic drug therapy may rarely have symptoms of blood dyscrasias, which can include infection, bleeding, and poor healing.
Consultations:
• In a patient with symptoms of blood dyscrasias, request a medical consult for blood studies and postpone dental treatment until normal values are reestablished.
• Medical consult may be required to assess disease control.
Teach patient/family:
• Importance of good oral hygiene to prevent soft tissue inflammation
• Caution to prevent injury when using oral hygiene aids
• To report oral lesions, soreness, or bleeding to dentist
When chronic dry mouth occurs, advise patient:
• To avoid mouth rinses with high alcohol content due to drying effects
• Of need for daily use of home fluoride products to prevent caries
• To use sugarless gum, frequent sips of water, or saliva substitutes

triazolam
(trye-ay′zoe-lam)
Halcion
✦ Apo-Triazo, Gen-Triazolam, Novo-Triolam, Nu-Triazo
Drug class.: Benzodiazepine, sedative-hypnotic

Controlled Substance Schedule IV, Canada F
Action: Produces CNS depression by interacting with a benzodiazepine receptor to facilitate the action of the inhibitory neurotransmitter γ-aminobutyric acid (GABA)
Uses: Insomnia; unapproved: oral sedation of anxious dental patients
Dosage and routes:
• *Adult:* PO 0.125-0.5 mg hs
• *Elderly:* PO 0.125-0.25 mg hs
Available forms include: Tabs 0.125, 0.25 mg
Side effects/adverse reactions:
▼ *ORAL:* Dry mouth
CNS: Headache, lethargy, drowsiness, daytime sedation, dizziness, confusion, light-headedness, anxiety, irritability, amnesia, poor coordination
CV: Chest pain, pulse changes
GI: Nausea, vomiting, diarrhea, heartburn, abdominal pain, constipation
HEMA: Leukopenia, granulocytopenia (rare)
Contraindications: Hypersensitivity to benzodiazepines, pregnancy category X, lactation, intermittent porphyria, ketoconazole, itraconazole, cisapride, ritonavir, indinavir, nelfinavir
Precautions: Anemia, hepatic disease, renal disease, suicidal individuals, drug abuse, elderly, psy-

chosis, child <15 yr, acute narrow-angle glaucoma, seizure disorders

Pharmacokinetics:

PO: Onset 30-45 min, duration 6-8 hr, half-life 2-3 hr; metabolized by liver; excreted by kidneys (inactive metabolites); crosses placenta; excreted in breast milk

Drug interactions of concern to dentistry:

• Increased effects: erythromycin
• Increased sedation: alcohol, CNS depressants, opioid analgesics, diltiazem, anesthetics
• Avoid use with ketoconazole, itraconazole, ritonavir, indinavir, nelfinavir
• Caution if used with fluvoxamine, reduce dose by 50%

DENTAL CONSIDERATIONS

General:

• Assess salivary flow as a factor in caries, periodontal disease, and candidiasis.
• If dizziness occurs, provide assistance when escorting patient to and from dental chair.
• When used for conscious sedation, have someone drive patient to and from dental office.
• Avoid the use of this drug in a patient with a history of drug abuse or alcoholism.
• Geriatric patients are more susceptible to drug effects; use a lower dose.
• Psychologic and physical dependence may occur with chronic administration.
• Determine why the patient is taking the drug.
• Patients on chronic drug therapy may rarely have symptoms of blood dyscrasias, which can include infection, bleeding, and poor healing.

Teach patient/family: *When chronic dry mouth occurs, advise patient:*

• To avoid mouth rinses with high alcohol content due to drying effects
• Of need for daily use of home fluoride products to prevent caries
• To use sugarless gum, frequent sips of water, or saliva substitutes

---

trifluoperazine HCl

(trye-floo-oh-per'a-zeen)

Stelazine

♣ Apo-Trifluoperazine, Novo-Flurazine, PMS-Trifluoperazine, Solazine, Terfluzine

Drug class.: Phenothiazine antipsychotic

Action: Blocks neurotransmission at dopaminergic synapses in the cerebral cortex, hypothalamus, and limbic system; exhibits strong peripheral α-adrenergic, anticholinergic blocking action; mechanism for antipsychotic effects is unclear

Uses: Psychotic disorders, nonpsychotic anxiety, schizophrenia

Dosage and routes:

Psychotic disorders

• *Adult:* PO 2-5 mg bid, usual range 15-20 mg/day, may require 40 mg/day or more; IM 1-2 mg q4-6h
• *Child >6 yr:* PO 1 mg qd or bid; IM not recommended for children, but 1 mg may be given qd or bid

Nonpsychotic anxiety

• *Adult:* PO 1-2 mg bid, not to exceed 5 mg/day; do not give longer than 12 wk

---

Available forms include: Tabs 1, 2, 5, 10 mg; conc 10 mg/ml; inj IM 2 mg/ml

Side effects/adverse reactions:

▼ *ORAL:* Dry mouth

CNS: Extrapyramidal symptoms: pseudoparkinsonism, akathisia, dystonia, tardive dyskinesia, seizures, headache, lichenoid reaction

CV: Orthostatic hypotension, hypertension, **cardiac arrest,** ECG changes, **tachycardia**

GI: Nausea, vomiting, anorexia, constipation, diarrhea, jaundice, weight gain

RESP: **Laryngospasm,** dyspnea, **respiratory depression**

HEMA: Anemia, **leukopenia, leukocytosis, agranulocytosis**

GU: Urinary retention, enuresis, impotence, amenorrhea, gynecomastia

EENT: Blurred vision, glaucoma, dry eyes

INTEG: Rash, photosensitivity, dermatitis

Contraindications: Hypersensitivity, cardiovascular disease, coma, blood dyscrasias, severe hepatic disease, child <6 yr, glaucoma

Precautions: Breast cancer, seizure disorders, pregnancy category C, lactation, diabetes mellitus, respiratory conditions, prostatic hypertrophy

Pharmacokinetics:

PO: Onset rapid, peak 2-3 hr, duration 12 hr

IM: Onset immediate, peak 1 hr, duration 12 hr

Metabolized by liver, excreted in urine, crosses placenta, excreted in breast milk

Drug interactions of concern to dentistry:

• Increased sedation: other CNS depressants, alcohol, barbiturate anesthetics, opioid analgesics

• Hypotension, tachycardia: epinephrine

• Increased extrapyramidal effects: phenothiazines and related drugs (haloperidol, droperidol), metoclopramide

• Additive photosensitization: tetracyclines

• Increased anticholinergic effects: anticholinergics

DENTAL CONSIDERATIONS

General:

• Monitor vital signs every appointment due to cardiovascular side effects.

• Patients on chronic drug therapy may rarely have symptoms of blood dyscrasias, which can include infection, bleeding, and poor healing.

• After supine positioning, have patient sit upright for at least 2 min before standing to avoid orthostatic hypotension.

• Assess salivary flow as a factor in caries, periodontal disease, and candidiasis.

• Avoid dental light in patient's eyes; offer dark glasses for patient comfort.

• Assess for presence of extrapyramidal motor symptoms, such as tardive dyskinesia and akathisia. Extrapyramidal motor activity may complicate dental treatment.

• Geriatric patients are more susceptible to drug effects; use lower dose.

• Use vasoconstrictors with caution, in low doses, and with careful aspiration.

Consultations:

• In a patient with symptoms of blood dyscrasias, request a medical consult for blood studies and postpone dental treatment until normal values are reestablished.

• Take precautions if dental surgery is anticipated and anesthesia is required.

• Physician should be informed if significant xerostomic side effects occur (increased caries, sore tongue, problems eating or swallowing, difficulty wearing prosthesis) so a medication change can be considered.

• If signs of tardive dyskinesia or akathisia are present, refer to physician.

Teach patient/family:

• Importance of good oral hygiene to prevent soft tissue inflammation

• Caution to prevent injury when using oral hygiene aids

• To use electric toothbrush if patient has difficulty holding conventional devices

When chronic dry mouth occurs, advise patient:

• To use daily home fluoride products for anticaries effect

• To avoid mouth rinses with high alcohol content due to drying effects

• To use sugarless gum, frequent sips of water, or saliva substitutes

---

triflupromazine HCl
(trye-floo-proe'ma-zeen)
Vesprin

Drug class.: Phenothiazine, antipsychotic

Action: Blocks neurotransmission at dopaminergic synapses in the cerebral cortex, hypothalamus, and limbic system; exhibits strong peripheral α-adrenergic, anticholinergic blocking action; mechanism for antipsychotic effects is unclear

Uses: Psychotic disorders, schizophrenia, acute agitation, nausea, vomiting

Dosage and routes:

Psychosis

• *Adult:* IM 60 mg; not to exceed 150 mg/day

• *Child >2.5 yr:* IM 0.2-0.25 mg/kg to max total dose of 10 mg/day

Nausea/vomiting

• *Adult:* IM 5-15 mg q4h, max 60 mg qd; IV 1 mg, max 3 mg/day

• *Child >2.5 yr:* IM 0.2 mg/kg, max 10 mg qd; do not give IV to child

Available forms include: Inj IM/IV 10, 20 mg/ml

Side effects/adverse reactions:

▼ *ORAL:* Dry mouth, metallic taste, lichenoid reaction

*CNS: Extrapyramidal symptoms: pseudoparkinsonism, akathisia, dystonia, tardive dyskinesia, drowsiness, headache, **seizures***

*CV: Orthostatic hypotension, hypertension, **cardiac arrest,** ECG changes, **tachycardia***

GI: Nausea, vomiting, anorexia, constipation, diarrhea, jaundice, weight gain

*RESP: **Laryngospasm,** dyspnea, **respiratory depression***

*HEMA: Anemia, **leukopenia, leukocytosis, agranulocytosis***

GU: Urinary retention, urinary frequency, enuresis, impotence, amenorrhea, gynecomastia

EENT: Blurred vision, glaucoma

INTEG: Rash, photosensitivity, dermatitis

Contraindications: Hypersensitivity, blood dyscrasias, coma, child <2.5 yr, brain damage, bone marrow depression

Precautions: Pregnancy category C, lactation, seizure disorders, hepatic disease, cardiac disease

---

bold italic = life-threatening conditions

Pharmacokinetics:

IV/IM: Onset erratic, peak 2-4 hr, duration 4-6 hr

IM: Onset 15-30 min, peak 15-20 min, duration 4-6 hr

Metabolized by liver; excreted in urine, feces; crosses placenta; excreted in breast milk

🦷 Drug interactions of concern to dentistry:

• Oversedation: other CNS depressants, opioid analgesics, alcohol, barbiturate anesthetics

• Hypotension, tachycardia: epinephrine

• Increased anticholinergic effects: anticholinergics

• Increased photosensitivity: tetracyclines

• Increased extrapyramidal effects: phenothiazines and related drugs (haloperidol, droperidol), metoclopramide

DENTAL CONSIDERATIONS

General:

• The primary use of this drug is to control nausea/vomiting, which may preclude elective dental therapy.

• Assess salivary flow as a factor in caries, periodontal disease, and candidiasis.

• Examine for evidence of blood dyscrasias (infection, bleeding, poor healing).

• After supine positioning, have patient sit upright for at least 2 min before standing to avoid orthostatic hypotension.

• Assess for the presence of extrapyramidal motor symptoms such as tardive dyskinesia and akathisia. Extrapyramidal motor activity may complicate dental treatment.

• Avoid dental light in patient's eyes; offer dark glasses for patient comfort.

• Monitor vital signs every appointment due to cardiovascular side effects.

• Geriatric patients are more susceptible to drug effects; use a lower dose.

• Use vasoconstrictors with caution, in low doses, and with careful aspiration.

• Take precautions if dental surgery is anticipated and anesthesia is required.

Consultations:

• Medical consult for blood studies (CBC); leukopenic and thrombocytopenic side effects may result in infection, delayed healing, and excessive bleeding. Postpone dental treatment until normal values are maintained.

• If signs of tardive dyskinesia or akathisia are present, refer to physician.

Teach patient/family:

• Importance of good oral hygiene to prevent soft tissue inflammation

• Use of electric toothbrush if patient has difficulty holding conventional devices

• Caution in use of oral hygiene aids to prevent injury

This drug will not be used chronically; however, *when chronic dry mouth occurs, advise patient:*

• To avoid mouth rinses with high alcohol content due to drying effects

• Of need for daily use of home fluoride products to prevent caries

• To use sugarless gum, frequent sips of water, or saliva substitutes

trifluridine (ophthalmic)

(trye-flure'i-deen)
Viroptic Ophthalmic Solution
Drug class.: Antiviral

Action: Inhibits viral DNA synthesis and replication
Uses: Primary keratoconjunctivitis, recurring epithelial keratitis, keratitis associated with herpes simplex virus types 1 and 2, and viccinia virus
Dosage and routes:
• *Adult and child >6 yr:* Instill 1 gtt q2h while awake, not to exceed 9 gtt/day, until corneal epithelium regrows; then 1 gtt q4h × 1 wk
Available forms include: Sol 1% in 7.5 ml container
Side effects/adverse reactions:
EENT: Burning, stinging, swelling, photophobia
Contraindications: Hypersensitivity
Precautions: Antibiotic hypersensitivity, pregnancy category C
🦷 **Drug interactions of concern to dentistry:**
• None reported
DENTAL CONSIDERATIONS
General:
• Protect patient's eyes from accidental spatter during dental treatment.
• Avoid dental light in patient's eyes; offer dark glasses for patient comfort.
Evaluate:
• Therapeutic response: absence of redness, inflammation, tearing
• Allergy: itching, lacrimation, redness, swelling

trihexyphenidyl HCl

(trye-hex-ee-fen'i-dil)
Trihexy-2
🍁 Apo-Trihex, Artane, PMS-Trihexyphenidyl

Drug class.: Antiparkinsonian, anticholinergic

Action: Blocks central muscarinic receptors, decreasing the severity of involuntary movements
Uses: Parkinson symptoms
Dosage and routes:
Parkinson symptoms
• *Adult:* PO 1 mg, increased by 2 mg q3-5d to a total of 6-10 mg/day
Drug-induced extrapyramidal symptoms
• *Adult:* PO 1 mg/day; usual dose 5-15 mg/day
Available forms include: Tabs 2, 5 mg; sus rel caps 5 mg; elix 2 mg/5 ml
Side effects/adverse reactions:
▼ *ORAL: Dry mouth,* soreness of mouth or tongue
CNS: Confusion, anxiety, restlessness, irritability, delusions, hallucinations, headache, sedation, depression, incoherence, dizziness, flushing, weakness
CV: Palpitation, tachycardia, postural hypotension
*GI: Constipation, **paralytic ileus,** nausea, vomiting, abdominal distress
GU: Hesitancy, retention
EENT: Blurred vision, photophobia, dilated pupils, difficulty swallowing
INTEG: Urticaria, rash
MS: Weakness, cramping
MISC: Suppression of lactation,

---

nasal congestion, decreased sweating, increased temperature

Contraindications: Hypersensitivity, narrow-angle glaucoma, myasthenia gravis, GI/GU obstruction, tachycardia, myocardial ischemia, unstable CV disease

Precautions: Pregnancy category C, children, gastric ulcer

Pharmacokinetics:

PO: Onset 1 hr, peak 2-3 hr, duration 6-12 hr; excreted in urine

👣 Drug interactions of concern to dentistry:

• Increased anticholinergic effects: scopolamine, atropine, phenothiazines, antihistamines, and other anticholinergics

• Increased CNS depression: alcohol, CNS depressants

• Decreased effects of phenothiazines

DENTAL CONSIDERATIONS

General:

• Assess salivary flow as a factor in caries, periodontal disease, and candidiasis.

• Place on frequent recall due to oral side effects.

• After supine positioning, have patient sit upright for at least 2 min before standing to avoid orthostatic hypotension.

• Avoid dental light in patient's eyes; offer dark glasses for patient comfort.

Teach patient/family:

• Importance of good oral hygiene to prevent soft tissue inflammation

• To use electric toothbrush if patient has difficulty holding conventional devices

When chronic dry mouth occurs, advise patient:

• To avoid mouth rinses with high alcohol content due to drying effects

• Of need for daily use of home fluoride products to prevent caries

• To use sugarless gum, frequent sips of water, or saliva substitutes

---

trimethadione

(trye-meth-a-dye′one)

Tridione

Drug class.: Anticonvulsant

Action: Increases the threshold for seizures initiated in the cortex, decreases CNS synaptic stimulation to low-frequency impulses

Uses: Refractory absence (petit mal) seizures

Dosage and routes:

• *Adult:* PO 300 mg tid; may increase by 300 mg/wk, not to exceed 600 mg qid

• *Child >6 yr:* PO 0.9 g/day in divided doses tid or qid

• *Child 2-6 yr:* PO 0.6 g/day in divided doses tid or qid

• *Child <2 yr:* PO 0.3 g/day in divided doses tid or qid

Available forms include: Caps 300 mg; chew tabs 150 mg

Side effects/adverse reactions:

▼ *ORAL: Bleeding gums*

CNS: Drowsiness, dizziness, fatigue, paresthesia, irritability, headache, insomnia, myasthenia gravis syndrome

CV: Hypertension, hypotension

GI: Nausea, vomiting, abnormal liver function tests

HEMA: **Thrombocytopenia, agranulocytosis, leukopenia, neutropenia, hemolytic anemia, eosinophilia, aplastic anemia,** increased pro-time

GU: **Fatal nephrosis,** vaginal bleeding, albuminuria, nephrosis, abdominal pain, weight loss

EENT: Photophobia, diplopia, epi-

---

staxis, retinal hemorrhage, scotomata, hemeralopia

INTEG: **Exfoliative dermatitis,** rash, alopecia, petechiae, erythema

Contraindications: Hypersensitivity, blood dyscrasias, pregnancy category D

Precautions: Hepatic disease, renal disease, retinal disease, porphyria, lactation, systemic lupus erythematosus

Pharmacokinetics:

PO: Peak 30 min-2 hr, half-life 10 days; excreted by kidneys

Drug interactions of concern to dentistry:

• Increased CNS depression: all CNS depressants

DENTAL CONSIDERATIONS
General:

• Short appointments and a stress reduction protocol may be required for anxious patients.

• Determine type of epilepsy, seizure frequency, and quality of seizure control. A stress reduction protocol may be required.

• Patients on chronic drug therapy may rarely have symptoms of blood dyscrasias, which can include infection, bleeding, and poor healing.

• Avoid dental light in patient's eyes; offer dark glasses for patient comfort.

• Place on frequent recall due to oral side effects.

• Monitor vital signs every appointment due to cardiovascular side effects.

Consultations:

• Obtain a medical consult for blood studies (CBC) because leukopenic and thrombocytopenic effects of drug may result in infection, delayed healing, and excessive bleeding. Dental treatment should be postponed until normal values are maintained.

• Medical consult may be required to assess disease control and patient's ability to tolerate stress.

Teach patient/family:

• Importance of good oral hygiene to prevent soft tissue inflammation

• To prevent trauma when using oral hygiene aids

---

trimethobenzamide
(trye-meth-oh-ben′za-mide)
Pediatric Triban, T-Gen, Tigan
Drug class.: Antiemetic

Action: Acts centrally by blocking chemoreceptor trigger zone, which in turn acts on vomiting center

Uses: Nausea, vomiting, prevention of postoperative vomiting

Dosage and routes:

Postoperative vomiting

• *Adult:* IM/rec 200 mg before or during surgery; may repeat 3 hr after

Discontinuing anesthesia

• *Child 13-40 kg:* PO/rec 100-200 mg tid-qid

• *Child <13 kg:* PO/rec 100 mg tid-qid

Nausea/vomiting

• *Adult:* PO 250 mg tid-qid; IM/rec 200 mg tid-qid

Available forms include: Caps 100, 250 mg; supp 100, 200 mg; inj IM 100 mg/ml

Side effects/adverse reactions:

▼ *ORAL:* Dry mouth

CNS: Drowsiness, restlessness, headache, dizziness, insomnia, confusion, nervousness, tingling, *vertigo,* extrapyramidal symptoms

CV: Hypertension, hypotension, palpitation

T

---

bold italic = life-threatening conditions

GI: Nausea, anorexia, diarrhea, vomiting, constipation

EENT: Blurred vision, diplopia, nasal congestion, photosensitivity

INTEG: Rash, urticaria, fever, chills, flushing

Contraindications: Hypersensitivity, shock, children (parenterally)

Precautions: Children, cardiac dysrhythmias, elderly, asthma, pregnancy category C, prostatic hypertrophy, bladder neck obstruction, narrow-angle glaucoma, stenosing peptic ulcer, pyloroduodenal obstruction

Pharmacokinetics:
PO: Onset 20-40 min, duration 34 hr
IM: Onset 15 min, duration 2-3 hr
Metabolized by liver, excreted by kidneys

🦷 Drug interactions of concern to dentistry:
• Increased effect: CNS depressants
• May mask ototoxic symptoms associated with antibiotics or large doses of salicylates

DENTAL CONSIDERATIONS
General:
• Nausea and vomiting may be accompanied by dehydration and electrolyte imbalance and should be corrected as part of treatment.
• Defer elective dental treatment when symptoms are present.

---

trimetrexate glucuronate
(tri-me-trex′ate)
Neutrexin
Drug class.: Folate antagonist

Action: Inhibits the enzyme dihydrofolate reductase, leading to interference with DNA, RNA, and protein synthesis in the *P. carinii* organism

Uses: Alternative therapy for *P. carinii* pneumonia in immunocompromised patients, including patients with AIDS; unapproved: lung, prostate, colon cancer

Dosage and routes:
Must be given concurrently with leucovorin
• *Adult:* IV inf 45 mg/m^2 once daily over 60-90 min; leucovorin is given IV 20 mg/m^2 over 5-10 min q6h for total dose of 80 mg/m^2; course of treatment is 21 days with trimetrexate and 24 days with leucovorin

Available forms include: IV 25 mg/5 ml vials with or without 50 mg leucovorin

Side effects/adverse reactions:
▼ *ORAL:* Oral ulceration if leucovorin is not used
*GI: Nausea, vomiting, **hepatotoxicity,** mucosal ulceration*
HEMA: Thrombocytopenia (<75,000/mm^3), anemia (Hgb <8 g/dl)
GU: Renal toxicity
INTEG: Rash, pruritus
MISC: Hyponatremia, hypocalcemia

Contraindications: Hypersensitivity to trimetrexate, methotrexate, or leucovorin

Precautions: Pregnancy category D, lactation, child <18 yr; impaired hematologic, renal, or hepatic function; serious bone marrow depression can occur if leucovorin is not used concurrently

Pharmacokinetics:
IV: Extended plasma levels up to 72 hr; highly plasma protein bound 95%-98%; hepatic metabolism; renal excretion

Drug interactions of concern to dentistry:

• Alteration of plasma levels: concurrent use with erythromycin, ketoconazole, and fluconazole
• Alteration in trimetrexate metabolites: acetaminophen

DENTAL CONSIDERATIONS
General:
• Examine for evidence of oral manifestations of blood dyscrasia (infection, bleeding, poor healing).
• Place on frequent recall due to oral side effects.
• Determine why the patient is taking the drug.
• Examine for oral manifestations of opportunistic infections.
• Consider local hemostasis measures to prevent excessive bleeding.
• Palliative treatment may be required for stomatitis.
• Refer to physician if oral ulcerative lesions occur.
• Consider semisupine chair position for patient comfort due to GI effects of disease.

Consultations:
• Obtain a medical consult for blood studies (CBC) because leukopenic or thrombocytopenic side effects may result in infection, delayed healing, and excessive bleeding. Postpone elective dental treatment until normal values are maintained.
• Medical consult may be required to assess disease control.

Teach patient/family:
• Importance of good oral hygiene to prevent soft tissue inflammation
• Caution to prevent injury when using oral hygiene aids
• That secondary oral infection may occur; must see dentist immediately if infection occurs

trimipramine maleate
(tri-mi'pra-meen)
Surmontil
♣ Apo-Trimip,　　Novo-Trimipramine, Rhotrimine

Drug class.: Antidepressant—tricyclic

Action: Inhibits both norepinephrine and serotonin (5-HT) uptake in the brain, although the precise antidepressant mechanism remains unclear
Uses: Depression, enuresis in children; unapproved: chronic pain, burning mouth syndrome
Dosage and routes:
• *Adult:* PO 75 mg/day in divided doses; may be increased to 200 mg/day
• *Child >6 yr:* PO 25 mg hs; may increase to 50 mg in children <12 yr or 75 mg in children >12 yr
Available forms include: Caps 25, 50, 100 mg
Side effects/adverse reactions:
▼ *ORAL: Dry mouth,* unpleasant taste
CNS: Dizziness, drowsiness, confusion, headache, anxiety, tremors, stimulation, weakness, insomnia, nightmares, EPS (elderly), increase in psychiatric symptoms
CV: Orthostatic hypotension, ECG changes, tachycardia, **hypertension,** palpitation
GI: Diarrhea, **paralytic ileus, hepatitis,** increased appetite, nausea, vomiting, cramps, epigastric distress, jaundice
HEMA: **Agranulocytosis, thrombocytopenia, eosinophilia, leukopenia**
GU: Retention, **acute renal failure**

---

bold italic = life-threatening conditions　　*For periodic updates, visit* **www.mosby.com**

EENT: Blurred vision, tinnitus, mydriasis

INTEG: Rash, urticaria, sweating, pruritus, photosensitivity

Contraindications: Hypersensitivity to tricyclic antidepressants, recovery phase of MI, convulsive disorders, prostatic hypertrophy

Precautions: Suicidal patients, severe depression, increased intraocular pressure, narrow-angle glaucoma, urinary retention, cardiac disease, hepatic disease, hyperthyroidism, electroshock therapy, elective surgery, pregnancy category C, MAO inhibitors

Pharmacokinetics:

PO: Steady state 2-6 days, half-life 7-30 hr; metabolized by liver; excreted by kidneys

Drug interactions of concern to dentistry:

• Increased anticholinergic effects: muscarinic blockers, antihistamines, phenothiazines

• Increased effects of direct-acting sympathomimetics (epinephrine, levonordefrin)

• Possible risk of increased CNS depression: alcohol, barbiturates, benzodiazepines, and other CNS depressants

• Decreased antihypertensive effects: clonidine, guanadrel, guanethidine

DENTAL CONSIDERATIONS
General:

• Take vital signs every appointment due to cardiovascular side effects.

• Assess salivary flow as a factor in caries, periodontal disease, and candidiasis.

• Patients on chronic drug therapy may rarely have symptoms of blood dyscrasias, which can include infection, bleeding, and poor healing.

• After supine positioning, have patient sit upright for at least 2 min to avoid orthostatic hypotension.

• Use vasoconstrictors with caution, in low doses, and with careful aspiration. Avoid use of gingival retraction cord with epinephrine.

• Place on frequent recall due to oral side effects.

Consultations:

• In a patient with symptoms of blood dyscrasias, request a medical consult for blood studies and postpone dental treatment until normal values are reestablished.

• Medical consult may be required to assess disease control.

• Physician should be informed if significant xerostomic side effects occur (increased caries, sore tongue, problems eating or swallowing, difficulty wearing prosthesis) so a medication change can be considered.

Teach patient/family:

• Importance of good oral hygiene to prevent soft tissue inflammation

• Caution to prevent injury when using oral hygiene aids

When chronic dry mouth occurs, advise patient:

• To avoid mouth rinses with high alcohol content due to drying effects

• Of need for daily use of home fluoride products to prevent caries

• To use sugarless gum, frequent sips of water, or saliva substitutes

---

tripelennamine HCl

(tri-pel-en'a-meen)
PBZ, PBZ-SR
Drug class.: Antihistamine, H$_1$-receptor antagonist

Action: Acts by competing with histamine for H$_1$-receptor sites; decreases allergic response by blocking histamine effects

Uses: Rhinitis, allergy symptoms

Dosage and routes:
• *Adult:* PO 25-50 mg q4-6h, not to exceed 600 mg/day; time rel 100 mg bid-tid, not to exceed 600 mg/day
• *Child >5 yr:* Time rel 50 mg q8-12h, not to exceed 300 mg/day
• *Child <5 yr:* PO 5 mg/kg/day in 4-6 divided doses, not to exceed 300 mg/day

Available forms include: Tabs 25, 50 mg; time rel tabs 100 mg

Side effects/adverse reactions:
▼ *ORAL:* Dry mouth
CNS: Dizziness, drowsiness, poor coordination, fatigue, anxiety, euphoria, confusion, paresthesia, neuritis
CV: Hypotension, palpitation, tachycardia
GI: Constipation, nausea, vomiting, anorexia, diarrhea
RESP: Increased thick secretions, wheezing, chest tightness
HEMA: **Thrombocytopenia, agranulocytosis, hemolytic anemia**
GU: Retention, dysuria, frequency
EENT: Blurred vision, dilated pupils, tinnitus, nasal stuffiness, dry nose/throat
INTEG: Rash, urticaria, photosensitivity

Contraindications: Hypersensitivity to H$_1$-receptor antagonist, acute asthma attack, lower respiratory tract disease

Precautions: Dental patients with chronic dry mouth, increased intraocular pressure, renal disease, cardiac disease, hypertension, bronchial asthma, seizure disorder, stenosed peptic ulcers, hyperthyroidism, prostatic hypertrophy, bladder neck obstruction, pregnancy category C

Pharmacokinetics:
PO: Onset 15-30 min, duration 4-6 hr; detoxified in liver; excreted by kidneys

Drug interactions of concern to dentistry:
• Increased CNS depression: CNS depressants, barbiturates, narcotics, hypnotics, tricyclic antidepressants, alcohol
• Increased photosensitization: tetracyclines
• Increased anticholinergic effects: muscarinic blockers

DENTAL CONSIDERATIONS
General:
• Assess salivary flow as a factor in caries, periodontal disease, and candidiasis.
• Patients on chronic drug therapy may rarely have symptoms of blood dyscrasias, which can include infection, bleeding, and poor healing.
• Consider semisupine chair position for patients with respiratory disease.
• Monitor vital signs every appointment due to cardiovascular side effects.

Teach patient/family: *When chronic dry mouth occurs, advise patient:*
• To avoid mouth rinses with high

---

bold italic = life-threatening conditions

alcohol content due to drying effects
• Of need for daily use of home fluoride products to prevent caries
• To use sugarless gum, frequent sips of water, or saliva substitutes

---

trovafloxacin mesylate/ alatrofloxacin mesylate

(troe′va-flox-a-sin) (ala-troe′flox-a-sin)

Trovafloxacin mesylate oral: Trovan

Alatrofloxacin mesylate injection: Trovan I.V.

Drug class.: A fluoronaphthyridone antiinfective (related to the fluoroquinolones)

Action: A broad-spectrum bactericidal agent that inhibits the enzymes topoisomerase II (DNA gyrase) and topoisomerase IV required for bacterial DNA replication, transcription repair, and recombination

Uses: For infections caused by susceptible microorganisms in nosocomial pneumonia, community-acquired pneumonia, acute bacterial exacerbated chronic bronchitis, acute sinusitis, abdominal infections, gynecologic infections, UTI, bacterial prostatitis, skin and skin structure infections, and selected STDs

Dosage and routes:
• *Adult >18 yr:* PO dose depends on type of infection; range 100-200 mg daily for 1-14 days; IV dose depends on type of infection; range 200-300 mg daily; single IV doses can be followed by appropriate oral doses for 10-14 days

Available forms include: Tabs 100, 200 mg; vials IV (alatrofloxacin for injection) 5 mg/ml in 40 and 60 ml

Side effects/adverse reactions:

▼ *ORAL:* Dry mouth, stomatitis, angular cheilitis

CNS: Dizziness, headache, lightheadedness, confusion, anxiety, hallucinations

CV: Hypotension, palpitation, flushing, peripheral edema, chest pain

GI: Vomiting, nausea, diarrhea, abdominal pain, flatulence, ***antibiotic-associated pseudomembranous colitis***

RESP: Dyspnea, bronchospasm, coughing

HEMA: Anemia, leukopenia, thrombocytopenia

GU: Vaginitis, frequency of urination, abnormal renal function

EENT: Rhinitis, sinusitis

INTEG: Pruritus, rash, photosensitization

META: Increased liver enzymes

MS: Arthralgia, myalgia, muscle cramps

MISC: Pain on injection, increased sweating, fatigue, fever, ***anaphylaxis***

Contraindications: Hypersensitivity and allergy to the fluoroquinolones

Precautions: Children <18 yr, mild to moderate cirrhosis, potential for liver damage, exposure to sunlight, visible or ultraviolet radiation, seizure disorders, cerebral atherosclerosis, pregnancy category C, lactation

Pharmacokinetics:

PO: Good oral absorption, bioavailability 88%, can be administered with food, peak serum levels 1.7 hr, plasma protein binding 76%, wide tissue distribution, excreted in breast milk, hepatic metabolism, excreted in feces and urine, 50% of dose is excreted unchanged in feces

IV: Alatrofloxacin is a prodrug converted to trovafloxacin

⚕ Drug interactions of concern to dentistry:

• Reduction in absorption: magnesium or aluminum antacid products, iron salts, sucralfate, and morphine within 30 min of oral trovafloxacin; separate doses by at least 2 hr

• Increases serum levels of caffeine

DENTAL CONSIDERATIONS
General:

• Determine why patient is taking the drug; specific infection.

• Do not use ingestible sodium bicarbonate products, such as the air polishing system (Prophy Jet), within 2 hr of drug use.

• Examine for oral manifestation of opportunistic infection.

• Avoid dental light in patient's eyes; offer dark glasses for patient comfort.

• Use caution in prescribing caffeine-containing analgesics.

Consultations:

• Medical consult may be required to assess disease control.

• Consult with patient's physician if an acute dental infection occurs and another antiinfective is required.

Teach patient/family:

• To prevent trauma when using oral hygiene aids

• Importance of good oral hygiene to prevent soft tissue inflammation

• To avoid mouth rinses with high alcohol content due to drying effects

unoprostone isopropyl
(yoo-noe-pros'tone)
Rescula
Drug class.: Prostaglandin agonist

Action: Reduces elevated intraocular pressure by increasing the outflow of aqueous humor; the precise mechanism is unknown

Uses: Indicated for lowering IOP in patients with open-angle glaucoma, or ocular hypertension who are intolerant to other medications or who failed to achieve a targeted IOP

Dosage and routes:

• *Adult:* TOP 1 gtt in affected eye(s) bid (caution with contact lens; may be inserted 15 min after applying drop)

Available forms include: Ophth sol 0.15% in 5 ml

Side effects/adverse reactions:

CNS: Dizziness, headache, insomnia

CV: Hypertension

RESP: Bronchitis, cough

EENT: Dry eyes, stinging, burning, itching, increased eyelash length, abnormal vision, lacrimation, foreign body sensation, rhinitis, sinusitis

MS: Back pain

MISC: Flulike syndrome, allergic reaction

Contraindications: Hypersensitivity to unoprostone isopropyl, benzalkonium chloride, or other ingredients contained in the solution

Precautions: Permanent changes in pigmented tissues of eye, bacterial keratitis, do not use while wearing contact lens, no data on

u

use in renal or hepatic failure or pediatric patients, pregnancy category C

Pharmacokinetics:

TOP: Little systemic absorption is reported; plasma T½ = 14 min, metabolites excreted in urine

Drug interactions of concern to dentistry:

• None reported; avoid use of anticholinergic drugs: atropine-like drugs, propantheline, diazepam, other benzodiazepines

DENTAL CONSIDERATIONS

General:

• Check compliance of patient with prescribed drug regimen for glaucoma.

• Protect patient's eyes from accidental spatter during dental treatment.

• Avoid dental light in patient's eyes; offer dark glasses for patient comfort.

Consultations:

• Medical consult may be required to assess disease control.

---

ursodiol

(er'soe-dye-ole)

Actigall

Drug class.: Gallstone solubilizing agent

Action: Suppresses hepatic synthesis, secretion of cholesterol; inhibits intestinal absorption of cholesterol

Uses: Dissolution of radiolucent, noncalcified gallbladder stones (<20 mm in diameter) in which surgery is not indicated; prevent gallstones in obese patients experiencing rapid weight loss

Dosage and routes:

• *Adult:* PO 8-10 mg/kg/day in 2-3 divided doses using gallbladder ultrasound q6mo; determine if stones have dissolved; if so, continue therapy and repeat ultrasound within 1-3 mo

Gallstone prevention

• *Adult:* PO 300 mg bid for 4-6 mo

Available forms include: Caps 300 mg

Side effects/adverse reactions:

▼ *ORAL:* Metallic taste, stomatitis

CNS: Headache, anxiety, depression, insomnia, fatigue

GI: Diarrhea, nausea, vomiting, abdominal pain, constipation, flatulence, dyspepsia, biliary pain

RESP: Cough, rhinitis

INTEG: Pruritus, rash, urticaria, dry skin, sweating, alopecia

MS: Arthralgia, myalgia, back pain

Contraindications: Calcified cholesterol stones, radiopaque stones, radiolucent bile pigment stones, chronic liver disease, hypersensitivity

Precautions: Pregnancy category B, lactation, children

Pharmacokinetics:

PO: 80% excreted in feces, 20% metabolized, excreted into bile, lost in feces

Drug interactions of concern to dentistry:

• Reduced action: aluminum-based antacids

DENTAL CONSIDERATIONS

General:

• Consider semisupine chair position for patient comfort due to GI effects of disease.

• Some opioids can cause spasm of bile duct leading to epigastric dis-

---

tress. Use caution in use for sedation or pain control. NSAIDs may be better choice.
• Consider drug as a factor in the diagnosis of altered taste.

---

valacyclovir HCl
(val-ay-sye′kloe-veer)
Valtrex, Zelitrex (Europe)
Drug class.: Antiviral

Action: Converted to acyclovir, which interferes with DNA synthesis required for viral replication
Uses: Herpes zoster in immunocompetent patients, genital herpes, recurrent genital herpes
Dosage and routes:
Initial herpes infection
• *Adult:* PO 1 g tid × 7 days with or without meals
Recurrent genital herpes treatment
• *Adult:* PO 500 mg bid × 5 days
Available forms include: Caps 500 mg, 1 g
Side effects/adverse reactions:
▼ *ORAL:* Glossitis, medication taste; although unknown for this drug, lichenoid drug reactions are reported with acyclovir
CNS: Headache, ***convulsions,*** tremors, confusion, lethargy, hallucinations, dizziness
GI: Nausea, vomiting, diarrhea, increased ALT/AST, abdominal pain, colitis
*HEMA: **Bone marrow depression, granulocytopenia, thrombocytopenia, leukopenia, megaloblastic anemia,*** anemia, increased bleeding time
*GU: Vaginitis, candidiasis, **glomer-ulonephritis, acute renal failure,*** oliguria, proteinuria, hematuria, changes in menses
INTEG: Rash, urticaria, pruritus
MS: Asthenia
Contraindications: Hypersensitivity to valacyclovir or acyclovir, avoid with patients with HIV or bone marrow or renal transplants due to risk of hemolytic uremic syndrome
Precautions: Pregnancy category B, renal impairment, lactation, children; reduce dose in renal impairment
Pharmacokinetics:
PO: Rapid absorption and conversion to acyclovir, renal excretion, extensive tissue distribution
⚡ Drug interactions of concern to dentistry:
• None reported in otherwise uncompromised patients
DENTAL CONSIDERATIONS
General:
• Determine why the patient is taking the drug.
• Be aware of general discomfort associated with shingles; acute symptoms may preclude patient's routine dental visit or mandate short appointments.
• Patients on chronic drug therapy may rarely have symptoms of blood dyscrasias, which can include infection, bleeding, and poor healing.
Consultations:
• Medical consult may be required to assess disease control.
• In a patient with symptoms of blood dyscrasias, request a medical consult for blood studies and postpone dental treatment until normal values are reestablished.

Teach patient/family:
• Importance of good oral hygiene to prevent soft tissue inflammation
• Caution to prevent trauma when using oral hygiene aids

---

valdecoxib

(val-de-kox'-ib)
Bextra

Drug class: Nonsteroidal antiinflammatory analgesic

Action: Mechanism of action is thought related to the inhibition of cyclooxygenase-2 (COX-2); appears to have antiinflammatory, analgesic, and antipyretic activity

Uses: Relief of signs and symptoms of osteoarthritis and adult rheumatoid arthritis, treatment of primary dysmenorrhea

Dosage and routes:
Osteoarthritis and adult rheumatoid arthritis
• *Adult:* PO 10 mg daily
Primary dysmenorrhea
• *Adult:* PO 20 mg bid
Available forms include: Tabs 10, 20 mg

Side effects/adverse reactions:
▼ *ORAL:* Dry mouth, taste alteration
CNS: Dizziness, headache, neuralgia, tremor, vertigo
CV: Peripheral edema, hypertension, some irregularities in heart rate
GI: Abdominal pain, diarrhea, dyspepsia, flatulence, nausea
RESP: URI
HEMA: Anemia, thrombocytopenia
GU: Menstrual irregularities
EENT: Sinusitis, ear ache
INTEG: Rash, dermatitis, pruritus
ENDO: Elevated liver enzymes, AST, ALT

MS: Back pain, myalgia
MISC: Flulike symptoms, allergic reactions

Contraindications: Hypersensitivity; patients who have experienced asthma, urticaria, or allergic reactions after taking aspirin or NSAIDs

Precautions: Hepatic impairment, presence or prior history of ulcers or GI bleeding; avoid in pregnancy; fluid retention, hypertension, CHF; asthma; may increase INR in patients taking warfarin; pregnancy category C, excreted in milk; no data to support use in lactating mothers or children <18 yr

Pharmacokinetics:
PO: Absolute bioavailability 83%; food does not appear to alter absorption; peak plasma levels in approximately 3 hr; high plasma protein binding (98%); hepatic metabolism (CYP 3A4 and CYP 2C9); active metabolite; excreted as metabolites in urine

⚕ Drug interactions of concern to dentistry:
• Increased plasma levels: fluconazole, ketoconazole
• Increased risk of GI side effects: aspirin
• Decreased antihypertensive effects: diuretics, calcium channel blockers
• Decreased renal clearance of lithium

DENTAL CONSIDERATIONS
General:
• Patients on chronic drug therapy may rarely have symptoms of blood dyscrasias, which can include infection, bleeding, and poor healing.
• Use aspirin or NSAIDs with caution.

• Consider altering chair position for comfort of arthritic patients.
• Assess salivary flow as a factor in caries, periodontal disease, and candidiasis.
• Monitor vital signs at each dental appointment due to cardiovascular side effects.

Consultations:
• In a patient with symptoms of blood dyscrasias, request a medical consult for blood studies and postpone treatment until normal values are reestablished.

Teach patient/family:
• Importance of good oral hygiene to prevent soft tissue inflammation
• Importance of updating health and drug history if physician makes any changes in evaluation or drug regimens

When chronic dry mouth occurs, advise patient:
• To avoid mouth rinses with high alcohol content due to drying effects
• To use fluoride products for anti-caries effects
• To use sugarless gum, frequent sips of water, or saliva substitutes

---

valganciclovir HCl
(val-gan-sye'kloh-veer)
Valcyte
Drug class.: Antiviral

Action: The L-valyl ester is a prodrug that is rapidly converted to ganciclovir; ganciclovir is initially phosphorylated by CMV protein kinase and further phosphorylated to ganciclovir triphosphate, which inhibits viral DNA synthesis
Uses: Treatment of CMV (cytomegalovirus) retinitis in patients with AIDS

Dosage and routes:
Active CMV retinitis
• *Adult:* PO 900 mg bid for 21 days with food; dose modification required in patients with renal impairment; do not crush or break tablets
Maintenance
• *Adult:* PO 900 mg qd with food; dose modification required in patients with renal impairment; do not crush or break tablets
Available forms include: Tabs 450 mg

Side effects/adverse reactions:
CNS: Headache, insomnia, convulsions, confusion, psychosis, hallucinations, sedation
GI: Diarrhea, nausea, hepatitis, liver function disorder, vomiting
HEMA: Anemia, pancytopenia, **granulocytopenia, neutropenia, aplastic anemia, bone marrow depression, thrombocytopenia**
GU: Decreased creatinine clearance
EENT: Retinal detachment
MISC: Pyrexia, peripheral neuropathy, infections
Contraindications: Hypersensitivity to ganciclovir or acyclovir, low neutrophil, platelet or hemoglobin, patients on hemodialysis, lactation
Precautions: Renal impairment (requires dose adjustment), preexisting cytopenias, cannot be substituted for ganciclovir capsules on a one-to-one basis, pregnancy category C, >65 yr, pediatric use
Pharmacokinetics:
PO: Well absorbed, absolute bioavailability (60%), prodrug rapidly converted by hepatic and intestinal esterases to ganciclovir, slowly metabolized intracellularly, excreted in the urine

---

bold italic = life-threatening conditions

Drug interactions of concern to dentistry:
• Increased risk of blood dyscrasias: dapsone, carbamazepine, phenothiazines
• Increased risk of seizures: imipenem/cilastatin (Primaxin)
• Low platelet counts may prevent the use of aspirin, NSAIDs

DENTAL CONSIDERATIONS
General:
• Patient on chronic drug therapy may present with symptoms of blood dyscrasias, which can include infection, bleeding, and poor healing.
• Examine for oral manifestation of opportunistic infection.
• Place on frequent recall to evaluate healing response.
• Consider local hemostasis measures to control excessive bleeding.
Consultations:
• Medical consult for blood studies (CBC); leukopenic or thrombocytopenic side effects may result in infection, delayed healing, and excessive bleeding. Postpone elective dental treatment until normal values are maintained.
• Medical consult may be required to assess disease control.
Teach patient/family:
• To prevent trauma when using oral hygiene aids
• Alert the patient to the possibility of secondary oral infection and the need to see dentist immediately if signs of infection occur
• Importance of good oral hygiene to prevent soft tissue inflammation

valproic acid/valproate sodium/divalprex sodium
(val-proe′ate)
Divalproex sodium: Depakote, Depakote ER, Depakote Sprinkle
♣ Epival
Valproate sodium: Depacon
Valproic acid: Depakene
♣ Alti-Valproic, Dom-Valproic, MedValproic, Novo-Valproic, Nu-Valproic, Penta-Valproic, PMS-Valproic Acid
Drug class.: Anticonvulsant

Action: Increased levels of γ-aminobutyric acid (GABA) in the brain
Uses: Simple, complex (petit mal) absence, mixed seizures; divalproex for manic episodes in bipolar disorder, complex partial seizures, migraine prophylaxis; unapproved: tonic-clonic (grand mal) seizures

Dosage and routes:
• *Adult and child:* PO 15 mg/kg/day divided in 2-3 doses; may increase by 5-10 mg/kg/day qwk, not to exceed 30 mg/kg/day in 2-3 divided doses
Manic episodes in bipolar disorder
• *Adult:* PO initially 75 mg in divided doses; increase dose to desired effect with max dose 60 mg/kg/day
Migraine prophylaxis
• *Adult and child >16 yr:* PO ext rel 250-500 mg bid, up to 1000 mg/day
Available forms include: Caps 250 mg; caps sprinkles 125 mg; de-

layed rel tabs 125, 250, 500 mg; syr 250 mg/5 ml; inj single dose vial 5 ml, 100 mg/ml

Side effects/adverse reactions:

▼ *ORAL:* Prolonged bleeding, delayed healing, gingival enlargement (rare)

CNS: Sedation, drowsiness, dizziness, headache, incoordination, paresthesia, depression, hallucinations, behavioral changes, tremors, aggression, weakness

*GI: Nausea, vomiting, abdominal pain, **severe hepatic failure, pancreatitis, toxic hepatitis,** anorexia, cramps, constipation, diarrhea, dyspepsia*

*HEMA: **Thrombocytopenia, leukopenia, lymphocytosis,*** increased prothrombin time

GU: Enuresis, irregular menses

INTEG: Rash, alopecia, bruising

MISC: Asthenia

Contraindications: Hypersensitivity, hepatic disease or significant hepatic dysfunction

Precautions: MI (recovery phase), hepatic disease, renal disease, Addison's disease, pancreatitis, pregnancy category D, lactation

Pharmacokinetics:

PO: Onset 15-30 min, peak 1-4 hr, duration 4-6 hr

REC: Absorption of enteric coated divalproex is delayed 1 hr

🐝 Drug interactions of concern to dentistry:

• Increased effects: CNS depressants; carbamazepine, phenobarbital levels may be increased; phenothiazines can lower the seizure threshold

• Increased bleeding and toxicity: salicylates, NSAIDs

• Increased serum levels of amitriptyline, nortriptyline (start with low dose and monitor)

DENTAL CONSIDERATIONS

General:

• Patients on chronic drug therapy may rarely have symptoms of blood dyscrasias, which can include infection, bleeding, and poor healing.

• Evaluate for clotting ability during gingival instrumentation because inhibition of platelet aggregation may occur.

• Consider semisupine chair position for patient comfort if GI side effects occur.

• Place on frequent recall if gingival overgrowth occurs.

• Ask about type of epilepsy, seizure frequency, and quality of seizure control.

Consultations:

• In a patient with symptoms of blood dyscrasias, request a medical consult for blood studies and postpone dental treatment until normal values are reestablished.

• Medical consult may be required to assess disease control.

Teach patient/family:

• Importance of good oral hygiene to prevent soft tissue inflammation and minimize gingival overgrowth

• Caution to prevent injury when using oral hygiene aids

• To use electric toothbrush if patient has difficulty holding conventional devices

• Need for frequent oral prophylaxis if gingival overgrowth occurs

• To report oral lesions, soreness, or bleeding to dentist

V

---

bold italic = life-threatening conditions   *For periodic updates, visit* **www.mosby.com**

valsartan

(val-sar'tan)
Diovan

Drug class.: Angiotensin II receptor (AT_1) antagonist

Action: Acts as a competitive antagonist for angiotensin II receptors, inhibiting both vasoconstrictor and aldosterone secreting effects

Uses: Hypertension as a single drug or in combination with other antihypertensive medications

Dosage and routes:
• *Adult:* PO initial dose 80 mg/day; adjust initial dose upward or add a diuretic; dose range 80-320 mg qd

Available forms include: Caps 80, 160 mg

Side effects/adverse reactions:

▼ *ORAL:* Taste alterations
CNS: Insomnia, dizziness, fatigue, vertigo
CV: Edema, palpitation
RESP: Cough, URI
GI: Diarrhea, dyspepsia, nausea
GU: Impotence
MS: Arthralgia, back pain, leg pain, muscle cramp

Contraindications: Hypersensitivity, second and third trimesters of pregnancy

Precautions: Pregnancy category C (first trimester), pregnancy category D (second and third trimesters), volume depletion, less effect in African-Americans, liver impairment, lactation, children <18 yr, elevated labs for liver function, BUN, and potassium

Pharmacokinetics:
PO: Bioavailability 25%, highly plasma protein bound (95%), peak plasma levels 2-4 hr, limited metabolism; excreted in feces 83%, urine 13%

⚕ Drug interactions of concern to dentistry:
• Possible reduction in effect: ketoconazole

DENTAL CONSIDERATIONS
General:
• Monitor vital signs every appointment due to cardiovascular side effects.
• Limit use of sodium-containing products such as saline IV fluids for those patients with a dietary salt restriction.
• Stress from dental procedures may compromise cardiovascular function; determine patient risk.
• Short appointments and a stress reduction protocol may be required for anxious patients.
• Use precaution if sedation or general anesthesia is required; risk of hypotensive episode.

Consultations:
• Medical consult may be required to assess disease control and patient's ability to tolerate stress.

vancomycin HCl

(van-koe-mye'sin)
Vancocin

Drug class.: Glycopeptide-type antiinfective

Action: Inhibits bacterial cell wall synthesis

Uses: Resistant staphylococcal infections, pseudomembranous colitis, staphylococcal enterocolitis, endocarditis

Dosage and routes:
Serious staphylococcal infections
- *Adult:* IV 500 mg q6h or 1 g q12h
- *Child:* IV 40 mg/kg/day divided q6h
- *Neonate:* IV 15 mg/kg initially followed by 10 mg/kg q8-12h

Pseudomembranous colitis/staphylococcal enterocolitis
- *Adult:* PO 500 mg-2 g/day in 3-4 divided doses for 7-10 days
- *Child:* PO 40 mg/kg/day divided q6h, not to exceed 2 g/day

Available forms include: Pulvules 125, 250 mg; powder for oral sol 1, 10 g; powder for inj IV 500 mg, 1, 5, 10 g

Side effects/adverse reactions:
▼ *ORAL:* Bitter taste sensation
CV: **Cardiac arrest, vascular collapse**
GI: Nausea
RESP: Wheezing, dyspnea
HEMA: **Leukopenia, eosinophilia, neutropenia**
GU: **Nephrotoxicity, fatal uremia,** increased BUN, creatinine, albumin
EENT: **Ototoxicity, permanent deafness,** tinnitus
INTEG: Chills, fever, rash, thrombophlebitis at injection site, urticaria, pruritus, necrosis
SYST: **Anaphylaxis**

Contraindications: Hypersensitivity, decreased hearing
Precautions: Renal disease, pregnancy category C, lactation, elderly, neonates

Pharmacokinetics:
PO/IV: Oral absorption poor; rapid peak plasma levels with IV infusion of repeated doses; little metabolism because most of drug is excreted by kidney; delayed clearance occurs with renal dysfunction

🦷 **Drug interactions of concern to dentistry:**
- Ototoxicity or nephrotoxicity: aminoglycosides and high-dose salicylates
- Increased effects of nondepolarizing muscle relaxants

DENTAL CONSIDERATIONS
General:
- Monitor vital signs every appointment due to cardiovascular side effects.
- Administer IV slowly over 1 hr; an administration that is too rapid can lead to a fall in blood pressure (monitor) and a red rash on the face, neck, and chest due to local histamine release. No specific treatment is required for this reaction; evaluate recovery progress.
- Determine why the patient is taking the drug.

Consultations:
- Medical consult may be required to assess disease control.

---

venlafaxine HCl
(ven'la-fax-een)
Effexor, Effexor XR
Drug class.: Bicyclic antidepressant

Action: Inhibits both norepinephrine and serotonin (5-HT) uptake and to a lesser extent uptake of dopamine, but the precise antidepressant mechanism remains unclear
Uses: Depression, prevention of major depressive disorder relapse

Dosage and routes:
• *Adult:* PO 75 mg/day in 2 or 3 divided doses; can increase dose 75 mg/day at no less than 4-day intervals; max dose 375 mg/day in 3 divided doses

Available forms include: Tabs 25, 37.5, 50, 75, 100 mg; ext rel caps 37.5, 75, 150 mg

Side effects/adverse reactions:
▼ *ORAL: Dry mouth,* glossitis (rare), cheilitis, gingivitis, candidiasis

CNS: Somnolence, dizziness, migraine, nervousness, anxiety, headache, anorexia, mania, hypomania

CV: Hypertension, tachycardia, vasodilation, postural hypotension

GI: Nausea, constipation, vomiting, dyspepsia

RESP: Dyspnea, bronchitis, yawning

HEMA: Ecchymosis, anemia, thrombocytopenia, leukopenia

GU: Abnormal ejaculation (male), male impotence, painful urination, decreased libido

EENT: Blurred vision, ear pain
INTEG: Sweating, rash, pruritus
MS: Asthenia, tremor, trismus
MISC: General body discomfort, asthenia

Contraindications: Hypersensitivity, concurrent use with an MAO inhibitor–type drug presents risk of severe reaction

Precautions: Pregnancy category C, lactation, children <18 yr, sustained hypertension with use, renal or hepatic impairment, elderly, long-term use (>4-6 wk), history of seizures, suicidal patients, mania

Pharmacokinetics:
PO: Good bioavailability (92%), metabolized in liver, active metabolite, renal excretion, plasma protein binding is low (27%)

⚘ Drug interactions of concern to dentistry:
• None currently reported; however, because this drug is similar in action to other antidepressants, it would be wise to avoid excessive amounts of vasoconstrictors, especially in gingival retraction cords
• Increased CNS depression: all CNS depressants

DENTAL CONSIDERATIONS
General:
• Monitor vital signs every appointment due to cardiovascular side effects.
• After supine positioning, have patient sit upright for >2 min before standing to avoid orthostatic hypotension.
• Assess salivary flow as a factor in caries, periodontal disease, and candidiasis.
• Examine for evidence of oral manifestations of blood dyscrasias (infection, bleeding, poor healing).
• Place on frequent recall to evaluate healing response.
• Consider semisupine chair position for patient comfort due to GI effects of disease.

Consultations:
• Medical consult may be required to assess disease control.
• Physician should be informed if significant xerostomic side effects occur (increased caries, sore tongue, problems eating or swallowing, difficulty wearing prosthesis) so a medication change can be considered.
• Obtain a medical consult for blood studies (CBC) because leukopenic or thrombocytopenic side effects may result in infection, delayed healing, and excessive bleeding. Postpone elective dental

treatment until normal values are maintained.

Teach patient/family:

• Importance of good oral hygiene to prevent soft tissue inflammation

• Caution to prevent injury when using oral hygiene aids

When chronic dry mouth occurs, advise patient:

• To avoid mouth rinses with high alcohol content due to drying effects

• Of need for daily use of home fluoride products to prevent caries

• To use sugarless gum, frequent sips of water, or saliva substitutes

---

verapamil/verapamil HCl

(ver-ap'a-mil)

Calan, Calan SR, Isoptin, Isoptin SR, Verelan, Verelan PM

♣ Apo-Verap, Novo-Veramil, Nu-Verap

Drug class.: Calcium channel blocker

Action: Inhibits calcium ion influx across cell membrane during cardiac depolarization; produces relaxation of coronary vascular smooth muscle; dilates coronary arteries; decreases SA/AV node conduction; dilates peripheral arteries

Uses: Chronic stable angina pectoris, vasospastic angina, dysrhythmias (class IV), hypertension; unapproved: migraine headache, cardiomyopathy

Dosage and routes:

• *Adult:* PO 80 mg tid or qid, increase qwk; ext rel PO 120-240 mg qd; IV bol 5-10 mg over >2 min, repeat if necessary in 30 min

• *Child 1-15 yr:* IV bol 0.1-0.3 mg/kg over >2 min, repeat in 30 min, not to exceed 10 mg in a single dose

• *Child <1 yr:* IV bol 0.1-0.2 mg/kg over >2 min with ECG monitoring, repeat if necessary in 30 min

Available forms include: Tabs 40, 80, 120; sus rel tabs 120, 180, 240 mg; ext rel caps 120, 180, 240, 360 mg; sus rel caps 100, 200, 300 mg; inj 2.5 mg/ml

Side effects/adverse reactions:

▼ *ORAL: Gingival enlargement,* dry mouth, ulcers

CNS: Headache, drowsiness, dizziness, anxiety, depression, weakness, insomnia, confusion, lightheadedness

CV: Edema, **CHF,** bradycardia, hypotension, palpitation, AV block

GI: Nausea, diarrhea, gastric upset, constipation, increased liver function studies

GU: Nocturia, polyuria

Contraindications: Sick sinus syndrome, second- or third-degree heart block, hypotension <90 mm Hg systolic, cardiogenic shock, severe CHF

Precautions: CHF, hypotension, hepatic injury, pregnancy category C, lactation, children, renal disease, concomitant β-blocker therapy

Pharmacokinetics:

IV: Onset 3 min, peak 3-5 min, duration 10-20 min

PO: Onset variable, peak 3-4 hr, duration 17-24 hr

Half-life 4 min (biphasic), 3-7 hr (terminal); metabolized by liver; excreted in urine (96% as metabolites)

☛ Drug interactions of concern to dentistry:

• Decreased effect: indomethacin,

---

possibly other NSAIDs, phenobarbital

• Increased effect: parenteral and inhalation general anesthetics or other drugs with hypotensive actions

• Increased effects of nondepolarizing muscle relaxants

• Increased effects of carbamazepine

DENTAL CONSIDERATIONS

General:

• Monitor cardiac status; take vital signs at each appointment because of CV side effects. Consider a stress reduction protocol to prevent stress-induced angina during the dental appointment.

• After supine positioning, have patient sit upright for at least 2 min before standing to avoid orthostatic hypotension at dismissal.

• Place on frequent recall to monitor gingival condition.

• Limit use of sodium-containing products, such as saline IV fluids, for patients with a dietary salt restriction.

• Assess salivary flow as a factor in caries, periodontal disease, and candidiasis.

• Use vasoconstrictors with caution, in low doses, and with careful aspiration. Avoid use of gingival retraction cord with epinephrine.

Consultations:

• In a patient with symptoms of blood dyscrasias, request a medical consult for blood studies and postpone dental treatment until normal values are reestablished.

• Medical consult may be required to assess disease control and patient's tolerance for stress.

Teach patient/family:

• Importance of good oral hygiene to prevent soft tissue inflammation and minimize gingival overgrowth

• Need for frequent oral prophylaxis if gingival overgrowth occurs

When chronic dry mouth occurs, advise patient:

• To avoid mouth rinses with high alcohol content due to drying effects

• Of need for daily use of home fluoride products to prevent caries

• To use sugarless gum, frequent sips of water, or saliva substitutes

---

vidarabine (ophthalmic)

(vye-dare′a-been)

Vira-A Ophthalmic

Drug class.: Antiviral

Action: Inhibits viral DNA synthesis by blocking DNA polymerase

Uses: Keratoconjunctivitis due to herpes simplex virus

Dosage and routes:

• *Adult and child:* TOP 0.5 inch oint into conjunctival sac q3h 5× daily

Available forms include: Oint 3%

Side effects/adverse reactions:

EENT: Burning, stinging, photophobia, pain, temporary visual haze

Contraindications: Hypersensitivity

Precautions: Antibiotic hypersensitivity, pregnancy category C

DENTAL CONSIDERATIONS

General:

• Protect patient's eyes from spatter during dental procedures.

• Avoid dental light in patient's eyes; offer dark glasses for patient comfort.

---

vitamin A

Aquasol A, Palmitate-A 500

Drug class.: Fat-soluble vitamin

Action: Vitamin A (retinol) combines with opsin to form rhodopsin necessary for visual adaptation to darkness and normal function of the retina; it is required for normal bone development and epithelial tissue growth; probably acts as a cofactor in many metabolic reactions

Uses: Vitamin A deficiency

Dosage and routes:

• *Adult and child >8 yr:* PO 100,000-500,000 IU qd × 3 days, then 50,000 qd × 2 wk; dose based on severity of deficiency; maintenance 10,000-20,000 IU for 2 mo

• *Child 1-8 yr:* IM 17,500-35,000 IU qd × 10 days

• *Infant <1 yr:* IM 7500-15,000 IU × 10 days

Maintenance

• *Child 4-8 yr:* IM 15,000 IU qd × 2 mo

• *Child <4 yr:* IM 10,000 IU qd × 2 mo

Available forms include: Caps 10,000, 25,000, 50,000 IU; tabs 500 IU; drops 5000 IU; inj 50,000 IU/ml

Side effects/adverse reactions:

▼ *ORAL: Gingival bleeding, dry/ cracked lips*

CNS: Headache, increased intracranial pressure, intracranial hypertension, lethargy, malaise

GI: Jaundice, nausea, vomiting, anorexia, abdominal pain

EENT: Papilledema, exophthalmos

INTEG: Drying of skin, pruritus, increased pigmentation, night sweats, alopecia

MS: Arthralgia, retarded growth, hard areas on bone

META: Hypomenorrhea, hypercalcemia

Contraindications: Hypersensitivity to vitamin A, malabsorption syndrome (PO), pregnancy category X

Precautions: Impaired renal function

Pharmacokinetics:

PO/INJ: Stored in liver, kidneys, fat; excreted (metabolites) in urine, feces

DENTAL CONSIDERATIONS

General:

• Oral manifestation of side effects could indicate hypervitaminosis.

• May cause dry/peeling skin around lips; provide lip lubricant for patient comfort during dental treatment.

vitamin D (calcifediol [D₃], calcitriol, ergocalciferol [D₂], dihydrotachysterol [vitamin D analog], and doxercalciferol)

Dihydrotachysterol (DHT): DHT, Hytakerol

Calcitriol (1alpha, 25 dihydrocalciferol): Calcijex, Rocaltrol

Calcifediol (25-hydroxycholecalciferol): Calderol

Ergocalciferol (D₂): Calciferol, Calciferol Drops, Disdol, Drisdol Drops

Cholecalciferol (D₃): Delta-D

♣ One-Alpha, Ostoforte, Radiostol Forte

Drug class.: Fat-soluble vitamin

Action: Needed for regulation of

calcium phosphate levels, normal bone development, parathyroid activity, neuromuscular functioning

Uses: Varies with the type of vitamin D selected but generally includes vitamin D deficiency, rickets, renal osteodystrophy, tetany, hypoparathyroidism, and hypophosphatemia; doxercalciferol is indicated for reduction of elevated intact parathyroid hormone (iPTH) levels for secondary hyperparathyroidism in patients receiving chronic renal dialysis

Dosage and routes:
• *Adult (vitamin D₂):* PO/IM 12,000 IU qd, then increased to 500,000 IU/day
• *Child:* PO/IM 1500/5000 IU qd × 2-4 wk; may repeat after 2 wk or 600,000 IU as single dose
• *Adult (DHT):* PO 0.75-2.5 mg for several days; maintenance 0.2-1.75 mg/day supplement with 10-15 g calcium lactate or gluconate
• *Adult and child >6 yr (calcitriol):* PO initial dose 0.25 μg/day; can increase at 2-4 wk intervals if required, usual dose 0.5-2 μg/day
• *Dialysis (calcifediol)* PO at dialysis 300-350 μg/wk
• *Cholecalciferol (D₃):* Vitamin D deficiency: usual dose range 400-1000 U daily

Hypoparathyroidism (vitamin D₂)
• *Adult and child:* PO/IM 200,000 IU given with 4 g calcium tabs
Doxercalciferol
• *Adult:* PO at dialysis depending on iPTH levels; initial dose 10 μg 3 × wk

Available forms include: DHT tabs 0.125, 0.2, 0.4 mg; sol 0.2 mg/ml; caps 0.125 mg; calcitriol caps 0.25, 0.5 μg; oral sol 1 μg/ml; inj 1 and 2 μg/ml; calcifediol caps 20, 50 μg; D₂ caps 50,000 IU; liq 8000 IU/ml; inj 500,000 IU/ml; D₃ tabs 400, 1000 IU

Side effects/adverse reactions:
▼ *ORAL:* Metallic taste, dry mouth can be early signs of toxicity
CNS: **Convulsions,** fatigue, weakness, drowsiness, headache, psychosis
CV: Hypertension, dysrhythmias
GI: Nausea, vomiting, anorexia, cramps, diarrhea, constipation, decreased libido
GU: **Hematuria, albuminuria, renal failure,** polyuria, nocturia
INTEG: Pruritus, photophobia
MS: Decreased bone growth, early joint pain, early muscle pain
Contraindications: Hypersensitivity, hypercalcemia, renal dysfunction, hyperphosphatemia
Precautions: Cardiovascular disease, renal calculi, pregnancy category C, hyperphosphatemia
Pharmacokinetics:
PO/INJ: Half-life 7-12 hr, duration 2 mo; stored in liver; excreted in bile (metabolites), urine
🦷 **Drug interactions of concern to dentistry:**
• None reported
DENTAL CONSIDERATIONS
General:
• Sensitivity of eyes to dental light may indicate late toxicity.
• Monitor vital signs every appointment due to cardiovascular side effects.
Teach patient/family:
• That oral side effects are associated with early symptoms of overdose

---

italic = common side effects

vitamin E (alpha tocopherol)

Aquavit-E, d'Alpha E, Dry E 400, Mixed E 400, VitaPlus E

Drug class.: Vitamin E (fat-soluble vitamin)

Action: Needed for digestion and metabolism of polyunsaturated fats, decreased platelet aggregation; decreases blood clot formation; promotes normal growth and development of muscle tissue, prostaglandin synthesis; antioxidant effect protects against free radicals

Uses: Vitamin E deficiency, hemolytic anemia in premature neonates, prevention of retrolental fibroplasia

Dosage and routes:

Prophylaxis
• *Adult and adolescent:* PO 30 IU qd

Treatment
• *Adult and adolescent:* PO 60-75 IU/day
• *Child:* PO 1 IU/kg/day or 4-5 times the RDA

Available forms include: Caps 100, 200, 400, 1000 IU; tabs 100, 200, 400, 500, 800 IU; drops 15 IU/0.3 ml

Side effects/adverse reactions:
CNS: Headache, fatigue
CV: Increased risk of thrombophlebitis
GI: Nausea, cramps, diarrhea
GU: Gonadal dysfunction
EENT: Blurred vision
INTEG: Sterile abscess, contact dermatitis
MS: Weakness
META: Altered metabolism of hormones (thyroid, pituitary, adrenal), altered immunity

Contraindications: None significant

Precautions: Pregnancy category A

Pharmacokinetics:
PO: Metabolized in liver, excreted in bile

🦷 **Drug interactions of concern to dentistry:**
• With doses >400 IU: increased action of oral anticoagulants

DENTAL CONSIDERATIONS
General:
• Determine why the patient is taking the drug.

---

warfarin sodium

(war'far-in)
Coumadin
🍁 Warfilone

Drug class.: Oral anticoagulant

Action: Interferes with blood clotting by indirect means; depresses hepatic synthesis of vitamin K–dependent coagulation factors (II, VII, IX, X)

Uses: Pulmonary emboli, deep vein thrombosis, MI, atrial dysrhythmias, to reduce risk of recurrent MI and thromboembolic events

Dosage and routes:
• *Adult:* PO/IV individualized for each patient depending on PT, can range from 1-10 mg

Available forms include: Tabs 1, 2, 2.5, 3, 4, 5, 6, 7.5, 10 mg; inj 2 mg/5 ml

Side effects/adverse reactions:
▼ *ORAL: Gingival bleeding,* stomatitis, salivary gland pain/swelling
CNS: Fever

w

---

*GI: Diarrhea, **hepatitis,** nausea, vomiting, anorexia, cramps*
*HEMA: **Hemorrhage, agranulocytosis, leukopenia, eosinophilia***
*GU: **Hematuria***
INTEG: Rash, dermatitis, urticaria, alopecia, pruritus
Contraindications: Hypersensitivity, hemophilia, leukemia with bleeding, peptic ulcer disease, thrombocytopenic purpura, hepatic disease (severe), severe hypertension, subacute bacterial endocarditis, acute nephritis, blood dyscrasias, pregnancy category D, eclampsia, preeclampsia
Precautions: Alcoholism, elderly
Pharmacokinetics:
PO: Onset 12-24 hr, peak 1.5-3 days, duration 3-5 days, half-life 1.5-2.5 days; 99% bound to plasma proteins; metabolized in liver; excreted in urine, feces (active/inactive metabolites); crosses placenta
⚘ Drug interactions of concern to dentistry:
• Increased action: diflunisal, salicylates, propoxyphene, metronidazole, erythromycin, clarithromycin, ketoconazole, itraconazole, fluconazole, NSAIDs, indomethacin, chloral hydrate, tetracyclines, fluoroquinolones, acetaminophen, ciprofloxacin, levofloxacin
• If NSAIDs must be used, monitor patients
• Decreased action: barbiturates, carbamazepine
• Possible increase in anticoagulant effects with celecoxib, rofecoxib (monitor INR levels)

DENTAL CONSIDERATIONS
General:
• Question patients about their recent use of acetaminophen, because acetaminophen has been shown to increase the INR to 4.0 or greater depending on the amount taken. Treatment may need to be delayed. Additional use of acetaminophen will require close monitoring of INR values. (*JAMA* 279: 657-662, 1998.)
• Patients on chronic drug therapy may rarely have symptoms of blood dyscrasias, which can include infection, bleeding, and poor healing.
• Consider local hemostasis measures to prevent excessive bleeding.
• Increase in bleeding with IM injections may occur.
Consultations:
• Medical consult should include partial prothrombin time, prothrombin time, or INR.
• For dental surgical procedures that may result in excessive bleeding, consider requesting dose reduction before dental treatment so that PT is no more than twice normal.
• In a patient with symptoms of blood dyscrasias, request a medical consult for blood studies and postpone dental treatment until normal values are reestablished.
Teach patient/family:
• Importance of good oral hygiene to prevent soft tissue inflammation
• Caution to prevent injury when using oral hygiene aids
• To report oral lesions, soreness, or bleeding to dentist

---

zafirlukast
(za-fir′loo-kast)
Accolate
Drug class.: Selective leukotriene receptor antagonist

Action: Competitive and selective

receptor antagonist of leukotriene LD_4 and LTE_3, resulting in inhibition of bronchospasm and airway edema

Uses: Prophylaxis and chronic treatment of asthma

Dosage and routes:
• *Adult and child >12 yr:* PO 20 mg bid at least 1 hr before or 2 hr after meals

Available forms include: Tabs 20 mg

Side effects/adverse reactions:
CNS: Headache, dizziness
GI: Nausea, diarrhea, abdominal pain, vomiting, dyspepsia
RESP: Infections
META: Elevation of ALT
MS: Asthenia, myalgia, back pain, arthralgia
MISC: Generalized pain, fever, accidental injury

Contraindications: Hypersensitivity, hepatic dysfunction with prior use of zafirlukast

Precautions: Not for acute bronchospasm, food decreases bioavailability, pregnancy category B, lactation, patients <7 yr, hepatic impairment, liver enzyme elevation, elderly (increased infection); if liver dysfunction suspected, discontinue use and measure liver enzymes, serum ALT

Pharmacokinetics:
PO: Rapid absorption, peak plasma levels 3 hr, extensively metabolized, 90% fecal excretion, 10% urinary excretion, 99% plasma protein bound

⚕ Drug interactions of concern to dentistry:
• Increased PT with concurrent use of warfarin
• Reduced plasma levels: erythromycin, terfenadine, theophylline
• Increased plasma levels with aspirin

DENTAL CONSIDERATIONS
General:
• Midday appointments and a stress reduction protocol may be required for anxious patients.
• Avoid prescribing aspirin-containing products.
• Acute asthmatic episodes may be precipitated in the dental office. Sympathomimetic inhalants should be available for emergency use. A stress reduction protocol may be required.
• Be aware that aspirin or sulfite preservatives in vasoconstrictor-containing products can exacerbate asthma.
• Consider semisupine chair position for patients with respiratory disease and if GI side effects are a problem.

Consultations:
• Medical consult may be required to assess disease control.

Teach patient/family:
• Use of electric toothbrush if patient has difficulty holding conventional devices
• Importance of updating health and drug history if physician makes any changes in evaluation or drug regimens

---

zalcitabine

(zal-site'a-been)
Hivid
Drug class.: Synthetic pyrimidine antiviral

Action: Converted by cellular enzymes to active drug; functions as antimetabolite to inhibit replication of HIV in vitro

Uses: Used in combination with

Z

zidovudine in advanced HIV infection

Dosage and routes:
• *Adult:* PO 0.75 mg q8h in combination with other antiretroviral agents

Available forms include: Tabs 0.375, 0.75 mg

Side effects/adverse reactions:

▼ *ORAL: Oral ulcers, dry mouth, glossitis*

CNS: Peripheral neuropathy, headache, nervousness, fatigue, Bell's palsy

*CV: **Hypertension, syncope palpitation, tachycardia, CHF***

*GI: **Pancreatitis,** nausea, dysphagia, diarrhea, GI pain, anorexia*

HEMA: Epistaxis

*GU: **Renal failure,** polyuria, renal calculus, abnormal renal function*

EENT: Abnormal vision

INTEG: Rash, sweating, pruritus, dermatitis

MS: Muscle pain

Contraindications: Hypersensitivity

Precautions: Pregnancy category C, lactation, children <13 yr, renal impairment, hepatic impairment

Pharmacokinetics:

PO: Peak plasma levels following oral doses in 0.8-1.6 hr; phosphorylated form excreted in urine (70%); food decreases rate of oral absorption

Drug interactions of concern to dentistry:
• Increased peripheral neuropathy: metronidazole, dapsone

DENTAL CONSIDERATIONS
General:
• Examine oral cavity for side effects if on long-term drug therapy.

• Monitor vital signs every appointment due to cardiovascular side effects.
• Palliative medication may be required for management of oral side effects.
• Assess salivary flow as a factor in caries, periodontal disease, and candidiasis.
• Prophylactic antibiotics may be indicated to prevent infection if surgery or deep scaling is planned.
• Patients may be more susceptible to infection and have delayed wound healing.

Consultations:
• Medical consult may be required to assess disease control and patient's ability to tolerate stress.

Teach patient/family:
• Importance of good oral hygiene to prevent soft tissue inflammation
• Caution to prevent injury when using oral hygiene aids
• That secondary oral infection may occur; must see dentist immediately if infection occurs

When chronic dry mouth occurs, advise patient:
• To avoid mouth rinses with high alcohol content due to drying effects
• Of need for daily use of home fluoride products to prevent caries
• To use sugarless gum, frequent sips of water, or saliva substitutes

---

zaleplon
(zal′e-plon)
Sonata
Drug class.: Hypnotic

Action: Interacts with the GABA benzodiazepine receptor complex binding to the omega-1 receptor subunit

Uses: Short-term treatment of insomnia

Dosage and routes:
• *Adult:* PO 10 mg immediately before bedtime; dose should not exceed 20 mg

Elderly, debilitated, or smaller patient
• *Adult:* PO 5 mg immediately before bedtime

Available forms include: Caps 5, 10 mg

Side effects/adverse reactions:
▼ *ORAL: Dry mouth*
CNS: Headache, dizziness, amnesia, anxiety, paresthesia, somnolence, depression, nervousness
CV: Palpitation, arrhythmia, tachycardia, syncope
GI: Nausea, constipation, abdominal pain, dyspepsia
RESP: Bronchitis
HEMA: Anemia
GU: Dysmenorrhea, bladder pain, dysuria
EENT: Abnormal vision, ear pain, eye pain, conjunctivitis, dry eyes
INTEG: Pruritus, rash
META: Weight gain, gout, hypercholesterolemia
MS: Myalgia, asthenia

Contraindications: Hypersensitivity

Precautions: Abuse potential similar to benzodiazepines, elderly, debilitated, smaller patients adjust dose downward; pregnancy category C, lactation, children

Pharmacokinetics:
PO: Rapid absorption, bioavailability 30%, peak plasma levels 1 hr, wide tissue distribution, rapid hepatic metabolism (CYP3A4), excretion in urine; heavy, high-fat meal delays absorption significantly

🦷 **Drug interactions of concern to dentistry:**
• Caution when using dental drugs that inhibit or induce cytochrome P-450 enzymes
• CNS depression: all CNS depressant drugs

DENTAL CONSIDERATIONS
General:
• Assess salivary flow as a factor in caries, periodontal disease, and candidiasis.
• Determine why patient is taking the drug.
• Consider semisupine chair position for patient comfort if GI side effects occur.

Consultations:
• Medical consult may be required to assess disease control and patient's ability to tolerate stress.

Teach   patient/family: *When chronic dry mouth occurs, advise patient:*
• To avoid mouth rinses with high alcohol content due to drying effects
• To use daily home fluoride products for anticaries effect
• To use sugarless gum, frequent sips of water, or saliva substitutes

---

zanamivir
(za-nam′a-veer)
Relenza
Drug class.: Antiviral

Action: Inhibits neuraminidase, which is essential for replication of influenza type A and B viruses
Uses: Uncomplicated influenza in adults and children >7 yr with

symptoms of no more than 2 days; more effective against influenza type A virus

Dosage and routes:

• *Adult and child >7 yr:* Inh 2 inhalations (total amount 10 mg) twice daily, 12 hr apart × 5 days; 2 doses should be given on day 1 if at least 2 hr apart, then q12h thereafter; doses must be given not more than 2 days after onset of flu symptoms

Available forms include: Oral inh rotadisks packaged as a unit with inhaler sufficient for 5-day therapy

Side effects/adverse reactions:

CNS: Headache, dizziness

GI: Diarrhea, nausea, vomiting

RESP: Bronchitis, cough, broncho-spasm (asthmatics)

HEMA: Lymphopenia, neutropenia

EENT: Sinusitis; ear, nose, and throat infections

INTEG: Urticaria

META: Elevation of liver enzymes, CPK

MS: Myalgia, arthralgia

MISC: Fever, malaise, fatigue

Contraindications: Hypersensitivity

Precautions: Teach use of inhaler to patient; chronic obstructive pulmonary disease or asthma does not preclude influenza vaccine, safety in high-risk medical conditions is unknown, pregnancy category B, lactation, children <12 yr

Pharmacokinetics:

▼ *ORAL INH:* 4%-17% of inhaled dose is absorbed, peak serum levels 1-2 hr, low plasma protein binding (<10%), excreted unchanged in urine

🦷 **Drug interactions of concern to dentistry:**

• None reported

DENTAL CONSIDERATIONS

General:

• Acute influenza patients are unlikely to be seen in the dental office except for dental emergencies.

---

zidovudine (AZT)

(zye-doe'vyoo-deen)

Retrovir

✿ Apo-Zidovine, Novo-AZT, Retrovir

Drug class.: Antiviral thymidine analog

Action: Inhibits replication of viral DNA

Uses: Symptomatic HIV infections (AIDS, ARC), confirmed *P. carinii* pneumonia, or absolute CD4 lymphocytes <200/mm^3

Dosage and routes:

• *Adult:* PO 100 mg q4h with adjustment for severity; must stop treatment if severe bone marrow depression occurs; restart after bone marrow recovery; also given IV; 600 mg daily limit

Available forms include: Tabs 300 mg; caps 100 mg; syr 50 mg/5 ml; inj 10 mg/ml

Side effects/adverse reactions:

▼ *ORAL: Taste changes, gingival bleeding,* mucosal ulceration, swelling of lips or tongue, delayed healing, opportunistic infection

CNS: Fever, headache, malaise, diaphoresis, dizziness, insomnia, paresthesia, somnolence, chills, tremor, twitching, anxiety, confusion, depression, lability, vertigo, loss of mental acuity

GI: Nausea, vomiting, diarrhea, anorexia, cramps, dyspepsia, constipation, dysphagia, flatulence, rectal bleeding

RESP: Dyspnea

italic = common side effects

HEMA: **Granulocytopenia, anemia**
GU: Dysuria, polyuria, frequency, hesitancy
EENT: Hearing loss, photophobia
INTEG: Rash, acne, pruritus, urticaria
MS: Myalgia, arthralgia, muscle spasm
Contraindications: Hypersensitivity
Precautions: Granulocyte count <1000/mm^3 or Hgb <9.5 g/dl, pregnancy category C, lactation, children, severe renal disease, severe hepatic function
Pharmacokinetics:
PO: Rapidly absorbed from GI tract, peak 0.5-1.5 hr; metabolized in liver (inactive metabolites); excreted by kidneys
☙ Drug interactions of concern to dentistry:
• Toxicity: data are very limited; however, drugs that undergo metabolism involving glucuronidation may possibly delay the metabolism and subsequent excretion of zidovudine; these drugs include aspirin, acetaminophen, and indomethacin; other drugs that can cause granulocytopenia could increase the risk of toxicity
• Decreased peak serum levels: clarithromycin
DENTAL CONSIDERATIONS
General:
• Examine for oral manifestations of opportunistic infections.
• Patients on chronic drug therapy may rarely have symptoms of blood dyscrasias, which can include infection, bleeding, and poor healing.
• Avoid dental light in patient's eyes; offer dark glasses for patient comfort.
• Place on frequent recall due to oral side effects.
Consultations:
• In a patient with symptoms of blood dyscrasias, request a medical consult for blood studies and postpone dental treatment until normal values are reestablished.
• Medical consult may be required to assess disease control.
Teach patient/family:
• Importance of good oral hygiene to prevent soft tissue inflammation
• Caution to prevent injury when using oral hygiene aids
• That secondary oral infection may occur; must see dentist immediately if infection occurs

---

zileuton
(zye-loo'ton)
Zyflo Filmtab
Drug class.: Leukotriene pathway inhibitor

Action: Inhibits the enzyme 5-lipoxygenase, thus interfering with synthesis of leukotrienes (LTB_4, LTC_4, LTD_4, and LTE_4), which contribute to inflammation, edema, mucous secretion, and bronchoconstriction
Uses: Prophylaxis and chronic treatment of asthma
Dosage and routes:
• *Adult:* PO 600 mg qid with meals and hs, daily dose 2400 mg
Available forms include: Tabs 600 mg
Side effects/adverse reactions:
CNS: **Headache**, dizziness, insomnia, somnolence, malaise
CV: Chest pain
GI: *Abdominal pain, dyspepsia, nausea,* constipation, flatulence, vomiting

---

bold italic = life-threatening conditions

z

HEMA: Lymphadenopathy, hyper-bilirubinemia
GU: UTI, vaginitis
EENT: Conjunctivitis
INTEG: Pruritus
MS: Asthenia, myalgia, arthralgia, neck pain
MISC: Generalized pain, malaise, elevation liver enzymes, fever

Contraindications: Hypersensitivity; active liver disease or transaminase elevations greater than or equal to 3 times the upper limit

Precautions: Not for acute bronchospasm, status asthmaticus; theophylline, warfarin, propranolol; hepatic impairment, pregnancy category C, lactation, children <12 yr, monitor ALT levels

Pharmacokinetics:
PO: Rapid absorption, peak plasma levels 1.7 hr, 93% bound to plasma proteins, metabolized, 94.5% excreted in urine

⚡ Drug interactions of concern to dentistry:
• Increased plasma levels of theophylline, propranolol
• Significant increase in PT when taking warfarin

DENTAL CONSIDERATIONS
General:
• Consider semisupine chair position for patient comfort due to GI side effects of disease.
• Acute asthmatic episodes may be precipitated in the dental office. Sympathomimetic inhalants should be available for emergency use.
• Midday appointments and a stress reduction protocol may be required for anxious patients.
• Be aware that aspirin or sulfite preservatives in vasoconstrictor-containing products can exacerbate asthma.

Consultations:
• Medical consult may be required to assess disease control.

Teach patient/family:
• Importance of updating health and drug history if physician makes any changes in evaluation or drug regimens

---

ziprasidone HCl
(zi-pray'si-done)
Geodon
Drug class.: Antipsychotic, atypical

Action: Unclear, but may be related to antagonism of dopamine (D_2) and serotonin (5-HT_2) receptors; also has affinity for D_3, 5-HT_{a2}, 5-HT_{2c}, 5-HT_{1d}, α_1-adrenergic receptors and histamine H_1 receptors

Uses: Schizophrenia

Dosage and routes:
• *Adult:* PO initial daily dose 20 mg bid with food; dosage adjustments (if indicated) should occur at intervals of not less than 2 days (although several weeks are preferred); doses up to 80 mg bid have been used

Available forms include: Caps 20, 40, 60, 80 mg

Side effects/adverse reactions:
▼ *ORAL: Dry mouth*
CNS: Dizziness, seizures, anorexia, extrapyramidal syndrome, somnolence, agitation, confusion
CV: Orthostatic hypotension, syncope, tachycardia, **increased QT interval**

GI: Nausea, constipation, dyspepsia, diarrhea
RESP: URI, cold symptoms
HEMA: Anemia (infrequent), **severe blood dyscrasias (rare)**
GU: Impotence, urinary retention, **priapism**
EENT: Abnormal vision
INTEG: Rash, urticaria, fungal dermatitis
ENDO: Elevated prolactin levels
META: Increased transaminase, increased creatinine phosphokinase, hypercholesteremia
MS: Myalgia, akathisia, dystonia, hypertonia
MISC: Asthenia, accidental injury, weight gain

Contraindications: Hypersensitivity, other drugs that prolong the QT interval (quinidine, pimozide, dofetilide, sotalol, thioridazine, moxifloxacin and sparfloxacin), recent MI, congenital long QT syndrome, heart failure

Precautions: May antagonize levodopa, dopamine agonists; QT prolongation and risk of sudden death, bradycardia, hypokalemia, hypomagnesemia, electrolyte depletion due to diarrhea, diuretics or vomiting, neuromalignant syndrome, tardive dyskinesia, seizures, suicide, pregnancy category C, lactation, pediatric use

Pharmacokinetics:
PO: Absolute bioavailability 60%, steady state plasma levels 2-3 days, plasma protein building 99%, hepatic metabolism by aldehyde oxidase (major) and CYP450 3A4 (minor) enzymes, excreted mostly in feces (66%) and in the urine (20%)

Drug interactions of concern to dentistry:
- Avoid use of any drug that prolongs the QT interval
- Caution in use of other CNS depressants: increased risk of CNS depressant effects
- Reduced plasma levels: carbamazepine
- Increased plasma levels: ketoconazole
- Drugs that lower BP: increased risk of hypotension
- Increased extrapyramidal effects: phenothiazines and related drugs (haloperidol, droperidol), metoclopramide

DENTAL CONSIDERATIONS
General:
- Monitor vital signs every appointment due to cardiovascular side effects.
- After supine positioning, have patient sit upright >2 min to avoid orthostatic hypotension.
- Assess salivary flow as a factor in caries, periodontal disease, and candidiasis.
- Consider semisupine chair position for patient comfort if GI side effects occur.
- Assess for presence of extrapyramidal motor symptoms such as tardive dyskinesia and akathisia. Extrapyramidal motor activity may complicate dental treatment.
- Use vasoconstrictor with caution, in low doses, and with careful aspiration; avoid use of epinephrine impregnated gingival retraction cord.

Consultations:
- Consultation with physician may be needed if sedation or general anesthesia is required.
- Physician should be informed if

z

significant xerostomic side effects occur (e.g., increased caries, sore tongue, problems eating or swallowing, difficulty wearing prosthesis) so a medication change can be considered.

• Medical consult may be required to assess disease control and patient's ability to tolerate stress.

Teach patient/family:

• Importance of good oral hygiene to prevent soft tissue inflammation

• To prevent trauma when using oral hygiene aids

• Use of electric toothbrush if patient has difficulty holding conventional devices

When chronic dry mouth occurs, advise patient:

• To avoid mouth rinses with high alcohol content due to drying effects

• To use daily home fluoride products for anticaries effect

• To use sugarless gum, frequent sips of water, or saliva substitutes

---

zoledronic acid

(zoe'le-dron-ik)

Zometa

Drug class.: Osteoporosis therapy adjunct, bisphosphonate

Action: Inhibits bone resorption but exact mechanism unclear; inhibits osteoclastic activity, induces osteoclast apoptosis, blocks osteoclastic resorption of mineralized bone and cartilage

Uses: Treatment of hypercalcemia of malignancy

Dosage and routes:

• *Adult:* IV maximum recommended dose for IV infusion is 4 mg given over no less than 15 min, at least 7 days must lapse between doses if retreatment is required

Available forms include: Vial 4 mg

Side effects/adverse reactions:

▼ *ORAL:* Candidiasis

CNS: Insomnia, anxiety, confusion, fatigue, agitation

CV: Hypotension

GI: Nausea, constipation, diarrhea, abdominal pain

RESP: Dyspnea, coughing

HEMA: Anemia

GU: UTI

META: Hypophosphatemia, hypokalemia, hypomagnesemia

MISC: Fever, skeletal pain, flulike symptoms

Contraindications: Hypersensitivity, risk of renal failure if dose rate is exceeded

Precautions: Data for use in children not available, monitor hypercalcemic parameters, ensure good hydration, renal impairment, bronchospasm in aspirin sensitive asthmatics, hypocalcemia, hypoparathyroidism, pregnancy category C, lactation

Pharmacokinetics:

IV INF: Shows triphasic half-life; plasma protein binding 22%; little to no metabolism; excreted mainly in urine; a high percentage of the dose remains bound to bone

🦷 **Drug interactions of concern to dentistry:**

• None reported

DENTAL CONSIDERATIONS

General:

• This drug is used in oncology units or hospitals only.

• Examine for oral manifestation of opportunistic infection.

- Consider semisupine chair position for patient comfort if GI side effects occur.
- Short appointments may be required.
- If oral candidiasis occurs, treat with suitable antifungal drug.

Consultations:
- Medical consult may be required to assess disease control.

---

zolmitriptan
(zole'my-trip-tan)
Zomig, Zomig ZMT
Drug class.: Serotonin agonist

Action: A selective serotonin agonist for 5-HT$_{1D}$ and 5-HT$_{1B}$ serotonin receptors on intracranial blood vessels, trigeminal sensory nerves (cranial vessel constriction), and inhibition of proinflammatory neuropeptide release

Uses: Acute treatment of migraine with or without aura in adults

Dosage and routes:
- *Adult:* PO initial 2.5 mg or lower; if headache returns repeat dose in 2 hr not to exceed 10 mg in 24 hr; lack of response to first dose requires physician consult before taking second dose; safe use in treating more than 3 headaches in 30 days has not been established; doses of 5 mg cause an increase in side effects

Available forms include: Tabs 2.5, 5 mg; tabs oral disintegrating 2.5 mg

Side effects/adverse reactions:

▼ *ORAL: Dry mouth* (5%)
CNS: Dizziness, somnolence, warm sensation, hyperesthesia, paresthesia, dizziness, vertigo, numbness
CV: Chest pain, chest tightness,
*palpitation, **serious cardiac events may occur (coronary artery spasm, myocardial ischemia, MI, ventricular tachycardia, ventricular fibrillation)***
GI: Nausea, dyspepsia, dysphagia
RESP: Bronchitis, hiccups
HEMA: Ecchymosis
GU: Hematuria, cystitis, frequency
EENT: Sweating, photosensitivity, pruritus, rash, dry eyes
MS: Myalgia, leg cramps, back pain; neck, jaw, and throat pain
MISC: Asthenia, allergy reaction

Contraindications: Hypersensitivity, ischemic heart disease (angina, MI), Prinzmetal's variant angina, uncontrolled hypertension, within 24 hr of use of ergotamine or other 5HT$_1$ agonist, hemiplegic or basilar migraine, prophylactic therapy of migraine, Wolff-Parkinson-White syndrome, accessory conduction arrhythmias, MAO inhibitors

Precautions: Renal impairment, hepatic impairment, may cause coronary vasospasm, pregnancy category C, lactation, children, geriatric

Pharmacokinetics:
PO: Good absorption, peak plasma levels 2 hr; bioavailability 40%, metabolized to active *N*-desmethyl metabolite; half-life of metabolite 2-3 hr; plasma protein binding 25%; excreted mainly in urine (65%) and less in feces (30%)

🐾 **Drug interactions of concern to dentistry:**
- Potential serotonin crises: selective serotonin reuptake inhibitors, ergot-containing drugs (avoid

---

z

use within 24 hr of taking this
drug)
• Decreased plasma levels: cimetidine

DENTAL CONSIDERATIONS
General:
• This is an acute-use drug; thus it
is doubtful that patients will come
to the office if acute migraine is
present.
• Be aware of patient's disease, its
severity, and frequency, when
known.
• Advise patient if dental drugs
prescribed have a potential for photosensitivity.
Consultations:
• If treating chronic orofacial
pain, consult with physician of
record.
• Medical consult may be required to assess disease control
and patient's ability to tolerate
stress.
Teach patient/family:
• That dryness of the mouth may
occur when taking this drug
• To avoid mouth rinses with high
alcohol content due to drying effects
• Importance of updating health
and drug history if physician
makes any changes in evaluation or
drug regimens

___

zolpidem

(zole-pi′dem)
Ambien

Drug class.: Nonbarbiturate, nonbenzodiazepine sedative-hypnotic

Action: Presumed to interact with
a subunit of the GABA-benzodiazepine receptor, binding only to the
omega-1 subunit
Uses: Insomnia

Dosage and routes:
• *Adult:* PO 10 mg before bedtime
• *Elderly and debilitated:* PO 5 mg
before bedtime
Available forms include: Tabs 5,
10 mg
Side effects/adverse reactions:
▼ *ORAL:* Dry mouth, taste alteration
CNS: Dizziness, daytime drowsiness, amnesia, headache
*CV: **Tachycardia, hypertension***
GI: Nausea, vomiting, dyspepsia
GU: Menstrual disorder, vaginitis,
cystitis
EENT: Double vision, tinnitus
INTEG: Urticaria, acne
MS: Muscle pain
Contraindications: Hypersensitivity, ritonavir
Precautions: Pregnancy category
B, lactation, altered reaction time,
elderly, limit duration of use
Pharmacokinetics:
PO: Half-life 2.5 hr, peak plasma
levels 1.6 hr; highly protein bound
🦷 **Drug interactions of concern
to dentistry:**
• Increased CNS depression: alcohol, all CNS depressants, fluconazole, ketoconazole, itraconazole
DENTAL CONSIDERATIONS
General:
• Assess salivary flow as a factor in
caries, periodontal disease, and
candidiasis.
• Monitor vital signs every appointment due to cardiovascular
side effects.
Consultations:
• Medical consult may be required
to assess disease control.
Teach patient/family: *When
chronic dry mouth occurs, advise
patient:*
• To avoid mouth rinses with high

alcohol content due to drying effects
• Of need for daily use of home fluoride products to prevent caries
• To use sugarless gum, frequent sips of water, or saliva substitutes

---

zonisamide
(zoe-nis'a-mide)
Zonegran
Drug class.: Anticonvulsant (sulfonamide derivative)

Action: Mechanism of action is unknown; has been shown to block sodium and T-type calcium channels; suppresses electroshock induced seizures in experimental models

Uses: Adjunctive therapy in partial seizures in adults with epilepsy

Dosage and routes:
• *Adult >16:* PO initial dose 100 mg/day; after 2 wk may increase the dose to 200 mg/day for at least 2 wk; recommended limit 400 mg/day; 2 wk must be allowed between increases in doses

Available forms include: Caps 100 mg

Side effects/adverse reactions:

▼ *ORAL:* Taste perversion, gingival overgrowth, stomatitis

CNS: Difficulty concentrating, mental slowness, somnolence, fatigue, anorexia, dizziness, headache, agitation, irritability, depression, psychiatric symptoms, psychomotor slowness

CV: (infrequent) Palpitation, bradycardia, hypotension

GI: Nausea, vomiting, abdominal pain, diarrhea, dyspepsia

RESP: Pharyngitis

HEMA: (rare) **Aplastic anemia, agranulocytosis, leukopenia, thrombocytopenia,** anemia

GU: Kidney stones, urinary frequency

EENT: Diplopia, rhinitis, increased cough

*INTEG: **Stevens-Johnson syndrome, toxic epidermal necrolysis,*** rash

META: Increase in serum creatinine, BUN, serum alk phosphatase

MS: Leg cramps, myalgia

Contraindications: Hypersensitivity to this drug or sulfonamides

Precautions: Discontinue if skin rash occurs, child <16 yr risk of oligohidrosis, hyperthermia; seizures with abrupt withdrawal; use contraception in women of childbearing age; pregnancy category C, hepatic or renal dysfunction; lactation, kidney stones

Pharmacokinetics:

PO: Peak plasma levels 2-6 hr, half-life >60 hr, steady state plasma levels reached in 14 days with stable doses, significant binding to erythrocytes, excreted unchanged or as metabolite in urine, metabolism involves CYP450 3A4 enzymes

🦷 **Drug interactions of concern to dentistry:**
• No dental drug interactions reported; drugs that either induce or inhibit CYP 3A4 enzymes may alter serum levels
• Carbamazepine increases renal clearance

DENTAL CONSIDERATIONS
General:
• Determine type of epilepsy, seizure frequency, and quality of seizure control.
• Patient on chronic drug therapy may rarely present with symptoms

---

z

of blood dyscrasias, which can include infection, bleeding, and poor healing.

• Short appointments and a stress reduction protocol may be required for anxious patients.

• Place on frequent recall to evaluate gingival condition and self-care.

• Consider semisupine chair position for patient comfort if GI side effects occur.

• Warn patient of increased CNS side effects when sedation is used. Advise not to drive a car to and from dental appointment.

Consultations:

• Consultation with physician may be needed if sedation or general anesthesia is required.

• In a patient with symptoms of blood dyscrasias, request a medical consult for blood studies and postpone treatment until normal values are reestablished.

• Medical consult may be required to assess disease control and patient's ability to tolerate stress.

Teach patient/family:

• Importance of good oral hygiene to prevent soft tissue inflammation

• To prevent trauma when using oral hygiene aids

• Importance of updating health and drug history if physician makes any changes in evaluation or drug regimens

• If rash develops due to drug, advise patients to see physician immediately

italic = common side effects

Appendixes

Appendix A

Abbreviations

ā	before	**ASHD**	arteriosclerotic heart disease
aa	of each	**AST**	aspartate aminotransferase, serum
abd	abdomen	**AV**	atrioventricular
ABGs	arterial blood gases	**BAL**	blood alcohol level
ac	before meals (*ante cibum*)	**BCG**	bicolor guiac test
ACE	angiotensin-converting enzyme	**bid**	twice a day (*bis in die*)
Ach	acetylcholine	**BM**	bowel movement
ACT	activated coagulation time	**BMR**	basal metabolic rate
ACTH	adrenocorticotropic hormone	**bol**	bolus
		BP	blood pressure
ad lib	as desired	**BPH**	benign prostatic hypertrophy
ADH	antidiuretic hormone		
ADP	adenosine diphosphate	**bpm**	beats per minute
AIDS	acquired immunodeficiency syndrome	**BS**	blood sugar
		BUN	blood urea nitrogen
aka	also known as	**Bx**	biopsy
ALT	alanine aminotransferase, serum	c̄	with
		C	Celsius (centigrade)
ama	against medical advice	**C section**	Cesarean section
amb	ambulation	**Ca**	cancer, calcium
amp	ampule	**CAD**	coronary artery disease
ANA	antinuclear antibody		
ant	anterior	**cAMP**	cyclic adenosine monophosphate
ANUG	acute necrotizing ulcerative gingivitis	**cap**	capsule
		cath	catheterization or catheterize
AP	anteroposterior		
APAP	acetaminophen	**CBC**	complete blood count
APB	atrial premature beats		
APTT	activated partial thromboplastin time	**CBS**	chronic brain syndrome
ARC	AIDS-related complex	**CC**	chief complaint
AROM	active range of motion	**cc**	cubic centimeter
ASA	acetylsalicylic acid (aspirin)	**cGMP**	cyclic guanosine monophosphate
asap	as soon as possible		

CHF	congestive heart failure
cm	centimeter
CML	chronic myeloid leukemia
CMV	cytomegalovirus
CNS	central nervous system
CO$_2$	carbon dioxide
CoA	coenzyme A
c/o	complains of
COMT	catechol-O-methyltransferase
con rel	controlled release
conc	concentration
COPD	chronic obstructive pulmonary disease
COX 2	cyclooxygenase 2
CPAP	continuous positive airway pressure
CPK	creatinine phosphokinase
CPR	cardiopulmonary resuscitation
CrCl	creatinine clearance
CRF	chronic renal failure
C&S	culture and sensitivity
crys	crystallinized
CSF	cerebrospinal fluid
CV	cardiovascular
CVA	cerebrovascular accident
CVP	central venous pressure
CysLT$_1$	cysteinyl leukotriene receptor
D&C	dilation and curettage
del rel	delayed release
DIC	disseminated intravascular coagulation
DM	diabetes mellitus
DOA	dead on arrival
DOB	date of birth
dr	dram
dsg	dressing
DVT	deep vein thrombosis
D$_5$W	5% glucose in distilled water

dx	diagnosis
ECG	electrocardiogram (EKG)
EEG	electroencephalogram
EENT	ear, eye, nose, and throat
elix	elixir, hydroalcoholic solution containing an active drug(s)
ENDO	endocrine systems
EPS	extrapyramidal symptoms
ESR	erythrocyte sedimentation rate
ext rel	extended release
F	Fahrenheit
FBS	fasting blood sugar
FHT	fetal heart tones
FIo$_2$	inspired oxygen concentration
FSH	follicle-stimulating hormone
fx	fracture
g	gram
GABA	γ-aminobutyric acid
gal	gallon
GERD	gastroesophageal reflux disease
GGT	gamma glutamyl transpeptidase
GHb	glycosylated hemoglobin
GI	gastrointestinal
G6PD	glucose-6-phosphate dehydrogenase
Ghb	glycosylated hemoglobin
gr	grain
GR	glucocorticoid receptor
gtt	drop
GTT	glucose tolerance test
GU	genitourinary
Gyn	gynecology
H	hydrogen

HbA1c	lab test for glycosylated hemoglobin	**IM**	intramuscular
Hct	hematocrit	**immed rel**	immediate release
HCG	human chorionic gonadotropin	**inf**	infusion
		inh	inhalation
HDL	high-density lipoprotein	**inj**	injection
		INR	international normalized ratio
HDCV	human diploid cell rabies vaccine	**INTEG**	relating to integumentary structures
HEMA	hematologic system		
Hgb	hemoglobin	**I&O**	intake and output
H&H	hematocrit and hemoglobin	**IOP**	intraocular pressure
H&P	history and physical exam	**IPPB**	intermittent positive-pressure breathing
5-HIAA	5-hydroxyindoleacetic acid	**IPTH**	intact parathyroid hormone
HMG-CoA	3-hydroxy-3-methylglutarylcoenzyme A reductase	**ITP**	idiopathic thrombocytopenic purpura
		IU	international units
5-HT	5-hydroxytryptamine (serotonin)	**IUD**	intrauterine contraceptive device
H_2O	water	**IV**	intravenous
HOB	head of bed	**IVAC**	intravenous controller
HR	heart rate		
hr	hour	**IVP**	intravenous pyelogram
hs	at bedtime *(hora somni)*	**IVPB**	intravenous piggyback
HSV	herpes simplex virus	**K**	potassium
		kg	kilogram
HSV-2	herpes genitalis	**L or l**	left
hypo	hypodermically	**L**	liter
Hx	history	**lat**	lateral
IBS	irritable bowel syndrome	**lb**	pound
ICP	intracranial pressure	**LDH**	lactic dehydrogenase
ICU	intensive care unit	**LDL**	low-density lipoprotein
I&D	incision and drainage	**LDL-C**	low-density lipoprotein–cholesterol
IgG	immunoglobulin G	**LE**	lupus erythematosus
IL-2	interleukin-2	**LFT**	liver function tests

LH	luteinizing hormone	**NPH**	neutral protamine Hagedorn
LHRH	luteinizing hormone-releasing hormone	**NPO**	nothing by mouth *(nil per os)*
liq	liquid		
LLQ	left lower quadrant	**NS**	normal saline
LMP	last menstrual period	**NSAID**	nonsteroidal antiinflammatory drug
LOC	loss of consciousness		
loz	lozenge	**NV**	neurovascular
LR	lactated Ringer's solution	**O₂**	oxygen
		OBS	organic brain syndrome
LRI	lower respiratory infection	**OD**	right eye *(oculus dexter)*
LUQ	left upper quadrant	**oint**	ointment
LVD	left ventricular dysfunction	**OOB**	out of bed
m	meter, minim	**ophth**	ophthalmic
m²	square meter	**OR**	operating room
MAC	*mycobacterium avium* complex	**ORIF**	open reduction, internal fixation
MAO	monoamine oxidase	**OS**	left eye *(ocular sinister)*
max	maximum		
MCA	motorcycle accident	**os**	mouth
META	metabolic	**OTC**	over the counter
mEq	milliequivalent	**OU**	each eye *(oculus uterque)*
mg	milligram		
μg	microgram	**oz**	ounce
MI	myocardial infarction	**p̄**	after (post)
		p	pulse
min	minute	**PABA**	para-aminobenzoic acid
mixt	mixture		
ml	milliliter	**PAC**	premature atrial contraction
mm	millimeter		
mo	month	**Paco₂**	arterial carbon dioxide tension (pressure tore)
MPA	mycophenolic acid		
MS	musculoskeletal		
MVA	motor vehicle accident	**Pao₂**	arterial oxygen tension (pressure tore)
n	nanogram		
Na	sodium	**PAT**	paroxysmal atrial tachycardia
NC	nasal cannula		
neg	negative	**PBI**	protein-bound iodine
NIDDM	non–insulin-dependent diabetes mellitus	**pc**	after meals *(post cibum)*
NKA	no known allergies	**PCA**	patient-controlled analgesia
NMI	no middle initial		
noc	nocturnal (night)	**PCN**	penicillin

PCWP	pulmonary capillary wedge pressure	**q4h**	every 4 hours
PE	physical examination	**q6h**	every 6 hours
		q12h	every 12 hours
PEEP	positive end-expiratory pressure	**qwk**	every week
		r	right
PERRLA	pupils equal, round, react to light and accommodation	**RAIU**	radioactive iodine uptake
		RAR	retinoic acid receptor
pH	hydrogen ion concentration	**RBC(s)**	red blood count or cell(s)
PMS	premenstrual syndrome	**RDA**	recommended dietary allowance
PNS	peripheral nervous system	**rec**	rectal
PO	by mouth *(per os)*	**REM**	rapid eye movement
postop	postoperatively	**RESP**	respiratory system
PP	postprandial		
PPAR-γ	proliferator-activated receptor gamma	**rhPDGF-BB**	recombinant human platelet-derived growth factor
ppm	parts per million		
preop	preoperatively		
prep	preparation		
prn	as needed *(pro re nata)*	**RLQ**	right lower quadrant
PSA	prostate specific antigen	**R/O**	rule out
PT	prothrombin time	**ROAD**	reversible obstructive airway disease
PTT	partial thromboplastin time		
PVC	premature ventricular contraction	**ROM**	range of motion
		RTI	respiratory tract infection
PVD	peripheral vascular disease	**RUQ**	right upper quadrant
q	every	**Rx**	therapy, treatment, or prescription
qam	every morning		
qd	every day		
qh	every hour	**s̄**	without
qid	four times a day	**SA**	sinoatrial
qod	every other day	**SAN**	sinoatrial node
qpm	every night	**SC**	subcutaneous
qsad	add a sufficient quantity	**sec**	second
		SERM	elective estrogen receptor modulator
qt	quart		
q2h	every 2 hours		
q3h	every 3 hours		

SGOT	serum glutamic-oxaloacetic transaminase
SGPT	serum glutamic pyruvate transaminase
SIADH	syndrome of inappropriate antidiuretic hormone
sig	patient dosing instructions on prescription label
SIMV	synchronous intermittent mandatory ventilation
SL	sublingual
SLE	systemic lupus erythematosus
slow rel	slow release
SMBG	self-monitored blood glucose
SMZ	sulfamethoxazole
SOB	short of breath
sol	solution
ss	one half
SSRI	serotonin selective reuptake inhibitor
stat	at once
surg	surgical
sus rel	sustained release dose form
supp	suppository
Sx	symptoms
syr	syrup, a highly concentrated sucrose solution containing a drug(s)
T	temperature
T$_3$	triiodothyronine
T$_4$	thyroxine
tab	tablet
TAH	total abdominal hysterectomy
TB	tuberculosis
TBG	thyroxine-binding globulin
tbsp	tablespoon
TD	transdermal
temp	temperature
TIA	transient ischemic attack
tid	three times daily (*ter in die*)
time rel	time release dose form
tinc	tincture, alcoholic solution of a drug
TMD	temporomandibular dysfunction
TMJ	temporomandibular joint
TMP	trimethoprim
TNF	tumor necrosis factor
top	topical
TPN	total parenteral nutrition
TPR	temperature, pulse, respirations
TSH	thyroid-stimulating hormone
tsp	teaspoon
TT	thrombin time
Tx	treatment
U	unit
UA	urinalysis
ULDL	ultra-low-density lipoprotein
URI	upper respiratory infection
USP	United States Pharmacopeia
UTI	urinary tract infection
UV	ultraviolet
vag	vaginal
visc	viscous
VD	venereal disease
VLDL	very-low-density lipoprotein
VO	verbal order
vol	volume
VPB	ventricular premature beats
VS	vital signs

WBC	white blood (cell) count	>	greater than
WHO	World Health Organization	<	less than
wk	week	≠	not equal
WNL	within normal limits	↑	increase
wt	weight	↓	decrease
yr	year	**2°**	secondary

Appendix B

Drugs causing dry mouth

Drug category	Brand name	Generic name
ANOREXIANT	Adipex-P, Fastin, Ionamin	phentermine
	Anorex	phendimetrazine
	Mazanor, Sanorex	mazindol
	Tenuate, Tepanil	diethylpropion
ANTIACNE	Accutane	isotretinoin
ANTIANXIETY	Atarax, Vistaril	hydroxyzine
	Ativan	lorazepam
	BuSpar	buspirone
	Equanil, Miltown	meprobamate
	Librium	chlordiazepoxide
	Paxipam	halazepam
	Serax	oxazepam
	Sonata	zalephon
	Valium	diazepam
	Xanax	alprazolam
ANTIARTHRITIC	Arava	leflunomide
ANTICHOLINERGIC/	Anaspaz	hyoscyamine
ANTISPASMODIC	Atropisol	atropine
	Banthine	methantheline
	Bellergal	belladonna alkaloids
	Bentyl	dicyclomine
	Darbid	isopropamide
	Daricon	oxyphencyclimine
	Ditropan	oxybutynin
	Donnatal, Kinesed	hyoscyamine atropine, phenobarbital, scopolamine
	Librax	chlordiazepoxide, clidinium
	Pamine	methscopolamine
	Pro-Banthine	propantheline
	Transderm-Scōp	scopolamine
ANTICONVULSANT	Felbatol	felbamate
	Lamictal	lamotrigine
	Neurontin	gabapentin
	Tegretol	carbamazepine

ANTIDEPRESSANT	Anafranil	clomipramine
	Asendin	amoxapine
	Celexa	citalopram
	Effexor	venlafaxine
	Elavil	amitriptyline
	Luvox	fluvoxamine
	Marplan	isocarboxazid
	Nardil	phenelzine
	Norpramin	desipramine
	Parnate	tranylcypromine
	Paxil	paroxetine
	Prozac	fluoxetine
	Sinequan	doxepin
	Tofranil	imipramine
	Wellbutrin	bupropion
	Zoloft	sertraline
ANTIDIARRHEAL	Imodium AD	loperamide
	Lomotil	diphenoxylate, atropine
	Motofen	difenoxin
ANTIHISTAMINE	Actifed	triprolidine with pseudoephedrine
	Atarax	hydroxyzine
	Benadryl	diphenhydramine
	Chlor-Trimeton	chlorpheniramine
	Claritin	loratadine
	Dimetane	brompheniramine
	Dimetapp	brompheniramine, phenylpropanolamine
	Phenergan	promethazine
	Pyribenzamine (PBZ)	tripelennamine
ANTIHYPERTENSIVE	Capoten	captopril
	Catapres	clonidine
	Coreg	carvedilol
	Ismelin	guanethidine
	Aceon	perindopril
	Minipress	prazosin
	Serpasil	reserpine
	Wytensin	guanabenz
	Vasotec	enalapril
ANTIINFLAMMATORY ANALGESIC	Dolobid	diflunisal
	Celebrex	celecoxib
	Feldene	piroxicam
	Motrin	ibuprofen
	Nalfon	fenoprofen
	Naprosyn	naproxen
	Vioxx	rofecoxib

ANTIINFLAMMA- TORY GI	Colazal	balsalazide
ANTINAUSEANT	Antivert	meclizine
	Dramamine	diphenhydramine
	Marezine	cyclizine
ANTIPARKINSONIAN	Akineton	biperiden
	Artane	trihexyphenidyl
	Cogentin	benztropine mesylate
	Larodopa	levodopa
	Marflex	orphenadrine HCl
	Parsidol	ethopropazine
	Sinemet	carbidopa, levodopa
	Tasmar	tolcapone
ANTIPSYCHOTIC	Clozaril	clozapine
	Compazine	prochlorperazine
	Eskalith	lithium
	Haldol	haloperidol
	Mellaril	thioridazine
	Navane	thiothixene
	Orap	pimozide
	Risperdal	resperidone
	Sparine	promazine
	Stelazine	trifluoperazine
	Thorazine	chlorpromazine
	Triavil	amitriptyline, perphenazine
	Zyprexa	olanzapine
ANTISECRETORY	Aciphex	rabeprazole
	Nexium	esomeprazole
ANTISPASMODIC	Detrol	tolterodine
ANTIVIRAL	Sustiva	efavirenz
BRONCHODILATOR		ephedrine (generic)
	Isuprel	isoproterenol
	Proventil, Ventolin	albuterol
	Xopenex	levalbuterol
CNS STIMULANT	Dexedrine	dextroamphetamine
	Desoxyn	methamphetamine
DECONGESTANT	Ornade	phenylpropanolamine, chlorpheniramine
	Sudafed	pseudoephedrine
DIURETIC	Aldactone	spironolactone
	Diuril	chlorothiazide
	Dyazide, Maxzide, Dyrenium	triamterene, hydrochlorothiazide

	HydroDIURIL, Esidrix	hydrochlorothiazide
	Lasix	furosemide
	Midamor	amiloride
MIGRAINE	Amerge	naratriptan
	Axert	almotriptan
	Maxalt	rizatriptan
MUSCLE RELAXANT	Flexeril	cyclobenzaprine
	Lioresal	baclofen
	Norflex, Disipal	orphenadrine
NARCOLEPSY	Provigil	modafinil
NARCOTIC ANALGESIC	Demerol	meperidine
	MS Contin	morphine
OPHTHALMIC	Azopt	brinzolamide
SEDATIVE	Dalmane	flurazepam
	Halcion	triazolam
	Restoril	temazepam

Appendix C

Controlled substances chart

Drugs	United States	Canada
Heroin, LSD, peyote, marijuana, mescaline, phencyclidine	Schedule I (CI)	Schedule H
Opium, fentanyl, morphine, meperidine, methadone, oxycodone (and its combinations), hydromorphone, codeine (single-drug entity), and cocaine	Schedule II (CII)	Schedule N
Short-acting barbiturates	Schedule II	Schedule C
Amphetamine and methylphenidate	Schedule II	Schedule G
Codeine combinations, hydrocodone combinations, glutethimide, paregoric, phendimetrazine, thiopental, testosterone, and other androgens	Schedule III (CIII)	Schedule F
Benzodiazepines (diazepam, midazolam, etc.), chloral hydrate, meprobamate, phenobarbital, propoxyphene (and combinations), pentazocine (and combinations), and methohexital	Schedule IV (CIV)	Schedule F
Antidiarrheals and antitussives with opioid derivatives	Schedule V (CV)	

Appendix D

FDA pregnancy categories

A   Studies have failed to demonstrate a risk to the fetus in any trimester

B   Animal reproduction studies fail to demonstrate a risk to the fetus; no human studies available

C   Given only after risks to the fetus are considered; animal reproduction stdies have shown adverse effects on fetus; no human studies available

D   Definite human fetal risks; may be given in spite of risks if needed in life-threatening conditions

X   Absolute fetal abnormalities; not to be used anytime during pregnancy because risks outweigh benefits

Appendix E

Drugs that affect taste

ALCOHOL DETOXIFICATION
disulfiram (Antabuse)

ALZHEIMER'S
donepezil (Aricept)

ANALGESICS (NSAIDs)
diclofenac (Voltaren)
etodolac (Lodine)
ketoprofen (Orudis)
meclofenamate (Meclofen)
sulindac (Clinoril)

ANESTHETICS (GENERAL)
midazolam (Versed)
propofol (Diprivan)

ANESTHETICS (LOCAL)
lidocaine transoral delivery
system (Dentipatch)

ANOREXIANTS
diethylpropion (Tenuate)
mazindol (Mazanor)
phendimetrazine (Adipost)
phentermine (Ionamin)

ANTACIDS
aluminum hydroxide (Amphojel)
calcium carbonate (Tums)
lansoprazole (Prevacid)
magaldrate (Riapan)
omeprazole (Prilosec)
sucralfate (Carafate)

ANTIARTHRITIC
leflunomide (Arava)

ANTICHOLINERGICS
clidinium (Quarzan)
mepenzolate (Cantil)
methantheline (Banthine)
propantheline (Pro-Banthine)

ANTICONVULSANTS
fosphenytoin (Cerebyx)
phenytoin (Dilantin)
topiramate (Topamax)

ANTIDEPRESSANTS
amitriptyline (Elavil)
clomipramine (Anafranil)
desipramine (Norpramin)
doxepin (Sinequan)
fluoxetine (Prozac)
imipramine (Tofranil)
nefazodone (Serzone)
nortriptyline (Pamelor)
protriptyline (Vivactil)
sertraline (Zoloft)

ANTIDIABETICS
metformin (Glucophage)
tolbutamide (Orinase)

ANTIDIARRHEALS
bismuth subsalicylate (Pepto-
Bismol)

ANTIEMETICS
dolasetron mesylate (Anazemet)

ANTIFUNGALS
griseofulvin (Fulvicin)
terbinafine (Lamisil)

ANTIGOUT
allopurinol (Zyloprim)
colchicine

ANTIHISTAMINE (H$_1$) ANTAGONISTS
azelastine (Astelin)
cetirizine (Zyrtec)

ANTIHISTAMINE (H$_2$) ANTAGONISTS
famotidine (Pepcid)

ANTIHYPERLIPIDEMICS
clofibrate (Atromid-S)
fluvastatin (Lescol)

ANTIINFECTIVES
ciprofloxacin (Ciloxan)
ethionamide (Trecator-SC)
levofloxacin (Levoquin)
lincomycin (Lincocin)
metronidazole (Flagyl)

ANTIINFLAMMATORY/ ANTIARTHRITIC
auranofin (Ridaura)
aurothioglucose (Solganal)
celecoxib (Celebrex)
rofecoxib (Vioxx)
sulfasalazine (Azulfidine)

ANTIMIGRAINE
almotriptan (Axert)

ANTIPARKINSON
entacapone (Comtan)
levodopa (Larodopa)
levodopa-carbidopa (Sinemet)
pergolide (Permax)
pramipexole dihydrochloride
(Mirapex)

ANTIPSYCHOTICS
lithium (Eskalith)
pimozide (Orap)
prochlorperazine (Compazine)
quetiapine fumarate (Seroquel)
risperidone (Risperdal)
triflupromazine (Vesprin)

ANTITHYROID
methimazole (Tapazole)
propylthiouracil

ANTIVIRALS
acyclovir (Zovirax)
amprenavir (Agenerase)
delavirdine mesylate
(Rescriptor)
didanosine (Videx)
efavirenz (Sustiva)
foscarnet (Foscavir)
indinavir (Crixivan)
penciclovir (Denavir)
rimantadine (Flumadine)
ritonavir (Norvir)
saquinavir (Invirase)
valcyclovir (Valtrex)
zidovudine (Retrovir)

ANXIOLYTIC/SEDATIVES
chloral hydrate (Noctec)
estazolam (ProSom)
quazepam (Doral)
zolpidem (Ambien)

ASTHMA PREVENTIVES
cromolyn (Intal)
nedocromil (Tilade)

BRONCHODILATORS
albuterol (Proventil)
bitolterol (Tornalate)
formoterol fumarate (Foradil)
ipratropium (Atrovent)
isoproterenol (Isuprel)
metaproterenol (Alupent)
pirbuterol (Maxair)
terbutaline (Brethine)

CALCIUM AFFECTING DRUGS
alendronate (Fosamax)
calcitonin (Calcimar)
etidronate (Didronel)

CANCER CHEMOTHERAPEUTICS
capecitabine (Xeloda)
fluorouracil (Efudex)
levamisole (Ergamisol)
tamoxifen (Nolvadex)

CARDIOVASCULAR
amiodarone (Cordarone)
amlodipine (Norvasc)
bepridil (Vascor)
captopril (Capoten)
clonidine (Catapres)
diltiazem (Cardizem)
enalapril (Vasotec)
flecainide (Tambocor)
fosinopril (Monopril)
guanfacine (Tenex)
labetalol (Trandate)
losartan (Cozaar)
mecamylamine (Inversine)
mexiletine (Mexitil)
moricizine (Ethmozine)
nadolol (Corgard)
nifedipine (Procardia XL)
penbutolol (Levabol)
perindopril (Aceon)
propafenone (Rythmol)
quinidine (Cardioquin)
valsartan (Diovan)

CNS STIMULANTS
dextroamphetamine (Dexedrine)
methamphetamine (Desoxyn)

DECONGESTANT
phenylephrine (Neo-Synephrine)

DIURETICS
acetazolamide (Diamox)
methazolamide (Naptazine)
polythiazide (Renese)

GLUCOCORTICOIDS
budesonide (Rhinocort)
flunisolide (Aerobid)
rimexolone (Vexol)

GALLSTONE SOLUBILIZATION
ursodiol (Actigall)

HEMORHEOLOGIC
pentoxifylline (Trental)

IMMUNOMODULATORS
interferon alfa (Roferon-A)
levamisole (Ergamisol)
tacrolimus (Protopic)

IMMUNOSUPPRESSANTS
azathioprine (Imuran)

METHYLXANTHINES
aminophylline (Somophyllin)
dyphylline (Dilor)
oxtriphylline (Choledyl)
theophylline (Theo-Dur)

NICOTINE CESSATION
nicotine polacrilex (Nicorette)

OPHTHALMICS
apraclonidine (Iopidine)
brimonidine (Alphagan)
brinzolamide (Azopt)
dorzolamide (Truspot)
olopatadine (Pantanol)

PROTON PUMP INHIBITORS
esomeprazole (Nexium)
lansoprazole (Prevacid)
omeprazole (Prilosec)

RETINOID, SYSTEMIC
  acitretin (Soriatane)

SALIVARY STIMULANT
  pilocarpine (Salagen)

SKELETAL MUSCLE RELAXANTS
  baclofen (Lioresal)
  cyclobenzaprine (Flexeril)
  methocarbamol (Robaxin)

VITAMINS
  calcifediol (vitamin D)
  calcitriol (vitamin D)
  dihydrotachysterol (vitamin D)
  phytonadione (vitamin K)

Appendix F

Combination products

Accuretic: quinapril 10 mg with hydrochlorothiazide 12.5 mg, or quinapril 20 mg with hydrochlorothiazide 12.5 mg, or quinapril 20 mg with hydrochlorothiazide 25 mg

Aceta with Codeine, Tylenol with Codeine No. 3: acetaminophen 300 mg with codeine phosphate 30 mg

Actagen, Actifed Cold and Allergy, Allercon, Allerfrim, Aprodine, Cenafed Plus, Genac, Triposed: pseudoephedrine HCl 60 mg with triprolidine HCl 2.5 mg

Activella: norethindrone acetate 0.5 mg with estradiol 1 mg

Adderall 5: amphetamine aspartate 1.25 mg, amphetamine sulfate 1.25 mg, dextroamphetamine saccharate 1.25 mg, and dextroamphetamine sulfate 1.25 mg

Adderall 10: amphetamine aspartate 2.5 mg, amphetamine sulfate 2.5 mg, dextroamphetamine saccharate 2.5 mg, and dextroamphetamine sulfate 2.5 mg

Adderall 20: amphetamine aspartate 5 mg, amphetamine sulfate 5 mg, dextroamphetamine sulfate 5 mg, and dextroamphetamine saccharate 5 mg

Adderall 30: amphetamine aspartate 7.5 mg, amphetamine sulfate 7.5 mg, dextroamphetamine sulfate 7.5 mg, and dextroamphetamine saccharate 7.5 mg

Advicor: niacin 500 mg and lovastatin 20 mg; niacin 750 mg and lovastatin 750 mg; niacin 1000 mg and lovastatin 20 mg

Advair Diskus: salmeterol 50 mcg and fluticasone propionate 100, 250, or 500 mcg

Aggrenox: aspirin 25 mg with dipyridamole 200 mg

Ak-Trol Ointment, Dexasporin Ointment, Dexacidin Ointment: dexamethasone 1 mg, polymyxin B sulfate 10,000 U, and neomycin sulfate 3.5 mg/g

Ak-Trol, Maxitrol, Dexacidin Suspension: dexamethasone 1 mg, polymyxin B sulfate 10,000 U, and neomycin sulfate 3.5 mg/ml of suspension

Aldactazide 25/25: spironolactone 25 mg with hydrochlorothiazide 25 mg

Aldactazide 50/50: spironolactone 50 mg with hydrochlorothiazide 50 mg

Aldoclor-150: methyldopa 250 mg with chlorothiazide 150 mg

Aldoclor-250: methyldopa 250 mg with chlorothiazide 250 mg

Aldoril-15: methyldopa 250 mg with hydrochlorothiazide 15 mg

Aldoril-25: methyldopa 250 mg with hydrochlorothiazide 25 mg

Aldoril D30: methyldopa 500 mg with hydrochlorothiazide 30 mg

Aldoril D50: methyldopa 500 mg with hydrochlorothiazide 50 mg

Allegra-D: fexofenadine 60 mg with pseudoephedrine HCl 120 mg

Allent, Bromfed, Bromfenex, Endafed, Ultrabrom: pseudoephedrine HCl 120 mg with brompheniramine maleate 12 mg

Allerest Maximum Strength 12 Hour, Contac Maximum Strength 12 Hour, Drize, Ornade Spansules, Resaid, Rhinolar-EX 12 Hour, Triaminic-12, Vanex Forte-R: phenylpropanolamine hydrochloride 75 mg with chlorpheniramine maleate 12 mg

Ambenyl Cough Syrup, Amgenal, Bromotuss/Codeine, Bromanyl Syrup: bromodiphenhydramine HCl 12.5 mg/5 ml with codeine phosphate 10 mg/5 ml

Anacin, P-A-C Analgesic: aspirin 400 mg with caffeine 32 mg

Anexsia 5/500, Bancap HC, Ceta-Plus, Co-Gesic, Dolacet, Duocet, Hydrocet, Hydrogesic, Hy-Phen, Lorcet-HD, Lortab 5/500, Margesic H, Panacet 5/500, Stagesic, T-Gesic, Vicodin: hydrocodone bitartrate 5.0 mg with acetaminophen 500 mg

Anexsia 7.5/650, Lorcet Plus: hydrocodone bitartrate 7.5 mg with acetaminophen 650 mg

Anexsia 10/660, Vicodin HP: hydrocodone bitartrate 10 mg with acetaminophen 660 mg

Antrocol Elixir: atropine sulfate 0.195 mg/5 ml with phenobarbital 16 mg/5 ml

Apresazide 25/25: hydralazine HCl 25 mg with hydrochlorothiazide 25 mg

Apresazide 50/50: hydralazine HCl 50 mg with hydrochlorothiazide 50 mg

Apresazide 100/50: hydralazine HCl 100 mg with hydrochlorothiazide 50 mg

Arthrotec: diclofenac 75 mg with misoprostol 200 µg; or diclofenac 50 mg with misoprostol 200 µg

Aspirin Free Excedrin, Premsyn PMS, Vitelle Lurline PMS, Pamprin Multi-Symptom Maximum Strength: acetaminophen 500 mg with caffeine 65 mg

Atacand HCT: candesartan cilexetil, hydrochlorothiazide

Azo-Sulfisoxazole: sulfisoxazole 500 mg with phenazopyridine HCl 50 mg

Barbidonna: belladonna alkaloids, atropine sulfate 0.025 mg, hyoscyamine sulfate 0.1286 mg, scopolamine hydrobromide 0.0074 mg and phenobarbital 16 mg

Barbidonna No. 2: belladonna alkaloids, atropine sulfate 0.025 mg, hyoscyamine sulfate 0.1286 mg, scopolamine hydrobromide 0.0074 mg, and phenobarbital 32 mg

Bayer Select Head Cold, Bayer Select Maximum Strength Sinus Relief, Contact Nondrowsy Sinus, Dristan Cold Tablets, Maximum Strength Ornex, Maximum Strength Sine-Aid, Maximum Strength Sinutab without Drowsiness, Maximum Strength Tylenol Sinus, Maximum Strength Sudafed Sinus, Maximum Strength Dynafed Plus, Tavist Sinus: pseudoephedrine HCl 30 mg with acetaminophen 500 mg

BC Powder Original Formula: aspirin 650 mg with caffeine 32 mg, salicylamide 145 mg

BC Powder Arthritis Strength: aspirin 742 mg with caffeine 36 mg, salicylamide 222 mg

Bellergal-S, Phenerbel-S: ergotamine tartrate 0.6 mg with levorotatory belladonna alkaloid maleates 0.2 mg and phenobarbital 40-mg tablets

Benylin Adult, Pertussin ES: dextromethorphan hydrobromide 15 mg/5 ml

Benylin DM, Diabetes CF: dextromethorphan hydrobromide 10 mg/5 ml

Bromfed Tablets, Rondec Chewable: pseudoephedrine HCl 60 mg with brompheniramine maleate 4 mg

Bromfenex-PD, Bromfed-PD, Dallergy-JR, ULTRAbrom PD: pseudoephedrine HCl 60 mg with brompheniramine maleate 6 mg

Bromo-Seltzer: acetaminophen 325 mg, citric acid 2.224 g, sodium bicarbonate 2.871 g/capful measure

Brontex: codeine phosphate 10 mg with guaifenesin 300 mg tablets

Brontex Liquid: codeine phosphate 2.5 mg with guaifenesin 75 mg/5 ml

Butibel: belladonna extract 15 mg (0.187 mg of alkaloids of belladonna leaf) with butabarbital sodium 15 mg

Butibel Elixir: belladonna extract 15 mg with butabarbital sodium 15 mg in each 5 ml

Cafergot, Ercaf, and **Wigraine:** ergotamine tartrate 1 mg with caffeine 100 mg

Cafergot Suppositories, Cafatine, Cafetrate, Wigraine: ergotamine tartrate 2 mg, caffeine 100 mg

Caladryl Lotion: diphenhydramine HCl 1% with calamine 8%, camphor 0.1%, alcohol 2.2%

Calcidrine Syrup: codeine 8.4 mg/5 ml with calcium iodide anhydrous 152 mg/5 ml

Capital with Codeine Suspension or **Tylenol with Codeine Elixir:** acetaminophen 120 mg/5 ml with codeine 12 mg/5 ml

Capozide 25/15: captopril 25 mg with hydrochlorothiazide 15 mg

Capozide 25/25: captopril 25 mg with hydrochlorothiazide 25 mg

Capozide 50/15: captopril 50 mg with hydrochlorothiazide 15 mg

Capozide 50/25: captopril 50 mg with hydrochlorothiazide 25 mg

Carisoprodol Compound, Sodol Compound, Soma Compound: carisoprodol 200 mg with aspirin 325 mg

Chardonna-2: belladonna extract 15 mg with phenobarbital 15 mg

Children's Cepacol Liquid: acetaminophen 160 mg/5 ml and pseudoephedrine 15 mg/5 ml

Claritin-D: loratadine 5 mg with pseudoephedrine sulfate 120 mg

Claritin-D 24 Hour: loratadine 10 mg with pseudoephedrine sulfate 240 mg

CombiPatch: estradiol 0.05 mg with norethindrone acetate 0.14 mg; estradiol 0.05 mg with norethindrone acetate 0.25 mg

Combipres 0.1: clonidine HCl 0.1 mg with chlorthalidone 15 mg

Combipres 0.2: clonidine HCl 0.2 mg with chlorthalidone 15 mg

Combipres 0.3: clonidine HCl 0.3 mg with chlorthalidone 15 mg

Combivent: albuterol sulfate 103 μg with ipratropium bromide 18 μg

Combivir: lamivudine 150 mg with zidovudine 300 mg

Comtrex Allergy-Sinus, Sine-off Sinus Medicine, Sinutab Maximum Strength Sinus Allergy: pseudoephedrine HCl 30 mg with chlorpheniramine maleate 2 mg and acetaminophen 500 mg

Comtrex Liqui-Gels, Cold Relief Tablets, Triaminicol Multi-Symptom Cough and Cold Tab-

lets: phenylpropanolamine HCl 12.5 mg with chlorpheniramine maleate 2 mg and dextromethorphan HBr 10 mg

Comtrex Max Strength Multi-Symptom Cold and Flu Relief, Maximum Strength Comtrex Liqui-Gels: phenylpropanolamine HCl 12.5 mg with chlorpheniramine maleate 2 mg, dextromethorphan HBr 15 mg and acetaminophen 500 mg

Contact Cough and Chest Cold: dextromethorphan hydrobromide 5 mg/5 ml, pseudoephedrine 15 mg/5 ml and guaifenesin 50 mg/5 ml

Contact 12 Hour Capsule, Gencold, Rhinolar-EX, Gold-Gest Cold, Teldrin-12 Hour Allergy Relief: phenylpropanolamine HCl 75 mg and chlorpheniramine 8 mg

Contuss Liquid: phenylpropanolamine HCl 20 mg, phenylephrine HCl 5 mg and guaifenesin 100 mg/5 ml

Corzide 40/5: bendroflumethiazide 5 mg with nadolol 40 mg

Corzide 80/5: bendroflumethiazide 5 mg with nadolol 80 mg

Cystex: methenamine 162 mg, sodium salicylate 162.5 mg, benzoic acid 32 mg

Darvocet-N 50, Propoxyphene Napsylate with Acetaminophen Tablets: acetaminophen 325 mg with propoxyphene napsylate 50 mg

Darvocet-N 100, Propacet 100: propoxyphene napsylate 100 mg with acetaminophen 650 mg

Darvon Compound-65 Pulvules: aspirin 389 mg with caffeine 32.4 mg, propoxyphene HCl 65 mg

Deconamine CX, Entuss-D: hydrocodone bitartrate 5 mg with pseudoephedrine HCl 30 mg and guaifenesin 300 mg

Deconamine CX Liquid, Detussin Expectorant, Cophene XP, SRC Expectorant, Tussafin Expectorant: hydrocodone bitartrate 5 mg with pseudoephedrine HCl 60 mg and guaifenesin 200 mg/5 ml

Deconamine SR, Rinade B.I.D, Kronofed-A, N D Clear, Novafed A, Time-Hist, Rescon ED, Pseudo-Chlor: pseudoephedrine hydrochloride 120 mg with chlorpheniramine maleate 8 mg

Demi-Regroton: chlorthalidone 25 mg with reserpine 0.125 mg

Dimacol, Sudafed Cold and Cough Liquid Caps: pseudoephedrine hydrochloride 30 mg with dextromethorphan hydrobromide 10 mg and guaifenesin 100 mg

Dimetane-DC Cough Syrup, Bromanate DC, Bromphen DC, Myphetane DC, Poly-Histine CS: phenylpropanolamine HCl 12.5 mg, brompheniramine maleate 2 mg and codeine phosphate 10 mg/5 ml

Dimetane-DX Cough Syrup, Bromatane DX, Bromophen DX, Bromarest DX, Bromfed DM, Myphetane DX: dextromethorphan hydrobromide 10 mg/5 ml with brompheniramine maleate 2 mg/5 ml, pseudoephedrine HCl 30 mg/5 ml

Dimetapp, Dimetapp 4 Hour Liqui-Gel, Dimaphen, Vicks DayQuil Allergy Relief 4 Hour: phenylpropanolamine HCl 25 mg, brompheniramine maleate 4 mg

Diutensin-R: methyclothiazide 2.5 mg with reserpine 0.1 mg

Donnagel Liquid or tablets: 600 mg attapulgite per 15 ml or per tablet

Donnatal, Hyosophen, Malatal, Spasmolin: atropine sulfate 0.0194 mg, hyoscyamine sulfate

0.1037 mg, scopolamine hydrobromide 0.0065 mg, and phenobarbital 16.2 mg

Donnatal, Bellacane, Hyosophen, Susano Elixirs: belladonna alkaloids, atropine sulfate 0.0194 mg/5 ml, hyoscyamine sulfate 0.1037 mg/5 ml, scopolamine hydrobromide 0.0065/5 ml and phenobarbital 16.2 mg/5 ml

Donnatal Extentabs: belladonna alkaloids, atropine sulfate 0.0582 mg, hyoscyamine sulfate 0.3111 mg, scopolamine hydrobromide 0.0195 mg, and phenobarbital 48.6 mg

Drixomed: pseudoephedrine sulfate 120 mg with dexbrompheniramine 6 mg

Drixoral Plus or Drixoral Cold and Flu Tablets: pseudoephedrine sulfate 60 mg, dexbrompheniramine maleate 3 mg and acetaminophen 500 mg

Drixoral Cough and Congestion Capsules, Vicks 44 Non-Drowsy Cold and Cough LiquiCaps, Thera-Flu Non-Drowsy Flu, Cold and Cough Maximum: pseudoephedrine HCl 60 mg, dextromethorphan hydrobromide 30 mg

DuoNeb Inh Sol: ipratropium HBr 0.5 mg and albuterol sulfate 3 mg

Duratuss, Entex PSE, Guai-Vent/PSE, Guaifenex PSE 120, Guaimax-D, Ru-Tuss DE, Sudal 120/600, Zephrex LA: pseudoephedrine HCl 120 mg with guaifenesin 600 mg

Duratuss-G: guaifenesin 1200 mg

Duratuss HD Elixir, Vanex Expectorant Liquid, Sutuss: pseudoephedrine HCl 30 mg with hydrocodone bitartrate 2.5 mg and guaifenesin 100 mg per 5 ml

Dyazide: hydrochlorothiazide 25 mg with triamterene 37.5 mg

Empirin with Codeine 30 mg (No. 3): aspirin 325 mg with codeine phosphate 30 mg

Empirin with Codeine 60 mg (No. 4): aspirin 325 mg with codeine phosphate 60 mg

Endocet: oxycodone HCl 5 mg and acetaminophen 325 mg

Enduronyl: deserpidine 0.25 mg with methyclothiazide 5 mg

Enduronyl-Forte: deserpidine 0.5 mg with methyclothiazide 5 mg

Entex LA, Ami-TexLA, Exgest LA, Guaipax, Guaitex LA, Partuss LA, Phenylfenesin LA, Rymed TR, Stamoist LA: guaifenesin 400 mg with phenylpropanolamine HCl 75 mg

E-Pilo and PE (products 1 through 6): epinephrine bitartrate 1% with pilocarpine HCl 1%, 2%, 3%, 4%, 6%

Equagesic, Micranin: meprobamate 200 mg with aspirin 325 mg

Esgic, Fioricet, Repan: acetaminophen 325 mg with butalbital 50 mg, and caffeine 40 mg

Esgic-Plus: butalbital 50 mg with acetaminophen 500 mg and caffeine 40 mg

Esimil: guanethidine monosulfate 10 mg with hydrochlorothiazide 25 mg

Etrafon 2-10, Triavil 2-10: perphenazine 2 mg with amitriptyline HCl 10 mg

Etrafon, Triavil 2-25: perphenazine 2 mg with amitriptyline HCl 25 mg

Etrafon-A, Triavil 4-10: perphenazine 4 mg with amitriptyline HCl 10 mg

Etrafon-Forte, Triavil 4-25: perphenazine 4 mg with amitriptyline HCl 25 mg

Excedrin Migraine, Excedrin Extra Strength: aspirin 250 mg with acetaminophen 250 mg and caffeine 65 mg

Excedrin PM Liquid: acetaminophen 167 mg and diphenhydramine HCl 8.3 mg/5 ml or acetaminophen 1000 mg and diphenhydramine HCl 50 mg/30 ml

Excedrin PM (caplets), **Extra Strength Tylenol PM, Aspirin Free Anacin PM, Sominex Pain Relief:** acetaminophen 500 mg with diphenhydramine citrate 38 mg

Excedrin PM (liquigels), **Extra Strength Tylenol PM** (gelcaps): acetaminophen 500 mg with diphenhydramine HCl 25 mg

Femhrt 1/5: norethindrone acetate 1 mg with ethinyl estradiol 5 μg

Fioricet with Codeine: acetaminophen 325 mg, butalbital 50 mg, caffeine 40 mg, and codeine phosphate 30 mg

Fiorinal, Butalbital Compound: aspirin 325 mg with butalbital 50 mg, caffeine 40 mg

Fiorinal with Codeine No. 3: aspirin 325 mg with butalbital 50 mg, caffeine 40 mg, codeine phosphate 30 mg

Flexaphen: chlorzoxazone 250 mg with acetaminophen 300 mg

Glucovance: glyburide 1.25 mg with metformin 250 mg; glyburide 2.5 mg with metformin 500 mg; glyburide 5 mg with metformin 500 mg

Goody's Extra Strength Headache Powders: aspirin 520 mg with acetaminophen 260 mg and caffeine 32.5 mg per powder

Helidac: bismuth subsalicylate 262.4 mg with metronidazole 250 mg (tabs) plus tetracycline 500 mg (caps)

Humibid DM, Fenesin DM, Guaifenex DM, Guaifenex Rx PM, Iobid DM, Monafed DM, Muco-Fen-DM, Respa DM: dextromethorphan hydrobromide 30 mg with guaifenesin 600 mg

Humibid DM Sprinkles: dextromethorphan hydrobromide 15 mg with guaifenesin 30 mg

Hycodan, Tussigon: hydrocodone bitartrate 5 mg with homatropine methylbromide 1.5 mg and acetaminophen 500 mg

Hydrap-ES, Ser-Ap-Es, Tri-Hydroserpine, Marpres, Unipres: hydrochlorothiazide 15 mg with hydralazine 25 and reserpine 0.1 mg

Hydropres-50, Hydro-Serp, Hydroserpine No. 2: reserpine 0.125 mg with hydrochlorothiazide 50 mg

Hydroserpine No. 1, Salutensin-Demi: reserpine 0.125 mg with hydrochlorothiazide 25 mg

Hydroserpine No. 2, Hydropnea-50, Hydro-Serp: reserpine 0.125 mg with hydrochlorothiazide 50 mg

Hyphed Syrup: hydrocodone bitartrate 2.5 mg with pseudoephedrine HCl 30 mg and chlorpheniramine maleate 2 mg in each 5 ml

Hyzaar: losartan potassium 50 mg with hydrochlorothiazide 12.5 mg or losartan potassium 100 mg with hydrochlorothiazide 25 mg

Iberet-500 Filmtabs, Generet-500: iron 105 mg, vitamins B_1 6 mg, B_2 6 mg, B_3 30 mg, B_5 10 mg, B_6 5 mg, B_{12} 25 μg, and C 500 mg

Iberet-500 Liquid: iron 78.75 mg, vitamins B_1 4.5 mg, B_2 4.5 mg, B_3

22.5 mg, B_5 7.5 mg, B_6 3.75 mg, B_{12} 18.75 µg, and C 375 mg

Inderide 40/25, Propranolol HCl, Hydrochlorothiazide Tablets 40/25: propranolol HCl 40 mg with hydrochlorothiazide 25 mg

Inderide 80/25, Propranolol HCl, Hydrochlorothiazide Tablets 80/25: propranolol HCl 80 mg with hydrochlorothiazide 25 mg

Inderide LA 80/50: propranolol HCl 80 mg with hydrochlorothiazide 50 mg

Inderide LA 120/50: propranolol HCl 120 mg with hydrochlorothiazide 50 mg

Inderide LA 160/50: propranolol HCl 160 mg with hydrochlorothiazide 50 mg

Iophen-C: codeine phosphate 10 mg/5 ml with iodinated glycerol 30 mg/5 ml

Iophen-DM, Tusso-DM: dextromethorphan hydrobromide 10 mg and iodinated glycerol 30 mg/5 ml

Legatrin PM: acetaminophen 500 mg with diphenhydramine hydrochloride 50 mg

Levsin with Phenobarbital Tablets, Bellacane: hyoscyamine sulfate 0.125 mg with phenobarbital 15 mg

Lexxel: enalapril maleate 5 mg with felodipine 5 mg

Lexxel 2: enalapril maleate 5 mg with felodipine 2.5 mg

Librax: clidinium bromide 2.5 mg with chlordiazepoxide HCl 5 mg

Lopressor HCT 50/25: metoprolol tartrate 50 mg with hydrochlorothiazide 25 mg

Lopressor HCT 100/25: metoprolol tartrate 100 mg with hydrochlorothiazide 25 mg

Lopressor HCT 100/50: metoprolol tartrate 100 mg with hydrochlorothiazide 50 mg

Lorcet-HD, Hydrogesic, Hy-Phen, Margesic H, Lortab 5/500, Anexsia 5/500, Panacet 5/500: hydrocodone bitartrate 5 mg with acetaminophen 500 mg

Lorcet Plus, Anexsia 7.5/650: hydrocodone bitartrate 7.5 mg with acetaminophen 650 mg

Lorcet 10/650: hydrocodone 10 mg with acetaminophen 650 mg

Lortab ASA, Alor 5/500, Azdone, Damason-P, Panasal 5/500: hydrocodone bitartrate 5 mg with aspirin 500 mg

Lortab 2.5/500: hydrocodone 2.5 mg with acetaminophen 500 mg

Lortab 7.5/500: hydrocodone bitartrate 7.5 with acetaminophen 500 mg

Lortab Elixir: 2.5 mg hydrocodone with 167 mg acetaminophen in 5 ml

Lotensin HCT: benazepril 10 mg and hydrochlorothiazide 12.5 mg

Lotensin HCT 5/6.25: benazepril 5 mg and hydrochlorothiazide 6.25 mg

Lotensin HCT 20/12.5: benazepril 20 mg with hydrochlorothiazide 12.5 mg

Lotensin HCT 20/25: benazepril 20 mg with hydrochlorothiazide 25 mg

Lotrel 2.5/10: amlodipine 2.5 mg with benazepril 10 mg

Lotrel 5/10: amlodipine 5 mg with benazepril 10 mg

Lotrel 5/20: amlodipine 5 mg with benazepril 20 mg

Lotrisone: clotrimazole 1% and betamethasone dipropionate 0.05%

Maxzide-25 MG: triamterene 37.5 mg with hydrochlorothiazide 25 mg

Maxzide: hydrochlorothiazide 50 mg with triamterene 75 mg

Melagesic PM: acetaminophen 500 mg with melatonin 1.5 mg

Mepergan: meperidine HCl 25 mg/ml with promethazine HCl 25 mg/ml injection

Mepergan Fortis caps: meperidine HCl 50 mg with promethazine HCl 25 mg

Metatensin No. 2: reserpine 0.1 mg with trichlormethiazide 2 mg

Metatensin No. 4: reserpine 0.1 mg with trichlormethiazide 4 mg

Midol Maximum Strength PMS Caplets: acetaminophen 500 mg with caffeine 60 mg, pamabrom 25 mg, and pyrilamine maleate 15 mg

Midol PM, Compoze NightTime Sleep Aid, 40 Winks, Maximum Strength Nytol, SnoozeFast, Sominex, Twilite: diphenhydramine 50 mg

Minizide 1: prazosin HCl 1 mg with polythiazide 0.5 mg

Minizide 2: prazosin HCl 2 mg with polythiazide 0.5 mg

Minizide 5: prazosin HCl 5 mg with polythiazide 0.5 mg

Moduretic: amiloride HCl 5 mg with hydrochlorothiazide 50 mg

Motrin IB Sinus, Sine-Aid IB: ibuprofen 200 mg, pseudoephedrine HCl 30 mg

Murocoll-2: scopolamine hydrobromide 0.3%, phenylephrine hydrochloride 10% drops

MycoLog II, Mycogen II, MycoTriacet, Mytrex: triamcinolone acetonide 0.1% and nystatin 100,000 units/gram (ointment or cream)

Mylanta Liquid: aluminum hydroxide 200 mg, magnesium hydroxide 200 mg, simethicone 20 mg

Naldecon CX Adult Liquid: codeine phosphate 10 mg/5 ml with guaifenesin 200 mg/5 ml and phenylpropanolamine HCl 12.5 mg/5 ml

Naldecon-DX Adult, Naldelate DX Adult: dextromethorphan hydrobromide 10 mg/5 ml with guaifenesin 100 mg/5 ml and phenylpropanolamine HCl 12.5 mg/5 ml

Naldecon-DX Children's Syrup, Pediacon DX Children's, Phenadex Children Cough and Cold: dextromethorphan hydrobromide 5.0 mg/5 ml with guaifenesin 100 mg/5 ml and phenylpropanolamine HCl 6.25 mg/5 ml

Naldecon EX Pediatric Drops: 50 mg/ml guaifenesin, 6.25 mg/ml phenylpropanolamine HCl and dextromethorphan HBr 5 mg/ml

Norco: hydrocodone bitartrate 10 mg with aspirin 325 mg

Norco 5/325: hydrocodone bitartrate 5 mg and acetaminophen 325 mg

Norgesic: orphenadrine citrate 25 mg with aspirin 385 mg, caffeine 30 mg

Norgesic Forte: orphenadrine citrate 50 mg with aspirin 770 mg, caffeine 60 mg

NyQuil Nighttime Cold/Flu Medicine, Nite Time Cold Formula, Nytcold, Genite: pseudoephedrine HCl 10 mg, doxylamine succinate 1.25 mg, dextromethorphan hydrobromide 5 mg, and acetaminophen 167 mg/5 ml

Ornex, Sinus Relief, Vicks DayQuil Sinus Pressure and Pain, No-Drowsiness Allerest: pseudoephedrine HCl 30 mg with acetaminophen 500 mg

Ortho-Prefest: estradiol and norgestimate

Orthoxicol Cough Syrup, Cheracol Plus Liquid: dextromethorphan hydrobromide 6.7 mg/5 ml with chlorpheniramine 1.3 mg/5 mg and phenylpropanolamine HCl 8.3 mg/5 ml

Palgic-D: pseudoephedrine HCl 90 mg with carbinoxamine maleate 8 mg

Pancof XP: hydrocodone bitartrate 2.5 mg with guaifenesin 100 mg and pseudoephedrine HCl 15 mg in each 5 ml

Parepectolin: attapulgite 600 mg/15 ml

Pediazole, Eryzole: erythromycin ethylsuccinate (equivalent to 200 mg of erythromycin) per 5 ml with sulfisoxazole acetyl (equivalent to 600 mg of sulfisoxazole) per 5 ml

Pepcid Complete: calcium carbonate 800 mg, magnesium hydroxide 165 mg, famotidine 10 mg

Percocet (note now available in several strengths): **Percocet 2.5/ 325:** oxycodone hydrochloride 2.5 mg with acetaminophen 325 mg; **Percocet 5/325:** oxycodone hydrochloride 5 mg with acetaminophen 325 mg; **Percocet 7.5/500:** oxycodone hydrochloride 7. 5 mg with acetaminophen 500 mg; **Percocet 10/650:** oxycodone hydrochloride 10 mg with acetaminophen 650 mg

Percodan, Roxiprin: oxycodone hydrochloride 4.5 mg, oxycodone terephthalate 0.38 mg, and aspirin 325 mg

Percodan-Demi: aspirin 325 mg with oxycodone HCl 2.25 mg, oxycodone terephthalate 0.19 mg

Percogesic, Aceta-Gesic, Major-Gesic, Phenylgesic: acetaminophen 325 mg with phenyltoloxamine citrate 30 mg

Peri-Colace, D-S-S Plus 100, Genasoft Plus, Peri-Dos: docusate sodium 100 mg with casanthranol 30 mg

Phenergan VC Syrup, Prometh VC Plain, Promethazine VC Plain: promethazine HCl 6.25 mg/5 ml with phenylephrine HCl 5 mg/5 ml

Phenergan VC with Codeine Syrup, Pentazine VC with Codeine Syrup, Prometh VC with Codeine Syrup, Pherazine VC with Codeine Syrup: promethazine hydrochloride 6.25 mg, codeine phosphate 10 mg and phenylephrine 5 mg/5 ml

Phenergan with Dextromethorphan, Pherazine DM, Prometh with Dextromethorphan, Phenameth DM: dextromethorphan hydrobromide 15 mg/5 ml with promethazine HCl 6.25 mg/ 5 ml

Premphase: conjugated estrogens 0.625 mg with medroxyprogesterone acetate 5 mg

Prempro: conjugated estrogens 0.625 mg with medroxyprogesterone acetate 2.5 mg

Prevpac: lansoprazole 30 mg (2 caps), amoxicillin 500 mg (4 caps), and clarithromycin 500 mg (2 tabs)

Primaxin IM: imipenem 500 mg with cilastatin 500 mg; imipenem 750 mg with cilastatin 750 mg for injection

Primaxin IV: imipenem 250 mg with cilastatin 250 mg; imipenem 500 mg with cilastatin 500 mg for injection

Profen LA, Coldloc-LA, Dura-Vent, Guaifenex PPA 75, SINU-vent: phenylpropanolamine HCl 75 mg with guaifenesin 600 mg

Pyridium Plus: phenazopyridine HCl 150 mg with hyoscyamine hydrobromide 0.3 mg and butabarbital 15 mg

Rauzide: bendroflumethiazide 4

mg with rauwolfia serpentina powdered 50 mg

Rebetron: ribavirin 200 mg and interferon alfa-2b 3 million IU

Regroton: reserpine 0.25 mg with chlorthalidone 50 mg

Renese-R: reserpine 0.25 mg with polythiazide 2 mg

Rhinocaps: phenylpropanolamine hydrochloride 20 mg with acetaminophen 162 mg and aspirin 162 mg

Rifamate: isoniazid 150 mg with rifampin 300 mg

Rifater: isoniazid 50 mg with rifampin 120 mg and pyrazinamide 300 mg

Robaxisal: methocarbamol 400 mg with aspirin 325 mg

Robitussin-DM, Cheracol-D, Genatuss DM, Halotussin DM, Halotussin DM Sugar Free, Mytussin DM, Tussin DM, Diabetic Tussin DM, Extra Action Cough Syrup, Guiatuss-DM, Glycotuss-DM, Robafen DM, Situssin DM, Phanatuss DM, Tolu-Sed DM: dextromethorphan hydrobromide 10 mg/5 ml with guaifenesin 100 mg/5 ml

Singlet for Adults Tablets, Simplet Tablets, TheraFlu Cough and Cold Medicine Powder: pseudoephedrine HCl 60 mg, chlorpheniramine maleate 4 mg, and acetaminophen 650 mg

Sinutab Without Drowsiness, Alka-Seltzer Plus Cold and Sinus, Allerest No Drowsiness, Coldrine, Ornex No Drowsiness, Sinus-Relief: pseudoephedrine HCl 30 mg with acetaminophen 325 mg

Sudafed 12 Hour Caplets: pseudoephedrine HCl 120 mg

Synalgos-DC: aspirin 356.4 mg with caffeine 30 mg and dihydrocodeine bitartrate 16 mg

Talacen: pentazocine HCl 25 mg with acetaminophen 650 mg

Talwin Compound Caplets: aspirin 325 mg with pentazocine HCl 12.5 mg

Tarka 1:240: trandolapril 1 mg with verapamil 240 ml

Tarka 2:180: trandolapril 2 mg with verapamil 180 ml

Tarka 4:240: trandolapril 4 mg with verapamil 240 ml

Tavist-D: phenylpropanolamine HCl 75 mg with clemastine fumarate 1.34 mg

Teczem: enalapril maleate 5 mg with diltiazem maleate 180 mg

Tenoretic 50: atenolol 50 mg with chlorthalidone 25 mg

Tenoretic 100: atenolol 100 mg with chlorthalidone 25 mg

Timentin Inj: ticarcillin disodium 3 g with clavulanate potassium 100 mg

Timolide 10/25: timolol maleate 10 mg with hydrochlorothiazide 25 mg

TracTabs 2X: methenamine 120 mg, methylene blue 6 mg, phenyl salicylate 30 mg, atropine 0.06 mg, hyoscyamine SO_4 0.03 mg, benzoic acid 7.5 mg

Triad, Esgic, Margesic, Medigesic: butalbital 50 mg with acetaminophen 325 mg and caffeine 40 mg

Triaminic-DM Syrup: dextromethorphan hydrobromide 5 mg/5 ml with phenylpropanolamine HCl 6.25 mg/5 ml

TriHemic 600: iron 115 mg, vitamin B_{12} 25 μg, vitamin C 600 mg, folic acid 1 mg, and intrinsic factor 75 mg

Trinalin Repetabs: pseudoephedrine HCl 120 mg with azatadine maleate 1 mg

Trinsicon, Ferotrinsic, Foltrin, Livitrinsic-F, Contrin: iron 110 mg, vitamin B$_{12}$ 15 µg, vitamin C 7.5 mg, folic acid 0.5 mg, and intrinsic factor 240 mg

Triple Sulfa, Gyne-Sulf, Sultrin Triple Sulfa, Trysul, Dayto Sulf, V.V.S.: sulfathiazole 3.42%, sulfacetamide 2.86%, and sulfabenzamide 3.7% vaginal cream

Tritec: ranitidine bismuth citrate 400 mg

Trizivir: abacavir sulfate 300 mg, lamivudine 150 mg and zidovudine 300 mg

Tussafed HC Syrup, Donatussin DC: hydrocodone bitartrate 2.5 mg with phenylephrine HCl 7.5 mg and guaifenesin 50 mg in each 5 ml

Tussionex Pennkinetic Suspension: chlorpheniramine (polistirex) 8 mg and hydrocodone (polistirex) 10 mg in 5 ml

Tylenol Flu Night Time Maximum Strength (powder): pseudoephedrine HCl 60 mg, diphenhydramine HCl 50 mg, and acetaminophen 1000 mg dissolved in 6 oz hot water

Tylenol Multi-Symptom Hot Medication (powder): pseudoephedrine HCl 60 mg, chlorpheniramine maleate 4 mg, dextromethorphan hydrobromide 30 mg with acetaminophen 650 mg dissolved in 6 oz hot water

Tylenol PM Extra Strength: acetaminophen 500 mg with diphenhydramine 25 mg

Tylenol with Codeine No. 2: acetaminophen 300 mg with codeine phosphate 15 mg

Tylenol with Codeine No. 3: acetaminophen 300 mg with codeine phosphate 30 mg

Tylenol with Codeine No. 4: acetaminophen 300 mg with codeine phosphate 60 mg

Tylox, Roxicet 5/500, Roxilox: acetaminophen 500 mg with oxycodone HCl 5 mg

Ultracet: acetaminophen and tramadol (doses not available)

Unasyn Inj: ampicillin sodium 1 g with sulbactam sodium 500 mg; ampicillin sodium 2 g with sulbactam sodium 1 g; ampicillin sodium 10 mg with sulbactam sodium 5 gm

Uniretic 7.5: moexipril 7.5 mg with hydrochlorothiazide 12.5 mg

Uniretic 15: moexipril 15 mg with hydrochlorothiazide 25 mg

Unisom Nighttime Sleep Aid: doxylamine succinate 25 mg

Unisom with Pain Relief: diphenhydramine HCl 50 mg with acetaminophen 650 mg

Urised, Uritin, Atrosept, Dolsed, UAA, Uridon Modified: methenamine 40.8 mg, phenyl salicylate 18.1 mg, atropine 0.03 mg, hyoscyamine 0.03 mg, and methylene blue 5.4 mg

Urisedamine: methenamine mandelate 500 mg with hyoscyamine 0.15 mg

Vanquish Caplets: aspirin 227 mg with acetaminophen 194 mg, caffeine 33 mg, and buffers

Vaseretic 5-12.5: enalapril maleate 5 mg with hydrochlorothiazide 12.5 mg

Vaseretic 10-25: enalapril maleate 10 mg with hydrochlorothiazide 25 mg

Vicks Children's NyQuil Nighttime Cough/Cold Liquid, Vicks Pediatric Formula 44 Cough and Cold Liquid: pseudoephedrine

HCl 10 mg, chlorpheniramine maleate 0.67 mg, dextromethorphan hydrobromide 5 mg/5 ml

Vicks Chloraseptic Sore Throat Lozenges, benzocaine 6 mg with 10 mg menthol: **Children's Throat Spray,** phenol 0.5%: **Mouthrinse,** phenol 1.4%: Children's Lozenges, benzocaine 5 mg

Vicks Cough Silencers: dextromethorphan hydrobromide 2.5 mg with benzocaine 1 mg lozenges

Vicks Formula 44D, Cough and Decongestant Liquid, Vicks 44D Cough and Head Congestion: dextromethorphan hydrobromide 10 mg/5 ml with pseudoephedrine HCl 20 mg/5 ml

Vicks Formula 44M, Cold, Flu and Cough Capsules, AlkaSeltzer Plus Cold and Cough: dextromethorphan hydrobromide 10 mg with chlorpheniramine 2 mg, pseudoephedrine HCl 30 mg, and acetaminophen 250 mg

Vicodin: acetaminophen 500 mg with hydrocodone bitartrate 5.0 mg

Vicodin-ES: acetaminophen 750 mg with hydrocodone bitartrate 7.5 mg

Vicodin-HP: acetaminophen 660 mg with hydrocodone bitartrate 10 mg

Vicoprofen: hydrocodone bitartrate 7.5 mg with ibuprofen 200 mg

Wigraine, Cafergot, Ercaf: ergotamine tartrate 1 mg and caffeine 100 mg

Wigraine Suppositories, Cafatine, Cafetrate: ergotamine tartrate 2 mg, caffeine 100 mg

Zestoretic 10/12.5, Prinzide: lisinopril 10 mg with hydrochlorothiazide 12.5 mg

Zestoretic 20/12.5, Prinzide 12.5: lisinopril 20 mg with hydrochlorothiazide 12.5 mg

Zestoretic 20/25, Prinzide 25: lisinopril 20 mg with hydrochlorothiazide 25 mg

Ziac 2.5: bisoprolol fumarate 2.5 mg with hydrochlorothiazide 6.25 mg

Ziac 5: bisoprolol fumarate 5.0 mg with hydrochlorothiazide 6.25 mg

Ziac 10: bisoprolol fumarate 10 mg with hydrochlorothiazide 6.25 mg

Ziradyl Lotion: diphenhydramine HCl 1% with zinc oxide 2%, alcohol 2%, camphor, and parabens

Zosyn: piperacillin 2 g with tazobactam 0.25 g; piperacillin 3 g with tazobactam 0.375 g, piperacillin 4 g with tazobactam 0.5 g and piperacillin 36 g with tazobactam 4.5 g in vials for IV administration

Zydone: hydrocodone bitartrate 5 mg and acetaminophen 400 mg; or hydrocodone bitartrate 7.5 mg and acetaminophen 400 mg; or hydrocodone bitartrate 10 mg and acetaminophen 400 mg

Appendix G

Dose calculations by weight

Manufacturer-recommended doses are based on extensive clinical trials and are usually intended for the average, healthy adult male of average weight and age. Thus age, sex, weight, and chronic diseases of the major organs of metabolism (liver) and excretion (kidney) may affect the usual safe and effective FDA-approved dose recommendations. Creatine clearance, peak and trough blood levels, and symptomatic patient response are often used to titrate doses for a given therapeutic effect. Dentists seldom treat infants, but doses for pediatric and geriatric patients require an adjustment downward from the usual adult dose. Geriatric patients may be particularly susceptible to effects produced by CNS depressants or drugs that affect renal function. No reliable general rule for dose calculations can supplant clinically derived doses, and many drug monographs now list doses for children based on a mg/kg or mg/lb basis. Children's doses are also based on a reduction of adult doses as determined by body surface area and weight. Clark's rule has been used for many years as a general guide for calculating children's doses.

Clark's Rule:

$$\frac{\text{Child's weight (lb)}}{150} \times \text{Adult dose} = \text{Child's dose}$$

weight lb/kg chart
1 kg = 2.2 lb

kilograms (kg)	pounds (lb)
10	22
20	44
25	55
30	66
35	77
40	88
45	99
50	110
55	121
60	132

Appendix H

Herbal and nonherbal remedies

Black cohosh
(Cimicifuga racemosa, Cimicifugae racemosae rhizoma)
Other names: Black snakeroot, baneberry
Class: Herbal remedy
Major ingredients: The active chemicals are described as triterpene glycosides (acetin, 27-deoxyacetin) along with tannins, a variety of acidic compounds, isoflavones, fatty acids, and a volatile oil. The fresh and dried rhizomes are the portion of the plant used.

Claimed actions: Estrogen-like action, suppression of luteinizing hormone release, and interaction with estrogen receptors.
Uses: It is used for the symptoms of premenstrual and dysmenorrhea disorders and menopause-associated hot flashes, vaginal dryness, water retention, and related complaints. Most of the pharmacologic studies are from the laboratory, but some clinical testing seems to support a role in reducing menopausal symptoms. Its use should be avoided in pregnancy and lactation.
Administration: Generally available in extracts for oral administration.
Side effects: GI complaints have been reported. Higher doses may cause more significant GI complaints, visual disturbances, lowered blood glucose levels, and CNS side effects such as dizziness. Use for longer than 6 months not recommended.
Dental considerations:
Ask why the product is being used. Evidence is lacking, but theoretically patients taking oral anticoagulants, aspirin, or NSAIDs could show increased bleeding times.
Drug interactions: No dental drug interactions are reported.

Chamomile
(Matricaria chamomilla, Matricaria recutita, Anthemis nobilis, and Matricariae flos)
Other names: common chamomile, German chamomile
Class: Herbal remedy
Major ingredients: Volatile oil containing alpha-bisabolol and other bisabolol derivatives (chamazulene, apigenin), various flavonoids, umbelliferone (a coumarin-like ingredient), and many other components. The portion of the plant used is the dried flower.

Claimed actions: Antiinflammatory, antispasmodic, antibacterial, carminative, and to promote wound healing.
Uses: It has been used to treat inflammation and spasm in the GI tract; topically for inflammation, burns, wounds, and infections of the skin and mucous membranes (including the oral cavity); topically for anogenital inflammation,

as a deodorant, and for a variety of other complaints. There are some data in laboratory models to support the antiinflammatory activity.
Administration: Available in a variety of dose forms, including teas, infusions (external use), a mouth rinse, and oral dose forms.
Side effects: Slight risk of contact dermatitis: possible cross allergies with ragweed.
Dental considerations:
Ask why the product is being used. Evidence is lacking, but theoretically patients taking oral anticoagulants could show increased bleeding times.
Drug interactions: Risk of increased sedation with CNS depressants. The GI activity of this herb may affect the absorption of some orally administered drugs.

Chaste tree, Chaste berry
(Vitex agnus-castus, angi casti fructrus)
Other names: Chaste tree fruit, monk's pepper, chaste tree
Class: Herbal remedy
Major ingredients: Iridoid glycosides (agnuide and aucubin), flavonoids, progestins, testosterone, and multiple essential oils. The portion of the plant used is the dried, ripe fruit.

Claimed actions: Inhibition of the release of prolactin through a proposed action on dopamine receptors, although not shown in human studies. It may also be antiandrogenic.
Uses: Premenstrual ailments, irregular menstrual cycle complaints, and breast pain. Also used in menopausal symptoms. There is a possible risk of increased ovulation and pregnancy in some women. Should be used with caution when other progestins/estrogens are used. Avoid use in pregnancy and lactation.
Administration: Extracts of the crushed fruit for oral administration.
Side effects: Usually minor but can include skin rashes, dry mouth, and headaches.
Dental considerations:
Ask why the product is being used.
Drug interactions: No dental drug interactions are reported. Dopamine receptor antagonists may block some herbal effects.

Chondroitin sulfate
Other names: Chondroitin
Class: Nonherbal remedy
Major ingredient: Chondroitin sulfate is a mucopolysaccharide, that is, a glycosaminoglycan (GAG). It is found in mammalian cartilaginous tissue and is believed to play a role in flexibility. It is highly viscous and related chemically to sodium hyaluronate.

Claimed actions: It has useful viscoelastic properties suitable for use in selected types of ocular surgery, usually in combination with sodium hyaluronate. Orally administered GAGs are believed to concentrate in cartilage. Chondrocytes use GAGs to form a new cartilage matrix. It may also inhibit leukocyte elastase where high concentrations are associated with rheumatoid arthritis. Other properties may include bringing synovial fluid into the joint. All of these may contribute to reduced inflammatory activity in joints. Serum lipid–lowering and antithrombogenic effects have also been suggested.

Uses: Chondroitin in an ophthalmic solution has been used to treat dry eyes. In combination with sodium hyaluronate it is used to support ocular surgery during cataract removal and lens implantation surgery. Its use in cardiovascular diseases remains in doubt. Its most popular use is in arthritis. Limited clinical studies seem to indicate that it is somewhat less effective than NSAIDs.

Administration: A variety of oral dose forms are available, many in combination with glucosamine. Professionally used ophthalmic preparations are also available.

Side effects: Long-term side effects are unknown. GI complaints may be reported on occasion.

Dental considerations:

Ask why the product is being used. Arthritic patients may also be taking aspirin, NSAIDs, or arthritic disease modifying drugs in addition to chondroitin. Question patient about other antiarthritic drugs used, including OTC drugs.

Drug interactions: None reported with dental drugs.

Dong quai
(Angelica sinensis)
Other names: Chinese angelica, dang-gui
Class: Herbal remedy
Major ingredients: It contains a variety of coumarins (oxypeucedain, osthol, and others), an essential oil, phytoestrogens, polysaccharides, lactones, and even vitamins E and B_{12}. The portion of the plant used is the root.

Claimed actions: Vasodilation, antispasmodic in blood vessels, CNS stimulation, and immunosuppressant and antiinflammatory properties. The mechanism of action of these effects is unclear.

Uses: It is used in Chinese herbal medicine in combination with other herbs. Uses include dysmenorrhea, other menstrual problems, and menopausal symptoms. Other uses include arthritis, hypertension, and ulcers. However, significant clinical studies are lacking. The remedy does not appear in the German Commission E Monographs. Avoid use during pregnancy and lactation.

Administration: Administered orally as in infusion, a tincture, or a chewable root.

Side effects: Photosensitization and some GI complaints including a laxative action are reported. Avoid during pregnancy and nursing.

Dental considerations:

Ask why the product is being used. Evidence is lacking, but theoretically patients taking oral anticoagulants, aspirin, or NSAIDs could show increased bleeding times.

Drug interactions: No dental drug interactions reported; its use with coumarin anticoagulants or calcium channel blockers is not recommended.

Echinacea
(Echinacea angustifolia, Echinacea purpurea, and Echinacea pallida)
Other names: American cone flower, Kansas snakeroot, purple cone flower
Class: Herbal remedy

Major ingredients: Caffeic acid glycoside (echinacoside), alkylamides (echinacein and others), essential oils (humulene and others), a variety of flavonoids, and many other components. As with any plant the contents vary with the species, the parts of the plant used, and whether dried or fresh. The portion of the plant used is the flower, other above-ground parts, and even the roots.

Claimed actions: Improved wound healing, stimulation of the immune system (some laboratory data suggest an increase in macrophage phagocytic activity and numbers of neutrophils), antibacterial, antiviral, and antiinflammatory activity. It may act as a nonspecific stimulator to the immune system, including macrophages and T-lymphocytes.

Uses: It has been used to enhance would healing, for *Candida* infections, as supportive therapy for common colds and upper respiratory infections, and lower urinary tract infections. Other uses include rheumatoid arthritis and as supportive use in colon cancer. Efficacy in prevention of colds and upper respiratory infections is not supported. Recent data do not support its use for common colds.

Contraindications: Should not be used in patients with autoimmune diseases or progressive infectious diseases, including tuberculosis, multiple sclerosis, leukocytosis, AIDS, HIV infection, and collagen diseases. *Caution:* Use beyond 8 consecutive weeks can suppress immunity.

Administration: Available in a variety of preparations for internal (oral administration) and external use. Parenteral dose forms are available in Germany. Products are intended for oral or topical administration.

Side effects: Generally limited to parenteral doses only. Fatigue, headache, and dizziness were reported with oral doses. Possible risk of cross-allergic reaction with chamomile or ragweed.

Dental considerations:
Ask why it is being used. Avoid use during immunosuppression. Use with caution in asthma, atopy, or allergic rhinitis.

Drug interactions: Use beyond 8 consecutive weeks could cause hepatic toxicity and should not be used with other hepatotoxic drugs (ketoconazole). May decrease effectiveness of immunosuppressants. Discontinue before use of general anesthetics.

Ephedra
Primary Botanical Source: *Ephedra sinica* Staph. (China)
Other Botanical Sources: *E. altissima, E. distachya, E. gerardiana* (India), *E. herba, E. intermedia* Shrenk et C.A. Mayer (India), *E. major* (India), and *E. vulgaris* are also used.

Other names: *Ma huang,* mahuang gen, epitonin, Sea Grape, Desert Herb, Yellow Horse, Squaw Tea, Popotillo, Teamster's Tea, Cao mahaung.

Class: Herbal remedy

Parts used: Entire plant, tops and dried stems from Asian shrub; however, botanical product compositions are not regulated by FDA.

Major ingredients: Sympathomimetic ephedrine alkaloids, pseudoephedrine alkaloids, tannins, and trace minerals.

Claimed actions: Ephedrine and pseudoephedrine have both direct and indirect agonist activity on the sympathetic nervous system, displacing noradrenaline from storage vesicles in nerve terminals. Ephedra is purported to promote the dilation of the small bronchioles of the lungs, promoting airway ventilation and oxygen exchange. Conversely, ephedra promotes vascular vasoconstriction, which increases blood pressure, heart rate, and peripheral vasoconstrictor activity. Diuretic action and hypoglycemic effects are reported in animals.

Uses: Ephedra appears to be effective as an adjunct for asthma, bronchospasm, and sinus allergies. It has also been used to treat nasal congestion and symptoms of colds and flu. The effectiveness of ephedra combined with caffeine, or in combination with the St. John's Wort, as an herbal weight-loss product has not been established. Ephedra is also used to treat arthritis, fever, hives, headache, and low blood pressure. No data are available to support anecdotal reports as an athletic performance enhancer.

Contraindications: Hypertension, anxiety, restlessness, glaucoma, cerebral circulation impairment, pheochromocytoma, hyperthyroidism, anorexia, angina, bulimia, prostate hypertrophy (BPH), diabetes, heart disease, myasthenia gravis, urinary retention; should not be used during pregnancy or in very young children

Administration: Products are found in tea, tablet, and tincture forms. Pharmaceutically standardized ephedrine and pseudoephedrine are available in OTC products. FDA wording indicates use should be limited to seven days. Maximum daily dose limit (as ephedrine) is 300 mg. For children over the age of 6 years, the daily limit is 2 mg/kg.

Side effects: Numerous deaths have been reported with use of ephedra. FDA proposed warning labels for all ephedra-containing products; some states have banned ephedra.

Warning: Numerous deaths have been reported with ephedra use. FDA proposed warning labels for all products containing ephedra. Many states have banned ephedra.

CNS: Dizziness, insomnia, irritability, headache, nervousness, seizure, *stroke,* tingling, hallucinations, psychosis

CV: Tachycardia, palpitation, significant blood pressure elevation, *heart failure*

ENT: Glaucoma

GI: Loss of appetite, nausea, vomiting

MS: Myalgia, rhabdomyolysis,

MISC: Anorexia, *brain hemorrhage, sudden death,* flushing, paleness

Dental considerations:

Although there is no data to support this statement, it would be prudent to have the patient discontinue this herbal remedy before general anesthesia procedures.

Determine why patient is taking the drug. Ask how long the product has been used.

Note: E. Nevadensis, Mormon tea (AKA American ephedra) does not contain ephedrine or pseudoephedrine and is minimally active.

Drug interactions:

• Risk of increased stimulatory effects: caffeine, coffee, cola nut, guarana

• Risk of increased arrhythmias: digitalis

• Decreased effects on raising blood pressure: tricyclic antidepressants

• Contraindicated with monoamine oxidase inhibitors

Evening Primrose Oil
(Oenothera biennis)
Other names: Evening primrose
Class: Herbal remedy
Major ingredients: The oil is a mixture of fatty acids, including linoleic acid (50%-80%), gamma-linolenic acid (GLA, 6%-11%), and smaller amounts of other fatty acids, including palmitic acid, oleic acid, and stearic acid. Other ingredients include tannin, sitosterol, and trace minerals. The portion of the plant used is the seed.

Claimed actions: Antiatherosclerotic, relief of premenstrual tension, relief of mastalgia, and antiinflammatory actions for arthritis and dermatologic conditions. The fatty acids contained in the oil may function like essential oils and act as precursors of prostaglandins that help regulate metabolic functions.
Uses: It is used for reduction of serum cholesterol and triglycerides. A single study using GLA appeared to show a significant lowering of serum cholesterol, but another study did not. Weight re-

duction claims are also made. Laboratory trials describing a decrease in platelet aggregation have not been clinically tested. Value in PMS shows some modest benefits after repeated use. Relief of cyclic breast pain may be better than placebo. Data do not support a reduction in rheumatoid disease destruction of tissues, but may have some effect in relieving symptoms. Claims are also made that GLA is effective in controlling symptoms of atopic dermatitis. This herb is not listed in the German Commission E monographs.
Administration: Available for oral administration in capsules.
Side effects: Few side effects are noted and occur only occasionally. They generally include GI complaints, including GI upset and nausea.
Dental considerations:
Ask why the product is being used.
Drug interactions: No dental drug interactions are reported. One reference recommended that the oil not be used in patients taking drugs that lower the seizure threshold (e.g., phenothiazines).

Feverfew
(Tanacetum parthenium, Chrysanthemum parthenium)
Other names: Feather few, Feverfew leaf, bachelor's button
Class: Herbal remedy
Major ingredients: Sesquiterpene lactones (parthenolide 85%), volatile oils (camphor, *trans*-chrysanthylacetate), flavonoids (luteolin, apigenin), and many other constituents. The portion of the plant used is the leaf.

Claimed actions: Antiinflammatory, may decrease platelet aggregation (laboratory studies), and reduces histamine release. Other actions include inhibition of prostaglandin synthesis and decrease in serotonin release from platelets. It is not listed in the German Commission E monographs.

Uses: Prophylactic use in migraine headaches, rheumatoid arthritis, stimulation of menstruation. It has also been used in folk medicine to control fever, as an external antiseptic, and even a mouth rinse following extractions. Avoid use during pregnancy and lactation.

Side effects: Oral products produce few complaints; chewing the leaves may lead to oral ulcerations, swelling of circumoral tissues. Potential risk of increased bleeding time.

Administration: Available in many oral dose forms or used to make an infusion.

Dental considerations:
Ask why product is being used.
In patients taking warfarin or other oral anticoagulant, inquire about bleeding history.
Inquire about unusual bleeding episodes following dental treatment.
Drug interactions: Avoid drugs that affect platelet action, such as aspirin and NSAIDs; they may reduce effectiveness. Advise patient not to take this herb for 2-3 weeks before surgery.

Garlic
(Allium Sativum)
Other names: Allium, poor man's treacle
Class: Herbal remedy
Major ingredients: A volatile oil containing several sulfur compounds, a sulfur-containing amino acid identified as alliin. With grinding allicin is converted to allicin (responsible for the typical odor of garlic). Many other constituents are also present, including minute quantities of trace minerals, beta-carotene, and vitamins. The portion of the plant used is whole, fresh or dried, garlic clove and oil of garlic.

Claimed action: Antibacterial, lipid-lowering activity, inhibition of platelet aggregation, antihypertensive, antioxidant, and a preventative for age-related vascular disorders.

Uses: It has been used to treat a wide array of bacterial, fungal, and viral infections. Data suggest it is about 1% as effective as penicillin in vitro. Use in oral fungal infections remains in doubt. Data show a limited reduction in cholesterol, reduction in blood pressure, and a decrease in platelet aggregation. The use of garlic in cancer prevention is controversial. Long-term effects are unknown.

Administration: Available in a variety of oral dose forms; however, the whole garlic clove is believed to contain the highest concentration of allicin, the major active ingredient.

Side effects: The taste and odor of garlic is by far the most common complaint. Rarely GI symptoms may occur with larger doses. Halitosis and burning of the mouth have been reported.

Dental considerations:
Ask why the product is being used.
Inquire about unusual bleeding episodes following dental treatment.

Drug interactions: Evidence is lacking, but there is always a chance that patients taking oral anticoagulants, aspirin, or NSAIDs could show increase bleeding time. Advise patient not to take this herb for 2-3 weeks before surgery. Discontinue 7 days before general anesthesia and general surgical procedures.

Ginger

(Zingiber Officinale, Zingiberis rhizoma)
Other names: Ginger root
Class: Herbal remedy
Major ingredients: The root contains a volatile oil and other chemicals termed *pungent principles*. These latter compounds are collectively known as gingerols, shogaols, and gingerdiols. The portion of the plant used is the root.

Claimed actions: Motion sickness prevention, promotion of salivary and gastric secretions, positive inotropic action, and antiinflammatory effects have all been claimed for this herb.
Uses: The most common uses include prevention of motion sickness and in dyspepsia. It has also been used for morning sickness of pregnancy and in rheumatoid arthritis. Gluonolactone, an active ingredient, has been reported to have serotonin (5-HT) antagonist activity, and gingerols may have a positive inotropic effect. There is a difference of opinion about its safe use in pregnancy and lactation with the German Commission E monographs warning against its use. Patients with gallstones should not take ginger.

Administration: Only the rhizome (root) of the plant is used. The German Commission E reference lists the dose at 2-4 g daily.
Side effects: Generally not reported except for toxic doses that could include CNS depression and arrhythmia.
Dental considerations:
Ask why the product is being used.
Drug interactions: None reported. Evidence is lacking, but there is theoretically a chance that patients taking oral anticoagulants, aspirin, or NSAIDs could show increased bleeding times.

Gingko

(Gingko biloba, Gingko folium)
Other names: Maidenhair tree, ginkyo
Class: Herbal remedy
Major ingredients: Common ingredients with claimed pharmacologic activity include multiple flavonoids (biobetin, ginkgetin), flavone glycosides (quercetin), bioflavones, terpenoids (gingkolides A, B, and C), and bilobalide. The portion of the plant used is the leaf.

Claimed actions: Improvement in blood flow in the microcirculation, inhibition of development of traumatically or toxic induced cerebral edema, improved hypoxic tolerance in cerebral tissues, reduction in retinal edema, increased memory performance, inhibition of age-related reduction in muscarinic receptors, and antagonism of platelet-activating factor (PAF). May also have monoamine oxidase inhibition properties.

Uses: It has been used to treat cerebral insufficiency, Alzheimer's dementia and other forms of dementia, circulatory disorders associated with diabetes, memory deficits, vertigo, tinnitus, and impotency associated with use of selective serotonin reuptake inhibitors. There are some data to support these uses. Benefits for exercise performance are not verified. It use is contraindicated during pregnancy and lactation.

Administration: Capsules and tablets of leaf extracts are available for use. Doses range from 120-240 mg of dry extract for 8 weeks for chronic diseases. Use for longer than 3 months requires reevaluation of benefits.

Side effects: May include GI complaints, headaches, and allergic reactions. Use with caution in patients with hypertension. One report of oral ulcerations is noted.

Dental considerations:
Ask why the product is being used. Inquire about unusual bleeding episodes following dental treatment.

Drug interactions: There is some evidence for anticoagulant activity with gingko; monitor or use antiplatelet drugs such as aspirin or NSAIDS with caution. Discontinue gingko use 2 weeks before surgery and general anesthesia. *Caution:* Concurrent use with MAO inhibitors and tricyclics. Possible interaction between ginkgo and trazodone (Desyrel) may cause excess stimulation of GABA receptors leading to CNS depression and possible coma. Discontinue 7 days before general anesthesia and general surgical procedures.

Ginseng
(Panax quinquefolium, Panax ginseng)
Class: Herbal remedy

Major ingredients: Constituents vary with the species of ginsing used. Contains steroid-like compounds called *ginsenosides* or *panaxosides.* Other ingredients include a volatile oil and flavonoids along with smaller quantities of other substances.

Claimed actions: Effects vary from CNS stimulation to depression. Improves resistance to stress in laboratory models, but there is a lack of evidence in humans. There are also claims of decreased platelet aggregation and increased memory and concentration.

Uses: Improvement of stamina and to enhance performance, a tonic and "adaptogen."

Administration: The root is use for teas and various other oral preparations.

Side effects: Not well documented but may include insomnia, diarrhea, and skin rash. However, adulterants included with ginsing products may increase risk for other side effects.

Dental considerations:
Ask why the product is being used.

Drug interactions: No specific dental drug interactions are reported, but ginsing may have monoamine oxidase inhibition properties. Discontinue 7 days before general anesthesia and general surgical procedures.

Glucosamine sulfate

Other names: Chitosamine, glucosamine

Class: Nonherbal remedy

Major ingredient: Glucosamine sulfate, an aminomonosaccharide (2-amino-2-deoxyglucose), is a component of mucopolysaccharides and mucoproteins. Other salt forms may also be used.

Claimed actions: Glucosamine is used in the synthesis of glycoproteins and glycosaminoglycans (GAGs). It is formed in the body from glucose through intermediary metabolic steps to be incorporated into GAGs, which are essential for cartilage function in joints.

Uses: It is used to treat the signs and symptoms of osteoarthritic disease. Other uses have included other inflammatory disorders, including tendinitis and rheumatoid arthritis. It has been clinically studied in comparison with NSAIDs. Some reports indicate equivalency with NSAIDs, but there is considerable doubt about its overall value in osteoarthritis. Nonetheless, patients indicated relief of pain and increased mobility. Oral, IV, IM, and intraarticular routes have been used to study glucosamine's effectiveness. These studies may lack rigid testing for effect in inflammatory joint diseases.

Administration: The usual dose is 500 mg three times daily.

Side effects: Side effects are uncommon but can include GI effects such as nausea, heartburn, diarrhea, and epigastric pain. CNS side effects are also rarely observed; they may include headache, insomnia, and drowsiness. However, arthritic patients may be taking aspirin, NSAIDs, or disease-modifying osteoarthritis drugs in addition to glucosamine and chondroitin. Question patient about other antiarthritic drugs used, including OTC drugs.

Dental considerations: Ask why the product is being used.

Drug interactions: No dental drug interactions are documented.

Goldenseal
(Hydrastis canadensis)

Other names: Eye root, yellow root, turmeric root

Class: Herbal remedy

Major ingredients: Contains the isoquinoline alkaloids hydrastine and berberine, other related alkaloids, and a volatile oil.

Claimed actions: Astringent and antiseptic. May also stimulate the secretion of bile and may have laxative action. Hydrastine has been shown to cause vasoconstriction in peripheral vessels. Berberine may have some antibacterial actions. This herb is not included in the German Commission E monographs.

Uses: It has been used in the treatment of eye infections or irritations, mucous membrane infections, and herpes labialis. It has also been used in the treatment of travelers' diarrhea and giardiasis. It is contraindicated for use in pregnancy and lactation.

Administration: Dose forms could not be documented, but it may be used in herbal product combinations.

Side effects: Safe in usual doses; adverse effects are more often observed with toxic doses (may include hypertension, convulsions, and breathing difficulties).

Dental considerations:
Ask why the product is being used.
Drug interactions: None reported.

Grape Seed Extract
Primary botanical source: *Vitis vinifera, Vitis coignetiae*
Others names: Grape Seed Extract, Grape Seed Oil, Muskat, De Pepins De Raisin.
Class: Herbal remedy
Parts used: Seed of grape, sometimes skin of grape
Major ingredients: The oil contains essential fatty acids, tocopherols (vitamin E), and procyanidolic oligomers (PCO's), also called *proanthocyanidins* (formerly called *pycnogenols*). *V. coignetiae* also contains epsilon-viniferin, oligostilbenes and amyelopsins, and 51-nucleotidase inhibitors. Resveratrol (3,5,41-trihydroxystilbene) is present when herbal preparations are mixed with grape skin extract.
Claimed actions: Grape seed extract provides nutritionally available fatty acids. The extract possesses molecules with potential free radical scavenging activity, antioxidant and antiperoxidant activity as noted in vascular injury, dose-dependent antilipoperoxidant activity, reported inhibition of xanthine oxidase enzymes; also inhibition of the enzymes: collagenase, elastase, hyaluronidase, and beta-glycuronidase; inhibition of 51-nucleotidase in snake venom
Uses: Dietary sources of fatty acids, suggested to be beneficial for Ehrlich ascites, prevention and treatment of cardiovascular, circulatory disorders, reported to have prevent cancer and dental caries (inhibits growth of *Streptococcus mutans*), improvement of ocular and night vision function. This remedy does not appear in the German Commission E monographs. There are insufficient data to support use during pregnancy or lactation.
Contraindications: Patients on warfarin and aspirin therapy. Grape seed extract is reported to increases the bleeding effects of warfarin and aspirin therapy. High doses of grape seed extract are reported to delay coagulation.
Administration: Administered orally in tablets or capsules. Doses range from 40 mg to 300 mg per day, with maintenance doses at 40-80 mg daily. No reliable dosage data are available for grape seed extract.
Side effects: *Hemat:* delayed coagulation and prolonged bleeding
Dental considerations:
Determine why the patient is taking botanical products.
"Pycnogenol," a trademarked and patented herbal product and vitamin supplement, contains proanthocyanidins from the maritime pine bark of *Pinus maritime,* sometimes called *Pinus nigra* var *maritime.*
Drug interactions: None reported

Hawthorn
(Crataegus oxyancantha, Crataegi folim cum flore, C. monogyna, and C. Laevigata)
Other names: English hawthorn, maybush
Class: Herbal remedy

Major ingredients: Flavonoids (hyperoside, vitexin-rhamnose, rutin, and proanthocyanidins) with vasodilating properties, as well as inhibition of vasoconstriction. Proanthocyanidins are reported to block angiotensin-converting enzyme (ACE). It also contains tyramine, a biogenic amine. The plant parts used include the flowers, leaves, fruits, and mixtures of other plant parts.

Claimed actions: Laboratory studies indicate positive inotropic effects, increased coronary and myocardial perfusion, and reduced peripheral vascular resistance. Dilation of coronary and peripheral blood vessels has also been reported. This information is based on laboratory studies only. Some ingredients may cause CNS depression.

Uses: Hypertension, reduction in anginal pain, decrease in cardiac sufficiency, and cardiotonic. It is approved in Germany as a prescription drug for mild cardiac insufficiency and bradyarrhythmias. Other uses include atherosclerosis.

Administration: Available in oral dose forms as an extract and plant parts for brewing teas.

Side effects: No contraindications or side effects are listed. At least one reference offered a caution when used with other drugs that may affect cardiac function.

Dental considerations: Ask why the product is being used.

Monitor vital signs in patients with cardiovascular disease.

Kava
(Piper methysticum, Piperis methystrici rhizoma)

Other names: Kava-Kava, kew, tonga

Class: Herbal remedy

Major ingredients: Kava lactones (kava alpha-pyrones), including methysticin, kawain, and others. The plant parts used are the dried rhizomes.

Claimed actions: These lactones have demonstrable pharmacologic activity on the CNS. Reported actions include sedation, muscle relaxation, and anticonvulsive and antispasmodic effects.

Uses: It has been used for a variety of complaints, including the relief of tension, stress, insomnia, and anxiety. An intoxicating effect has also been reported. Mechanism of actions range from GABA receptor modification to dopamine antagonist activity. It has also been used for a variety of other applications ranging from promotion of wound healing to gonorrhea treatment. There is little doubt the lactones are pharmacologically active, but the therapeutic value remains to be established. A local anesthetic action is also claimed.

Administration: Products for oral administration are available; in some areas the kava-kava is chewed. Use should be limited to no more than 3 months. It should not be used in patients with endogenous depression or Parkinson's disease or during pregnancy and lactation.

Side effects: Continued use results in discoloration of hair, skin, and nails. GI complaints may occasionally accompany use. Chewing kava-kava can result in circumoral numbness. Patients using kava-kava may have reduced alertness. **Warning:** Deaths associated with liver toxicity have been reported in Europe. Patients with liver impairment should be warned to avoid this herbal product.

Dental considerations:

Ask why the product is being used.

Drug interactions: Use caution when other CNS depressants are given, including other herbal remedies with antidepressant or sedative activity. One report suggests avoiding benzodiazepines in patients using Kava. Discontinue 24 hours prior to general anesthesia and general surgical procedures.

Ma-Huang

(Ephedra Sinica, Ephedra herba)
Other names: Ephedra, Desert herb

Class: Herbal remedy

Major ingredients: Contains ephedrine; some species also contain pseudoephedrine. Other components may include norepinephrine. The plant parts used are the dried young branches harvested in the fall, although some species may not contain these active alkaloids.

Claimed actions: Ephedrine has both direct and indirect actions on the sympathetic nervous system. It has direct effects on adrenergic receptors, and its indirect action is one of releasing stored catecholamines (norepinephrine) from presynaptic nerve terminals. This is well established, and ephedrine is used as a sympathomimetic. It is orally effective with a longer dura-

tion of action than epinephrine. CNS-stimulating effects are also suggested with ephedrine.

Uses: It is used for bronchospasm in asthma and other bronchospastic diseases. It acts as a cardiac stimulant with increases in blood pressure. It is also used to decrease appetite (anorexiant) and in the treatment of narcolepsy.

Administration: Various oral preparations are available, and it is also used in teas. Doses should be carefully controlled and followed to avoid excessive sympathomimetic effects.

Side effects: Hypertension, tachycardia, restlessness, headache, irritability, arrhythmias, hyperglycemia, and other related actions due to excessive or prolonged sympathetic stimulation. It should not be used in combination with St. John's Wort.

Dental Considerations:

Ask why this product is being used. If it is being used to treat asthma or bronchitis, the same precautions as for any asthmatic patient should be observed. If it is being used as an appetite suppressant, ask the patient if he or she has previously taken Fen-Phen and follow appropriate guidelines for management. Monitor vital signs every appointment due to cardiovascular side effects.

Drug interactions: Patients on high doses of Ma-Huang could possibly show exaggerated responses to injected catecholamines. Avoid the use of drugs that enhance the action of epinephrine on the cardiovascular system. Patients should avoid combinations of Ma-Huang with cardiac glycosides, halothane, guanethidine, and MAO inhibitors. Discontinue use 24 hours prior to general surgical procedures and general anesthesia. Reduced indinavir and cyclosporine concentrations.

SAMe

Others names: Ademethionine, adenosylmethionine, S-adenosylmethionine, S-adenosyl-L-methionine, Sammy.
Class: Nonherbal remedy
Major ingredients: S-adenosylmethionine

Claimed actions: A naturally occurring molecule found in most body tissues. SAMe is an active methyl carrier playing an essential role in transmethylation. It is involved in the synthesis, metabolism, and activation of hormones, neurotransmitters, phospholipids, proteins, nucleic acids, and some medications. SAMe is intimately linked to Vitamin B_{12} and folic acid metabolism. When these vitamins are absent, reduced levels of SAMe can result. As a result, SAMe affects serotonin and many body tissues, including cartilage and membranes. It functions as an antidepressant via an unknown mechanism, but is associated with increased levels of serotonin, dopamine, and norepinephrine.
Uses: Symptomatic relief of swelling and pain associated with inflammation (reported effects similar to ibuprofen), osteoarthritis, fibromyalgia, intrahepatic cholestasis, AIDS-related myelopathy, alcoholic liver cirrhosis, chronic liver disease associated with drug use, some forms of depression.

SAMe is also advocated by some practitioners as a substitute for tricyclic antidepressants.
Contraindications: None reported, however there is a possible risk of hypomania in patients with bipolar disorder.
Administration: Most positive results have come from IV administration. Oral dose forms are available but have a low bioavailability; doses range from 400-1600 mg daily. Back pain dosage is reported to be 200 mg tid. IM preparations are also available.
Side effects:
GI: Diarrhea, nausea, vomiting
CNS: Hypomania in bipolar disorder, anxiety
Dental considerations:
Determine why patient is taking the drug.
Drug interactions: None reported

Saw Palmetto
(Serenoa repens, Sabal fructus)
Other names: Sabal, cabbage palm, saw palmetto berry
Class: Herbal remedy
Major ingredients: Contains various sitosterols (phytosterols) such as beta-sitosterol and other sitosterol compounds, flavonoids, polysaccharides, and free fatty acids. The portion of the plant used is the ripe, dried fruit.

Claimed actions: Reported to be antiandrogenic, antiinflammatory, and may have some low-level estrogenic activity. The antiandrogenic activity is suggested to occur by inhibition of the enzyme testosterone-5-alpha-reductase. This action prevents the conversion of testosterone to dihydrotestosterone, the active androgenic hormone. Some data support blockade of dihydrotestosterone to receptors in the cell nucleus. Limited data seem to support the estrogenic effects. The antiinflammatory effects remain doubtful.

Uses: This herbal product has been used in the treatment of symptoms associated with benign prostatic hypertrophy, in particular urinary difficulties. Clinical trials show better results than placebo with claims of comparative results to prescription medications. There is no direct effect on reduction of the size of the prostate gland. Improvement in urinary symptoms may be somewhat similar to finasteride (Proscar).

Administration: Available for oral administration as the herb, in teas, or in extracts.

Side effects: Few side effects are reported with usual doses. Headache and GI side effects, including diarrhea with higher doses, may occur. Whether it can influence other androgens or even show estrogenic effects in women is not clear. Avoid use in pregnancy and in women of childbearing age.

Dental considerations:
Ask why the product is being used.
Drug interactions: No dental drug interactions are reported.

St. John's wort
(Hypericum perforatum, Hyperici herba)
Other names: Hypericum, kaimath weed, John's wort
Class: Herbal remedy
Major ingredients: Contains quinoids (hypericin, pseudohypericin), flavonoids (hyperoside, quercitin, rutin), bioflavonoids, and a volatile oil. The pharmacologically active component is established as hypericin. The portions of the plant used are the aboveground parts harvested during the flowering season.

Claimed actions: The primary actions are antidepressant, antiinflammatory, and antimicrobial. Hypericin may act as a selective serotonin reuptake inhibitor or a monoamine oxidase inhibitor.

Uses: It is used for the treatment of symptoms of depression; data indicate that it may be equal to or slightly less effective than the tricyclic antidepressant amitriptyline. Hypericin is soon to be evaluated as a drug for depression. The volatile oil seems to increase the healing of burns. It has been suggested to have some effect against herpes simplex viruses and HIV; efficacy remains to be established. Extracts may have some antibacterial properties. It has also been used for symptoms of dyspepsia.

Administration: A variety of oral preparations are available, and it is also used as an infusion.

Side effects: Side effects are generally minimal, but photosensitization, headache, nervousness, restlessness, hypomania, and constipation have been noted. It should be used with caution in severely depressed patients. Its safety during pregnancy and lactation is unknown. Avoid use in patients with a history of seizure disorders or migraine.

Dental considerations:
Ask why the product is being used.
Drug interactions: Should be used only with caution in patients taking

other antidepressive medications, including MAO inhibitors, tricyclic antidepressants, and selective serotonin reuptake inhibitors. It has been suggested that a risk of serotonin syndrome could occur with these antidepressants. Avoid indirect-acting sympathomimetics. Discontinue use 2 weeks before general anesthesia. Other drugs suggested to interact include metronidazole, caffeine, theophylline, digoxin, warfarin, cyclosporine, indinavir, possibly other HIV drugs, oral contraceptives, losartan and iron salts. Possibly interacts with some cancer chemotherapy medications. Avoid dental drugs with a potential for photosensitivity.

Valerian
(*Valeriana officinalis, Valerianae radix*)
Other names: Valerian root, Indian valerian
Class: Herbal remedy
Major ingredients: Valepotriates (isovaltrate and others), a volatile oil (bornyl isovalerenate and isovalerenic acid), sesquiterpenes, and multiple other substances. Pharmacologically active components are not identified with any certainty. The portions of the plant used are the fresh underground parts and roots.

Claimed actions: Sedation, reduction in nervousness, sleep promoting, and antispasmodic.
Uses: It is used for restlessness, sleeping disorders, and insomnia. Other uses include agitation associated with menstrual activity, colic, stomach cramps, and uterine spasticity. Laboratory data suggest that it may increase GABA levels at synapses. Antispasmodic properties are not well defined. Limited clinical evidence suggests some improvement in sleep. It has also been used externally by adding to bath water.
Administration: Available for oral use in a variety of oral products, including tinctures, infusions, and extracts.
Side effects: Generally not observed in usual doses. GI complaints, headache, sleeplessness, mydriasis, excitability, and cardiac disturbances may occur with long-term use.
Dental considerations:
Ask why the product is being used.
Drug interactions: Although no interactions are reported, monitor patients for increased sedation when using other CNS depressants. May potentiate CNS depressants.

Yohimbe bark
(*Pausinystalia yohimbe*)
Other names: Yohimbe cortex
Class: Herbal remedy
Major ingredients: The principal alkaloid is yohimbine (quebrachine) with lesser amounts of stereoisomers of yohimbine along with other alkaloids, including corynantheidine and allo-yohimbine. It also contains a variety of plant tannins. The portion of the plant used is the dried bark of the trunk and branches of the tree.

Claimed actions: The major effects of this drug are due to yohimbine. Do not confuse the prescription drug yohimbine with yohimbe. Yohimbine has α_2-adrenergic antagonist activity. Presynaptic α_2-receptors regulate norepinephrine release. In a feedback-type action, antagonism of these receptors is associated with greater norepinephrine release. It may also dilate blood vessels; claims are made for a calcium channel blocking action and inhibition of monoamine oxidase enzymes.

Uses: It has been used to treat erectile dysfunction, as an aphrodisiac, for exhaustion, and even for orthostatic hypotension. Limited data concern yohimbine and not yohimbe. Yohimbine has not been approved for this application. According to the German Commission E monographs, yohimbe's effectiveness is not documented and it is not recommended.

Administration: Limited products are available and usually in combination with other ingredients.

Side effects: Usual doses produce few side effects; however, in large doses significant adverse effects are reported. These include increased salivation, anxiety, hallucinations, exanthema, nervousness, irritability, tachycardia, and sweating. Other effects may also be observed. Cardiac failure, which could be fatal, is reported. Contraindicated in patients with hepatic or renal impairment and psychiatric disorders.

Dental considerations:
Ask why the product is being used.

Drug interactions: No specific dental drug interactions are reported, but it may have MAO inhibitory action. Avoid use of indirect-acting sympathomimetics and tricyclic antidepressants.

BIBLIOGRAPHY

Blumenthal M et al: *The complete German Commission E monographs,* Austin, 1998, American Botanical Council.

DerMarderosian A, editor: *The review of natural products,* St Louis, 1996, Facts and Comparisons.

Miller LG: Herbal medicinals: selected clinical considerations focusing on known or potential drug-herb interactions, *Arch Intern Med* 158(20):2200-2211, 1998.

Natural medicines comprehensive database, Stockton, CA, 1999, Pharmacist's Letter/Prescriber's Letter, Therapeutic Research Faculty.

Nonherbal dietary supplements, *Pharmacist's Letter* 98(4), 1998.

O'Hara MA et al: A review of 12 commonly used medicinal herbs, *Arch Fam Med* 7:523-536, 1998.

PDR for herbal remedies, Montvale, NJ, 1998, Medical Economics.

Therapeutic use of herbs, continuing education booklets part 1 and part 2, Stockton, CA, 1998, Pharmacist's Letter.

Appendix I

Drugs affecting the cytochrome P450 isoenzymes

The cytochrome P450 (CYP 40) families of isoenzymes act as major enzyme systems for the oxidative metabolism of a wide spectrum of drugs. The highest concentrations of CYP450 are found in the liver and intestine, with lesser amounts in other tissues. They are distinguished from one another by family names using letters and numbers; for example, CYP 1A2, CYP 2D6, or CYP 3A4. A number of drugs and foods can induce or inhibit specific isoenzymes and, in some instances, this has resulted in serious drug interactions. It is also true that one drug may be a substrate for CYP 450 and at the same time cause induction or inhibition of the same enzyme. Because enzymes are substrate specific, each CYP 450 isoenzyme will catalyze the metabolism of only selected drugs. On the other hand, more than one CYP 450 enzyme may participate in metabolism of a drug.

An example of a drug interaction involving CYP 3A4 is provided. Lovastatin (Mevacor, a drug that interferes with cholesterol synthesis) is a substrate for CYP 3A4. Erythromycin (a macrolide antiinfective) is an inhibitor of CYP 3A4. Thus erythromycin inhibits the metabolism of lovastatin if the drugs are taken concurrently by the same patient. This results in increased plasma levels of lovastatin. Significant increases in the plasma levels of lovastatin increase the risk of a potentially serious adverse effect known as *rhabdomyolysis*. Thus erythromycin is contraindicated when a patient is also taking lovastatin. In some cases, inhibition of CYP450 in the intestines will result in altered drug absorption. This can mean either too little drug is absorbed or more drug is absorbed than expected. Either effect will modify the anticipated response. When a drug is both a substrate and inducer of CYP 450 enzymes, the anticipated response of a second dose will be less than expected. For some drugs, this can be overcome by giving higher than normal doses. Grapefruit juice is an example of a food that is an inhibitor of CYP 3A4.

The following table lists a number of enzymes and drugs that function either as substrates, inhibitors, or inducers of one or more of the CYP450 isoenzymes. It is almost impossible to list all of the potential or established drug interactions, but some involve commonly used dental drugs. When the notation of dental drug interaction appears, please refer to the individual monographs for each drug to see the specific drug interactions. (Hint: Select the generic name and use the colored tabs on the side of the book to quickly locate a drug.)

Isoenzyme
CYP 1A2

acetaminophen	substrate	
caffeine	substrate	
ciprofloxacin (Cipro)	inhibitor	dental drug interactions
clozapine (Clozaril)	substrate	
cimetidine (Tagamet)	inhibitor	
cyclobenzaprine (Flexeril)	substrate	
erythromycin	inhibitor	
estradiol	substrate	
fluvoxamine (Luvox)	inhibitor	dental drug interactions
naproxen (Naprosyn)	substrate	
norfloxacin (Noroxin)	inhibitor	
rifampin (Rifadin)	inducer	
theophylline	substrate	dental drug interactions
tacrine (Cognex)	substrate and inhibitor	
ticlopidine (Ticlid)	inhibitor	
verapamil (Calan)	substrate	
warfarin (Coumadin)	substrate	

Nondrug substance

Cigarette smoke	inducer

CYP 2C8-10

cimetidine (Tagamet)	inhibitor
diazepam (Valium)	substrate
diclofenac (Cataflam)	substrate
omeprazole (Prilosec)	inhibitor
phenobarbital	inducer
rifampin (Rifadin)	inducer

CYP 2C9

amitriptyline (Elavil)	substrate
bosentan (Tracleer)	substrate
celecoxib (Celebrex)	substrate
diclofenac	substrate
fluconazole (Diflucan)	inhibitor
fluvastatin (Lescol)	substrate
glipizide (Glucotrol)	substrate
ibuprofen	substrate
imipramine (Tofranil)	substrate
ketoconazole (Nizoral)	inhibitor
metronidazole (Flagyl)	inhibitor
naproxen	substrate
phenytoin (Dilantin)	substrate
piroxicam (Feldene)	substrate
rifampin	inducer
ritonavir (Norvir)	inhibitor
secobarbital	inducer

valdecoxib (Bextra)	substrate	
warfarin (Coumadin)	substrate	
CYP 2C19		
diazepam (Valium)	substrate	
felbamate (Felbatol)	inhibitor	
fluoxetine (Prozac)	inhibitor	
fluvoxamine (Luvox)	inhibitor	
lansoprazole (Prevacid)	substrate	
omeprazole (Prilosec)	substrate	
propranolol (Inderal)	substrate	
rifampin	inducer	
CYP 2D6		
amitriptyline (Elavil)	substrate	
cevimeline (Evoxac)	substrate	
chlorpheniramine (Chlor-Trimeton)	inhibitor	
codeine	substrate	
desipramine (Norpramin)	substrate	
dextromethorphan	substrate	
diphenhydramine (Benadryl)	inhibitor	dental drug interactions
fluoxetine (Prozac)	inhibitor	
haloperidol (Haldol)	substrate	
mexiletine (Mexitil)	substrate	
oxycodone	substrate	
propoxyphene	substrate	
ritonavir (Norvir)	inhibitor	
timolol (Blocadren)	substrate	
tramadol (Ultram)	substrate	
CYP 2E1		
acetaminophen	substrate	
chlorzoxazone (Paraflex)	substrate	
disulfiram	inhibitor	
ethanol	substrate and inducer	
isoniazid	inducer	
CYP 3A3		
alprazolam (Xanax)	substrate	
cimetidine (Tagamet)	inhibitor	
erythromycin	substrate	
midazolam (Versed)	substrate	
ranitidine (Zantac)	inhibitor	
CYP 3A4		
alprazolam (Xanax)	substrate	dental drug interactions
amprenavir (Agenerase)	substrate and inhibitor	dental drug interactions
atorvastatin (Lipitor)	substrate	dental drug interactions

buspirone (BuSpar)	substrate	dental drug interactions
bosentan (Tracleer)	substrate and inducer	
carbamazepine (Tegretol)	substrate and inducer	dental drug interactions
clorazepate (Tranxene)	substrate	dental drug interactions
chlordiazepoxide (Librium)	substrate	dental drug interactions
cimetidine (Tagamet)	inhibitor	
clarithromycin (Biaxin)	substrate and inhibitor	dental drug interactions
cyclosporine (Sandimmune)	substrate	
diazepam (Valium)	substrate	dental drug interactions
diltiazem (Cardizem)	substrate	
erythromycin	substrate and inhibitor	dental drug interactions
estazolam (ProSom)	substrate	dental drug interactions
felodipine (Plendil)	substrate	dental drug interactions
dexamethasone (Decadron)	substrate and inhibitor	dental drug interactions
indinavir (Crixivan)	substrate and inhibitor	dental drug interactions
itraconazole (Sporanox)	inhibitor	dental drug interactions
ketoconazole (Nizoral)	inhibitor	dental drug interactions
lovastatin (Mevacor)	substrate	dental drug interactions
lidocaine	substrate	
metronidazole (Flagyl)	inhibitor	dental drug interactions
midazolam (Versed)	substrate	dental drug interactions
nefazodone (Serzone)	inhibitor	dental drug interactions
nelfinavir (Viracept)	substrate and inhibitor	dental drug interactions
nifedipine (Procardia)	substrate	
nisoldipine (Sular)	substrate	
omeprazole (Prilosec)	inhibitor	
phenobarbital	substrate and inducer	dental drug interactions
quazepam (Doral)	substrate	dental drug interactions
ritonavir (Norvir)	substrate and inhibitor	dental drug interactions
saquinavir (Invirase, Fortovase) interactions	substrate and inhibitor	dental drug interactions
sertraline (Zoloft)	inhibitor	dental drug interactions
sildenafil (Viagra)	substrate	dental drug interactions
simvastatin (Zocor)	substrate	dental drug interactions
tacrolimus (Prograf)	substrate	

triazolam (Halcion)	substrate	dental drug interactions
valdecoxib (Bextra)	substrate	
verapamil (Calan)	substrate	
warfarin (Coumadin)	substrate	dental drug interactions
zolpidem (Ambien)	substrate	dental drug interactions
Nondrug products		
grapefruit juice	inhibitor of enteric	

CYP 3A4

St. John's Wort	inducer	dental drug interactions

CYP 3A5

lovastatin (Mevacor)	substrate	
midazolam (Versed)	substrate	
nifedipine (Procardia)	substrate	

Appendix J

Prescription examples

This appendix illustrates a number of prescriptions that can be used as a guide to help you write prescriptions for dental patients. They can be used as written or modified to address each patient's specific needs and your personal preferences. They are not a substitute for your clinical judgment. The process of selecting and prescribing a medication for a patient is usually rather straightforward, but can be challenging in some cases. It is important for the prescribing dentist to be completely knowledgeable about any drug prescribed. Complete prescribing information should be consulted before selecting a drug. This means knowing how the drug acts, its intended use, the dose and dose forms, how frequently the drug should be taken, and adverse effects and drug interactions. These essential drug facts are tools for the profession. The better a dentist knows the tools and the patient, the more competent the therapy. In the following examples, prescriptions for brand name drugs are for illustrative purposes only and do not constitute a recommendation for that particular product. Generic products are generally the least expensive way to prescribe medications, but in some cases (especially for new drugs or specialty products) only brand name products are available.

Before prescribing or recommending (in the case of OTC products) a medication for a patient, it is strongly suggested the dentist adhere to the following protocol:

a. Examine and evaluate the patient, leading to a diagnosis
b. Obtain the patient's medical and drug history (including the use of OTC drugs, illegal drugs, and herbal or nonherbal remedies)
c. Calculate the duration of drug therapy and required number of doses
d. Assess the patient's prior experience with drugs, including drug allergy
e. Research the potential side effects and drug interactions
f. Adhere to all federal and state laws regulating drug use in practice
g. Consider the cost to the patient if less expensive alternatives are available
h. Consider the patient's ability to use more complex dose forms or to follow complex instructions for use
i. Have an alternative selection in mind in the event a patient cannot tolerate the prescribed drug

I. ANALGESICS

Controlled substances (requires state and DEA registration to prescribe with DEA number included on the prescription)

Prescription examples are for acute pain without regard to intensity of pain. Because acute pain is generally managed within 3-4 days, prescriptions should limit the number of doses to be dispensed. In given situations, more than 10 or 12 doses may be required. *If the analgesic product you are using is not illustrated, don't worry. These are merely examples provided for guidance in prescription writing and are not inclusive of all analgesic products, which number into the hundreds.* For illustrative purposes, both brand and generic names are used. Notice the directions for use indicate a specific time interval for optimum response; prn use is avoided to ensure more appropriate dosing intervals for the analgesic. The cautions of sedation and avoidance of alcohol are appropriate for each product.

Rx

Darvocet-N 100*

Disp: 12 (twelve) tabs
Sig: Take one (1) tab p.o. q 4 hours for pain relief.

*(The maximum recommended dose for propoxyphene napsylate is 600 mg/day. Do not take with alcohol, and reduce the dose or select another drug if significant liver or renal failure is present or select another drug.)

Rx

Empirin with Codeine #4*

Disp: 12 (twelve) tabs
Sig: Take one (1) tab p.o. q 4 hours for pain relief.

*(This product contains 60 mg of codeine phosphate, a preferable oral adult dose; the No. 3 product contains 30 mg of codeine phosphate.)

Rx

Fiorinal with Codeine 30 mg*

Disp: 12 (twelve) caps
Sig: Take one (1) cap p.o. q 4-6 hours for pain relief.

*(This product contains a short-acting barbiturate; Fioricet with Codeine 30 mg contains acetaminophen instead of aspirin.)

Rx

Lortab 5/500

Disp: 12 (twelve) tabs
Sig: Take one (1) tab p.o. q 6 hours for pain relief.

Rx

Percodan

Disp: 10 (ten) tabs
Sig: Take one (1) tab p.o. q 6 hours for pain relief.

Rx

Phenaphen with Codeine #4*

Disp: 12 (twelve) caps
Sig: Take one (1) cap p.o. q 4 hours for pain relief.

*(This product contains 60 mg of codeine phosphate, a preferable oral adult dose; the No. 3 product contains 30 mg of codeine phosphate.)

Rx
Tylenol with Codeine Elixir*
Disp: 90 ml (volume may vary with duration and patient's age)
Sig: Take 5 ml (one teaspoonful) every 6-8 hours for pain relief.
*(This is an example for a child 3-6 yr. For a child 7-12 yr the dose is 10 ml, and for adults the dose is 15 ml. Be sure you know the quantities of acetaminophen and codeine phosphate contained in each 5-ml dose. This product also contains alcohol. Your pharmacist can increase the amount of codeine in each 5-ml dose unit; consult your pharmacist for instructions.)

Rx
Tylenol with Codeine #4*
Disp: 12 tabs
Sig: Take one (1) tab p.o. q 4 hours for pain relief.
*(This product contains 60 mg of codeine phosphate, a preferable oral adult dose; the No. 3 product contains 30 mg of codeine phosphate.)

Rx
Vicodin
Disp: 10 (ten) tabs
Sig: Take one (1) tab p.o. q 6 hours for pain relief.

Rx
Zydone 5/400*
Disp: 10 (ten) tabs
Sig: Take one (1) or two (2) tabs p.o. q 4-6 hours for pain relief.
*(Because Zydone is available in several strengths, the prescription must be specific as shown in the example.)

Nonnarcotics or analgesics not classified as controlled substances

Doses for aspirin and acetaminophen for both adults and children are given in the respective monographs. For consistent dose levels and effects, it is important to prescribe NSAIDs by the clock rather than prn.

Rx
diclofenac sodium 50-mg tabs (immediate release type)
Disp: 9 tabs
Sig: Take one (1) tab p.o. q 8 hours for pain relief.

Rx
diflunisal 500-mg tabs*
Disp: 7 tabs
Sig: Take two (2) tabs p.o. the first dose; then one (1) tab p.o. q 12 hours for pain relief.
*(The 250-mg tabs may be sufficient for some patients. The initial dose is 500 mg; do not exceed doses of 1.5 g/day.)

Rx
etodolac 400-mg tabs*
Disp: 16 tabs
Sig: Take one (1) tab p.o. q 6-8 hours for pain relief.
*(The 200-mg tabs may be sufficient for some patients. Dose limit is 1200 mg/day.)

Rx

ibuprofen* 400-mg tabs†

Disp: 24 tabs

Sig: Take 1 tab p.o. q 4 hours for pain relief.

*(Special preparations for children, such as Children's Motrin with specified doses, are available for toothaches; doses are printed on the package.)

†(If larger doses are preferred, the time interval between doses must be adjusted to reflect the larger dose; for example 600 mg every 6 hours. Another option is to recommend OTC ibuprofen in 200-mg tablets and tell the patient to take 2 tabs every 4 hours. For some patients, a prescription may be required to ensure a desirable patient benefit. Ibuprofen also can be used for chronic pain.)

Rx

ketoprofen 25-mg caps (or 50-mg caps)*

Disp: 12 caps

Sig: Take one (1) cap p.o. q 6-8 hours for pain relief.

*(The larger dose may be required for some patients. Select the smaller dose for the elderly and patients with severe renal or hepatic disease; also available OTC in 12.5-mg tabs.)

Rx

meclofenamate sodium* 50-mg caps

Disp: 18 caps

Sig: Take one (1) cap p.o. q 4-6 hours for pain relief.

*(Total daily dose is limited to 400 mg.)

Rx

naproxen sodium tabs 550-mg tabs

Disp: 10 tabs

Sig: Take one (1) tab p.o. q 12 hours for pain relief.

(Naproxen sodium also can be used for chronic pain.)

Rx

Ultram 50-mg tabs*

Disp: 12 tabs

Sig: Take one (1) tab p.o. q 4-6 hours for pain relief.

*(For more severe pain, the 100-mg tabs can be prescribed. Do not exceed the daily dose limit of 400 mg.)

Rx

Vioxx 50-mg tabs

Disp: 5 tabs

Sig: Take one (1) tab p.o. daily for pain relief.

II. ANTIINFECTIVES

The primary considerations when selecting an antiinfective drug include potential causative organisms, the severity of the infection, the age of the infection (cellulitis vs. pus formation), the patient's prior history of antiinfective drug use, and the immunologic status of the patient. The duration of antiinfective drug therapy differs somewhat among clinicians, ranging from 5-10 days. Certainly surgical intervention or removal of a necrotic pulp makes a significant difference not only in resolution, but also the duration of the infection. The examples provided for illustration purposes show doses calculated to cover the patient for 7-10 days. Examples include both generic and brand name products. One or two examples of prescriptions for children are shown; doses were calculated using mg per kg of body weight and reflect manufacturers' or USP recommended doses. Antiinfectives should be prescribed to take at specific intervals, such as every 6 hours. Using symbols, such as qid for four times a day, may not allow for proper intervals between doses. However, for some drugs, such as rinses or lozenges, abbreviations such as qid or tid are satisfactory. *Please note these prescriptions are intended to help you develop your own prescription as dictated by the patient's need and circumstance.*

Rx

amoxicillin trihydrate 500-mg caps*

Disp: 21 caps

Sig: Take one (1) cap p.o. q 8 hours for infection until all are taken.

*(Some may prefer to give an initial loading dose of 1000 mg followed by the 500-mg doses.)

Rx

penicillin V potassium 500-mg tabs*

Disp: 28 tabs

Sig: Take one (1) tab p.o. q 6 hours for infection until all are taken.

*(Some may prefer to give an initial loading dose of 1000 mg followed by the 500-mg doses.)

Rx for prophylaxis against bacterial endocarditis for three different appointments

---

Rx

amoxicillin trihydrate 500-mg caps

Disp: 12 caps

Sig: Take four (4) caps p.o. 1 hour before each dental appointment.

Rx for a child weighing 30 kg (66 lb)

The package insert dose for children is 20 mg/kg/day (in equal doses given every 8 hours) for mild/moderate infections and 40 mg/kg/day (in equal doses given every 12 hours) for severe infections. The example chosen is 20 mg/kg/day; this means the total daily dose will be 600 mg, or 200 mg every 8 hours in individual doses.

Rx

amoxicillin for oral suspension 200 mg/5 ml

Disp: 150 ml*

Sig: Take 5 ml p.o. every 8 hours for infection until all is taken.

*(This is enough volume to provide doses for 10 days.)

Rx

cefadroxil 500-mg caps

Disp: 14 caps

Sig: Take one (1) cap p.o. q 12 hours for infection until all are taken.

Rx for prophylaxis against bacterial endocarditis for a single appointment

Rx

cefadroxil 1-gram tabs*

Disp: 2 tabs

Sig: Take two (2) tabs p.o. 1 hour before appointment.

*(Alternatively, 500-mg caps could also be used, noting that 4 caps are required for a single use.)

Rx

clindamycin hydrochloride 300-mg caps*

Disp: 28 caps

Sig: Take one (1) cap p.o. q 6 hours for infection until all are taken.

*(Doses of 150 mg also are used depending on severity of the infection.)

Rx

azithromycin 250-mg caps

Disp: 6 caps

Sig: Take two (2) caps p.o. the first day, then one (1) cap daily for infection until all are taken. Take 1 hour a.c. or 2 hours p.c.

Rx

Biaxin 250-mg tabs*

Disp: 20 tabs

Sig: Take one (1) tab p.o. q 12 hours for infection until all are taken.

*(The 500-mg dose may be required for some infections, such as maxillary sinusitis subsequent to loss of root tip in the sinus cavity.)

Rx for prophylaxis against bacterial endocarditis for six appointments

Rx

clindamycin hydrochloride 300-mg caps

Disp: 12 caps

Sig: Take two (2) caps p.o. 1 hour before each appointment.

Rx

doxycycline 100-mg caps

Disp: 11 caps

Sig: Take one (1) cap p.o. q 12 hours the first day, then take one (1) cap p.o. daily for infection until all are taken.

Rx

Ery-Tab 250-mg tabs*

Disp: 40 tabs

Sig: Take one (1) tab p.o. q 6 hours for infection until all are taken.

*(This is an erythromycin base; other dose options depending on the dose form selected include 333 mg q 8 hours or 500 mg q 12 hours.)

Rx

erythromycin ethyl succinate 400-mg tabs

Disp: 40 tabs

Sig: Take one (1) tab p.o. q 6 hours for infection until all are taken.

Rx

metronidazole 250-mg tabs

Disp: 21 tabs

Sig: Take one (1) tab p.o. q 8 hours for infection until all are taken; avoid use of alcohol products.

III. ANTIFUNGAL ANTIINFECTIVES

These are examples (not all products are illustrated) of prescriptions for drugs for *Candida* infections of the oral cavity, which are usually prescribed for use over 14 days. Remember patient evaluation, history, and diagnosis always precede drug selection.

Rx
clotrimazole 10-mg troches
Disp: 70 troches
Sig: Slowly dissolve one (1) troche in your mouth 5 times a day while awake until all are used.

Rx
fluconazole 50-mg tabs*
Disp: 15 tabs
Sig: Take two (2) tabs p.o. the first day, then take one (1) tab p.o. daily for infection until all are taken.
*(The 100-mg dose size may be required for more severe infections or in immunocompromised patients.)

Rx
Fungizone Oral Suspension 100 mg/ml
Disp: 24 ml
Sig: Rinse with 1 ml qid and then spit.

Rx
nystatin ointment*
Disp: 15 grams
Sig: Apply a small amount to affected areas after each meal and at bedtime.
*(Possible use in angular cheilitis associated with candidiasis.)

Rx
nystatin oral suspension (100,000 u/ml)
Disp: 320 ml
Sig: Rinse for 1 min with 5 ml of solution q 6 hours while awake and then expectorate. One rinse should be used just before bedtime.*
*(Dentures also should be carefully cleaned and then soaked in the oral solution for approximately 15 min each day during treatment.)

Although some sugar is contained in the commercial preparation of nystatin oral suspension, it is still effective against candidiasis. An alternative choice for oral nystatin rinse when sugar is not desirable for the patient is shown in the following example. Be sure to check labels for sugar content in all locally acting oral products.

Rx
nystatin extemporaneous powder
Disp: 50 million units*
Sig: Add 1/8 tsp (500,000 U) to 1/2 cup water (8 oz) and rinse qid for 2 weeks.
*(This is the smallest container of powder available; it supplies enough powder for 25 days of use.)

Rx
Sporanox Oral Solution 10 mg/ml
Disp: 150 ml
Sig: Rinse with 20 ml once a day and swallow.*
*(Unlike other antifungal rinses, itraconazole [Sporanox] is systemically absorbed and has a therapeutic effect.)

IV. OTHER DENTAL PRESCRIPTIONS

The following prescriptions are examples for a variety of dental diseases. They are grouped according to their usual applications. *Again, there may be many choices for treatment that are not shown; these are examples for assistance in prescription writing.*

Recurrent aphthous stomatitis

Rx
Aphthasol Oral Paste 5%
Disp: 5 grams
Sig: Dab a small amount of paste on ulcer qid, pc, and hs.

Rx
Benadryl Elixir 40 ml*
Kaopectate 80 ml
Water q.s. ad. 240 ml
Sig: Rinse with 5 ml for 1-2 min prn for comfort and then expectorate.
*(A 50/50 mixture of Benadryl/Kaopectate also can be used. Benadryl Elixir alone also serves as a palliative rinse, but contains alcohol; may use Children's Benadryl, which is alcohol free.)

Rx
chlorhexidine rinse 0.12% or write Peridex
Disp: 16 ounces
Sig: Rinse with 1 ml twice daily.*
*(Optional application route: moisten a cotton-tipped applicator and dab on ulcer bid.)

Rx
fluocinonide gel 0.05% or write Lidex Gel
Disp: 15 grams
Sig: Apply (dab on or use cotton-tipped applicator) to ulcers bid.

Rx
Zylocaine Viscous 2%
Disp: 100 ml
Sig: Rinse with 5 ml for 1-2 min q 4 hours.
(Optional choice: rinse before meals and at bedtime.)

Desquamative lesions (lichen planus, phemphigoid)

Rx
Diprolene gel 0.05%*
Disp: 15 grams
Sig: Apply a small amount to lesions tid. Apply the last dose at bedtime.
*(This is a very-high-potency glucocorticoid; consider switching to a high-potency gel once severe lesions are under control.)

Rx
Lidex gel 0.05%*
Disp: 30 grams
Sig: Apply a small amount to lesions tid. Apply the last dose at bedtime.
*(This is a high-potency topical glucocorticoid. Alternatively, if the lesions are small, dab a small amount directly on the lesions.)

Rx
prednisone 5-mg tabs
Disp: 44 tabs
Sig: Take two (2) tabs p.o. AM and PM × 2 days, then reduce by one (1) tab each day until all are taken.

Drugs affecting salivary flow
Prescriptions to reduce salivary flow (using four appointments as an example, because the number of tablets to dispense depends on the number of appointments):

Rx
atropine sulfate 0.4-mg tabs
Disp: 4 tabs
Sig: Take 1 tab p.o. 30-60 min before appointment.

Rx
Pro-Banthine 15-mg tabs
Disp: 4 tabs
Sig: Take one (1) tab p.o. 45-60 min before appointment.
*(Many pharmacies may no longer stock this particular drug.)

Prescription to stimulate salivary flow in selected patients:

Rx
Evoxac 30-mg caps
Disp: 42 caps*
Sig: Take one (1) cap p.o. three times a day.
*(Larger doses increase risk of side effects; enough doses are ordered for a 2-week period to evaluate patient response.)

Drugs for herpes labialis

Rx
acyclovir 200-mg caps
Disp: 35 caps
Sig: Take one (1) cap p.o. 5 times a day.

Rx
acyclovir ointment 5%
Disp: 3 grams
Sig: At the first sign of lesion, apply a small amount to affected areas 6 × daily for 1 week.

Rx
Denavir Cream 1%
Disp: 2 grams
Sig: At first sign of lesion, apply a small amount to affected area q 2 hours (while awake) × 4 days.

Mild allergic reactions

Rx
Benadryl 25-mg caps*
Disp: 15 caps
Sig: Take one (1) cap q 4-8 hours for symptom relief.
Caution: sedation.
*(Adults can take up to 50 mg per dose. Alternative long-acting and nonsedating antihistamines also are available as well as other rapid-onset, short-acting, sedating antihistamines. However, for immediate hypersensitive reactions, rapid-acting drugs are preferred.)

Rx
Medrol Dosepak 4-mg tabs
Disp: 1 unit
Sig: Follow labeled directions on package for use.
(Note: A pack contains 21 tabs.)

Fluoride toothpaste

Rx
1.1% neutral sodium fluoride toothpaste*
Disp: two (2) tubes
Sig: Apply thin ribbon to dry toothbrush and brush for 2 min. Spit out excess; do not eat, drink, or rinse for 30 min after use.
*(You may prefer to write Previ-Dent 5000 Plus.)

Appendix K

Selected references

Advisory Statement: Antibiotic prophylaxis for dental patients with total joint replacements, *JADA* 128:1004-1008, July 1997.

Borea G et al: Tranexamic acid as a mouthwash in anticoagulant-treated patients undergoing oral surgery, *Oral Surg Oral Med Oral Pathol* 75:29-31, 1993.

Cohen DM, Bhattacharyya I, Lydiatt WM: Recalcitrant oral ulcers caused by calcium channel blockers: diagnosis and treatment considerations, *JADA* 130:1611-1618, November 1999.

Cupp MJ, Tracy TS: Role of the cytochrome P450 3A subfamily, *US Pharmacists* 22:HS9-HS21, 1997.

Dajani AS et al: Prevention of bacterial endocarditis: recommendations by the American Heart Association, *JADA* 128:1142-1151, August 1997.

Drug interaction facts, updated quarterly, St Louis, Facts and Comparisons.

Facts and comparisons, updated monthly, St Louis, Facts and Comparisons.

Fye KH et al: Celecoxib-induced Sweet's syndrome, *J Am Acad Dermatol* 45:300-302, August 2001.

Gahart BL: *2000 Intravenous medications,* ed 16, St Louis, 1999, Mosby.

Halevy S, Shai A: Lichenoid drug eruptions, *J Am Acad Dermatol* 29:249-255, 1993.

Hardman JG et al: *Goodman and Gilman's the pharmacological basis of therapeutics,* ed 9, New York, 1996, McGraw-Hill.

Little JW, Falace DA: *Dental management of the medically compromised patient,* ed 6, St Louis, 2002, Mosby.

Mancano MA: Drug interactions with protease inhibitors Part I, *Pharmacy Times* 67:14-17, June 2001.

The medical letter, handbook of adverse drug interactions, New Rochelle, NY, 1999, The Medical Letter.

Mosby's Drug Consult 2002, St Louis, 2002, Mosby.

Pharmacist's Letter 16: 2000.

Pharmacist's Letter 17: 2001.

Physicians' desk reference, ed 54, Montvale, NJ, 2000, Medical Economics.

Rees TD: Oral effects of drug abuse, *Crit Rev Oral Biol Med* 3(3):163-184, 1992.

Rees TD: Systemic drugs as a risk factor for periodontal disease initiation and progression, *Compendium* 16:20-42, 1995.

Shulman JD, Wells LM: Acute fluoride toxicity from ingesting home-use dental products in children birth to 6 years of age, *J Public Health Dent* 57(3):150-158, 1997.

Skidmore-Roth L: *Mosby's 2002 nursing drug reference,* St Louis, 1999, Mosby.

Taylor SE, Gage TW: New drugs and products approved from 2000. *Texas Dental Journal* 118:1070-1081, 2001.

United States Pharmacopeial Convention: *Drug information for the health care professionals USPDI,* ed 21, Englewood, Colo, 2001, Micromedex.

United States Pharmacopeial Convention: *USP Dictionary of USAN and International Drug Names 2001,* Rockville, Md, 2001, The Convention.

Valsecchi R, Cainelli T: Gingival hyperplasia induced by erythromycin, *Acta Derm Venereol (Stockh)* 72:157, 1992.

Westbrook P et al: Reversal of nifedipine-induced gingival hyperplasia by the calcium channel blocker, isradipine, *J Dent Res* 74(S1):208, 1995.

Whal MJ: Altering anticoagulant therapy: a survey of physicians, *JADA* 127:625-638, 1996.

Whal MJ: Myths of dental surgery in patients receiving anticoagulant therapy, *JADA* 131:77-81, 2000.

Wright JM: Oral manifestations of drug reactions, *Dent Clin North Am* 28:529-543, 1984.

Zelickson BD, Rogers RS: Oral drug reactions, *Dermatol Clin* 5:695-708, 1987.

Generic and Trade
Name Index

Index

Entries can be identified as follows: generic name, Trade Name, DRUG CATEGORY, *Combination Product.*

Entries can be identified as follows: generic name, Trade Name, DRUG CATEGORY, *Combination Product.*

Entries can be identified as follows: generic name, Trade Name, DRUG CATEGORY, *Combination Product.*

Entries can be identified as follows: generic name, Trade Name, DRUG CATEGORY, *Combination Product.*

Entries can be identified as follows: generic name, Trade Name, DRUG CATEGORY,
Combination Product.

Entries can be identified as follows: generic name, Trade Name, DRUG CATEGORY, *Combination Product.*

Entries can be identified as follows: generic name, Trade Name, DRUG CATEGORY, *Combination Product.*

Entries can be identified as follows: generic name, Trade Name, DRUG CATEGORY, *Combination Product.*

Entries can be identified as follows: generic name, Trade Name, DRUG CATEGORY,
Combination Product.

Entries can be identified as follows: generic name, Trade Name, DRUG CATEGORY,
Combination Product.

Entries can be identified as follows: generic name, Trade Name, DRUG CATEGORY,
Combination Product.

Entries can be identified as follows: generic name, Trade Name, DRUG CATEGORY, *Combination Product.*

Entries can be identified as follows: generic name, Trade Name, DRUG CATEGORY, *Combination Product.*

Entries can be identified as follows: generic name, Trade Name, DRUG CATEGORY, *Combination Product.*

Entries can be identified as follows: generic name, Trade Name, DRUG CATEGORY, *Combination Product.*

Entries can be identified as follows: generic name, Trade Name, DRUG CATEGORY,
Combination Product.

Entries can be identified as follows: generic name, Trade Name, DRUG CATEGORY, *Combination Product.*

Entries can be identified as follows: generic name, Trade Name, DRUG CATEGORY, *Combination Product.*

Entries can be identified as follows: generic name, Trade Name, DRUG CATEGORY, *Combination Product.*

Entries can be identified as follows: generic name, Trade Name, DRUG CATEGORY,
Combination Product.

Entries can be identified as follows: generic name, Trade Name, DRUG CATEGORY, *Combination Product.*

Entries can be identified as follows: generic name, Trade Name, DRUG CATEGORY, *Combination Product.*

Entries can be identified as follows: generic name, Trade Name, DRUG CATEGORY, *Combination Product.*

Entries can be identified as follows: generic name, Trade Name, DRUG CATEGORY, *Combination Product*.

Entries can be identified as follows: generic name, Trade Name, DRUG CATEGORY, *Combination Product.*

Entries can be identified as follows: generic name, Trade Name, DRUG CATEGORY, *Combination Product.*

Entries can be identified as follows: generic name, Trade Name, DRUG CATEGORY, *Combination Product.*

Entries can be identified as follows: generic name, Trade Name, DRUG CATEGORY, *Combination Product.*

Entries can be identified as follows: generic name, Trade Name, DRUG CATEGORY, *Combination Product.*

Entries can be identified as follows: generic name, Trade Name, DRUG CATEGORY,
Combination Product.

Entries can be identified as follows: generic name, Trade Name, DRUG CATEGORY, *Combination Product.*

Entries can be identified as follows: generic name, Trade Name, DRUG CATEGORY, *Combination Product.*

Entries can be identified as follows: generic name, Trade Name, DRUG CATEGORY, *Combination Product.*

Entries can be identified as follows: generic name, Trade Name, DRUG CATEGORY, *Combination Product.*

Entries can be identified as follows: generic name, Trade Name, DRUG CATEGORY, *Combination Product.*

Entries can be identified as follows: generic name, Trade Name, DRUG CATEGORY,
Combination Product.

Entries can be identified as follows: generic name, Trade Name, DRUG CATEGORY, *Combination Product.*

Entries can be identified as follows: generic name, Trade Name, DRUG CATEGORY, *Combination Product.*

New Drug Updates 2003

Following are monographs for 11 new drugs that have received FDA approval since the publication of *Mosby's Dental Drug Reference*, sixth edition. These monographs follow the same format as those in the book. They are arranged in alphabetical order by generic name, and trade names are given for all medications in common use. Each monograph contains the same subsections as those listed and described on pages ix through xi of the Preface to this book.

Drug monographs included in this insert

Generic	Trade
atomoxetine HCl	Strattera
cefditoren pivoxil	Spectracef
dexmethylphenidate HCl	Focalin
dutasteride	Avodart
eplerenone	Inspra
escitalopram oxalate	Lexapro
ezetimibe	Zetia
fondaparinux sodium	Arixtra
olmesartan medoxomil	Benicar
pimecrolimus	Elidel
tegaserod maleate	Zelnorm

atomoxetine HCl

(a-to-mox'e-teen)

Strattera

Drug class.: Selective norepinephrine reuptake inhibitor

Action: Proposed to enhance noradrenergic function by selective inhibition of the presynaptic norepinephrine transporter; has little or no affinity for other neuronal transporters or receptor sites; mechanism of action in ADHD is unknown

Uses: Treatment of attention deficit hyperactivity disorder

Dosage and routes:

• *Child and adolescent ≤70 kg:* PO initial dose 0.5 mg/kg/day and increased after 3 days to target daily dose of ≈1.2 mg/kg either as a single AM dose or in two equally divided doses AM and PM; daily dose limit 1.4 mg/kg or 100 mg

• *Adult and child or adolescent >70 kg:* PO initial dose 40 mg/day and increased after 3 days to total daily dose of ≈80 mg either as a single AM dose or in two equally divided doses AM and PM; after 2 to 4 more wk, the dose may be increased to 100 mg; daily dose limit 100 mg

Available forms include: Caps 10, 18, 25, 40, 60 mg

Side effects/adverse reactions:

▼ *ORAL:* Dry mouth

CNS: Aggression, irritability, somnolence, mood swings, anorexia, dizziness, headache, crying

CV: Increased blood pressure, tachycardia, palpitation, chest pain

GI: Vomiting, dyspepsia, nausea, abdominal pain, constipation

RESP: Cough, UTI, rhinorrhea, nasal congestion

GU: Urinary retention, impotence, dysmenorrhea, prostatitis

EENT: Ear infection, mydriasis

INTEG: Dermatitis, pruritus

MS: Arthralgia

MISC: Fatigue, decreased appetite, flu, weight loss

Contraindications: Hypersensitivity, MAO inhibitor use concurrently or within 2 wk of taking MAO inhibitor, narrow-angle glaucoma

Precautions: Hypertension, tachycardia, CV disease, monitor weight and growth changes, urinary retention, pregnancy category C, nursing, use in geriatric patients not established, use of herbals, poor metabolizers of CYP2D6 drugs, hepatic impairment

Pharmacokinetics:

PO: Absolute bioavailability 63%-94%, peak plasma levels in 1-2 hr, half-life 5 hr, plasma protein binding 98%; metabolized primarily by CYP2D6 to active metabolite (4-hydroxyatomoxetine); excreted as glucuronide mainly in urine (80%) and some in feces (17%)

⚡ Drug interactions of concern to dentistry:

• No dental drug interactions reported; however, drugs that inhibit CYP2D6 enzymes (paroxetine, fluoxetine) can increase plasma levels

• Albuterol and other β_2-agonists should be used with caution because of potential effects on the cardiovascular system

DENTAL CONSIDERATIONS

General:

• Assess salivary flow as a factor in caries, periodontal disease, and candidiasis.

• Monitor vital signs every appointment because of cardiovascular side effects.

• Consider semi-supine chair position for patient comfort if GI side effects occur.

• Use vasoconstrictor with caution, in small doses, and with careful aspiration.

Consultations:

• Medical consult may be required to assess disease control and patient's ability to tolerate stress.

Teach patient/family:

• Importance of good oral hygiene to prevent soft tissue inflammation/infection

When chronic dry mouth occurs, advise patient:

• To avoid mouth rinses with high alcohol content because of drying effects

• To use daily home fluoride products for anticaries effect

• To use sugarless gum, frequent sips of water, or saliva substitutes

---

cefditoren pivoxil

(sef'di-toe-reen)

Spectracef

Drug class.: Cephalosporin, third generation

Action: Inhibits bacterial cell wall synthesis, rendering cell wall osmotically unstable

Uses: Mild to moderate infections in adults and children >12 yr; for susceptible microorganisms causing (1) acute bacterial exacerbation of chronic bronchitis (*H. influenzae, H. parainfluenzae, S. pneumoniae* [penicillin susceptible only] or *M. catarrhalis*), (2) pharyngitis/tonsillitis (*S. pyogenes*), (3) uncomplicated skin and skin-structure infections (*S. aureus* and *S. pyogenes*)

Dosage and routes:

Acute bacterial exacerbation of chronic bronchitis:

• *Adult and child >12 yr:* PO 400 mg bid × 10 days

Pharyngitis, tonsillitis, uncomplicated skin and skin-structure infections

• *Adult and child >12 yr:* PO 200 mg bid × 10 days

Severe renal failure:

• *Adult and child >12 yr:* PO not to exceed 200 mg/day

Moderate renal impairment:

• *Adult and child >12 yr:* PO not to exceed 200 mg bid

Available forms include: Tabs 200 mg

Side effects/adverse reactions:

▼ *ORAL:* Dry mouth, ulceration, candidiasis, stomatitis, taste perversion

CNS: Headache, abnormal dreams, anorexia, dizziness, insomnia

CV: Peripheral edema

*GI: Diarrhea, nausea, abdominal pain, dyspepsia, vomiting, **pseudomembranous colitis***

HEMA: Leukopenia, thrombocytopenia, increased coagulation time

GU: Vaginal candidiasis, urinary frequency

EENT: Pharyngitis, rhinitis, sinusitis

*INTEG: **Toxic epidermal necrosis,*** pruritus, rash, urticaria, Stevens-Johnson syndrome, erythema multiforme

META: Hyperglycemia, altered liver function tests

MS: Asthenia, myalgia

*MISC: **Anaphylaxis,*** fever

Contraindications: Hypersensitivity to this drug or known allergy to other cephalosporins, carnitine deficiency, milk protein hypersensitivity (tablets contain sodium caseinate)

Precautions: Penicillin-allergic patients, diarrhea, not for prolonged treatment, risk of resistance emergence, alteration of normal GI flora, decrease in prothrombin activity (long-term use, renal/hepatic impairment, patients taking anticoagulants), take with meals, pregnancy category B, lactation, safety and efficiency have not been established in children <12 yr, elderly patients with impaired renal function, reduce dosage in severe renal impairment

Pharmacokinetics:
PO: Absorption enhanced by a fatty meal, peak plasma levels (fasting) 1.5-3 hr, hydrolyzed by esterases on absorption, low plasma protein (serum albumin) binding, parent drug excreted by glomerular filtration and tubular secretion

⚖ Drug interactions of concern to dentistry:
• Reduced absorption: concurrent use with antacids, H_2 receptor antagonist
• Increased and prolonged serum levels: probenecid
• Does not alter pharmacokinetics of ethinyl estradiol

DENTAL CONSIDERATIONS
General:
• Precaution regarding allergy to medication.
• Assess salivary flow as a factor in caries, periodontal disease, and candidiasis.
• Determine why patient is taking the drug.
• Consult with patient's physician

if an acute dental infection occurs and another antiinfective is required.
• Examine for oral manifestation of opportunistic infection.
• Patient receiving chronic drug therapy may rarely present with symptoms of blood dyscrasias, which can include infection, bleeding, and poor healing.

Consultations:
• Medical consult may be required to assess disease control.
• In a patient with symptoms of blood dyscrasias, request a medical consult for blood studies and postpone treatment until normal values are reestablished.

Teach patient/family:
• Importance of good oral hygiene to prevent soft tissue inflammation/ infection
When chronic dry mouth occurs, advise patient:
• To avoid mouth rinses with high alcohol content due to drying effects
• To use daily home fluoride products for anticaries effect
• To use sugarless gum, frequent sips of water, or saliva substitutes

---

dexmethylphenidate HCl

(dex-meth-il-fen'-i-date)
Focalin

Drug class.: CNS stimulant; related to the amphetamines

Controlled Substance Schedule II
Action: Blocks the reuptake of norepinephrine and dopamine in the presynaptic neuron and is presumed to increase the release of these neurotransmitters

italic = common side effects

Uses: Treatment of attention deficit hyperactivity disorder (ADHD)

Dosage and routes:

Patients new to methylphenidate:
• *Adult and child >6 yr:* PO 2.5 mg bid; dosage may be adjusted at weekly intervals in 2.5- to 5-mg increments up to 20 mg/day

Patients currently using methylphenidate:
• *Adult and child >6 yr:* PO starting dose is half the dose of racemic methylphenidate, not to exceed 20 mg/day

Available forms include: Tabs 2.5, 5, 10 mg

Side effects/adverse reactions:

▼ *ORAL:* Dry mouth

CNS: Anorexia, insomnia, mood alteration

CV: Tachycardia, angina, arrhythmias, palpitation

GI: Abdominal pain, nausea

*HEMA: **Thrombocytopenia purpura, leukopenia***

EENT: Blurred vision

*INTEG: **Exfoliative dermatitis,*** skin rash, urticaria, erythema multiforme

MS: Twitching (includes vocal tics), arthralgia

MISC: Fever, weight loss

Contraindications: Hypersensitivity to methylphenidate, glaucoma, marked anxiety, tension, agitation, tics, Tourette's syndrome, MAO inhibitor use

Precautions: Long-term effect on growth in children unknown, exacerbation of psychotic behavior, history of seizures, hypertension, heart failure, recent MI, hyperthyroidism, use in child <6 yr not established, drug dependence, pregnancy category C, lactation

Pharmacokinetics:

PO: Readily absorbed, peak plasma levels 1-1.5 hr; mean plasma half-life 2.2 hr; readily metabolized, excreted in urine (80%)

🦷 **Drug interactions of concern to dentistry:**
• May inhibit metabolism of phenobarbital, tricyclic antidepressants, and selective serotonin reuptake inhibitors
• Increased effects of anticholinergics, CNS stimulants, tricyclic antidepressants, and sympathomimetics

DENTAL CONSIDERATIONS

General:
• Stress importance of updating health and drug history if physician makes any changes in evaluation/drug regimens.
• Monitor vital signs every appointment because of cardiovascular side effects.
• Assess salivary flow as a factor in caries, periodontal disease, and candidiasis.
• Patient receiving chronic drug therapy may rarely present with symptoms of blood dyscrasias, which can include infection, bleeding, and poor healing.
• Use vasoconstrictor with caution, in small doses, and with careful aspiration.
• Determine why patient is taking the drug.
• Consider semi-supine chair position for patient comfort if GI side effects occur.

Consultations:
• In a patient with symptoms of blood dyscrasias, request a medical consult for blood studies and postpone treatment until normal values are reestablished.

• Medical consult may be required to assess disease control.

Teach patient/family:

• Importance of good oral hygiene to prevent soft tissue inflammation/infection

• To prevent injury when using oral hygiene aids

• Importance of updating health and drug history if physician makes any changes in evaluation/drug regimens

When chronic dry mouth occurs, advise patient:

• To avoid mouth rinses with high alcohol content because of drying effects

• To use daily home fluoride products for anticaries effect

• To use sugarless gum, frequent sips of water, or saliva substitutes

---

dutasteride

(doo-tas'teer-ide)

Avodart

Drug class.: Synthetic steroid

Action: Selectively inhibits steroid 5α-reductase enzymes (types 1 and 2), thereby inhibiting the conversion of testosterone to 5α-dihydrotestosterone (DHT)

Uses: Treatment of benign prostate hyperplasia (BPH) in men to improve symptoms, reduce the risk of urinary retention, and reduce the need for BPH-related surgery

Dosage and routes:

• *Adult:* PO 0.5 mg/day with or without food

Available forms include:

Caps 0.5 mg

Side effects/adverse reactions:

GU: Impotence, ejaculation disorder

MISC: Decreased libido, gynecomastia

Contraindications: Hypersensitivity to this drug or other 5α-reductase inhibitors, women and children; women who are pregnant or might be pregnant should not handle capsules, potential risk of fetal abnormality for male fetus

Precautions: Hepatic impairment, men cannot donate blood until at least 6 mo after last dose, drug also found in semen, no data on use in patients <18 yr or in renal impairment, pregnancy category X, nursing mothers (not used in women)

Pharmacokinetics:

PO: Absolute bioavailability ≈60%, peak plasma levels 2-3 hr, highly bound to plasma proteins (99%), extensively metabolized mainly by CYP3A4 isoenzymes; one metabolite (6B-hydroxydutastride) in active, unchanged dutasteride and metabolites excreted in the feces

💊 Drug interactions of concern to dentistry:

• No drug interaction studies have been conducted; however, caution should be observed when used in combination with potent and chronically used CYP3A4 inhibitors (see Appendix I)

• Opioids and anticholinergic drugs may enhance urinary retention; use alternative analgesics (NSAIDs)

DENTAL CONSIDERATIONS

General:

• Determine why patient is taking the drug.

Consultations:

• Medical consult may be required to assess disease control.

Teach patient/family:
• Importance of updating health and drug history if physician makes any changes in evaluation/ drug regimens

---

eplerenone

(e-pler'en-one)

Inspra

Drug class.: Antihypertensive, aldosterone antagonist

Action: Acts as a selective aldosterone receptor antagonist, thereby inhibiting aldosterone's effects on blood pressure and sodium reabsorption; it is chemically related to spironolactone

Uses: Treatment of hypertension as a single drug or in combination with other antihypertensive drugs

Dosage and routes:
• *Adult:* PO starting dose 50 mg/ day; for patients with an inadequate response after a trial period, dose can be increased to 50 mg bid

Available forms include:
Tabs 25, 50, 100 mg

Side effects/adverse reactions:
CNS: Headache, dizziness, fatigue
*CV: Angina pectoris, **myocardial infarction***
GI: Diarrhea, abdominal pain
RESP: Cough
GU: Albuminuria, abnormal vaginal bleeding
META: Increased GGT; hypercholesterolemia; hypertriglyceridemia; hyperkalemia; increased ALT, BUN, creatinine, uric acid
MISC: Influenza-like symptoms, gynecomastia

Contraindications: Hypersensitivity, serum potassium >5.5 mEq/L, type 2 diabetes with microalbuminuria, serum creatinine >2.0 mg/dl in males or >1.8 mg/dl in females, creatinine clearance <50 ml/min; potassium supplements, potassium-sparing diuretics, ketoconazole, itraconazole

Precautions: Hyperkalemia, monitor serum potassium periodically, impaired hepatic/renal function, ACE inhibitors, angiotensin II antagonists, pregnancy category B, lactation, use in children has not been established

Pharmacokinetics:
PO: Bioavailability unknown, peak plasma levels 1.5 hr, plasma protein binding 50%, metabolized by CYP450 3A4 isoenzymes, no active metabolites, excreted in urine (67%) and feces (32%)

Drug interactions of concern to dentistry:
• See Contraindications; use with caution in patients taking strong inhibitors of CYP3A4 isoenzymes (erythromycin) (see Appendix I)
• Monitor blood pressure if NSAIDs are required

DENTAL CONSIDERATIONS
General:
• Monitor vital signs every appointment because of cardiovascular side effects.
• Short appointments and a stress reduction protocol may be required for anxious patients.
• Precaution if dental surgery is anticipated, general anesthesia required.
Consultations:
• Medical consult may be required to assess disease control and patient's ability to tolerate stress.
• Consultation with physician may be needed if sedation or general anesthesia is required.

Teach patient/family:
• Importance of updating health and drug history if physician makes any changes in evaluation/drug regimens

---

escitalopram oxalate

(es-sye-tal'oh-pram)
Lexapro
Drug class.: Antidepressant, selective serotonin reuptake inhibitor

Action: Inhibits CNS neuronal reuptake of serotonin; minimal effects on reuptake of norepinephrine or dopamine

Uses: Treatment of major depressive disorder; maintenance treatment of major depressive disorder

Dosage and routes:
• *Adult:* PO 10 mg/day; dose may be increased to 20 mg/day after a minimum of 1 wk; dose limit in elderly is 10 mg/day

Available forms include: Tabs 5, 10, 20 mg

Side effects/adverse reactions:
▼ *ORAL: Dry mouth*
CNS: Insomnia, dizziness, somnolence, anorexia, headache
GI: Nausea, diarrhea, abdominal pain, constipation, indigestion
RESP: Rhinitis, sinusitis
GU: Ejaculation disorder, decreased libido, impotence
META: Hyponatremia
MISC: Sweating, fatigue, influenza-like symptoms

Contraindications: Hypersensitivity to this drug or citalopram, concurrent use of MAO inhibitors and up to 2 wk after discontinuing use of MAO inhibitors

Precautions: Hyponatremia, activation of mania/hypomania, seizures, suicide, hepatic/renal impairment, concurrent use of citalopram, pregnancy category C, lactation, use in children has not been established

Pharmacokinetics:
PO: Absolute bioavailability 80%, plasma protein binding 56%, hepatic metabolism (CYP3A4, CYP2D6, and CYP2C19); renal excretion

⚡ Drug interactions of concern to dentistry:
• Increased sedation: alcohol and other CNS depressants
• Drugs that inhibit CYP3A4 or other CYP isoenzymes may or may not affect plasma levels but should be used with observation and caution
• A modest inhibitor of CYP2D6

DENTAL CONSIDERATIONS
General:
• Assess salivary flow as a factor in caries, periodontal disease, and candidiasis.
• Consider semi-supine chair position for patient comfort if GI side effects occur.
• Question patient about tolerance of NSAIDs or aspirin related to GI disease.
• Evaluate respiration characteristics and rate.

Consultations:
• Medical consult may be required to assess disease control and patient's ability to tolerate stress.
• Physician should be informed if significant xerostomia side effects occur (increased caries, sore tongue, problems eating or swallowing, difficulty wearing prosthesis) so that a medication change can be considered.

Teach patient/family:
• Importance of good oral hygiene to prevent soft tissue inflammation/infection

When chronic dry mouth occurs, advise patient:
• To avoid mouth rinses with high alcohol content due to drying effects
• To use daily home fluoride products for anticaries effect
• To use sugarless gum, frequent sips of water, or saliva substitutes
• Importance of stressing compliance with recommended regimes for oral care

---

ezetimibe
(ez-et'i-mibe)
Zetia

Drug class.: Cholesterol-lowering agent

Action: Selectively inhibits the intestinal absorption of cholesterol and chemically related phytosterols
Uses: Adjunctive therapy to diet for reduction of cholesterol in patients with primary hypercholesterolemia
Dosage and routes:
• *Adult:* PO 10 mg/day with or without food; can also be taken with an HMG-CoA reductase inhibitor
Available forms include: Tabs 10 mg
Side effects/adverse reactions:
CNS: Fatigue
GI: Abdominal pain, diarrhea
RESP: Coughing, pharyngitis, sinusitis
META: Increase in serum transaminases (combo with HMG-CoA reductase inhibitor)

MS: Arthralgia, back pain
MISC: Viral infection
Contraindications: Hypersensitivity; concurrent use with an HMG-CoA reductase inhibitor in patients with active liver disease or in patients with unexplained, persistent increase in serum transaminases; hepatic impairment
Precautions: When used with an HMG-CoA reductase inhibitor, must follow all precautions for use (including pregnancy risk, risk of increased serum transaminase or myopathy); pregnancy category C, pregnancy, lactation and children <10 yr not established
Pharmacokinetics:
PO: Absorbed with or without food; peak plasma levels 4-12 hr, primarily metabolized in small intestine and liver; extensive glucuronide conjugation, highly plasma protein bound (>90%); excreted in feces (78%) and urine (11%)
Drug interactions of concern to dentistry:
• No dental drug interactions have been reported

DENTAL CONSIDERATIONS
General:
• Consider semi-supine chair position for patient comfort if GI, respiratory, or musculoskeletal side effects occur.
• Monitor vital signs every appointment because of possible cardiovascular disease.
Teach patient/family:
• Importance of updating health and drug history if physician makes any changes in evaluation/drug regimens

fondaparinux sodium
(fon-da'-pa'rin'no)
Arixtra

Drug class.: Synthetic anticoagulant

Action: Selectively binds to antithrombin III (ATIII) to inhibit activation of factor Xa, resulting in inhibition of thrombus formation and development

Uses: Prophylaxis of deep vein thrombosis in patients undergoing hip fracture surgery, hip replacement surgery, or knee replacement surgery

Dosage and routes:
• *Adult:* SC After establishment of hemostasis, 2.5 mg once daily beginning 6-8 hr after surgery; duration of use 6-9 days

Available forms include: Single-dose syringe 2.5 mg/0.5 ml

Side effects/adverse reactions:
CNS: Insomnia, dizziness, confusion, headache
CV: Edema, hypotension
GI: Nausea, constipation, vomiting, diarrhea, dyspepsia
HEMA: Hemorrhage, injection site bleeding, anemia, hematoma, postoperative bleeding, major bleeding events
GU: UTI
INTEG: Rash, pruritus, bullous eruption
META: Increase in AST, ALT, hypokalemia
MISC: Fever, pain

Contraindications: Hypersensitivity, renal impairment, body weight <50 kg, major bleeding problems, endocarditis, thrombocytopenia

Precautions: Neuroaxial (spinal/epidural) anesthesia, avoid IM use, anticoagulant effects persist for 2-4 days after administration, elderly patients, pregnancy category B, no data available for nursing mothers, use in children has not been established

Pharmacokinetics:
SC: Absolute bioavailability 100%, peak levels ≈2 hr; excreted unchanged in urine (77% over 72 hr)

⚡ Drug interactions of concern to dentistry:
• Avoid concurrent use of aspirin and NSAIDs

DENTAL CONSIDERATIONS
General:
• Determine why patient is taking the drug.
• Monitor vital signs every appointment because of cardiovascular side effects.
• Consider local hemostasis measures to prevent excessive bleeding.
• Antibiotic prophylaxis before dental treatment may be required for joint prosthesis. (See 1997 ADA guidelines.)
• Delay elective dental treatment until patient completes anticoagulant therapy.

Consultations:
• Medical consult should include routine blood counts, including platelet counts and bleeding time.

Teach patient/family:
• Importance of good oral hygiene to prevent soft tissue inflammation/infection
• To prevent injury when using oral hygiene aids
• To report oral lesions, soreness, or bleeding to dentist

olmesartan medoxomil
(ol-me-sar′tan)
Benicar
Drug class.: Angiotensin II (AT$_1$)
receptor antagonist

Action: Blocks the vasoconstrictor
and aldosterone-releasing effects
of angiotensin II

Uses: Hypertension, as a single
drug or in combination with other
antihypertensives

Dosage and routes:
• *Adult:* PO 20 mg/day as monotherapy in patients who are not
volume contracted; after 2 wk the
dose may be increased to 40 mg/
day; for patients with volume depletion (taking diuretics or impaired renal function), use lower
starting dosage

Available forms include: Tabs 5,
20, 40 mg

Side effects/adverse reactions:
▼ *ORAL:* Facial edema (angio-
edema)
CNS: Dizziness, vertigo, insomnia
CV: Tachycardia
GI: Diarrhea, headache, dyspepsia,
abdominal pain, nausea
RESP: Bronchitis, URT infection,
cough
GU: Hematuria, UTI
EENT: Pharyngitis, rhinitis, sinus-
itis
INTEG: Rash
META: Increased creatine phospho-
kinase, increased bilirubin, hyper-
lipidemia, hyperuricemia, hyper-
cholesterolemia, hyperglycemia,
hypertriglyceridemia
MS: Back pain, arthralgia, myalgia
MISC: Influenza-like symptoms,
fatigue

Contraindications: Hypersensitivity

Precautions: Discontinue drug if
pregnancy occurs, pregnancy category C, volume- or salt-depleted
patients, use in nursing mothers or
pediatric patients has not been established, impaired renal function,
CHF, renal artery stenosis

Pharmacokinetics:
PO: Absolute bioavailability
≈26%, steady-state levels are
achieved in 3-5 days, peak plasma
levels 1-2 hr, ester hydrolysis occurs on absorption with no further
metabolism of olmesartan, highly
bound to plasma proteins (99%),
excreted in urine and feces

**⚕ Drug interactions of concern
to dentistry:**
• No significant drug interactions
have been reported, but there is
always a chance of increased hypotensive effects when used with
other antihypertensives or sedatives

DENTAL CONSIDERATIONS
General:
• Monitor vital signs every appointment because of cardiovascular side effects.
• Consider semi-supine chair position for patient comfort if GI side
effects occur.
• Limit use of sodium-containing
products such as saline IV fluids
for patients with a dietary salt
restriction.
• Stress from dental procedures
may compromise cardiovascular
function, determine patient risk.
• Patients with hypertensive disease may be taking more than one
drug to control blood pressure;
although not specifically noted for
this drug, postural hypotension is

---

bold italic = life-threatening conditions   *For periodic updates, visit* **www.mosby.com**

always a possibility. After supine positioning, have patient sit upright for ≥2 min to avoid orthostatic hypotension.

• Short appointments and a stress reduction protocol may be required for anxious patients.

• Use precaution if sedation or general anesthesia is required; risk of hypotensive episode.

Consultations:

• Medical consult may be required to assess disease control and patient's ability to tolerate stress.

Teach patient/family:

• Importance of updating health and drug history if physician makes any changes in evaluation/drug regimens

---

pimecrolimus

(pim-e-koe'li-mus)
Elidel

Drug class.: Topical antiinflammatory

Action: Mechanism in atopic dermatitis is unknown; however, it does inhibit calcineurin and inflammatory cytokine release

Uses: Short-term and intermittent long-term treatment of mild to moderate atopic dermatitis in nonimmunocompromised patients ≥2 yr in which conventional therapies cannot be used because of potential risks or in patients with an inadequate response or patients who are not responsive to conventional therapies

Dosage and routes:

• *Adult and child >2 yr:* TOP Apply thin layer to affected area bid, rub in gently and completely; reevaluate after 6 wk if symptoms persist

Available forms include: Cream 1% in 15-, 30-, 100-g tubes

Side effects/adverse reactions:

CNS: Headache

EENT: Nasopharyngitis, pharyngitis, cough

INTEG: Burning, cutaneous infection, folliculitis, other localized symptoms

MISC: Influenza, viral infections, fever

Note: In clinical trials other side effects reported were not distinguished from placebo or vehicle. No long-term trials were reported.

Contraindications: Hypersensitivity to drug or vehicle components

Precautions: Do not use for active cutaneous viral infections, infected dermatitis, natural or artificial sunlight exposure, pregnancy category C, data on excretion in human milk are not available, children <2 yr

Pharmacokinetics:

TOP: Low levels of absorption (below assay limits), any absorbed drug is metabolized by CYP3A enzymes, excreted in feces (81%) as metabolites

Drug interactions of concern to dentistry:

• Drug interactions have not been evaluated; low blood levels were measured in some patients; use drugs that inhibit CYP3A cytochrome enzymes with caution in patients with widespread and erythrodermic disease

DENTAL CONSIDERATIONS
General:

• Determine why patient is taking this drug.

---

italic = common side effects

tegaserod maleate

(teg-a-ser′od)
Zelnorm

Drug class.: Serotonin agonist, a prokinetic drug

Action: A partial agonist that binds to 5-HT$_4$ receptors, resulting in stimulation of the peristaltic reflex and intestinal secretions

Uses: Short-term treatment of irritable bowel syndrome in women whose primary bowel symptom is constipation

Dosage and routes:
• *Adult:* PO (women only) 6 mg bid before meals × 4-6 wk; for patients who respond to therapy an additional 4-6 wk can be considered

Available forms include: Tabs 2, 6 mg

Side effects/adverse reactions:
▼ *ORAL:* Facial edema
CNS: Headache, dizziness, migraine, vertigo
CV: Flushing, hypotension, angina, syncope, arrhythmias
GI: Abdominal pain, diarrhea, nausea, flatulence, irritable colon, cholecystitis, appendicitis
RESP: Asthma
GU: Menorrhagia, albuminuria, polyuria, renal pain
INTEG: Pruritus, sweating
META: Increased ALT, increased AST, bilirubinemia, increased creatine phosphokinase
MS: Back pain, arthropathy
MISC: Accidental trauma, leg pain

Contraindications: Hypersensitivity, severe renal impairment, moderate or severe hepatic impairment, history of bowel obstruction, gallbladder disease, suspected sphincter of Oddi obstruction or abdominal adhesions

Precautions: Avoid use in patients with diarrhea, pregnancy category B, lactation (discontinue drug or discontinue nursing), safety and usefulness in children <18 yr are not established

Pharmacokinetics:
PO: Absolute bioavailability in fasting patients is ≈10%, peak plasma levels ≈1 hr; plasma protein binding 98%; undergoes presystemic acid hydrolysis in stomach, then oxidation and conjugation to inactive metabolites; excreted in feces (67%) and in urine (33%)

🦷 **Drug interactions of concern to dentistry:**
• No dental drug interactions reported; does not induce CYP450 enzymes
• Avoid use of drugs (opioids, anticholinergics) that could lead to risk of constipation
• Use NSAIDs or acetaminophen for mild or moderate pain

DENTAL CONSIDERATIONS
General:
• Monitor vital signs every appointment because of cardiovascular side effects.
• Consider semi-supine chair position for patient comfort if GI side effects occur.
• Short appointments and a stress reduction protocol may be required for anxious patients.
• Avoid drugs with anticholinergic activity, such as antihistamines, opioids, benzodiazepines, propantheline, atropine, and scopolamine.

Consultations:
• Consult with physician before prescribing drugs that can cause constipation (opioids).

---

bold italic = life-threatening conditions

• Consultation with physician may be needed if sedation or general anesthesia is required.
• Medical consult may be required to assess disease control and patient's ability to tolerate stress.

Teach patient/family:
• Importance of updating health and drug history if physician makes any changes in evaluation/drug regimens